CLINICAL NUTRITION

Parenteral Nutrition

CLINICAL NUTRITION
Parenteral
Nutrition

THIRD EDITION

John L. Rombeau, MD
Professor of Surgery
Hospital of the University of Pennsylvania
Department of Surgery
Philadelphia, Pennsylvania

Rolando H. Rolandelli, MD
Professor of Surgery
Chief, Section of General Surgery
Temple University Hospital
Department of Surgery
Philadelphia, Pennsylvania

W.B. SAUNDERS COMPANY
A Harcourt Health Sciences Company
Philadelphia London New York St. Louis Sydney Toronto

W.B. SAUNDERS COMPANY
A Harcourt Health Sciences Company

The Curtis Center
Independence Square West
Philadelphia, Pennsylvania 19106

Library of Congress Cataloging-in-Publication Data

Clinical nutrition: parenteral nutrition / [edited by] John L. Rombeau,
Rolando H. Rolandelli.—3rd ed.

p.   cm.

Includes bibliographical references and index.

ISBN 0–7216–8120–4

1. Enteral feeding.   2. Tube feeding.   I. Title: Parenteral nutrition.
   II. Rombeau, John L.   III. Rolandelli, Rolando.   [DNLM: 1. Nutrition.
   2. Parenteral Nutrition.   WB 410 C64151 2000]

RM222.C58 2000   615.8′54—dc21

DNLM/DLC   99–050227

Acquisitions Editor: Ray Kersey
Project Manager: Amy Norwitz
Illustration Specialist: Bob Quinn

CLINICAL NUTRITION: Parenteral Nutrition   ISBN 0–7216–8120–4

Printed in the United States of America.

Last digit is the print number: 9   8   7   6   5   4   3   2   1

◆ Contributors

Michael Adolph, M.D.
Chief Physician, Clinic of Anesthesiology, Surgical Intensive Care and Emergency Medicine; Teaching Hospital of the University of Goettingen Hospital Wolfsburg, Wolfsburg, Germany
Lipid Emulsions in Parenteral Nutrition

Jorge E. Albina, M.D.
Professor of Surgery, Brown University School of Medicine; Director, Surgical Research Director, Nutritional Support Service, Rhode Island Hospital, Department of Surgery, Providence, Rhode Island
Metabolic Response to Illness and Its Mediators

David B. Allison, Ph.D.
Associate Professor of Medical Psychology, Columbia University; Associate Research Scientist, Obesity Research Center; St. Luke's–Roosevelt Hospital Center, New York, New York
Nutritional Support of the Obese Patient

Michael C. Allwood, Ph.D.
Head, Pharmacy Academic Practice Unit, University of Derby, Derby, United Kingdom
Trace Elements and Vitamins in Adult Intravenous Nutrition

Roberto Anaya-Prado, M.D.
Chief of General Surgery, Adjunct Professor of Surgery, Mexican Institute for Social Security, Guadalajara, Jalisco, México
Gastrointestinal Fistulas: Clinical and Nutritional Management

Humberto Arenas-Marquez, M.D.
Chief of General Surgery, Professor of Surgery, Specialized Surgical and Nutritional Clinic, Guadalajara, Jalisco, México
Gastrointestinal Fistulas: Clinical and Nutritional Management

Robin Bankhead, C.R.N.P., M.S., C.N.S.N.
Coordinator of Nutritional Support Service, Temple University Hospital, Department of Surgery, Philadelphia, Pennsylvania
Parenteral Nutrition in Short Bowel Syndrome

Luis M. Barrera-Zepeda, M.D.
Surgical Resident, Specialized Surgical and Nutritional Clinic, Guadalajara, Jalisco, México
Gastrointestinal Fistulas: Clinical and Nutritional Management

Mette M. Berger, M.D., Ph.D.
University of Lausanne Medical School, Lausanne, Switzerland
Trauma and Burns

Glen F. Bergman, M.M.Sc., R.D., C.N.S.D.
Clinical Nutritionist, Nutrition and Metabolic Support Service, Emory University Hospital, Atlanta, Georgia
Nutrient Pharmacotherapy

Bruce R. Bistrian, M.D., Ph.D.
Professor of Medicine, Harvard Medical School; Chief, Clinical Nutrition; Chief, Laboratory of Nutrition/Infection, BI Deaconess Medical Center, Boston, Massachusetts
Lipid Emulsions in Parenteral Nutrition

Eugene E. Cepeda, M.D.
Pediatrician, Hutzel Hospital, Detroit Medical Center, Detroit, Michigan
Parenteral Nutrition in Neonates

Glenn M. Chertow, M.D., M.P.H.
Assistant Professor of Medicine in Residence, University of California, San Francisco; Director of Clinical Services, Divisions of Nephrology, Moffit–Long Hospitals and UCSF–Mt. Zion Medical Center, San Francisco, California
Metabolic Assessment

René L. Chioléro, M.D.
Chief of Medicine, University of Lausanne Medical School, Lausanne, Switzerland
Trauma and Burns

Patricia S. Choban, M.D.
Adjunct Professor of Human Nutrition and Food Management, College of Human Ecology, Ohio State University, Columbus, Ohio
Nutritional Support of the Obese Patient

Jesus M. Culebras, M.D., Ph.D.
Professor of Surgery, Department of
Physiology, University of Leon; Chief of
Surgery, Hospital de Leon, Leon, Spain
Peripheral Parenteral Nutrition

David F. Driscoll, Ph.D.
Assistant Professor of Medicine, Harvard
Medical School; Senior Researcher,
Nutrition/Infection Laboratory, Department
of Medicine, BI Deaconess Medical Center,
Boston, Massachusetts
Lipid Emulsions in Parenteral Nutrition

Barbara Ehrenpreis
Home Parenteral Nutrition (HPN)
Consumer
*Home Parenteral Nutrition: Clinical
Outcome*

Richard A. Falcone, Jr., M.D.
Surgical Resident, University of Cincinnati
College of Medicine, Department of
Surgery, Cincinnati, Ohio
Pediatric Parenteral Nutrition

**Sheung-Tat Fan, M.S., M.D., F.R.C.S.
(Ed & Glasg), F.A.C.S.**
Professor of Surgery, Department of
Surgery, The University of Hong Kong
Medical Centre, Queen Mary Hospital,
Hong Kong, China
Liver Disease and Parenteral Nutrition

Louis Flancbaum, M.D.
Associate Professor of Clinical Surgery,
Columbia–Presbyterian Medical Center;
Chief, Division of Bariatric Surgery, St.
Luke's–Roosevelt Hospital Center, New
York, New York
Nutritional Support of the Obese Patient

R. Armour Forse, M.D., Ph.D.
Laszlo Nando Tauber Professor of Surgery
and Vice-Chairman, Department of Surgery,
Boston Medical Center, Boston University
School of Medicine, Boston, Massachusetts
Perioperative Nutritional Support

Steven Fukuchi, M.D.
Surgical Resident, Temple University
Hospital, Department of Surgery,
Philadelphia, Pennsylvania
*Parenteral Nutrition in Short Bowel
Syndrome*

A. Garcia-de-Lorenzo, M.D., Ph.D.
Associate Professor, Faculty of Medicine,
Autonomous University; Intensive Care

Medicine Specialist, Hospital Universitario
la Paz, Madrid, Spain
Peripheral Parenteral Nutrition

Alejandro Gonzalez-Ojeda, M.D.
Associate Researcher, Clinical Research
Unit at Western Medical Center, Mexican
Institute for Social Security, Guadalajara,
Jalisco, México
*Gastrointestinal Fistulas: Clinical and
Nutritional Management*

John P. Grant, M.D.
Professor of Surgery, Duke University
Medical Center, Durham, North Carolina
Parenteral Access

Daniel P. Griffith, R.Ph., B.C.N.S.P.
Clinical Coordinator, Nutrition and
Metabolic Support Service, Emory
University Hospital, Atlanta, Georgia
Nutrient Pharmacotherapy

Jose L. Gutierrez de la Rosa, M.D.
Attending Surgeon, Specialized Surgical
and Nutritional Clinic, Guadalajara, Jalisco,
México
*Gastrointestinal Fistulas: Clinical and
Nutritional Management*

Raymond M. Hakim, M.D., Ph.D.
Professor of Medicine, Vanderbilt
University School of Medicine, Nashville,
Tennessee
Renal Failure and Parenteral Nutrition

**Jeanette Hasse, Ph.D., R.D., L.D.,
F.A.D.A., C.N.S.D.**
Transplant Nutrition Specialist, Baylor
Institute of Transplantation Sciences,
Baylor University Medical Center, Dallas,
Texas
Transplantation

W. Scott Helton, M.D.
Professor of Surgery, University of Illinois
at Chicago; Chief, Division of General
Surgery, University of Illinois at Chicago
Hospital, Chicago, Illinois
*Intravenous Nutrition in Patients with
Acute Pancreatitis*

Steven B. Heymsfield, M.D.
Professor of Medicine, Columbia University
College of Physicians and Surgeons;
Deputy Director, New York Obesity
Research Center, St. Luke's–Roosevelt
Hospital Center, New York, New York
Nutritional Support of the Obese Patient

Allison Hilf
Home Parenteral Nutrition (HPN)
Consumer
*Home Parenteral Nutrition: Clinical
Outcome*

Lyn Howard, M.B. (Oxon), F.R.C.P.
Professor of Medicine, Associate Professor
of Pediatrics and Head, Division of Clinical
Nutrition, Albany Medical College;
Attending Physician, Albany Medical
Center, Albany, New York
*Home Parenteral Nutrition: Clinical
Outcome*

T. Alp Ikizler, M.D.
Assistant Professor of Medicine and
Medical Director, Vanderbilt University
School of Medicine, Nashville, Tennessee
Renal Failure and Parenteral Nutrition

Danny O. Jacobs, M.D., M.P.H.
Professor and Chairman, Department of
Surgery, Creighton University School of
Medicine; Chairman, Department of
Surgery, Saint Joseph Hospital, Omaha,
Nebraska
Metabolic Assessment

Carolyn R. Jonas, Ph.D., R.D.
Department of Medicine, Emory University
School of Medicine, Atlanta, Georgia
Nutrient Pharmacotherapy

F. Jorquera, M.D., Ph.D.
Associate Professor of Medicine, School of
Nursing, University of Leon;
Gastroenterologist, Hospital de Leon, Leon,
Spain
Peripheral Parenteral Nutrition

John M. Kinney, M.D., F.A.C.S.
Visiting Professor, Rockefeller University,
New York, New York
*History of Parenteral Nutrition, with Notes
on Clinical Biology*

Gordon L. Klein, M.D.
Professor, Department of Pediatrics and
Preventive Medicine and Community
Health, Division of Pediatric
Gastroenterology, University of Texas
Medical Branch, Galveston, Texas
*Hepatobiliary Complications of Parenteral
Nutrition*

**Winston W. K. Koo, M.B.B.S.,
F.R.A.C.P.**
Professor of Pediatrics, Obstetrics and
Gynecology, Wayne State University;

Neonatologist, Hutzel Hospital, Detroit
Medical Center, Detroit, Michigan
Parenteral Nutrition in Neonates

Donald P. Kotler, M.D.
Professor of Medicine, Columbia
University; College of Physicians and
Surgeons, New York, NY; Senior Attending
Physician, St. Luke's–Roosevelt Hospital
Center, New York, New York
*Acquired Immunodeficiency Syndrome and
Parenteral Nutrition*

Michael E. Kupferman, M.D.
Surgical Resident, Hospital of the
University of Pennsylvania, Department of
Surgery, Philadelphia, Pennsylvania
*Parenteral Nutrition in Inflammatory Bowel
Disease*

Nancy Lau, M.D.
Clinical Fellow, St. Luke's–Roosevelt
Hospital, Department of Gastroenterology,
Columbia University College of Physicians,
New York, New York
*Acquired Immunodeficiency Syndrome and
Parenteral Nutrition*

Lorraine M. Leader, M.D., C.N.S.P.
Assistant Professor of Medicine, Division of
Digestive Diseases, Emory University
School of Medicine, Atlanta, Georgia
Nutrient Pharmacotherapy

Edward W. Lipkin, M.D., Ph.D.
Associate Professor, Medicine, University
of Washington School of Medicine;
Attending Physician, University of
Washington Medical Center, Seattle,
Washington
Metabolic Bone Disease

Timothy O. Lipman, M.D.
Professor of Medicine, Georgetown
University School of Medicine; Chief, GI-
Hepatology-Nutrition Section, Department
of Veterans Affairs Medical Center,
Washington, DC
Ethical Issues and Parenteral Nutrition

**Margaret Malone, Ph.D., B.C.N.S.P.,
F.C.C.P.**
Professor, Department of Pharmacy
Practice, Albany College of Pharmacy;
Adjunct Associate Professor of Medicine,
Albany Medical College, Albany, New York
*Home Parenteral Nutrition: Clinical
Outcome*

Manoj K. Maloo, M.D.
Clinical Fellow, Harvard Medical School, and Fellow, Department of Surgery, Beth Israel Deaconess Medical Center, Boston, Massachusetts
Perioperative Nutritional Support

Catherine McIsaac, M.S., R.D.
University of Illinois at Chicago Hospital, Chicago, Illinois
Intravenous Nutrition in Patients with Acute Pancreatitis

Jay M. Mirtallo, M.S., R.Ph.
Clinical Associate Professor, The Ohio State University College of Pharmacy; Specialty Practice Pharmacist, Nutrition Support/Surgery, The Ohio State University Medical Center, Department of Pharmacy, Columbus, Ohio
Parenteral Formulas

Juan M. Palma-Vargas, M.D.
Attending Surgeon, Specialized Surgical and Nutritional Clinic, Guadalajara, Jalisco, México
Gastrointestinal Fistulas: Clinical and Nutritional Management

Ronnie Tung-Ping Poon, M.S., F.R.C.S.(Ed)
Assistant Professor, Department of Surgery, The University of Hong Kong Medical Centre, Queen Mary Hospital, Hong Kong, China
Liver Disease and Parenteral Nutrition

Susan Roberts, M.S., R.D., L.D., C.N.S.D.
Clinical Dietitian for Marrow/Stem Cell Transplantation Area, Baylor University Medical Center, Dallas, Texas
Transplantation

Rolando H. Rolandelli, M.D.
Professor of Surgery, Chief, Section of General Surgery, Temple University Hospital, Department of Surgery, Philadelphia, Pennsylvania
Parenteral Nutrition in Short Bowel Syndrome

John L. Rombeau, M.D.
Professor of Surgery, Hospital of the University of Pennsylvania, Department of Surgery, Philadelphia, Pennsylvania
Parenteral Nutrition in Inflammatory Bowel Disease

Harry C. Sax, M.D., F.A.C.S.
Associate Professor of Surgery, University of Rochester Medical Center, Rochester, New York
Total Parenteral Nutrition: Effects on the Small Intestine

Karen E. Shattuck, M.D.
Associate Professor of Pediatrics, Division of Neonatology, University of Texas Medical Branch, Galveston, Texas
Hepatobiliary Complications of Parenteral Nutrition

Alan Shenkin, F.R.C.P., F.R.C.Path.
Professor of Clinical Chemistry, University of Liverpool; Clinical Director of Clinical Chemistry, Royal Liverpool University Hospital, Liverpool, United Kingdom
Trace Elements and Vitamins in Adult Intravenous Nutrition

Michael S. Sherman, M.D.
Associate Professor of Medicine; Director, Pulmonary Diagnostic Laboratory, Division of Pulmonary and Critical Care Medicine, Hahnemann University Hospital, School of Medicine, Philadelphia, Pennsylvania
Parenteral Nutrition and Cardiopulmonary Disease

Elaine B. Trujillo, M.S., R.D.
Senior Clinical and Research Dietitian, Metabolic Support Service, Brigham & Women's Hospital, Boston, Massachusetts
Metabolic Assessment

Enrique Sánchez-Perez Verdia, M.D.
Surgical Resident, Specialized Surgical and Nutritional Clinic, Guadalajara, Jalisco, México
Gastrointestinal Fistulas: Clinical and Nutritional Management

Carolyn D. Viall, R.N., M.S.N.
Clinical Director of Pediatrics, University of North Carolina Hospitals, Chapel Hill, North Carolina
Home Parenteral Nutrition: Finances

Matthew D. Vrees, M.D.
Clinical Research Fellow, Brown University Program in Surgery; Department of Surgery, Rhode Island Hospital, Providence, Rhode Island
Metabolic Response to Illness and Its Mediators

Howard T. Wang, M.D.
Resident, General Surgery, University of Rochester Medical Center, Rochester, New York
Total Parenteral Nutrition: Effects on the Small Intestine

Brad W. Warner, M.D.
Associate Professor of Surgery, University of Cincinnati College of Medicine; Attending Surgeon, Children's Hospital Medical Center, Cincinnati, Ohio
Pediatric Parenteral Nutrition

James M. Watters, M.D., F.R.C.S.C.
Professor, Department of Surgery, University of Ottawa; Active Staff, Division of General Surgery, Ottawa Hospital, Civic Site, Ottawa, Ontario, Canada
Parenteral Nutrition in the Elderly Patient

A. Zarazaga, M.D., Ph.D.
Associate Professor, Faculty of Medicine, Autonomous University; Surgeon, Hospital Universitario la Paz, Madrid, Spain
Peripheral Parenteral Nutrition

Thomas R. Ziegler, M.D., C.N.S.P.
Assistant Professor of Medicine, Division of Endocrinology and Metabolism, Emory University School of Medicine; Associate Director, Nutrition and Metabolic Support Service, Emory University Hospital, Atlanta, Georgia
Nutrient Pharmacotherapy

◆ Preface

Fifteen years have elapsed since the first edition of *Clinical Nutrition* and 8 years since its second edition. In various capacities I have been associated with all editions of this book. Every one was very challenging and very rewarding as well, and each one was special in a certain way. This one, however, is particularly special to me because it is the last edition by Dr. John L. Rombeau. This textbook was Dr. Rombeau's idea and the product of his 25 years of experience in the field of nutritional support. Dr. Caldwell first, and I most recently, were privileged to learn the art of crafting a book from one of the masters.

"Dr. Rombeau's book" has evolved from a compilation of early concepts in nutritional support to the standard review textbook used by multiple disciplines throughout the world to achieve board certification in nutritional support. Editing a textbook with such a scope has become an enormous responsibility. Fortunately, Dr. Rombeau has established very clear rules for this book. First, the main goal of each edition is to help patients in need of nutritional support by providing practitioners with state-of-the-art scientific information regarding nutritional support. Second, the authorship should include physicians and other health care professionals providing nutritional support and should represent all physician specialties caring for patients receiving nutritional support. Third, each edition should include new chapters representing the changes and advances observed between editions.

I believe this third edition of *Clinical Nutrition: Parenteral Nutrition* follows "Dr. Rombeau's rules" quite well. This edition has incorporated many recent developments in nutritional support and still can provide the beginner in the field with the basic principles for the care of patients in need of parenteral nutrition. The authorship includes pharmacists, nutritionists, and nurses; and among physicians there are surgeons, internists, pediatricians, endocrinologists, intensivists, and nephrologists. We have added chapters on nutrient pharmacotherapy, transplantation, finances of home parenteral nutrition, and peripheral parenteral nutrition. One other innovation in this edition was the Medline search for authors with publications in the topics covered by each chapter. Although many of the authors were already well known to us, we did find some new authors who bring an entirely new perspective to this edition.

In keeping pace with the progress in scientific knowledge, topics previously discussed in separate chapters were merged into one chapter; for example, discussions of trace elements and vitamins are now in one chapter (Chapter 4), as are discussions of cardiac and pulmonary diseases (Chapter 16). Other topics have been divided from one into two chapters; for example, hepatobiliary complications (Chapter 8) and metabolic bone disease (Chapter 9). A new chapter has been devoted to a topic of recent controversy, the effect of parenteral nutrition on the intestine (Chapter 17). We have also invited new authors to write chapters on classic topics such as parenteral nutrition and gastrointestinal fistulas (Chapter 13) and parenteral nutrition and renal failure (Chapter 18). Overall, the book continues to provide all of the core competencies to practice nutritional support while updating the practitioner on new scientific developments.

On the reader's behalf, I wish to acknowledge Dr. Rombeau for his contribution to this edition and for the creation and the growth of this textbook. On my behalf, I would like to express my personal gratitude to Dr. Rombeau for inviting me to contribute to this textbook early in my career and then for giving me the honor of co-editing the book with him. If I have captured only a small proportion of all the wisdom Dr. Rombeau tried to impart to me, I believe I will be able to meet the high standards he set for my professional career.

I wish to thank Debbie Muto, my loyal administrative assistant, for her sustained support. I also would like to express my gratitude to many individuals who helped me in editing galley proofs. These include Robin Bankhead, Nurse Coordinator of the Nutrition Support Service at Temple; Joan Ullrich, Nutritionist Coordinator of Home Enteral Nutrition Services at UCLA; Nancy Hood, Social Worker; and Dr. Steve Fukuchi,

Surgery Resident at Temple, previously a research fellow in my laboratory. Ray Kersey and Catherine Stamato, from W.B. Saunders, deserve my special thanks for "keeping me on track" through this entire process.

I sincerely hope the knowledge gained by health care practitioners from the reading of this book can alleviate the suffering of patients unable to sustain their nutritional needs by the enteral route.

ROLANDO H. ROLANDELLI, M.D.

NOTICE

Medicine is an ever-changing field. Standard safety precautions must be followed, but as new research and clinical experience broaden our knowledge, changes in treatment and drug therapy may become necessary or appropriate. Readers are advised to check the most current product information provided by the manufacturer of each drug to be administered to verify the recommended dose, the method and duration of administration, and contraindications. It is the responsibility of the treating physician, relying on experience and knowledge of the patient, to determine dosages and the best treatment for each individual patient. Neither the Publisher nor the editor assumes any responsibility for any injury and/or damage to persons or property arising from this publication.

THE PUBLISHER

◆ Contents

1

◆ History of Parenteral Nutrition, with Notes on Clinical Biology

John M. Kinney, M.D., F.A.C.S.

The history of parenteral nutrition is sometimes devoted to the introduction of total parenteral nutrition (TPN) during the 1960s. However, one may ask how TPN came to be introduced at that particular time and also what its influence on clinical nutrition was in the decades that immediately followed.

This chapter has been divided into six arbitrary sections whose contents overlap to some degree. First discussed, in sections one through three, are the early history before 1800; the definition of the major nutrients, which occurred up to the early 1900s; and the establishment of modern biochemistry and physiology from 1920 onward. The introduction of parenteral nutrition may be considered to span from 1937 to 1968. It was during the 1930s that clinicians, particularly surgeons, acknowledged the hazards of operating on the seriously malnourished patient, who frequently experienced failure of wound healing, developed infection, and had a prolonged convalescence that might end in death. In addition to a lack of nutritional knowledge, many other milestones had to be achieved before effective intravenous nutrition could be provided, such as the conquest of pyrogens, learning procedures for asepsis, gaining access to the central circulation, and devising methods for blood banking, all of which contributed to the introduction of modern TPN in the 1960s. The final two sections of this chapter are devoted to the evolution of TPN as it achieved a role in clinical nutrition and its own transformation with new medical knowledge and changing patterns of clinical practice. This material has been selected from publications up to the early 1990s.

◆ EARLY HISTORY—17TH AND 18TH CENTURIES

The 1500s included the growth of the study of human anatomy and the famous work of the Belgian anatomist Vesalius.[1] Such careful description of the human body in death led to theories of function during life consistent with the construction of the body. In 1614, Sanctorius examined the influence of metabolic balance on body weight measured by an ingenious beam balance.[2] In 1628, Harvey discovered the circulation of the blood.[3] In addition to this monumental contribution, Harvey attracted a large group of English investigators, known as the Oxford physiologists, two of whom made early experiments related to parenteral nutrition. One of these was Sir Christopher Wren, who studied the intravenous infusion of ale, opium, and beer into animals in 1656. Six years later, Richard Lower transfused blood from one animal to another. By 1670, various European investigators attempted transfusion of blood into patients with such dire results that the practice was formally outlawed.

The period from 1750 to 1800 established the scientific basis for the role of food as the fuel for the human body. Black discovered CO_2,[4] and Priestley and Scheele discovered O_2 but failed to understand oxidation.[5] Lavoisier established in the 1770s that gas exchange in the human body is the same as combustion and is quantitatively related to the amount of oxidation of food with resultant heat production.[6] He has sometimes been referred to as the "father of chemistry" because of his textbook *Elements of Chemistry*, published in 1793. He could equally well be considered the scientific father of nutritional biochemistry and physiology.

◆ KNOWLEDGE OF NUTRIENTS—1820 to 1920

Boussingault, an Alsatian farmer, miner, and chemist, during the 1830s ran an experimental farm where he explored various nutritional programs for farm animals and is credited with the first nitrogen balance studies.[7] Prominent French biochemists were involved in arguments with Liebig and others in Germany over issues such as whether animal fat could arise from carbohydrate ingestion. Claude Bernard struggled with the variety of nutritional theories being offered without substantiation.[8] He declared that he would accept no explanation that he could not verify in his own laboratory. The rigor of his physiologic studies did much to establish the role of carbohydrate metabolism, particularly in relation to liver glycogen and the recognition of diabetes mellitus.

During the early years of the 1800s, the chemical composition of the three major foodstuffs was determined. The landmark studies of Liebig guided research in the metabolism of food and developed data proving that carbohydrate could be converted to fat in the animal body.[9]

Voit and his graduate student Pettenkofer built the famous Pettenkofer-Voit calorimeter in the 1850s. This device provided the first careful measurements of the amounts of carbohydrate and fat oxidized in the animal body at rest.[10] It then became clear that the process of oxidation and heat production, which Harvey thought occurred in the heart and Lavoisier thought occurred in the lungs, was actually occurring in tissues throughout the body.

These ideas were advanced by the brilliant investigations of Voit, Rubner, and their colleagues.[11] Rubner, in particular, provided the studies that bridged the earlier work in gas exchange with the chemical reactions of nutrient oxidation. He established the standard caloric values of foods that are still in use today. In addition to the caloric equivalent of foods, he discovered the specific dynamic action of foods and the fact that energy expenditure appeared to be proportional to the surface area of animals and humans.[12]

The students of Voit and Rubner, particularly Graham Lusk[13] and Eugene DuBois[14] in New York City, spread their influence to many countries. The most extensive studies of the basal metabolic rate (BMR) in various medical illnesses were published by DuBios in 1924.[15] The period 1930 to 1950 was one in which BMR measurements were central to the management of thyroid disease. Thereafter, chemical measurements in the blood and urine replaced the BMR, and a generation of hospital patients was treated

on the basis of assumed levels of energy expenditure, which were never measured.

Nutritional biochemistry at the beginning of the 1900s developed in university departments and was perceived to be of economic importance to the agricultural, dairy, and meat industries. Two outstanding biochemists came from hospital laboratories and are now considered by many to be the fathers of clinical biochemistry: Otto Folin (McLean Hospital, Waltham, Mass, later chairman at Harvard)[16] and Donald van Slyke (Hospital of the Rockefeller Institute—later the Rockefeller University).[17] Both individuals and their associates contributed important measurement techniques that allowed new understanding of normal metabolism and alteration associated with human disease.

The development of nutritional science depended on the development of specific measurements for individual nutrients. However, a measurement of a nutrient could not be attempted until the nutrient was identified. During the first 40 years of the 20th century, the laboratories of biochemistry departments commonly included facilities for animal diet preparation. A defined diet of supposedly complete composition would be fed to an animal, usually a rodent, and growth rate, activity, and appearance carefully followed. When growth was inadequate, extracts of foods would be added to the diet until proper growth was obtained. Then the successful extract would be chemically analyzed in search of the hidden factor. Micronutrients were often discovered by means of the "deficiency disease" route. Dudrick has written of the early days of hyperalimentation, which provided a human counterpart to this search for unexpectedly important nutrients.[18]

◆ MODERN BIOCHEMISTRY AND PHYSIOLOGY—1920 ONWARD

After World War I, the modern phase of biochemistry and physiology began to develop. A transition in nutritional science was particularly evident with the publication of two famous textbooks that became classics in their time. One was *The Science of Nutrition* by Lusk, which went through four editions between 1906 and 1928.[19] This was in contrast to *The Newer Knowledge of Nutrition* by E. V. McCollum, which went through five editions between 1918 and 1939.[20] The books by Lusk provided a broad summary of nutritional knowledge at the whole-body level together with early findings on macronutrients and vitamins. In particular, Lusk included extensive data from calorimetric studies. A major change in nutrition research is seen in the books by McCollum, in which the major focus had become enzymes and vitamins, and whole-body calorimetry was ignored.

The interval from 1920 to 1940 was a particularly exciting period in nutritional biochemistry that allowed one to relate gas exchange in the whole body to the handling of a food within the cell. Individual enzymatic reactions in carbohydrate chemistry became known as steps in the glycolytic pathway.[21] Next came the concept of metabolic cycles such as the tricarboxylic acid cycle.[22] The introduction of the central role of coenzyme A served to connect glycolysis and other substrates to the tricarboxylic acid cycle.[23] The release of CO_2 in the tricarboxylic acid cycle of oxidation coupled with phosphorylation was seen to produce ATP (the energy currency used for work), while yielding heat and O_2 uptake for the formation of water.[24] This allowed molecular confirmation of Rubner's caloric equivalent of food from nearly a century before.

Metabolic Response to Starvation

At an earlier time in the 20th century, one occasionally heard that the weight loss seen after injury was simply a severe case of starvation. The similarities and differences between the metabolic response to starvation and to severe illness or injury have gradually become evident over the last 50 years. This differentiation between metabolic responses will ultimately establish whether nutritional support can be central therapy for any given patient.

Malnutrition, with or without edema, has been the subject of progressive reports from developing countries since the beginning of the 1900s. A shift from protein deficiency to calorie deficiency in the etiology of kwashiorkor versus marasmus occurred from 1950 to 1975.[25] This background may be significant when using these terms for patients in an urban hospital who are candidates for nutritional support.[26]

Studies of experimental starvation, total or partial, have shown that dietary restric-

tion causes a reduction in energy expenditure. One of the most complete studies of prolonged human starvation was conducted by Benedict and his associates at the Carnegie Institute of Nutrition in Boston in 1912.[27] A normal, 40-year-old man received continuous metabolic study for 31 days with intake of only distilled water. This period of fasting caused a weight reduction of 22%. Perhaps the most striking feature of these extensive measurements was the starting BMR of 1432 kcal/24 h, which dropped to 1002 calories per day by the end of the third week and remained near this level for the last 10 days. One of the professional staff later remarked that the subject wished to continue the study for religious reasons, but the staff became alarmed that he might be near death and thus stopped the experiment.

The weight loss in the prolonged total starvation of a group was not available until the tragic case in 1992 of the 30 Irish hunger strikers.[28] Their weight loss was nearly linear up to 70 days, when it averaged 38% of the starting weight. The first death occurred at 26% weight loss in 47 days in an individual who suffered a gunshot wound. Nine others died in the subsequent 23 days before the fast was terminated.

The decrease in both BMR and weight loss is, of course, slower with semistarvation than with total starvation. Thirty-two healthy young men were studied in the 1940s at the University of Minnesota in an effort to learn the consequences of partial starvation in countries under the Nazi occupation. These men underwent 24 weeks of semistarvation, which resulted in an average loss of 23% of body weight.[29] During this time, the average BMR decreased by 39%. However, when the BMR was calculated per kilogram of actual body weight, the decrease was only half as much. These data are consistent with the loss of fat and a selective portion of lean tissue during semistarvation; the remaining lean tissue maintained an energy expenditure that amounted to approximately 60% of that of the normal human body. Elia has summarized the organ and tissue contribution to the BMR and how this may be influenced in various pathologic states.[30, 31]

World War II shifted medical research to problems of immediate concern to combat troops stationed around the world. James Gamble, a Boston pediatrician, undertook to determine the minimal intake of food and fluid to allow survival in a life raft if a person was forced down at sea.[32] These findings highlighted that an intake of only 100 g of carbohydrate per day exerted a marked effect on reducing nitrogen excretion.

Cahill and associates conducted extensive metabolic studies that provided much new data on human starvation.[33] In particular, this involved key interorgan reactions, particularly in regard to muscle release of amino acids, gluconeogenic precursors in the liver, and the mechanisms to guarantee a continuous supply of glucose for the brain (until ketones could begin to serve as fuel) as well as tissues depending on glycolysis for energy.

Metabolic Response to Injury and Illness

Infectious fevers were characterized in the early 1900s by a "toxic" destruction of body protein. Shaffer and Coleman reported that acute typhoid patients needed large protein intakes and twice-normal calorie intakes to achieve nitrogen balance.[34] This was confirmed by Coleman and DuBois, who showed minimal specific dynamic action with such diets in the presence of the acute febrile state.[35] Clinicians found particular interest in the work of DuBois[35a] regarding the BMR during fever (the BMR increased by 7% for each degree Fahrenheit of fever, sometimes reaching increases of 50%) and the BMR in association with thyroid disease (which could increase by 80% or more in "thyroid storm").

Cuthbertson studied the metabolic response to long bone fracture in healthy young males and observed an increase in energy expenditure and nitrogen excretion that lasted from 1 to 3 weeks after the injury.[36] These studies were misinterpreted by some to mean that the increased energy expenditure exceeded the availability of energy from fat, and hence the body turned to the hydrolysis of protein for two-carbon fuel, which accounted for the increase in nitrogen excretion.

Surgical metabolism made major advances with the work of F. D. Moore and associates in Boston beginning in 1941. The normal pattern of convalescence after surgical operation became a framework for exploring changes in blood volume, fluid and electrolyte shifts, endocrine responses, loss of tissue, and the unique metabolic features of fractures and burns.[37] Weight loss was analyzed by combining metabolic balance studies[38] with body composition using tracers for the simultaneous measure of various body compartments.[39] These studies established that the rapid weight loss after injury and infection is associated with the simultaneous loss of lean tissue and the expansion of the extracellular space. Moore comented that "the engine shrinks within the chassis."

The marked weight loss seen with severe illness or injury was often explained by the extreme increases in energy expenditure thought to accompany such conditions. During the late 1950s Kinney and associates undertook to combine metabolic balance studies with the study of resting energy expenditure (REE) in various types of acute surgical disease and injury. This began with serial measurements of gas exchange, using the tight-fitting mouthpiece or face mask commonly employed in BMR measurements. This equipment was often not tolerated by an acutely ill patient, or it produced a clearly abnormal pattern of breathing with questionable values for gas exchange.[40] A clear plastic head canopy was designed to allow the patient to lie comfortably and breathe in a relaxed manner for 39 to 60 minutes with nothing attached to the face or upper airway.[41] The downstream air could be continuously analyzed for O_2, CO_2, and $^{14}CO_2$ if a ^{14}C-labeled nutrient had been infused. Multiple measurements each day were used to calculate the REE.

There was considerable surprise when actual measurements revealed much lower increases in the REE than had been assumed.[42] Major operations were seldom followed by the increases in REE that had been shown by DuBois during fever and thyroid disease. However, if the fever involved an extensive inflammatory response such as acute peritonitis, the REE might be increased by 30 to 50% with correspondingly large increases in nitrogen excretion consistent with the earlier findings of Shaffer and Coleman.[34] Major thermal burns were found to have the highest REE (up to 100% above normal) when treated with the open application of antibacterial preparations, a common practice in the 1960s. (However, these extreme degrees of resting hypermetabolism are seldom seen today. One may speculate that modern care in a heated environment, early tangential excision, and closed dressings all have contributed to this reduction in the REE elevations seen in the patient with a major burn.)

These measurements allowed the study of the caloric equivalent of fever[43, 44] and the relation of the REE to the total exchangeable potassium.[45] When combined with metabolic balance studies, the method allowed calculation of the tissue composition of weight loss and the contribution of protein to the REE in various acute surgical conditions.[46]

◆ **CLINICAL INTRODUCTION OF TOTAL PARENTERAL NUTRITION**

Much of the early attention to the intravenous administration of fluids and drugs was to make use of the lifesaving quality of supplying needed elements rapidly and directly into the bloodstream. Therefore, much of the early intravenous use of saline and glucose had to do with the treatment of shock states. Successful blood transfusion had to await Landsteiner's discovery of the major blood groups in 1901.[47] Yet the transfusion of human blood was seldom used until the advent of blood donation and blood banking during the 1940s. Plasma was found to be more effective than saline or glucose for treating shock. The intravenous fluid was administered through bottles and rubber tubing, which were washed and reused up to the early 1940s. Such infusions were frequently associated with chills and fever. Seribert discovered in 1923 that these reactions were caused by organic substances, termed *pyrogens*, which later were identified as endotoxin from bacteria.[48] A rabbit assay was developed to test for such pyrogens.

Carl Walter published in 1933 a detailed account of the problems associated with intravenous infusions and transfusions of blood.[49] (The chairman of medicine at the Peter Bent Brigham Hospital in Boston had established a rule against *any* intravenous treatment because of the frequency and severity of pyrogenic reactions.) Walter's article presents the technical steps in sterilization, which he employed to produce sterile, pyrogen-free water and thus safe intravenous solutions of saline, glucose, and other additives. Subsequently, he founded the Fenwal Laboratories, which pioneered in sterile disposable infusion equipment, directed one of the first blood banks in the country, and became an international authority on hospital infection.

The role of industry in making sterile, pyrogen-free solutions and disposable sterile infusion equipment readily available in the hospital is an advance that is frequently overlooked when considering the development of parenteral nutrition. Cody has reviewed these developments in the history of one company.[50]

Intravenous Infusion of Protein Hydrolysates

The Harrison Department of Surgical Research at the University of Pennsylvania during the 1930s became increasingly interested in the biochemical aspects of surgical care[51] and, in particular, the nutritional aspects of convalescence from illness or injury. Ravdin, Rhoads, and others were particularly impressed with the hazards associated with a patient's having hypoproteinemia. There was growing attention to the importance of low plasma protein levels in producing tissue edema, delayed gastric emptying, poor wound healing, and delayed tissue regeneration after chemical, physical, or thermal injury. Ravdin and associates explored these effects of protein depletion in various ways, including the influence of nutrition on hepatic regeneration in animals after injury from chloroform.[52] In other institutions, Whipple studied protein depletion in the dog using plasmapheresis,[53] and Cannon and coworkers reported experimental animal studies that linked a decrease in immune function with protein depletion.[54]

The requirements and metabolism of individual amino acids were only partially known in the 1930s. W. C. Rose, professor of biochemistry at the University of Illinois, and colleagues had just completed the list of essential amino acids for animals in 1935 after they had discovered threonine.[55] Rose's laboratory published from 1942 to 1952 extensive studies on the relative amounts of essential amino acids required in adult humans.[56] He kept student volunteers on rigid dietary control and used nitrogen balance as a way of identifying when an essential amino acid was missing or provided in inadequate amounts. It is worth noting that this monumental work was performed despite inadequate knowledge of the B vitamins, no availability of isotopic amino acids, and only limited knowledge concerning the essential amino acids.

The clinical introduction of modern parenteral nutrition came in three phases: (1) in 1937, Elman's use of protein hydrolysates with glucose infused into a peripheral vein followed by (2) in 1962, Wretlind's use of balanced intravenous nutrition that included lipid in a peripheral vein and (3) in 1968, Dudrick and associates' use of lipid-free hyperalimentation in a central vein.

Elman reported the provision of amino acids to patients in the form of an infusion of a casein hydrolysate supplemented by tryptophan and methionine or cystine.[57] Many scientists were ambivalent about Elman's approach to providing intravenous amino acids. This skepticism resulted from the knowledge that all amino acids are normally absorbed from the intestinal tract and pass via the portal vein to the liver. The administration of amino acids in a peripheral vein was necessarily unphysiologic.[58] The amino acids were thought to be improperly utilized and perhaps toxic to the brain. Not until studies by Lindstrom counteracted such concerns by showing that the metabolic utilization of casein hydrolysate was the same using either the intravenous or the intraportal route was this method accepted.[59]

Elman published his experience in 1947 in a book entitled *Parenteral Alimentation in Surgery*. His preface is an entertaining review of historical efforts at parenteral nutrition. Intravenous protein hydrolysates lessened the negative nitrogen balance in surgical patients but did not reliably produce a positive balance. The variable results were thought to be because the solutions did not have a uniform amino acid composition. There was variable in vitro digestion of the source protein, which might leave an excess of the acid or enzyme together with an excess of undigested protein, either of which might cause fever or an allergic reaction. Despite the limitations of this form of therapy, it has been suggested that Elman should be honored as "the father of intravenous nutrition."[58]

Wretlind visited Elman and other investigators in the United States during the late 1940s and returned to Stockholm to work on producing a more uniform protein hydrolysate for intravenous use. However, trials with an improved solution did not readily produce a positive nitrogen balance, and Wretlind concluded that this goal would never be possible without the provision of adequate calories. The University of Pennsylvania investigators experimented with the use of protein hydrolysates that had been introduced by Elman in St. Louis. However, they concluded that without an adequate supply of calories, the amino acid intake appeared to be oxidized to meet energy requirements and not incorporated into new tissue.

The glucose calories that could be given into a peripheral vein were restricted by the volume of fluid that could be given if isotonic solutions were used, and damage to the vein occurred with more concentrated solutions. Extensive research was devoted to examining the balance between the fluid loads that could be tolerated and the increase in glucose concentration that could still avoid serious damage to the vein wall. Rhoads sought to include one of the newer diuretics along with the large fluid volumes needed to infuse an adequate supply of glucose.[61] Unfortunately, the response to the diuretic was too unpredictable for it to be used in this manner. Alcohol by intravenous infusion had been shown to be unsatisfactory in prolonged use.

At Vanderbilt in the 1940s, Meng and Early had developed an olive oil emulsion that was successful in the dog but was not satisfactory in humans.[62] Therefore, the search went on for a fat preparation that was stable, nontoxic, and readily utilized as a calorie source. Geyer and Stare conducted extensive work in Boston to develop and study a cottonseed oil emulsion, which was marketed until the late 1960s under the name of Lipomul.[63] The incidence of side effects from the cottonseed oil emulsion prevented its general acceptance for clinical nutrition and resulted in its withdrawal from the market in the late 1960s, causing some unintended results (presented later). Thompson in 1974 published an extensive review of the pathology of parenteral nutrition with lipids.[64] He traced reports of functional changes and histologic findings in organs and tissues as successive lipid preparations were tested for over five decades.

Investigators in both Europe and the United States were united in their conviction that effective parenteral nutrition had to provide adequate calories to produce effective utilization of protein intake. However, they had to either solve the problem of the intravenous toxicity of lipids or learn to successfully handle the water volume needed to infuse sufficient glucose calories.

Balanced Intravenous Nutrition Without Complications

During the late 1950s, Wretlind experimented with a wide variety of lipid preparations in the dog until he developed a soybean oil emulsion using an egg yolk phosphatide.[65] This provided excellent growth in puppies with no evidence of organ dysfunction. Extensive studies in patients were performed with his surgical colleagues Schuberth and Hallberg, demonstrating an impressive freedom from side effects.[66, 67]

The triglyceride particles were shown by Hallberg and associates to have an in vivo decay rate comparable to that of normal chylomicrons.[68] The particles rapidly assumed an apoprotein envelope from circulating proteins.[69] Changes in the respiratory quotient and tracer studies confirmed that the lipid preparation was promptly utilized as a calorie source. For the first time, it was possible to infuse patients with an amount of carbohydrate, amino acids (by hydrolysate), and lipid that simulated the dietary intake of a normal individual without fear of fever, chills, or abnormal metabolic reactions.

Lipid-Free Hyperalimentation

Jonathan Rhoads encouraged Dudrick and associates to undertake a project to determine whether it was possible for puppies to grow normally with the entire nutrition provided by the intravenous route.[70] Vars and colleagues designed a special swivel apparatus that allowed the dogs and later unrestrained rats to move about without disturbing the flow of nutrients.[71, 72] Midway in this study, the Food and Drug Administration forced the withdrawal of Lipomul, which was the only lipid emulsion available in the United States. Rhoads urged that the project not be terminated, but rather that researchers find out whether the missing calories from fat could be provided by extra glucose calories. To the surprise of the investigators, the animals grew at a normal rate and appeared to be entirely healthy.[73] At the time of sacrifice, small amounts of pigment were seen in the Kupffer cells of the liver but did not appear to have any functional significance. The original intention had been to give the animals an increased amount of water to lower the osmolality of the nutrient solution.

Catheterization of the central circulation and the right side of the heart had been considered too hazardous to undertake in humans during the 1930s. Around 1940, Dickinson Richards started this experimental procedure at a major university hospital, leading to a departmental prohibition of such catheterization due to its presumed hazard. Richards then joined forces with André Cournand, who was investigating shock by this procedure at the Columbia Service at Bellevue Hospital.[74] This work was awarded a Nobel Prize shortly after. Catheterization of the central circulation opened a new chapter in cardiology, followed by popularization of central venous pressure measurements in the intensive care unit during the early 1960s. Thus, such catheterization of a central vein was an accepted procedure when Dudrick and coworkers introduced hyperalimentation with its need for sufficient blood flow to dilute the nutrients and prevent damage to the vessel walls. These investigators proposed the subclavian approach from the report of Aubaniac.[75]

The opportunity to find out whether a human infant could grow with only intravenous nutrition was presented by an infant who was born with massive atresia of the small bowel.[76] She underwent surgery on the day of her birth, and most of the small bowel was resected. Ten days later, she was doing poorly, and a contrast study showed that the stomach had no motility. A catheter was passed into the external jugular vein, and a mixture of protein hydrolysate and glucose with vitamins and electrolytes was started. Within 48 hours, the vital signs were normal, and her weight steadily increased from 4 to 7.5 lb in the next 45 days. Efforts to discontinue the hyperalimentation were unsuccessful, and therefore the patient continued receiving intravenous feeding for the 22 months of her life. She did well for the first 16 months but then appeared to reach a plateau and died 6 months later. Studies were than undertaken in puppies with extensive resection of the small bowel to determine the extent of intestinal loss that could be sustained if adequate nutrition allowed sufficient time for adaptation.[77]

The rapid acceptance in the United States of the lipid-free hyperalimentation was a tremendous stimulus to medical interest in nutrition and provided new horizons in the clinical care of a wide variety of clinical conditions.[78] However, the differences of opinion between U.S. advocates of lipid-free hyperalimentation and those elsewhere who believed in providing lipid as part of parenteral nutrition continued throughout the 1970s, even after lipid products reached the U.S. market in 1976 and 1978. These differences provided stimulus for research into both carbohydrate and fat metabolism as well as amino acid metabolism, as noted in the following section.

◆ APPLICATION OF PARENTERAL NUTRITION—1972 TO 1985

Nutritional Assessment

Malnutrition was formerly considered a problem only in the underdeveloped world. Butterworth published a classic paper, "Skeleton in the Hospital Closet," in 1976 in which he called attention to the mortality and morbidity associated with malnutrition in hospital patients.[79] This was followed by multiple reports in the U.S. and European literature reporting the prevalence of hospital malnutrition to be from 25 to 65%, depending on the patient population.[80–83] The medical community became aware that although weight loss was the primary feature of malnutrition, the actual weights of patients in the hospital were frequently neglected. The problems associated with single body-weight measurements have been reviewed.[84] The new attention to hospital malnutrition gave impetus to nutritional assessment.

Major problems became evident with measurements for nutritional assessment: (1) a wide range of normal values in some measurements meant that a person might start at the top of the range and develop considerable deficit before dropping below the range of normal; (2) the relationship between abnormal measurements and loss of function of tissues and organs was often not clear; therefore, (3) measurements of malnutrition provided only a general approximation to the outcome, and (4) this led to controversy over just how soon and how much nutritional support to provide for a given patient.

Nutritional assessment in the 1970s usually related to body composition, plasma protein concentrations, and immune competence. Bedside anthropometry became popular, particularly the estimate of fat stores from skin folds[85] and estimate of muscle from forearm circumference.[86] Plasma proteins, such as transferrin, with a short half-life were considered along with the serum albumin concentration.[87] Immune status was measured by skin tests of delayed hypersensitivity.[88]

Increasing the sensitivity of assessment would be expected to increase the number of patients who might benefit from nutritional support while helping to exclude some patients who might receive unnecessary support. Therefore, efforts were made to combine various measurements such as the prognostic nutritional index developed at the University of Pennsylvania.[89] It depended largely on the serum albumin and transferrin concentrations. A clinical assessment of nutritional status, termed *subjective global assessment*, was designed to provide a focused history and physical examination that emphasized aspects of nutritional significance.[90] This was combined with specific laboratorty tests to evaluate clinical abnormalities already noted. Bedside anthropometry, attention to fluid status, and simple muscle function were included. This same group reported that the subjective global assessment was a better predictor of postoperative complications than serum albumin levels, serum transferrin levels, delayed cutaneous hypersensitivity, the creatinine-height index, or the prognostic nutritional index.[91]

Determining the Indications

The introduction of TPN forced many clinicians to face the prevalence of malnutrition in their patients and to consider when this new therapy would be of benefit. The question "What is malnutrition?" became "How severe should the changes in malnutrition become before it affects the outcome of my patient?" The first question was more involved than the attention it usually received, and information regarding the second question is only slowly emerging. Initial worry over septic complications with intravenous nutrition was decreased with the demonstration that meticulous catheter care and the expertise of a multidisciplinary team could sharply reduce the rate of complications and enhance the effectiveness of care.[92, 93]

There was early excitement over the widespread benefits that might accrue from the application of parenteral nutrition to hospitalized patients as diverse as those undergoing elective operation for benign disease to those with advanced cancer. Buzby and associates conducted a large study in Veterans Administration hospitals to assess the preoperative use of TPN.[94] Patients with no evidence of malnutrition failed to show benefit from using preoperative TPN. There was even a suggestion that the treated patients had a small chance of infection not present in the untreated group. The time when postoperative use of TPN should be started remained controversial, although many clinicians felt that it should be started if a period without adequate oral intake exceeded 7 days. TPN was thought important for patients with inflammatory bowel disease, to allow a period of "bowel rest"; however, this approach is no longer a primary means of therapy.[95] Studies by Brennan and coworkers are consistent with the idea that the use of TPN in cancer patients does not appear to improve the outcome unless the nutritional support allows time for some form of effective cancer therapy to be provided.[96]

Moderating the Calorie Intake

The REE of acute injury was frequently overestimated during the 1950s and 1960s. When actual measurements established unexpectedly modest levels of hypermetabolism, it became apparent that the increases due to disease or injury were seldom enough to offset the lack of energy expenditure resulting from inactivity during a period of hospitalization, particularly with constant bed rest.

During the first decade of hyperalimentation, the recommended calorie intakes were relatively high by current standards. Factors

contributing to these high initial calorie (and carbohydrate) intakes were as follows:

1. There was a persistent belief that the rapid weight loss of acute catabolic conditions was associated with a large increase in REE.
2. When the increases in REE were estimated, an additional requirement or "stress factor" was added to ensure effectiveness.
3. The high glucose loads were usually reduced as intravenous lipid became available, but lipid was sometimes added to the usual glucose intake as a sort of calorie "bonus."
4. There was a delayed recognition that a strongly positive calorie balance might be associated with undesirable side effects. One of the most common problems that could arise during chronic TPN therapy was hepatic dysfunction, particularly abnormal liver chemistries, which were often assumed to be associated with some degree of hepatic steatosis.[97–99] A study of the hepatic histologic appearance by needle biopsy in patients receiving TPN with and without liver disease revealed that an abnormal histologic appearance was correlated with abdominal sepsis, renal failure, or preexisting liver disease but not with the TPN.[100]

Large glucose loads were shown by Nordenstrom and coworkers to be associated with a stimulus to the sympathetic nervous system, as evidenced by increases in norepinephrine excretion.[101] This was associated with increased ventilatory drive[102] as reported by Barcroft and associates.[103] These undesirable side effects of "calorie loading" were most frequently evident with rapid infusions during the acute catabolic phase and less evident or absent during the later anabolic phase of recovery. As time has passed, the recommended calorie intake during the acute catabolic phase has changed toward giving only the requirement for energy equilibrium and gradually increasing the intake to a positive balance during the subsequent anabolic phase. In other words, the goal of a positive balance of calories and nitrogen was recognized to be tissue synthesis, and it was recognized that this is not a major priority for the body (and sometimes may not even be possible) during the acute catabolic phase.

The need for intravenous lipids in TPN was a controversial subject in the United States after a commercial preparation became available in 1976. However, it became evident that apart from providing a concentrated, isotonic source of energy, the lipid emulsion also supplied essential fatty acids for synthesis of significant cellular constituents.[104] Without an exogenous supply, the long-term patient becomes deficient, with potential complications.

Malnutrition is accepted to be associated with reduced host defense and increased incidence or severity of certain infections.[105, 106] During the 1970s and 1980s, concern was expressed that TPN, given in order to replete or maintain energy and nutritional stores and to support host defense mechanisms in critical illness, might have the opposite effect and cause further impairment of host defenses. Interest was focused on possible detrimental effects of parenterally administered lipids. Palmblad has reviewed this evidence and concluded that host defense considerations are not adequate justification for withholding intravenous lipid therapy, but that much more research is needed to understand how lipids modulate immunity.[107]

Patient-Oriented Research

The period 1970 to 1985 was one of rapid growth in the study of energy and nutrient metabolism. Measurements of body composition, indirect calorimetry, metabolic balance, regional catheterization, and isotopic studies were employed in healthy subjects and gradually introduced to the study of hospitalized patients.

Early studies with isotopic glucose revealed that the hyperglycemia associated with acute catabolic conditions is not associated with decreased oxidation, as had been suggested.[108] Other studies showed that there is an upper limit to the rate of glucose oxidation.[109] High and low infusion rates of glucose indicated that rates of glucose oxidation are lower and fat oxidation higher in acutely ill patients than in healthy controls.[110] However, hyperalimentation often produced a respiratory quotient over 1 on the basis of increased CO_2 excretion associated with lipogenesis.[111] The ventilatory response to the increased CO_2 was to increase both dead space and alveolar ventilation.[112] This response was abolished as lipid was substituted for some of the glucose calories.[113] Subsequent studies indicated that the nitrogen intake had a specific influence on ventilatory drive.[114, 115]

The malnourished patient displays weakness and fatigue that seem consistent with prolonged negative nitrogen balance, being in large part at the expense of skeletal muscle. The study of muscle metabolism was advanced by the needle biopsy technique of Bergstrom, which allowed changes to be studied in various surgical conditions.[116] A decrease in muscle glutamine levels was seen with short-term starvation, and a marked drop was seen in various stress states.[117] One of the indices for the effectiveness of various types of parenteral nutrition has been the degree to which this drop in muscle glutamine levels could be attenuated.[118]

Infusions of glycerol or free fatty acids in healthy humans show a linear relationship between the concentration of these lipid materials and their turnover rate. After injury, this correlation no longer exists and the turnover rate is faster than predicted from the plasma concentration.[119] Isotopic palmitate studies in such patients showed higher rates of turnover and oxidation than would be expected from circulating concentrations.[120] These findings are consistent with respiratory quotient measurements indicating higher fat oxidation than suggested by plasma concentrations of fatty acids in acutely ill patients.

Many clinicians and scientists have been involved in research directed toward understanding the metabolic response of the patient at nutritional risk and the optimal application of nutritional support. Space does not permit the proper acknowledgment of many contributors. However, certain individuals were actively involved in the initial years of parenteral nutrition and have continued over the subsequent 30 years to make important contributions that have shaped the modern approach to nutritional support.

Josef Fischer developed one of the first national nutritional support services in a large urban hospital and has continued to write authoritative books on parenteral nutrition and to develop a progressive research program with particular emphasis on the pathophysiology of amino acid metabolism.[121] George Blackburn did much to establish the American Society of Parenteral and Enteral Nutrition (ASPEN) as an effective nutritional organization. He has since directed an active research program in clinical nutrition[122] and maintained a popular postgraduate educational series in nutritional support while providing continued leadership in national nutritional organization. Wesley Alexander has combined leadership in clinical infection and transplantation with a continuing interest in nutrition,[123] where novel ideas in the laboratory have undergone clinical trials and have influenced patient care. Michael Meguid has conducted nutritional investigation while developing extensive opportunities to foster nutritional support through education and research throughout the world.

Robert Wolfe and his associates have explored the altered kinetics of nutrients in various pathologic conditions, particularly in the burned patient. During the 1970s, some investigators stressed that TPN with large amounts of both calories and nitrogen should be administered to realize the full benefits of nutritional support. Wolfe and associates showed that an upper limit for glucose oxidation exists beyond which benefit is not expected.[124] Later his group demonstrated that the administration of amino acids beyond a specific amount resulted in a faster turnover rate of nitrogen with no improvement in nitrogen balance.[125] He has extended these research techniques to normal humans and the metabolism associated with conditions including bed rest,[126] fasting,[127] and exercise.[128] He and his associates have extended their investigations with stable isotopes to the mathematics of modeling systems[129] and to many sophisticated studies in the injured patient. He is responsible for a definitive text on the methodology of radioactive and stable isotopes and has provided unique training opportunities for a number of visiting investigators.[130]

Formation of ASPEN and ESPEN

The enthusiasm surrounding TPN was a great stimulus to nutritional support of all kinds and attracted the interest of not only physicians but also dieticians, nurses, and pharmacists. In 1978, a multidisciplinary organization, ASPEN, was formed and its 20th anniversary was celebrated at the group's clinical congress in Washington in 1998.[131] The organization is dedicated to the optimal nutritional support of patients during hospitalization and throughout covalescence. It also represented the growing recognition that multidisciplinary teams could enhance the provision of nutritional support.

A parallel interest was growing during the 1970s in Europe, resulting in the formation of the European Society of Parenteral and Enteral Nutrition (ESPEN).[132] Although a formal meeting was held in Stockholm in 1979, the society was not formally established until the following year. The 20th anniversary of ESPEN was celebrated in Stockholm in 1999.

Home Parenteral Nutrition— The Oley Foundation

Several investigators during the 1970s demonstrated that TPN could be effectively administered in the home setting.[133, 134] Increased use of home TPN was made, particularly in patients with severe short bowel syndrome, or inflammatory bowel disease, or who were undergoing therapy for selected malignant disease. ASPEN published guidelines for home TPN in 1987 in which the need for proper selection and monitoring was emphasized.[135] Specific contraindications were also noted, particularly whenever the responsible family member was unable to learn the techniques required, whenever such home support was not desired by the patient or family, or when the risks were judged to exceed the potential benefits.

The Oley Foundation was established through the leadership of Lynn Howard to provide a network of support for such patients and to track the national experience with this therapy. The foundation is now over 15 years old and is performing a much-needed service for the field of TPN.[136]

◆ SHARPENING THE FOCUS— 1985 ONWARD

Form Versus Function

Hill and Beddoe have presented the dimensions of the human body including neutron activation data for body nitrogen content.[137] Pierson, Heymsfield, and associates have further refined the models of human body composition using current research techniques.[138] Elia has analyzed various models of body composition in comparison with bedside techniques, suggesting the important developments needed to better utilize our research knowledge in treating the malnourished patient.[139]

Windsor and Hill have reported that the important measures of physiologic function are those that correlate with clinical outcome.[140] These investigators have sought to correlate the changes in body composition with weight loss in adults and the associated physiologic impairment (respiratory function, muscle strength, wound healing, and immune function). These investigators reported that preoperative protein loss in surgical patients influences clinical outcome only when it is accompanied by physiologic impairment. From their work in body composition, they considered that the "critical protein loss" is approximately 20% of the protein in the predicted healthy state. This appeared to approximate a weight loss of 10%, which might be considered a threshold for starting nutritional support.

Kursheed Jeejeebhoy is a gastroenterologist who has shown an unusual capacity to bridge the clinical and research aspects of nutritional support. He used metabolic balance studies to demonstrate the time course of the protein-sparing effects of fat versus carbohydrate. He was one of the earliest to write a book that outlined the principles of TPN in the hospital and in the home.[141] He urged the use of physiologic and statistical approaches to measure the outcome of this new therapy.[142]

Jeejeebhoy stressed that changes in body weight or in body composition must be correlated with function because function determines outcome.[143] The adverse functional effects of malnutrition on muscle function, that is, weakness and fatigue, could not be equated to a simple loss of lean body mass, nor could restoration of muscle function be equated with a positive nitrogen balance. This concept led to a standardized examination of muscle contraction (stimulation of the adductor pollicis) to reveal functional evidence of malnutrition.[144] It was postulated that similar changes occur in the stimulated malnourished muscle as occur after exercise-induced fatigue, perhaps involving calcium accumulation and slow relaxation. Thus, malnutrition would be associated with limited energy sources for muscle force on stimulation.

Insulin Resistance

Insulin is the central hormone for metabolic regulation and particularly for anabolic processes.[145] This involves all three macronutrients. Many of the metabolic events after injury or infection may be related to a loss or reduction of the tissue sensitivity to insulin. The catabolic response includes a modest hyperglycemia and a decreased uptake of glucose by insulin-sensitive tissues.[146] There is an increase in circulating levels of free fatty acids and glycerol, indicating a reduced antilipolytic effect of insulin and associated with increased fat oxidation.[119] The insulin resistance has been shown to develop postoperatively in close association with the increase in nitrogen loss, perhaps indicating a reduced sensitivity to the inhibitory effects of insulin on protein breakdown.[147] The changes in insulin action in stress states have been attributed to the combined action of the catabolic hormones,[148] although cytokine actions may contribute to these effects.[149] There are different types of insulin resistance, and it remains to be determined whether that seen after injury is the same as that in infection. There is evidence that acute starvation promptly results in insulin resistance, raising the possibility of another factor in postoperative insulin resistance.[150]

It has been traditional to consider metabolic regulation by insulin to occur in the membrane or within the cell. During the early 1990s, there was growing interest in whether the metabolic regulation of these "intracellular" events may, in part, be regulated through changes in the microcirculatory blood flow and pericellular fluid. Baron and coworkers have shown that insulin influences the microcirculation in human muscle.[151] Thus, insulin appears to be a vasoactive peptide that may play an extracellular regulatory role in metabolism.[152]

Cytokines and Inflammation

Cuthbertson introduced the study of metabolic response to injury by the study of long bone fractures in previously healthy young males,[36] yet the findings were frequently considered to be common to both injury and infection with the exception of fever in the latter. Atkins studied fever for decades and along with coworkers identified a product of white blood cells important in the etiology of fever.[153] Kluger has developed scientific evidence for the beneficial effects of fever.[154] Beisel and Sobocinski in 1979 published a hypothesis that the leukocyte endogenous mediator is a central mediator of nonspecific and specific immunity, facilitates wound healing, and places metabolic demands on the host leading to a negative nutrient balance and malnutrition.[155] LEM, leukocyte endogenous mediator, also known as endogenous pyrogen or lymphocyte-activating factor, represents a factor that induces fever and evokes profound cellular, organ, and systemic alterations in nitrogen metabolism, trace metal metabolism, and hormonal distribution. Leukocyte endogenous mediator was later named interleukin 1.

Much of the initial attention to the metabolic and nutritional aspects of cytokines was devoted to tumor necrosis factor and interleukin 1. The biologic roles of these two cytokines were found to involve many functions. Dinarello presented interleukin 1 as having metabolic, hematologic, vascular, and neural effects.[156] Tumor necrosis factor was found to be the same as "cachectin," a macrophage-secreted hormone released in response to invasive stimuli, and is central to the production of inflammation with associated fever.[157] When tumor necrosis factor was given acutely to animals, it would produce lethal shock, whereas chronic low-dose administration led to cachexia.[158] This has led to intense efforts to develop blocking agents that interrupt the effects of tumor necrosis factor. A major challenge on the research frontier has been to understand the interaction between cytokines and the conventional catabolic hormones, as well as the interaction among the many emerging growth factors such as insulin-like growth factor I and the anabolic hormones such as insulin and growth hormone.[159]

Parenteral Versus Enteral Nutrition and Gut Function

It has been accepted by nearly everyone that "if the gut works, use it." However, the opinions have been in conflict regarding whether the atrophy of the intestinal mucosa that accompanies TPN carries any significant meaning in regard to absorptive capacity, immune function, or even vulnerability to bacterial translocation.[160] Therefore, studies from various disciplines are directing attention to the function of the atrophic gut and to which enteral nutrients may prevent or restore the mucosa to normal.[161] This questions assumes particular significance when treating patients with short bowel conditions.

The study of immunity and inflammation has increased attention on the intestinal tract as an immune organ. The intestine is a central player in immunity with an extensive antigen-presenting area, a large traffic of lymphocytes in and out of the organ, and sophisticated neural connections, such that it has been called "the small brain."[162, 163] The numerous ways that enteral nutrition may support these functions and maintain the gut barrier function presents an obvious challenge to those interested in the proper balance between enteral and parenteral nutrition in nutritional support.

Douglas Wilmore was a collaborator with Dudrick in the initial development of hyperalimentation. Subsequently, he and his associates have made numerous contributions to the understanding of the metabolic response to injury, particularly the interorgan traffic of nutrients.[164] He and his coworkers emphasized that the healing wound requires glucose because of the need for energy from glycolysis, thus leading to the recognition that the wound places specific metabolic requirements on the body economy as though it were another organ.[165] His group conducted studies to differentiate the response to infection from that of injury. They then extended the observation of decreased muscle glutamine after injury to develop the therapeutic role of glutamine for selected tissues such as the intestinal mucosa.[166, 167] This has stimulated extensive work on nutrition for the enterocyte as well as the role of glutamine and trophic factors in adaptation after intestinal loss.

Nutritional Pharmacology and Oxidative Stress

The term *nutritional pharmacology* has had at least two definitions. The older one was the addition of drugs to the administration of nutrients. However, the more common usage relates to adding specific nutrients (or related compounds) in amounts beyond conventional requirements to achieve pharmacologic actions.

The branched-chain amino acids[168] and medium-chain triglycerides[169] represent early efforts to modify conventional parenteral solutions. The most common specific nutrients currently under consideration for their pharmacologic effects are glutamine,[170] arginine,[171] the short-chain fatty acids,[172] and the n-3 fatty acids.[173] Furst and colleagues have emphasized the potential importance of dipeptides to provide particular amino acids in increased amounts or when solubility prevents their inclusion in conventional parenteral solutions.[174] Dahlan and associates have demonstrated changes in the cell membrane with an intravenous lipid emulsion.[175]

The concept of disease-specific solutions, marketed for the specific treatment of one or another condition, is still in an early phase. It seems obvious that success in this area will progress only as fast as our fundamental knowledge of the underlying physiologic and metabolic abnormalities can be developed.

The concept of tissue damage from *free radicals* or *reactive oxygen species* has gained rapid momentum during the late 1980s and has been implicated in conditions as diverse as hemorrhagic shock, acquired immunodeficiency syndrome, arthritis, and aging.[176] Oxidative stress is said to result when these free radicals are generated in excess in the human body, causing cell injury or death by damage to DNA, proteins, and/or lipids. Cells can tolerate mild oxidative stress and may respond by increased synthesis of antioxidant defense enzymes.[177] Oxidative stress may occur by either an excessive production or a decrease in the concentration of normal antioxidant materials. Malnutrition may be associated with decreased levels of antioxidants such as α-tocopherol, vitamin C, and glutathione. There is major interest in whether specific antioxidants or their precursors should be included as part of future nutrition in various stress states.

Studies on the inflammatory response have led to our understanding of an unexpected confluence of amino acid metabolism, cellular inflammation, and free radical pharmacology in the form of nitric oxide. Stuehr and Marketta announced in 1985 that mouse macrophages could produce nitrate and nitrite in response to endotoxin.[178] This led to an explosion of interest in nitric oxide when it became evident that it was involved in signal transduction in essentially every major physiologic system in the body. The sole source appears to be arginine. Its diversity of molecular targets relates to its ability to rapidly react with other reactive compounds that have unpaired electrons. In addition to regulating vascular tone, it is a mediator of cytotoxicity, and induction of its synthesis is central to immune response, leading to inflammation and tissue injury.[179] The present knowledge is so incomplete that attempting to manipulate production from arginine or block its peripheral actions has produced negative as well as positive effects.

Outcomes and Evidence-Based Medicine

Medical progress through the first half of the 1900s depended largely on a process of carefully observing groups of patients given a new and promising therapy. The outcome was then compared with that previously observed in groups undergoing conventional treatment. This approach was effective if therapeutic effects were dramatic or the pathophysiology was relatively uncomplicated. The era of randomized trials began in the 1950s, and the methods have been refined since then despite objections on ethical grounds.[179] The importance of objective data supporting any particular therapy has become more urgent as various strategies are being employed to restrict the growth of costs for health care. Nowhere is this more relevant that in nutritional support.

Providing nutritional support seems intuitively correct if there is doubt about a patient's receiving an adequate oral intake. The risks are small in qualified hands; hence, why should a purified mixture of established nutrients have to go through the same testing and regulatory steps in production and then have to prove efficacy as if it were a strange new drug for a poorly understood disease?

Koretz has written,[180] "Since the introduction of nutritional support (NS) as a specific therapeutic entity in the 1960s, a number of claims have been made, and widely believed, regarding its ability to improve the natural history of many diseases. However, these claims have been disseminated in the absence of supportive data prospective randomized controlled trials (PRCTs); in fact, when such studies have been performed, they have by and large not been able to demonstrate that NS does improve morbidity and/or mortality."

The prospective randomized controlled trials pose ethical problems because the physician is sworn to treat the individual patient, whereas the clinical scientist is concerned with answering questions, that is, determining the validity of formally constructed hypotheses, not delivering therapy. Thus, some have argued that techniques appropriate to the laboratory may not be applied to humans.[181] Others have argued that prospective randomized controlled trials are the most scientifically sound and ethically correct means of evaluating new therapies. There is potential conflict between the roles of physician and physician-scientist; therefore, society has created mechanisms to ensure the interests of individual patients who elect to participate in a clinical trial.[182]

Critics of current medical care state that all too often physicians rely on custom, hearsay, and dogma in choosing treatments. Ten centers around the world are cooperating in the Cochrane Collaboration, with the objective of searching the world literature to find and review all the prospective randomized controlled trials ever published and republish the findings in an electronic form. It is hoped that this will bring a new force to clinical decision making by using current best evidence. However, such ambitious ventures are not limited to demonstrating that popular forms of therapy are not effective; it hopes also to highlight positive evidence for therapies that have been overlooked. A new journal in England entitled *Evidence-Based Medicine* and its U.S. counterpart, the American College of Physicians *Journal Club,* are designed to publicize the actual evidence about which therapies work and which do not.[183]

Nutrition is not primary therapy except for conditions in which the problem is limited to inadequate food intake. For most clinical conditions, nutritional support is not intended to be primary but rather to support the nutritional needs of the patient so that primary therapy may be effective. The pharmacologic use of nutrients may bring a different perspective to nutritional support, requiring a more fundamental understanding of normal homeostasis and the underlying mechanisms by which stress states induce catabolism, before we address the particular anabolic requirements for recovery.

REFERENCES

1. Saunders JB de CM: The Illustrations from the Works of Vesalius. World Publishing, 1950.
2. Winslow CEA, Herrington LP: Temperature and Human Life. Princeton University Press, 1949.
3. Frank RG Jr: Harvey and the Oxford Physiologists. University of California Press, 1980.
4. Read J: Joseph Black, MD. Glasgow, Jackson Son, 1950.
5. Clark JR: Joseph Priestley "a Comet in the System." The Friends of Joseph Priestley House, 1994.
6. Holmes FL: Lavoisier and The Chemistry of Life. University of Wisconsin Press, 1985.
7. McCosh FWJ: Boussingault, Chemist and Agriculturist. D Reidel, 1984.
8. Holmes FL: Claude Bernard and Animal Chemistry. Cambridge, Harvard University Press, 1974.
9. Thomas K: Justus von Liebig. In Darby WJ, Jukes TH (eds): Founders of Nutrition Science, Vol 2. American Institute of Nutrition, 1992, pp 619–628.
10. Mitchell HH: Carl von Voit. In Darby WJ, Jukes TH (eds): Founders of Nutrition Science, Vol 2. American Institute of Nutrition, 1992, pp 1081–1091.
11. Lusk G: The regulation of temperature and basal metabolism. In The Science of Nutrition, 4th ed. Johnson Reprint, 1976, pp 118–143.
12. Chambers WH: Max Rubner. In Darby WJ, Jukes TH (eds): Founders of Nutrition Science, Vol 2. American Institute of Nutrition, 1992.
13. Deuel H Jr: Graham Lusk. In Darby WJ, Jukes TH (eds): Founders of Nutrition Science, Vol 2. American Institute of Nutrition, 1992, pp 655–664.
14. Pollack H: Eugene Floyd DuBois—A biographical sketch. In Darby WJ, Jukes TH (eds): Founders of Nutrition Science, Vol 1. American Institute of Nutrition, 1992, pp 269–272.
15. DuBois EF: Basal Metabolism in Health and Disease. Philadelphia, Lea & Febiger, 1924.
16. Meites S: Otto Folin: America's First Clinical Biochemist. American Association for Clinical Chemistry, 1989.
17. Astrup P, Severinghaus JW: The History of Blood Gases, Acids and Bases. Munksgaard, 1986, pp 252–256.
18. Dudrick SJ: Intravenous nutrition in the high risk infant. In Winters Hesselmeyer (eds): Wiley & Sons, pp 7–30.
19. Lusk G: The Science of Nutrition, 4th ed. Philadelphia, WB Saunders, 1931.
20. McCollum EV: The Newest Knowledge of Nutrition, 5th ed. New York, Macmillan, 1939.
21. Peters JP, Slyke DD: Chemistry nature and classification. In Quantitative Clinical Chemistry Interpretations, Vol 1, 2nd ed. Baltimore, Williams & Wilkins, 1946, pp 97–154.
22. Krebs HA: The intermediary stages in the biological oxidation of carbohydrate. Adv Enzymol 191:3, 1943.

23. Lipman F: Metabolic generation and utilization of phosphate bond energy. Adv Enzymol 99:1, 1941.
24. Harold FM: The Vital Force: A Study of Bioenergetics. WH Freeman, 1986.
25. Waterlow JC: Protein-Energy Malnutrition. London, Edward Arnold, 1992.
26. McClave SA, Mitoraj TE, Thielmeier KA, Greenburg RA: Differentiating subtypes (hypoalbuminemia vs marasmic) of protein-calorie malnutrition: Incidence and clinical significance in a university hospital setting. JPEN J Parenter Enteral Nutr 16:337–342, 1992.
27. Benedict FG: A Study of Prolonged Fasting. Washington, DC, Carnegie Institute, 1915. Publication No. 203.
28. Allison SP: The uses and limitations of nutritional support. Clin Nutr 11:319–330, 1992.
29. Keys A, Brozek J, Henschel A, et al: The Biology of Human Starvation, Vols 1 and 2. University of Minnesota Press, 1950.
30. Elia M: Energy expenditure in the whole body. In Kinney JM, Tucker HN (eds): Energy Metabolism. New York, Raven Press, 1992, pp 19–59.
31. Elia M: Tissue distribution and energetics in weight loss and undernutrition. In Kinney JM, Tucker HN (eds): Physiology, Stress, and Malnutrition. New York, Lippincott-Raven, 1997, pp 383–411.
32. Gamble JL: Physiological information gained from studies on the life raft ration. Harvey Lect 42:247–273, 1947.
33. Cahill GF Jr: Starvation in man. N Engl J Med 282:668–675, 1970.
34. Shaffer PA, Coleman W: Protein metabolism in typhoid fever. Arch Intern Med 4:538, 1909.
35. Coleman W, DuBois EF: Calorimetric observations in typhoid patients with and without food. Arch Intern Med 15:887, 1915.
35a. DuBois EF: Basal Metabolism in Health and Disease. Philadelphia, Lea & Febiger, 1924, pp 311–340.
36. Cuthbertson DP: The disturbance of metabolism produced by bony and non-bony injury, with notes on certain abnormal conditions of bone. Biochem J 24:1244–1263, 1930.
37. Moore FD: Metabolic Care of the Surgical Patient. Philadelphia, WB Saunders, 1959.
38. Moore FD, Ball MR: The Metabolic Response to Surgery. Springfield, Ill, Charles C Thomas, 1952.
39. Moore FD: The Body Cell Mass and Its Supporting Environment. Philadelphia, WB Saunders, 1963.
40. Kinney JM: The effect of injury upon human protein metabolism. In Protein Metabolism, a Ciba Symposium, Leyden 1962. Berlin, Springer-Verlag, 1962, pp 275–296.
41. Kinney JM: Energy deficits in acute illness and injury in energy metabolism and body fuel utilization. Cambridge, MA, Harvard University Printing Office, 1966, pp 167–179.
42. Kinney JM: Tissue fuel and weight loss after injury. J Clin Pathol 23 (Suppl 4):65–72, 1970.
43. Kinney JM, Roe CF: Caloric Equivalent of Fever. I: Patterns of postoperative response. Ann Surg 156:610–622, 1962.
44. Roe CF, Kinney JM: The caloric equivalent of fever. II: The influence of major trauma. Ann Surg 161:140–147, 1965.
45. Kinney JM. Lister J, Moore FD: Relationship of energy expenditure to total exchangeable potassium. Ann N Y Acad Sci 110:711–722, 1963.

46. Duke JH, Jorgensen SB, Broell JR, et al: Contribution of protein to caloric expenditure following injury. Surgery 68:168–174, 1970.
47. Williams JT, Moravec DF: Intravenous Therapy. Hammond, Ind., Clissold, 1967, pp 41–42.
48. Siebert FB: Fever producing substances in some distilled water. Am J Physiol 67:90–104, 1923.
49. Walter CW: Finding a better way. JAMA 263:1675–1678, 1990.
50. Cody TG: Innovating for health: The story of Baxter International Inc. Deerfield, Ill, Baxter International Inc., 1994.
51. Ravdin IS, Rhoads JE: Certain problems illustrating the importance of knowledge of biochemistry by the surgeon. Surg Clin North Am 15:85–100, 1935.
52. Goldschmidt S, Vars H, Ravdin IS: Influence of foodstuffs upon susceptibility of liver to injury by chloroform and probable mechanism of their action. J Clin Invest 18:277–289, 1939.
53. Whipple GH: Hemoglobin, Plasma Protein and Cell Protein. Springfield, Ill, Charles C Thomas, 1948.
54. Cannon PR, Humphreys EM, Wissler RW, Frazier LE: Chemical, clinical and immunological studies on the products of human plasma fractionation. J Clin Invest 23:601, 1944.
55. McCoy RH, Meyer CE, Rose WC: Feeding experiments with mixtures of highly purified amino acids. VIII: Isolation and identification of a new essential amino acid. J Biol Chem 112:283, 1935.
56. Rose WC, Haines WJ, Johnson JE: Letter to the Editor. J Biol Chem 146:683, 1942.
57. Elman R: Amino acid content of the blood following intravenous injection of hydrolyzed casein. Proc Soc Exp Biol Med 37:437–440, 1937.
58. Wretland A: Parenteral Nutrition Support. Lecture, XV International Nutrition Congress in Adelaide, Australia. Stockholm, 1993.
59. Lindstrom F: I: The effect of intraportal administration of a dialyzed enzymatic casein hydrolysate (Aminosol) on the urinary excretion of amino acids and peptides. II: Amino acid concentration in the hepatic vein and a peripheral vein after intravenous infusion of Aminosol. Acta Chir Scand Suppl 186, 1954.
60. Elman R: Parenteral Alimentation in Surgery. New York: Paul B Hoeber, 1947.
61. Rhoads JE: Diuretics as an adjuvant in disposing of extra water as a vehicle in parenteral hyperalimentation [Abstract]. Fed Proc 21:389, 1962.
62. Meng HC, Early F: Study of complete parenteral alimentation in dogs. J Lab Clin Med 34:1121–1132, 1949.
63. Geyer RP: Parenteral nutrition. Physiol Rev 40:150–186, 1960.
64. Thompson SW: The Pathology of Parenteral Nutrition with Lipids. Springfield, Ill, Charles C Thomas, 1974.
65. Wretland A: Complete intravenous nutrition. Theoretical and experimental background. Nutr Metab 14(Suppl):1–57, 1972.
66. Hallberg D, Holm I, Obel AL, et al: Fat emulsions for complete intravenous nutrition. Postgrad Med J 43:307–316, 1967.
67. Wretland A: Current Status of Intralipid and other fat emulsions. In Meng HC, Wilmore DW (eds): Fat Emulsions in Parenteral Nutrition. Chicago, American Medical Association, 1976, pp 109–122.

68. Hallberg D, Schuberth O, Wretlind A: Experimental and clinical studies with fat emulsion for intravenous nutrition. Nutr Dieta 8:245–281, 1966.

69. Havel RJ, Kane JP, Kashyap ML: Interchange of apolipoproteins between chylomicrons and high density lipoproteins during alimentary lipemia in man. J Clin Invest 52:32–38, 1973.

70. Rhoads JE, Dudrick SJ: History of intravenous nutrition. In Rombeau JL, Caldwell MD (eds): Clinical Nutrition: Parenteral Nutrition, 2nd ed. Philadelphia, WB Saunders, 1993, pp 64–74.

71. Rhode CM, Parkins W, Tourtellotte D, Vars HM: Method for continuous intravenous administration of nutritive solutions suitable for prolonged metabolic studies in dogs. Am J Physiol 159:409–414, 1949.

72. Steiger E, Vars HM, Dudrick SJ: A technique for long-term intravenous feeding in unrestrained rats. Arch Surgery 104:330–332, 1972.

73. Dudrick S, Wilmore DW, Vars HM, Rhoads JE: Long-term total parenteral nutrition with growth, development, and positive nitrogen balance. Surgery 64:134–142, 1968.

74. Cournand A: Measurement of the cardiac output in man using the right heart catheterization. Description of technique, discussion of validity and of place in the study of the circulation. Fed Proc 4:207, 1945.

75. Aubaniac R: L'injection intraveineuse sous-claviculaire: Avantages et technique. Presse Med 60:1456, 1952.

76. Wilmore DW, Dudrick SJ: Growth and development of an infant receiving all nutrients exclusively by vein. JAMA 203:140–144, 1968.

77. Wilmore DW, Dudrick SJ, Daly JM, Vars HM: The role of nutrition in the adaptation of the small intestine after massive resection. Surg Gyn Obstet 132:673, 1971.

78. Dudrick SJ, Rhoads JE: New horizons for intravenous feeding. JAMA 215:939–949, 1971.

79. Butterworth CE: Skeleton in the hospital closet. Nutr Today 9:4, 1976.

80. Bistrian BR, Blackburn GL, Vitale J, et al: Prevalence of malnutrition in general medical patients. JAMA 235:1567, 1976.

81. Bistrian BR, Blackburn GL, Hallowell E, et al: Protein status of general surgical patients. JAMA 230:858, 1974.

82. Hill GL, Blackett RL, Pickford I, et al: Malnutrition in surgical patients: An unrecognized problem. Lancet 1:689, 1977.

83. Weinsier RL, Humber EM, Krumdieck CL, et al: Hospital malnutrition: A prospective evaluation of general medical patients during the course of hospitalization. Am J Clin Nutr 32:418, 1979.

84. Morgan DB, Hill GL, Gurkinshaw L: The assessment of weight loss from a single measurement of body weight: The problems and limitations. Am J Clin Nutr 33:2110–2115, 1980.

85. Durnin JVGA, Womersley J: Body fat assessed from total body density and its estimation from skinfold thickness: Measurements on 481 men and women aged from 16 to 72 years. Br J Nutr 37:77, 1974.

86. Collins JP, McCarthy ID, Hill GL: Assessment of protein nutrition in surgical patients: The value of anthropometrics. Am J Clin Nutr 32:1527, 1979.

87. Kelleher PC, Phinney SD, Sims EAH, et al: Effects of carbohydrate-containing and carbohydrate-restricted hypocaloric and eucalorie diets on serum concentrations of retinol-binding protein, thyroxine-binding prealbumin and transferrin. Metabolism 32:95, 1983.

88. Brown R, Bancewicz J, Hamid J, et al: Failure of delayed hypersensitivity skin testing to predict postoperative sepsis and mortality. BMJ 284:851, 1982.

89. Buxby GP, Mullen JL, Matthews DS, et al: Prognostic nutritional index in gastrointestinal surgery. Am J Surg 139:160, 1980.

90. Detsky AS, McLaughlin JR, Baker JP, et al: What is subjective global assessment of nutritional status? JPEN J Parenter Enteral Nutr 11:8–13, 1987.

91. Baker JP, Detsky AS, Whitwell J, et al: A comparison of the predictive value of nutritional assessment techniques. Human Nutr Clin Nutr 36c:233–241, 1982.

92. Dudrick SJ, Wilmore DW, Vars HM: Long-term venous catheterization — An adjunct to surgical care and study. Curr Top Surg Res 1:325, 1969.

93. Goldmann DA, Maki DG: Infection control in total parenteral nutrition. JAMA 223:1360, 1973.

94. The Veterans Affairs Total Parenteral Nutrition Cooperative Study Group: Perioperative total parenteral nutrition in surgical patients. N Engl J Med 325:525–532, 1991.

95. Silberman H, Eisenberg D: Nutrition therapy: Clinical applications. In Silberman H, Eisenberg D (eds): Parenteral and Enteral Nutrition for the Hospitalized Patient. Norwalk, CT, Appleton-Century-Crofts, 1982, pp 230–286.

96. Sclafani LM, Brennan MF: Nutritional support in the cancer patient. In Fischer JE (ed): Total Parenteral Nutrition, 2nd ed. Boston, Little, Brown, 1991, pp 323–346.

97. Grant JP, Cox CE, Kleinman LM et al: Serum hepatic enzyme and bilirubin elevations during parenteral nutrition. Surg Gynecol Obstet 145:573–580, 1977.

98. Baker AL, Rosenberg IH: Hepatic complications of total parenteral nutrition. Am J Med 82:489–497, 1987.

99. Sheldon GF, Petersen SR, Sanders R: Hepatic dysfunction during hyperalimentation. Arch Surg 113:504–508, 1978.

100. Wolfe BM, Walker BK, Shaul DB, et al: Effect of total parenteral nutrition on hepatic histology. Arch Surg 123:1084–1090, 1988.

101. Nordenstrom J, Jeevanandam M, Elwyn DH, et al: Increasing glucose intake during total parenteral nutrition increases norepinephrine excretion in trauma and sepsis. Clin Physiol 1:525–534, 1981.

102. Askanazi J, Rosenbaum SH, Hyman AI, et al: Respiratory changes induced by the large glucose loads of total parenteral nutrition. JAMA 243:1444–1447, 1980.

103. Barcroft H, Basnayake V, Celander O, et al: The effect of carbon dioxide on the respiratory response to noradrenaline in man. J Physiol 137:3665, 1957.

104. Wene JD, Connor WE, DenBesten L: The development of essential fatty acid deficiency in healthy men fed fat-free diets intravenously and orally. J Clin Invest 56:127–134, 1975.

105. Palmblad J: Malnutrition associated immune deficiency syndrome—Clues to mechanisms. Acta Med Scand 222:1–3, 1987.

106. Chandra RK: Nutrition, immunity and infection. Lancet 1:688–691, 1983.

107. Palmblad J: Intravenous lipid emulsions and host defense—A critical review. Clin Nutr 10:303–308, 1991.

108. Long CL, Spencer JL, Kinney JM, et al: Carbohydrate metabolism in man: Effect of elective operations and of major injury. J Appl Physiol 31:110, 1971.

109. Wofe RR, O'Donnell TF, Stone MD, et al: Investigation of factors determining the optimal glucose infusion rate in total parenteral nutrition. Metabolism 29:892–900, 1980.

110. Robin AP, Nordenstrom J, Askanazi J, et al: Influence of parenteral carbohydrate on fat oxidation in surgical patients. Surgery 95:608–618, 1983.

111. Askanazi J, Carpentier YA, Elwyn DH, et al: Influence of total parenteral nutrition on fuel utilization in injury and sepsis. Ann Surg 191:40, 1980.

112. Askanazi J, Rosenbaum SH, Hyman AI, et al: Respiratory changes induced by the large glucose loads of total parenteral nutrition. JAMA 243:1444–1447, 1980.

113. Rodriguez J, Askanazi J, Weissman C, et al: Ventilatory and metabolic effects of glucose infusions. Chest 88:512–518, 1985.

114. Askanazi J, Weissman C, LaSala PA, et al: Effect of protein intake on ventilatory drive. Anesthesiology 60:106–110, 1984.

115. Takala J, Askanazi J, Weissman C, et al: Changes in respiratory control induced by amino acid infusions. Crit Care Med 16:465–469, 1988.

116. Bergstrom JP, Fürst P, Larsson J, et al: Influence of injury and nutrition on muscle water and electrolyes: Effect of severe injury, burns and sepsis. Acta Chir Scand 153:261–266, 1987.

117. Askanazi J, Fürst P, Michelsen CB, et al: Muscle and plasma amino acids after injury: Hypocaloric glucose vs amino acid infusion. Ann Surg 191:465–472, 1980.

118. Vinnars E, Holmstrom B, Schildt R, et al: Metabolic effects of four intravenous nutritional regimens in patients undergoing elective surgery. II—Muscle amino acids and energy-rich phosphates. Clin Nutr 2:3–11, 1983.

119. Carpentier YA, Jeevanandam M, Robin AP, et al: Measurement of glycerol turnover by infusion of nonisotopic glycerol in normal and injured subjects. Am J Physiol 247:Endocrinol Metab 10:E405–E411, 1984.

120. Nordenstrom J, Carpentier YA, Robin AP, et al: Free fatty acid mobilization and oxidation during total parenteral nutrition in trauma and infection. Ann Surg 198:725–735, 1983.

121. Fischer JE: Metabolism in surgical patients: Protein, carbohydrate and fat utilization by oral and parenteral routes. In Sabiston D (ed): Textbook of Surgery. Philadelphia, WB Saunders, 1986, pp 116–150.

122. Blackburn GL, Grant JP, Young VR (eds): Amino Acids—Metabolism and Medical Applications. Boston, John Wright–PSG, 1983.

123. Mochizuki H, Trocki O, Domioni L, et al: Mechanisms of prevention of postburn hypermetabolism and catabolism by early enteral feeding. Ann Surg 200:297–310, 1984.

124. Wolfe RR, O'Donnell TF, Stone MD, et al: Investigations of factors determining the optimal glucose infusion rate in total parenteral nutrition. Metabolism 29:892–900, 1980.

125. Wolfe RR, Goodenough RD, Burke JF, Wolfe MH: Response of protein and urea kinetics in burn patients to different levels of protein intake. Ann Surg 197:163–171, 1983.

126. Ferrando AA, Wolfe RR: Effects of bed rest with or without stress. In Kinney JM, Tucker HN (eds): Physiology, Stress, and Malnutrition: Functional Correlates, Nutritional Intervention. Philadelphia, Lippincott-Raven, 1997, pp 413–430.

127. Klein S, Young VR, Blackburn GL, et al: Palmitate and glycerol kinetics during brief starvation in normal weight young adult and elderly subjects. J Clin Invest 78:928–933, 1986.

128. Romijn JA, Coyle EF, Sidossis LS, et al: Regulation of Endogenous Fat and Carbohydrate Metabolism in Relation to Exercise Intensity and Duration. Bethesda, MD, American Physiological Society, 1993, pp 380–391.

129. Rosenblatt J, Wolfe RR: Calculation of substrate flux using stable isotopes. Am J Physiol 254:526–531, 1988.

130. Wolfe RR: Radioactive and stable isotope tracers in biomedicine. New York, Wiley-Liss, 1992.

131. ASPEN Board of Directors: Guidelines for use of total parenteral nutrition in the hospitalized adult patient. JPEN J Parenteral Enteral Nutr 10:441–445, 1986.

132. Clark R, Vinnars E: Early history of ESPEN. 13:57–61, 1994.

133. Fleming CR, Beart RW Jr, Berkner S: Home parenteral nutrition for management of the severely malnourished adult patient. Gastroenterology 79:11, 1980.

134. Grundfest S, Steiger E: Home parenteral nutrition. JAMA 244:1701, 1980.

135. ASPEN Board of Directors: Guidelines for use of home total parenteral nutrition. JPEN J Parenter Enteral Nutr 11:342–344, 1987.

136. Lifeline Letter. The Oley Foundation, 214 Hun Memorial, Albany Medical Center, A-23, Albany, NY 12208.

137. Hill GL, Beddoe AH: Dimensions of the human body and its compartments. In Kinney JM, Jeejeebhoy KN, Hill GL, Owen OE (eds): Nutrition and Metabolism in Patient Care. Philadelphia, WB Saunders, 1988, pp 89–118.

138. Wang Z-M, Pierson RN, Heymsfield SB: The five-level model: A new approach to organizing body-composition research. Am J Clin Nutr 56:19–28, 1992.

139. Elia M: Body composition analysis: An evaluation of two component models, multicomponent models and bedside techniques. Clin Nutr 11:114–127, 1992.

140. Windsor JA, Hill GL: Weight loss with physiologic impairment—A basic indicator of surgical risk. Ann Surg 207:290–296, 1988.

141. Jeejeebhoy KN: Total Parenteral Nutrition in the Hospital and at Home. Boca Raton, FL, CRC Press, 1983.

142. Jeejeebhoy KN: Assessment of nutritional status: The relative merits of anthropometry, plasma proteins and muscle function in the scientific basis for the care of the critically ill. In Little RA, Frayn KN (eds): The Scientific Basis for Care of the Critically Ill. Manchester, England, Manchester University Press, 1986.

143. Jeejeebhoy KN: The functional basis of assessment. In Kinney JM, Jeejeebhoy KN, Hill GL,

Owen OE (eds): Nutrition and Metabolism in Patient Care. Philadelphia, WB Saunders, 1988, pp 739–751.

144. Jeejeebhoy KN: Muscle function and energetics. *In* Wilmore DW, Carpentier YA (eds): Metabolic Support of the Critically Ill Patient (update in Intensive Care and Emergency Medicine, Vol 17). Berlin, Springer-Verlag, 1993, pp 46–62.

145. Moller DE, Flier JS: Insulin resistance—Mechanisms, syndromes and implication. N Engl J Med 325:938–947, 1991.

146. Frayn KN: Hormonal control of metabolism in trauma and sepsis. Clin Endocrinol 24:577–599, 1986.

147. Nair KS, Adey D, Charlton M, Ljungqvist O: Protein metabolism in diabetes mellitus. Diabes Nutr Metab 8:113–122, 1995.

148. Black PR, Brooks DC, Bessey PO, Wilmore DW: Mechanisms of insulin resistance following injury. Ann Surg 196:420–435, 1982.

149. Okkusawa S, Gelfland JA, Ikejima T: Interleukin I induces a shock-like state in rabbits: Synergism with tumor necrosis factor and the effect of cyclooxygenase inhibitor. J Clin Invest 81:1162–1172, 1988.

150. Newman W, Brodows R: Insulin action during acute starvation: Evidence for selective insulin resistance in normal man. Metabolism 32:590–596, 1983.

151. Baron AD, Laakso M, Brechtel G, et al: Reduced postprandial skeletal muscle blood flow contributes to glucose intolerance in human obesity. J Clin Endocrinol Metab 70:1525–1533, 1990.

152. Baron AD: Hemodynamic actions of insulin. Am J Physiol 267:E187-E202, 1994.

153. Atkins E, Bodel P, Francis L: Release of an endogenous pyrogen in vitro from rabbit mononuclear cells. J Exp Med 101:519–528, 1967.

154. Kluger MJ: Fever: Metabolic asset or liability. *In* Kinney JM, Tucker HN (eds): Organ Metabolism and Nutrition. New York, Raven Press, 1994, pp 91–106.

155. Beisel WR, Sobocinski PZ: Endogenous mediators of fever-related metabolic and hormonal responses. *In* Lipton JM (ed): Fever. New York, Raven Press, 1979, pp 39–48.

156. Dinarello CA: Role of interleukin-1 and tumor necrosis factor in systemic responses to infection and inflammation. *In* Gallin J, Goldstein JM, Snyderman R (eds): Inflammation—Basic Principles and Clinical Correlates, 2nd ed. New York, Raven Press, 1992, pp 181–195.

157. Beutler BA, Milsark IW, Cerami A: Cachectin/tumor necrosis factor: Production, distribution and metabolic fate in vivo. J Immunol 135:3972–3977, 1985.

158. Tracey KJ, Lowry SF, Cerami A: Cachectin: A hormone that triggers shock and chronic cachexia. J Infect Dis 157:413–420, 1988.

159. Moldawer LL, Lowry SF: Interactions among pro-inflammatory cytokines and the classic macroendocrine system in sepsis and inflammation. *In* Kinney JM, Tucker HN: Organ Metabolism and Nutrition. New York, Raven Press, 1994.

160. Clifford WL, Walker WA: Changes in the gastrointestinal tract during enteral or parenteral feeding. Nutr Rev 47:193–198, 1989.

161. Dechelotte P, Darmaun D, Rongier M, et al: Absorption and metabolic effects of enterally administered glutamine in humans. Am J Physiol 260:677–682, 1991.

162. Castro GA: Immunological regulation of epithelial function. *In* Walker WA, Harmatz PA, Wershil BK (eds): Immunophysiology of the Gut. New York, Academic Press, 1993.

163. Brandtzaeg P, Halstensen TS, Helgeland L, Kett K: The mucosal immune system in inflammatory bowel disease. *In* MacDonald TT (ed): Immunology of Gastrointestinal Disease. Dordrecht, Netherlands, Kluwer Academic, 1992, p 19.

164. Wilmore DW: Homeostasis: Bodily changes in trauma and surgery. *In* Sabiston DC (ed): Textbook of Surgery—The Biological Basis of Modern Surgical Practice. Philadelphia, WB Saunders, 1986, p 23.

165. Wilmore DW: The wound as an organ. *In* Little RA, Frayn KN (eds): The Scientific Basis for the Care of the Critically Ill. Manchester, England, Manchester University Press, 1986, pp 45–60.

166. Suoba WW: Glutamine—A key substrate for the splanchnic bed. Annu Rev Nutr 11:285–308, 1991.

167. Ardawi MSM: Effect of glutamine-supplemented total parenteral nutrition on the small bowel of septic rats. Clin Nutr 11:207–215, 1992.

168. Marchesini G, Fabbri A, Bianchi G, Bugianesi E: Branched-chain amino acids in liver disease. *In* Cynober L (ed): Amino Acid Metabolism and Therapy in Health and Nutritional Disease. New York, CRC Press, 1995, pp 337–348.

169. Johnson RC, Young SK, Cotter R, et al: Medium-chain triglyceride emulsion: Metabolism and tissue distribution. Am J Clin Nutr 52:502–508, 1990.

170. Glutamine transport in muscle protein economy. Nutr Rev 47:215–217, 1989.

171. Barbul A: The use of arginine in clinical practice. *In* Cynober L (ed): Amino Acid Metabolism and Therapy in Health and Nutritional Disease. New York, CRC Press, 1995, pp 351–378.

172. Koruda MJ, Rolandelli RH, Settle RG, et al: Effect of parenteral nutrition supplemented with short-chain fatty acids on adaptation to massive small bowel resection. Gastroenterology 95:715–720, 1988.

173. Spielmann D: Metabolism of unsaturated fatty acids: Role of n-3 and n-6 fatty acids in clinical nutrition. *In* Kinney JM, Borum PR (eds): Perspectives in Clinical Nutrition. Baltimore, Urban & Schwarzenberg, 1989.

174. Treml H, Kienle B, Weilemann LS, et al: Glutamine dipeptide–supplemented parenteral nutrition maintains intestinal function in the critically ill. Gastroenterology 107:1594–1601, 1994.

175. Dahlan W, Richelle M, Kulapongse S, et al: Modification of erythrocyte membrane lipid composition induced by a single intravenous infusion of phospholipid-triacylglycerol emulsions in man. Clin Nutr 11:255–261, 1992.

176. Halliwell B, Evans PJ, Kaur H, Aruoma II: Free radicals, tissue injury, and human disease: A potential for therapeutic use of antioxidants? *In* Kinney JM, Tucker HN (eds): Organ Metabolism and Nutrition, Ideas for Future Critical Care. New York, Raven Press, 1994, pp 425–445.

177. Frank L: Developmental aspects of experimental pulmonary oxygen toxicity. Free Radic Biol Med 11:463–494, 1991.

178. Hyskop PA, Hinshaw DB, Halsey WR Jr, et al: Mechanisms of oxidant mediated cell injury. J Biol Chem 263:1665–1675, 1988.

179. Donabedian A: The quality of care—How can it be assessed? JAMA 260:1743–1748, 1988.

180. Koretz R: What supports nutritional support? Dig Dis Sci 29:577–588, 1984.

181. Hellman S, Hellman DS: Of mice but not men—Problems of the randomized clinical trial. N Engl J Med 324:1585–1592, 1991.

182. Passamani E: Clinical trials—Are they ethical? N Engl J Med 324:1589–1592, 1991.

183. Looking for the Evidence in Medicine. Science [News and Comment]. 272:22–24, 1996.

2

◆ Metabolic Response to Illness and Its Mediators

Matthew D. Vrees, M.D.
Jorge E. Albina, M.D.

Major injuries or severe systemic infections trigger a stereotypic host response consisting of physiologic and metabolic changes presumably coordinated and directed toward enhancing the possibility of survival. Prominent among these changes are fever and increased heat production, anorexia and lassitude, neutrophilia, increased gluconeogenesis and net protein catabolism, activation of complement and coagulation cascades, alterations in immune responsiveness, induction of acute-phase protein synthesis, and changes in the distribution of body minerals. Although variable in magnitude, the response repertoire of the organism to external (traumatic or infectious) or internal (i.e., a myocardial or enteric infarction) injury appears to qualitatively deviate little among diverse pathologic conditions in terms of its individual components. For the most part, the response appears to be proportional to the magnitude of the injury. The capacity of the organism to generate such response is, in turn, proportional to the size of its body cell mass, with younger, well-fed, and more muscled individuals mounting a more robust metabolic response. Over the years, the physiologic and metabolic alterations that follow injury have been designated by different names that describe similar phenomena, including the *stress response* and the *general adaptation syndrome* of Hans Selye, the *flight-or-fight mechanism* of Walter Cannon, or the *alarm response*.

Although the understanding of the individual components of the metabolic response to injury has been progressively refined over the last 50 years, the process of defining its intimate mechanisms, identifying its mediators, and clarifying its value in preserving the organism is not yet finished. As more potential inducers and modulators of the ultimate genetic response of cells to distant injury are being described,

reductionistic attempts to model the role of multiple mediators in the whole-body response to injury must contend with an increasingly complex information base. Deviating from a simple linear model in which neural or hormonal factors fully accounted for all responses to injury, current explanations of these response phenomena must consider the participation of cytokines and growth factors (together with their inhibitors and competitors), reactive oxygen and nitrogen intermediates, products of arachidonic acid metabolism, ion fluxes, and other potential initiators, regulators, or terminators of the response. In this connection, it must be kept in mind that many of these mediators need not transit through the vasculature to reach their cellular target, but rather elicit their effects through paracrine or autocrine mechanisms. Moreover, externally imposed conditions, such as voluntary or involuntary nutritional support, bed rest, the ambient temperature, pain or its control, anti-infectious therapy, or the artificial support of individual or multiple organs in the context of contemporary medical care, can substantially modify the natural history of the alterations induced by the initial injury.

Current interpretation of the events that follow injury and infection may be to some extent biased by a "wisdom-of-the-body" mindset that considers the consequences of injury an evolved "response," with implied adaptive and prosurvival teleologic connotations, rather than an "effect" of injury, with pathologic corollaries quite distinct from a primacy of survival as a physiologic imperative. Under this different and less flattering light, then, changes observed in severely injured individuals could be seen as unwelcome reflections of metabolic illness leading to progressive disease characterized by what has been termed the *systemic inflammatory response syndrome* and its consequential multiple-system organ failure, rather than as a purposefully integrated adaptive response. Arthur Baue indicated the multiple-system organ failure syndrome to be a consequence of medical and surgical progress,[1] in that it appears in individuals who would probably not have survived their injuries were it not for current sophisticated life-support systems. The perpetuation in time and magnitude of a metabolic response to injury evolved to preserve life could lead, paradoxically, to the subject's demise.

The purpose of this chapter is to describe in some detail the metabolic alterations that follow tissue injury or infection and to present a brief and current snapshot of the principal endogenous mediators thought to determine such alterations. As in other areas of science, knowledge in this area has progressed dramatically on the basis of clinical and laboratory studies performed by a multitude of investigators. Probably unfairly skipping over two centuries of stuttering progress in the field, we begin a historical description of the understanding of the metabolic response to injury by summarizing the work of Sir David P. Cuthbertson. In a series of landmark publications starting in 1930, Cuthbertson described a biphasic response to injury.[2-5] If the organism survives the initial insult, an *ebb* or *necrobiotic* phase of hypometabolism with decreased oxygen consumption, decreased cardiac output, and shock occurs, followed by a *flow* phase of increased metabolic reactions. The flow phase was characterized by Cuthbertson as an accelerated rate of loss of nitrogen, phosphorus, sulfur, and other elements that is directly proportional to the magnitude of the injury and the subject's previous nutritional status and is inversely proportional to the age of the subject.

Walter B. Cannon in turn provided evidence for the release of catecholamines after injury and for their central involvement in maintaining homeostasis after a variety of insults.[6] Working with denervated heart preparations, Cannon showed that circulating factors, the catecholamines, released from the adrenal glands, induced tachycardia after stimulation through cold, pain, fright, hypoxia, or muscular activity. Animals subject to sympathectomy lived normally unless challenged with hemorrhage, hypoxia, or cold, to which they were unable to respond, and died. The flight-or-fight response physiologically defined by tachycardia, capillary dilation, piloerection, and an increased respiratory rate also includes metabolic alterations such as abrupt hyperglycemia, increased plasma free fatty acid concentrations, and marked water and sodium conservation by the kidneys.

The initiation of the response to injury through neural pathways and the interaction of afferent signals with catecholamine responses have been well established through experiments in which injury to anatomically or pharmacologically denervated tissue resulted in markedly blunted adrenal and systemic responses. In this regard, Hume and Egdahl first described the decreased production of adrenal steroids when burn injuries are produced on denervated limbs of animals after transection of the spinal cord above the level of the injury or after transection of the medulla oblongata.[7] Neural input appears to be relevant to the initiation of the stress response but not to its persistence, because neural blockade during the flow phase of the response is without effect, at least in regard to whole-body thermogenesis.[8]

The concept that catecholamines and other canonical hormones could fully explain the alterations seen after injury and infection took flight on the wings of a plethora of experimental data.[9] It probably culminated in the experimental work in the laboratory of Douglas W. Wilmore, where it was shown that the simultaneous infusion of cortisol, glucagon, and epinephrine in healthy volunteers resulted in hypermetabolism, negative nitrogen and potassium balances, glucose intolerance, hyperinsulinemia with insulin resistance, sodium retention, and leukocytosis.[10]

A qualitative shift in the understanding of the mediators of the metabolic response to injury took place after the identification of cytokines as products of inflammatory cells capable of inducing systemic alterations. Distinct from classic endocrine products, cytokines were shown to be synthesized and released primarily by cells of the immune system and to be able to modify responses in adjacent cells and distant organs. Work by multiple investigators demonstrated systemic effects of these mediators and established the triad of interleukin 1 (IL-1), tumor necrosis factor-α (TNF-α) (or cachectin), and IL-6 as sufficient and necessary to initiate most of the changes associated with the metabolic response to injury.[11, 12] In a landmark study in 1988,

Michie and colleagues infused TNF-α into cancer patients for 24 hours and demonstrated the induction of fever and increased plasma concentrations of stress-related hormones and acute-phase proteins.[13] Moreover, they compared the responses obtained using TNF-α with those found after the administration of endotoxin to the subjects and found them to be practically indistinguishable.[13] In a similar vein, others showed that the administration of TNF-α, this time to healthy volunteers, resulted in hyperglycemia, increased plasma free fatty acid and glycerol concentrations, and increased thermogenesis, thus resembling changes induced by injury or infection.[14]

It appears relevant to point out that cytokines do not, by themselves and directly, mediate all components of the metabolic response to injury. Indeed, substantial interaction exists between the cytokine system and other mediators of the stress response. For example, the effects of TNF-α on protein metabolism may be mediated through glucocorticoids, and this cytokine has been shown to induce the release of corticotropin. Moreover, TNF-α–induced shock, which greatly resembles gram-negative sepsis, may result from the overproduction of arachidonic acid metabolites because it is prevented and reversed in animals by the administration of prostaglandin synthesis inhibitors. Lastly, although IL-1 has been shown to mediate febrile responses, its effects on thermoregulation appear to be mediated through its induction of the release of corticotropin-releasing factor or arginine vasopressin.[15]

Crosstalk between the cytokine and endocrine systems also encompasses the regulation of cytokine production or activity by classic hormones. In this regard, glucocorticoids have been shown to down-regulate cytokine expression by multiple mechanisms including binding to and inactivation of transcription factors such as AP-1 and NF-κB, up-regulation of suppressive nuclear factors including IκB through glucocorticoid-responsive elements, and reductions in the cytokine messenger RNA half-life.[16] The suppressive effects of glucocorticoids on cytokine production are not restricted to the *proinflammatory* cytokines (e.g., TNF-α, IL-1, IL-6) but also to the *anti-inflammatory* cytokine set that includes IL-4 and IL-10.[16] Apparently spared from the suppressive effects of glucocorticoids are some growth factors associated with wound healing and maturation such as transforming growth factor-β and platelet-derived growth factor.[16]

In summary, the changes in physiology and metabolism that follow major injury or infection appear to be determined by multiple interacting layers of effectors, each contributing directly or indirectly to the observed clinical alterations. In addition, although the stereotypic nature of the response to injury and infection has been highlighted, there are quantitative and maybe qualitative differences in some aspects of the metabolic response to traumatic or infectious illness. These differences are, however, difficult to elucidate clinically because injury and infection frequently coincide. For the purpose of this discussion, alterations associated with infection and major injury are described together.

◆ ALTERATIONS IN THERMOGENESIS

A well-known effect of significant injury is noninfectious fever. Even in the absence of fever, major trauma and burns are followed by increases in resting thermogenesis that are mostly proportional to the severity of the injury in both magnitude and duration. The metabolic rate, and thus oxygen consumption, increases during the flow phase of injury and returns to predicted normal values with its resolution. Classic work by Kinney and colleagues established approximate ranges of increases in resting thermogenesis of zero to 30% after elective surgery, 15 to 45% after accidental severe injury, 10 to 60% in sepsis, and 50 to 100% after major burns.[17, 18] The duration of hypermetabolism reported by these authors was remarkable, with long bone fractures resulting in increased thermogenesis for over 20 days and peritonitis for 1 month. Others, however, have questioned these results. Quebbeman and associates, for example, failed to find significant increases in resting thermogenesis in patients with diverse medical and surgical diseases, including major trauma and sepsis.[19] Our own clinical experience agrees mostly with that of Quebbeman in that in nonburned critically ill patients we rarely observe increases in basal thermogenesis of the magnitude and duration indicated by others. In this regard, Kinney[20] and others[21] have reported that, probably because of changes in patient care practices, recent determinations of thermogenesis in burns demonstrate that the increases in resting energy expenditure are in the range of 20 to 40%, rather than the almost doubling that was measured three decades ago. It must also be remembered that the subject's prior state of nutrition affects the resting thermogenesis. The co-incidence of injury and starvation in patients has opposite effects on thermogenesis, determining that individual patients may exhibit hypo-, normo-, or hypermetabolism during the course of their illnesses.

It is clear, however, that severely injured or infected patients do exhibit increased basal thermogenesis. In this regard, work by Wilmore and others demonstrated that in the burn patient, thermogenesis increases in proportion to burn size up to 40 to 50% of body surface area and then plateaus, indicating that a maximal level of heat production is achieved with burns of this magnitude.[8] Moreover, work by the same investigators showed that hypermetabolism in burns does not depend on the cooling effect of increased water loss from the wound, concluding that these patients are "internally warm, not externally cold."[8]

The mediators and cellular mechanisms for the hypermetabolism of injury at the cellular level remain mostly unexplained. Many of the neural, endocrine, and cytokine components of the metabolic response to injury can induce increases in thermogenesis. In doing so, these compounds must somehow impact directly or indirectly on heat-generating pathways at the cellular level to elicit an increase in heat production. In this regard, it appears that most energy consumption, and thus heat production, in cells without uncoupled oxidative phosphorylation is associated with the regulation of cell volume and with protein turnover.[22] In regard to the latter, and as discussed later, multiple mediators of the stress response have been shown to result in increased protein synthesis and breakdown and thus determine increased heat production through this mechanism. In regard to the former, it has been reported that cells increase their intracellular sodium concentration($[Na^+_I]$) after severe injury and in sepsis. This increase in $[Na^+_I]$ is accompanied by decreases in the intracellular potassium concentration $[K^+_I]$[23] that are disproportionate to the decrease in intracellular protein[24] and

that could be in part secondary to increased levels of circulating glucocorticoids and aggravated by glucose feedings.[25] Although it was proposed originally that these alterations in intracellular cation concentrations are due to a decrease in Na^+,K^+-ATPases,[23] more recent work has proposed an increased rate of Na^+-pump activity in muscle, which is in turn fueled by glycolysis.[26–29] The relationship between Na^+-pump activity and aerobic glycolysis, confirmed in two studies in skeletal muscle,[26, 27] provides additional potential connections to the whole-body metabolic response. Increased Na^+,K^+-ATPase activity results in increased thermogenesis. Increased glycolytic flux to supply energy to the ATPase results in increased pyruvate and lactate production. Enhanced pyruvate production in turn facilitates its transamination by glutamate to alanine, explaining, at least in part, the increased alanine release from muscle in injury and, potentially, the reported decrease in muscle glutamine content. An increase in lactate production and release dependent on increased Na^+,K^+-ATPase activity and resulting from aerobic glycolysis would explain observations of increased circulating lactate in injury independent of tissue hypoxia. Moreover, the resynthesis of glucose from lactate or from amino acids in the liver in the context of the accelerated gluconeogenesis of injury would add to the metabolic cost of the process.

Although the hypothesis that alterations of Na^+ influx into cells or of Na^+,K^+-ATPase could be the ultimate mediator of the thermogenic and protein catabolic responses to injury was cogently presented by Flear more than 20 years ago,[28] it has to contend with more recent opinion by Häussinger and others, who have demonstrated increased cell volume as a potent inhibitor of proteolysis,[30] and that of Hotchkiss and coworkers, who, using very sensitive analytic techniques, failed to detect alterations in $[Na^+_I]$ or in glucose metabolism in red blood cells isolated from septic animals.[31]

Although the flow phase of the response to injury is, then, characterized by variable increases in thermogenesis, in contrast, catastrophic disease can be accompanied by hypometabolism. In this connection, uncontrolled sepsis is associated with a progressive decline in energy metabolism potentially resulting from mitochondrial dysfunction.[32–34]

In regard to the mediators of the thermogenic response to injury, it has been well established that it does not result from increased thyroid function. Indeed, it has been repeatedly shown that bound and free serum triiodothyronine (T_3) levels are reduced and serum thyroxine (T_4) levels are maintained after injury, and that there is a reduced rate of conversion of T_4 to T_3 and elevated serum levels of reverse T_3. The circulating thyroid-stimulating hormone level is found to be reduced, rather than increased, despite this environment of relative hypothyroidism. Catecholamines in turn are known to have substantial thermogenic effects. Infusion of epinephrine or norepinephrine in humans results in hypermetabolism, a response suppressed by β-adrenergic blockade.[8] Wilmore and coworkers demonstrated that β-adrenergic blockade in severely burned patients decreased, but did not fully normalize, their basal metabolic rate.[35] Supporting the role of classic endocrine mediators in the thermogenic response to injury, Bessey and associates[10] reported increased basal thermogenesis, along with other components of the metabolic response to injury including hyperglycemia, hyperinsulinemia, and negative nitrogen and potassium balances, in healthy subjects injected with cortisol, glucagon, and epinephrine.

The potential thermogenic effects of cytokines have also been studied. IL-1 is considered to be the most important endogenous pyrogen.[15] Local production of IL-1 in the brain, rather than its transit from the general circulation across the blood-brain barrier, has been proposed to be required for its thermogenic effects.[36] Supporting this concept, systemic injection of endotoxin results in increased IL-1β messenger RNA and protein in the hypothalamus.[15] The thermogenic effects of IL-1 at the hypothalamic level are thought to be mediated through the release of corticotropin-releasing factor and ultimately through prostaglandins.[15] IL-6 has also been implicated in determining the increased thermogenesis of injury at the hypothalamic level, because central injections of IL-6 increase the metabolic rate of animals.[15] Lastly, TNF-α is thought to be directly and indirectly involved in the control of thermogenesis. Although the injection of TNF-α does indeed result in fever, its potential role in the thermogenic alterations that follow injury could also be mediated at the cellular level. In this regard, it has been shown that TNF-α increases $[Na^+_I]$ through the disruption of the cellular membrane and enhances lactate production.[37, 38] TNF-α could then mediate the enhanced thermogenesis associated with the increased Na^+,K^+-ATPase activity discussed earlier.

◆ ALTERATIONS IN GLUCOSE METABOLISM

Hyperglycemia with insulin resistance is a consistent finding in injury. Work from Robert R. Wolfe's laboratory has contributed significantly to the understanding of the mechanisms for these alterations and the effects of nutritional support in trauma, sepsis, and burns.[39] It is because of the integrated vision of the alterations in metabolism that follow injury provided by this author that the discussion that follows relies heavily on his publications.

In regard to the hyperglycemia of injury, evidence indicates that elevations in blood glucose concentrations occur as a consequence of increased hepatic glucose production from amino acids predominantly released from skeletal muscle, from glycerol released during the hydrolysis of triglycerides, and from lactate generated by peripheral tissues and converted to glucose in the liver in completion of the Cori cycle.[40] Endogenous rates of glucose production in traumatized patients have been shown to be elevated by more than 100%, with glucose recycling though enhanced Cori cycle flux being responsible for a substantial portion of the gluconeogenesis.[40] The increased gluconeogenesis of injury results, at least in relation to the amino acids as gluconeogenic precursors, primarily from an enhanced capacity of the liver for glucose production and not from the increased availability of gluconeogenic precursors that results from the accelerated release of alanine and glutamine from skeletal muscle.[41]

In addition to the increased glucose production just described, insulin resistance, defined both by the reduced ability of insulin to suppress hepatic glucose production and by the blunting of the effects of this hormone to increase glucose uptake by muscle and adipose tissue, contributes to the elevated blood glucose concentration found in injury.

The coincident finding of elevated blood glucose and normal or elevated serum insulin concentrations in injury confirms the inability of insulin to reduce glucose production in these circumstances.[41] This inability is not absolute, because the infusion of insulin to obtain supraphysiologic plasma concentrations of the hormone can completely abrogate hepatic glucose production even in infected and noninfected severely burned patients.[42]

Additional evidence points to the reduced sensitivity of insulin-responsive tissues to the hormone. In this connection, Wolfe and coworkers demonstrated that five times as much insulin was required to maintain euglycemia in the context of constant intravenous glucose infusion in severely burned patients than in healthy controls.[43] Interestingly, the resistance to insulin's effect on glucose metabolism does not extend to its effects on K^+ uptake by cells.[44] Because insulin must bind to its receptor and signal intracellularly to promote K^+ influx, these findings support the concept of an altered processing of glucose by cells. In this regard, work by Black and associates confirmed the presence of insulin resistance in burn patients using an insulin clamp technique, in which the amount of glucose required to maintain euglycemia during a constant insulin infusion is determined, and they demonstrated in addition a significant increase in the rate of insulin clearance in the patients.[45] Moreover, these authors also proposed that burn patients exhibit a postreceptor defect in their response to insulin.[45] This conclusion would predict alterations in the metabolic pathways followed by glucose once in the cell. However, it has been shown that the actual rate of glucose oxidation as a percentage of glucose uptake is only modestly depressed in burned patients.[43] Additional studies in burned children equally failed to detect alterations in the rate of pyruvate oxidation, thus arguing against significant alterations in pathways of glucose oxidation.[46]

Despite data discussed previously regarding the relative insulin unresponsiveness of injury, the basal rate of glucose clearance (glucose uptake/serum glucose concentration) is actually increased in severely ill patients.[43] This counterintuitive observation is probably explained on the basis of the ongoing glucose clearance by insulin-independent tissues, and to some extent by the equally insulin-independent uptake of glucose into inflammatory cells at a site of injury. This latter conclusion was supported by the demonstration of increased glucose uptake across burned legs in humans.[47] It must be kept in mind, however, that increased glucose clearance does not imply increased glucose oxidation. The majority of glucose uptake in injury is processed through glycolysis, and glucose carbon is returned to the circulation as lactate.

The alterations in glucose metabolism seen in injury can be mostly explained by the effects of classic hormones. To some extent, these alterations, most specifically those related to insulin resistance, do not fully depend on injury because they are observed in healthy individuals during bed rest with ample access to food.[44, 48] In terms of the accelerated rate of glucose production in illness, results indicate the preponderance of glucagon as the mediator of gluconeogenesis.[49] In addition, evidence has been presented for the markedly enhanced release of glucagon in injury and the lack of suppression of its secretion by glucose.[50] Glucose production was decreased in experiments where the production of glucagon was blocked with somatostatin in burned patients.[49] Catecholamines, which are known to induce rapid glycogenolysis, do not appear to be particularly important in maintaining a rapid rate of gluconeogenesis.[51] The role of glucocorticoids in regulating glucose metabolism, as well as their role in all other metabolic alterations seen after injury, is thought to be primarily permissive. In this regard, it has been shown that adrenalectomized animals respond as well as intact animals to stress if pretreated with basal amounts of glucocorticoids.[52] In the context of glucose metabolism, adrenal steroids are thought to facilitate the gluconeogenic effects of glucagon.[53] Cortisol, in this regard, increases the activity of key gluconeogenic enzymes in the liver[54] and promotes glucagon secretion.[55] In addition to their effect on gluconeogenesis, the adrenal steroids antagonize the effects of insulin by multiple mechanisms including decreasing the affinity and number of insulin receptors in cells,[56, 57] reducing the production of glucose transporters and inducing their intracellular sequestration,[57] and, potentially, altering intracellular pathways of glucose utilization.[58]

◆ ALTERATIONS IN PROTEIN METABOLISM

Of all metabolic derangements following injury, those of protein metabolism have attracted the most attention and are probably those of most significant clinical relevance. Resolving years of debate regarding the existence of a "labile protein pool" available for utilization in circumstances of decreased intake or increased requirements, the current nutrition paradigm indicates that there are no storage forms of protein (see Irwin and Hegsted[59] for a historical review). Each protein in the body has one or more specific functions. Decreases in total body protein must, therefore, result in decreased function. Whether the impacted function is decreased muscle strength, altered immune responsiveness, diminished gut integrity, or any other, the unavoidable corollary is diminished ability to cope with persistent illness. Clinical observation suffices to evidence the rapid rate of muscle wasting in acute, severe illness. The rate of lean tissue loss in severe trauma can exceed 1 kg/day, leading to pronounced decreases in muscle mass and the consequential weakness and reduced work capacity. Elwyn pointed out that the negative nitrogen balance in severe burns during the infusion of 5% dextrose is eight times greater than that in a healthy individual.[20] Identical calculations in severe trauma indicate a negative nitrogen balance sixfold higher than in healthy controls.

Based on the ratios among the increased nitrogen, sulfur, and phosphorus losses in the urine, early work by Cuthbertson indicated that skeletal muscle breakdown accounts for the bulk of protein catabolism in injury. This conclusion was fully supported by other investigators.[60–62] Work in burn patients confirmed that the accelerated rate of net protein catabolism occurs systemically and is not limited to the injured area.[63] In this connection, Aulick and Wilmore demonstrated the accelerated release of amino acids (primarily of alanine) from the legs of severely burned patients.[63] Most importantly, they showed the increased amino acid flux not to depend on the presence of local burn injury, thus establishing the systemic nature of the enhanced protein catabolism of injury. Although the accelerated rate of amino acid release from muscle in injury is an indicator of the rate of net protein breakdown, the qualitative profile of amino acids released under these conditions does not reflect muscle protein composition. Alanine and glutamine are released from muscle disproportionately to their relative abundance in muscle protein. The specific source of the carbon skeleton for alanine has been debated and appears to be pyruvate. Glutamine released from muscle arises through the activity of glutamine synthase on glutamic acid. In addition, it appears that not all muscles respond equally in terms of net protein breakdown after injury and that fast-twitch, fiber-rich muscles (i.e., gastrocnemius and psoas) suffer the greatest rates of loss.[64]

One should note that total body protein is in constant turnover, with proteins of different half-lives and pool size being simultaneously broken down and resynthesized. The rather modest requirements for dietary protein in humans witnesses the efficiency of the turnover process for amino acid recycling. This perpetual cycle of protein catabolism and anabolism makes it possible that profound alterations in total body protein content can occur as a consequence of minor changes in catabolic or synthetic rates that are maintained over time. It is obvious that if both components of the turnover process move in opposite directions (i.e., an increase in catabolism simultaneous with a decrease in synthesis), major reductions in total body protein can take place in a relatively short period of time. Alterations in both protein breakdown and protein synthesis have been detected as consequence of injury. It has been shown, for example, that changes in protein metabolism following mild or moderate stress, such as that resulting from elective surgery, are mostly restricted to reductions in the rate of total body protein synthesis, without increases in total body protein breakdown.[65, 66] The resulting net protein breakdown is thus mild and self-limiting. The decrease in protein synthesis associated with mild injury appears to be an extremely sensitive marker of stress, because it has been documented after reconstructive surgery when no simultaneous alterations in body weight or even in nitrogen balance were found.[66] In this regard, Kinney has indicated that the negative nitrogen balance that follows major elective surgery proceeds without increases in whole-body thermogenesis.[20] As the magnitude of the injury increases, total protein breakdown increases to an extent not compensated by increases in total body protein synthesis.[67] Rates of net protein breakdown in severely septic patients have been measured at greater than 2 ± 0.1 g/kg/day.[67] Nutritional support, at least when provided in the form of parenteral nutrition, has been shown to be capable of increasing total body protein synthesis rates but unable to reduce protein catabolism in severely septic individuals.[67]

The intimate mechanism for the accelerated rate of protein breakdown (and the decrease in the synthesis of proteins not related to the acute-phase response) in severe injury remains obscure. The roles of the counter-regulatory hormones glucagon, cortisol, and epinephrine are consistently highlighted in all reviews on this topic. Their combined infusion, however, although sufficient to induce increased net protein breakdown, determines changes that are minor in comparison to those seen clinically.[10] In this regard, glucagon is not known to alter rates of protein synthesis or breakdown in muscle, with its most important property probably being the acceleration of gluconeogenesis in the liver.[68] Glucocorticoids, in turn, enhance net muscle protein breakdown, as witnessed by changes found in patients with Cushing's syndrome. This effect is thought to be mediated mainly through the inhibition of protein synthesis associated with reductions in total ribosomal mass.[69] It has been debated, however, whether alterations in protein turnover found in critical illness can be attributed to increased circulating glucocorticoids, because protein synthesis has been shown to be decreased in models of injury without increases in levels of plasma adrenal steroids and because it appears that the mechanism for the decreased protein synthesis in injury depends more on reduced translational efficiency than on reductions in ribosomal mass.[64] In addition, there is evidence that glucocorticoids may accelerate muscle protein breakdown through the stimulation of the nonlysosomal, ATP-dependent, ubiquitin-mediated proteolytic pathway, an effect well documented in fasting.[70] In this connection, glucocorticoid receptor blockade markedly reduced protein breakdown in septic experimental animals.[71] In regard to the effects of catecholamines on protein kinetics, it has been shown that these compounds can actually increase protein synthesis, an effect mediated through their β_2-receptor,[72] and also can suppress protein breakdown.[73] Indeed, adrenergic blockade was found to have little effect on whole-body protein kinetics in burn patients.[74]

In addition to the impact of procatabolic hormones on protein kinetics in injury, it has been proposed that the effects of proanabolic mediators are attenuated in injury. For example, the ability of insulin to promote protein synthesis in muscle is somewhat diminished after severe trauma.[75] It has been shown, however, that induced hyperinsulinemia in burned or septic patients decreases leucine appearance and oxidation rates, as well as urea production.[76] Moreover, it was demonstrated through the use of somatostatin infusions that the basal rate of insulin production in septic patients contributes to reduce their rapid rate of net protein breakdown.[77] The reductions in levels of growth hormone and insulin-like growth factor I frequently found in critical illness may in addition favor net protein catabolism.[78, 79]

In regard to the role of cytokines on protein metabolism after severe injury, it is thought that the incremental effects of some of these compounds (mainly TNF-α) on the whole-body proteolytic rate depend on the stimulation of cortisol production, because they are greatly attenuated in adrenalectomized animals and in animals treated with glucocorticoid receptor antagonists.[71, 80, 81] In this connection, it must be remembered that the profound anorexia thought to be mediated by TNF-α cannot but contribute to the whole-body net protein catabolic state of illness.[82]

In contrast to observations mentioned earlier regarding the lack of direct effects of TNF-α on muscle protein kinetics, results using cultured muscles demonstrated a direct effect of IL-1 on protein degradation, without changes in protein synthesis.[83] These proteolytic effects of IL-1 were shown to depend on prostaglandin E_2 production, accelerated by muscle culture at 39° C (rather than at 37° C), and to be mediated by lysosomal proteases.[83]

Interestingly, although the hormonal and cytokine responses to injury are relatively short lived, there is evidence of persistent alterations in protein kinetics well into the patient's recovery. In this regard, studies on burn patients detected significantly increased rates of total protein breakdown even when the patients were convalescing and ready to leave the hospital.[84] The potential contributions of decreased physical activity and reduced food intake to this finding were not clarified.

Although the metabolic response to injury is characterized by increased whole-body net protein catabolism, some organs, most prominently the liver, exhibit enhanced synthesis and release into the circulation of a specific set of proteins termed the *acute-phase response proteins*. These proteins, whose increase in plasma concentrations during stress can exceed by three orders of magnitude those detected in health, include some associated with hemostatic function (fibrinogen), microbicidal and prophagocytic activity (complement components, C-reactive protein), protease inhibitors (α_2-macroglobulin, α_1-antitrypsin), metal binders (haptoglobin, hemopexin, ceruloplasmin), and others with less well defined functions (serum amyloid A).[85–87] Simultaneous with the increase in the circulating concentrations of these acute-phase proteins, there is a marked and sustained suppression of albumin synthesis that in part explains the persistent decrease in its circulating concentration found in a variety of disease states independent of the nutritional status of the patient.

In terms of the regulation of the acute-phase response, in vitro studies with hepatocyte cultures and in vivo data suggest that the primary mediators of the acute-phase response are IL-1, TNF-α, and members of the IL-6 family including oncostatin-M, leukemia inhibitory factor, and IL-11.[88] Injection of IL-1, TNF-α, and IL-6 into experimental animals reproduces the acute-phase response found in acute inflammation.[88, 89] Because TNF-α induces the production of IL-1 and IL-6, and IL-1 can in turn induce IL-6, it is not surprising that the administration of single cytokines or their combinations leads to similar acute-phase response protein synthesis. Members of the IL-6 family, sharing the ability to bind and signal through the gp130 complex, are particularly strong promoters of the acute-phase response.[88, 90]

Substantial information on the specific role of individual cytokines in determining acute-phase protein synthesis has accumulated over the past few years. Blockage of the functional type I IL-1 receptor in mice with monoclonal antibody reduces by at least 90% the circulating levels of the main acute-phase response proteins amyloid A, amyloid P, C3, and seromucoid.[91] Interestingly, treatment with the antibody did not prevent the increase in circulating corticosterone levels or the decrease in serum albumin levels found in the model. Results with

knockout mice for IL-1β[42] or IL-1 receptor type I[92] support those obtained with antibodies by demonstrating a markedly attenuated acute-phase response. In contrast with the results just discussed, blocking TNF-α with specific antibodies, although efficient in preventing endotoxemic shock, failed to prevent the acute-phase response.[93]

Anti-IL-1 therapy reduced circulating IL-6 levels after turpentine injection in animals,[91] an effect not shared by anti–TNF-α therapy. Supporting the hypothesis that the acute-phase response (and the weight loss and cachexia) that follows injury is mediated mainly by IL-6, experiments using anti–IL-6 antibodies, as well as those using animals deficient in this cytokine,[94] demonstrated complete suppression of these responses.[95]

Interestingly, some components of the acute-phase response seem to be capable of feedback regulating those cytokines implicated in the induction of the response.[85–87] For example, native α_2-macroglobulin can bind IL-1, IL-6, TNF-α, transforming growth factor-β, and platelet-derived growth factor and can serve as a cytokine and growth factor reservoir. Protease-activated α_2-macroglobulin in turn appears to serve as a cytokine scavenger because it is recognized by specific cellular receptors and removed by endocytosis. Additionally, α-1 acid glycoprotein protects against TNF-α–induced lethality.[96] Serum amyloid A and α-1 acid glycoprotein sequester circulating IL-1 and decrease TNF-α expression. Lastly, injections of serum amyloid A prevent IL-1– and TNF-α–induced fever and prostaglandin E_2 production in experimental animals.[97]

Demonstrating one more level of complexity in the regulation of the stress response, it has been shown that IL-6, canonically considered a proinflammatory cytokine, can act as an anti-inflammatory agent. In this regard, it was shown that the injection of IL-6 in humans promotes the appearance of IL-1 receptor antagonist and of soluble TNF-α receptor p55 in the circulation.[98]

◆ ALTERATIONS IN LIPID METABOLISM

Mediated mainly through β_2-adrenergic stimulation,[74, 99, 100] lipolysis with the release of fatty acids and glycerol from adipose tissue is markedly enhanced after injury. Glycerol thus released into the circulation adds to the pool of gluconeogenic precursors. Most fatty acids are re-esterified to triglycerides in the liver. The bulk of the triglycerides thus formed are released into the circulation as very low density lipoprotein (VLDL).[101] This accelerated rate of interorgan lipid traffic, the *triglyceride–fatty acid cycle*, has an intracellular counterpart that involves the in situ re-esterification of fatty acids in the adipocyte after triglyceride hydrolysis. Both the intracellular and the interorgan components of the cycle are accelerated in injury, consume energy, and thus contribute to overall thermogenesis in illness.[99] Interestingly, the accelerated release of VLDL from the liver may prove to have a function distinct from fat's role as an energy source in view of the potential role of VLDL and other lipoproteins[102] as binders and inactivators of endotoxin.[103, 104] In this regard, hypolipemic animals have been shown to have increased sensitivity to lipopolysaccharides.[102]

Interestingly, in trauma,[40] sepsis,[105] and critical illness,[106] the rate of lipolysis (measured as glycerol appearance) is substantially greater than the measured fat oxidation rate, suggesting an accelerated rate of fatty acid oxidation at the tissue site where lipolysis occurs. The fasting rate of fatty acid oxidation was found to be twice as high in traumatized patients as in healthy controls.[40] Calculations performed using data from Shaw and Wolfe indicate that fat oxidation meets most energy requirements in injury, providing roughly 1800 kcal/day in a 70-kg patient.[40] Comparable studies performed in subjects with severe acute pancreatitis failed to reveal enhanced rates of fatty acid turnover but confirmed that fat oxidation contributes significantly to total energy production.[107]

Although catecholamines appear to suffice in explaining the accelerated lipolysis of injury, cytokines may also contribute to this phenomenon. It has been proposed that TNF-α can accelerate lipolysis though the stimulation of hormone-sensitive lipase in the adipocyte and promote hypertriglyceridemia by inhibiting lipoprotein lipase.[14, 108] Interestingly, TNF-α has also been shown to decrease the synthesis of apolipoprotein A-I.[109] Since the overexpression of this apolipoprotein has been shown to be protective against endotoxin,[110] TNF-α may prove to be detrimental to the host in infectious diseases by indirectly increasing its sensitivity to lipopolysaccharide. IL-6 administration in humans results in enhanced fatty acid and ketone body production and accelerated fat oxidation.[111] It is unclear at this time whether these effects are directly mediated through this cytokine or are secondary to its function as a secretagogue for catecholamines and cortisol.

◆ ALTERATIONS IN VITAMIN METABOLISM

Remarkably little has been published in the particularly interesting area of alterations in vitamin metabolism in response to injury. Although the increased metabolic rate of injury must determine alterations in vitamin turnover and requirements, information on its impact on specific vitamins is lacking. It has been well documented that acute infectious disease determines the accelerated utilization and redistribution of most vitamins and that severe infections can precipitate the appearance of clinical signs of vitamin deficiency.[112]

In terms of specific alterations in individual vitamins, classic work of Levenson and colleagues and others indicated that a dramatic decrease in plasma and urine ascorbic acid follows injury.[113, 114] These alterations appear to be more severe in burns, with evidence for decreased tissue saturation with vitamin C revealed by intravenous loading tests.[113, 114] The same authors described similar changes in urinary excretion and tissue saturation for thiamine and nicotinamide.[113, 114] Circulating vitamin A concentrations are transiently decreased in hospitalized patients and most particularly during infectious complications.[115] The decrease in serum retinol levels that is found under these conditions depends in part on reductions in circulating retinol-binding protein.[116] The corresponding increase in unbound retinol determines its enhanced urinary excretion.[117]

Cobalamin (vitamin B_{12}) metabolism is also significantly altered in injury and infection. Biologically active cobalamin is transported in plasma bound to transcobalamin II.[118] Present in plasma, however, are other transcobalamins (I and III) or R proteins that do not appear to have a physiologic role in cobalamin transport but are expressed in high concentrations in leukocytes, where they have been proposed to exert an antibacterial role.[119] Markedly elevated plasma concentrations of vitamin B_{12} associated with the increased appearance of its binding proteins is not uncommon in injury and sepsis.

◆ ALTERATIONS IN MINERAL METABOLISM

Although better described in relation to infectious challenges, stress of any nature causes profound changes in mineral metabolism. Alterations in sodium and potassium metabolism dependent on antidiuretic factors and proposed disruptions in the cellular content of these elements were discussed earlier. Of clinical relevance is the disproportionate loss of K^+ seen after injury. Under normal conditions, potassium is held in cells at a fixed ratio to cellular protein. The stability of this ratio of 3 mEq of potassium per gram of protein nitrogen constitutes the basis for defining the body cell mass by total body potassium that is the cornerstone for multiple models of body composition.[120–122] Balance studies have shown that potassium and nitrogen accretion during refeeding and their respective losses in long-term fasting are constrained to the ratio just described.[25] Changes in total body potassium have thus been equated with changes in total body protein.[122] These concepts do not fully explain findings in injury, where there appears to be a selective cellular potassium depletion, resulting in urinary potassium-to-nitrogen loss ratios higher than the predicted 3 mEq/g. Indeed, Bessey and associates reported a urinary potassium-to-nitrogen ratio of 7 in their healthy volunteers infused with triple hormones.[10] Because dextrose infusion, even at low rates, additionally promotes urinary potassium loss,[123] injured patients can suffer severe total body potassium loss that may not be reflected in clinical hypokalemia. Lehr and coworkers demonstrated total body potassium depletion in a variety of surgical patients, most prominently in those with high-output gastrointestinal fistulas or inflammatory bowel disease.[124] These patients reveal significant potassium avidity on recovery. Failure to provide substantial quantities of this cation during convalescence and refeeding can precipitate clinically relevant hypokalemia.

Iron metabolism is altered in injury as a result of the release of lactoferrin from activated neutrophils.[125] Unsaturated lactoferrin in the circulation binds iron, and the complex is then cleared by the liver, with resultant hypoferremia.[125] Serum zinc concentrations also decline in injury through the increased synthesis of the metal-binding protein metallothionein in liver cells[126] and through increased urinary losses of this metal that depend in part on the decreased serum albumin concentration. In contrast, circulating levels of copper increase in infection and stress due to elevations in the plasma level of the copper-containing ferroxidase ceruloplasmin.[127]

REFERENCES

1. Baue AE: Physiology of shock and injury. *In* Geller E (ed): Shock and Resuscitation. New York, McGraw-Hill, 1993, pp 67–126.
2. Cuthbertson DP: The disturbance of metabolism produced by bony and non-bony injury, with notes on certain abnormal conditions of bone. Biochem J 24:1244–1263, 1930.
3. Cuthbertson DP: The distribution of nitrogen and sulphur in the urine during conditions of increased catabolism. Biochem J 25:236–244, 1931.
4. Cuthbertson DP: Observations on the disturbance of metabolism produced by injury to the limbs. QJM 25:233–246, 1932.
5. Cuthbertson DP: Post-shock metabolic response. Lancet 1:433–437, 1942.
6. Cannon WB: The Wisdom of the Body. New York, WW Norton, 1967.
7. Hume DM, Egdahl RH: The importance of the brain in the endocrine response to injury. Ann Surg 150:692–712, 1959.
8. Wilmore DW: Hormonal responses and their effect on metabolism. Surg Clin North Am 56:999–1018, 1976.
9. Wilmore DW, Long JM, Mason AD Jr, et al: Catecholamines: Mediator of the hypermetabolic response to thermal injury. Ann Surg 180:653–669, 1974.
10. Bessey PQ, Watters JM, Aoki TT, et al: Combined hormonal infusion simulates the metabolic response to injury. Ann Surg 200:264–281, 1984.
11. Tracey KJ, Cerami A: Tumor necrosis factor: A pleiotropic cytokine and therapeutic target. Annu Rev Med 45:491–503, 1994.
12. Tracey KJ, Lowry SF: The role of cytokine mediators in septic shock. Adv Surg 23:21–56, 1990.
13. Michie HR, Spriggs DR, Manogue KR, et al: Tumor necrosis factor and endotoxin induce similar metabolic responses in human beings. Surgery 104:280–286, 1988.
14. Van der Poll T, Romijn JA, Endert E, et al: Tumor necrosis factor mimics the metabolic response to acute infection in healthy humans. Am J Physiol 261:E457–E465, 1991.
15. Rothwell NJ: Hypothalamus and thermogenesis. *In* Kinney JM, Tucker HN (eds): Energy Metabolism: Tissue Determinants and Cellular Corollaries. New York, Raven Press, 1992, pp 229–245.

16. Bratts R, Linden M: Cytokine modulation by glucocorticoids: Mechanisms and actions in cellular studies. Aliment Pharmacol Ther 10:81–90, 1996.

17. Kinney JM, Duke JH, Long CL, et al: Tissue fuel and weight loss after injury. J Clin Pathol 23 (Suppl 4):65–72, 1970.

18. Long CL, Schaffel N, Geiger JW, et al: Metabolic response to illness. Estimation of energy and protein needs from indirect calorimetry and nitrogen balance. JPEN J Parenter Enteral Nutr 3:452–456, 1979.

19. Quebbeman EF, Ausman RK, Schneider TC: A reevaluation of energy expenditure during parenteral nutrition. Ann Surg 195:283–286, 1982.

20. Kinney JM, Fürst P, Elwyn DH, Carpentier YA: The intensive care patient. In Kinney JM, Jeejeebhoy KN, Hill GL, Owen OE (eds): Nutrition and Metabolism in Patient Care. Philadelphia, WB Saunders, 1988, pp 656–671.

21. Cunningham JJ, Hegarty MT, Meara PA, et al: Measured and predicted calorie requirements of adults during recovery from severe burn trauma. Am J Clin Nutr 49:404–408, 1989.

22. Hirsch J, Leibel RL, Edens NK: Overview: Cellular corollaries of energy expenditure. In Kinney JM, Tucker HN (eds): Energy Metabolism: Tissue Determinants and Cellular Corollaries. New York, Raven Press, 1992, pp 525–532.

23. Curreri PW, Wilmore DW, Mason AD Jr, et al: Intracellular cation alterations following major trauma: Effect of supranormal caloric intake. J Trauma 11:390–396, 1971.

24. Abbott WE, Albertson K: The effect of starvation, infection and injury on the metabolic processes and body composition. Ann N Y Acad Sci 110:941–964, 1963.

25. Gamble JL, Ross SG, Tisdall G: The metabolism of fixed base during fasting. J Biol Chem 57:633–695, 1923.

26. James JH, Fang CH, Schrantz SJ, et al: Linkage of aerobic glycolysis to sodium-potassium transport in rat skeletal muscle. J Clin Invest 98:2388–2397, 1996.

27. Luchette FA, Friend LA, Brown CC, et al: Increased skeletal muscle Na^+/K^+-ATPase activity as a cause of increased lactate production after hemorrhagic shock. J Trauma 44:796–803, 1998.

28. Flear CTG, Bhattacharya SS, Singh CM: Solute and water exchanges between cells and extracellular fluids in health and disturbances after trauma. JPEN J Parenter Enteral Nutr 4:98–120, 1980.

29. Jacobs DO, Kobayashi T, Imagire J, et al: Sepsis alters skeletal muscle energetics and membrane function. Surgery 110:318–326, 1991.

30. Häussinger D, Lang F, Gerok W: Regulation of cell function by the cellular hydration state. Am J Physiol 267:E343–E355, 1994.

31. Hotchkiss RS, Song SK, Ling CS, et al: Sepsis does not alter red blood cell glucose metabolism or Na^+ concentration: a ^{2}H-, ^{23}Na-NMR study. Am J Physiol 258:R21–R31, 1990.

32. Tanaka J, Sato T, Kamiyama Y: Bacteremic shock: Aspects of high energy metabolism of rat liver following living Escherichia coli injection. J Surg Res 33:49–57, 1982.

33. McGivney A, Bradley SG: Action of bacterial endotoxin and lipid A on mitochondrial enzyme activities of cells in culture and subcellular fraction. Infect Immun 25:664–671, 1979.

34. Greer G, Epps W, Vail W: Interaction of lipopolysaccharides with mitochondria. I: Quantitative assay of Salmonella typhimurium lipopolysaccharides with isolated mitochondria. J Infect Dis 127:551–556, 1973.

35. Wilmore DW, Long JM, Mason AD Jr: Catecholamines: Mediator of the hypermetabolic response to thermal injury. Ann Surg 4:653, 1974.

36. Breder CD, Dinarello CA, Saper CB: Interleukin-1 immunoreactive innervation of human hypothalamus. Science 240:321–324, 1988.

37. Kagan BL, Baldwin RL, Munoz D, et al: Formation of ion-permeable channels by tumor necrosis factor-alpha. Science 255:1427–1430, 1992.

38. Zentella A, Manogue K, Cerami A: Cachectin/TNF-mediated lactate production in cultured myocytes is linked to activation of a futile substrate cycle. Cytokine 5:436–447, 1993.

39. Wolfe RR: Regulation of glucose metabolism. In Burke JF (ed): Surgical Physiology. Philadelphia, WB Saunders, 1983, pp 75–97.

40. Shaw JHF, Wolfe RR: An integrated analysis of glucose, fat, and protein metabolism in severely traumatized patients. Studies in the basal state and the response to total parenteral nutrition. Ann Surg 209:63–72, 1989.

41. Wolfe RR: Glucose metabolism in burn injury: A review. J Burn Care Rehabil 6:408–418, 1985.

42. Fantuzzi G, Dinarello CA: The inflammatory response in interleukin-1 beta-deficient mice: Comparison with other cytokine-related knock-out mice. J Leukoc Biol 59:489–493, 1996.

43. Wolfe RR, Durkot MJ, Allsop JR, et al: Glucose metabolism in severely burned patients. Metabolism 28:1031–1039, 1979.

44. Shangraw RE, Jahoor F, Miyoshi H, et al: Differentiation between septic and postburn insulin resistance. Metabolism 38:983–989, 1989.

45. Black PR, Brooks DC, Bessey PQ, et al: Mechanisms of insulin resistance following injury. Ann Surg 196:420–435, 1982.

46. Wolfe RR, Jahoor F, Herndon DN, et al: Isotopic evaluation of the metabolism of pyruvate and related substrates in normal adult volunteers and severely burned children: Effect of dichloroacetate and glucose infusion. Surgery 110:54–67, 1991.

47. Wilmore DW, Aulick LH, Mason AD Jr, et al: Influence of the burn wound on local and systemic responses to injury. Ann Surg 186:444–458, 1977.

48. Lipman RL, Raskin P, Love T, et al: Glucose intolerance during decreased physical activity in man. Diabetes 21:101–107, 1972.

49. Wolfe RR, Burke JF: Somatostatin infusion inhibits glucose production in burn patients. Circ Shock 9:521–527, 1982.

50. Wilmore DW, Moylan JA, Pruitt BA, et al: Hyperglucagonaemia after burns. Lancet 1:73–75, 1974.

51. Durkot MJ, Wolfe RR: Effects of adrenergic blockade on glucose kinetics in septic and burned guinea pigs. Am J Physiol 241:R222–R227, 1981.

52. Ingle DJ: Permissive action of hormones. J Clin Endocrinol Metab 14:1772, 1954.

53. Einstein AB, Strack I: Effects of glucagon on carbohydrate synthesis and enzyme activity in rat liver. Endocrinology 83:1337–1348, 1968.

54. Wicks WD, Barnett CA, McKibbin JB: Interaction between hormones and cyclic AMP in regulating specific hepatic enzyme synthesis. Fed Proc 33:1105–1111, 1974.

55. Wise JK, Hendler R, Felig PJ: Influence of gluco-corticoids on glucagon secretion and plasma amino acid concentrations in man. J Clin Invest 52:2774–2782, 1973.

56. Olefsky JM, Johnson J, Liu F, et al: The effects of acute and chronic dexamethasone administration on insulin binding to isolated rat hepatocytes and adipocytes. Metabolism 24:517–527, 1975.

57. Kahn BB, Flier JS: Regulation of glucose-transporter gene expression in vitro and in vivo. Diabetes Care 13:548–564, 1990.

58. Nosadini R, Del Prato S, Tiengo A, et al: Insulin resistance in Cushing's syndrome. J Clin Endocrinol Metab 57:529–536, 1983.

59. Irwin MI, Hegsted DM: A conspectus of research on protein requirements of man. *In* Irwin MI (ed): Nutritional Requirements of Man: A Conspectus of Research. Washington, DC, Nutrition Foundation, 1980, pp 1–45.

60. Long CL, Schiller WR, Blakemore WS, et al: Muscle protein catabolism in the septic patient as measured by 3-methylhistidine excretion. Am J Clin Nutr 30:1349–1352, 1977.

61. Wannemacher RW Jr, Dinterman RE, Pekarek RS, et al: Urinary amino acid excretion during experimentally induced sandfly fever in man. Am J Clin Nutr 28:110–118, 1975.

62. Williamson DH, Farrell R, Kerr A, et al: Muscle-protein catabolism after injury in man, as measured by urinary excretion of 3-methylhistidine. Clin Sci Mol Med 52:527–533, 1977.

63. Aulick LH, Wilmore DW: Increased peripheral amino acid release following burn injury. Surgery 85:560–565, 1979.

64. Vary TC, Kimball SR: Sepsis-induced changes in protein synthesis: Differential effects on fast- and slow-twitch muscles. Am J Physiol 262:C513–C519, 1992.

65. Crane CW, Picou D, Smith R, et al: Protein turnover in patients before and after elective orthopaedic operations. Br J Surg 64:129–133, 1977.

66. Kien CL, Young VR, Rohrbaugh DK, et al: Whole-body protein synthesis and breakdown rates in children before and after reconstructive surgery of the skin. Metabolism 27:27–34, 1978.

67. Shaw JHF, Wildbore M, Wolfe RR: Whole body protein kinetics in severely septic patients. Ann Surg 205:288–294, 1987.

68. Wolfe BM, Culebras JM, Aoki TT, et al: The effects of glucagon on protein metabolism in normal man. Surgery 86:248–257, 1979.

69. Rannels SR, Jefferson LS: Effects of glucocorticoids on muscle protein synthesis in perfused rat hemocorpus. Am J Physiol 238:E564–E572, 1980.

70. Wing SS, Goldberg AL: Glucocorticoids activate the ATP-ubiquitin-dependent proteolytic system in skeletal muscle during fasting. Am J Physiol 264:E668–E676, 1993.

71. Hall-Angeras M, Angeras U, Zamir O, et al: Effect of the glucocorticoid receptor RU 38486 on muscle protein breakdown in sepsis. Surgery 109:468–473, 1991.

72. Choo JJ, Horan MA, Little RA, et al: Anabolic effects of clenbuterol on skeletal muscle are mediated by beta $_2$-adrenoreceptor activation. Am J Physiol 263:E50–E56, 1992.

73. McElligott MA, Barreto A, Chaung LY: Effect of continuous and intermittent clenbuterol feeding on rat growth rate and muscle. Comp Biochem Physiol 92C:135–138, 1989.

74. Herndon DN, Nguyen TT, Wolfe RR, et al: Lipolysis in burned patients is stimulated by the beta 2-receptor for catecholamines. Arch Surg 129:1301–1305, 1994.

75. Herndon DN, Nguyen TT, Wolfe RR: Effects of physiological hyperinsulinemia on muscle protein kinetics in severely burned patients. Clin Nutr 13:23–27, 1994.

76. Jahoor F, Herndon DN, Wolfe RR: Role of insulin and glucagon in the response of glucose and alanine kinetics in burn-injured patients. J Clin Invest 78:807–814, 1986.

77. Zhang XJ, Kunkel KR, Jahoor F, et al: Role of basal insulin in the regulation of protein kinetics and energy metabolism in septic patients. JPEN J Parenter Enteral Nutr 15:394–399, 1991.

78. Wolfe RR, Jahoor F, Hartl WH: Protein and amino acid metabolism after injury. Diabetes Metab Rev 5:149–164, 1989.

79. Jeffries MK, Vance ML: Growth hormone and cortisol secretion in patients with burn injury. J Burn Care Rehabil 13:391–395, 1992.

80. Tiao G, Fagan J, Roegen V: Energy-ubiquitin-dependent muscle proteolysis during sepsis in rats is regulated by glucocorticoids. J Clin Invest 97:339–348, 1996.

81. Zamir O, Hasselgren PO, Higashiguchi T, et al: Tumor necrosis factor (TNF) and interleukin-1 (IL-1) induce muscle proteolysis through different mechanisms. Mediat Inflam 1:247–250, 1992.

82. Michie HR, Sherman ML, Spriggs DR, et al: Chronic TNF infusion causes anorexia but not accelerated nitrogen loss. Ann Surg 209:19–24, 1989.

83. Baracos V, Rodemann P, Dinarello CA, et al: Stimulation of muscle protein degradation and prostaglandin E_2 release by leukocytic pyrogen (interleukin-1). N Engl J Med 308:553–558, 1983.

84. Jahoor F, Desai M, Herndon DN, et al: Dynamics of the protein metabolic response to burn injury. Metabolism 37:330–337, 1988.

85. Moshage H: Cytokines and the hepatic acute phase response. J Pathol 181:257–266, 1997.

86. Pannen BHJ, Robotham JL: The acute-phase response. New Horiz 3:183–197, 1995.

87. Steel DM, Whitehead AS: The major acute phase reactants: C-reactive protein, serum amyloid P component and serum amyloid A protein. Immunol Today 15:81–88, 1994.

88. Moldawer LL, Copeland EM III: Proinflammatory cytokines, nutritional support, and the cachexia syndrome. Interactions and therapeutic options. Cancer 79:1828–1839, 1997.

89. Moldawer LL, Andersson C, Gelin J, et al: Regulation of food intake and hepatic protein synthesis by recombinant-derived cytokines. Am J Physiol 254:G450–G456, 1988.

90. Benigni F, Fantuzzi G, Sacco S, et al: Six different cytokines that share GP130 as a receptor subunit, induce serum amyloid A and potentiate the induction of interleukin-6 and the activation of the hypothalamus-pituitary-adrenal axis by interleukin-1. Blood 87:1851–1854, 1996.

91. Gershenwald JE, Fong YM, Fahey TJ: Interleukin 1 receptor blockade attenuates the host inflammatory response. Proc Natl Acad Sci U S A 87:4966–4970, 1990.

92. Solorzano CC, Kaibara A, Pruitt JH: Mice lacking a functional IL-1 type I but not a TNF type I

receptor exhibit an attenuated acute phase response in acute inflammation. Surg Forum 47:72–73, 1996.

93. Sherry BA, Gelin J, Fong Y: Anticachectin/tumor necrosis factor-alpha antibodies attenuate development of cachexia in tumor models. FASEB J 3:1956–1962, 1989.

94. Fattori E, Cappelletti M, Costa P, et al: Defective inflammatory response in interleukin 6–deficient mice. J Exp Med 180:1243–1250, 1994.

95. Oldenburg HS, Rogy MA, Lazarus DD: Cachexia and the acute-phase protein response in inflammation are regulated by interleukin-6. Eur J Immunol 23:1889–1894, 1993.

96. Libert C, Brouckaert P, Fiers W: Protection by alpha 1-acid glycoprotein against tumor necrosis factor–induced lethality. J Exp Med 180:1571–1575, 1994.

97. Shainkin-Kestenbaum R, Berlyne G, Zimlichman S, et al: Acute phase protein, serum amyloid A, inhibits IL-1- and TNF-induced fever and hypothalamic PGE_2 in mice. Scand J Immunol 34:179–183, 1991.

98. Tilg H, Trehu E, Atkins MB, et al: Interleukin-6 (IL-6) as an anti-inflammatory cytokine: Induction of circulating IL-1 receptor antagonist and soluble tumor necrosis factor receptor p55. Blood 83:113–118, 1994.

99. Wolfe RR, Herndon DN, Jahoor F, et al: Effect of severe burn injury on substrate cycling by glucose and fatty acids. N Engl J Med 317:403–408, 1987.

100. Wolfe RR, Herndon DN, Peters EJ, et al: Regulation of lipolysis in severely burned children. Ann Surg 206:214–221, 1987.

101. Wolfe RR: Assessment of substrate cycling in humans using tracer methodology. In Kinney JM, Tucker HN (eds): Energy Metabolism: Tissue Determinants and Cellular Corollaries. New York, Raven Press, 1992, pp 495–523.

102. Feingold KR, Funk JL, Moser AH, et al: Role for circulating lipoproteins in the protection from endotoxin toxicity. Infect Immun 63:2041–2046, 1995.

103. Hardardottir I, Grunfeld C, Feingold KR: Effects of endotoxin and cytokines on lipid metabolism. Curr Opin Lipidol 5:207–215, 1994.

104. Hardardottir I, Grunfeld C, Feingold KR: Effects of endotoxin on lipid metabolism. Biochem Soc Trans 23:1013–1018, 1995.

105. Shaw JHF, Wolfe RR: Free fatty acid and glycerol kinetics in severely septic patients and in patients with early and advanced gastrointestinal cancer. Ann Surg 205:368–376, 1987.

106. Klein S, Peters EJ, Shangraw RE, et al: Lipolytic response to metabolic stress in critically ill patients. Crit Care Med 19:776–779, 1991.

107. Shaw JHF, Wolfe RR: Glucose, fatty acid, and urea kinetics in patients with severe pancreatitis. The response to substrate infusion and total parenteral nutrition. Ann Surg 204:665–672, 1986.

108. Cooney RN, Owens E, Slaymaker D, et al: Prevention of skeletal muscle catabolism in sepsis does not impair visceral protein metabolism. Am J Physiol 270:E621–E626, 1996.

109. Grunfeld C, Feingold KR: Effects of TNF, IL-1, and the combination of both cytokines on cholesterol

metabolism in Syrian hamsters. Lymph Cytol Res 13:161–166, 1994.

110. Levine DM, Parker TS, Donnelly TM, et al: In vivo protection against endotoxin by plasma high density lipoprotein. Proc Natl Acad Sci U S A 90:12040–12044, 1993.

111. Stouthard JML, Romijn JA, Van der Poll T, et al: Endocrinologic and metabolic effects of interleukin-6 in humans. Am J Physiol 268:E813–E819, 1995.

112. Beisel WR: Infectious diseases: Effects on food intake and nutrient requirements. In Hodges RE, Alfin-Slater RB, Kritchevsky D (eds): Human Nutrition, a Comprehensive Treatise. Vol 4: Nutrition: Metabolic and Clinical Applications. New York, Plenum Press, 1979, pp 329–346.

113. Lund CC, Levenson SM, Green RW, et al: Ascorbic acid, thiamine, riboflavin and nicotinic acid in relation to acute burns in man. Arch Surg 55:557–583, 1947.

114. Levenson SM, Green RW, Taylor FHL, et al: Ascorbic acid, riboflavin, thiamin, and nicotinic acid in relation to severe injury, hemorrhage, and infection in the human. Ann Surg 124:840–856, 1946.

115. Mitra AK, Alvarez JO, Wahed MA, et al: Predictors of serum retinol in children with shigellosis. Am J Clin Nutr 68:1088–1094, 1998.

116. Beisel WR: Infection-induced depression of serum retinol. Am J Clin Nutr 68:993–994, 1998.

117. Mitra AK, Alvarez JO, Guay-Woodford L, et al: Urinary retinol excretion and kidney function in children with shigellosis. Am J Clin Nutr 68:1095–1103, 1998.

118. Seetharam B, Alpers DH: Absorption and transport of cobalamins. Ann Rev Nutr 2:243–269, 1982.

119. Gilbert HS: Proposal of a possible function for granulocyte vitamin B12 binding proteins in host defense against bacteria. Blood 44:926 (abstract 65), 1974.

120. Cohn SH, Vartsky D, Yasumura S, et al: Compartmental body composition based on total body nitrogen, potassium and calcium. Am J Physiol 239:E524–E530, 1980.

121. Moore FD: Energy and the maintenance of the body cell mass. JPEN J Parenter Enteral Nutr 4:228–260, 1980.

122. Spanier AH, Shizgal HM: Caloric requirements of the critically ill patient receiving intravenous hyperalimentation. Am J Surg 133:99–104, 1977.

123. Gamble JL: Chemical Anatomy: Physiology and Pathology of the Extracellular Fluid, 6th ed. Cambridge, Harvard University Press, 1960.

124. Lehr L, Schober O, Hundeshagen H: Total body potassium depletion and the need for preoperative nutritional support in Crohn's disease. Ann Surg 196:709–714, 1982.

125. Klempner MS, Dinarello CA, Gallin JI: Human leukocytic pyrogen induces release of specific granule contents from human neutrophils. J Clin Invest 61:1330–1336, 1978.

126. Sobocinski PZ, Canterbury WJ Jr, Mapes CA, et al: Involvement of hepatic metallothioneins in hypozincemia associated with bacterial infection. Am J Physiol 234:E399–E406, 1978.

127. Keusch GT, Farthing MJG: Nutrition and infection. Annu Rev Nutr 6:131–154, 1986.

3

◆ Lipid Emulsions in Parenteral Nutrition

David F. Driscoll, Ph.D.
Michael Adolph, M.D.
Bruce R. Bistrian, M.D., Ph.D.

The safe use of intravenous lipid emulsion (IVLE) has been a therapeutic challenge to clinicians in the 20th century. The motivation to develop such a product was the need for a calorically dense source of energy that was iso-osmotic and could be given daily by way of a peripheral vein. In the early part of the 20th century, the infusion of IVLE in patients met with variable degrees of success.[1] A large amount of this work was carried out between 1945 and 1960 at the Harvard School of Public Health under the direction of Drs. Frederick Stare and Robert Geyer, and much attention focused on a cottonseed oil–based lipid emulsion known as Lipomul IV.[2] Unfortunately, although the use of this preparation was more successful than earlier attempts, the adverse reactions encountered were at times severe. These adverse reactions consisted of a constellation of symptoms, manifesting either acutely as an immune-mediated anaphylactic reaction or subacutely as a fall in hematocrit, thrombocytopenia, hemoptysis, fever, and diffuse abdominal pain that was suggestive of fat overload syndrome. By the mid-1960s Lipomul IV was removed from the U.S. market. Then in the mid-1970s, a soybean oil–based product that had been developed in Sweden by Dr. Arvid Wretlind seemed to avoid the earlier problems and, after significant clinical experience in Europe, was approved by the U.S. Food and Drug Administration as Intralipid.[3] However, its primary use in the clinical setting was for the prevention of essential fatty acid deficiency in patients receiving parenteral nutrition for protracted periods of time. The soybean oil–based lipid emulsion is replete in the two essential fatty acids, linoleic and linolenic acid.

Shortly after its approval, a landmark study by Jeejeebhoy and colleagues demonstrated the safety and efficacy of administering this product as a daily caloric source.[4] These data, coupled with the emerging clinical experience by Solassol and Joyeax and associates using lipids as a daily caloric source in the form of a total nutrient admixture (TNA),[5, 6] established the role of lipids as a safe source of dense calories that could be given on a daily, rather than on an intermittent, basis in both hospitalized (metabolically stressed) and home care (metabolically unstressed) patients. Substituting a portion of the daily glucose calories with lipids to produce a mixed-fuel system avoids an excess of either energy source and its attendant complications.

◆ PHARMACEUTICAL REVIEW OF INTRAVENOUS LIPID EMULSIONS

Pharmaceutical-grade IVLE is a complex dispersion of oil droplets that has been carefully homogenized to produce a high-quality dispersion, safe for intravenous administration, with particles of a mean dimension approximately 0.3 μm or 300 nm in diameter. Commercial IVLEs are highly concentrated dispersions and are available in final lipid concentrations of 10, 20, and 30%. Both the 10% and the 20% IVLEs can be given as separate infusions or as a TNA formulation. The 30% IVLE is only indicated for pharmaceutical compounding purposes as a TNA and is not recommended for direct intravenous administration in its undiluted form. Just how concentrated IVLEs are can be estimated by making some elementary mathematical assumptions, and then the relative concentrations of lipid droplets can be calculated in order to illustrate the magnitude of lipid droplets per milliliter of these undiluted dispersions.[7] For most commercially available IVLEs, the phospholipid emulsifying agent is held constant, irrespective of the final lipid concentration. This would suggest that there exists an amount of emulsifier in excess of that necessary to stabilize the emulsion, at least in the lower concentrations of IVLE formulations. The proportion of emulsifier to triglyceride is greatest in the 10% IVLE formulation (Table 3–1). This ratio has been suggested to underlie the hypertriglyceridemia seen with the separate administration of 10% IVLE to neonates[8] and to adults at very high infusion rates.[9]

The mean lipid droplet size of 300 nm is within the typical range of the dimensions of endogenous chylomicrons (range, 80 to 500 nm),[10] and the formulations are manufactured in this way so as to behave in a similar manner with respect to their metabolic fate.[11] Chylomicrons are composed of a core of reconstituted triglycerides surrounded by a surface-active layer of phospholipids and small amounts of cholesterol and apoprotein B; they assist in the digestion of fats, facilitated through the process of emulsification. Pharmaceutical IVLEs consist of a relatively homogeneous dispersion of lipid droplets as triglycerides that are similarly surrounded by a phospholipid surfactant in a continuous aqueous phase, forming an oil-in-water emulsion system. The most common IVLE emulsifying agent or surfactant used is a purified mixture of egg yolk phospholipids.

All lipid emulsions intended for intravenous administration must be oil-in-water mixtures in order to avoid introducing potentially fatal lipid emboli into the intravascular compartment, which may occur with water-in-oil mixtures or "cracked" oil-in-water emulsions. A *cracked oil-in-water emulsion* is another term for the terminal phase of emulsion destabilization, in which finely dispersed lipid droplets progress through a stage of aggregation and coarsening of fat globules, resulting in the separation of the two immiscible phases oil and water. The degree to which this occurs in the clinical setting is variable and is not always visually apparent. A 1995 study employed a single-particle optical sensing technique using light extinction to identify the subvisible changes associated with globule size coarsening that occur in the upper size range of the lipid droplet size distribution of the emulsion (i.e., globules >1 μm).[12] From this work involving 90 admixtures using a fractional factorial design, it is clear that when 0.4% or greater of the total fat present exceeds 5 μm in diameter using the single-particle optical sensing technique, the emulsion can be considered pharmaceutically unstable and therefore unsuitable for intravenous administration. Although the precise toxic dose of unstable and enlarged fat globules is unknown, a pharmaceutically unstable lipid emulsion should be considered unsafe and therefore unfit for human administration.

Thus, three principal components affect the final stability and subsequent safety of parenteral lipid emulsions: the "internal" or dispersed oil phase, the emulsifying agent, and the "external" or continuous aqueous phase. Any assessment of the physicochemi-

Table 3–1. Concentration of Lipid Droplets in Intravenous Lipid Emulsions

MDD	Lipid Concentration (droplets/ml)		
	10%	20%	30%
0.3 μm	7.77×10^{12}	1.55×10^{13}	2.33×10^{13}
0.4 μm	3.27×10^{12}	6.55×10^{12}	9.83×10^{12}
0.5 μm	1.67×10^{12}	3.35×10^{12}	5.03×10^{12}

$$\text{Droplet Number} = \frac{\text{Total Mass}}{\text{Mass of Individual Droplet}}$$

where

Total Mass = lipid concentration in g/ml
Mass of Individual Droplet = density (of oil) × volume (of sphere)
Droplet Number = Lipid concentration in g/ml/oil density × 4/3 π r^3

Example:

where

Total Mass = 0.1 g/ml, 0.2 g/ml, or 0.3 g/ml
Density of Oil = 0.91 (soybean oil)
Volume of Sphere = 4/3 π r^3
Radius of Droplet = ½ diameter in centimeters (MDD = 0.3 μm or 0.15 × 10^{-4} cm)

MDD, mean droplet diameter.

cal stability and safety of IVLE must consider these vital constituents that form the emulsion system.

Dispersed Oil Phase

The commercial emulsions provide a wide array of lipids used, including the polyunsaturated fatty acids (PUFAs) as either n-3 or n-6 long-chain triglycerides (LCTs), such as fish oil and soybean oil, respectively; monounsaturated fatty acids as n-9 LCTs, such as olive oil; and saturated fatty acids, such as medium-chain triglycerides (MCTs). The commercially available parenteral emulsion products intended for intravenous administration include these oils either alone or in combination with others as mixtures (Table 3–2). When combinations of these oils are produced, they are prepared by physically blending or mixing the lipid components (known as *physical* mixtures), or by transesterification of the MCTs and LCTs to chemical mixtures (known as *structured* lipids).[13]

Combinations of oils can reduce the adverse reaction profile of an individual oil by decreases in dosage and may even enhance the metabolic clearance, and subsequent safety, of the IVLE. For example, from studies assessing the differences in plasma clearance between certain lipid emulsions, the differences have been explained by changes in the physical characteristics of lipid droplets from an MCT-LCT *physical* mixture.[14] Nuclear magnetic resonance studies performed on the dispersed phase identified MCT at the surface of the LCT droplets, which might explain the superior clearance from plasma seen with pure MCT and MCT-LCT mixtures compared with pure LCT lipid emulsions. Additional evidence of similar droplet behavior has also been shown in an in vitro study evaluating the effect of different lipid emulsions on neutrophilic adhesion.[15] Again, MCT-LCT emulsions acted similarly to pure MCT emulsions in that they stimulated neutrophilic adhesion, whereas pure LCT did not. In fact, neither did a *structured* MCT-LCT mixture, which suggests that the dominant action of the *structured* lipid droplet was similar to that of a pure LCT emulsion. Thus, it would appear from these preliminary findings that the pharmaceutical and physiologic actions of *physical* mixtures of MCT and LCT behave similarly to those of pure MCT emulsions, and that *structured* mixtures of MCT and LCT behave more like pure LCT dispersions. These findings might also explain the differences in the physicochemical stability between IVLEs either alone or as a TNA,[16] yet it will require further study to confirm and possibly extend the implications of these findings.

Finally, the dispersed oil phase of IVLEs is used as a drug vehicle for compounds that

Table 3–2. Commercially Available Lipid Emulsions*

Product	Company (Country)	Lipid Composition†	Concentration (%)	Size (ml)‡
Liposyn II	Abbott (USA)	Soybean-safflower 50:50	10, 20	100, 200, 500
Liposyn III		Soybean oil 100%	10, 20, 30	100, 200, 500
Intralipid	Fresenius/Kabi	Soybean oil 100%	10, 20, 30	50, 100, 250, 500
Structolipid	(Sweden)	Soybean-MCT 64:36	20	500
Lipofundin N	B. Braun	Soybean oil 100%	10, 20	100, 250, 500
Lipofundin MCT/LCT	(Germany)	Soybean-MCT 50:50	10, 20	100, 250, 500
Lipoplus		MCT-soybean–fish oil 50:40:10	10, 20	100, 250, 500
Lipovenous	Fresenius	Soybean oil 100%	10, 20, 30	100, 250, 500
Lipovenous MCT	(Germany)	Soybean-MCT 50:50	10, 20	250, 500
Omegaven		Fish oil 100%	10	50, 100
Clinoleic	Baxter (France)	Olive oil–soybean 80:20	20	100, 250, 500
Critilip	Baxter (USA)	MCT–soybean oil 75:25	20	500

*Not meant to be an inclusive list.
†Proportion by weight.
‡Not all intravenous lipid emulsions are available in all sizes listed.
MCT, medium-chain triglyceride.

have poor water solubility and/or stability in aqueous media. Compared with the unique formulation characteristics of specifically designed drug liposomes, IVLEs may offer a simpler and cost-effective alternative drug dosage form. Two examples of IVLEs being used in this manner in the United States include propofol (Diprivan)[17] and diazepam (Dizac)[18] parenteral emulsions. However, not all such drugs can be successfully incorporated into IVLEs, as their potential toxicity may be increased.[19] Toxicities may arise from incomplete incorporation of the drug into the lipid droplet and/or destabilization of the lipid emulsion vehicle. Thus, specifically designed drug liposomes are not bioequivalent with IVLE-based drug delivery systems.

Emulsifier

The principal emulsifying agent used to stabilize IVLEs is a purified mixture of egg yolk phosphatides. From a physicochemical standpoint, the phospholipid emulsifier possesses some ideal characteristics for producing a stable dispersion and forms the basis of the emulsion system. The amphophilic characteristics of the emulsifier are critical to its ability to adsorb at the oil-water interface and therefore make the two immiscible phases miscible.

The hydrophilic head occurs at position 3 of the glycerol backbone, which is esterified with phosphoric acid linked through another ester bond to an alcohol such as choline. The head is composed of polar phosphate groups that extend into the continuous aqueous phase, whereas the hydrophobic tails orient toward the dispersed oil phase of the emulsion. Ionization of the polar phosphate group in the hydrophilic head produces a net negative charge on the individual droplets (also known as *zeta potential*). This electronegative potential, along with its corresponding counterions (required for electroneutrality), forms a complex electric double layer that provides a formidable electrostatic barrier against droplet coalescence. These layers of ions form two types of ionic atmospheres. A dense inner ionic core of electrostatic charges surrounding each lipid droplet (Stern layer) is accompanied by a less dense outer ionic atmosphere of electrolytes (Gouy-Chapman layer).

The hydrophobic tails comprise principally nonpolar fatty acid residues, such as palmitic (a saturated fatty acid), which occupies position 1 of the glycerol moiety; position 2 is generally occupied by an unsaturated fatty acid, such as oleic acid. Coupled with the position opposite the hydrophilic head, the closely packed alignment of the emulsifier along the oil-water interface forms a molecular film around each submicron lipid droplet that forms an effective mechanical barrier against the coalescence of fat globules. This barrier may be viewed as a defense against the attractive forces between nonpolar molecules or lipid droplets known as London van der Waals dispersion forces. In essence, the phospholipid-emulsifying agent confers emulsion stability by producing a highly proficient electromechanical barrier against coalescence of lipid droplets and the emulsion's ultimate destruction into the two original immiscible phases.

Continuous Aqueous Phase

The continuous phase of IVLEs is of less importance as a drug vehicle than the dispersed oil phase. From a physiologic perspective, however, the aqueous attributes of the continuous phase are vitally important for safe intravenous administration. The continuous, or external, phase of the emulsion dictates its physicochemical characteristics; thus, all parenteral emulsions intended for intravenous administration must be aqueous to be miscible with blood. Inadvertent intravenous administration of a water-in-oil emulsion or other water-insoluble formulations could have disastrous consequences.[20, 21]

In terms of IVLEs and TNAs, the composition of the continuous aqueous phase has major implications for the physicochemical stability of the dispersion. It is the *ion-rich* phase of the emulsion. The relative concentrations of prescribed electrolytes will greatly influence the otherwise stabilizing forces of electrostatic repulsion (i.e., net negative charge imparted by the emulsifier) between lipid droplets and may adversely affect the subsequent stability of the emulsion system. For example, high concentrations of electrolyte salts, especially higher-valence cations such as calcium and magnesium, tend to make the emulsion less stable by reducing the efficacy of the electronegative surface charge of the phospholipid-emulsifying agent on the lipid droplets.[12, 22] In addition, low final concentrations of ionic amino acids also decrease stability.[23] Although dextrose is a nonelectrolyte, in low final concentrations it too makes for a less stable emulsion.[24, 25] In essence, formulations with the combination of low final concentrations of both amino acids and dextrose, as occurs in formulations intended for peripheral vein administration, tend to be less stable than formulations with higher final concentrations of these macronutrients, such as those intended for central venous alimentation.

Alteration of the dispersion medium, such as a compositional change of the IVLE that occurs during the extemporaneous compounding of TNA formulations, influences the molecular forces that interact at the oil-water interface, as well as the balance of ionic charges within the bulk, or continuous aqueous phase, of the emulsion. The variable compositions of TNA formulations, particularly those used in acutely ill patients to treat severe metabolic disorders, compared with the stable home total parenteral nutrition (TPN) patient, provide an extraordinary array of physicochemical challenges to the integrity of the barriers against coalescence and thus the stability and subsequent safety of the parenteral nutrient admixture. The effects of forming a TNA product may promote destabilization and coalescence, or a net repulsive energy to stabilize the system may be maintained. For any parenteral pharmaceutical formulation, destabilization is an expected outcome of the extemporaneous manipulations of the original container, whether it is an emulsion or not. What is important is the assurance of a reasonably assigned "new" shelf life by the compounding pharmacist that ensures the administration of a stable and compatible formulation during the infusion period.

◆ ASSESSING THE RISKS OF SINGLE-FUEL (GLUCOSE-ONLY) VERSUS MIXED-FUEL (GLUCOSE-LIPID) PARENTERAL NUTRITION SYSTEMS

Clinically Relevant Glucose Infusion Issues

The rate of glucose infusion has a significant effect on the risk of one's developing metabolic complications. Intravenous glucose may follow one of three principal metabolic pathways. Oxidation of infused glucose to meet the energy demands of the body is the most desirable. The infused glucose may also proceed through nonoxidative pathways. The nonoxidative disposal to replete glycogen stores is also desirable and occurs at limited cost and metabolic risk to the host. However, the glycogen storage capacity of the human body is limited, leaving the alternative nonoxidative fate of glucose to the production of fat from glucose, a process known as *de novo lipogenesis*, to prevail, and this can produce clinically significant adverse effects. Finally, the circulating glucose level also increases when excessive infusion rates are used, and this can produce significant impairments in immune function, particularly in activated monocytes.[26] Optimizing the amount of glucose metabolized by the oxidative pathway, controlling its level in the circulation, and minimizing its metabolism to fat improve the clinical care of patients receiving nutritional support. The use of a mixed-fuel system fosters this balance.

Basal Versus Optimal Versus Maximal Glucose Infusion Rates

To meet the obligate glucose needs of the body (e.g., brain, kidney, red blood cells), the normal endogenous hepatic production rate for glucose approximates 2 mg/kg/min as the *basal* glucose production rate.[27] Thus, for example, the basal glucose production for the reference 70-kg man is approximately 200 g/day. During acute metabolic stress, and in an effort to meet heightened energy demands, the rate of production and consumption increases dramatically. Assuming that the patient is adequately nourished before the acute stressful event (trauma, sepsis, major abdominal surgery), these increased needs are met by the rapid depletion of glycogen stores, which can be exhausted within 24 hours.[28] Additional energy needs are derived from increased muscle proteolysis with the release of gluconeogenic amino acids, such as alanine. Of course, this occurs at the expense of lean tissue and cannot be sustained for an indefinite period of time, as the reparative processes to injury will become significantly impaired, which may lead to additional complications, such as wound dehiscence and immune dysfunction. The time course to develop these impairments is variable and is much longer in the well-nourished patient than in the moderate to severely malnourished patient.[29] In general, it can be stated that acutely ill patients should receive in the parenteral nutrition admixture glucose that at least meets basal production rates. Obvious exceptions to this would include those patients with significant glucose intolerance, in whom lesser quantities are given until normoglycemia is attained.

The *optimal* glucose infusion rate is that at which the ratio of glucose oxidized is high, but not maximal, in relation to the amount that is disposed of by nonoxidative pathways and the ratio is at the inflection of the parabolic curve relating these two functions. In this range, the efficiency in terms of the percentage and the total amount oxidized is optimized. As the nonoxidative disposal of glucose underlies the occurrence of most of the significant complications, it is important to modulate the flow of glucose through this metabolic pathway. In elaborate studies performed by Burke and colleagues[30, 31] the optimal glucose infusion rate was approximately two times the basal rate, or 4 mg/kg/min, which approximates the basal energy expenditure. This rate is not a goal but rather should be viewed as a ceiling dose in order to avoid the increased risk of metabolic complications associated with the continuous administration of excessive parenteral glucose, especially in patients with critical illness. The infusion rate of glucose should generally be between 2 and 4 mg/kg/min. If a mixed-fuel system is used, then the amount of glucose infused is usually slightly less than the optimal glucose infusion rate, but the addition of fat at 10 to 30% of nonprotein calories improves net protein utilization over glucose alone when both regimens are provided at energy requirement levels.

Finally, the *maximal* glucose infusion rate is the amount of parenteral glucose administered that results in the greatest quantity oxidized, which is clearly above the optimal infusion rate yet does so at an incrementally increased fraction being disposed of by the nonoxidative pathways.[31] In essence, although more glucose can be given, resulting in greater amounts of glucose oxidation, this increase occurs at the expense of increasing the rate of nonoxidative clearance and thus, potentially, metabolic complications. The maximal glucose infusion rate has been demonstrated to be nearly two times the optimal infusion rate, or approximately 7 mg/kg/min. There is no obvious clinical benefit associated with such high glucose infusion rates, and there are substantial risks at this level of intake. Moreover, the risk of significant metabolic complications is magnified in patients who are malnourished, have significant comorbid disease or diseases, or are severely stressed. In adults, infusion of continuous glucose at the maximal infusion rate of 7 mg/kg/min is generally not recommended, even though it can be tolerated in some individuals.

Table 3–3 illustrates the various carbohydrate intakes possible in a variety of adult patient weights at the different glucose infusion rates.

Specific Adverse Consequences Associated with the Nonoxidative Disposal of Parenteral Glucose

Metabolic complications associated with excessive glucose intakes commonly develop in severely stressed patients receiving parenteral nutrition. Critically ill patients with comorbid diseases involving major organ

Table 3–3. Amounts of Glucose at Various Infusion Rates in Adults

Weight (kg)	Basal (g/day) (2 mg/kg/min)	Optimal (g/day) (4 mg/kg/min)	Maximal (g/day) (7 mg/kg/min)*
40	115	230	403
50	144	288	504
60	173	346	605
70	202	403	706
80	230	460	806

*Not recommended.

systems and accompanied by moderate to severe malnutrition are at the greatest risk of developing clinically significant adverse events. Ironically, these are the same patients who can be expected to derive the greatest clinical benefits from expert nutritional support. Of the various complications of excessive glucose administration in the critically ill, the development of hyperglycemia (>220 mg/dl), hepatic steatosis, respiratory decompensation, and severe electrolyte disturbances are most notable. Of these, hyperglycemia can be the most difficult to manage[32] and also has the greatest implications for infectious complications and patient outcomes.

Hyperglycemia

Increasing the amount of glucose that must be cleared during a critical illness ultimately produces hyperglycemia. Subsequently, the rate of administration or dose must be adjusted to reflect more appropriately the capacity for oxidation and nonoxidative clearance. Even then, seemingly modest doses of glucose may still produce hyperglycemia due to the hormonal milieu arising from the metabolic response to injury and the unique hormonal response to parenteral glucose administration. In addition, insulin resistance due to the systemic inflammatory response, as well as that due to hyperglycemia or obesity if present, occurs at the level of the liver, in terms of limiting glucose production, and in muscle, in terms of fostering glucose uptake. Thus, the combination of these effects plus the exogenous infusion of glucose can result in pronounced hyperglycemia in susceptible patients.

A sustained blood glucose level that exceeds 220 mg/dl impairs key elements of the actions of white blood cells to perform their vital immune functions such as granulocyte adherence, chemotaxis, phagocytosis, and microbicidal activity. Interference with these processes during critical illness has been associated with an increase in infectious complications. The clinical significance of hyperglycemia during acute illness has been reviewed.[26]

De Novo Lipogenesis

As the glucose infusion rate increases, a greater fraction is committed to the formation of fat in the liver. As de novo lipogenesis continues, hepatic steatosis that may affect vital liver cell functions ensues. Hyperbilirubinemia[33] arising from impairment in hepatocyte function, and immune incompetence from Kupffer cell dysfunction,[34] are two examples of the clinical consequences of severe fat accumulation in the liver. Controlling the total amount of glucose administered, the infusion rate, and the provision of exogenous fat minimizes de novo lipogenesis.

Respiratory Decompensation

The consequences of de novo lipogenesis also have implications for respiratory function, as the endogenous metabolic conversion of glucose to fat is energy yielding, which reduces the energy derived from glucose oxidation for other vital functions and thereby increases energy expenditure. Energy derived from the metabolism of nutrients such as protein, carbohydrate, and fat is ultimately derived from oxygen consumption and carbon dioxide production. For example, under normal circumstances during glucose oxidation, the amount of carbon dioxide produced is equal to the amount of oxygen consumed. This ratio is known as the *respiratory quotient* and is thus 1 for carbohydrate oxidation. By way of comparison, this balance is considerably altered by de novo lipogenesis. Although the respiratory quotient by stoichiometry can be as high as 8 mol of carbon dioxide produced for each mol of oxygen consumed, in humans, de novo lipogenesis is accomplished by reductive biosynthesis. Reducing equivalents for this process are provided by glucose oxidation, leading to an actual respiratory quotient of about 2.4 for de novo lipogenesis. In critically ill patients receiving artificial ventilation, overfeeding with glucose can prolong the need for mechanical ventilatory assistance by dramatically increasing carbon dioxide production, thus lengthening intensive care unit stays and increasing the risk for iatrogenic complications and the cost of clinical care.

Hyperinsulinemia, Fluid Retention, and Electrolyte Disorders

The continuous intravenous administration of hypertonic glucose is unphysiologic and produces a continuous and profound hyperinsulinemic state. Under normal conditions

Table 3–4. Daily Lipid Infusions in Adults at 15% and 30% and at the Toxic Threshold

Weight (kg)	15% of kcal† (g)	30% of kcal† (g)	0.11 g/kg/h* (g)
40	17	34	106
50	21	42	132
60	25	50	158
70	29	58	185
80	33	66	211

*Not recommended and is the threshold at which toxicities are reported.[39] Although these represent very high doses if given over 24 hours, it is the rate that is important. Therefore, giving ¼ the dose, equivalent to a typical 6-hour intermittent infusion, may have similar adverse consequences in susceptible patients.
†Assumes feeding at 25 kcal/kg/day as total calories.

in the fasting state, serum insulin concentrations are typically in the range of 1 to 5 μU/ml. In the postabsorptive state, and depending on the amount and type of carbohydrate ingested, serum insulin levels may rise to 30 to 50 μU/ml. However, when hypertonic glucose is given continuously by intravenous administration, serum insulin levels may reach 80 to 100 μU/ml.[32] The metabolic effects of such high insulin levels in the serum have major implications for the malnourished, critically ill patient. For example, insulin is a potent antinatriuretic and antidiuretic hormone in terms of its effects on sodium and fluid balance at the level of the kidney.[35] Coupled with increased levels of aldosterone and antidiuretic hormone that occur in critical illness, there may be severe consequences in patients with cardiopulmonary dysfunction. Moreover, insulin's potent anabolic action can result in acute and dramatic shifts in serum electrolyte levels. Most notably, potassium and phosphorus (along with magnesium and nitrogen, as other major components of lean tissue) are driven intracellularly, and acute, even life-threatening, deficiencies may occur if their replacement is inadequate.[36] In fact, deaths associated with the "refeeding syndrome" are, in part, related to these acute metabolic changes.[37]

Clinically Relevant Long-Chain Triglyceride Infusion Issues

As with glucose, the rate and quantity of LCT emulsions infused in patients has a significant impact on their tolerance and adverse reaction profile. These effects are magnified in the presence of critical illness and comorbid disease. Perturbations in reticuloendothelial system function, hypertriglyceridemia, and adverse impacts on pulmonary gas diffusion have been associated with the rapid, intermittent infusion of IVLEs. However, when given in sufficiently high doses, even continuous administration of IVLEs can produce pathologic effects.[38] In an editorial by Klein and Miles in which they reviewed the complication rates associated with LCT emulsions in humans, they concluded that the adverse effects reported with LCT administration occurred when lipid infusion rates were greater than 0.11 g/kg/h.[39] Table 3–4 illustrates variable lipid infusion rates in a series of adult patient weights.

Reticuloendothelial System Dysfunction

The reticuloendothelial system (RES) is a network of mononuclear cells that provides an important means of immune defense that includes phagocytosis and the secretion of cytokines. Approximately 90% of RES function is accomplished by cells resident in the liver, with the remainder of the network of fixed macrophages present in the lungs, bone marrow, spleen, and lymph nodes.[40] The administration of LCT lipid emulsions has been shown to interfere with RES function in the liver, principally by impairing Kupffer cell activity in animals[41] and in humans[42] when measured by technetium Tc 99m sulfur colloid (TSC) clearance.

When LCT lipid emulsions were given as a discontinuous infusion in humans, the RES clearance of TSC was unchanged after 1 day of infusion but was significantly reduced after 3 consecutive days of infusion at a dose of 0.13 g/kg/h, suggesting significant impairment in function.[42] This finding suggested a specific dose-response relationship with respect to LCT emulsions and RES function. In a separate study,[43] the same daily dose of lipid was given, but as a continuous infusion over 3 days as a TNA admixture, and no changes in RES function were detected. Thus, for example, in a 70-kg patient, the intermittent infusion of 91 g of IVLE over 10 hours (0.13 g/kg/h) for 3 consecutive days resulted in fat overload as evidenced by a halving of the clearance of TSC, whereas the same daily dose given over 24 hours (equivalent to 0.054 g/kg/h, or approximately half the intermittent infusion rate) had no effects on RES function. These findings, along with that of Abbott and coworkers[44] suggest that IVLEs provided by continuous administration are better metabolized and therefore represent a safer method of providing parenteral lipid calories.

Hypertriglyceridemia

Factors in the development of hypertriglyceridemia include the total daily dose and rate of infusion and underlie the problems associated with tolerance to IVLEs in susceptible patients. However, an additional factor affecting hypertriglyceridemia has emerged. Specifically, the phospholipid-emulsifying agent has been implicated in the development of elevated plasma levels of triglycerides by interfering with actions of lipoprotein lipase.[45] These effects have been demonstrated only when the phospholipid concentration is highest in proportion to the number of triglyceride droplets (see Table 3–1). This occurs when the standard concentration of egg yolk phospholipid surfactant (12 g/L) is used with the lowest IVLE concentration (10%). Hypertriglyceridemia with 10% IVLE has been reported in infants,[8] and in adults[9] at high infusion rates (0.1 to 0.3 g/kg/h). The 10% IVLE formulations that have a reduced phospholipid surfactant concentration or the higher concentrations of lipid products (i.e., 20%) have not been shown to produce hypertriglyceridemia in unstressed patients.

Pulmonary Gas Diffusion Abnormalities

The IVLEs in broadest use are a rich source of essential fatty acids that may influence prostaglandin metabolism. It is well known that the pulmonary microcirculation is critically dependent on endogenous prostanoids in order to adapt appropriately to changes in blood flow that may occur during acute metabolic stress. Therefore, exogenous supplementation of prostaglandin precursors, such as linoleic acid, which leads to arachidonic acid may induce vasoactive changes in pulmonary blood flow that have clinical consequences. The prostaglandins produced in response to the exogenous provision of IVLEs may favor either vasodilation or vasoconstriction. The differential effects of the types of prostaglandins produced have been shown to vary with the infusion rate of the precursors.[46] More recently, the clinical consequences of altering the rate of prostaglandin precursors, supplied from IVLE, have been described.[47, 48] In the study by Mathru and coworkers, 15 patients were randomly assigned to receive 500 ml of 20% IVLE (100 g) over 5 hours (termed the *fast infusion*) or over 10 hours (termed the *slow infusion*).[48] For example, in the 70-kg reference man, the fast-infusion rate used in this study would provide IVLE at 0.285 g/kg/h and at the slow-infusion rate, approximately half that, or 0.142 g/kg/h, both of which exceed the threshold lipid infusion rate of 0.11 g/kg/h at which adverse effects occur.[39] Patients receiving the fast infusion had increases in mean pulmonary artery pressure, suggesting a dominant vasoconstrictive influence principally mediated by thromboxane A_2, whereas those receiving the slow infusion had an increase in their shunt fraction, suggesting a dominant vasodilatory effect principally mediated by prostaglandin E_2 and prostacyclin I_2. These effects could serve to override the normal compensatory respiratory responses such as hypoxic vasoconstriction that occur during acute ventilation-perfusion mismatches. The consequences of either of these effects in critically ill patients with acute respiratory distress syndrome are potentially serious and could lead to clinically significant hypoxemia and cardiac failure.[47]

Clinical Application of a Mixed-Fuel Regimen

IVLE administration is intended to supply essential fatty acids and/or provide a dense source of calories. As a supplement of essential fatty acids, IVLEs are generally given in the long-term setting to patients who are on full parenteral nutrition support, have little to no capacity to absorb nutrients via oral intake, and have reduced fat stores as a consequence of their disease. With adequate fat stores, at least in the early stages of the disease process leading to malnutrition, cycling the IVLE-free parenteral nutrition admixture over a discontinuous infusion period affords mobilization of endogenous adipose tissue stores of the essential fatty acids, which prevents a deficiency state.[49] Clearly, however, TPN-dependent patients with chronic intestinal malabsorption will eventually require routine exogenous lipid administration in order to prevent essential fatty acid deficiency.

In the acute care setting, IVLEs are generally given as a daily caloric source, often to reduce the amount of carbohydrate calories and their potential for producing complications when given in excess to susceptible patients. Moreover, as lipids are a preferred source of fuel for skeletal muscle, substitution of a portion of the glucose calories has resulted in better nitrogen balance.[50] Given the acute metabolic stress of such patients, excessive administration of either fat or carbohydrates can be harmful. In this setting, the composition of the TNA formulation is intended to provide a balance of nonprotein calories. Generally, 15 to 30% of the daily calories are administered as fat, with the balance as carbohydrate. Exceeding 30% of calories as fat in the acute care setting has not been shown to confer additional clinical benefits.[51] IVLEs can be administered either as a TNA formulation or as a separate infusion of lipid emulsion. Providing IVLEs as TNA not only simplifies nutritional therapy but affords additional safety benefits related to better utilization when given continuously,[44] reduced potential for microbial growth,[52, 53] and a reduction in the hyperinsulinemic state and its attendant complications.[54]

It is clear from the previous discussion that the rate and quantity of energy supplied are crucial to the safety of either intravenous glucose or intravenous lipids. The likelihood and consequence of these adverse effects are heightened when acute metabolic stress is present. Critically ill patients, particularly those with pre-existing malnutrition and organ dysfunction, are most susceptible to the adverse consequences of excessive energy intakes. Thus, two important clinical points emerge from these issues: first, the dose of nutrients provided must be consistent with the energy needs of the patient; and second, the rate of infusion must be compatible with the ability of the

patient to metabolize the nutrients supplied. If either of these conditions is not met, nutrition-related complications may occur and thereby diminish or obviate any potential clinical benefit that may derive from nutritional support.

As a first principle, the appropriate feeding weight of the patient must be obtained from the outset in order to determine the correct dose of macronutrients. In patients who are malnourished or obese, the feeding weight must be adjusted between these weight extremes, and often a compromise is made between the patient's ideal body weight and usual body weight. However, during critical illness, it is prudent initially to provide mildly (most patients) to moderately (obese patients) hypocaloric nutrition with a "do-no-harm" objective, with the principal role of nutritional intervention designed to be the support of the metabolic response to injury rather than energy balance. In critically ill patients with severe malnutrition and a marked reduction in lean body mass, it may be difficult to predict the actual caloric needs, since the energy expenditure may be substantially different from the estimated values. This has been attributed in part to a disproportionate loss of skeletal muscle over visceral organs in protein-calorie malnutrition with severe weight loss, since visceral organs have basal expenditures far in excess of muscle on a weight basis.[55] Under such circumstances, and to avoid overfeeding in critically ill, ventilator-dependent patients, the early use of indirect calorimetry is recommended.

As a second principle, once the appropriate feeding weight has been determined, the rate of infusion should be concordant with the patient's ability to metabolize the type and amount of energy supplied. Excessive rates of infusion of either carbohydrate or lipid can produce serious metabolic disturbances and attendant complications. Moreover, providing a mixture of glucose and lipids in net quantities that do not exceed energy needs not only is a more physiologic regimen but also reduces the likelihood of complications from either substrate. A daily mixed-fuel parenteral nutrition regimen can be accomplished in a number of ways, including providing the lipids as a separate infusion; providing lipids, glucose, and amino acids mixed in one container for immediate use; and adding lipid in one container but in a separate compartment for later admixing by the clinician, patient, or caregiver.

Separate Infusion of Lipids

The separate infusion of IVLEs has been the historical means of providing parenteral lipids and can be done safely, bearing in mind the attendant risks associated with this method of administration. Essentially, there are two potential problems with the intermittent administration of IVLEs. First, as discussed extensively in previous sections, the discontinuous infusion of parenteral lipids may increase the risk of metabolic complications if the infusion rate is excessive. These complications are perhaps viewed by some to be of lesser importance, since the exposure to IVLE is limited in time and therefore effectively cleared in the postinfusion setting. However, it is clear that in susceptible patients receiving large amounts over brief intervals, such infusions can be harmful. The IVLE threshold of 0.11 g/kg/h to produce metabolic complications is applicable in all infusion conditions, irrespective of whether it is a continuous or a discontinuous infusion.

A second problem associated with the separate administration of IVLEs is the risk of inadvertent microbial contamination, especially in prolonged infusion conditions. The Centers for Disease Control and Prevention has historically recommended an infusion period, or "hang time," for a bottle of lipids not to exceed 12 hours[56] and recommended that the administration set be changed every 24 hours.[57] The hang time recommendation arises from the ability of IVLEs to support an array of typical nosocomial pathogens and a recognition that the microbial growth profiles reach logarithmic proportions between 12 and 24 hours.[58, 59] The more recent recommendation for administration set changes is in response to the outbreak of postoperative infections with an anesthetic agent that is in the equivalent of a 10% IVLE drug vehicle.[60]

Thus, if IVLEs are given separately, three criteria should be met to ensure their safe and efficacious administration to acutely ill patients. First, the discontinuous infusion rate should not exceed 0.11 g/kg/h. In the 70-kg reference man receiving 25 kcal/kg and 20% of the total calories as fat, a 200-ml bottle of 20% lipids should not be given over an infusion period of less than 6 hours

(0.095 g/kg/h). Second, no manufacturer's container of lipids, ready for infusion, should be infused for a period exceeding 12 hours. If greater quantities of lipids are desired and the infusion rate over 12 hours would exceed 0.11 g/kg/h, then the IVLE is given as two containers, changed at 12-hour intervals, over 24 hours. There is no minimal infusion rate for lipid administration, only a maximal rate. Third, the intravenous administration set should be changed every 24 hours when lipids are given by separate infusion, consistent with the 1996 Centers for Disease Control and Prevention recommendation. Moreover, diethylhexylphthalate-free administration sets should be used, as IVLE efficiently extracts this potential carcinogen from the plastic that makes up the set. These sets have been referred to as *fat infusion sets* or *nitroglycerin sets*. The diethylhexylphthalate-free sets are generally provided by the lipid manufacturer, although they are also available from brand-specific administration sets that are dedicated to certain commercial infusion pumps.

Combined Infusion of Intravenous Lipid Emulsions as Total Nutrient Admixture

TNAs offer a number of advantages compared with the separate infusion of lipids, and these have been described.[53] With respect to the infusion-related issues, like fat emulsion–free TPN admixtures, TNAs are less able to support the growth of typical nosocomial pathogens than IVLEs alone.[52] This is likely due to two major physicochemical differences between native IVLEs and TNAs. Specifically, IVLEs are iso-osmotic and have a mean pH of 7.5, whereas TNAs for central venous alimentation are hypertonic (i.e., often exceeding 1500 mOsm/L) and have a typical final pH of 5.8 to 6 after compounding the all-in-one dosage form. With regard to their safe hang time, the typical 24-hour infusion applies as it would for fat emulsion–free TPN.[61] Finally, because TNAs behave like fat emulsion–free TPN with respect to concerns about microbial growth potential, a study has questioned the need for administration set changes every 24 hours and suggests that set changes every 72 hours would confer no additional risks than those of TPN without IVLEs.[62] Thus, TNAs should be treated in the same manner as fat emulsion–free TPN with the obvious exception of the size of the in-line filter. Fat emulsion–free TPN should be filtered through a 0.22-μm filter, whereas TNAs should be administered through a 1.2-μm filter,[63] which is consistent with the Food and Drug Administration recommendations.[20]

Combined Infusion of Intravenous Lipid Emulsions in Compartmentalized Infusion Containers

The addition of IVLEs to a compartmentalized infusion container is generally done when the infusions are intended for later use. In the United States, the addition of IVLE to compartmentalized infusion containers is accomplished in two ways. They can be added, along with the other nutrients in an extemporaneous fashion, to an empty dual-chamber bag. This method is generally used when providing parenteral nutrition to the patient in a home care setting when the entire formula is prepared by the pharmacist. The upper chamber is reserved for the addition of lipids, and the lower chamber is used for all the other nutritional components (amino acids, glucose, electrolytes, and so forth). The addition of IVLEs in this manner allows an extended shelf life of the product compared with a TNA made ready for infusion. Generally, IVLEs added to dual-chamber bags have an assigned expiration date of 1 week or more. The nonpharmacy personnel (clinician, patient, or caregiver) are instructed to "activate" the bag by removing the *separator* to allow the complete mixing of the IVLE with the other admixture components to produce a TNA formulation. This task is performed immediately before infusion. The new expiration date for the TNA after mixing by nonpharmacy personnel generally does not exceed 24 hours. From a physicochemical stability perspective, this is viewed as the safest way to provide TNAs in the home care setting.[64]

There are other types of compartmentalized bags that are commercially available for admixture activation. In the United States, only fat emulsion–free compartmentalized parenteral nutrition bags are available (Table 3–5). The other way of making a TNA formulation in a compartmentalized bag is to add just the IVLE to a manufacturer's premade bag of parenteral nutrition. This method of parenteral compounding is generally performed in the institutional setting because of the uncertainty of assigning prolonged expiration dates for ready-to-use TNA formulations. In addition, it may offer a cost-effective alternative for some institutions not able to devote dedicated pharmacy personnel to the tasks of extemporaneous compounding of parenteral nutrition admixtures. Although this method of compounding could be accomplished by nonpharmacy personnel in the home care setting, it would be performed under nonsterile conditions, and the risk of contamination probably outweighs any benefit that could be gained from this practice, which can be avoided by the use of dual-chamber bags previously described.

Finally, multicompartmental containers that can accommodate the separation of amino acids, carbohydrate, and lipids (i.e., three-compartment bags) are available in Europe (Table 3–6). Clearly, a major benefit of this dosage form is in allowing the activation (versus compounding) of the parenteral nutrition admixture by nonpharmacy personnel without compromising the pharmaceutical integrity of the formulation.

◆ CLINICAL REVIEW OF PURE LONG-CHAIN TRIGLYCERIDE MIXTURES

As energy donors, lipid emulsions are an integral element of parenteral nutrition regimens for critically ill patients. Moreover, lipids are not only structural building blocks of cells and tissues but carriers of essential fatty acids and fat-soluble vitamins. In addition, certain fatty acids are precursors of prostaglandins and other eicosanoids and thereby serve important metabolic functions.

Fatty acids can be divided into three groups: saturated, monounsaturated, and polyunsaturated fatty acids.[65] Each class of fatty acids has a preferential specific role (Table 3–7). Saturated fatty acids (medium- or long-chain) are more devoted to energy supply, but one should not forget their specific structural role. The PUFAs of the n-3 and n-6 families have very important structural and functional roles and ideally should not be extensively used for energy purposes. This section provides a brief overview of the evolution of different types of lipid emulsions (Table 3–8) that are already in wide-

Table 3–5. Intravenous Lipid Emulsions in Compartmentalized Infusion Containers

Product	Size (ml)	Company (Country)	Amino Acid–Glucose Mixtures			
			Amino Acids (g)	Glucose (g)	Lipids (g)	Electrolytes
Nutrimix	1000	Abbott	17.5	125.0	—	—
	1000	(USA)	25.0	125.0	—	—
	1000		17.5	25.0	—	+
	1000		21.3	50.0	—	+
	1500		31.9	187.5	—	—
	1500		37.5	187.5	—	—
	2000		35.0	50.0	—	—
	2000		42.5	100.0	—	—
	2000		42.5	200.0	—	—
	2000		42.5	250.0	—	—
	2000		50.0	250.0	—	—
	2000		35.0	50.0	—	+
Clinimix	2000	Baxter	55.0	100.0	—	±
	2000	(USA)	55.0	200.0	—	±
	2000		55.0	500.0	—	±
	2000		55.0	100.0	—	±
	2000		85.0	100.0	—	±
	2000		85.0	200.0	—	±
	2000		85.0	400.0	—	±
	2000		85.0	500.0	—	±
	2000		100.0	200.0	—	±
	2000		100.0	300.0	—	±
	2000		100.0	400.0	—	±
	2000		100.0	500.0	—	±
	2000		100.0	750.0	—	±

—, No lipids or electrolytes; +, contains electrolytes; ±, available with or without electrolytes.

Long-Chain Triglycerides in Parenteral Nutrition

Since the 1970s, lipid emulsions based on LCTs from soybean or safflower oil have been used in parenteral nutrition. For many years, lipid supply has been considered as a means of preventing or correcting essential fatty acid deficiency and of providing an efficient fuel to many tissues of the body. In the 1970s, the first reports of an interference with the immune system were published[66, 67] and were confirmed by further observations in the 1980s[68] and 1990s.[69] Obviously, these effects are related to the dose and infusion rate of lipid emulsions. The mechanisms are not totally clear, but an excessive intake of linoleic acid seems to be one of the major reasons for interference with immune function.[70] Therefore, efforts at further developing and optimizing lipid emulsions have focused on replacing part of

spread clinical use or are in the final stages of development.

the LCTs by MCTs synthesized from coconut oil.

◆ MEDIUM-CHAIN TRIGLYCERIDES IN PARENTERAL NUTRITION

An MCT-LCT–containing lipid emulsion has been available on the European market since 1984 and later worldwide. Numerous research teams have studied the parenteral application of this physical MCT-LCT mixture in a clinical environment and during long-term home parenteral nutrition (HPN). MCTs have several advantages in comparison with LCTs.[71] Because of their physical and chemical properties, MCTs have better solubility and are more readily hydrolyzed by lipases. They are more quickly eliminated from the circulation and taken up by peripheral tissues. They are not stored as body fat but are oxidized more rapidly than LCTs. MCTs are ketogenic, and both medium-chain fatty acids and ketone bodies are carnitine-independent substrates. For

Table 3–6. Intravenous Lipid Emulsion in Compartmentalized Infusion Containers

Product	Size (ml)	Company (Country)	Amino Acid–Glucose–Lipid Mixtures			
			Amino Acids (g)	Glucose (g)	Lipids (g)	Electrolytes
NuTRIflex		B. Braun (Germany)				
Version						
Peri	1250		40	80	50*	+
	1875		60	120	75	+
	2500		80	160	100	+
Plus	1250		48	150	50	±
	1875		72	225	75	±
	2500		96	300	100	±
Special	1250		72	180	50	±
	1875		108	270	75	±
Clinomel		Baxter (France)				
Version						
N5-800	1000		28	100	40†	+
	1500		42	150	60	+
	2000		56	200	80	+
N6-900	1000		34	120	40	+
	1500		51	180	60	+
	2000		68	240	80	+
N6-900	1000		40	160	40	+
	1500		60	240	60	+
	2000		80	320	80	+
Compleven	2500	Fresenius (Germany)	75	240	100	+

*Medium-chain triglyceride–long-chain triglyceride intravenous lipid emulsion.
†Long-chain triglyceride emulsion.
+, with electrolytes; ±, with and without electrolytes.

Table 3–7. Role of Different Classes of Fatty Acids

	Energy	Structure	Function
Medium-chain saturated fatty acids	+ + +	0	0
Long-chain fatty acids			
Saturated	+ +	+ +	(+)
Monounsaturated	+ +	+ +	(+)
Polyunsaturated			
Linoleic or n-6 family	+	+ + +	+ + +
Linolenic or n-3 family	+	+ + +	+ + +

Adapted from Spielmann D, Bracco U, Traitler H, et al: Alternative lipids to usual ω6, PUFAs: γ-linolenic, α-linolenic, stearidonic acid, EPA, etc. JPEN J Parenter Enteral Nutr 12:1115–1235, 1988.

Table 3–8. Evolution in Parenteral Lipid Emulsions

Conventional Lipid Emulsion	Lipid Emulsions with a Reduced Amount of PUFA Pattern	Lipid Emulsions with a Specific FA
LCT	MCT-LCT	MCT-LCT-FO
LCT rich in α-tocopherol	MCT-LCT rich in α-tocopherol	FO
	Olive oil–containing emulsion	
	Structured triglycerides	

LCT, long-chain triglyceride; MCT, medium-chain triglyceride; FO, fish oil; FA, fatty acids; PUFA, polyunsaturated fatty acids.

these and other reasons, the comparison of LCTs and MCTs with respect to several effects is of interest.

Oxidative Utilization

For many years, the oxidative utilization of MCTs and LCTs in total parenteral nutrition of severely injured patients was unknown. Therefore, our own group investigated the oxidation rates of trioctanoin (C 8:0) and triolein (C 18:1) in an MCT-LCT emulsion, as well as the oxidative utilization of triolein in a pure LCT emulsion in severely injured patients. We used the technique of ^{13}C-isotope labeling in combination with the method of indirect calorimetry.[72–74] The highest oxidative utilization was seen in the labeled-MCT group (study A: 32.27 ± 6.84%, [1-^{13}C]trioctanoin in MCT-LCT emulsion). The corresponding values were 11.18 ± 3.96% (study B: [^{13}C]triolein in MCT-LCT emulsion) and 16.29 ± 3.78% (study C: [^{13}C]triolein in LCT emulsion), respectively. Therefore we concluded that during simultaneous parenteral supply, the oxidative utilization of MCTs is three times as high as that of LCTs. Compared with pure LCT emulsions, the oxidation rate of MCTs is twice as high as that of labeled LCTs.[72, 75]

Protein-Sparing Effect

Further benefits of MCTs include their less pronounced tendency for deposition in tissues and their favorable effect on protein metabolism. Ball investigated the effect of MCT-LCT versus LCT emulsions on plasma ketone levels and nitrogen balance in intensive care unit patients.[76] The rise in ketones during lipid infusion was greater for the MCT-LCT emulsion on day 1. The gradually increasing difference in nitrogen balance between the two treatment groups, and the better balance in the group receiving MCT-LCT emulsion on day 6, may reflect the need for several days' treatment with fat and protein before the optimal protein-sparing effects of fat are manifest. Improved nitrogen balance with MCT-LCT emulsion has been shown in a previous study on less ill patients,[77] and improved protein synthesis and reduced catabolism have been observed in stressed animals. In another study, thyroxine-binding prealbumin levels were in-

creased, and the authors postulated a beneficial effect on visceral protein metabolism.[78]

Hepatic Function

In a prospective crossover study,[79] eight patients with inflammatory bowel disease on HPN were randomized to receive 50% of nonprotein calories as exclusively LCT or MCT-LCT emulsion for 3 months and then to receive the other emulsion during a second period of 3 months. The other HPN components remained unchanged. Three patients with inflammatory bowel disease showed an increase in plasma levels of liver transaminases, γ-glutamyl transferase, and alkaline phosphatase while receiving HPN with LCTs. After a second measurement confirming the alteration, these three patients were switched to the mixed emulsion, and the abnormalities resolved in 2 to 8 weeks. No alteration of liver function occurred during nutritional support with the mixed MCT-LCT emulsion. This beneficial effect of MCT-LCT emulsion was confirmed in a subsequent long-term (3 to 60 months) study on 24 HPN patients.[80] Even after liver transplantation, critically ill patients experienced no adverse effects of MCT-LCT emulsion on liver function tests.[81] Liver size and density remained unchanged in patients receiving MCT-LCT emulsion.[82]

No direct explanation can be offered concerning the protective effect of MCT-LCT emulsion on liver function.[79, 80] However, the difference between MCT-LCT and LCT emulsions could be because

1. Medium-chain fatty acids released in high amounts during MCT-LCT infusion are a better substrate for hepatocytes than long-chain fatty acids; medium-chain fatty acids are oxidized in greater proportion than long-chain fatty acids and induce less fat deposition.

2. Ketone bodies, produced in higher amounts during MCT-LCT than in LCT infusion, are known to be a good substrate for the intestinal mucosa;[83] hence, TPN with MCT-LCT emulsion may better protect the integrity of the gut barrier, which would result in less periportal inflammation by reducing the egress of toxins and bacteria from the intestine.

3. MCT-LCT emulsions have a lower ability to acquire and transport cholesteryl es-

ters and may induce fewer alterations in bile composition.

Immunology and Reticuloendothelial Function

The effect of parenteral lipid emulsions on the immune system has been studied widely and seems to be controversial. Several reports suggest that parenteral fat may depress immunologic function and increase the patient's susceptibility to septic complications,[67, 68, 84] whereas others suggest that this is not the case.[85, 86] The immunologic effects of different types of unsaturated fatty acids have been investigated in relation to their effect on phospholipid fatty acids and eicosanoid synthesis.[87] A number of differences between n-6 and n-3 PUFAs in their effects on several aspects of immune function have been well described. MCTs have been reported to possess certain advantages compared with LCTs, and they might be superior in avoiding the suppression of immune and phagocytic functions in severely stressed patients.

In patients undergoing preoperative parenteral nutrition, Sedman and associates examined the effects of different lipid emulsions on lymphocyte function.[69] Thirty-three patients with gastrointestinal cancer were randomized to receive TPN with either no lipid, 50% of the total calories as LCTs, or 50% MCT-LCT emulsion. No alterations in lymphocyte transformation occurred with any regimen. There was a significant reduction in lymphokine-activated killer cell activity with LCT administration, whereas MCT-LCT administration was associated with a significant increase in lymphokine-activated killer cell and natural killer cell activities. Interleukin 2 (IL-2) production was significantly increased in patients receiving 50% LCT emulsion. These results suggest that the prolonged administration of TPN regimens with 50% LCTs leads to immunosuppressive effects that may be mediated through increased release of IL-2 from activated lymphocytes.

Others have tried to investigate the impact of different chain lengths of fatty acids (C_6 to C_{12} versus C_{16} to C_{20}) on the production of tumor necrosis factor (TNF) by peripheral blood mononuclear cells of patients under short- or long-term TPN therapy.[88] The TPN formula containing the MCT-LCT emulsion had no impact on cell-associated plus secreted TNF production, whereas that containing the LCT emulsion resulted in a significant increase in the production of the monokine 30 days after TPN was begun.

In patients with acquired immunodeficiency syndrome, TPN including LCTs revealed significant abnormalities in lymphocyte function. Such abnormalities were not observed with MCT-LCT emulsion. In addition, there was a tendency to higher CD4/CD8 lymphocyte ratios with MCT-LCT emulsion.[89]

MCT-LCT versus LCT emulsions were evaluated for their ex vivo effects on human neutrophil and monocyte functions.[90] Cell functions were examined during preoperative TPN in malnourished patients with gastric cancer. Bacterial killing activity was decreased in neutrophils with LCT emulsion, whereas there was no negative effect with MCT-LCT emulsion.

The RES functions in the phagocytosis of microorganisms as well as in the secretion of chemical mediators of the inflammatory response. It has been also implicated in the clearance of lipid particles associated with the infusion of lipid emulsion.[91, 92] Animal studies suggest that the intravenous administration of LCT emulsion may impair RES function and clearance of bacteremia.[41, 93]

Seidner and colleagues examined the RES function by measuring the clearance rates of intravenously injected TSC while the subject received TPN containing only protein and dextrose, and again after 3 days of fat infusion (0.13 g/kg of body weight).[42] Mean ($\pm$ SEM) clearance rate constants before and after continuous LCT infusion (24 hours) were 0.38 ± 0.09 and 0.41 ± 0.08 min^{-1}, respectively, whereas those before and after intermittent MCT-LCT infusion (10 hours) were 0.23 ± 0.06 and 0.38 ± 0.10 min^{-1}, respectively. In contrast to intermittent LCT infusion, the administration of continuous LCT or an intermittent MCT-LCT mixture does not impair TSC clearance by the RES. Thus, the provision of fat principally as MCT-LCT emulsion may enable adequate metabolism of lipid emulsion without RES dysfunction and thus may be of particular benefit in critically ill or septic patients.

Pulmonary Hemodynamics and Gas Exchange

MCT-LCT fat emulsions, compared with those containing only LCT in calorically equivalent amounts, contain less linoleic and linolenic acid. These differences may be important because a major contribution to the gas exchange effects of intravenous fat use is attributed to the increased production of prostaglandins (thromboxane A_2, prostacyclin)[94–96] since fat emulsions provide precursors of prostaglandins.[97]

Radermacher and colleagues investigated the pulmonary vascular and gas exchange effects of an infusion with fat emulsions containing MCT in patients with the sepsis syndrome receiving TPN.[98] The intravenous fat administration did not cause any significant alterations in systemic or pulmonary hemodynamics. The respiratory gas exchange was analyzed using a multiple inert gas elimination technique. There was no change in the shunt fraction (Q_S/Q_T), perfusion of lung regions with low V_A/Q ratios, or in dead space (V_D/V_T).

The lack of changes in pulmonary hemodynamics and gas exchange contrasts with data from other authors[99, 100] who reported increased mean pulmonary artery pressure and a fall in arterial P_{O_2} due to an increased mean venous admixture, in particular in patients with septic acute respiratory failure.[100] In these studies, the infusion rate of the fat emulsion as well as the patients' baseline physiologic data were similar to those in the previous study.[98] The rise in plasma triglyceride levels, which in the past has been suggested to be responsible for the reported hemodynamic and gas exchange response,[101, 102] was comparable to that of the infusion of LCTs at equivalent infusion rates as well. Therefore, the different composition of the fat emulsion may explain the discrepancy between these studies and the previous one. Although equivalent gram weights of lipids were administered in the study by Radermacher and colleagues,[98] half the triglycerides consisted of MCTs, which are oxidized faster than LCTs[72, 73] without acting as a precursor for prostaglandin formation. In addition to altered prostaglandin synthesis, a dose dependency as an underlying mechanism for different effects on pulmonary hemodynamics and gas exchange has been discussed.[103] In a short-term period the authors infused equal amounts of lipid emulsions, MCT-LCT versus LCT, in patients after open heart surgery. Although there were no alterations in the MCT-LCT group, parenteral administration of LCT reduced cardiac output and Pa_{O_2} with significant increases in both

pulmonary artery pressures and vascular resistances. The changes in pulmonary hemodynamics and gas exchange associated with LCT administration[99, 100] are consistent with later findings,[47, 48] discussed previously.

Peroxidation in Parenteral Nutrition

Unless prevented by antioxidants, peroxidation reactions in lipid emulsions may lead to clinical complications. Apart from its implications in chronic diseases, lipid peroxidation leads to tissue damage and an inflammatory response, together with an impairment of immune defenses. It may markedly alter the function of several major organs including the lungs, liver, heart, and kidneys.

The relationship between breath pentane, evolved from the peroxidation of linoleic acid, and plasma levels of α-tocopherol have been evaluated.[104] This study demonstrated that patients receiving long-term TPN (including 45 mg of α-tocopherol per day) had a higher rate of breath pentane output and presumably, therefore, an increase in lipid peroxidation. There was a significant inverse correlation between the plasma α-tocopherol level and pentane output, suggesting that vitamin E deficiency is responsible for the increased output of pentane in the breath. Wispe and associates demonstrated that the intravenous administration of vitamin E counteracted this LCT-induced peroxidation.[105]

In contrast to a conventional LCT lipid emulsion, a lipid emulsion enriched with α-tocopherol produced adequate plasma α-tocopherol levels.[106] Thus, it is possible to prevent vitamin E depletion and lipid peroxidation by following this approach. Moreover, supplements of 200 mg of α-tocopherol daily, in order to prevent peroxidative damage, have been investigated in patients on HPN.[107] The rise in serum α-tocopherol concentration was accompanied by a decrease in the number of enlarged low-density lipoprotein particles, a sign of reduced peroxidative damage to these lipoproteins.

Medium-Chain Triglyceride– Long-Chain Triglyceride Versus Long-Chain Triglyceride Emulsion—Conclusion

Directly compared with pure LCT emulsions, MCT-LCT emulsions are a more efficient fuel, put less strain on the liver, and have significantly less impact on the immune system and RES function. MCT-LCT emulsions appear to be of particular benefit to patients with the systemic inflammatory response syndrome or sepsis because, containing only half the amount of LCTs, they supply a significantly smaller amount of n-6 fatty acids and hence of the precursors of potentially immunosuppressive prostaglandins.

◆ STRUCTURED TRIGLYCERIDES

An alternative to a physical mixture of MCTs and LCTs can be obtained by interesterifying medium- and long-chain fatty acids to create a mixed triglyceride molecule called a *structured triglyceride* (STG). One must clearly differentiate between chemically defined and randomized STGs. The latter can be synthesized by mixing MCT and LCT oils and heating the mixture in the presence of a catalyst. During this process, fatty acids of different chain lengths can be esterified into one triglyceride molecule. The individual STG molecule within the emulsion is composed of three fatty acids in which the proportion of medium- and long-chain fatty acids varies randomly, that is, the structure of the individual triglyceride is heterogeneous and depends on the initial proportion of LCT and MCT oils.[13, 108] Chemically defined STGs, in contrast, are made by enzymatic re-esterification. As a consequence of the positional specificity of the lipase used, these triglycerides contain, for example, medium-chain fatty acids in the 1,3 positions and long-chain fatty acids in the 2 position.[109]

Several groups have demonstrated a positional specificity of lipoprotein lipase.[109, 110] Therefore, one can conclude that only some of the different STG molecules in a so-called randomized STG emulsion may result in a metabolic improvement. Chemically defined STG molecules may act more efficiently, but the costs of the synthesis are very high. This is why most of the research work in animals and patients was done with randomized STG emulsions.

Magnusson and coworkers examined protein and energy metabolism in 34 partially hepatectomized rats.[111] The TPN contained either LCTs or triglycerides comprising both medium- and long-chain fatty acids on the same carbon skeleton. In conclusion, structured lipid emulsions (randomized) exerted a stimulatory effect on muscle protein synthesis and preserved body weight better than a pure LCT emulsion.

STGs (random) and pure LCT-containing fat emulsions, infused at equimolar doses, have been studied in healthy volunteers.[108] No distinct differences were found. The capacity of healthy subjects to hydrolyze STGs was at least as high as that to hydrolyze LCTs. Plasma fatty acid profiles during fat infusion were similar to the fatty acid compositions of the infused emulsions.

Sandström and associates designed a study to evaluate the safety of and tolerance to an STG fat emulsion compared with that of a standard LCT emulsion in postoperative patients requiring TPN.[112] Twenty patients were included and treated for 5 to 7 days. Safety and tolerance variables demonstrated no major difference between the study and the control groups. In a subsequent study, the same group used the method of indirect calorimetry in order to show that the intravenous provision of STG versus pure LCT emulsions is associated with increased whole-body fat oxidation in stressed postoperative patients.[113]

In 1997, the effect of randomized STGs with a physical mixture of MCTs and LCTs on the nitrogen balance of moderately catabolic postoperative patients was compared.[114] Twelve patients operated for placement of an aortic prosthesis received STGs and 13 patients received the physical mixture in a randomized, double-blind, parallel study. TPN was infused for 5 days. Over this period the cumulative nitrogen balance was less negative in the STG group. The full spectrum of methods and results is still not published, making it difficult to discuss the study protocol and to find a possible explanation for this difference in nitrogen balance. In the same trial, the effects of STGs and the physical mixture of MCT-LCT emulsion on the mononuclear phagocyte system measuring TSC clearance was also studied.[114] Before the start of the trial and after 5 days of parenteral nutrition, TSC clearance had not changed significantly in both groups. The authors concluded that in contrast to LCT emulsions, lipid emulsions containing STGs did not alter the functioning of the mononuclear phagocyte system. In this respect, there was no difference between STGs and the physical mixture.

In conclusion, STGs have been proved to be safe as classic LCT soybean oil emulsions. Compared with LCTs, random STGs have shown similar advantages to the benefits proved for the physical mixture of MCT-LCT emulsions. Further studies are necessary to investigate the potential benefits of STG compared with MCT-LCT emulsions in clinical settings.

◆ LIPID EMULSIONS CONTAINING OLIVE OIL

As pointed out earlier, soybean oil emulsions provide PUFAs in excess of requirements, causing the development of abnormal fatty acid profiles, augmentation of peroxidation, and the creation of eicosanoid imbalances. To reduce these risks of TPN in critically ill patients, substitution of parts of the soybean oil–based lipid emulsions by other lipid components is strongly recommended. Meanwhile, the concept of a physical mixture with MCTs and LCTs has been well proved. Another concept is based on the idea of mixing 20% soybean oil with 80% olive oil, the latter being rich in the monounsaturated fatty acid oleic acid.

Granato and coworkers compared the effect of this new lipid emulsion with two conventional soybean oil–based lipid emulsions on phytohemagglutinin-stimulated human lymphocytes in vitro.[115] Their results indicate that olive oil–based emulsions, unlike soybean oil–based lipid emulsions, do not inhibit lymphocyte function in vitro. They concluded that changes in membrane fatty acid composition may contribute to the differential effects of emulsions on immune function.

Soybean oil emulsions contain predominantly γ-tocopherol, which affords little protection against lipid peroxidation. The newly developed olive oil–based lipid emulsion contains the more biologically active α-tocopherol. In an animal experiment, the plasma α-tocopherol levels can be maintained at a normal level with olive oil emulsion, whereas there is an accumulation of the less active γ-tocopherol with soybean oil.[116] They concluded that olive oil emulsions are a better source of antioxidants and should contribute to decreased peroxidation.[117] A controversial statement was given by Arborati and coworkers, who evaluated both the lipid peroxide content and the per-

oxidability of fat emulsions under oxidative conditions.[118] Fat emulsions manufactured exclusively from soybean oil, from coconut and soybean oils, and from soybean and olive oils were studied. Although the highest values for lipid peroxide content were found in a 20% soybean emulsion, the peroxidability was significantly increased in the soybean–olive oil mixture. Lowest levels were found in a physical mixture of MCT-LCT emulsion. Therefore, they concluded that reduction of the PUFAs by simultaneous substitution with MCTs constitutes the best approach to the reduction of the susceptibility of fat emulsions to peroxidative modification.

Compared with conventional LCT emulsions, olive oil–based lipid emulsions show benefits regarding peroxidation and immune function. No data are available demonstrating any clinical advantage with regard to MCT-LCT or other lipid emulsions.

◆ LIPID EMULSIONS CONTAINING FISH OIL

The virtual absence of heart disease or myocardial infarction among Greenland Inuits was a key epidemiologic observation leading to the focus on n-3 fatty acids. Studies comparing the diet, blood and tissue lipids, bleeding times, and various aspects of platelet aggregation among Greenland Inuits, Inuits living in Denmark, and Danes have supported the view that diet, in particular the long-chain n-3 fatty acids, rather than genetics, accounts for the striking advantage Greenland Inuits have over the other two groups with respect to heart disease.[119, 120] Following these first reports, there was an exponential increase in the number of publications focusing on the metabolic and clinical effects of fish oils. Preliminary clinical trials have shown certain beneficial effects of fish oil intakes in diseases associated with inflammatory reactions such as rheumatoid arthritis or inflammatory bowel disease; in conditions with impaired immune competence such as burns, postoperative situations, and cyclosporine treatment after renal transplants; and in conditions with enhanced platelet aggregation such as after coronary angioplasty.

Dietary supplementation with n-3 fatty acids was shown to have a beneficial influence on the pathophysiologic response to endotoxins and to exert important modulations on eicosanoid and cytokine biology.[121, 122] These include inducing changes in the substrate availability for eicosanoid synthesis, altering membrane fluidity, and altering the production of noneicosanoid secondary messengers.[123] Indeed, inflammatory symptoms of rheumatoid arthritis, psoriasis, Crohn's disease, and ulcerative colitis are all ameliorated by fish oil preparations whether or not directly related to cytokine production. Consumption of eicosapentaenoic acid (EPA) reduces the production of IL-1α and IL-1β as well as TNF-α and TNF-β in response to an endotoxin stimulus. The anti-inflammatory effects of fish oil also may include decreased production of inflammatory substances such as leukotriene B_4 and platelet-activating factors released by the action of cytokines, as well as a large reduction in cytokine-induced synthesis of prostaglandin E_2 and thromboxane B_2 in the colonic mucosa.[124] These findings are in line with a decrease in the arachidonic-to-EPA ratio in blood mononuclear cell membranes as well as a decrease in neutrophil chemotaxis to leukotriene B_4.[125] The combined observations may be explained partly by the finding that leukotriene B_4 enhances blood monocyte IL-1 production after lipopolysaccharide exposure.[126]

The possibility to rapidly influence compositional changes by parenteral application of lipid emulsions containing n-3 fatty acids is of great interest. Reports suggest that parenteral fish oil emulsions are obviously well tolerated by healthy volunteers,[122] and their prolonged infusion into postoperative patients was without side effects.[127] Parenteral application of a physical mixture with 85% soybean oil and 15% fish oil was associated with considerable increases in EPA and docosahexaenoic acid in leukocyte membrane phospholipids, the maximal incorporation being observed after 5 days of fish oil nutrition.

As reported previously,[128] lipid emulsions containing fish oil (n-3 fatty acids) are poor substrates for lipoprotein lipase and triglycerides, and they tend to accumulate in the circulation. In contrast to most triglyceride fatty acids, triglycerides containing n-3 fatty acids are taken up by tissues mainly via remnant endocytosis, followed by intracellular triglyceride hydrolysis. Even the addition of n-3–containing triglycerides to classic LCT emulsions inhibits the release of free fatty acids from the soybean oil emulsion.[128] In contrast, the combination in the same particle of MCTs together with fish oil triglycerides appears to completely normalize triglyceride hydrolysis by lipoprotein lipase[129] and to rapidly produce small remnants enriched with n-3 fatty acids. Furthermore, Carpentier and coworkers obtained evidence that the presence of both MCT and fish oil triglycerides in remnant particles enhances their uptake by different types of cells.[130] In healthy subjects, the infusion of an emulsion containing 50% MCT, 40% soybean, and 10% fish oil triglycerides is associated with a rapid triglyceride elimination and completely avoids lipid accumulation in plasma.

Cukier and associates performed a study in rats in order to assess the impact of TPN regimens including different lipid emulsions on the mononuclear phagocyte system.[131] Although the glucose-based parenteral nutrition indicated inhibitory effects, TPN regimens including a physical mixture of MCTs, LCTs, and fish oils improved liver and lung macrophage phagocytosis.

After parenteral n-3 fatty acid nutrition in 40 patients undergoing major intestinal surgery, the ability of leukocytes to release leukotrienes from whole blood leukocytes and from circulating cytokines was investigated.[132] The TPN regimen was isonitrogenous and isoenergetic with a conventional MCT-LCT emulsion, containing a physical mixture of MCTs, LCTs, and fish oils. During the study period, a significant increase in 5-series leukotrienes was observed after cellular stimulation in the EPA-enriched nutrition group with a concomitant significant decrease in 4-series leukotrienes. They concluded that the lower ratio of 4-series leukotrienes to 5-series leukotrienes may lead to an attenuation of inflammatory reaction. In contrast to IL-1β, IL-6, and IL-10, the systemic levels of TNF-α were postoperatively decreased in the EPA-enriched group.

Obviously, such new preparations seem promising not only for metabolic care but also for hemodynamic stability in different organ systems of intensive care unit patients. There is evidence that n-3 fatty acids can also modulate regional blood flow and therefore prevent intestinal ischemia. Pscheidl and associates demonstrated in a low-dose endotoxin rat model that chemically defined structured lipids with n-3 fatty acids in the sn-2 position (medium-chain fatty acid–n-3 fatty acid–medium-chain fatty acid) can improve splanchnic circulation by a shift in prostaglandin production.[133] This beneficial aspect has been confirmed with a physical mixture of MCTs, LCTs, and fish oils.[134] The results of this subsequent study indicate that improvement in regional blood flow did not significantly diminish bacterial translocation but significantly decreased viable bacteria in splanchnic organs.

Finally, not only n-6 but also n-3 PUFAs are prone to lipid peroxidation, and inadequate control by associated antioxidants may counterbalance their beneficial effects.[135] Therefore, a well-balanced enrichment of this new generation of lipid emulsion with α-tocopherol is strongly recommended.[136]

SUMMARY

Lipid emulsions derived from soybean or safflower oil contain excessive quantities of PUFAs and insufficient amounts of α-tocopherol. Their parenteral use can rapidly lead to an unbalanced pattern of eicosanoid production and is associated with an increased production of peroxidative catabolites. In order to avoid negative effects from these metabolic products, it is recommended to use preparations with a reduced content of PUFAs in combination with an enrichment in α-tocopherol. Indeed, the physical mixture of MCTs and LCTs is a well-proven concept in parenteral nutrition of critically ill patients. Having a demonstrably higher utilization rate, MCT-containing lipid emulsions do not impair liver function, produce less immune and no RES function compromise, and do not interfere with pulmonary hemodynamics or gas exchange.

Newer preparations based on structured triglycerides or olive oil appear to achieve the same goal, that is, reducing the n-6 PUFA intake. These new lipid emulsions are safe and well tolerated. Further studies are necessary to investigate potential benefits compared with the physical mixture of MCT-LCT emulsion in a clinical environment.

A promising substrate in the evolution of parenteral lipid emulsions can be seen in fish oils (n-3 fatty acids). Their fixed combination in a physical mixture of MCT-LCT emulsion displays a number of interesting aspects. With regard to current literature, n-3 fatty acids have a beneficial influence on the pathophysiologic response to endotoxins and exert important modulations on eicosanoid and cytokine biology. Furthermore, their intravenous use may improve organ perfusion in different critical situations.

REFERENCES

1. Levenson SM, Hopkins BS, Waldron M, et al: Early history of parenteral nutrition. Fed Proc 43:1391–1406, 1984.
2. Geyer R: Parenteral nutrition. Physiol Rev 40:150–186, 1960.
3. Wretlind A: Development of fat emulsions. JPEN J Parenter Enteral Nutr 5:230–235, 1981.
4. Jeejeebhoy KN, Anderson GH, Nakhooda AF, et al: Metabolic studies in total parenteral nutrition in man. J Clin Invest 57:125–136, 1975.
5. Solassol C, Joyeax H, Etco L, et al: New techniques for long-term intravenous feeding: An artificial gut in 75 patients. Ann Surg 179:519–522, 1974.
6. Solassol C, Joyeax H, Astruc B, et al: Complete nutrient mixtures with lipids for total parenteral nutrition in cancer patients. Acta Chir Scand 498(Suppl):151–154, 1980.
7. Driscoll DF: Physicochemical assessment of total nutrient admixture stability and safety: Quantifying the risk. Nutrition 12:166–167, 1997.
8. Haumont D, Richelle M, Deckelbaum R, et al: Effect of liposomal content of lipid emulsions on plasma lipids in low birth weight infants receiving parenteral nutrition. J Pediatr 121:759–763, 1992.
9. Carpentier YA, Richelle M, Bury J, et al: Phospholipid excess of fat emulsions slows triglyceride removal and increases lipoprotein remodelling. Arteriosclerosis 7:541a, 1987.
10. Lipid metabolism. In Guyton AC (ed): Textbook of Medical Physiology, 10th ed. Philadelphia, WB Saunders, 2000.
11. Wretlind A: Recollections of pioneers in nutrition: Landmarks in the development of parenteral nutrition. J Am Coll Nutr 11:366–373, 1992.
12. Driscoll DF, Bhargava HN, Li L, et al: Physicochemical stability of total nutrient admixtures. Am J Health Syst Pharm 52:623–634, 1995.
13. Babayan VK: Medium chain triglycerides and structured lipids. Lipids 22:417–420, 1987.
14. Hamburger L, Carpentier Y, Keyserman F, et al: More efficient clearance of intravenous (I.V.) lipid emulsions containing medium chain triglyceride (MCT) and fish oil triglycerides as compared to traditional long chain triglyceride (LCT) lipid emulsions in in vitro models and humans. FASEB J 2988:a514, 1998.
15. Wanten GJA, Geijtenbeek TB, Raymakers R, et al: LCT/MCT- and MCT emulsions increase human neutrophil β2-integrin expression, degranulation and adhesion to ICAM-1, contrary to LCT- and structured lipid emulsions. JPEN J Parenter Enteral Nutr 23:S8(30a), 1999.
16. Driscoll DF, Bacon MN, Bistrian BR: Physicochemical stability of two different brands of lipid

emulsion for total nutrient admixtures. JPEN J Parenter Enteral Nutr 22:S6(21), 1998.

17. Diprivan package insert. *In* Physicians' Desk Reference, 52nd ed. Medical Economics Company, Inc., Montvale, NJ, 1998, pp 3157–3163.

18. Dizac package insert. *In* Physicians' Desk Reference, 52nd ed. Medical Economics Company, Inc., Montvale, NJ, 1998, p 1935.

19. Trissel LA: Amphotericin B does not mix with fat emulsion. Am J Health Syst Pharm 52:1463–1464, 1995.

20. Kennelly C, Barnes S: Inadvertent i.v. administration of enteral formula causes adverse sequelae ranging from microembolism and hypersensitivity reactions to increased production of stool. Am J Crit Care 7:80, 1998.

21. Food and Drug Administration safety alert: Hazards of precipitation associated with parenteral nutrition. Am J Hosp Pharm 51:427–428, 1994.

22. Burnham WR, Hansrani PK, Knotts S, et al: Stability of fat emulsion–based intravenous feeding admixture. Int J Pharmaceutics 13:9–22, 1983.

23. Washington C, Connolly MA, Manning R, et al: The electrokinetic properties of phospholipid-stabilized fat emulsions. V: The effect of amino acids on emulsion stability. Int J Pharmaceutics 77:57–63, 1991.

24. Washington C, Athersuch A, Kynoch DJ: The electrokinetic properties of phospholipid-stabilized fat emulsions. IV: The effect of glucose and of pH. Int J Pharmacol 77:57–63, 1991.

25. Li L, Sampogna TP: A factorial design on the physical stability of 3-in-1 admixtures. J Pharm Pharmacol 45:985–987, 1993.

26. Khaodhiar L, McCowen K, Bistrian B: Perioperative hyperglycemia, infection or risk? Curr Opin Clin Nutr Metab Care 7:79–82, 1999.

27. Cahill GF: Starvation in man. N Engl J Med 282:668–675, 1970.

28. Wolfe RR: Carbohydrate metabolism in critically ill patients. Crit Care Clin 3:11–24, 1987.

29. Daley BJ, Cahill S, Driscoll DF, Bistrian BR: Parenteral and enteral nutrition. *In* Wolfe MM (ed): Gastrointestinal Pharmacotherapy. Philadelphia, WB Saunders, 1993, pp 293–316.

30. Wolfe R, Durkot M, Allsop J, et al: Glucose metabolism in severely burned patients. Metabolism 28:1031–1039, 1979.

31. Wolfe R, O'Donnell T, Stone M, et al: Investigation of factors determining the optimal glucose infusion rate in total parenteral nutrition. Metabolism 29:892–900, 1980.

32. McMahon M, Nanji N, Driscoll DF, Bistrian BR: Parenteral nutrition in patients with diabetes mellitus: Theoretical and practical considerations. JPEN J Parenter Enteral Nutr 13:545–553, 1989.

33. Sheldon GF, Petersen SR, Sanders R: Hepatic dysfunction during hyperalimentation. Arch Surg 113:504–508, 1978.

34. Pomposelli JJ, Moldawer LL, Palombo JD, et al: Short-term administration of parenteral glucose-lipid mixtures improves protein kinetics in portacaval shunted rats. Gastroenterology 91:306–312, 1986.

35. DeFronzo RA, Cooke CR, Andres R, et al: The effect of insulin on renal handling of sodium, potassium, calcium and phosphate in man. J Clin Invest 55:845–855, 1975.

36. Bistrian BR, Bothe A, Blackburn GL: Complica-tions of total parenteral nutrition. Clin Anaesthesiol 1:693–705, 1983.

37. Apovian CM, McMahon MM, Bistrian BR: Guidelines for refeeding the marasmic patient. Crit Care Med 18:1030–1033, 1990.

38. Kollef MH, McCormack MT, Caras WE, et al: The fat overload syndrome: Successful treatment with plasma exchange. Ann Intern Med 112:545–546, 1990.

39. Klein S, Miles JM: Metabolic effects of long-chain and medium-chain triglycerides in humans. JPEN J Parenter Enteral Nutr 18:396–397, 1994.

40. Saba TM: Physiology and pathophysiology of the reticuloendothelial system. Arch Intern Med 126:1031–1052, 1970.

41. Hamawy KJ, Moldawer LL, Georgieff M, et al: The effect of lipid emulsions on reticuloendothelial system function in the injured animal. JPEN J Parenter Enteral Nutr 9:559–565, 1985.

42. Seidner DL, Mascioli EA, Istfan NW, et al: Effects of long-chain triglyceride emulsions on reticuloendothelial system function in humans. JPEN J Parenter Enteral Nutr 13:614–619, 1989.

43. Jensen GL, Mascioli EA, Seidner DL, et al: Parenteral infusion of long and medium-chain triglycerides and reticuloendothelial system function in man. JPEN J Parenter Enteral Nutr 14:467–471, 1990.

44. Abbott WC, Grakauskas AM, Bistrian BR, et al: Metabolic and respiratory effects of continuous and discontinuous lipid infusions. Arch Surg 119:1367–1371, 1984.

45. Carpentier YA, Van Gossum A, Dubois DY, Deckelbaum RJ: Lipid metabolism in parenteral nutrition. *In* Rombeau JL, Caldwell MD (eds): Parenteral Nutrition. Philadelphia, WB Saunders, 1993, pp 35–74.

46. Kadowitz PJ, Spannhake EW, Levin JL, et al: Differential effects of prostaglandins on the pulmonary vascular bed. Prostaglandin Thromboxane Res 7:731–744, 1980.

47. Hwang TL, Huang SL, Chen MF: Effects of intravenous fat emulsion on respiratory failure. Chest 97:934–938, 1990.

48. Mathru M, Dries DJ, Zecca A, et al: Effect of fast vs slow Intralipid infusion on gas exchange, pulmonary hemodynamics, and prostaglandin metabolism. Chest 99:426–429, 1991.

49. Mascioli EA, Smith MF, Trerice MS, et al: Effect of total parenteral nutrition with cycling on essential fatty acid deficiency. JPEN J Parenter Enteral Nutr 3:171–173, 1979.

50. MacFie J, Smith RC, Hill GL: Glucose or fat as a non-protein energy source? Gastroenterology 80:103–107, 1981.

51. Delafosse B, Viale JP, Tisot S, et al: Effects of glucose-to-lipid ratio and type of lipid on substrate oxidation rate in patients. Am J Physiol 267(5 pt 1):E775–E780, 1994.

52. Rowe CE, Fukuyama TT, Martinoff JT: Growth of microorganisms in total nutrient admixtures. Drug Intell Clin Pharm 21:633–638, 1987.

53. Driscoll DF: Clinical issues regarding the use of total nutrient admixtures. DICP, Ann Pharmacother 24:296–303, 1990.

54. MacFie J, Courtney DF, Brennan TG: Continuous versus intermittent infusion of fat emulsions during total parenteral nutrition: Clinical trial. Nutrition 7:99–103, 1991.

55. Ahmad A, Duerksen DR, Munroe S, Bistrian BR: An evaluation of resting energy expenditure in hospitalized, severely underweight patients. Nutrition, in press.

56. Simmons BP, Hooten TM, Wong ES, et al: Guidelines for the prevention of intravascular infections. Centers for Disease Control: Guidelines and control of nosocomial infections. NITA 5:40–46, 1982.

57. Pearson ML, Hospital Infection Control Practices Advisory Committee: Guidelines for prevention of intravascular device-related infections. Infect Control Hosp Epidemiol 17:438–473, 1996.

58. Melly MA, Meng HC, Schaffner W: Microbial growth of lipid emulsions used for parenteral nutrition. Arch Surg 110:1479–1481, 1975.

59. Crocker KS, Noga R, Filibeck DJ, et al: Microbial growth comparisons of five commercial parenteral lipid emulsions. JPEN J Parenter Enteral Nutr 8:391–395, 1984.

60. Bennett SN, McNeil MM, Bland LA, et al: Postoperative infections traced to contamination of an intravenous anesthetic, propofol. N Engl J Med 333:147–154, 1995.

61. Brown DH, Simkover RA: Maximum hang times for i.v. fat emulsions. Am J Hosp Pharm 44:282, 284, 1987.

62. Didier ME, Fischer S, Maki DG: Total nutrient admixtures appear safer than lipid emulsion alone as regards microbial contamination: Growth properties of microbial pathogens at room temperature. JPEN J Parenter Enteral Nutr 22:291–296, 1998.

63. Driscoll DF, Bacon MN, Bistrian BR: Effects of inline filtration on lipid particle size distribution in total nutrient admixtures. JPEN J Parenter Enteral Nutr 20:296–301, 1996.

64. Driscoll DF: Total nutrient admixtures: Theory and practice. Nutr Clin Pract 10:114–119, 1995.

65. Spielmann D, Bracco U, Traitler H, et al: Alternative lipids to usual ω6 PUFAS: γ-linolenic acid, α-linolenic acid, stearidonic acid, EPA, etc. JPEN J Parenter Enteral Nutr 12(Suppl):111s–123s, 1988.

66. Jarstrand C, Berghem L, Lahnborg G: Human granulocyte and reticuloendothelial system function during Intralipid infusion. JPEN J Parenter Enteral Nutr 2:663–670, 1978.

67. Nordenström J, Jarstrand C, Wiernick A: Decreased chemotaxis and random migration of leukocytes during Intralipid infusion. Am J Clin Nutr 32:2416–2422, 1979.

68. Fisher GW, Hunter KW, Wilson SR, Mease D: Diminished bacterial defenses with Intralipid. Lancet 2:819–820, 1980.

69. Sedman PC, Somers SS, Ramsden CW, et al: Effects of different lipid emulsions on lymphocyte function during total parenteral nutrition. Br J Surg 78:1396–1399, 1991.

70. Wan MF, Teo TC, Babayan VK, Blackburn GL: Lipids and the development of immune dysfunction and infection. JPEN J Parenter Enteral Nutr 12:43S–48S, 1983.

71. Wolfram G: The use of lipid infusions in postoperative nutrition. Chirurg Gastroenterol 10:173–176, 1994.

72. Adolph M: Fett als Energieträger in der parenteralen Ernährung. In Adolph M (ed): Fett in der parenteralen Ernährung, Vol 5. Munich, W Zuckschwerdt-Verlag, 1998.

73. Adolph M, Eckart J, Metges C, et al: Oxidation of long and medium chain triglycerides during total parenteral nutrition of severely injured patients [Abstract]. Clin Nutr 7(Suppl):78, 1988.

74. Adolph M, Eckart J, Metges C, et al: Is there an influence of MCT on the LCT oxidation rate during total parenteral nutrition of trauma patients [Abstract]? JPEN J Parenter Enteral Nutr 14(Suppl):21, 1989.

75. Adolph M, Hailer S, Eckart J: Serum phospholipid fatty acids in severely injured patients on total parenteral nutrition with medium chain/long chain triglyceride emulsions. Ann Nutr Metab 39:251–260, 1995.

76. Ball MJ: Parenteral nutrition in the critically ill: Use of a medium chain triglyceride emulsion. Int Care Med 19:89–95, 1993.

77. Dennison A, Ball M, Crowe P, et al: Total parenteral nutrition using conventional and medium chain triglycerides. JPEN J Parenter Enteral Nutr 4:360–366, 1988.

78. Calon B, Poltecher T, Frey A, et al: Long chain versus medium and long chain triglyceride-based fat emulsion in parenteral nutrition of severe head trauma patients. Infusionsther Transfusionsmed 17:246–248, 1990.

79. Carpentier YA, Richelle M, Haumont D, Deckelbaum RJ: New developments in fat emulsion. Proc Nutr Soc 49:375–380, 1990.

80. Carpentier YA, Dubois DY, Siderova VS, Richelle M: Exogenous lipids and hepatic function. In Kinney JM, Tucker HN (eds): Organ Metabolism and Nutrition. New York, Raven Press, 1994, pp 349–367.

81. Kuse ER, Kemnitz J, Kotzerke J, et al: Fat emulsions in parenteral nutrition after liver transplantation: The recovery of the allografts RES function and histological observations. Clin Nutr 9:331–336, 1990.

82. Baldermann H, Wicklmayr M, Rett K, et al: Changes of hepatic morphology during parenteral nutrition with lipid emulsion containing LCT or MCT/LCT quantified by ultrasound. JPEN J Parenter Enteral Nutr 15:601–603, 1991.

83. Stein TP, Yoshida S, Schluter MD, et al: Comparison of intravenous nutrients on gut mucosal protein synthesis. JPEN J Parenter Enteral Nutr 18:447–452, 1994.

84. Ota DM, Copeland EM, Corriere JM: The effects of 10% soybean emulsion on lymphocyte transformation. JPEN J Parenter Enteral Nutr 2:112–115, 1978.

85. Monson JRT, Ramsden CW, MacFie J, et al: Immunorestorative effect of lipid emulsions during total parenteral nutrition. Br J Surg 73:843–846, 1986.

86. Ota DM, Jessup MM, Babcock GF, et al: Immune function during intravenous administration of a soybean oil emulsion. JPEN J Parenter Enteral Nutr 9:23–27, 1985.

87. Kinsella JE, Lokesh B, Broughton S, Whelan J: Dietary polyunsaturated fatty acids and eicosanoids: Potential effects on the modulation of inflammatory and immune cells: An overview. Nutrition 6:24–44, 1990.

88. Gogos CA, Zoumbos NC, Makri M, Kalfarentzos FE: Medium- and long-chain triglycerides have different effects on the synthesis of tumor necrosis factor by human mononuclear cells in patients under total parenteral nutrition. J Am Coll Nutr 13:40–44, 1994.

89. Gelas P, Cotte L, Poitevin-Later F, et al: Effect of parenteral medium- and long-chain triglycerides on lymphocytes subpopulations and functions in patients with acquired immunodeficiency syndrome: A prospective study. JPEN J Parenter Enteral Nutr 22:67–71, 1998.

90. Waitzberg DL, Bellinati-Pires R, Salgado MM, et al: Effect of total parenteral nutrition with different lipid emulsions on human monocyte and neutrophil functions. Nutrition 13:128–132, 1997.

91. Dutoid DF, Villet WT, Heydenrych J: Fat emulsion deposition in mononuclear phagocyte system. Lancet 2:898–902, 1978.

92. Meurling S, Roos KA: Liver changes in rats on continuous and intermittent parenteral nutrition with and without fat. Acta Chir Scand 147:475–480, 1981.

93. Sobrado J, Moldawer LL, Pomposelli JJ, et al: Lipid emulsions and reticuloendothelial system function in healthy and burned guinea pigs. Am J Clin Nutr 42:855–863, 1985.

94. Hageman JR, McCulloch KE, Gora P, et al: Intralipid alterations in pulmonary prostaglandin metabolism and gas exchange. Crit Care Med 11:794–798, 1983.

95. Hageman JR, Hunt CE: Fat emulsions and lung function. Clin Chest Med 7:69–77, 1986.

96. Hammermann C, Aramburo MJ: Intravenous lipids in newborn lungs. Thromboxane-mediated effects. Crit Care Med 17:430–436, 1989.

97. Hunt CE, Cora P, Inwood RJ: Pulmonary effects of Intralipid: The role of Intralipid as a prostaglandin precursor. Prog Lipid Res 20:199–204, 1981.

98. Radermacher P, Santak B, Strobach H, et al: Fat emulsions containing medium chain triglycerides in patients with sepsis syndrome: Effects on pulmonary hemodynamics and gas exchange. Intensive Care Med 18:231–234, 1992.

99. Venus B, Prager R, Patel CB, et al: Cardiopulmonary effects of Intralipid infusion in critically ill patients. Crit Care Med 16:587–590, 1988.

100. Venus B, Prager R, Patel CB, et al: Hemodynamic and gas exchange alterations during Intralipid infusion in patients with adult respiratory distress syndrome. Chest 95:1278–1281, 1989.

101. Greene HL, Hazlett D, Demaree R: Relationship between Intralipid-induced hyperlipemia and pulmonary function. Am J Clin Nutr 29:127–135, 1976.

102. Branemark PI, Lindstrom J: Microcirculatory effect of emulsified fat in infusions. Circ Res 15:124–130, 1964.

103. Fiaccadori E, Tortorella G, Gonzi GL, et al: Hemodynamic and respiratory effects of medium-chain and long-chain triglyceride fat emulsions: A prospective, randomized study. Riv Ital Nutriz Parent Ent 15:6–14, 1997.

104. Lemoyne M, Van Gossum A, Kurian R, et al: Plasma vitamin E and selenium and breath pentane in home parenteral nutrition patients. Am J Clin Nutr 48:1310–1315, 1988.

105. Wispe JR, Bell EF, Roberts RJ: Lipid peroxidation in newborn rabbits: Effects of oxygen, lipid emulsions, and vitamin E. Pediatr Res 20:505–507, 1986.

106. Traber MG, Carpentier YA, Kayden HJ, et al: Alterations in plasma α- and γ-tocopherol concentrations in response to intravenous infusion of lipid emulsions in humans. Metabolism 42:701–709, 1993.

107. Siderova AC, Richelle M, Dubois D, et al: Intravenous α-tocopherol supplementation in patients receiving long-term home parenteral nutrition. Clin Nutr 14:47–48, 1995.

108. Nordenström J, Thörne A, Olivecrona A: Metabolic effects of infusion of a structured-triglyceride emulsion in healthy subjects. Nutrition 11:269–274, 1995.

109. Hultin M, Müllertz A, Zundel MA, et al: Metabolism of emulsions containing medium- and long-chain triglycerides or interesterified triglycerides. J Lipid Res 35:1850–1860, 1994.

110. Lutz O, Lave T, Frey A, et al: Activities of lipoprotein lipase and hepatic lipase on long- and medium-chain triglyceride emulsions used in parenteral nutrition. Metabolism 38:507–513, 1989.

111. Magnusson Borg IK, Göran Sandberg L, Wennberg AK, et al: Effects of a fat emulsion containing medium chain fatty acids and long chain fatty acids on protein and energy metabolism in partially hepatectomized rats. Clin Nutr 14:23–28, 1995.

112. Sandström R, Hyltander A, Körner U, et al: Structured triglycerides to postoperative patients: A safety and tolerance study. JPEN J Parenter Enteral Nutr 17:153–157, 1993.

113. Sandström R, Hyltander A, Körner U, et al: Structured triglycerides were well tolerated and induced increased whole body fat oxidation compared with long-chain triglycerides in postoperative patients. JPEN J Parenter Enteral Nutr 19:381–386, 1995.

114. Kruimel JW, Naber AHJ: Structured triglycerides. In Educational Program, XIX ESPEN Congress, Amsterdam, 1997, pp 102 104.

115. Granato D, Blum S, Zbinden I, et al: Effect of ClinOleic®, an olive oil-based parenteral lipid emulsion, on lymphocyte function in vitro [Abstract]. Clin Nutr 15(Suppl 1):3, 1996.

116. Dutot G, Melin C: Assessment of lipid peroxidation during lipid infusion: Influence of fatty acid composition of fat emulsion [Abstract]. Clin Nutr 10(Suppl 2):50, 1991.

117. Dutot G, Trimbo S, Melin C: Vitamin E intake can be optimized in parenteral nutrition by using a new olive oil based fat emulsion [Abstract]. 15th International Congress of Nutrition, Adelaide, Australia, 1993.

118. Arborati M, Ninio E, Chapman MJ, et al: Comparison of lipoperoxide content and lipoperoxidability in parenteral fat emulsions with different triglyceride content [Abstract]. Clin Nutr 16(Suppl 2):O.18, 1997.

119. Bang HO, Dyerberg J, Sinclair HM: The composition of the Eskimo food in northwestern Greenland. Am J Clin Nutr 33:2657–2661, 1980.

120. Dyerberg J, Bang HO, Hjorne N: Fatty acid composition of the plasma lipids in Greenland Eskimos. Am J Clin Nutr 28:958–966, 1975.

121. Chan S, McCowen KC, Bistrian BR: Medium-chain triglycerides and n-3 polyunsaturated fatty acid–containing emulsions in intravenous nutrition. Curr Opin Clin Nutr Metab Care 1:163–169, 1998.

122. Fürst P: Old and new substrates in clinical nutrition. J Nutr 128:789–796, 1998.

123. Grimble RF: Dietary manipulation of the inflammatory response. Proc Nutr Soc 51:285–294, 1994.

124. Endres S, Ghorbani R, Kelley VE, et al: The effect

of dietary supplementation with n-3 polyunsaturated fatty acids on the synthesis of interleukin-11 and tumor necrosis factor by mononuclear cells. N Engl J Med 320:265–271, 1989.

125. Lowry SF, Thompson WA: Nutrient modification of inflammatory mediator production. New Horiz 2:164–174, 1994.

126. Rola-Plezcynski M: Differential effects of leucotriene B_4 and T_4 and T_8 lymphocyte phenotype and immunoregulatory functions. J Immunol 135:1357–1360, 1985.

127. Morlion BJ, Torwesten E, Lessire H, et al: The effect of parenteral fish oil on leucocyte membrane fatty acid composition and leukotriene-synthesizing capacity in patients with postoperative trauma. Metabolism 45:1208–1213, 1996.

128. Oliveira T, Carpentier YA, Hansen I, et al: Triglyceride hydrolysis of soy vs fish oil LCT emulsions. Clin Nutr 11(Suppl):44, 1992.

129. Hamberger L, Carpentier YA, Hansen I, et al: In vitro lipolysis of MCT and fish oil containing emulsions: Evidence that longer chain fatty acids must be cleared as intact triglycerides in emulsion remnants. Clin Nutr 15(Suppl):23, 1996.

130. Carpentier YA, Siderova VS, Richelle M, et al: Does the presence of fish oil in emulsion particles affect the elimination of MCT/LCT emulsion? Clin Nutr 15(Suppl):2, 1996.

131. Cukier C, Waitzberg DL, Logullo AF, et al: Fish oil enriched TPN improves liver and lung phagocytosis in rats. Clin Nutr 16(Suppl 2):42, 1997.

132. Wachtler P, König W, Senkal M, et al: Influence of a total parenteral nutrition enriched with ω-3 fatty acids on leukotriene synthesis of peripheral leukocytes and systemic cytokine levels in patients with major surgery. J Trauma 42:191–198, 1997.

133. Pscheidl E, Reisch S, Rügheimer E: Chemically defined structured lipids with omega-3 fatty acids maintain splanchnic blood flow in a low-dose continuous endotoxin model. Infusionsther Transfusionsmed 21:380–387, 1994.

134. Pscheidl E, Böke-Pröls T: Omega-3 fatty acids enriched fat emulsions modulate splanchnic blood flow and microbial translocation in a low dose endotoxin rat model. Clin Nutr 16(Suppl 2):16, 1997.

135. Schjøtt J, Brekke O-L, Jynge P, et al: Infusion of EPA and DHA lipid emulsions: Effects on heart lipids and tolerance to ischaemia-reperfusion in the isolated rat heart. Scand J Clin Lab Invest 53:873–877, 1993.

136. Dupont I, Siderova VS, Vanweyenberg V, et al: Incorporation of alpha-tocopherol in plasma lipoproteins during and after infusion of fish oil containing emulsions. Clin Nutr 16(Suppl 2):2, 1997.

4

◆ Trace Elements and Vitamins in Adult Intravenous Nutrition

Alan Shenkin, F.R.C.P., F.R.C.Path.
Michael C. Allwood, Ph.D.

◆ MICRONUTRIENTS IN NUTRITIONAL SUPPORT

There has been a surge of interest in characterizing the requirements of trace elements and vitamins in clinical nutrition. This is a direct result of the recognition that most micronutrients are necessary not only to prevent obvious deficiency syndromes but also because they have a subtle role in metabolic processes that may not be immediately apparent in terms of structure or function but that contributes to overall well-being and to the outcome of disease.

Many of the general principles regarding micronutrient requirements relate to all forms of nutritional support; hence, relevant aspects of the equivalent review in the companion volume *Enteral and Tube Feeding*[1] are repeated here, modified as necessary for intravenous nutrition (IVN). Studies of patients receiving IVN, especially for prolonged periods, have taught much about nutritional requirements for micronutrients. This not only has permitted the recognition of rare micronutrient deficiencies—for example, deficiency of chromium or molybdenum—but also has enabled the study of requirements and metabolism in long-term stable patients. This is of special relevance now, with many patients receiving home IVN.

◆ CLINICAL DEFICIENCY SYNDROMES AND SUBCLINICAL DEFICIENCY STATES

"Classic" nutritional deficiency usually results in a complex syndrome of typical signs and symptoms, and these have now been fully characterized for each of the vitamins and trace elements.[2-4] These syndromes were the basis on which the essential micronutrients were initially identified, and careful dietary studies on both animals and humans have permitted a reasonable understanding of the nutritional consequences of severe deficiency as well as understanding of the intake necessary to prevent clinically obvious deficiency from developing.

However, it is now clear that as an individual develops progressively more severe depletion in the micronutrient status, the person passes through a series of stages with biochemical or physiologic consequences. The metabolic or physiologic penalty of such suboptimal nutritional status is usually not clear, but the assumption remains that this impaired metabolism is likely to have detrimental effects. Similarly, although the concentration of a micronutrient may be adequate in the blood or in many tissues, specific and localized tissue deficiencies can occur and can lead to pathologic changes;[5] for example, folic acid may be locally deficient in bronchopulmonary, esophageal, or cervical tissue,[6] and vitamin A may be deficient only in lung tissue.[7] Such situations can be defined as subclinical deficiency.[4] One study of subclinical deficiency in critically ill patients is shown in Figure 4–1, in which the vitamin B_1 and B_2 status at the time of admission to the intensive care unit was plotted in relation to the outcome. Those patients who subsequently died had a greater incidence of abnormal vitamin B_1 status and a poorer biochemical vitamin B_2 status despite being within the reference range.[8, 9] None of the patients had clinical signs of deficiency. Although it is not possible to assess the extent to which the vitamin status contributed to the outcome, these results led to a protocol for subsequent patients to receive a bolus injection of water-soluble vitamins on admission to the intensive care unit.

The time course for the development of a subclinical deficiency state varies for each

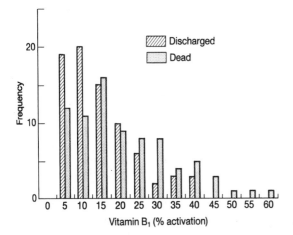

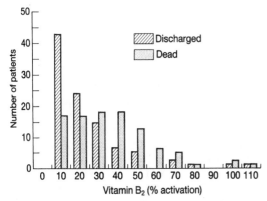

Figure 4–1. Vitamin B_1 and B_2 status in relation to outcome in patients admitted to an intensive therapy unit. An abnormal vitamin B_1 status is defined as an activation of red blood cell transketolase of greater than 25%, and abnormal vitamin B_2 status as activation of glutathione reductase of greater than 60%. (From Payne-James J, Grimble G, Silk D [eds]: Artificial Nutrition Support in Clinical Practice. London, Edward Arnold, 1995, pp 151–166.)

individual micronutrient and depends on the nature and amount of tissue or body stores.[10] Moreover, the extent of depletion necessary before there are significant biochemical, physiologic, or histologic changes is poorly characterized. It is tempting to speculate that there might be a linear relationship between the rate of depletion of a micronutrient and the reduction in function of that micronutrient. However, it is probable that the early period of depletion of nutrients will result in compensatory mechanisms that protect the organism, and it will only be when the depletion becomes more severe that even these subclinical effects become apparent (Fig. 4–2).

The consequences of an inadequate in-

take are more clearly delineated in Figure 4–3. This shows the progression from the optimal tissue status through a period of initial depletion until the period of subclinical deficiency is reached, with a variety of biochemical and nonspecific physiologic deficits and nonspecific histologic changes for certain micronutrients, until eventually the full-blown clinical deficiency state can be recognized.

An important concept is that a subclinical deficiency state can be either absolute or relative. Thus, an intake less than the requirement in normal health leads to subclinical deficiency or to a typical clinical deficiency state. However, certain patients have significantly increased requirements as a result of their disease process, and hence an intake normally regarded as adequate may be relatively insufficient and lead to a subclinical deficiency state (see later). Most of the recommendations for vitamin and trace element supplements in IVN include an allowance for an increased requirement in disease. Despite this, it is surprising how frequently case reports still appear of patients receiving IVN who have developed frank vitamin or trace element deficiency. Close examination of these cases usually reveals that the patients have had both a low intake of the vitamin in question and an increased requirement because of disease.[11, 12] Chemical degradation after compounding but before or during administration may also ac-

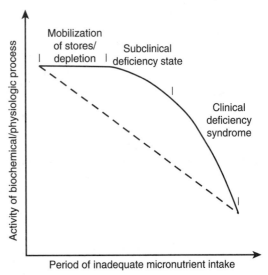

Figure 4–2. The dotted line shows the linear reduction in function that would probably only occur in in vitro reactions. In vivo, the solid line is expected.

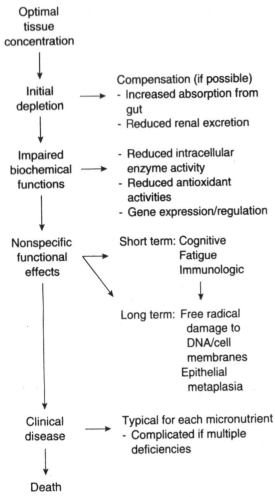

Figure 4–3. The consequences of inadequate micronutrient intake.

count for the low intake of vitamins. The rate of progression through subclinical deficiency to clinical deficiency is rapid in such patients. One of the major challenges in clinical nutrition is to clarify the extent of the increased need for each micronutrient in particular disease states, possibly by the use of better laboratory methods, and to ensure an optimal intake to meet the requirement.

◆ FUNCTIONS OF MICRONUTRIENTS

Micronutrients can be classified as having two main types of function. First, they are required for optimal enzyme activity. Thus, many trace elements are essential as activators of particular enzyme systems, for exam-

ple, zinc or manganese, or indeed may be part of the prosthetic group of particular enzymes, for example, selenium or molybdenum. Similarly, most vitamins are coenzymes, or are part of coenzymes, which are essential for enzyme activity, for example, the coenzymes of the electron transport chain.

Second, certain micronutrients are involved directly in metabolic or regulatory activities. Thus, vitamin E and vitamin A (and β-carotene) have antioxidant activity, whereas vitamin D, vitamin A, and zinc (as *zinc fingers*) are involved in the control of DNA transcription. There is, however, no simple system for classifying the increasingly wide range of reactions in which micronutrients are directly involved.

Those micronutrients especially important in free radical metabolism are vitamin A (β-carotene) and vitamin E, which, being fat soluble, are involved in protection of cell membranes; and vitamin C, superoxide dismutase (zinc, copper), and glutathione peroxidase (selenium) in the protection of the aqueous phase of the cell.[13, 14]

Given the range of functions of micronutrients, and especially the fact that most micronutrients take part in more than one reaction, it is inevitable that an intake that achieves adequate function in one reaction may not be optimal for another; for example, the intake of vitamin A necessary to prevent night blindness may not be ideal to prevent epithelial metaplasia.[7] Similarly, zinc binds to prosthetic groups of many enzymes and to cross-linking sites of other proteins, and the concentration of free zinc in the cytoplasm (10^{-9} to 10^{-10} M) required to bind to cytoplasmic enzymes is much lower than the concentration in cell vesicles (e.g, 10^{-4} M) necessary for binding to proteins such as insulin.[15] Even if the biochemical reactions are similar, concentrations necessary to achieve the optimal effect might be different. For example, vitamin K is necessary to achieve γ-carboxylation of glutamic acid in the synthesis of certain proteins, such as blood coagulation proteins, and osteocalcin in the bone matrix.[16] Different concentrations of vitamin K may well be necessary to optimize these reactions in different tissues.[17]

An even more complex situation exists for an element such as selenium. It is clear that severe deficiency can lead to myopathy, either cardiomyopathy in endemic deficiency[18] or skeletal myopathy[19, 20] or cardio-myopathy[21] in artificial nutrition. However, only a relatively small proportion of all those who develop biochemically proven selenium deficiency while on long-term selenium-deficient IVN or in population studies also develop clinical signs of deficiency.[22] Whether this depends on the requirement for some precipitating agent, for example, a viral infection or some other environmental stress, is not known. However, an intriguing observation is that deficiency of a micronutrient (Se) may lead to the mutation of a nonvirulent form of coxsackievirus B3 to a virulent form, which might then cause cardiomyopathy.[23] There may also be an interaction with vitamin E, which has similar antioxidant activity and can compensate for selenium in some animal conditions.[24]

The effect of selenium in these myopathies has been found to be due to the action of the selenoenzyme glutathione peroxidase. A further function for selenium is as part of the enzyme tyrosine deiodinase, which is required for triiodothyronine biosynthesis.[25] The interaction of selenium and iodine in sustaining thyroid metabolism is an area of special interest.[26] Thus, the optimal intake of selenium may depend not only on the selenium status but also on the vitamin E and iodine status and on other physiologic or pathologic factors.

◆ FACTORS AFFECTING THE MICRONUTRIENT REQUIREMENT OF INDIVIDUAL PATIENTS

Although it is possible to suggest for each trace element and vitamin an intake that is likely to meet the requirements of the majority of patients, it is essential for clinicians to be aware of circumstances that lead to an increased requirement, so that individual or multiple supplements can be considered. This is especially relevant to patients requiring IVN, since the time course of the disease process, and the possibly protracted treatment before beginning IVN, may well mean that some patients will require greater amounts of intravenous micronutrients.

Micronutrient Status at the Onset of Disease or on Admission to the Hospital

The typical diet or lifestyle of a patient in relative health may already have compro-mised the patient's micronutrient status at the time of admission to the hospital. Since many individuals have poor dietary habits, with an excessive intake of refined carbohydrate, inadequate fiber, and variably inadequate intake of fruit, vegetables, and milk, they are already at risk of inadequate intake, especially of B vitamins and iron. This is particularly the case in adolescence, when the anabolism associated with rapid growth puts demands on the provision of all nutrients. At the same time, adolescents frequently follow food fads or undergo atypical reducing diets, further exacerbating the situation. Studies have suggested that adolescent girls are particularly at risk of inadequate folate and vitamin A intake.[27, 28]

Elderly individuals also have a high frequency of nutritional problems relating to the inadequacy of the diet itself, dental problems, interactions of drugs with nutrient metabolism, chronic illness, and economic factors. The high incidence of abnormalities, especially in micronutrient status, is therefore not surprising, and studies have shown a high prevalence of vitamin C, iron, zinc, and folate deficiency in such populations.[29]

An excess intake of alcohol or cigarette smoke also alters the micronutrient status. Individuals who derive a high proportion of their energy from alcohol are likely to have inadequate intake of most water-soluble vitamins as well as phosphate and magnesium. Moreover, there may be impaired metabolism of vitamin A in cirrhosis, possibly related to inadequate zinc status.[30] Vitamin B_1 deficiency in particular should be sought in this group of individuals.

There is also good evidence for an increased requirement of vitamin C in smokers, possibly due to altered metabolic turnover.[31] Similarly, the status of β-carotene and vitamin E is impaired relative to nonsmokers, suggesting a link with oxidative damage due to free radical production.[32]

Effects of the Underlying Disease Process

The micronutrient status at the time of presentation may also be impaired because of the effects of the disease process itself. Any condition causing malabsorption affects the absorption of trace elements and vitamins; inflammatory bowel disease, celiac disease, chronic pancreatitis, biliary cirrhosis, and other forms of small bowel disease affect all micronutrients, but particularly the fat-soluble vitamins. When considering the possibility of malabsorption, the effect of antagonistic supplements should always be remembered—individual oral supplements of iron, zinc, or copper or other ligands such as phytate may lead to reduced absorption of other trace elements.[33, 34]

Similarly, the underlying disease may cause increased loss of elements in body fluids, especially in chronic diarrhea. Although this mainly affects the major minerals (sodium, potassium, and magnesium), patients with chronic diarrhea lose large amounts of zinc and other water-soluble trace elements.

Moreover, the disease state itself may cause an inflammatory or acute-phase response with increased protein turnover in tissues such as skeletal muscle, leading to release of intracellular elements, especially zinc, which are then excreted in the urine.[35] Such a deficit must be corrected during the phase of recovery from illness.

Increased Requirements Due to Illness or the Effects of Treatment or Surgery

Effects of Illness

The increases in metabolic rate and in protein turnover associated with an illness, infection, or trauma inevitably lead to increased involvement of micronutrients as cofactors of the metabolic processes. As long as patients have an increased intake within a balanced regimen, so that the amount of micronutrient provided increases proportionally with protein and energy substrates, metabolic requirements should be adequately met. It is, however, unlikely that this will be the case in patients receiving their nutrition by the parenteral route because it is common practice to provide a similar amount of vitamins and trace elements to most adult patients. An example of unbalanced supplementation is in hypermetabolic patients with a high carbohydrate intake as part of their energy requirement, in whom there is an increased likelihood of water-soluble vitamin deficiency, especially vitamin B_1.[8, 11]

Effects of Surgery

Complications of surgery frequently alter micronutrient status. Inevitably, short gut syndrome reduces the absorption of most micronutrients, although some may be absorbed throughout the whole length of the small bowel. Hence, the total length of gut remaining is critical in determining the proportion of the micronutrient intake that can be absorbed. Special care is necessary if the terminal ileum has been resected, because of the absorption of vitamin B_{12} from this region.

Small bowel or pancreatic fistula fluids have a high content of micronutrients, especially zinc, whereas biliary fistula fluid is rich in copper and manganese, and thus these micronutrients are lost along with the fluid.

There is also a theoretical risk of loss of water-soluble vitamins and trace elements in patients who receive peritoneal dialysis or hemodialysis. This is usually not a major problem, although such patients are at higher risk for deficiencies of folic acid, pyridoxine, vitamin C, zinc, and iron.[36]

An important source of loss of micronutrients during treatment of patients with severe burns is through the damaged skin. The losses of zinc, copper, and selenium, and probably also other micronutrients, are much greater in burn exudate fluid than are the losses in urine or feces.[37, 38] A major deficit of these elements can accumulate quickly, and the best method of replacing such elements and the amounts required are not known. Some studies have suggested that increasing trace element provision by a factor of about four to six may be beneficial,[39] and an intravenous supplement of zinc (400 μmol/day; 26.5 mg/day), copper (42 μmol/day; 2.6 mg/day), and selenium (2.9 μmol/day; 229 μg/day) designed to replace the extensive losses through the skin has led to reduced pulmonary infectious complications.[40] The optimal intake of such additional micronutrients and whether they are better provided intravenously or enterally need to be established.

Effects of Anabolism

Patients who have lost a significant amount of lean body mass because of catabolic illness may develop an acute deficiency state when there is a change to net anabolism and tissue regeneration. This point in the progress of a patient generally occurs when the stimulus to the release of catabolic mediators (interleukins and tumor necrosis factor) and of catabolic hormones (especially catecholamines and cortisol) has been resolved (e.g., by drainage of an abscess, or by coverage of a burn area). Deficiency states are therefore more likely to occur during the anabolic phase that follows the resolution of a catabolic illness.[41] Well-recognized examples of this are the rash of zinc deficiency[35] and skeletal muscle myopathy due to selenium deficiency.[20]

◆ OPTIMIZATION OF THE PROVISION OF MICRONUTRIENTS

Defining the optimal intake of micronutrients is therefore far from ideal. On one hand, it is possible to make a reasonable assessment of the requirements of an individual based on the requirements in health, the likely underlying nutritional state of the patient at the time of presentation, and the ongoing effects of the disease process. For patients receiving IVN, estimates of absorption from the oral diet have permitted calculation of the likely intravenous requirements. Such a level of provision has been proved to be adequate in most cases to prevent the development of a deficiency state. On the other hand, the provision of micronutrients to ensure the best possible tissue function remains a much more desirable yet distant goal. Possible methods of trying to optimize their provision in relation to function can be considered with respect to the free radical scavenging system and also to the immune system.

The role of micronutrients in limiting the oxidative damage caused by free radicals is now well established. The key issue, however, is whether the increased provision of free radical scavengers such as vitamin E; of micronutrients directly involved in free radical metabolic pathways, such as vitamin C, selenium, zinc, or copper; or of the metalloenzyme superoxide dismutase may influence outcomes.[42] Increased provision of these nutrients alters the fatty acid content of cell membranes and also the production of end-products of oxidative metabolism, such as malonyl dialdehyde. Correlations between these biochemical markers and outcomes, however, tend to be rather tenuous

and may be more coincidental than "cause and effect." Free radical damage has been related especially to pancreatitis. There is clear biochemical evidence of oxidative stress in experimental models of acute pancreatitis,[43, 44] although pretreatment with antioxidants seems necessary to achieve a clinically beneficial effect.[43, 45] Biochemical and clinical benefit of an oral cocktail of antioxidant nutrients has also been shown in recurrent pancreatitis.[46] There is growing interest in the potential value of folic acid supplements in reducing the blood concentration of homocysteine, which is an independent risk factor for atherosclerosis.[46a]

It is to be expected that in the next few years, well-controlled clinical trials will help to clarify the situations in which the increased provision of these micronutrients is or is not helpful, both in reducing the biochemical effects of free radicals and in altering complication rates and outcomes in serious illness. Many of the disease states thought to be associated with free radicals are chronic degenerative conditions, such as atherosclerosis and neoplastic disease.[42] The increasing number of patients dependent on lifelong IVN makes the long-term provision of adequate amounts of micronutrients an important part of nutritional therapy.

Micronutrient deficiencies have been associated with impairment of various aspects of immune function. However, controlled evidence of efficacy in vivo is limited. Most studies have involved oral rather than intravenous supplements. A study of the effect of a mixture of vitamins and trace elements in free-living, healthy elderly individuals demonstrated a marked reduction in episodes of infection over a 1-year period.[29] This was found to correlate with an increase in T4 lymphocyte cell numbers, improved lymphocyte responsiveness to phytohemagglutinin, and an increase in natural killer cells. A small proportion of patients was found to have biochemical evidence of deficiency for individual or multiple micronutrients at the start of the trial, and supplementation improved the biochemical status for these nutrients.

Supplementation with zinc alone in elderly individuals with mild zinc deficiency has been shown to increase lymphocyte nucleotidase activity and serum thymulin levels, together with an improved response to skin test antigens.[47] Improved taste acuity is also observed. Similarly, zinc supplements in patients with Crohn's disease lead to increased plasma thymulin levels.[48]

There has been a long-standing interest in the potential value of vitamin A supplementation in infectious diseases, and a meta-analysis of 20 trials has confirmed that such supplements to children in developing countries do have anti-infective properties. In community studies of children with measles,[49] supplements have led to a significant reduction in mortality from diarrheal disease and also a reduction in respiratory disease.

Studies have been performed on the value of intakes higher than recommended daily allowances, but few studies have had a convincing overall effect. Large doses of vitamin E might improve immunity in elderly persons. Various aspects of cell-mediated immunity, including skin tests, mitogenic responses, and interleukin 2 production, have been shown to respond to vitamin E, either alone or in combination with vitamin C and vitamin A.[50]

An interesting study on university students has shown that a selenium supplement of 200 µg/day in individuals with an apparently healthy diet led to an increase in markers of immune function.[51, 52] These markers included interleukin 2 receptor expression and T lymphocyte function.

Because of the difficulty of studying effects on immune status independently from the disease process itself, it remains to be established whether these findings are relevant to patients receiving IVN.

◆ RISK OF TOXICITY OF MICRONUTRIENTS

Although water-soluble vitamins are generally regarded as being virtually free of toxic effects when given in large amounts, fat-soluble vitamins and trace elements have a much narrower range of safe yet adequate dosage.[34, 53]

Excess vitamin D provision not only causes hypercalcemia but also has been linked to the metabolic bone disease of long-term IVN.[54, 55] Vitamin A toxicity has been observed during IVN in patients with renal failure.[56] There is also concern regarding the toxicity of added manganese, neurologic disturbances having been observed in some children[57] and adults[58] with manganese deposition in the brain, although patient susceptibility is variable. Overprovision of manganese and copper is more likely in pa-

tients with cholestatic liver disease because these elements are normally excreted in the bile.

Trace elements are also present as contaminants in IVN solutions. Aluminium toxicity is well documented, although because this has now been addressed by the manufacturers, it should no longer be a major problem.[55] However, some additives such as calcium gluconate may still contain significant amounts of aluminum. Chromium is a persistent contaminant of amino acid solutions leading to high blood concentrations,[22] although these have not been shown to be harmful.

◆ MONITORING MICRONUTRIENT STATUS IN PATIENTS RECEIVING INTRAVENOUS NUTRITION

Ideally, micronutrient provision would be matched to requirements by monitoring with laboratory tests. Unfortunately, such tests are generally fairly poor in terms of accuracy in reflecting the nutritional state; sensitivity to small changes in status; and specificity, that is, being affected only by nutritional status and not by other effects of disease. Hence, at best, laboratory tests can only be used as a guide toward substantial underprovision or overprovision of particular nutrients but in most cases cannot be used to "fine tune" the provision to meet the requirements of individual patients.

Measurement of micronutrient concentrations in plasma or serum provides a reasonable index of the status of only a few nutrients (e.g., vitamin B_{12}), and for certain micronutrients (e.g., folate or selenium) it may reflect the adequacy of recent intake. An excessive provision of elements such as manganese and chromium may also be detected by high serum concentrations.

For most other micronutrients, serum measurement is seriously limited in value. This reflects the lack of correlation between the amount of the nutrient in the plasma compartment and the amount within the intracellular compartment in most body tissues. For example, there may be substantial stores of particular nutrients in individual tissues (e.g., vitamin A or vitamin B_{12} in the liver), but their mobilization into the plasma is affected by the availability of appropriate binding proteins or by metabolism. Moreover, there are differences in the content of individual micronutrients between tissues, and hence the serum concentration will not reflect these different concentrations.

Furthermore, the concentration in plasma can alter rapidly when an acute-phase response to trauma or infection leads to the redistribution of metals between body compartments.[59] For example, during an acute-phase response, there is increased synthesis of metallothionein, leading to uptake of zinc into the liver,[60] and increased synthesis of ferritin, causing uptake of iron;[61] the result is a fall in the plasma concentration of both zinc and iron. These changes in plasma concentration clearly do not reflect changes in whole-body status.[62] Moreover, there may be changes in the binding proteins in plasma as a result of the disease process. The serum albumin concentration falls in association with any acute illness,[63] and this inevitably leads to a fall in the plasma zinc concentration. Similarly, a reduction in retinol-binding protein concentration as part of the acute-phase response or protein malnutrition also leads to a fall in serum retinol levels, whatever the content of retinol stores within the liver.[64]

However, patients receiving long-term IVN, especially at home, may well be stable, with relatively little acute-phase response to injury, infection, or other inflammation. If this is the case, it may be possible to interpret the plasma concentrations of elements such as zinc, copper, and iron.[65] In a patient with no evidence of an acute-phase reaction, a low plasma concentration of zinc is indicative of poor status. Of particular relevance is the trend in concentration of the trace element as the magnitude of the acute-phase response changes. Repeated measurements of a rapid-response acute-phase protein such as C-reactive protein may therefore be helpful in assessing changes in the acute-phase response and the validity of some of these plasma measurements.[59, 66]

Increasingly, attempts are being made to relate blood cell concentrations to micronutrient status and to the requirements for individual micronutrients. It is well established that the concentration of certain intracellular enzymes gives a good index of the micronutrient status, for example, red cell transketolase as an index of the thiamine status or red cell glutathione peroxidase as an indication of the selenium status.[10] Alternatively, whole blood thiamine or selenium analysis probably yields better precision for comparative studies. Similarly,

red cell folate is widely used as an index of the whole-body folate status. Because the acute-phase response causes significant alterations in the distribution of vitamin C and zinc between body compartments, leukocyte studies have been performed, and these have been shown to provide a better index of body status for these nutrients.[67, 68] Preparation of white blood cells is technically difficult, and such methods are likely to be used only in the research environment.

A summary of some tests commonly used to assess micronutrients is included in Tables 4–1 and 4–2. Because of the limitations in interpretation of these data, it is common practice, especially in patients receiving IVN, to assess on a regular basis only the status of zinc, copper, selenium (mainly in long-term nutritional problems), iron, and folic acid. The other laboratory tests that are available to assess micronutrients are usually used only when there is a particular clinical problem in which confirmation of micronutrient deficiency is necessary. If such tests are not available and a deficiency is suspected, a therapeutic trial, especially of increased water-soluble vitamins, can be safely given. In patients receiving IVN, some intestinal absorptive capacity may still be present, and hence an oral or enteral multimineral or multivitamin supplement may also be provided. A 2-week course of a well-balanced micronutrient supplement is unlikely to cause any harm and may occasionally be beneficial. Alternatively, an increased intravenous supply can be given for a limited period, with careful clinical monitoring. In such cases, a blood or plasma sample at the beginning of supplementation should be stored for possible analysis at a later date. Documentation of patients who benefit clinically in this way could, in the long term, help to clarify the increased micronutrient requirements of certain types of patients.

◆ PHARMACEUTICAL ASPECTS OF PROVISION OF VITAMINS AND TRACE ELEMENTS IN INTRAVENOUS NUTRITION

Fat-Soluble Vitamins

Vitamin A

Chemistry

Vitamin A (retinol) comprises a number of β-ionone derivatives of β-carotene, the most

Text continued on page 72

Table 4–1. Essential Inorganic Micronutrients (Trace Elements)

	Function(s)	Biochemical Modes of Action	Effects of Deficiency	Recommended Oral Intake (Men)		Recommended IV Supply[101-105]	Assessment of Status[102, 106, 107, 107a]	Comments
				USA[53]	UK[34]			
Zinc	Protein synthesis Control of differentiation	Enzyme cofactor "Zinc fingers" in DNA[108]	Growth ↓[30] Hair loss[35] Skin rash Immune function ↓[109]	15 mg	9.5 mg	3.2–6.5 mg	Plasma zinc* With albumin and C-reactive protein† Leukocyte zinc‡ Alkaline phosphatase* Hair zinc*	Plasma Zn falls in acute-phase reaction
Iron	O$_2$ transport Electron transport	Hemoglobin and myoglobin Cytochromes	Hypochromic anemia Possibly increased resistance to infection[110]	10 mg	8.7 mg	1.2 mg + blood transfusion as required	Serum iron or IBC* Serum ferritin with CRP† Bone marrow iron† Soluble transferrin receptor‡	Serum Fe falls and ferritin increases in APR—care needed not to exceed IBC
Copper	Collagen and elastin synthesis Antioxidant	Lysyl oxidase Zn and Cu superoxide dismutase Ceruloplasmin	Subperiosteal bleeding[111] Cardiac arrhythmia Anemia Neutropenia[112]	1.5–3 mg	1.2 mg	0.3–1.3 mg	Plasma copper or ceruloplasmin with CRP† Liver copper‡	Plasma Cu increases in acute-phase reaction

Element	Function	Biochemical role	Deficiency features				Tests for status	Comments
Selenium	Antioxidant Thyroid function Immune function	Glutathione peroxidase Tyrosine deiodinase[25] T lymphocyte receptor expression	Cardiomyopathy[21] Skeletal myopathy[19, 20] Nail abnormalities Macrocytosis[113] Neoplastic risk ↑	70 µg	75 µg	30–60 µg	Plasma Se† RBC glutathione peroxidase† Urine Se* Whole blood Se‡ Platelet glutathione peroxidase‡	Preillness Se status varies depending on total Se intake Se depletion may be asymptomatic
Manganese	Not clear Some antioxidant	Enzyme cofactor Mitochondrial superoxide dismutase	Cholesterol ↓[114] Red blood cells ↓ Possibly mucopolysaccharide abnormalities	2–5 mg	1.4 mg	0.2–0.3 mg	Plasma Mn‡ Whole blood Mn‡	Deficiency state not confirmed in humans
Chromium	Carbohydrate metabolism	Insulin activity Lipoprotein metabolism Gene expression	Glucose intolerance[115] Weight loss Peripheral neuropathy[116]	50–200 µg	>25 µg	10–20 µg	Plasma Cr‡ Glucose tolerance*	Contamination-free blood sampling required Cr is present as contaminant of most TPN solutions Rarely measured
Molybdenum	Amino acid metabolism Purine metabolism	Sulfite oxidase Xanthine oxidase	Intolerance to S amino acids:[117] Tachycardia Visual upset	75–250 µg	50–400 µg	19 µg	Urine xanthine‡ Hypoxanthine‡ Sulfite‡ Plasma Mo‡	
Iodine	Energy metabolism	Thyroid hormones	Hypothyroidism	150 µg	140 µg	131 µg	Serum T$_4$† Serum T$_3$† Serum TSH†	
Fluoride	Bone and tooth mineralization	Calcium fluorapatite	Dental caries	1.5–4.0 mg	0.05 mg/kg (infants)	0–0.95 mg	Urine excretion‡	Provision in nutritional support is controversial

*Test of little value in assessing status.
†Test widely available and clinically useful.
‡Good marker of status but of limited availability.
APR, acute-phase reaction; CRP, C-reactive protein; IBC, iron-binding capacity; RBC, red blood cell; TPN, total parenteral nutrition; TSH, thyroid-stimulating hormone.

Table 4–2. Essential Organic Micronutrients (Vitamins)

	Function(s)	Biochemical Modes of Action	Effects of Deficiency	Recommended Oral Intake (Men) USA[53]	Recommended Oral Intake (Men) UK[34]	IV Requirements or Recommendations per Day[102, 105, 118]	Assessment of Status[10, 102, 107a]	Comments
Vitamin A	Visual acuity Antioxidant Growth and development Immune function	Rhodopsin in retina[119] Free radical scavenger Induction of DNA transcription	Xerophthalmia[119] Night blindness[120] Increased risk of some neoplasms[4]	1000 µg	700 µg	1000 µg RE/day as retinol or retinol palmitate	Plasma retinol* Plasma retinol-binding protein* Liver biopsy retinol‡	Fall in retinol during acute-phase response due to fall in retinol-binding protein
Vitamin D	Calcium absorption Macrophage differentiation	Receptor-mediated transcription	Osteomalacia (adults) Rickets (children) Immune status ↓[121]	5 µg	—	5 µg as ergocalciferol	Serum Ca or P or alkaline phosphatase† Serum 25-hydroxyvitamin D† Rarely required, 1,25-dihydroxyvitamin D‡	
Vitamin E	Antioxidant in membranes	Free radical scavenger	Hemolytic anemia in infants[122] Central or peripheral neuropathy[123] Myopathy[124] Increased risk of atherosclerosis, certain neoplasias[4]	10 mg	>4 mg	10 mg as α-tocopherol equivalents	Plasma tocopherol or cholesterol† Hydrogen peroxide hemolysis‡	Vitamin E is transported in LDL
Vitamin K	Blood coagulation Bone calcification	γ-Glutamyl carboxylation Coagulation proteins and osteocalcin[16]	Bleeding disorders ? Bone disorders[17]	80 µg	1 µg/kg/day	150 µg	Prothrombin time† Plasma phylloquinone‡	Time-consuming assay Results should be expressed per mmol triglyceride
B₁ (thiamine)	Carbohydrate and fat metabolism	Decarboxylation reactions as TPP	Beriberi with neurologic, cardiac effects[125] Wernicke-Korsakoff syndrome[126] Immune function ↓[127]	1.2 mg	0.9 mg	3 mg	RBC transketolase† Blood thiamine† Urine thiamine or creatinine‡	Deficiency may occur and is reversed rapidly

B$_2$ (riboflavin)	Oxidative metabolism	Coenzyme as FAD or FMN	Lesions of lips, tongue, skin[128] Possibly immune function ↓[127]	1.4 mg	1.3 mg	3.6 mg	RBC glutathione reductase† Blood FAD‡ Urine riboflavin or creatinine†	
B$_6$ (pyridoxine)	Amino acid metabolism	Transamination reactions	Anemia (children) Lesions of lips and skin Premenstrual symptoms[129] Carpal tunnel syndrome	2 mg	1.4 mg	4 mg	RBC transaminase† Blood pyridoxal phosphate‡ Urine 4-pyridoxic acid‡	Less interference by disease than for transaminase
Niacin	Oxidative metabolism	Coenzyme as NAD or NADP	Pellagra—rash, weakness, diarrhea	15 mg	16 mg	40 mg	Urine N-methylnicotinamide‡ Blood niacin‡	Rarely measured
B$_{12}$	DNA metabolism	Recycling folate coenzymes Valine metabolism	Megaloblastic anemia Demyelination of neurons	2 μg	1.5 μg	5 μg	Serum vitamin B$_{12}$†	
Folate	Purine and pyrimidine metabolism	Single-carbon transfer	Megaloblastic anemia Growth retardation Pancytopenia[130] Hyperhomocysteinemia[131] Neural tube defects in pregnancy[132]	200 μg	200 μg	400 μg	Serum folate† RBC folate†	Recent intake Whole-body status
Biotin	Lipogenesis and gluconeogenesis	Carboxylase reactions	Scaly dermatitis[133] Hair loss	30–100 μg	10–200 μg	60 μg	Serum biotin‡ Urine biotin‡	Rarely assayed
Vitamin C (ascorbic acid)	Collagen synthesis Antioxidant Absorption of iron	OH proline and OH lysine synthesis Reduction reactions Fe^{3+}→Fe^{2+}	Scurvy Impaired wound healing ?Impaired immune function[134] ?Oxidative damage	60 mg	40 mg	100 mg	Leukocyte vitamin C‡ Plasma vitamin C*	Plasma vitamin falls in injury or infection

*Test of little value in assessing status.
†Test widely available and clinically useful.
‡Good marker of status but of limited availability.
FAD, flavin adenine dinucleotide; FMN, flavin mononucleotide; LDL, low-density lipoprotein; NAD, nicotinamide adenine dinucleotide; NADP, nicotinamide adenine dinucleotide phosphate; RBC, red blood cell; RE, retinol equivalents; TPP, thiamine pyrophosphate.

biologically active of which is all-*trans*-retinol. This compound is a primary alcohol with five conjugated bonds, all in the trans configuration. The vitamin A employed in parenteral nutrition (PN) multivitamin additives is usually an ester, acetate, or palmitate. Vitamin A esters are available in liquid form.

Stability in Parenteral Nutrition

Vitamin A is relatively stable after addition to PN mixtures provided that it is protected from light.[69] However, losses of vitamin A may be caused by sorption to the plastic container[70] and exposure to daylight.[71] Retinol acetate is relatively more lipophilic and migrates into polyvinyl chloride (PVC) film, accounting for up to a 30% loss during storage and administration if PVC-containing materials are used.[72] Possible losses to ethyl vinyl acetate (EVA) have not been evaluated. In contrast, retinol palmitate does not absorb to PVC, and no losses to plastic are observed during storage.[69, 73] Retinol is highly sensitive to ultraviolet radiation,[71] with exposure to daylight leading to rapid degradation by a photolytic reaction. Losses can amount to more than 90% during infusion in daylight conditions if no light-protecting precautions are taken.[72] However, because artificial light emits negligible ultraviolet radiation, retinol is unaffected by normal room lighting. The presence of fat emulsion provides substantial photoprotection in daylight.[74] Nonetheless, it is essential to cover the infusion container with light-protecting overwrap when infusing in daylight.

Vitamin D

Chemistry

Ergocalciferol (vitamin D_2) and cholecalciferol (D_3) have similar chemical sterol-like structures, differing only in the structure of the side chain. Ergocalciferol contains an unsaturated bond between C-22 and C-23 and an additional methyl group. Vitamins D_2 and D_3 are considered to be biologically equivalent in humans, and both are used in parenteral multivitamin products. Ergocalciferol and cholecalciferol consist of white powders and are usually solubilized in the fat emulsion.

Stability in Parenteral Nutrition

The stability of vitamin D in PN mixtures has received little attention. Gillis and colleagues reported significant losses in the delivery of vitamin D (cholecalciferol) from a non–fat-containing PN mixture in PVC bags during simulated administration using radiolabeled compound.[75] The authors speculated that these losses were as a result of binding to the bag and set. In contrast, Dahl and associates reported no losses during infusion in a fat emulsion.[76] Bioavailability studies in children have suggested that vitamin D status is maintained during long-term IVN.[77]

Vitamin E

Chemistry

Vitamin E activity can be identified in eight naturally occurring compounds, all comprising a six-chromanol ring structure. Four tocopherol isomers contain a phytol side chain, whereas four tocotrienols have similar side chains with three additional double bonds. The biologic activity of the tocopherol isomers, the usual artificial source of vitamin E, decreases over the sequence α to δ, although the extent varies depending on the assay of activity used.[78] α-Tocopherol, as the *d* or *dl* form, is an oily liquid, whereas the acetate or acid succinate esters are powders. The form usually in PN is *dl* α-tocopherol.

Stability in Parenteral Nutrition

After addition to PN mixtures, tocopherols are relatively stable during storage and also during administration, at least when protected from light or exposed only to fluorescent (artificial) light.[79] The presence of fat emulsion also appears to offer protection.[80]

Tocopherols are degraded by exposure to daylight (ultraviolet radiation), by a photooxidative reaction that requires the presence of oxygen. Therefore, the rate and extent of reaction vary in PN mixtures, depending on factors directly influencing the amount of dissolved oxygen. This probably accounts for the wide variations in chemical losses reported. Losses amounting to 30 to 50% during administration have been observed.[77, 79]

Vitamin K

Chemistry

Naturally occurring vitamin K_1, phytomenadione (phylloquinone), is a naphthoquinone-like compound in the all-trans isomer form. The synthetic derivative is a mixture of cis and trans isomers, but with not more than 20% of the former. Phytomenadione exists as an oily liquid and is therefore usually supplied in intravenous vitamin supplements. Fat emulsions for IVN also contain significant amounts of vitamin K_1.[81]

Stability in Parenteral Nutrition

Phytomenadione is stable in PN mixtures during storage in EVA bags for periods of at least 20 days at 4° C.[82] Some losses (between 5 and 17%) during infusion have been reported, probably due to daylight exposure that causes some photodegradation.[83]

Water-Soluble Vitamins

Biotin (Vitamin H)

Chemistry

Biotin has three asymmetric carbon atoms, making eight potential isomers. Only D-biotin possesses biologic activity. Biotin is a white powder that is only slightly soluble in water.

Stability in Parenteral Nutrition

Biotin is relatively stable in aqueous solution and is unaffected by weak oxidizing or reducing agents, heat, or normal light.[83] Information on the stability of biotin in PN mixtures is sparse. Only Dahl and associates report any data, which indicate that biotin is stable for at least 4 days at 2 to 8° C in the all-in-one mixture tested.[80] Indirect evidence from vitamin status studies suggests that blood biotin levels are maintained during long-term PN administration.[84]

Thiamine (Vitamin B₁)

Chemistry

Thiamine consists of a pyrimidine ring linked to thiazole by a methylene bridge. The hydrochloride salt is very soluble in water. Thiamine diphosphate (cocarboxylase), employed in some multivitamin additives, is the actual coenzyme form of vitamin B_1. Both consist of white powders. Solutions of thiamine diphosphate are less stable than those of thiamine hydrochloride because of their hydrolysis to thiamine monophosphate.[83]

Stability in Parenteral Nutrition

Thiamine is relatively stable in most PN mixtures.[69] However, thiamine is sensitive to strong reducing agents and in particular to bisulfite. Sodium bisulfite is still included in some commercial amino acid products, and therefore losses of thiamine can be expected when multivitamin additions are made to PN mixtures containing such amino acid preparations.[85] There is some loss of thiamine on exposure to sunlight but not to fluorescent light.[86] Degradation rates are such that losses may reduce the shelf-life to only 1 to 3 days,[86] depending on the final volume and therefore the concentration of bisulfite after compounding.[87]

Riboflavin (Vitamin B₂)

Chemistry

Riboflavin comprises an isoalloxazine ring attached to a ributyl side chain. It is an orange-yellow crystalline powder. Riboflavin is sparingly soluble in water, but the sodium phosphate salt is far more soluble and is used in PN. Riboflavin is stable in acid conditions but less stable in alkali.

Stability in Parenteral Nutrition

Studies suggest that riboflavin is stable in IVN mixtures during refrigerated storage. Greater than 80% of the riboflavin originally supplied remains after 8 weeks in a range of IVN mixtures.[88] Like most vitamins, riboflavin is sensitive to daylight, and significant losses have been reported during administration in daylight conditions, although these are substantially less than losses of vitamins A and E.[86]

Nicotinamide (Nicotinic Acid, Niacin)

Chemistry

Nicotinic acid is a 3-pyridinecarboxylic acid. Nicotinamide, the physiologically active compound, is the amide derivative. It can also be generated from tryptophan by biotransformation in the liver. Nicotinamide is a freely soluble white powder.

Stability in Parenteral Nutrition

Nicotinamide is one of the most stable vitamins and is insensitive to light or oxidizing or reducing agents.[83] This vitamin would therefore be expected to be stable after addition to PN mixtures, and this was confirmed over a 4-day period at least.[76]

Pyridoxine (Vitamin B₆)

Chemistry

Pyridoxine is the generic name for 3-hydroxy-2-methylpyridine derivatives with biologic activity, pyridoxine (alcohol), pyridoxal (aldehyde), and pyridoxamine (amine). The hydrochloride salt is freely soluble and stable in water.

Stability in Parenteral Nutrition

Pyridoxine is a relatively stable compound. Dahl and coworkers reported that pyridoxine was stable for at least 4 days at 20° C in PN mixtures,[76] and the relative stability has been confirmed over 8 weeks of storage in PN mixtures at 5° C.[88] Pyridoxine exhibits sensitivity to direct sunlight but is relatively insensitive to indirect daylight and is not degraded by artificial light exposure.[89]

Cyanocobalamin (Vitamin B₁₂)

Chemistry

Cyanocobalamin is a complex molecule, comprising four pyrrole groups joined in a large ring containing six conjugated double bonds. A cobalt atom is attached to a cyanide group and linked to a nitrogen of 5,6-dimethylbenzamidazole. This red crystalline compound is only poorly soluble in water.

Stability in Parenteral Nutrition

Cyanocobalamin is relatively stable in solution, although it may be sensitive to strong light. The only data available suggest that the vitamin is also stable in PN mixtures, at least for 4 days.[76]

Ascorbic Acid (Vitamin C)

Chemistry

Ascorbic acid is a hexose-like compound, comprising an almost-planar five-membered ring, with four possible stereoisomers. The biologically active form consists of L(+)-ascorbic acid. It is water soluble but relatively unstable in solution because of its rapid oxidation.[90]

Stability in Parenteral Nutrition

Ascorbic acid is the least stable vitamin in solution.[88] The compound reacts directly with oxygen to form dehydroascorbic acid, this reaction being catalyzed by heavy metals, in particular copper and iron.[90] This in turn is rapidly hydrolyzed to 2,3-diketogulonic acid. The final stage of the degradation pathway leads to oxalate formation.

Both the rate and the extent of losses of ascorbic acid in PN mixtures after compounding depend on a number of factors, most of which relate to the quantity of oxygen present or entering the mixture during storage and administration.[91] These include the volumes of dextrose and other infusions, but not the amino acid or fat emulsion volumes (which are essentially oxygen-free), the nature of the filling process used during compounding, the head space remaining after filling, the nature of the amino acids (some products contain reducing agents that compete for oxygen, thus reducing ascorbate degradation), and the type of bag used. Since multilayered bags are largely impermeable to oxygen under normal conditions, losses due to this process are prevented, and mixtures prepared in such containers may be assigned extended shelf-lives.[92] In summary, some loss of ascorbic acid after addition to a PN mixture is inevitable, and the reaction with dissolved oxygen is complete in 6 to 24 hours. This usually accounts for a loss of at least 50 mg in a standard adult PN mixture. Some further losses also occur during administration. PN mixtures filled into EVA bags should be infused within 2 to 3 days of compounding, although most mixtures in multilayered bags can be assigned shelf-lives of beyond 7 days.[92]

Pantothenic Acid (Vitamin B₅)

Chemistry

Pantothenic acid is an amide consisting of pantoic acid joined to β-alanine by a peptide bond. Only the D(+) enantiomer is biologically active. It consists of a viscous liquid, soluble in water but unstable in solution. It is usually used as the alcohol form, D-pantothenyl alcohol (dexpanthenol).

Stability in Parenteral Nutrition

Pantothenic acid is expected to be relatively stable in neutral solutions. Only one report describes the stability of pantothenic acid in PN mixtures. Dahl and colleagues have shown that the vitamin is stable for at least 4 days when stored at 2 to 8° C.[76]

Folic Acid (Pteroylglutamic Acid)

Chemistry

Folic acid consists of pteridine linked through a methylene bridge to *p*-aminobenzoic acid, which is linked as an amide to glutamic acid. Folic acid is a yellowish crystalline powder that is poorly soluble in water. The addition of sodium hydroxide causes the formation of the soluble disodium salt, but the insoluble free acid is formed below approximately pH 7.

Stability in Parenteral Nutrition

Folic acid can be degraded by reducing agents (for example, ascorbic acid), hydrolysis, and light.[83] Riboflavin also has adverse effects on stability. It is therefore not surprising that the stability of folic acid in PN mixtures remains poorly defined. Conflicting reports have been published, indicating poor chemical stability[93] and the possibility of absorption to the container walls, but in some studies extended excellent chemical stability during storage was found.[94] Available evidence indicates that folic acid is probably relatively stable in most PN mixtures.[88]

Trace Elements

Stability in Parenteral Nutrition

Trace elements are added to PN mixtures in relatively small amounts, and the final concentrations are consequently of a very low order.

As trace elements are usually supplied as inorganic salts, with the possible exception of iron (one form used is iron dextran), in practice their addition to PN mixtures is unlikely to cause their loss of stability. One possible exception to this is iodine. However, some trace elements could interact with specific PN mixture components, causing physical incompatibilities to develop and resulting in precipitates. Some specific examples have been identified in the literature, involving in particular copper and iron.

Some amino acid formulations contain cysteine, which can partially degrade during sterilization to produce small amounts of hydrogen sulfide.[95, 96] After the addition of trace elements, insoluble copper sulfide precipitates. Because hydrogen sulfide is a gas, the precipitate is more likely in reduced–gas-permeable multilayered "big bags."[96]

Iron phosphate precipitates have been reported in high-phosphate-containing regimens after storage for periods greater than a few days.[97] This precipitate can be prevented by formulating mixtures with vitamins in multilayered bags.[98]

The reduction of selenite to elemental selenium by high concentrations of ascorbic acid has been proposed,[99] but this is unlikely to occur in clinical practice, since it occurs only in acid solution.[100]

◆ PROVISION OF MICRONUTRIENTS IN INTRAVENOUS NUTRITION

Micronutrient requirements can generally be obtained from commercially available mixtures designed for intravenous use. The composition of these additives has changed over the years with increased understanding of trace elements and vitamin requirements. The availability of these has, however, been erratic because of supply problems and in some countries because of a lack of licensing and/or marketing agreements. Where supply problems exist, it is necessary to try to arrange either for suitable, safe, local production or for an oral or enteral preparation to be attempted in the short term.

SUMMARY

The provision of adequate amounts of vitamins and trace elements involves more than just the prevention of clinical deficiency states. An inadequate supply may lead to subclinical, yet important, effects that may have long-lasting consequences to health—for example, free radical damage or failure or delay of tissue repair. An adequate intake is therefore necessary in all patients requiring IVN. Parenteral preparations are now available with well-balanced amounts of all essential vitamins and trace elements.

However, since the doses of these micronutrients are rarely adjusted in adult patients receiving IVN, additional amounts of one micronutrient, or indeed all micronutrients, may be required.

A knowledge of the stability of micronutrients when mixed with the other components of an IVN regimen, and of the effects of the type of container and conditions of storage, is essential in ensuring that patients actually receive the micronutrients they require.

Controversy exists regarding whether the provision of larger amounts of individual micronutrients will improve outcomes, particularly for those micronutrients known to affect the free radical scavenging mechanisms or immune function. Controlled clinical trials of different amounts of micronutrients in different diseases are required, in both short- and long-term studies and by both enteral and intravenous routes. Such studies should relate outcomes to the best available markers of micronutrient status. This should ultimately lead to the better matching of nutritional provision to the patient's requirements.

REFERENCES

1. Shenkin A: Micronutrients. *In* Rombeau JL, Rolandelli RH (eds): Enteral and Tube Feeding, 3rd ed. Philadelphia, WB Saunders, 1997, pp 96–111.
2. Shils ME, Olson JA, Shike M, Ross AC: Modern Nutrition in Health and Disease, 9th ed. Baltimore, Williams & Wilkins, 1999.
3. O'Dell BL, Sunde RA: Handbook of Nutritionally Essential Mineral Elements. New York, Marcel Dekker, 1997.
4. Gaby SK, Bendich A, Singh VN, Machlin LJ: Vitamin Intake and Health—A Scientific Review. New York, Marcel Dekker, 1991, pp 1–217.
5. Sauberlich HE, Machlin LJ: Beyond deficiency. New views on the function and health effects of vitamins. Ann N Y Acad Sci 669:1–404, 1992.
6. Heimburger DC: Localized deficiencies of folic acid in aerodigestive tissues. Ann N Y Acad Sci 669:87–96, 1992.
7. Biesalski HK, Stofft E: Biochemical, morphological and functional aspects of systemic and local vitamin A deficiency in the respiratory tract. Ann N Y Acad Sci 669:325–331, 1992.
8. Cruickshank AM, Telfer ABM, Shenkin A: Thiamine deficiency in the critically ill. Intensive Care Med 14:384–387, 1988.
9. Shenkin SD, Cruickshank AM, Shenkin A: Subclinical riboflavin deficiency is associated with outcome of seriously ill patients. Clin Nutr 8:269–271, 1989.
10. Fidanza F, Brubacher GB: Vitamin nutritive methodology. *In* Fidanza F (ed): Nutritional Status Assessment. London, Chapman & Hall, 1991, pp 186–191.
11. Nakasaki H, Ohta M, Soeda J, et al: Clinical and biochemical aspects of thiamine treatment for metabolic acidosis during total parenteral nutrition. Nutrition 13:110–117, 1997.
12. Carlin A, Walker WA: Rapid development of vitamin K deficiency in an adolescent boy receiving total parenteral nutrition following bone marrow transplantation. Nutr Rev 49:179–183, 1991.
13. Dreosti IE: The physiological biochemistry and antioxidant activity of the trace elements copper, manganese, selenium and zinc. Clin Biochem Rev 12:127–129, 1991.
14. Halliwell B, Gutteridge JMC: Free Radicals in Biology and Medicine, 2nd ed. Oxford, Clarendon Press, 1989.
15. Williams RJP: An introduction to the biochemistry of zinc. *In* Mills CF (ed): Zinc in Human Biology. London, Springer-Verlag, 1989, pp 15–31.
16. Shearer MJ: Vitamin K metabolism and nutriture. Blood Rev 6:92–104, 1992.
17. Vermeer C, Knapen MHJ, Jie K-SG, Grobbee DE: Physiological importance of extra hepatic vitamin-K dependent carboxylation reactions. Ann N Y Acad Sci 669:21–33, 1992.
18. Diplock AT: Metabolic and functional defects in selenium deficiency. Philos Trans R Soc Lond 294:105–117, 1981.
19. Mansell PI, Rawlings J, Allison SP, et al: Reversal of skeletal myopathy with selenium supplementation in a patient on home parenteral nutrition. Clin Nutr 6:179–183, 1987.
20. Van Rij AM, Thompson CD, McKenzie JM, Robinson MF: Selenium deficiency in total parenteral nutrition. Am J Clin Nutr 32:2076–2085, 1979.
21. Johnson RA, Baker SS, Fallon JT, et al: An occidental case of cardiomyopathy and selenium deficiency. N Engl J Med 304:1210–1212, 1981.
22. Shenkin A, Fell GS, Halls DJ, et al: Essential trace element provision to patients receiving home intravenous nutrition in the United Kingdom. Clin Nutr 5:91–97, 1986.
23. Beck M, Shi Q, Morris VC, Levander OA: Rapid genomic evolution of a non-virulent Coxsackie virus B$_3$ in selenium deficient mice results in selection of identical isolates. Nat Med 1:433–436, 1995.
24. Combs GF, Combs SB: Biochemical functions of selenium. *In* The Role of Selenium in Nutrition. London, Academic Press, 1986, pp 205–263.
25. Arthur JR, Nicol F, Beckett GJ: Selenium deficiency, thyroid hormone metabolism, and thyroid hormone deiodinases. Am J Clin Nutr 57(Suppl):236S–239S, 1993.
26. Vanderpas JB, Contempre B, Duale NL, et al: Selenium deficiency mitigates hypothyroxinemia in iodine-deficient subjects. Am J Clin Nutr 57:271S–275S, 1993.
27. Clark AJ, Mossholder S, Gates R: Folinic status in adolescent females. Am J Clin Nutr 46:302–306, 1987.

28. Sumner SK, Liebman M, Wakefield LM: Vitamin A status of adolescent girls. Nutr Rep Int 35:423–431, 1987.

29. Chandra RK: Effect of vitamin and trace element supplementation on immune response and infection in elderly subjects. Lancet 340:1124–1127, 1992.

30. Aggett PJ: Severe zinc deficiency. In Mills CF (ed): Zinc in Human Biology. London, Springer-Verlag, 1989, pp 259–279.

31. Kallner AB, Hartmann D, Hornig DH: On the requirements of ascorbic acid in man: Steady state turnover and body pool in smokers. Am J Clin Nutr 34:1347–1355, 1981.

32. Stryker WS, Kaplan LA, Stein EA, et al: The relation of diet, cigarette smoking, and alcohol consumption to plasma β carotene and α-tocopherol levels. Am J Epidemiol 127:283–296, 1988.

33. Solomons NW, Pideda O, Viteri F, Standstead HH: Studies in the bioavailability of zinc in humans: Mechanisms of the intestinal interactions of nonheme iron and zinc. J Nutr 113:337–349, 1983.

34. Panel of Dietary Reference Values, Department of Health: Dietary Reference Values for Food Energy and Nutrients for the United Kingdom. London, HMSO, 1991.

35. Kay RG, Tasman-Jones C, Pybus J, et al: A syndrome of acute zinc deficiency during total parenteral alimentation in man. Ann Surg 183:331–340, 1976.

36. Kopple JD: Renal disorders and nutrition. In Shils ME, Olson JA, Shike M, Ross AC (eds): Modern Nutrition in Health and Disease, 9th ed. Baltimore, Williams & Wilkins, 1999, pp 1439–1472.

37. Berger MM, Cavadini C, Bart A, et al: Cutaneous copper and zinc losses in burns. Burns 18:373–380, 1992.

38. Berger MM, Cavadini C, Bart A, et al: Selenium losses in 10 burned patients. Clin Nutr 11:75–82, 1992.

39. Berger MM, Cavadini C, Chiolero R, et al: Influence of large intakes of trace elements on recovery after major burns. Nutrition 10:327–334, 1994.

40. Berger MM, Spertini F, Shenkin A, et al: Trace element supplementation modulates pulmonary infection rates after major burns: A double-blind, placebo-controlled trial. Am J Clin Nutr 68:365–371, 1998.

41. Tasman-Jones C, Kay RG, Lee SP: Zinc and copper deficiency with particular reference to parenteral nutrition. Surg Annu 10:23–52, 1978.

42. Furst P: The role of antioxidants in nutritional support. Proc Nutr Soc 55:945–961, 1996.

43. Niederau C, Niederau M, Borchard F, et al: Effects of antioxidants and free radical scavengers in three different models of acute pancreatitis. Pancreas 7:486–496, 1992.

44. Schulz HU, Niederau C: Oxidative stress–induced changes in pancreatic acinar cells: Insights from in vitro studies. Hepatogastroenterology 41:309–312, 1994.

45. Schoenberg MH, Buchler M, Younes M, et al: Effect of antioxidant treatment in rats with acute hemorrhagic pancreatitis. Dig Dis Sci 39:1034–1040, 1994.

46. McCloy R: Chronic pancreatitis at Manchester, UK. Digestion 59(Suppl 4):36–48, 1998.

46a. Ward M, McNulty H, McPartlin J, et al: Plasma homocysteine, a risk factor for cardiovascular disease, is lowered by physiological doses of folic acid. Q J Med 90:519–524, 1997.

47. Prasad AS, Fitzgerald JT, Hess JW, et al: Zinc deficiency in elderly patients. Nutrition 9:218–224, 1993.

48. Brignola C, Belloli C, De-Simone G, et al: Zinc supplementation restores plasma concentrations of zinc and thymulin in patients with Crohn's disease. Aliment Pharmacol Ther 7:275–280, 1993.

49. Glasziou PP, Mackerras DEM: Vitamin A supplementation in infectious diseases; a meta-analysis. BMJ 306:366–370, 1989.

50. Meydani SN, Hayek M, Coleman L: Influence of vitamin E and B₆ on immune response. Ann N Y Acad Sci 669:125–140, 1992.

51. Kiremidjian-Schumacher L, Roy M, Wishe HI, et al: Supplementation with selenium and human immune cell functions—Effect on cytotoxic lymphocytes and natural killer cells. Biol Trace Elem Res 41:115–127, 1994.

52. Roy M, Kiremidjian-Schumacher L, Wishe HI, et al: Supplementation with selenium and human immune cell functions—Effect on lymphocyte proliferation and interleukin 2 receptor expression. Biol Trace Elem Res 41:103–114, 1994.

53. Food and Nutrition Board, National Research Council: Recommended Dietary Allowances, 10th ed. Washington, DC, National Academy Press, 1989.

54. Verhage A, Cheong WK, Allard JP, Jeejeebhoy KN: Increase in lumbar spine bone mineral content in patients on long-term parenteral nutrition without vitamin D supplementation. JPEN J Parenter Enteral Nutr 19:431–436, 1995.

55. Klein GL: Metabolic bone disease of total parenteral nutrition. Nutrition 14:149–152, 1998.

56. Gleghorn EE, Eisenberg LD, Hack S, et al: Observations of vitamin A toxicity in three patients with renal failure receiving parenteral alimentation. Am J Clin Nutr 44:107–112, 1986.

57. Fell JME, Reynolds AP, Meadows N, et al: Manganese toxicity in children receiving long term parenteral nutrition. Lancet 347:1218–1221, 1996.

58. Reynolds N, Blumsohn A, Baxter JP, et al: Manganese requirement and toxicity in patients on home parenteral nutrition. Clin Nutr 17:227–230, 1998.

59. Shenkin A: Trace elements and inflammatory response: Implications for nutritional support. Nutrition 11:100–105, 1995.

60. Schroeder JJ, Cousins RJ: Interleukin 6 regulates metallothionein gene expression and zinc metabolism in hepatocyte monolayer cultures. Proc Nat Acad Sci U S A 87:3137–3141, 1990.

61. Konijn AM, Carmel N, Levy R, Hershko C: Ferritin synthesis in inflammation. II: Mechanisms of increased ferritin synthesis. Br J Haematol 49:361–370, 1981.

62. Fraser WD, Taggart DP, Fell GS, et al: Changes in iron, zinc and copper concentrations in serum and in their binding to transport proteins after cholecystectomy and cardiac surgery. Clin Chem 35:2243–2247, 1989.

63. Fleck A: Plasma proteins as nutritional indicators in the perioperative period. Br J Clin Pract 42(Suppl 63):20–24, 1988.

64. Olson JA: New approaches to methods for the assessment of nutritional status of the individual. Am J Clin Nutr 36:1160–1168, 1982.

65. Malone M, Shenkin A, Fell GS, Irving MH: Evaluation of a trace element preparation in patients receiving home intravenous nutrition. Clin Nutr 8:307–312, 1989.

66. Louw JA, Werbeck A, Louw MEJ, et al: Blood vitamin concentrations during the acute phase response. Crit Care Med 20:934–937, 1992.

67. Goode HF, Kelleher J, Walker BE: The effects of acute infection on indices of zinc status. Clin Nutr 10:55–59, 1991.

68. Schorah CJ, Habibzadeh N, Hancock M, et al: Changes in plasma and buffy layer vitamin C concentration following major surgery: What do they reflect? Ann Clin Biochem 23:566–570, 1986.

69. Allwood MC: Stability of vitamins in TPN solutions in 3 litre bags. Br J Intraven Ther 3:22–26, 1982.

70. Moorhatch P, Chiou WL: Interactions between drugs and plastic intravenous fluid bags. 1: Sorption studies on 17 drugs. Am J Hosp Pharm 31:72–78, 1974.

71. Allwood MC, Plane JH: The wavelength-dependent degradation of vitamin A exposed to ultraviolet light. Int J Pharmaceutics 31:1–7, 1986.

72. Howard L, Ohu R, Feman S, et al: Vitamin A deficiency from long-term parenteral nutrition. Ann Intern Med 93:576–577, 1980.

73. Billion-Rey F, Guillaumont M, Frederich A, Aulanger G: Stability of fat-soluble vitamins A (retinol palmitate), E (tocopherol acetate) and K₁ (phylloquinone) in total parenteral nutrition at home. JPEN J Parenter Enteral Nutr 17:56–60, 1993.

74. Smith JH, Canham JE, Wells PA: Effect of phototherapy light, sodium bisulfite, and pH on vitamin stability in total parenteral nutrition admixtures. JPEN J Parenter Enteral Nutr 12:394–402, 1988.

75. Gillis J, Jones G, Penchary P: Delivery of vitamins A, D and E in total parenteral nutrition solutions. JPEN J Parenter Enteral Nutr 7:11–14, 1983.

76. Dahl GB, Jeppson RI, Tengborn HJ: Vitamin stability in a TPN mixture stored in an EVA plastic bag. J Clin Hosp Pharm 11:271–279, 1986.

77. Davis AT, Franz FP, Coutney DA, et al: Plasma vitamin and mineral status in home parenteral nutrition patients. JPEN J Parenter Enteral Nutr 11:480–485, 1987.

78. Traber MG: Vitamin E. *In* Shils ME, Olson JA, Shike M, Ross AC (eds): Modern Nutrition in Health and Disease, 9th ed. Baltimore, Williams & Wilkins, 1999, pp 347–362.

79. McGee CD, Mascarwnhas MG, Ostro MJM, et al: Selenium and vitamin E stability in parenteral solutions. JPEN J Parenter Enteral Nutr 5:568–570, 1985.

80. Dahl GB, Svensson L, Kinnander NJG, et al: Stability of vitamins in soybean oil fat emulsion under conditions simulating intravenous feeding of neonates and children. JPEN J Parenter Enteral Nutr 18:234–239, 1994.

81. Lennon C, Davidson KW, Sadowski JA, Mason JB: The vitamin K content of intravenous lipid emulsions. JPEN J Parenter Enteral Nutr 17:142–144, 1993.

82. Schmutz CW, Martinelli E, Muhlebach S: Stability of vitamin K assessed by HPLC in total parenteral nutrition. Clin Nutr 12(Suppl):169, 1992.

83. Buhler V: Vademecum for Vitamin Formulations. Stuttgart, Wissenschaftliche Verlagsgesellschaft, 1988.

84. Hariz MB, De Potter S, Carriol O, et al: Home parenteral nutrition in children: Bioavailability of vitamins in binary mixtures for 8 days. Clin Nutr 12:147–152, 1993.

85. Bowman B, Nguyen P: Stability of thiamine in parenteral nutrition solutions. JPEN J Parenter Enteral Nutr 7:567–568, 1983.

86. Smith JL, Canham JE, Kirkland WD, Wells PA: Effect of intralipid, amino acids, container, temperature and duration of storage on vitamin stability in total parenteral nutrition admixtures. JPEN J Parenter Enteral Nutr 12:478–483, 1988.

87. Kearney MCJ, Allwood MC, Hardy G: The stability of thiamine in TPN mixtures stored in EVA and multilayered bags. Clin Nutr 14:295–301, 1995.

88. Allwood MC, Kearney MCJ: Compatibility and stability of additives in parenteral nutrition admixtures. Nutrition 14:697–706, 1998.

89. Chen MF, Boyce W, Triplett L: Stability of B vitamins in mixed parenteral nutrition solution. JPEN J Parenter Enteral Nutr 7:462–464, 1983.

90. Davies MB, Austin J, Partridge DA: Vitamin C: Its Chemistry and Biochemistry. Royal Society of Chemistry paperback. Letchworth, England, Royal Society of Chemistry, 1991.

91. Allwood MC: Factors influencing the stability of ascorbic acid in total parenteral nutrition infusion. J Clin Hosp Pharm 9:75–85, 1984.

92. Allwood MC, Brown PE, Ghedini C, Hardy G: The stability of ascorbic acid in TPN mixtures stored in a multilayered bag. Clin Nutr 11:284–288, 1992.

93. Nordfjeld K, Pederson JL, Rasmussen M, Jensen VG: Storage of mixtures for parenteral nutrition. III: Stability of vitamins in TPN mixtures. J Clin Hosp Pharm 9:293–301, 1984.

94. Barker A, Hebron BS, Beck PR, Ellis B: Folic acid and total parenteral nutrition. JPEN J Parenter Enteral Nutr 8:3–13, 1984.

95. Bates CG, Greiner G, Gegenheimer A: Precipitate in admixtures of new amino acid injection. Am J Hosp Pharm 41:1316, 1984.

96. Chatterji DC, Kapoo J: Precipitate in admixtures of new amino acid injection [Reply]. Am J Hosp Pharm 41:1316–1317, 1984.

97. Wan KK, Tsallas G: Dilute iron dextran formulation for addition to parenteral nutrient solutions. Am J Hosp Pharm 37:206–210, 1980.

98. Allwood MC, Martin HM, Greenwood M, Maunder M: Precipitation of trace elements in parenteral nutrition mixtures. Clin Nutr 17:223–226, 1998.

99. Levander OA: Considerations in the design of selenium bioavailability studies. Fed Proc 42:1721–1725, 1983.

100. Ganther HE, Kraus RJ: Chemical stability of selenious acid in total parenteral nutrition solutions containing ascorbic acid. JPEN J Parenter Enteral Nutr 13:185–188, 1989.

101. Jacobson S, Wester PO: Balance study of twenty trace elements during total parenteral nutrition in man. Br J Nutr 37:107–126, 1977.

102. Shenkin A: Clinical aspects of vitamin and trace element metabolism. Baillieres Clin Gastroenterol 2:765–798, 1988.

103. American Medical Association: Guidelines for essential trace element preparations for parenteral use. JAMA 241:2051–2054, 1979.

104. American Medical Association, Department of

Food and Nutrition: Working conference on parenteral trace elements. Bull N Y Acad Med
60:1115–1212, 1984.

105. Shils ME, Brown RO: Parenteral nutrition. *In*
Shils ME, Olson JA, Shike M, Ross AC (eds): Modern Nutrition in Health and Disease, 9th ed. Baltimore, Williams & Wilkins, 1999, pp 1657–1688.

106. Fidanza F: Nutritional Status Assessment. London, Chapman & Hall, 1991.

107. O'Dell BL, Sunde RA: Handbook of Nutritionally
Essential Mineral Elements. New York, Marcel
Dekker, 1997.

107a. Sauberlich HE: Laboratory Tests for the Assessment of Nutritional Status, 2nd ed. Boca Raton,
CRC Press, 1999.

108. Klug A, Rhodes D: Zinc fingers. Trends Biochem
Sci 121:464–469, 1987.

109. Fraker PJ, Gershwin ME, Good RA, Prasad AS:
Interrelationship between zinc and immune function. Fed Proc 45:1474–1479, 1986.

110. Weinberg EB: Iron and infection. Microbiol Rev
42:45–66, 1978.

111. Karpel JT, Peden VH: Copper deficiency in long-
term parenteral nutrition. J Pediatr 80:32–36,
1972.

112. Dunlap WM, James GW, Hume DM: Anaemia and
neutropenia caused by copper deficiency. Ann Intern Med 80:470–476, 1974.

113. Vinton N, Dahlstrom K, Strobel C, Ament M: Macrocytosis and pseudoalbinism: Manifestations of
selenium deficiency. J Paediatr 111:711–717,
1988.

114. Friedman BJ, Freeland-Graves JH, Bales CW, et al:
Manganese balance and clinical observations in
young men fed a manganese deficient diet. J Nutr
117:133–143, 1987.

115. Offenbacher EG, Pi-Sunger FX, Stroecker BJ: Chromium. *In* O'Dell BC, Sunde RA (eds): Handbook
of Nutritionally Essential Mineral Elements. New
York, Marcel Dekker, 1997, pp 389–412.

116. Jeejeebhoy KN, Chu RC, Marliss EB, et al: Chromium deficiency, glucose intolerance and neuropathy reversed by chromium supplementation in a
patient receiving long-term parenteral nutrition.
Am J Clin Nutr 30:531–538, 1977.

117. Abumrad NN, Schneider AJ, Steel D, Rogers LS:
Amino acid intolerance reversed by molybdate
therapy. Am J Clin Nutr 34:2551–2559, 1981.

118. American Medical Association, Department of
Food and Nutrition: Multivitamin preparations
for parenteral use: A statement by the Nutrition
Advisory Group. JPEN J Parenter Enteral Nutr
3:258–265, 1979.

119. Watson NJ, Hutchinson CH, Atta HR: Vitamin A
deficiency and xerophthalmia in the United Kingdom. BMJ 310:1050–1051, 1995.

120. Main ANH, Mills PR, Russell RI, et al: Vitamin A
deficiency in Crohn's disease. Gut 24:1169–1175,
1983.

121. Manolagas SC, Hustmeyer FG, Yu XP: 1,25 dihydroxy vitamin D_3 and the immune system. Proc
Soc Exp Biol Med 191:238–245, 1989.

122. Ritchie JH, Fish MB, Mc Masters V, et al: Edema
and hemolytic anemia in premature infants: A
vitamin E deficiency syndrome. N Engl J Med
279:1185–1190, 1968.

123. Howard L, Oversen L, Satya-Marti S, Chu R: Reversible neurological symptoms caused by vitamin E deficiency in a patient with short bowel
syndrome. Am J Clin Nutr 36:1243–1249, 1982.

124. Bieri JG, Farrell PM: Vitamin E. Vitam Horm
34:31–75, 1976.

125. La Selve P, Demolin P, Holzapfel L, et al: Shoshin
beriberi: An unusual complication of prolonged
parenteral nutrition. JPEN J Parenter Enteral Nutr
10:102–103, 1986.

126. Nadel AM, Burger PC: Wernicke encephalopathy
following prolonged intravenous therapy. JAMA
235:2403–2405, 1976.

127. Chandra RK: Immunology of nutritional disorders. London, Edward Arnold, 1980, pp 1–110.

128. Duhamel JF, Ricour C, Dufier JL, et al: Deficit en
vitamin B_2 et nutrition parenteral exclusive. Arch
Fr Pediatr 36:342–346, 1979.

129. Gaby SK: Vitamin B_6. *In* Gaby SK, Bendich A,
Singh VN, Machlin LJ (eds): Vitamin Intake and
Health. New York, Marcel Dekker, 1991, pp 163–
174.

130. Tennant GB, Smith RC, Leinster SJ, et al: Amino
acid infusion induced depression of serum folate
after cholecystectomy. Scand J Haematol 27:333–
338, 1981.

131. Naurath HJ, Joosten E, Riezler R, et al: Effects of
vitamin B_{12}, folate and vitamin B_6 supplements in
elderly people with normal serum vitamin concentrations. Lancet 346:85–89, 1995.

132. Czeizel AE, Dudas I: Prevention of the first occurrence of neural-tube defects by periconceptional
vitamin supplementation. N Engl J Med 327:1832–
1835, 1992.

133. Innis SM, Allardyce DB: Possible biotin deficiency in adults receiving long-term total parenteral nutrition. Am J Clin Nutr 37:185–187, 1983.

134. Gaby SK, Singh VN: Vitamin C. *In* Gaby SK, Ben-
dich A, Singh VN, Machlin LJ (eds): Intake and
Health—A Scientific Review. New York, Marcel
Dekker, 1991, pp 103–161.

5

◆ Metabolic Assessment

Elaine B. Trujillo, M.S., R.D.
Glenn M. Chertow, M.D., M.P.H.
Danny O. Jacobs, M.D., M.P.H.

As emphasized in a 1997 consensus review of clinical practice, the field of nutritional support is based on the tenets that nutrient depletion increases morbidity and mortality and that the prevention or correction of nutrient deficiencies can minimize or eliminate the adverse effects of malnourishment.[1] In consideration of these principles, the primary goals of nutritional support, therefore, have been to (1) identify patients who have, or are likely to develop, protein-energy or other nutrient deficiencies; (2) quantify the risk that the patients will develop complications related to these nutritional deficiencies; and (3) monitor the patients' response to nutritional therapy and assess its efficacy.

Nutritional assessment techniques were historically based on tests for changes in body composition. The purpose of these tests was to identify malnourished patients and to monitor their response to refeeding. Therefore, changes in body composition were traditionally assessed by measuring changes in body anthropometry, nitrogen balance, and circulating concentrations of various hepatic secretory proteins, including albumin and transferrin.

However, it is now clear that for most critically ill patients, the administration of parenteral or enteral nutrition over the course of their hospitalization does not significantly alter body composition. As the resources of most hospitals are increasingly absorbed in the care of the critically ill, the assessment of chronic deficits or long-term responses is becoming far less urgent and, as some argue, probably less important. Furthermore, at least in the case of parenteral nutritional support, it is clear that the risks of using the therapy in unselected patients may outweigh its benefits. Despite the nature of the discussion that follows, it is important to note that these observations do not negate the ultimate association between malnutrition and outcome and, therefore, the indication for nutritional support for many patients during their hospital stays.

These issues were highlighted in a 1993 report by Sandstrom and colleagues,[2] and their observations are echoed in reports by Brennan and coworkers.[3, 4] Sandstrom and colleagues reported a prospective study of 300 unselected patients randomized to receive total parenteral nutrition (TPN) or peripheral hydration providing 250 to 300 g of dextrose daily. Sixty percent of their patients were able to eat within 9 days after operation. Furthermore, the administration of peripheral hydration solutions alone for *more than 14 days* was associated with increased mortality. However, 20% of the patients who received TPN *and who could not be identified by standard preoperative evaluation* also had higher mortality rates compared with patients who received peripheral hydration for less than 14 days, although this difference did not reach statistical significance. Based on their findings, the authors concluded that

1. For most surgical patients, semistarvation does not adversely affect the clinical outcome.
2. Undernutrition imposes different kinds of complications than TPN.
3. Whereas "inadequate" nutritional support is associated with increased morbidity and mortality, overfeeding may currently pose the greatest threat to hospitalized patients.
4. Although TPN is clearly lifesaving in 20% of unselected patients, these individuals are difficult to identify preoperatively.

The importance of patient selection and monitoring is also highlighted in a meta-analysis.[5] The authors collated data from 26 randomized trials of 2211 critically ill patients reported in the literature between

1980 and 1998. In these studies, TPN was compared with standard care, which was the use of intravenous dextrose in peripheral hydration solutions along with oral diet. Their analyses revealed that the administration of TPN had no effect on mortality but did *tend* to lower complication rates—the latter was not significant at the chosen significance level of .05. Several a priori hypotheses that are highly relevant to this discussion were also evaluated in specific patient groups. The hypothesis testing of these subsets suggested that (1) malnourished patients who received TPN had fewer complications but no differences in mortality and (2) the relative risk of morbidity or mortality (more complications and higher death rates) was incrementally increased in critically ill nonsurgical patients.

These reports and others lend credence to a theoretical construct that is displayed graphically in Figure 5–1. In this depiction, the large, curved arrow represents the risk of morbidity or mortality that can be attributed to malnutrition. The left-hand y-axis represents the relative risk of a poor outcome. In the family of malnutrition risk curves that can be drawn, all would show a positive correlation between time in days and the likelihood of adverse events. However, the conceptual framework allows curves with significantly greater slopes, for example, for patients with elevated energy expenditures or those who enter the hospital with pre-existing malnutrition. Two hori-

zontal bars are depicted that relate to the y-axis on the right. These bars represent the risks associated with providing parenteral or enteral alimentation, that is, the risk of the therapies themselves. In both instances, it is assumed that parenteral or enteral feeding is provided at levels sufficient to meet the patient's metabolic requirements.

The bulk of current evidence suggests that there is an increased morbidity secondary to the administration of parenteral alimentation for many, if not most, hospitalized patients—including those who have recently undergone major operative procedures. The gray band represents the uncertainty of the magnitude of this risk. However, barring the development of organ dysfunction that might complicate the delivery of parenteral nutritional support or problems that would make central venous access more difficult—for example, sepsis, thrombocytopenia, or coagulopathy—the risk of parenteral alimentation can be assumed to be constant or near-constant.

Current opinion suggests that in the absence of aspiration, problems related to tube placement such as sinusitis, or, rarely, tube feeding–induced intestinal necrosis (that is, if the gastrointestinal tract is intact and can be used safely), the risk of complications is *not* increased by enteral alimentation.

If one accepts these caveats, then as the malnutrition risk curve shifts to the left according to the presence of pre-existing malnutrition and its severity, the risks associ-

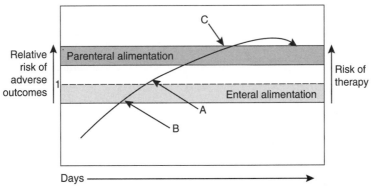

Figure 5–1. Comparative risks of malnutrition and alimentation. The large, curved arrow represents the risk of morbidity or mortality that can be attributed to malnutrition. The left-hand y-axis represents the relative risk of a poor outcome. The two horizontal bands represent the risks associated with providing parenteral or enteral alimentation. The dark gray band represents the uncertainty about the magnitude of the risk of increased morbidity secondary to the administration of parenteral alimentation. Arrow A identifies a region beyond which the risk of malnutrition increases and would have measurable effects on the outcome by increasing morbidity and mortality. Arrow B indicates the risk reduction that may be recognized by the institution of enteral feeding, or administration of specific nutrients, growth factors, or other agents. Arrow C refers to a region where the risks of malnutrition outweigh the risk of parenteral alimentation.

ated with enteral alimentation are always less than the risks of parenteral nutritional support and enteral feeding. Furthermore, this theoretical construct allows the possibility that enteral feeding, when instituted early in the course of hospitalization, may *decrease* the risk of adverse outcomes secondary to malnourishment.

Several points along this malnutrition risk curve are of interest. Arrow A identifies a region beyond which the risk of malnutrition increases and would have measurable effects on the outcome by increasing morbidity or mortality. Arrow B, therefore, indicates the risk reduction that may be recognized by the institution of enteral feeding appropriate to the patient's estimated needs. This arrow also identifies a risk reduction that may be attained by the administration of specific nutrients, growth factors, or other agents that reduce risk without necessarily affecting body composition. Arrow C refers to a region where the risks of malnutrition outweigh the risks of parenteral alimentation and where it would therefore be appropriate to institute intravenous feedings.

But arrow C also illustrates the critical question that nutrition and metabolic support professionals must answer: How long can my patient go underfed before the risk of malnourishment outweighs the risks of parenteral alimentation? More precisely stated, this question is: How can one assess when a patient has reached or will reach this portion of the malnutrition risk curve?

For clinicians, it would also be important to be able to assess when an intervention has *reduced* the risk of morbidity or mortality secondary to underfeeding. These questions are the subject of this brief review.

New methods are needed to assess the nutritional and metabolic status of the critically ill patient. The ideal assessment technique or techniques must be fluid and capable of detecting alterations in metabolism associated with both the structure and the function of organ systems. Furthermore, the ideal technique would also confer the ability to detect responses to treatment and to direct nutritional or metabolic therapy (Table 5–1). This chapter reviews nutritional and assessment techniques that can be used for these purposes. By necessity, our discussion includes a brief review of some techniques that have historical or contextual importance before proceeding to discuss briefly more dynamic assessment tools and some experimental technologies.

◆ TRADITIONAL NUTRITIONAL INDICES: STATIC, FLUID, AND GLOBAL NUTRITIONAL ASSESSMENT TECHNIQUES

The body comprises 35 components, which are classified into five levels of increasing complexity: atomic (e.g., nitrogen, potassium); molecular (e.g., water, protein); cellular (e.g., body cell mass, intracellular and

Table 5–1. Advantages and Limitations of Different Assessment Methods

Method	Accuracy	Costs	Radiation	Time	Patient Convenience
Carcass analysis	+ + +	− −			
Neutron activation	+ + +	− −	− −	+ +	+ +
Densitometry	+ +	+		+ +	+/−
Dilution method	+ +	+/−	(−)	+	+
^{40}K method	+ +	−		+ +	+ +
Dual-energy x-ray absorptiometry	+ +	−	−	+ +	+ +
Computed tomography	+ +(+)	− −	− −	+ +	+ +
Nuclear magnetic resonance imaging	+ +	− −		+(+)	+
Anthropometry	+	+ + +		+ +	+
Infrared interaction	+	+ +		+ +	+(+)
Ultrasound measurements	+	+ +		+ +	+ +
Bioelectric impedance	+	+		+ + +	+ + +
Total body electric conductivity	+	−		+ + +	+ + +
Creatinine and *N*-methylhistidine excretion	+	+ +		−	−

+ + +, excellent; + +, very good; +, good; +/−, reasonable; −, bad; − −, very bad.
From Deurenberg P, Schutz Y: Body composition: Overview of methods and future directions of research. Ann Nutr Metab 39:330, 1995. Reproduced by permission of S. Karger AG, Basel.

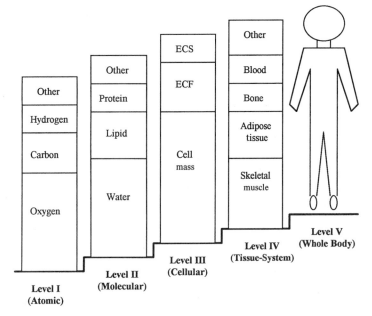

Figure 5–2. The five levels of body composition and their respective components. ECS, extracellular solids; ECF, extracellular fluid. (Adapted from Wang Z, Pierson RN Jr, Heymsfield SB: The five level model: A new approach to organizing body composition research. Am J Clin Nutr 56:19–28, 1992. © Am J Clin Nutr. American Society for Clinical Nutrition.)

extracellular fluid); tissue (e.g., skeletal muscle, adipose tissue); and whole body (e.g., weight, height) (Fig. 5–2).[6] Each level and component is distinct. If all the components at each level are summed, the total is equivalent to body weight. For example, at the molecular level:

$$Body\ Weight = Fat + Water + Protein + Mineral + Glycogen$$

The levels and the components within each level are distinct; however, there are associations within and between levels. For instance, fatness can be characterized by total body carbon, fat, fat cells, and adipose tissue at the atomic, molecular, cellular, and tissue-system levels, respectively.[7, 8]

Although modern technology now allows the measurement of all major body components in vivo, these methodologies are not readily available for clinical use. Accordingly, the nutritional state of patients is routinely based on clinical judgment in conjunction with the most commonly used nutritional indicators, such as clinical history, particularly weight change and physiologic function; biochemical markers such as albumin and transferrin levels; and upper arm anthropometry, such as triceps skin fold thickness and arm circumference.[9, 10] The correlation between anthropometric measures of body composition and nutritional status led to the early emphasis on using

changes in body composition to assess the severity of malnutrition and the response to nutritional intervention. Although a statistically significant association exists between these indices and the patient's nutritional status, the variance of the association is quite large. Therefore, these measurements have proved most useful when they are used for epidemiologic surveys rather than for assessing the nutritional status of individual patients.[11]

More dynamic indices such as the measurement of changes in nitrogen balance or 3-methylhistidine levels, or the concentration of serum proteins with shorter half-lives, may be more useful for monitoring patients who are actually receiving enteral or parenteral nutrition.[10] However, it is unclear if the measurement of these indices individually or in combination confers an advantage over evaluation by a skilled physician in the detection or monitoring of patients who require specialized nutritional support. For example, the subjective global assessment, in which patients are nutritionally assessed based on a combination of parameters, including history, symptoms, and physical examination, gives reproducible results regarding the ranking of nutritional status and is a good predictor of complications.[12–14]

Although clinical evaluation may function as well as any individual test or battery of tests, neither technique is particularly accurate. Misclassification rates may be as high as 30%, even under optimal conditions.[15] It is not clear which of the commonly used nutritional assessment techniques is the most reliable because of the lack of comparative data. Most current nutritional assessment techniques are based on their ability to predict the clinical outcome. However, the validity of any of these techniques to truly measure "nutritional risk" has not been proved, and the effect of nutritional therapy to influence the outcome in patients judged to be "malnourished" has not been consistent.[6]

The other major difficulty has been that most nutritional assessment techniques are influenced by non-nutritional factors. For example, the administration of intravenous fluids or blood products or the excessive loss of fluid or protein through diarrhea, various enteric tubes, fistulas, or ostomies may invalidate anthropometric and serum protein measurements. In addition, the synthesis of plasma proteins varies according to the degree of expansion of total body water, liver function, and the effects of cytokines. Thus, assessment tools based on these indices may be unreliable, especially in patients with injury and sepsis.[16, 17]

Anthropometry

Anthropometry uses simple measurements of body thicknesses, such as skin fold measurements and arm circumferences, to estimate fat and lean-tissue mass. Early studies showed that the total body energy content as determined by anthropometry correlates relatively well with the same quantity as estimated by underwater weighing; however, it does not correlate with measurements of changes in total body potassium or to changes in total body nitrogen as measured by neutron activation analysis.[11, 18, 19] Anthropometry may detect large shifts in body composition over months or years; however, changes in energy and protein stores in the short term are not accurately detected. The major advantages of anthropometry are that it is simple, safe, and inexpensive and that it can be easily applied at the bedside. These relative advantages are offset by errors inherent in the method, such as inter-rater variability and the potentially confounding influence of age, hydration status, and physical activity.[6, 10, 20] Since the measurements are usually compared with those of a reference population and the reference measurements are not available for elders or ethnic minorities, the use of anthropometry in these population groups is problematic.[21] Finally, the validity of these measurements for estimating body composition in very obese or heavily muscled subjects is questionable because of the technical difficulties of performing the measurements. Generally, body fat is overestimated by skin folds in very lean subjects and underestimated in obese subjects.[21, 22] Nevertheless, markedly abnormal anthropometric values (below the 5th percentile) are often associated with poor clinical outcome.[6]

Anthropometric methods, including skin fold thickness, circumference measurements, the creatinine-height index, and 3-methylhistidine, are considered doubly indirect methods for determining body composition (Table 5–2). They are generally based on a statistical relationship between easily measurable body parameters and data obtained by direct (i.e., neutron activation analysis) or indirect (i.e., densitometry, ^{40}K measurements, and dilution techniques) methods.[22] Anthropometry may provide useful information for most epidemiologic stud-

Table 5–2. Assessment Methods

Direct	Indirect	Doubly Indirect
Carcass analysis	Densitometry	Anthropometry
Neutron activation	Dilution techniques	Infrared absorptiometry
	^{40}K scanning	Ultrasound measurements
	Computed tomography	Bioelectric impedance
	Nuclear magnetic resonance imaging	Creatinine excretion
	Dual-photon absorptiometry	N-methylhistidine excretion

From Deurenberg P, Schutz Y: Body composition: Overview of methods and future directions of research. Ann Nutr Metab 39:326, 1995. Reproduced by permission of S. Karger AG, Basel.

ies and about the nutritional status of patients with chronic diseases such as hepatic cirrhosis[23, 24] and anorexia nervosa.[25] However, in the severely ill hospitalized patient who is subject to major shifts in body water, anthropometric measurements may be especially hazardous. Anthropometry functions best as a measure of the amount and rate of change in total body energy stores and nitrogen mass over extended periods of observation. It does not perform well as an index of the functional capacity of lean tissues, especially in diseased patients.

Measurement of Energy Expenditure

The major components associated with daily energy expenditure include the basal metabolic rate (BMR), the thermic effect of exercise, and the thermogenesis of food intake. The BMR is the amount of energy expended under complete rest, shortly after awakening, having fasted during the previous 12 to 18 hours.[26] The BMR is dependent on age, sex, and body size and correlates roughly with the body surface area. Normally, the basal energy expenditure ranges from roughly 0.8 to 1.2 kcal/min in healthy adults and is most closely associated with lean body mass, not fat. Approximately two thirds of the basal energy expenditure represents the energy needed for the maintenance of cell membrane pumps and for protein synthesis in the liver, brain, heart, and kidney.[27] The resting energy expenditure (REE), which is often used synonymously with the BMR, represents the amount of energy expended 2 hours after a standard meal under conditions of rest and thermal neutrality. It is generally 10% higher than the BMR.[26]

A patient's energy expenditure may increase 10 to 30% with major fractures, 20 to 60% with severe infections, and 40 to 110% with severe third-degree burns.[28] In addition, fever accelerates chemical reactions. For this reason, the REE rises approximately 14% for each degree Celsius increase in temperature. Clinically, the goal is to administer sufficient energy to malnourished patients to prevent negative energy balances. In practice, this may be accomplished by using a variety of standard formulas that are available to calculate the BMR. The difficulty is that in order to assess the optimal level of caloric intake, a percentage increase in caloric needs over the predicted BMR is added according to the metabolic stress level of the patient (e.g., the severity of the injury or infection). This approach may be very inaccurate, since the range of thermogenic responses to injury, trauma, and infection is very large. In these circumstances, measurement of the REE by direct or indirect calorimetry may be more accurate.

Direct calorimetry measures heat production as the temperature change produced in a medium. As such, it quantitates the amount of heat dissipated by the body and requires little patient cooperation. However, the equipment required for the measurements is expensive, large, and immobile. Furthermore, during the measurements the patient is placed in a chamber and is not readily accessible. Thus, direct calorimetry is almost never used in the clinical setting. Indirect calorimetry measures gas exchange by means of oxygen consumption and carbon dioxide production. It allows the heat produced by oxidative processes to be determined. It can be readily performed at the bedside using small, mobile, closed- or open-circuit units. In open-circuit methods, the subject breathes air from the environment while the expired air is collected for volumetric measurements. This gas volume is corrected to standard conditions and is analyzed for its oxygen and carbon dioxide content. These figures are then used to calculate oxygen consumption and carbon dioxide production. In the closed-circuit method, the subject is isolated from outside air and typically breathes from a reservoir that contains pure oxygen. As gas is expired by the subject, carbon dioxide is removed. In this closed system, the decrease in gas volume is directly related to the rate of oxygen consumption and therefore can be used to calculate the metabolic rate.[29]

Under appropriate conditions, the measurement of energy expenditure over short periods may accurately estimate the REE. Estimates of the total energy expenditure have been derived by multiplying the REE by a factor of 1 to 2. This obviates the need to estimate the effects of changes in body composition, nutritional status, disease processes, trauma, or other clinical events on the metabolic rate. The BMR is best measured early in the morning, with the patient in a supine position in a thermoneutral environment, after at least 30 minutes of skeletal muscle rest and a 12- to 18-hour fast. In contrast, the REE is measured in a thermoneutral environment after the nonfasting subject has rested in a supine position for at least 30 minutes. It can be determined throughout the day and repeatedly during nutritional therapy. When measured in this manner, the REE, which increases on awakening, includes the contribution of the BMR and encompasses the thermic effects of food.

Gas exchange has been used to measure the influence of various metabolic conditions as well as the effects of disease and injury. In addition to measuring energy expenditure, indirect calorimetry has been used to calculate the oxidation rates of carbohydrates, lipids, and proteins as reflected in the respiratory quotient.[30] Net substrate utilization can be calculated from oxygen consumption, carbon dioxide production, and metabolized protein as urea nitrogen excretion. In calculating substrate utilization, there is a general assumption that the substrates being used have a similar chemical composition and calorie equivalent. Although this assumption is generally true for most typical carbohydrate and lipid substrates, it is probably not true for proteins. Proteins are composed of many amino acids in varied concentrations, and individual amino acids have notably different oxidation values. Hence, the deamination of some atypical protein sources (e.g., solutions with high levels of branched-chain amino acids, glutamine, or other parenteral amino acids, and some disease-specific enteral feedings) may not correspond to oxidation of more common proteins. Furthermore, nitrogen excretion in the urine may not exactly correspond to the rate of amino acid oxidation, and there may be inaccuracies due to the normal fluctuation in blood urea nitrogen concentrations and changes in urea clearance.[29]

Nevertheless, indirect calorimetry plays an important role in nutritional support. Changes in body weight and oxygen consumption are closely correlated. As a person loses weight, oxygen consumption decreases in a predictable fashion. Moreover, the rate of oxygen consumption rises in concert with refeeding. For these reasons, measurements of the oxygen consumption of malnourished patients may be used to determine the severity of their depletion relative to their normal body weight and composition.[31] Indirect calorimetry can accurately estimate the daily energy expenditure of the critically ill patient when standard formulas are inaccurate. This may be very helpful in the care of the hospitalized patient who has lost a significant amount of weight and is still suffering catabolic stress from infection or trauma.

Immunologic Tests

Specific nutrient deficiencies and protein-calorie malnutrition lead to consistent and reproducible changes in immunologic function. Malnutrition decreases the synthesis of acute-phase proteins that help the organism to survive during times of stress, infection, or injury. Almost all of the body's defense mechanisms are damaged by nutritional deficiencies. The systems affected include immunoglobulin and antibody production, phagocytosis, complement activity, and secretory and mucosal immunity. Of the many immunologic tests that could be used for nutritional assessment, only the total lymphocyte count and skin tests are sufficiently simple and reproducible to be used for routine nutritional and metabolic assessment. Unfortunately, many disease processes and drug treatments can alter immune competence in a nonspecific fashion. In addition, changes in body cell mass and immunosuppression as suggested by anergy may occur in the same patient without a direct cause-and-effect relationship. Thus, changes in one of these variables do not necessarily reflect changes in the other. Consequently, given our current armamentarium, traditional immunologic function tests are not useful measures of metabolic status. In addition, scientists are increasingly interested in studying lymphocyte function ex vivo. Changes in proliferation rate, cytotoxicity, cytokine production, or elaboration in response to nutritional intervention may ultimately be useful measures of immunologic potency.

Other in Vitro Tests: Biologic and Biochemical Markers

Traditionally, measurement of levels of the serum transport proteins albumin and transferrin has been used to detect and monitor protein and energy deficits. Changes in the circulating concentrations of these proteins are highly variable and may not identify patients whose protein and energy deficits are mild to moderate. Furthermore, changes in albumin and transferrin levels are relatively insensitive to the effects of refeeding, given their half-lives of 20 and 8 days, respectively.[32, 33] To date, there is not an ideal nutritional marker that is both sensitive and specific. However, serum prealbumin and retinol-binding protein come the closest. Prealbumin is a rapid-turnover protein. It has a half-life of 1.9 days, and its serum concentration is a sensitive indicator of protein-calorie malnutrition. The prealbumin level is not significantly influenced by fluctuations in hydration status and is not affected by liver disease as early as or to the same extent as other serum protein markers, such as albumin. Retinol-binding protein, also a rapid-turnover protein, has a very short half-life of 20 to 25 hours, and although its concentration is comparable to that of prealbumin in sensitivity, it is excreted in the urine, and its level is affected to a greater degree by renal and liver disease than the level of prealbumin.[34–36]

In response to stress and trauma, the liver increases the production of acute-phase proteins and decreases the production of constitutive proteins. This phenomenon has been shown to be principally under the control of various cytokines such as interleukin 1, interleukin 6, tumor necrosis factor, interleukin 11, interleukin 13, oncostatin-M, and leukemia inhibitory factor. Measurements of acute-phase proteins are of value in the assessment of the activity and response to therapy in several diseases. The inflammatory stimulus may be infection, tissue injury, chemical or physical trauma, or neoplasia.[37] C-reactive protein (CRP) in particular has been found to be a useful marker of inflammation, and its measurement may allow the earlier diagnosis of bacterial sepsis.[38] In healthy people, levels of CRP are low. Levels rise exponentially with the onset of infection and return to normal or near-normal after the elimination of infection. Serial measurements of CRP levels are beneficial for monitoring a patient's response to therapy after the initial insult, and an increase in CRP levels may be the first indicator of disease recrudescence, a secondary process, or ineffective therapy.[39] Serum amyloid A (SAA) is also a sensitive marker of the acute-phase response and has been used in conjunction with CRP as a means of discriminating between bacterial and viral in-fections.[40] A direct correlation between SAA levels and the metastatic stage of tumor has been proposed with the suggestion that the SAA level has prognostic significance.[41] Although no clinician should base the likelihood of a significant infection solely on serum CRP or SAA levels, the determination of CRP in conjunction with prealbumin levels may help distinguish between a depressed prealbumin level secondary to an acute-phase response and a depressed prealbumin level secondary to malnutrition.

The measurement of serum insulin-like growth factor I (IGF-I) levels may offer a sensitive index of short-term changes in nutritional status. Previously referred to as somatomedin C, IGF-I is stimulated by growth hormone and promotes the growth of most cell types. Food intake and nutritional status are major regulators of IGF-I levels, which are reduced in chronic undernutrition and protein-calorie malnutrition.[42, 43] Hence, the magnitude of IGF-I reduction relates to the severity of the nutritional insult,[44] and IGF-I levels consistently increase with nutritional repletion.[42, 45] In adults, IGF-I levels decline within 24 hours of the start of fasting, reach 10 to 15% of prefast values by 10 days, and return toward normal with refeeding.[42] Changes in circulating IGF-I levels may be more responsive to nutritional therapy than changes observed in the levels of transferrin, prealbumin, and retinol-binding protein.[46, 47] Furthermore, changes in IGF-I levels correlate with changes in nitrogen balance.[48, 49] Both the quality of dietary protein and the amount of energy are important for the restoration of serum IGF-I levels after fasting.[48, 50, 51] Like other nutritional markers, IGF-I levels are also independently affected by liver and renal disease. In addition, the confidence levels for serum IGF-I concentrations in healthy subjects are quite large, which makes the identification of malnourished patients more difficult.[52] In obese persons, serum IGF-I concentrations are moderately decreased and correlate negatively with the abdominal fat mass.[42, 53]

Leptin may mediate changes in appetite and metabolic rate. Leptin is a 16-kd protein that is secreted by adipose tissue;[54] it is the product of the *ob* gene.[55] It is thought that leptin acts as a marker of fat stores under steady-state conditions but also increases or decreases with changes in energy balance. Hence, there is a set-point that is determined by an individual's fat stores, but changes from that set-point may still occur and contribute to the regulation of metabolism and appetite.[56] Most of the work on leptin's role in energy balance regulation has been in animals, and the relationship between changes in circulating leptin concentrations, energy intake, and hunger in humans has not been fully ascertained.[57]

◆ NEUTRON ACTIVATION, WHOLE-BODY COUNTING, AND OTHER NUCLEAR-BASED TECHNIQUES

Potassium, nitrogen, phosphorus, hydrogen, oxygen, carbon, sodium, chloride, and calcium can be measured with a group of techniques referred to as *whole-body counting* and *in vivo neutron activation analysis.* Shielded whole-body counters count the γ-ray decay of naturally occurring ^{40}K. The ^{40}K counts can be used to determine the total body potassium, which then can be used to calculate the body cell mass and the fat-free body mass.[10]

In vivo total body neutron activation analysis is a direct analytic technique based on nuclear reactions rather than on chemical reactions. The subject receives a moderated beam of fast neutrons. Capture of neutrons by atoms of the target elements creates unstable isotopes such as ^{49}Ca and ^{15}N. The isotopes revert to their stable baseline condition by emission of one or more γ-rays of characteristic energy. The energy emitted identifies the particular element, and the level of activity shows its abundance. The total body bone and cellular mineral, protein, and fat content can then be derived from these measurements. The neutron activation systems are calibrated against various phantoms, which are used to evaluate the precision of the instruments. If the isotope has a very short half-life (e.g., ^{15}N, with a half-life of 10 to 15 seconds), then the γ-ray counting proceeds simultaneously and is referred to as *prompt gamma neutron activation analysis* and can be used to measure the total body nitrogen and hydrogen. The total body nitrogen can be used to calculate the total body protein. If the γ-ray emissions are longer (e.g., ^{49}Ca, half-life of 8.7 minutes), the technique is referred to as *delayed gamma neutron activation analysis*[58] and can be used to measure the total body calcium, sodium, chloride, and phosphorus.

These elements can be used to calculate the bone mineral mass and extracellular fluid volume. Finally, inelastic neutron-scattering methods measure the total body carbon. Carbon is useful in models designed to quantify the total body fat.[10]

Few facilities are available to measure neutron activation, and the technique is expensive because it requires a cyclotron and equipment for total body counting. Like many techniques that measure body composition, neutron activation analysis is not particularly sensitive to short-term fluxes. It may be best suited for static measurements of body compartments. Cohn and associates[59] first suggested a model that treats the whole body as a four-compartment system composed of fat, water, protein, and bone mineral (M_O).[59] Since then, six-component systems have been described[60, 61] that also include tissue mineral (M_S) and glycogen (G) where

$$\text{Body Fat} = \text{Body Mass} - (\text{Water} + \text{Protein} + M_O + M_S + G)$$

Water is measured by tritium dilution; the protein measurement is based on the total body nitrogen; M_O is calculated from the total body calcium; M_S is calculated from the total body potassium, total body sodium and chlorine, and total body calcium; and G is estimated from the total body nitrogen, assuming a known and constant glycogen-to-nitrogen ratio in skeletal muscle and liver.[61] This technique has at least one distinct advantage. All the individual components of the model are determined independently, except for glycogen, which is typically less than 1% of the total body weight. This avoids potential complications and difficulties in interpretation inherent to methods in which the lean body mass is not determined directly but is rather assumed to be a fixed fraction of the total body water (TBW). In addition, this model has no assumptions that are known to be influenced by age, gender, race, and disease (Table 5–3).

Although malnourished patients have a proportionately greater loss of whole-body potassium than nitrogen, compared with control subjects, changes in whole-body nitrogen measured during short periods are quite variable, with large error terms. Whole-body nitrogen determinations are often combined with measurements of whole-body potassium since the latter is an index

Table 5–3. Assumptions of the Multicompartment Neutron Activation Chemical Model

Compartment	Assumption
Total body water (TBW)	TBW = ^3H_2O dilution space × 0.95 (hydrogen-exchange correction).
Total body protein	Protein is 16% nitrogen.
Total body mineral	
Bone	Bone mineral (ash) is 36.4% calcium.
Soft tissue	Derived from potassium, sodium, calcium, and chlorine.
Total body lipid	Carbon remaining after adjustment of total body carbon for carbon in glycogen, protein, and mineral is in lipid. The lipid compartment is 77.4% carbon.
Total body glycogen	Estimated known and constant glycogen-to-nitrogen ratio in skeletal muscle and liver.

From Heymsfield SB, Wang Z, Baumgartner RN, et al: Body composition and aging: A study by in vivo neutron activation analysis. J Nutr 123:434, 1993. © American Society for Nutritional Sciences.

of the body cell mass and is thought to be largely proportional to the cellular protein in many disease states.[59] However, wasting may decrease the whole-body potassium more than the whole-body nitrogen because of an exaggerated loss of cell-rich muscle or a loss of cells from other tissues[6] and thus disrupt the normal proportionality; that is, changes in intracellular potassium may occur independently of changes in protein concentration.[7]

Photon absorptiometry systems direct photons of defined energy at the subject under evaluation. As the beam passes over the patient, its energy decreases as some photons are absorbed by the body. The amount of beam attenuation depends on the nature of the tissue through which it passes. These changes in attenuation can be used to quantify the mineral, fat, and lean-tissue compartments of the body. Typically, a dual-energy system is used when variable body thicknesses such as the trunk are being analyzed because this technique improves the ability to distinguish bone from soft tissues. Gotfredsen and colleagues used dual-photon absorptiometry (DPA) to measure lean body mass and total body fat.[62] The accuracy of

their method for measuring lean body mass was 2.5%. Therefore, it is a very reliable method for measuring body compositional changes in vivo. The radiation dose is small (about 5 mrad), which means that DPA can be used to follow changes in body composition over time.

Dual-energy x-ray absorptiometry (DEXA) is a two-dimensional projection system similar in concept to DPA but is different in that an x-ray tube replaces the isotopic source of photons.[7, 63, 64] The x-ray tube produces a higher radiation flux than the isotope source used in DPA, greatly increasing the speed and precision. Like DPA systems, DEXA systems are used to measure the bone mineral density of the lumbar spine, the hip, and the total body. It is also possible to estimate the fat body mass and the lean mass defined as the nonfat-nonbone body mass. DEXA is mainly used to measure the bone mineral content and density in studies of aging, ethnicity, and various clinical conditions.[63, 65] However, it is also used to evaluate the effect of calcium and vitamin D supplementation on the bone mineral status in postmenopausal women and in patients on long-term parenteral nutrition. It has also been used to monitor changes in body composition in obese women during weight loss and in patients with acquired immunodeficiency syndrome and cystic fibrosis.[66, 67] The DEXA technique allows the measurement of the total body mass, bone mineral body mass, and percentage body fat in an accurate (±3%) and reproducible fashion.[63, 66–68]

◆ MULTIPLE-ISOTOPE DILUTION TECHNIQUES

Body composition can also be quantified using multiple-isotope dilution. A fixed known amount of tritiated water and ^{22}Na are administered simultaneously. The TBW is determined at equilibrium from the plasma tritium concentration at specific time points after administration,[69] and the total exchangeable sodium (Na_e) is determined from the specific activity of ^{22}Na. The total exchangeable potassium (K_e) is then calculated from measurement of the TBW multiplied by a constant, R, which is the ratio of the sum of the sodium and potassium in a sample of whole blood divided by its water content. The Na_e content is then subtracted from this quantity to yield K_e. Thus

$$K_e = (TBW \times R) - Na_e$$

The validity of determining exchangeable potassium using this method has been demonstrated in humans and animals.[70] Once these quantities are derived, other measurements of body composition can be calculated using other equations:

$$Body\ Cell\ Mass = K_e \times 0.00833$$

$$Lean\ Body\ Mass = TBW/0.73$$

$$Extracellular\ Mass = Lean\ Body\ Mass - Body\ Cell\ Mass$$

$$Body\ Fat = Body\ Weight - Lean\ Body\ Mass$$

To compare the body composition of individuals with different body sizes, the data are usually corrected for body size by expressing the components of body composition relative to the TBW. The body cell mass represents the total cellular mass and is the living metabolically active component of the body.[71] As such, it performs all the work done by the body and is responsible for all the oxygen consumption and carbon dioxide production.[72] In the average or typical healthy individual, the body cell mass accounts for 50% of the lean body mass. The extracellular mass is metabolically inactive, and its major functions are transport and support.

The predictive value of these formulas is poor in subjects with an abnormal body composition. As shown previously, the TBW content is used to calculate the size of other body compartments. However, in individuals with an abnormal body composition, the characteristic relationship between the body cell mass and the TBW may no longer exist. Thus, the TBW accurately predicts the size of the body cell mass in healthy individuals but not necessarily in individuals whose body composition is abnormal, such as patients who are catabolic (for example, after stress or injury), who typically have weight loss, a negative potassium and nitrogen balance, and a positive salt and water balance. Thus, a characteristic response to severe malnutrition, catabolic stress, or both is expansion of the extracellular mass relative

to the body cell mass, which is contracted.[73] The Na_e/K_e ratio, which is a dynamic expression of the extracellular mass expressed as a function of the body cell mass, increases significantly under various conditions, including in sepsis, in malnutrition, and after major abdominal surgery.[69, 74]

Shizgal showed that the Na_e/K_e ratio is a very sensitive index of nutritional status, compared with the usual anthropometric and biochemical measurements (e.g., percentage of recent weight loss, triceps skin fold thickness, midarm muscle circumference, serum albumin and transferrin levels, delayed hypersensitivity skin test response, and total lymphocyte count).[74] Tellado and colleagues showed that the Na_e/K_e ratio more accurately identifies which patients with sepsis and malnutrition or a variety of surgical diseases are at risk for dying during hospitalization[75] than do the traditional indices. In their study, depending on the cutoff point chosen, accuracy rates ranged from 52 to 91%. A cutoff point of 2 yielded an accuracy rate of approximately 79%, with acceptably low false-positive and false-negative fractions (20% and 16%, respectively).

The techniques required to measure the Na_e/K_e ratio accurately are complex and time-consuming, and they require specialized laboratory facilities and specially trained personnel. Consequently, they are not suited for routine patient management but should be reserved for research purposes.

As mentioned previously, there are inherent difficulties in using the total body potassium as an index of cellular depletion and repletion. Estimates of body cell mass that use total body potassium measurements generally assume that 3.6% of the cell is nitrogen.[76] The ability to determine the body cell mass varies as the potassium content of the cell changes because of changes in intracellular water (ICW). These techniques may also be inaccurate, as alluded to previously, if the composition of the cell changes because of alterations in nitrogen content that occur independently of changes in intracellular potassium and ICW. In other words, a fall in total body potassium is usually interpreted as a change in lean body mass of normal composition. However, this is true only if changes in body composition are proportional to changes in body cell mass. In fact, as discussed earlier, changes in intracellular potassium concentrations may occur independently of changes in lean body mass. Therefore, a fall in total body potassium may not accurately reflect changes in body cell mass, but a fall in intracellular potassium may be an index of cellular health, membrane function, or ionic integrity.

The relationship between global shifts in the distribution of body cations and changes in membrane integrity is poorly understood. What is the association, if any, between changes in membrane pump activity and transmembrane potential, cation balance, and measurements of K_e and Na_e? The studies reviewed previously raise an interesting possibility of a relative or absolute increase in intracellular sodium that could be related to decreased membrane pump activity or efficiency. Clearly, patients with a variety of catabolic illnesses have an abnormal Na_e/K_e ratio; but it is not as clear whether short-term nutritional repletion (10 to 14 days) is associated with normalization of this index. Studies of the effects of starvation and stress on the transmembrane potential of myocytes report findings that are similar to those reported in studies of the effects of these conditions on Na_e/K_e ratios.[77–79] After 10 days of starvation, the transmembrane potential difference of skeletal muscle falls significantly. A 10-day refeeding period using a standard parenteral nutritional solution with crystalline amino acids and dextrose does not restore a normal potential difference, even if nitrogen equilibrium or a positive nitrogen balance is restored.

Pichard and colleagues measured free intracellular potassium ion activity, membrane potential, and total potassium and calculated intracellular potassium concentrations in predominantly slow- and fast-twitch muscles of rats after dietary restriction and subsequent refeeding.[80] Several interesting findings were revealed: (1) intracellular potassium activity and membrane potential decreased only in the predominantly slow-twitch muscle and returned to normal with refeeding, (2) calculated intracellular potassium concentrations decreased in both fast- and slow-twitch muscle and did not increase significantly after refeeding, and (3) potassium supplementation did not significantly change these indices or the ratio of free to total intracellular potassium. As the authors note, these experiments demonstrate that changes in intracellular potassium ion activity may be dissociated from

changes in intracellular potassium concentration. Thus, the changes in total body potassium and intracellular potassium that occur during various dietary manipulations are not necessarily secondary to changes in muscle mass as assessed by measurements of total body nitrogen but may be due to changes in cell energetics or in membrane characteristics such as permeability and selectivity.

Thus, very different methodologies suggest a persistent defect in cellular membrane function in patients with catabolic illnesses that is not restored by a typical course of intravenous nutritional support. All point toward a fruitful area for future research in metabolic and nutritional assessment—namely, methods that are directed at cellular function and integrity or at the final outcome of alterations in membrane integrity (e.g., shifts in the ratios of ICW and extracellular water [ECW] or in the intracellular or extracellular distribution of the major cations). Both raise the same quandary for clinical nutritionists. Given that the severely malnourished patient benefits from a short course of preoperative intravenous nutritional support, as evidenced by a decrease in mortality and morbidity, and given that a significant accretion of lean body tissue does not occur over this period, what is the best means of identifying this beneficial effect? Which techniques are relevant to the care of malnourished, critically ill patients and are accessible to the clinical nutritionist? One might argue that what is needed is a measure of cellular health.

◆ BIOELECTRIC IMPEDANCE ANALYSIS

The body's electrical resistance may provide a diagnostic element in the diseased and might be useful to identify certain affections.

Vigouroux 1888

Retention of sodium and water is a characteristic consequence of injury and is thought to result from the enhanced release of hormones such as vasopressin[81] and aldosterone.[82] This hormonal response is proportional to the severity of injury and appears to be more pronounced after shock and severe infection.[83] The hydration of the body's tissues may be further increased by exogenous fluid administered during the resuscitation phase. The quantity of fluid thus retained predicts survival in burn patients.[84] Conversely, early mobilization of extracellular fluid and associated diuresis heralds an impending recovery. Therefore, a precise determination of the body fluid volume and distribution could help the physician monitor the severity of illness.

The traditional method of determining the volume and distribution of body fluids is based on the dilutional principle.[71] Substances such as Evans' dye, bromide, and heavy water are known to distribute exclusively in the plasma, TBW, and ECW compartment, respectively. For example, if a measured quantity of heavy water is administered and allowed to attain equilibrium with the body's fluids, concentrations of this tracer determined in venous blood are inversely proportional to the TBW volume.[85] Although these techniques are accurate, multiple blood samples and extensive processing are required. Therefore, a noninvasive method that provides information on the body's hydration status instantaneously may be a useful tool in the assessment of fluid balance.

The impedance technique has become increasingly popular as a noninvasive method of determining volumes of body fluids and associated changes in lean body mass.[86] However, it should be realized that electric impedance reflects fluid volumes, such as the TBW and possibly the ECW. As has been discussed, various disease processes may alter the relationship between the body's total fluid content and the lean body mass that is more constant during health (TBW = lean body mass $\times$ 0.73). Prediction of the lean body mass using impedance techniques may be unreliable in patients, particularly if regression equations derived from healthy populations are used.[87]

In the next portion of this chapter, the rationale, history, present use, and future potential of impedance measurements as a tool for analyzing body composition and for metabolic assessment are discussed, as are factors that may influence their accuracy.

Rationale

Measurement of impedance (in ohms, Ω) consists of the determination of two electric characteristics of the human body: electric resistance and reactance. A model of a cylinder containing fluid usually serves to explain the rationale of an impedance measurement. When an alternating electric current is applied to a cylinder, conduction of the current is opposed by its contents; the ability to oppose current is termed *electric resistance*. Resistance (R) is defined as the pure opposition to the flow of alternating current and is expressed in ohms. A value of R determined across a cylinder is related to its length and inversely related to its diameter (Fig. 5–3).[88] If the length and diameter are known, R reflects the volume of the cylinder's fluid contents. When a portion of the fluid is replaced by fat, which is a poor conductor, R determined across the cylinder increases. The human body resembles a set of serially connected cylinders (arm, trunk, and leg) with a known length (height) and a relatively constant diameter. Thus, R measured across the body reflects its total fluid content.[89, 90] In healthy humans, R usually constitutes 98% of the impedance signal; these parameters are therefore frequently described interchangeably.

Reactance (X_c) is the second component of impedance and is thought to reflect capacitive elements in the body. X_c contributes very little to whole-body impedance (~2%) and is also expressed in ohms. Cell walls

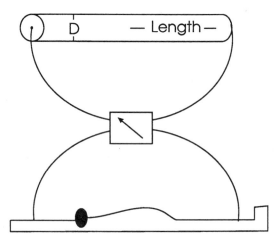

Figure 5–3. Rationale of impedance measurements. The resistance following conduction of an alternating electric current measured across a cylinder filled with fluid is related to its length and inversely related to its diameter (D). If the length and diameter are known, the resistance reflects the fluid volume. The body is analogous to a cylinder in that its resistance reflects its fluid contents.

and membranes possess electric capacity similar to that observed in electric condensors.[88, 91, 92] Some investigators have suggested that a single cell acts as a parallel plate condenser. In this construct, the electrolyte solutions are conducting plates, and membrane hydrocarbons serve as the nonconducting component.[93, 94] Cole demonstrated that the increased area of the cellular membrane of an egg after osmotic swelling was associated with a fall in the membrane's capacitance.[93] Although X_c has attracted less attention in the past than R, X_c may represent cellular health and reflect the ICW, or the body cell mass, the compartment responsible for the vast majority of metabolic activity.[95] X_c or the angular transformation of the X_c/R ratio (phase angle, see later) has been associated with altered fluid distribution and clinical disease.[96] The phase angle has been defined as "the degree by which the body differs from a pure resistor."[97]

History

During the 19th century, the application of direct electric current was a preferential method of treating subjects with mental disorders. The French psychiatrist Vigouroux postulated that associated R values "may provide a diagnostic element in the diseased and might be useful to identify certain affections."[98] However, almost half a century elapsed before body impedance was measured by passing alternating electric current between two attached electrodes. This novel method was claimed to provide a means of monitoring thyroid disease.[97] Unfortunately, polarization between electrodes and skin and additional unpredictable skin effects rendered this two-electrode configuration inaccurate. In contrast, a four-electrode configuration minimized the influence of the skin, and impedance determined from this electrode arrangement was thought to reflect exclusively subcutaneous and deeper tissue.[88, 99]

Early on, investigators learned that impedance measurements were dependent on the frequency of the alternating current.[100–102] Thomasset realized that electric pathways in the human body were extremely complex and affected by circulation and ventilation.[103] He postulated that the body should be considered a combination of frequency-dependent resistors and capacitors that were arranged as parallel and serial circuits. As a result of his original studies, alterations in body R were used to guide fluid management in patients with cardiac conditions and cirrhosis.[104]

Validation of impedance analysis against a generally accepted method (criterion or "gold standard") of body fluid determination such as an isotope dilution technique had not yet occurred. In 1965, a significant relationship was demonstrated between the ECW volume measured by bromide dilution and the body's impedance after conduction of a 1-kHz alternating current in healthy and edematous subjects.[105] Shortly thereafter, body impedance after conduction of high-frequency (100-kHz) current was related to the TBW as determined by tritium (heavy-water) dilution.[89]

Technique

Impedance measurements for body compositional analysis should be performed with the subject in a supine position. The arm (preferably the right) and the leg (right) should not touch other body parts, since this leads to a disturbance of the electric field that may result in falsely low values. Two sets of two electrodes are used for one measurement of impedance.

A first set of "outer" electrodes, attached to a hand and a foot, serve as transmitters of the current. Specifically, one electrode is positioned on the skin of the right hand overlying the third metacarpal bone, while a second electrode is placed on the third metatarsal bone close to the third toe. A second set of "inner" electrodes, attached to the right wrist and ankle, measures impedance. A wrist electrode is placed on the dorsal surface between protruding portions of the ulnar and radial bones. The ankle electrode is attached to skin on the level of protruding parts of the tibial and fibular bone.[86]

When alternating current generated by a plethysmograph is introduced by way of the first set of electrodes, this current flows through the arm, the trunk, and the leg, and back in the opposite direction (Fig. 5–4). The body opposes the flow of current, and the total impedance signal is determined by electrodes positioned on the wrist and ankle: whole-body impedance. The plethysmograph measures impedance and separates

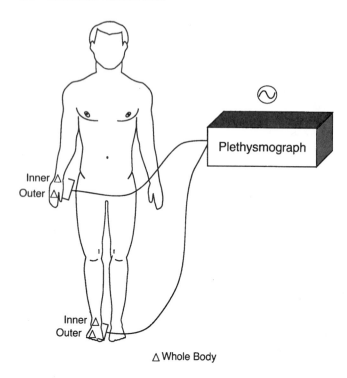

Figure 5–4. Whole-body impedance. The body opposes conduction of current generated by a plethysmograph when the current is introduced at a set of outer electrodes. The impedance signal is determined by inner electrodes positioned on a wrist and an ankle.

the signal into R and X_c. Impedance plethysmographs employ either a single alternating current of high frequency (usually at 50 kHz) or multiple frequencies (1 kHz to 1 MHz).

Impedance During Health

Hoffer and colleagues were the first to find that the body's R and its fluid contents during a steady state were highly related.[89] Scheltinga and coworkers also demonstrated a close relationship between these parameters in a heterogeneous group of healthy volunteers.[106] Acute changes in the body's state of hydration were also found to affect an impedance signal. For example, a constant infusion of Ringer's solution caused a drop in whole-body impedance values.[107] Similarly, a bolus infusion of 1 L of 0.9% sodium chloride over 15 minutes resulted in an instantaneous fall in R determined across the whole body and its various segments; a new equilibrium was attained after 15 to 45 minutes. The drop in the electric signal was inversely related to the TBW content as determined by heavy-water dilution.[106] Conversely, hemodialysis caused an increase in impedance that was closely correlated with changes in body weight.[108] Orally administered fluids may not be detected, which is probably related to a slow absorption and subsequent redistribution with the ongoing production of urine. When using whole-body impedance, the influence of the bladder contents is small since the trunk itself contributes only approximately 15% to the whole-body impedance signal.

The impedance technique has been validated with a number of other body compositional methods such as dilution of tracers,[89, 109] underwater weighing,[110] anthropometrics,[111] total body electric conductivity,[112] computed tomographic scanning,[113] magnetic resonance imaging,[114] total body potassium,[86] and DEXA[115] in healthy populations of all ages.[116, 117] Although in most studies a tight correlation was demonstrated between techniques, several variables should be considered that determine the accuracy and reliability of a prediction of body composition with bioelectric impedance analysis (BIA).

Position of Electrodes

Impedance analysis performed with a four-electrode configuration is a popular technique[88, 99] since the two-electrode method may be subject to erratic skin effects and therefore requires the transdermal introduction of small needles.[118, 119] However, standardized positioning of the R-detecting set of electrodes is essential when four electrodes are used. For instance, positioning an R-detecting set close to an elbow and a knee while a current-introducing set is maintained on traditionally used spots of the hand and foot diminishes the body's R by approximately 60%.[106] Indeed, the majority of body R is present in body portions with small diameters, such as a forearm and a lower leg.[120, 121] This can be understood by realizing that R is inversely related to diameter.[99] When knee and elbow electrodes were used, R values were more closely related to those predicted and measured.[106] Schell and Gross found that repositioning R-detecting electrodes from their standard positions on the wrist and the ankle toward the trunk in 1-cm increments resulted in a drop of 10Ω/cm.[122] Thus, if serial impedance measurements are anticipated, the position of the electrodes should be marked with indelible ink to diminish lead placement error.

Some investigators have proposed performing segmental measurements by changing the positions of current-transmitting electrodes simultaneously with the positions of the detecting set. However, a discrepancy of as much as 15% was reported between measured and calculated (by adding individual measures of an arm, a trunk, and a leg) values of total body R.[123, 124] Altering the standard position of current-transmitting electrodes (hand and foot) results in a distortion of the electric field and subsequently changes an R signal. When appropriate adjustments were made to ensure a constant electric field, this error was reduced to 3%.[106] In addition, significant interference between current-transmitting and R-detecting electrodes may occur if the interelectrode distance is less than the diameter of a limb.[99, 125]

Body Position and Geometry

Body position is one of the determinants of an R signal. This can be understood by recognizing that R is inversely related to diameter. An R signal determined across a leg increases significantly for at least 2 hours after the transition from a standing to a supine position. This observation is thought to result from a shift of blood and extracellular fluids from the peripheral to the central circulation.[107, 126] This shifting phenomenon is accompanied by a progressive decrease in the diameter of a lower leg. The observation that R determined across a trunk diminishes over this time provides further support for the "shifting" hypothesis. Therefore, R values determined in supine individuals (e.g., hospitalized patients) may be high when compared with R measured in volunteers who were upright just before the impedance measurement.

The body geometry may also affect the determination of impedance.[92] Alterations in the position of an arm or a leg relative to the trunk are thought to distort the lines of current and orientation of the electric field.[127] For example, increasing the angle between an arm and a trunk from 30 degrees to 90 degrees causes an increase in the whole-body impedance signal.[122] Thus, the error of an impedance measurement is minimized if tests are performed at a constant limb-trunk angle.

Temperature

A strong direct correlation ($r = .99$) is present between the fall in temperature and the increase in R measured across a 1-F cylinder containing a 0.9% sodium chloride solution. Similarly, the R of cow and human blood is reported to change in a linear fashion with temperature.[128] However, the effects of alterations in skin and core temperature on an in vivo impedance signal are less well understood.[129] The body impedance of healthy subjects measured during low environmental temperatures appeared higher than values obtained in a room with a high temperature; these effects probably resulted from an associated alteration in blood flow and limb diameter.[130] An increase in core temperature results in sweating, which in turn may cause shunting of the electric current. In addition, the area of contact between the electrodes and the skin may be diminished. For these and other reasons, measurements performed immediately after exercise are unreliable.[122] The effects of fever on impedance parameters are unknown. Additional confounding variables, such as alterations in blood flow and fluid retention, may influence the interpretation of an in vivo impedance measurement in febrile subjects.

Other Factors

Several other factors can affect the accuracy of impedance analysis. In vitro studies have suggested that the hematocrit is an important determinant of the impedance signal.[131, 132] Animals with a high hematocrit demonstrated a larger drop in impedance after a standard challenge of 250 ml of 0.9% saline than did animals with a low hematocrit.[125] The vascular tree may form a low-impedance pathway "preferable" to electric current (the "path of least resistance"). Since an elevated hematocrit represents a large number of red blood cells per unit of plasma, a standard intravenous load of 0.9% sodium chloride is thought to lead to a more pronounced shunting of the electric current than in the low-hematocrit scenario. Increased shunting may in turn lead to a marked fall in impedance. Indeed, a significant relationship was present between impedance and hematocrit in a group of healthy volunteers.[133]

Daily variation of impedance values in weight-stable individuals is reported to range from 2% (expressed as a coefficient of variation, defined as the standard deviation divided by the mean) to 2.8%.[86, 122, 134] Kushner and Schoeller performed impedance measurements in a group of five subjects and found a week-to-week variability of 2.2%.[90] Weekly measurements in five healthy, weight-stable (± 1 kg) volunteers were performed for 10 weeks, and it was found that the week-to-week variability approximated 2.5%.[135]

Impedance During Illness

The altered intake of nutrients and release of cytokines and other humoral factors associated with inflammation and other disease states may disrupt the steady-state relation between R and the TBW. A disease itself may also affect the conduction of the electric current.[136, 137] However, the body's drive for homeostasis could result in the maintenance of a constant number of conducting particles (electrolytes) per fluid volume. If this were the case, the close relationship between the body R and the fluid contents would persist during illness. For example, Hoffer and colleagues found that these parameters were closely related in both healthy volunteers and patients with various degrees of hydration.[89] Incorporation of the ionic mass (an approximation of the total number of electrolytes in the body) did not improve this relationship. Kushner and

Schoeller demonstrated correlation coefficients ranging from 0.93 to 0.97 between the TBW predicted from body impedance and heavy-water dilution in patients suffering from diabetes, inflammatory bowel disease, and obesity.[90] Furthermore, the results from patients with malignant hematologic disorders awaiting bone marrow transplantation and healthy volunteers were uniformly distributed along the regression line.[138] Schols and colleagues also found a strong correlation between the body fluid contents and impedance in a population of patients with chronic obstructive pulmonary disease.[139] In contrast, the impedance technique did not accurately predict the fat-free mass in cardiopulmonary and surgical patients.[87] However, these studies used regression equations derived from a healthy population, which may not be applicable in a specific patient population. The development of disease-specific impedance equations will most likely increase the accuracy of a TBW prediction.[140]

Although a relationship between R and the TBW can be maintained during disease, profound changes in X_c have been reported in patients. Malnourished[109] and overhydrated[141–143] subjects demonstrated low values of X_c compared with individuals with a normal fluid status. Diminished values of X_c were also observed in stable, critically ill patients who had retained 4 L of ECW. Moreover, an inverse correlation was present between X_c and the volume of ECW.[98] The relationship between critical illness, cellular function, X_c, and ECW is fascinating. Critical illness is known to affect electric characteristics of a cell such as its transmembrane potential; these events are associated with cellular dysfunction and electrolyte redistribution.[144] Unfortunately, X_c and transmembrane potential have not been studied simultaneously, although they may prove to be different expressions of an identical characteristic of a cellular membrane. X_c is hypothesized to fall during critical illness as a result of accumulating ECW, which in turn causes the intercellular distance to increase and subsequently alters the ability of overhydrated tissue to store electric charge.

Prognostic Implications

Several studies have suggested that the body's impedance may be useful as a predictor of health and illness. Furthermore, a diminished lean body mass, as estimated by impedance techniques, was related to the occurrence of postoperative complications in a group of cancer patients.[145] We also observed that the phase angle measured across a leg was a sensitive indicator of health and disease and may predict recovery.[95] Conversely, a narrowing (fall) in the phase angle was related to the length of hospital stay, the total number of TPN days, and the cumulative dose of steroids and antibiotics in a group of bone marrow transplantation patients.[138]

Ott and coworkers found that the phase angle was the most potent predictor of death (more so than age, CD4 lymphocyte count, serum albumin levels, and other parameters) in 75 patients positive for the human immunodeficiency virus.[146] In a study of more than 3000 hemodialysis patients who had undergone BIA, Chertow and colleagues showed that a phase angle less than 4 degrees was an independent determinant of death, after adjustment for age, sex, race, dialysis intensity, and several biochemical indicators of nutritional status.[147] Among patients with a phase angle less than 3 degrees, the unadjusted relative risk was 4.3 (2.9 to 6.2); the adjusted relative risk was 2.2 (1.6 to 3.1), indicating at least of doubling of the death risk for these patients.

Regional and Segmental Impedance Analysis

The forearm and lower leg "cylinders" contribute the vast majority (>90%) of the body's total impedance, despite accounting for less than one quarter of the fat-free mass. Hence, impedance methods tend to be insensitive to changes in the trunk or abdominal cavity.[148] This has led to an interest in regional ("proximal" electrode placement) and segmental (e.g., limb-only) BIA.

The TBW of healthy subjects as measured by heavy-water dilution was more accurately predicted when these "high-impedance cylinders" were bypassed and an impedance value of the "proximal body" was obtained.[135] In addition, proximal electrode placement detected a fall in impedance after saline administration more precisely than did distal electrodes in both a dog and a human model.[95, 125]

Limbs resemble a cylinder very closely and may serve as a representative body segment. For example, R measured across an arm and a leg allowed an accurate prediction of the total fluid contents in healthy individuals[123, 124] and in hemodialysis patients.[149] Further research is required to determine whether regional or segmental BIA is sensitive to change and whether "part-body" BIA is a better or worse predictor of clinical outcomes.

Serial Bioelectric Impedance Analysis

Few investigators have performed serial BIA measurements. Kotler and associates evaluated changes in body weight, body fat, and body cell mass (estimated by BIA) in 23 human immunodeficiency virus–infected patients with malabsorption.[150] Changes in body weight were mirrored by changes in the estimated body cell mass. Quirk and coworkers performed serial BIA in 31 children with cystic fibrosis and found that impedance predicted the change in total body potassium, whereas weight, height, and fat-free mass by caliper anthropometry did not.[151] These studies indicate that BIA is sensitive to change. More studies are required to determine the sensitivity of impedance techniques to changes in the natural history of acute and chronic diseases, and to gauge responses to the administration of nutritional support, growth factors, or other nutrition-directed therapies.

Present State of Knowledge

In 1994, the National Institutes of Health (NIH) sponsored a technology assessment conference dedicated to the evaluation of single-frequency impedance technology as a method of body composition analysis. A summary of the NIH statement has been published.[152] A complete text of the draft conference statement is also available online at http://text.nlm.nih.gov.

Briefly, although the NIH conference expert panel concluded that height-adjusted R (ht^2/R) was related to the TBW, assumptions underlying the R-TBW relation, particularly the assumption of uniform hydration of tissues, were felt to weaken the application of BIA for body composition analysis. However, since 1994, there have been two major advances (one mathematic, the other technological) that should improve and minimize the errors associated with BIA measurements. First, the replacement of the original series model with a parallel R model has improved the prediction of more complex body compartments. Applications of the parallel R model have provided better estimates of fat-free mass and body cell mass than series models previously employed.[153] Indeed, the parallel model is more consistent with human physiology (i.e., the ICW or body cell mass exhibits capacitive properties, whereas the ECW does not, and the ICW and ECW are in parallel).

Second, multifrequency bioelectric impedance analysis (MFBIA) has become widely available. At the 1994 NIH conference, most of the reported work with MFBIA was preliminary. MFBIA should provide a more accurate view of the TBW distribution.[154] In theory, current flows around cells at low frequency (i.e., through the ECW) and encounters few (if any) capacitive elements. At high frequency, the current penetrates the cells, generating a view of the TBW. MFBIA offers tremendous promise in helping to distinguish the distribution, as well as volume, of body water.

Future Directions

Impedance analysis is a noninvasive, safe, and painless method of estimating TBW. In addition, it may (1) provide a window into the distribution of body water (particularly with MFBIA), (2) approximate body composition, and (3) have prognostic value, at least in certain chronic diseases (acquired immunodeficiency syndrome), end-stage renal disease). There are several additional potential applications that should be explored.

Application in Critically Ill Patients

There have been relatively few applications of impedance methods in the hospital (and intensive care unit) setting, particularly among critically ill patients. Since these patients are among those most prone to disturbances in the distribution of body water, impedance may help surgeons, intensivists, and other critical care personnel rationalize the administration of fluids and may help to guide nephrologic therapy (e.g., dialysis, ultrafiltration). MFBIA may be particularly

helpful in this regard, if these methods prove superior in identifying aberrant ECW/ICW ratios. Favorable changes in the distribution of body water may herald recovery, perhaps before other clinical parameters (e.g., urine output, recovery from respiratory failure).

In our experience, patients consulted by our metabolic support service (inpatients in need of nutritional support) exhibited phase angles several degrees below the population norm[155] and well below levels observed in stable, chronically ill outpatients. Whether impedance can be used to monitor the response to nutritional support is unknown but worthy of study.

Finally, drug kinetics and disposition may be assisted by information derived by BIA. In addition to improving the prediction of creatinine clearance from serum creatinine values,[156] impedance has been used to help predict the clearance of aminoglycosides[157] and theophylline.[158] This innovative approach is promising, since tailoring a regimen of drug prescription has been reported to improve the outcome of critically ill patients.[151]

Prescription of Intravenous Feedings

Body impedance, instead of body weight, has been proposed as the basis for prescribing total parenteral nutrition. Schroeder and colleagues warned that prescribing calories for a hypothetical patient based on weight may result in an overprescription of 57% or an underprescription of 10%.[87] In contrast, when body impedance was used as the basis for prescription, these figures were reduced to 11% and 14%, respectively. Obese patients who are at risk for overprescription of calories and associated morbidity might particularly benefit from such an approach.

◆ MUSCLE FUNCTION AND ENERGY METABOLISM

Skeletal muscle is the largest store of endogenous amino acids. During periods of total or partial starvation, body protein is catabolized to provide the necessary amino acids and carbon skeletons for gluconeogenesis, fuel for the gut, and fuel for the synthesis of acute-phase proteins. All body protein that is proteolyzed has served an important role, either functional or structural. These observations have led various investigators to hypothesize that nutritional or metabolic deficiencies may alter the metabolic status and thereby the function of an organ, such as skeletal muscle, before a change in body composition can be detected. Similarly, normalization of functional abnormalities may be a more accurate reflection of the effects of refeeding than are the findings of other assessment techniques based on static measurements. Numerous studies have shown that skeletal muscle function, including that of the diaphragm, can be rapidly altered by nutrient deprivation and restored by refeeding.[10, 159–163]

Early studies showed that a reduction in grip strength was more sensitive in detecting postoperative complications than body weight, midarm muscle circumference, or serum albumin levels and correlated with the risk of morbidity in medical and surgical patients.[164–166] Muscle function analysis using electric nerve stimulation has allowed objective nutritional assessment. It is nonvolitional and therefore is not limited or influenced by the patient's motivation. Electromyographic electrodes are placed over the abductor pollicis longus to record the action potential and on the wrist at the ulnar nerve to deliver electric stimuli of typically 10, 20, 30, and 50 Hz. The stimulus causes the abductor pollicis longus to contract. The maximal relaxation rate and the force-to-frequency ratio is then determined. The maximal relaxation rate is determined at the maximal slope during the relaxation phase of the tension-time curve; force-to-frequency ratios are calculated using the maximal amplitude of the tension-time curve generated by different frequencies.[164]

As malnutrition develops, the rate of relaxation is slowed and the maximal relaxation rate decreases. Also, there is a decrease in the maximal amplitude as frequency is increased, thus increasing force-to-frequency ratios. In contrast, the well-nourished individual experiences an incremental increase in maximal amplitude as the frequency of stimulation increases, resulting in a small force-to-frequency ratio.[164] This method has been found to be more sensitive and specific than traditional nutritional assessment techniques. In obese patients and patients with anorexia nervosa, Russell and colleagues showed that starvation causes the ratio of the force at 10 Hz to that at 50 to 100 Hz to double and the relax-

ation rate to slow from a mean of about 10% of maximal force lost/10 msec to 5 to 6%. The development of fatigue was also demonstrated. Refeeding corrected these changes before a gain in body nitrogen.[165–168] The combination of an abnormal force-frequency curve and a slow relaxation rate in a group of preoperative surgical patients was found to be the most specific and sensitive predictor of nutritionally associated complications when compared with other nutritional parameters, such as hand grip strength, arm muscle circumference, and albumin and transferrin levels.[169] It has also been shown that protein deprivation with adequate caloric intake in a group of elderly women impairs muscle function with significant decreases in adductor pollicis muscle function by 3 weeks.[170] However, muscle function analysis using electric stimulation of the adductor pollicis muscle may be too sensitive. Shizgal and colleagues did not detect a correlation in body composition using this technique and multiple-isotope dilution techniques.[171] In this study of healthy volunteers, changes in muscle function were evident by 24 hours of starvation but returned to normal within 6 hours of a single normal meal. This observation led the authors to hypothesize that the reaction of skeletal muscle to electric stimulation does not directly reflect nutritional status but may be more closely related to energy availability and production.

With respect to skeletal muscle and perhaps to other organ systems as well, major changes in energy substrates occur with starvation and in other catabolic states. Changes in these energy stores may be very closely related to changes in muscle function and may influence the functional changes observed in the skeletal muscle of malnourished subjects. During exercise, muscle glycogen is rapidly depleted, and its subsequent repletion depends on the availability of substrate.[172] Chronic semistarvation is associated with a 54.2% decrease in muscle mass concomitant with a 90.3% decrease in muscle glycogen and a 59.6% reduction in total muscle energy content. There appears to be a linear relationship between the amount of energy administered intravenously as glucose and the skeletal muscle glycogen content.[173]

Indeed, alterations in muscular energy metabolism may explain many of the abnormalities noted in the nerve stimulation and muscle contraction studies, including the decrease in the muscle relaxation rate reported in many studies of the effects of malnutrition.[174] A reduction in adenosine triphosphate (ATP) turnover or a decrease in the free energy available from ATP hydrolysis might result if the energy stores, substrates, or enzymatic processes responsible for ATP resynthesis and utilization are compromised. Both actin-myosin cross-bridge detachment[175] and calcium uptake into the sarcoplasmic reticulum[176] are rate-limiting determinants of skeletal muscle relaxation and require ATP hydrolysis, and the muscle relaxation rate correlates with ATP turnover in contracting muscle.[177] Therefore, it is likely that the slowing of the muscle relaxation rate observed in malnourished patients is a manifestation of diminished ATP turnover. Thus, one end result of an alteration in muscle energetics is a change in muscle function.

These findings suggest an important but poorly defined physiologic process by which muscle function is altered according to changes in energy metabolism and substrate availability. ATP is synthesized from oxidative metabolism in the mitochondria by breakdown of the high-energy phosphate storage compound phosphocreatine (PCr), by anaerobic glycolysis, or by both processes. In healthy persons under nonstressful conditions, ATP synthesis is not self-limiting. However, under stressful condition, such as after trauma or infection with fever, tissue anoxia, and increased muscular work and other metabolic alterations, mitochondrial ATP synthesis may become rate limiting and fall below the rate of ATP utilization. In these instances, glycolysis, a less efficient form of ATP production, becomes prominent. In this process, glucose is metabolized to lactic acid, and two ATP molecules are produced per mole of glucose consumed. In contrast, the complete metabolism of lactate to carbon dioxide and water within the mitochondrion and the subsequent oxidation by the electron transport system of the reduced nicotinamide adenine dinucleotide produces 36 molecules of ATP. In addition, the increased production of lactic acid, in contrast to the genesis of neutral water rapidly exchanging carbon dioxide, causes an intracellular acidosis. Either a decrease in substrate or precursor availability or a decrease in the production of high-energy phosphate compounds, in the presence of

constant or increased need, could alter muscle energy metabolism and depress muscle energy stores.[178]

Many studies using biopsy techniques to obtain tissue specimens for in vitro analysis have detected changes in skeletal muscle energy metabolism associated with malnutrition and severe illness. Typically, markedly decreased concentrations of skeletal muscle adenine nucleotides, PCr, and glycogen are noted.[179–181] More severely ill patients who are hemodynamically unstable and catabolic may have markedly decreased ATP, decreased PCr, normal adenosine diphosphate (ADP), increased creatine, and slightly increased AMP concentrations.[182] Morbidly obese patients who have undergone jejunoileal bypass and who suffer from chronic protein depletion have an ongoing loss of muscle ATP and PCr.[178] Metcoff and associates found reduced pyruvate kinase and dehydrogenase activities in muscle biopsy tissue from malnourished patients.[183] Hypocaloric fasting increases the intracellular calcium content of skeletal muscle and decreases phosphofructokinase and succinate dehydrogenase concentrations.

Thus, a large body of evidence suggests that muscle energy metabolism and function are altered by malnutrition. Although the specific findings vary somewhat from one study to another, the following general conclusions can be drawn: (1) muscle function is altered and muscle strength decreases with malnutrition, (2) muscle strength is a crude predictor of the postoperative outcome, (3) muscle high-energy phosphate metabolism is altered by malnutrition, and both oxidative and glycolytic processes are disturbed, (4) the alterations in high-energy phosphate metabolism are associated with reproducible changes in muscle function, and (5) nutritional repletion normalizes biochemical indices of malnutrition and muscle function. The advent of magnetic resonance spectroscopy (MRS) has provided a new and powerful tool with which to examine changes in muscle energy metabolism in vivo. The technique has the potential to improve our understanding of how muscle energetics vary with metabolic or nutritional status and of how they influence changes in muscle function.

◆ MAGNETIC RESONANCE SPECTROSCOPY

When an organism is placed in a strong magnetic field, the atomic nuclei containing an odd number of nuclear particles (e.g., ^1H, ^{13}C, ^{19}F, ^{23}Na, ^{31}P, and ^{39}K), by virtue of their angular momentum or spin, behave like bar magnets and tend to align their poles in the direction of the applied magnetic field. When the orientation of the nuclei is flipped by the temporary application of energy as a radiofrequency pulse and then allowed to relax to its original orientation, the number of precessing or spinning nuclei is given by the signal strength at that given frequency. The computer-assisted capture and analysis of this relaxation or dissipation of energy is the basis of MRS and magnetic resonance imaging.[184]

Because of its nondestructive nature, MRS investigations may study single-celled organisms, isolated cells in culture, perfused organs, organ slices, and in vivo organs in their fully functional or diseased state within a living organism. Organ systems that have been studied with this technique include the brain, heart, liver, and skeletal muscle.

Many investigations relevant to metabolic assessment have been performed on skeletal muscle. Comprising over 50% of the total body mass, skeletal muscle is the largest "organ" in the body. As such, it is quantitatively and metabolically one of the most important tissues in the body. During illness or periods of starvation, skeletal muscle is catabolized, resulting in the loss of both structural and functional proteins, impaired muscle function, and body composition alterations that typify these disease states. Changes in skeletal muscle energetics may be intimately associated with these abnormalities. For example, serial MRS using ^{31}P was performed on the hind limb of rats over 8 days of starvation and 4 days of refeeding.[185] During this time, the ratio of ATP to inorganic phosphate (P_i), ratio of PCr to P_i, and intracellular pH were unchanged. In contrast, the PCr/ATP ratios were significantly lower by the fourth day of complete starvation but had returned to normal by the fourth day of refeeding. This study demonstrated that ^{31}P MRS could be used to detect and monitor changes in muscle energy metabolism associated with both starvation and refeeding, and it was hypothesized that resting PCr/ATP ratios may correlate with nutritional depletion and repletion. It also suggested that during periods of starvation, intracellular ATP concentrations were maintained at the expense of PCr.

The importance of skeletal muscle PCr in a model of sepsis was illustrated using ^{31}P MRS and the poorly metabolized creatine analogue β-guanidinopropionic acid (β-GPA).[186] After rats were fed a control diet or β-GPA to replace 70% of their PCr stores for 14 days, they underwent sham or cecal-ligation-and-puncture (CLP) operations followed by ^{31}P MRS of their gastrocnemius muscle 24 hours later. All β-GPA fed rats had altered cellular energetics; however, CLP rats fed β-GPA experienced the greater deterioration compared with CLP rats fed control diets. Both the phosphorylation potentials and the free energy of ATP hydrolysis were significantly lower in the CLP rats fed β-GPA compared with the other three groups. This study showed that there is an overall decrease in energy availability associated with sepsis that is worsened by PCr depletion, thus supporting the contention that PCr plays an important role as an energy buffer during systemic infection. It also demonstrated the ability of ^{31}P MRS to study the effects of sepsis and dietary replacement of PCr on cellular energetics.

^{31}P MRS may also be used to evaluate the effects of starvation on the distribution of water in skeletal muscle using ^{31}P MRS-visible water space markers. After intravenous infusion of dimethyl methylphosphonate (DMMP, a marker for the TBW) and phenylphosphonate (PPA, a marker for the ECW), ^{31}P-MRS gastrocnemius muscle spectra were obtained from rats at baseline and after 4 days of starvation.[187] This study revealed that starvation significantly increased the ratio of ECW to total water in the gastrocnemius muscle as measured by the PPA/DMMP ratio. Because muscle water contents were comparable between groups, this expansion of the extracellular space was accompanied by contraction of the intracellular compartment. Furthermore, the decline in the PCr/ATP ratio after starvation was inversely related to changes in the PPA/DMMP ratio. Thus, changes in cellular bioenergetics and water distribution can be measured noninvasively using in vivo ^{31}P MRS and MRS-visible water space markers in starvation and other pathologic conditions.

^{31}P MRS is useful in assessing the impact of nutritional therapies on stress states. For example, in a rat model of hind limb ischemia-reperfusion, ascorbate was administered for a period of 30 minutes before the induction of a 4-hour ischemic period and 15 minutes before and 15 minutes into a 2.5-hour period of reperfusion.[188] The ischemic period was associated with a decline in the PCr/(PCr + P_i) ratio, ATP concentration, and intracellular pH in both treated animals and nontreated controls. Treatment with ascorbate had a significantly positive effect on the recovery of high-energy phosphates—PCr/(PCr + P_i) was 86% higher and ATP concentration was 40% higher compared with controls—and intracellular pH at the end of the reperfusion period. This study demonstrates how ^{31}P MRS may be used to continuously monitor PCr recovery as well as provides in vivo evidence of the salvage effects of ascorbate after ischemia-reperfusion injury, likely due to ascorbate's antioxidant function.

^{31}P-MRS studies have shown significant changes in hepatocellular energetics associated with hepatic oxidant stress,[189] sepsis,[190] and hind limb ischemia-reperfusion injury.[191] These studies suggest that decreases in energy availability as measured by increases in the P_i/ATP ratio, and hepatocellular membrane damage as measured by increases in the ratios of phosphomonoester (PME) to ATP that occur in various disease or stress states, may be useful indices of the metabolic status of the liver and potential monitors of response to specific therapies.

There are several human studies relevant to nutritional support that report on the metabolic changes induced by diseases. The effects of malnutrition on adult human muscle energetics assessed by ^{31}P MRS found that compared with healthy control subjects, PCr/ATP and P_i/ATP ratios were significantly lower, whereas the PCr/P_i ratio was not significantly different.[192] There were also significant correlations between the body mass index and the PCr/ATP and P_i/ATP ratios, suggesting that the progressive loss of body mass index is associated with a loss of muscle creatine and phosphorus in relation to ATP. A liver ^{31}P-MRS study performed in elderly patients with differing nutritional statuses and inflammatory states revealed that protein-deprivation patients had higher ratios of PME to nucleoside triphosphate (NTP) than controls, in contrast to hypoalbuminemic patients associated with an inflammatory syndrome, who demonstrated no significant differences from control patients.[193] The significance of these findings is not entirely clear, although increases in

PME/NTP ratios have been related to hepatocellular injury or increased cell turnover. There have been similar increases in PME/NTP ratios as well as the ratio of PME to phosphodiester in patients with liver metastases.[194]

^{13}C MRS may have wide application in the study of organ and tissue metabolism of compounds such as glycogen, fats, and triglycerides. ^{13}C MRS has been used in the evaluation of malnourished patients with hepatic failure before and after liver transplantation.[195] The study revealed a significant increase in saturated fatty acids and a significant decrease in unsaturated fatty acids after liver transplantation, suggesting that there may be a differential uptake of fats before and after transplantation. The authors further suggest that ^{13}C MRS may be useful in optimizing the dietary management of severely malnourished, chronic liver failure patients before liver transplantation. ^{13}C MRS has also been used to assess liver glycogen storage and the regulation of glucose homeostasis after a mixed meal in healthy subjects.[196] Using this technique, the authors were able to provide a comprehensive picture of normal human carbohydrate metabolism after the ingestion of a mixed meal.

It is evident from these human MRS studies that we are at the threshold of a new technology that has vast implications for the metabolic assessment of patients. At present, ^{1}H MRS is able to demonstrate the resonances of aspartate, glutamine, and lactate in the brain of a rat. The ability to monitor changes in intracellular glutamine in concert with cellular energetic changes may prove to be informative in future human nutrient-deprivation studies as well as in the assessment of nutritional and metabolic therapies.

SUMMARY

Although no one technique is available that will meet all the needs of nutritional support professionals, the future is promising. This chapter reviews various methods and techniques that are used to assess metabolic and nutritional status. Technological advances in bioengineering, molecular biology, and physiology are providing exciting new tools that may eventually replace or supplement traditional static indices of metabolic assessment. At the very least, an increased understanding of the cellular abnormalities associated with various diseases will likely change our view of illness and our approaches to nutritional and metabolic intervention.

REFERENCES

1. Klein S, Kinney J, Jeejeebhoy K, et al: Nutrition support in clinical practice: Review of published data and recommendations for future research direction. JPEN J Parenter Enteral Nutr 21:133–156, 1997.
2. Sandstrom R, Drott C, Hyltander A, et al: The effect of postoperative intravenous feeding (TPN) on outcome following major surgery evaluated in a randomized study. Ann Surg 217:185–195, 1993.
3. Brennan MF, Pisters PW, Posner M, et al: A prospective randomized trial of total parenteral nutrition after major pancreatic resection for malignancy. Ann Surg 220:436–441, 1994.
4. Heslin MJ, Latkany L, Leung D, et al: A prospective, randomized trial of early enteral feeding after resection of upper gastrointestinal malignancy. Ann Surg 226:567–577, 1997.
5. Heyland DK, MacDonald S, Keefe L, Drover JW: Total parenteral nutrition in the critically ill patient: A meta analysis. JAMA 280:2013–2019, 1998.
6. Klein S, Kinney J, Jeejeebhoy K, et al: Nutrition support in clinical practice: Review of published data and recommendations for future research directions. JPEN J Parenter Enteral Nutr 21:133–156, 1997.
7. Heymsfield SB, Matthews D: Body composition: Research and clinical advances—1993 A.S.P.E.N. Research Workshop. JPEN J Parenter Enteral Nutr 18:91–103, 1994.
8. Wang ZM, Heshka S, Pierson RN Jr, Heymsfield SB: Systematic organization of body-composition methodology: An overview with emphasis on component-based methods. Am J Clin Nutr 61:457–65, 1995.
9. Stack JA, Babineau TJ, Bistrian BR: Assessment of nutritional status in clinical practice. Gastroenterologist 4(Suppl 1):S8–S15, 1996.
10. Jeejeebhoy KN: Nutritional assessment. Gastroenterol Clin North Am 27:347–369, 1998.
11. Forse RA, Shizgal HM: The assessment of malnutrition. Surgery 88:17–24, 1980.
12. Detsky AS, McLaughlin JR, Baker JP, et al: What is subjective global assessment of nutritional status? JPEN J Parenter Enteral Nutr 11:8–13, 1987.
13. Pikul J, Sharpe MD, Lowndes R, et al: Degree of preoperative malnutrition is predictive of postoperative morbidity and mortality in liver transplant recipients. Transplantation 57:469–472, 1994.
14. Enia G, Sicuso C, Alati G, et al: Subjective global assessment of nutrition in dialysis patients. Nephrol Dial Transplant 8:1094–1098, 1993.
15. Thuluvath PJ, Triger DR: How valid are our reference standards of nutrition? Nutrition 11:731–733, 1995.
16. Prealbumin in Nutritional Care Consensus Group: Measurement of visceral protein status in assessing protein and energy malnutrition: Standard of care. Nutrition 11:169–171, 1995.
17. Hedlund JU, Hansson LO, Örtquist AB: Hypoalbuminemia in hospitalized patients with community-acquired pneumonia. Arch Intern Med 155:1438–1442, 1995.
18. Hill GL: Fat-free body mass from skinfold thickness: A close relationship with total body nitrogen. Br J Nutr 39:403–408, 1978.
19. Frisancho AR: Triceps skinfold and upper arm muscle norms for assessment of nutritional status. Am J Clin Nutr 27:1052–1057, 1974.
20. Shenkin A: Impact of disease on markers of macronutrient status. Proc Nutr Soc 56:433–441, 1997.
21. Howell WH: Anthropometry and body composition analysis. In Matarese LE, Gottschlich MM (eds): Contemporary Nutrition Support Practice. Philadelphia, WB Saunders, 1998, pp 33–46.
22. Deurenberg P, Schutz Y: Body composition: Overview of methods and future directions of research. Ann Nutr Metab 39:325–333, 1995.
23. Loguercio C, Sava E, Marmo R, et al: Malnutrition in cirrhotic patients: Anthropometric measurements as a method of assessing nutritional status. Br J Clin Pract 44:98–101, 1990.
24. Loguercio C, Sava E, Sicolo P, et al: Nutritional status and survival of patients with liver cirrhosis: Anthropometric evaluation. Minerva Gastroenterol Dietol 42:57–60, 1996.
25. Moreiras-Varela O, Nunez C, Carbajal A, Morande G: Nutritional status and food habits assessed by dietary intake and anthropometric parameters in anorexia nervosa. Int J Vitam Nutr Res 60:267–274, 1990.
26. Trujillo EB, Robinson MK, Jacobs DO: Nutritional assessment in the critically ill. Crit Care Nurse 19:67–78, 1999.
27. Porter C, Cohen NH: Indirect calorimetry in critically ill patients: Role of the clinical dietitian in interpreting results. J Am Diet Assoc 96:49–57, 1996.
28. Long CL, Schaffel N, Geiger JW, et al: Metabolic response to injury and illness: Estimation of energy and protein needs from indirect calorimetry and nitrogen balance. JPEN J Parenter Enteral Nutr 3:452–456, 1979.
29. Frankenfield D: Energy dynamics. In Matarese LE, Gottschlich MM (eds): Contemporary Nutrition Support Practice. Philadelphia, WB Saunders, 1998, pp 79–95.
30. McClave SA, Snider HL: Use of indirect calorimetry in clinical nutrition. Nutr Clin Pract 7:207–221, 1992.
31. Caldwell FT: Measurement of oxygen consumption and CO_2 production in clinical nutritional assessment. In Levenson SM (ed): Nutritional Assessment: Present Status, Future Directions and Prospects. Columbus, Ohio, Ross Laboratories, 1981, pp 19–24.
32. Brose L: Prealbumin as a marker of nutritional status. J Burn Care Rehabil 11(4):372–375, 1990.
33. Winkler MF, Gerrior SA, Pomp A, Albina JE: Use of retinol-binding protein and prealbumin as indicators of the response to nutrition therapy. J Am Diet Assoc 89:684–687, 1989.
34. Prealbumin in Nutritional Care Consensus Group: Measurement of visceral protein status in assessing protein and energy malnutrition: Standard of care. Nutrition 11:169–171, 1995.
35. Mears E: Outcomes of continuous process im-

provement of a nutritional care program incorporating serum prealbumin measurements. Nutrition 12:479–484, 1996.

36. Church JM, Hill GL: Assessing the efficacy of intravenous nutrition in general surgical patients: Dynamic nutritional assessment with plasma proteins. JPEN J Parenter Enteral Nutr 11:135–139, 1987.

37. Malle E, DeBeer FC: Human serum amyloid A (SAA) protein: A prominent acute-phase reactant for clinical practice. Eur J Clin Invest 26:427–435, 1996.

38. Mustard RA, Bohnen JMA, Haseeb S, Kasina R: C-reactive protein levels predict postoperative septic complications. Arch Surg 122:69–73, 1987.

39. Jaye DL, Waites KB: Clinical applications of C-reactive protein in pediatrics. Pediatr Infect Dis J 16:735–746, 1997.

40. Nakayama T, Sonoda S, Urano T, et al: Monitoring both serum amyloid protein A and C-reactive protein as inflammatory markers in infectious diseases. Clin Chem 39:293–297, 1993.

41. Biran H, Friedman N, Neumann L, et al: Serum amyloid A (SAA) variations in patients with cancer: Correlation with disease activity, stage, primary site, and prognosis. J Clin Pathol 39:794–797, 1986.

42. Ketelslegers JM, Maiter D, Maes M, et al: Nutritional regulation of insulin-like growth factor-I. Metabolism 44(Suppl 4):50–57, 1995.

43. Soliman AT, Hassan AE, Aref MK, et al: Serum insulin-like growth factor I and II concentrations and growth hormone and insulin responses to arginine infusion in children with protein-energy malnutrition before and after nutritional rehabilitation. Pediatr Res 20:1122–1130, 1986.

44. Harris TB, Kiel D, Roubenoff R, et al: Association of insulin-like growth factor-I with body composition, weight history, and past health behaviors in the very old: The Framingham heart study. J Am Geriatr Soc 45:133–139, 1997.

45. Counts DR, Gwirtsman H, Carlsson LM, et al: The effect of anorexia nervosa and refeeding on growth hormone–binding protein, the insulin-like growth factors (IGF's), and the IGF-binding proteins. J Clin Endocrinol Metab 75:762–767, 1992.

46. Clemmons DR, Underwood LE, Dickerson RN, et al: Use of plasma somatomedin-C/insulin-like growth factor I measurements to monitor the response to nutritional repletion in malnourished patients. Am J Clin Nutr 41:191–198, 1985.

47. Donahue SP, Phillips LS: Response of IGF-I to nutritional support in malnourished hospital patients: A possible indicator of short-term changes in nutritional status. Am J Clin Nutr 50:962–969, 1989.

48. Isley WL, Underwood LE, Clemmons DR: Dietary components that regulate serum somatomedin-C concentrations in humans. J Clin Invest 71:175–182, 1983.

49. Clemmons DR, Klibanski A, Underwood LE, et al: Reduction of plasma immunoreactive somatomedin-C during fasting in humans. J Clin Endocrinol Metab 53:1247–1250, 1981.

50. Isley WL, Underwood LE, Clemmons DR: Changes in plasma somatomedin-C in response to ingestion of diets with variable protein and energy content. JPEN J Parenter Enteral Nutr 8:407–411, 1984.

51. Clemmons DR, Seek M, Underwood LE: Supplementary essential amino acids augment the somatomedin-C/insulin-like growth factor I response to refeeding after fasting. Metabolism 34:391–395, 1985.

52. Thissen JP, Ketelslegers JM, Underwood LE: Nutritional regulation of the insulin-like growth factors. Endocr Rev 15:80–101, 1994.

53. Merimée TJ, Zapf J, Froesch ER: Insulin-like growth factors in the fed and fasted states. J Clin Endocrinol Metab 55:999–1002, 1982.

54. MacDougald DA, Hwang CS, Fan HY, et al: Regulated expression of the obese gene product (leptin) in white adipose tissue and 3T3-L1 adipocytes. Proc Natl Acad Sci U S A 92:9034–9037, 1995.

55. Zhang Y, Proenca R, Maffei M, et al: Positional cloning of the mouse obese gene and its human homologue. Nature 372:425–432, 1994.

56. Johansen KL, Mulligan K, Tai V, Schambelan M: Leptin, body composition, and indices of malnutrition in patients on dialysis. J Am Soc Nephrol 9:1080–1084, 1998.

57. Stratton RJ, Stubbs RJ, Elia M: Interrelationship between circulating leptin concentrations, hunger, and energy intake in healthy subjects receiving tube feeding. JPEN J Parenter Enteral Nutr 22:335–339, 1998.

58. Kanaley J: Body composition and in vivo neutron activation. J Lab Clin Med 127:414–415, 1996.

59. Cohn SH, Vaswani AH, Yasumura S, et al: Improved models for determination of body fat by in vivo neutron activation. Am J Clin Nutr 40:255–259, 1984.

60. Heymsfield SB, Waki M, Kehayias J, et al: Chemical and elemental analysis of humans in vivo using improved body composition models. Am J Physiol 261:E190–E198, 1991.

61. Wang ZM, Deurenberg P, Guo SS, et al: Six-compartment body composition model: Inter-method comparisons of total body fat measurement. Int J Obes Relat Metab Disord 22:329–337, 1998.

62. Gotfredsen A, Jensen J, Borg J, et al: Measurement of lean body mass and total body fat using dual photon absorptiometry. Metabolism 35:88–93, 1986.

63. Plourde G: The role of radiologic methods in assessing body composition and related metabolic parameters. Nutr Rev 55:289–296, 1997.

64. Kellie SE: Measurement of bone density with dual energy x-ray absorptiometry. JAMA 267:286–294, 1992.

65. Lukaski HC: Soft tissue composition and bone mineral status: Evaluation by dual-energy x-ray absorptiometry. J Nutr 123:438–443, 1993.

66. Reference deleted.

67. Rochat T, Slosman DO, Pichard C, Belli DC: Body composition analysis by dual-energy x-ray absorptiometry in adults with cystic fibrosis. Chest 106:800–805, 1994.

68. Slosman DO, Casez JP, Pichard C, et al: Assessment of whole body composition with dual-energy x-ray absorptiometry. Radiology 185:593–598, 1992.

69. Shizgal HM, Milne CA, Spanier AH: The effect of nitrogen sparing intravenously administered fluids on post-operative body composition. Surgery 85:496–481, 1979.

70. Shizgal HM, Spanier AH, Humes J, et al: Indirect measurement of total exchangeable potassium. Am J Physiol 233:F253–F258, 1977.

71. Moore FD, Oleson KH, McMurphy JD, et al: The body cell mass and its supporting environment. *In* Body Composition in Health and Disease. Philadelphia, WB Saunders, 1963, pp 1–43.
72. Shizgal HM, Martin MF: Caloric requirement of the critically ill septic patient. Crit Care Med 16:312–317, 1988.
73. Guirao X, Franch G, Gil MJ, et al: Extracellular volume, nutritional status, and refeeding changes. Nutrition 10:558–561, 1994.
74. Shizgal HM: Body composition. *In* Fischer J (ed): Surgical Nutrition. Boston, Little, Brown, 1983, pp 3–17.
75. Tellado JM, Garcia-Sabrido JL, Hanley JA, et al: Predicting mortality based on body composition analysis. Ann Surg 209:81–87, 1989.
76. Moore FD: Energy and the maintenance of body cell mass. JPEN J Parenter Enteral Nutr 4:228–260, 1980.
77. Legaspi A, Robets JP, Horowitz GD, et al: Effect of starvation and total parenteral nutrition on electrolyte homeostasis in normal man. JPEN J Parenter Enteral Nutr 12:109–115, 1988.
78. Legaspi A, Roberts JP, Albert JD, et al: The effect of starvation and total parenteral nutrition on skeletal muscle amino acid content and membrane potential difference in normal man. Surg Gynecol Obstet 166:233–240, 1988.
79. Fantini GA, Roberts JP, Lowry SF, et al: Effect of hormonal and substrate backgrounds on cell membrane function in normal males. J Appl Physiol 63:1107–1113, 1987.
80. Pichard C, Hoshino E, Allard JP, et al: Intracellular potassium and membrane potential during malnutrition and subsequent refeeding. Am J Clin Nutr 54:489–498, 1991.
81. Dudley HF, Boling EA, Lequesne LP, et al: Studies on antidiuresis in surgery: Effects of anesthesia and posterior pituitary antidiuretic hormone on water metabolism in man. Ann Surg 140:354–367, 1954.
82. Llaurado JG: Increased excretion of aldosterone immediately after operation. Lancet 1:1295–1298, 1955.
83. Flear CT, Bhattacharya SS, Singh CM: Solute and water exchanges between cells and extracellular fluids in health and disturbances after trauma. JPEN J Parenter Enteral Nutr 4:98–120, 1980.
84. Carlson RG, Miller SF, Finley RK, et al: Fluid retention and burn survival. J Trauma 27:127–135, 1987.
85. Schloerb PR, Friis-Hansen BJ, Edelman IS, et al: The measurement of total body water in the human subject by deuterium oxide dilution. J Clin Invest 29:1296–1310, 1950.
86. Lukaski HC, Johnson PE, Bolunchuk WW, et al: Assessment of fat-free mass using bioelectrical impedance measurements of the human body. Am J Clin Nutr 41:810–817, 1985.
87. Schroeder D, Christi PM, Hill GL: Bioelectrical impedance analysis for body composition: Clinical evaluation in general surgical patients. JPEN J Parenter Enteral Nutr 14:129–133, 1990.
88. Nyboer J: Electrical Impedance Plethysmography. Springfield, Ill, Charles C Thomas, 1970, pp 3–49.
89. Hoffer EC, Meador CK, Simpson DC: Correlation of whole-body impedance with total body water volume. J Appl Physiol 27:531–534, 1969.
90. Kushner RF, Schoeller DA: Estimation of total body water by bioelectrical impedance analysis. Am J Clin Nutr 44:417–424, 1986.
91. Sapegno E: Über die Impedanz und Kapazitat des quergestreiften Muskels in Langs- und Querrichtung. Pflugers Arch 224:186–205, 1930.
92. Barnett A: The basic factors involved in proposed electrical methods for measuring thyroid function. I: The effect of body size and shape. West J Surg Obstet Gynecol 45:322–326, 1937.
93. Cole KS: Membranes, Ions and Impulses. Berkeley, University of California Press, 1968, pp 6–103.
94. Ti Tien H: Bilayer Lipid Membranes. New York, Marcel Dekker, 1974, pp 117–161.
95. Scheltinga MR, Jacobs DO, Kimbrough TD, et al: Alterations in body fluid content can be detected by bioelectrical impedance analysis. J Surg Res 50:461–468, 1991.
96. Mattar JA: Application of total body bioimpedance to the critically ill patient. Brazilian Group for Bioimpedance Study. New Horiz 4:493–503, 1996.
97. Brazier MAB: The impedance angle test for thyrotoxicosis. West J Surg Obstet Gynecol 43:429–441, 514–527, 1935.
98. Vigouroux R: Sur la résistance électrique considérée comme signe clinique. Progr Medicale 16:45–47, 1888.
99. Horton JW, van Ravenswaay AC: Electrical impedance of the human body. J Franklin Inst 20:557–572, 1935.
100. Hober R: Messungen der inneren Leitfahigkeit von Zellen. Pflugers Arch 150:15–45, 1913.
101. Philippson M: Sur la résistance électrique des cellules et des tissus. C R Seances Soc Biol Fil 83:1399–1402, 1920.
102. Pauly H, Schwan HP: Dielectric properties and ion mobility in erythrocytes. Biophys J 6:621–639, 1966.
103. Thomasset MA: Proprietes bio-electriques des tissus: Appreciation par la mésure de l'impedance de la teneur ionique extra-cellulaire et de la teneur ionique intra-cellulaire en clinique. Lyon Med 209:1325–1350, 1963.
104. Danaoui M, Joly R, Thomasset MA: Surveillance de l'equilibre électrolytique au cours des traitements diuretiques majeurs par la méthode de l'impédance. Lyon Med 210:5–35, 1963.
105. Thomasset MA: Mesure du volume des liquides extra-cellulaires par la méthode électro-chimique: Signification biophysique de l'impédance a 1 kilocycle du corps humain. Lyon Med 214:131–143, 1965.
106. Scheltinga MR, Jacobs DO, Kimbrough TD, et al: Alterations in body fluid content can be detected by bioelectrical impedance analysis (BIA). J Surg Res 50:461–468, 1991.
107. Tedner B, Jacobson HS, Linnarsson D, et al: Impedance fluid volume monitoring during intravenous infusion in healthy subjects. Acute Care 10:200–206, 1983/1984.
108. Bohm D, Odaischi M, Beyerlein C, et al: Total body water: Changes during dialysis estimated by bio-impedance analysis. Infusiontherapie (Basel) 17(Suppl 3):75–78, 1990.
109. McDougall D, Shizgal HM: Body composition measurements from whole body resistance and reactance. Surg Forum 37:42–44, 1986.
110. Segal KR, Van Loan M, Fitzgerald PI, et al: Lean

body mass estimation by bioelectrical impedance analysis: A four-site cross validation study. Am J Clin Nutr 47:7–14, 1988.

111. Houtkooper LB, Lohman TG, Going SB, et al: Validity of bioelectrical impedance for body composition assessment in children. J Appl Physiol 66:814–821, 1989.

112. Segal KR, Gutin B, Presta E, et al: Estimation of human body composition by electrical impedance methods: A comparative study. J Appl Physiol 58:1565–1571, 1985.

113. Brown BH, Karatzas T, Nakielny R, et al: Determination of upper arm muscle and fat areas using electrical impedance measurements. Clin Phys Physiol Meas 9:47–55, 1988.

114. Chan YL, Leung SS, Lam WW, et al: Body fat estimation in children by magnetic resonance imaging, bioelectrical impedance, skinfold and body mass index: A pilot study. J Paediatr Child Health 34:22–28, 1998.

115. Wattanapenpaiboon N, Lukito W, Strauss BJ, et al: Agreement of skinfold measurement and bioelectrical impedance analysis (BIA) methods with dual energy x-ray absorptiometry (DEXA) in estimating total body fat in Anglo-Celtic Australians. Int J Obes Relat Metab Disord 22:854–860, 1998.

116. Steen B, Bosaeus I, Elmstîhl S, et al: Body composition in the elderly estimated with an electrical impedance method. Comp Gerontol Section A 1:102–105, 1987.

117. Davies PSW, Preece MA, Hicks CJ, et al: The prediction of total body water using bioelectrical impedance in children and adolescents. Ann Hum Biol 15:237–240, 1988.

118. Thomasset MA: Propriétés bio-électriques des tissus. Mesures de l'impédance en clinique: Signification des courbes obtenues. Lyon Med 208:107–118, 1962.

119. Boulier A, Fricker J, Thomasset A-L, et al: Fat-free mass estimation by the two-electrode impedance method. Am J Clin Nutr 52:581–585, 1990.

120. Settle RG, Foster KR, Epstein BR, et al: Nutritional assessment: Whole body impedance and body fluid compartments. Nutr Cancer 2:72–80, 1980.

121. Chumlea WC, Baumgarter RN, Roche AF: Specific resistivity used to estimate fat-free mass from segmental body measures of bioelectrical impedance. Am J Clin Nutr 48:7–15, 1988.

122. Schell B, Gross R: The reliability of bioelectrical impedance measurements in the assessment of body composition in healthy adults. Nutr Rep Int 36:449–459, 1987.

123. Baumgarter RN, Chumlea WC, Roche AF: Estimation of body composition from bioelectric impedance of body segments. Am J Clin Nutr 50:221–226, 1989.

124. Fuller NU, Elia M: Potential use of bioelectrical impedance of the "whole body" and of body segments for the assessment of body composition: Comparison with densitometry and anthropometry. Eur J Clin Nutr 43:779–791, 1989.

125. Scheltinga MR, Helton WS, Rounds J, et al: Impedance electrodes positioned on proximal portions of limbs quantify fluid compartments in dogs. J Appl Physiol 70:2039–2045, 1991.

126. Hargens AL, Pipton CL, Gollnick PD, et al: Fluid shifts and muscle function in humans during acute simulated weightlessness. J Appl Physiol 54:1003–1009, 1983.

127. Kim OW, Baker LE, Pearce JA, Kim WK: Origins of the impedance change in impedance cardiography by a three-dimensional finite element model. IEEE Trans Biomed Eng 35:993–1000, 1988.

128. Burger HC, van Dongen R: Specific electrical R of body tissues. Phys Med Biol 5:431–447, 1961.

129. Klein JJ, Sedensky JA: Relation of total body resistive impedance to body temperatures [Abstract P5.12]. Proc 31st Annu Conference Eng Med Biol 20:351, 1978.

130. Caton JR, Mole PA, Adams WC, et al: Body composition analysis by bioelectrical impedance analysis: Effect of skin temperature. Med Sci Sports Exerc 20:489–491, 1988.

131. Geddes LA, Baker LE: The specific R of biological material—A compendium of data for the biomedical engineer and physiologist. Med Biol Eng 5:271–293, 1967.

132. De Vries PMJM, Meijer JH, Vlaanderen K, et al: Measurement of transcellular fluid shift during haemodialysis. 2: In vitro and clinical evaluation. Med Biol Eng Comput 27:152–158, 1989.

133. Lukaski HC: Personal communication, 1989.

134. Deuenberg P, Weststrate JA, Paymans I, et al: Factors affecting bioelectrical impedance measurements in humans. Eur J Clin Nutr 42:1017–1022, 1988.

135. Scheltinga MR, Jacobs DO, Wilmore DW: Unpublished observations.

136. Souweine G, Lenoir J, Lachanat J, et al: Determination of body fluid compartments by impedance measurements: Differences in the repartitioning of water between Duchenne muscular dystrophy and some neurological diseases. J Neurol 226:199–203, 1981.

137. Cardus D, Wesley G, McTaggart G: Electric impedance measurements in quadriplegia. Arch Phys Med Rehabil 69:186–187, 1988.

138. Scheltinga MR, Young LS, Benfell K, et al: Glutamine-enriched intravenous feedings attenuate extracellular fluid expansion following a standard stress. Ann Surg 214:385–395, 1991.

139. Schols AMWJ, Wouters EFM, Soeters PB, et al: Body composition by bioelectrical-impedance analysis compared with deuterium dilution and skinfold anthropometry in patients with chronic obstructive pulmonary disease. Am J Clin Nutr 53:421–424, 1991.

140. Chertow GM, Lazarus JM, Lew NL, et al: Development of a population-specific regression equation to estimate total body water in hemodialysis patients. Kidney Int 51:1578–1582, 1997.

141. Nyboer J, Sedensky JA: Bioelectrical impedance during renal dialysis. Proc Dial Trans Forum 4:214–219, 1974.

142. Subramanian R, Manchada SC, Nyboer J, et al: Total body water in congestive heart failure: A pre and post treatment study. J Assoc Physicians India 28:257–262, 1980.

143. Scheltinga MR, Kimbrough TD, Jacobs DO, et al: Altered cellular membrane function can be characterized by measuring body reactance. Surg Forum 41:43–44, 1990.

144. Cunningham JJN, Carter NW, Rector JFC, et al: Resting transmembrane potential difference of skeletal muscle in normal subjects and severely ill patients. J Clin Invest 50:49–59, 1971.

145. Fritz T, Hollwarth I, Ramaschow M, et al: The predictive role of bioelectrical impedance analy-

sis (BIA) in postoperative complications of cancer patients. Eur J Surg Oncol 16:326–331, 1990.

146. Ott M, Fischer H, Polat H, et al: Bioelectrical impedance analysis as a predictor of survival in patients with human immunodeficiency virus infection. J Acquir Immune Defic Syndr Hum Retrovirol 9:20–25, 1995.

147. Chertow GM, Jacobs DO, Lazarus JM, et al: Phase angle predicts survival in hemodialysis patients. J Renal Nutr 7:204–207, 1997.

148. Rallison LR, Kushner RF, Penn D, Schoeller DA: Errors in estimating peritoneal fluid by bioelectrical impedance analysis and total body electrical conductivity. J Am Coll Nutr 12:66–72, 1993.

149. Zhu F, Schneditz D, Wang E, et al: Validation of changes in extracellular volume measured during hemodialysis using a segmental bioimpedance technique. ASAIO J 44:M541–M545, 1998.

150. Kotler DP, Fogleman L, Tierney AR: Comparison of total parenteral nutrition and an oral, semi-elemental diet on body composition, physical function, and nutrition-related costs in patients with malabsorption due to acquired immunodeficiency syndrome. JPEN J Parenter Enteral Nutr 22:120–126, 1998.

151. Quirk PC, Ward LC, Thomas BJ, et al: Evaluation of bioelectrical impedance for prospective nutritional assessment in cystic fibrosis. Nutrition 13:412–416, 1997.

152. Bioelectrical impedance analysis in body composition measurement: National Institutes of Health Technology Assessment Conference Statement. Am J Clin Nutr 64:524S–532S, 1996.

153. Kotler DP, Burastero S, Wang J, Pierson RN Jr: Prediction of body cell mass, fat-free mass, and total body water with bioelectrical impedance analysis: Effects of race, sex, and disease. Am J Clin Nutr 64:489S–497S, 1996.

154. Cha K, Chertow GM, Gonzalez J, et al: Multifrequency bioelectrical impedance estimates body water distribution. J Appl Physiol 79:1316–1319, 1995.

155. Chertow GM, Trujillo EB, Jacobs DO: Unpublished observations.

156. Smythe MA, Baumann TJ, Zarowitz BJ, et al: Relationship between values of bioelectrical impedance and creatinine clearance. Pharmacotherapy 10:42–46, 1990.

157. Zarowitz BJ, Peterson EL, Robert S: Characterization of drug disposition and dosing using bioelectrical impedance. Med Prog Technol 19:193–198, 1993–94.

158. Zaske DE, Bootman JL, Solem MB, Strate RG: Increased burn patient survival with individual dosages of gentamycin. Surgery 91:142–149, 1982.

159. Brough W, Horne G, Blount A, et al: Effects of nutrient intake, surgery, sepsis, and long term administration of steroids on muscle function. BMJ 293:983–988, 1986.

160. Christie PM, Hill GL: Effect of intravenous nutrition on nutrition and function in acute attacks of inflammatory bowel disease. Gastroenterology 99:730–736, 1990.

161. Dureuil B, Viires N, Veber B, et al: Acute diaphragmatic changes induced by starvation in rats. Am J Clin Nutr 49:738–744, 1989.

162. Hanning RM, Blimkie CJR, Bar-Or O, et al: Relationship among nutritional status and skeletal and respiratory muscle function in cystic fibrosis:

Does early dietary supplementation make a difference? Am J Clin Nutr 57:580–587, 1993.

163. Windsor JA, Hill GL: Weight loss with physiologic impairment: A basic indicator of surgical risk. Ann Surg 207:290–296, 1988.

164. Brooks SD, Kearns PF: Muscle function analysis: An alternative nutrition assessment technique. Support Line 19:12–15, 1997.

165. Hunt DR, Rowland BJ, Johnston D: Hand grip strength—A simple prognostic indicator in surgical patients. JPEN J Parenter Enteral Nutr 9:701–704, 1985.

166. Klidjian AM, Foster KJ, Kammereling, et al: Relation of anthropometric and dynamometric variables to serious postoperative complications. BMJ 2:899–901, 1980.

167. Russell DM, Leiter LA, Whitwall J, et al: Skeletal muscle function during hypocaloric diets and fasting: A comparison with standard nutritional assessment parameters. Am J Clin Nutr 37:133–138, 1983.

168. Russell DM, Prendergast PJ, Darby PL, et al: A comparison between muscle function and body composition in anorexia nervosa: The effect of refeeding. Am J Clin Nutr 38:229–237, 1983.

169. Zeiderman MR, McMahon MJ: The role of objective measurement of skeletal muscle function in the preoperative patients. Clin Nutr 8:161–166, 1989.

170. Castaneda C, Charnley JM, Evans WJ, Crim MC: Elderly women accommodate to a low-protein diet with losses of body cell mass, muscle function, and immune response. Am J Clin Nutr 62:30–39, 1995.

171. Shizgal HM, Vasilevsky CA, Gardiner PF, et al: Nutritional assessment and skeletal muscle function. Am J Clin Nutr 44:761–771, 1986.

172. Hultman E, Bergstrom J, Roch-Norlund AE: Glycogen storage in human skeletal muscle. Adv Exp Med Biol 11:273–286, 1971.

173. King R, Macfie J, Hill G, et al: Effect of intravenous nutrition with glucose as the only calorie source on muscle glycogen. JPEN J Parenter Enteral Nutr 5:226–228, 1981.

174. Jewel Brand Wilkie DR: The mechanical properties of relaxing muscle. J Physiol 152:30–38, 1960.

175. Edwards RHT, Hill DK, Jones DA: Metabolic changes associated with slowing of relaxation in fatigued mouse muscle. J Physiol 251:287–301, 1975.

176. Dawson MJ, Gadian DG, Wilkie DR: Mechanical relaxation rate and metabolism studied in fatiguing muscle by phosphorus nuclear magnetic resonance. J Physiol 299:465–469, 1980.

177. Sjoholm H, Sahlin K, Edstrom L, et al: Quantitative estimation of anaerobic and oxidative energy metabolism and contraction characteristics in intact human skeletal muscle in response to electrical stimulation. Clin Physiol 3:227–230, 1983.

178. Bergstrom J, Bostrom H: Preliminary studies of energy-rich phosphagens in muscle from severely ill patients. Crit Care Med 4:197–202, 1976.

179. Lennmarken C, Larsson J: Skeletal muscle function and energy metabolites in malnourished surgical patients. Acta Chir Scand 152:169–174, 1986.

180. Lennmarken C, Sandstedt S, Crover S, et al: Muscle metabolic changes in severe malnutrition—Effect of total parenteral nutrition. Clin Nutr 3:41–44, 1984.

181. Symreng T, Larsson J, Schildt BO, et al: Nutritional assessment reflects muscle energy metabolism in gastric carcinoma. Ann Surg 198:146–150, 1983.

182. Furst P, Bergstrom J, Hultman E, Vinnars E: Intermediary energy metabolism for the catabolic state with special regard to muscle tissue. *In* Wilkinson AW, Cuthbertson D (eds): Metabolism and the Response to Injury. London, Pitman Medical, 1976, pp 194–220.

183. Metcoff J, Frank S, Yoshida T: Cell composition and metabolism in kwashiorkor (severe protein-calorie malnutrition in children). Medicine 45:365–370, 1966.

184. Bore PJ: Principles and applications of phosphorus magnetic resonance spectroscopy. *In* Kressel HY (ed): Magnetic Resonance Annual. New York, Raven Press, 1985, pp 45–69.

185. Jacobs DO, Whitman G, Maris J, et al: ^{31}P nuclear magnetic resonance spectroscopy of rat skeletal muscle during starvation [Abstract]. JPEN J Parenter Enteral Nutr 9:107a, 1985.

186. Lara TM, Wong MS, Rounds J, et al: Skeletal muscle phosphocreatine depletion depresses myocellular energy status during sepsis. Arch Surg 133:1316–1321, 1998.

187. Mizobata Y, Rounds JD, Prechek D, et al: ^{31}P magnetic resonance spectroscopy demonstrates expansion of the extracellular space in the skeletal muscle of starved rats. J Surg Res 56:491–499, 1994.

188. Lagerwall K, Daneryd P, Schersten T, Soussi B: In vivo ^{31}P nuclear magnetic resonance evidence of the salvage effect of ascorbate on the postischemic reperfused rat skeletal muscle. Life Sci 56:389–397, 1995.

189. Kobayashi T, Robinson MK, Robinson V, et al: Glutathione depletion alters hepatocellular high-energy phosphate metabolism. J Surg Res 54:189–195, 1993.

190. Kobayashi T, Robinson MK, Rounds JD, et al: Depression of hepatocyte energy status during systemic infection. Surg Forum 43:11–13, 1992.

191. Wong MS, Robinson MK, Lara TM, et al: Hindlimb ischemia-reperfusion impairs hepatocellular energetics and function via the complement system. Surg Forum 49:181–183, 1998.

192. Thompson A, Damyanovich A, Madapallimattam A, et al: ^{31}P magnetic resonance studies of bioenergetic changes in skeletal muscle in malnourished human adults. Am J Clin Nutr 67:39–43, 1998.

193. Bourdel-Marchasson I, Biran M, Thiaudiero E, et al: ^{31}P magnetic resonance spectroscopy of human liver in elderly patients: Changes according to nutritional status and inflammatory state. Metabolism 45:1059–1061, 1996.

194. Brinkmann G, Melchert UH, Muhle C, et al: Influence of different fasting periods on P-31-MR-spectroscopy of the liver in normals and patients with liver metastases. Eur Radiol 6:62–65, 1996.

195. Thomas EL, Taylor-Robinson SD, Barnard ML, et al: Changes in adipose tissue composition in malnourished patients before and after liver transplantation: A carbon-13 magnetic resonance spectroscopy and gas-liquid chromatography study. Hepatology 25:178–183, 1997.

196. Taylor R, Magnusson I, Rothman DL, et al: Direct assessment of liver glycogen storage by ^{13}C nuclear magnetic resonance spectroscopy and regulation of glucose homeostasis after a mixed meal in normal subjects. J Clin Invest 97:126–132, 1996.

6

◆ Parenteral Access

John P. Grant, M.D.

Solutions used in total parenteral nutrition (TPN), which provides all nutrients, including carbohydrate, protein, electrolytes, minerals, and vitamins, are by necessity very hypertonic: they are three to eight times the normal serum osmolality. Infusion of such solutions into small vessels or into vessels with a low blood flow results in severe burning and rapid thrombosis of the vein. Hemolysis has also been observed. The development of TPN has therefore required techniques to gain access to veins with high blood flow, such as the superior vena cava, the right atrium, the inferior vena cava, or a surgically created arteriovenous fistula. In addition to the requirement of rapid dilution by high blood flow, vascular access for TPN should be easily established, well tolerated by the patient, and capable of remaining in place for long periods of time, and it should not restrict joint mobility or otherwise interfere with physical activity.

◆ HISTORY

The most common vascular access used for TPN is a percutaneously placed subclavian vein catheter. This technique was first introduced in 1952 by Aubaniac, who found that the technique provided rapid access to the central venous system with minimal complications in patients suffering from military injuries.[1] The use of the technique was first reported in the United States by Wilson and associates in 1962.[2] Over the next 5 years, experience with the subclavian catheter was gained primarily from its use for central venous pressure monitoring. The catheters were seldom left in place for more than 14 days and were usually left for only 3 to 4 days. When prolonged central venous measurements were required, it was suggested that the catheter be changed every 2 to 5 days to avoid subclavian vein thrombosis and infection.[3, 4] The use of the subclavian catheter for intravenous nutritional support was first proposed by Dudrick and col-

leagues in their early work at the University of Pennsylvania in 1969.[5] Since then, the percutaneous subclavian vein catheterization technique has gained widespread use for TPN because of its ease of placement and dressing management and its low complication rate.

In 1965, Yoffa described a supraclavicular approach to the subclavian vein, claiming it was a safer technique with a higher percentage of successful catheterizations.[6] Since 1969, others have used the internal jugular vein, the external jugular vein, the basilic vein, and even the right atrial appendage. First described in 1949 by Duffy,[7] the use of an inferior vena caval catheter via the femoral vein has found clinical application[7] in selected patients with superior vena caval thrombosis. This chapter discusses placement of the more commonly used central venous catheters, with some comments on particular clinical situations requiring specialized catheter placement.

◆ BASIC PRINCIPLES

The four basic principles that must be observed to ensure optimal safety and success in the placement of central venous catheters are (1) proper preparation of the patient, (2) proper timing of catheterization, (3) proper preparation of the skin, and (4) the availability of proper equipment and supplies.

Proper Patient Preparation

Before the placement of a central venous catheter, the nurse and the physician should thoroughly explain to the patient the reason for the catheter placement and the technique to be used in order to allay any fears or misconceptions of the procedure that the patient might have. When properly informed, the patient rarely requires sedation. The patient should be cautioned to expect some discomfort, even though a local anesthetic will be used. Although some prefer placing the patient in the Trendelenburg position, this position has no advantage, and a supine position in bed is optimal. The placement of a rolled towel between the scapulae is also no longer advocated.[8] It is helpful to instruct the patient to "reach for the toes" to bring the clavicle into a horizontal position and to establish the normal curve of the axillary and subclavian veins from the thoracic outlet into the arm. If the shoulders are in a shrugged position, the vein will be at a variable distance below the lower edge of the clavicle and may take a tortuous course. If the bed is particularly soft, it may be necessary to place a wooden board under the patient to allow proper positioning.

It has been proposed that proper head positioning is important for passing a catheter from the subclavian vein into the superior vena cava. Some claim that if the head is turned away from the cannulation site, there will be a higher incidence of successful cannulation of the superior vena cava than of the internal jugular vein. Others have suggested that turning the head toward the cannulation site is of value. However, there has been no documentation of any significant change in the angle between the internal jugular vein and the subclavian vein with turning of the head. The patient's head should be positioned in the most comfortable angle for cannulation—usually slightly turned away from the side of cannulation.

Proper Timing of Catheterization

The placement of a central venous catheter for TPN should always be done on an elective basis, when proper preparation of the patient can best be established. Proper time should be taken in skin preparation, definition of landmarks, and catheter insertion. Placement of catheters in emergency situations has been shown to be associated with a significantly increased complication rate because of suboptimal conditions.[9]

Proper Skin Preparation

The area of proposed cannulation is first shaved carefully to assist in the sterile prep-

aration and subsequent placement of a bandage. Since it is desirable for these catheters to remain in place for extended periods, strict attention must be paid to aseptic technique during catheter placement. A wide area around the proposed cannulation site should be thoroughly cleansed with an antiseptic soap; the skin should then be defatted with ether, acetone, or trichlorotrifluoroethane; a povidone-iodine solution should then be applied; and sterile draping should follow (Fig. 6–1). The physician should cleanse the hands with antiseptic soap and should wear a mask and gown. Earlier practice was to perform the procedure in the operating room only, but this has been found to be unnecessary. Instead, cannulations should be performed in the patient's room. The number of people in the room should be limited to avoid airborne contamination, and all those present should wear masks.

Availability of Proper Equipment and Supplies

The placement of central venous catheters is facilitated with the help of a trained assistant, such as a hyperalimentation nurse, and appropriate instruments. Most institutions have found it cost-effective to develop a catheter insertion tray, which consists of basins, clamps, syringes, and sponges (Fig. 6–2). I have found the use of reusable material preferable to the use of disposable kits; however, others have been satisfied with the disposable kits. In addition to the tray materials, a cart containing the various preparation solutions, gowns, gloves, masks, and catheters greatly assists in catheterization (Fig. 6–3). A wide variety of catheters are available for use in central venous catheterization. Selection of a catheter depends on personal preference and familiarity. New materials are continually being investigated in hopes of discovering a material with significantly lower thrombogenicity. Currently available materials include the standard polyvinyl chloride, silicone elastomer (Silastic), polytetrafluoroethylene (Teflon), polyurethane, and heparin-coated catheters. Of all the materials, polyurethane is currently preferred.

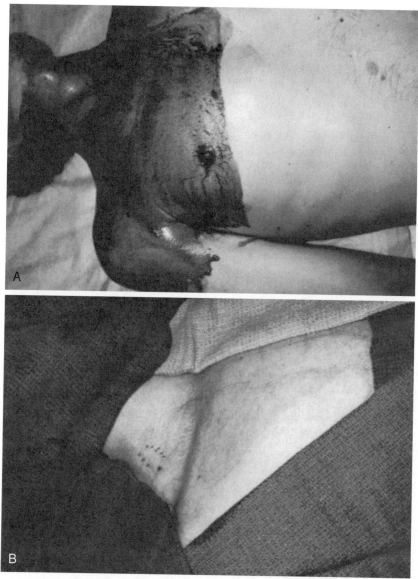

Figure 6–1. Preparation of chest skin for percutaneous placement of subclavian catheters. *A*, All hair is removed by shaving, and the skin is prepared with an antiseptic soap, followed by a defatting agent and then a povidone-iodine solution. *B*, The area is draped with sterile towels.

◆ CENTRAL VENOUS CANNULATION

Percutaneous Infraclavicular Subclavian Vein Cannulation

Landmarks used in subclavian vein catheterization by the infraclavicular route should be based on anatomic relationships (Fig. 6–4). The axillary vein passes obliquely across the axilla toward the middle third of the clavicle, at which point it becomes the subclavian vein at the lateral border of the

first rib. The subclavian vein arches behind the clavicle over the first rib anterior to the insertion of the anterior scalene muscle. At this point just medial to the midpoint of the clavicle, the vein reaches its most cephalic portion in its arch over the rib, and it is at this point that the safest cannulation can be achieved. At the medial border of the anterior scalene muscle, the subclavian vein joins the internal jugular vein to form the brachiocephalic vein. It is therefore suggested that the appropriate landmark for subclavian vein cannulation is the insertion

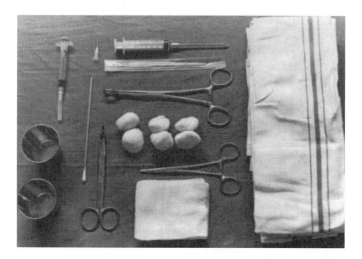

Figure 6–2. Materials included on a tray for percutaneous placement of subclavian catheters. (From Grant JP: Handbook of Total Parenteral Nutrition. Philadelphia, WB Saunders, 1980, p 49.)

of the anterior scalene muscle on the tubercle of the first rib, which lies just posterior to the clavicle. This postage stamp–sized area contains no other major structures, and cannulation at this point should be entirely safe. Advancement of the needle more medially can result in pneumothorax, advancement more posteriorly can result in arterial puncture, and advancement more superiorly and posteriorly can result in brachial plexus injury.

After adequate preparation of the patient,

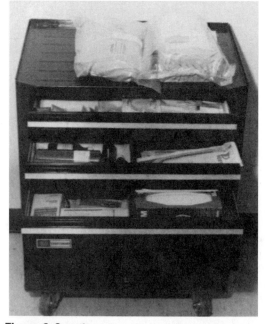

Figure 6–3. Catheter insertion cart containing preparation solutions, gowns, gloves, masks, and catheters.

a small wheal of local anesthetic should be placed at the proposed puncture site, which should be approximately 2 cm below the clavicle at a point that allows access to the target area. Usually this allows placement of the barrel of the syringe and needle in the deltopectoral groove, further reducing the difficulties if a patient cannot extend the shoulders fully back onto the bed, such as might occur in uncooperative patients or those with marked arthritis. The needle is then advanced through the anesthetized skin toward the target area, with the barrel of the syringe maintained horizontal to the floor, which ensures no penetration into the area of the artery or lung. As the needle is advanced, intermittent aspiration on the syringe confirms passage into the subclavian vein by a rapid rush of blood into the barrel of the syringe. Once the needle has been advanced into the subclavian vein, a guidewire is advanced through the needle, and the needle is subsequently removed. Care must be taken during this procedure to avoid air aspiration. Failure of the guidewire to advance easily usually means that the needle is no longer within the vein or that it is against the wall at the junction of the internal jugular vein and the subclavian vein (Fig. 6–5). In the latter case, withdrawing the needle a short distance often allows passage of the wire farther into the venous system. Once the guidewire is in place, the catheter is passed over the wire and the wire is removed. Documentation that the catheter is in a large-bore vein can be done by free aspiration of blood.

Easy and rapid confirmation that the cath-

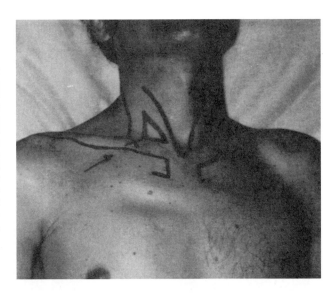

Figure 6–4. Landmarks used in the placement of a percutaneous subclavian catheter by the infraclavicular route. A postage stamp–sized area is defined by the superior and inferior margins of the clavicle, a line extended from the lateral head of the sternocleidomastoid muscle inferiorly across the clavicle, and the completion of the square medially. The posterior border is marked by the insertion of the anterior scalene muscle on the tubercle of the first rib, and the anterior border is marked by the posterior surface of the clavicle. (From Grant JP: Handbook of Total Parenteral Nutrition, 2nd ed. Philadelphia, WB Saunders, 1992, p 113.)

eter has not been passed into the internal jugular vein can be accomplished by gently aspirating blood from the catheter while firmly pressing along the course of the internal jugular vein with the tip of the finger. If the tip of the catheter lies within the internal jugular vein, occlusion of the vein by pressure of the finger will result in a sudden stoppage of blood flow into the syringe during aspiration. If blood cannot be aspirated, the catheter should be partially withdrawn, rotated, and reinserted, and this procedure should be repeated until one is certain that

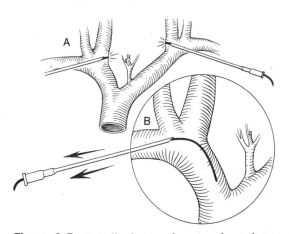

Figure 6–5. *A*, Difficulty in advancing the catheter into the subclavian vein may be due to its abutment against the wall of the internal jugular vein. *B*, *Inset* shows the technique of slightly withdrawing the needle from the vein to allow the catheter to curve and advance distally into the superior vena cava. (From Grant JP: Handbook of Total Parenteral Nutrition, 2nd ed. Philadelphia, WB Saunders, 1992, p 116.)

the catheter does not lie in the internal jugular vein. Experience from thousands of subclavian vein catheterizations and antecubital placements of central venous catheters has demonstrated that approximately 4% of these catheters will pass into the internal jugular vein; some testing of the catheter's position, therefore, is mandatory before chest roentgenography to avoid the cost of an unnecessary roentgenogram.[10]

After the presumed proper placement of the subclavian catheter, chest roentgenography is necessary to document the position of the catheter as well as to rule out the presence of pneumothorax (Fig. 6–6). Roentgenography should be performed before the catheter is connected to any hypertonic solution. Until a roentgenogram is obtained, a 5% dextrose solution, with or without electrolytes, should be connected to the catheter to maintain its patency, or a heparin lock should be established. After proper catheter placement, a sterile dressing should be applied using either gauze or plastic.

Supraclavicular Percutaneous Approach to the Subclavian Vein

The landmarks used in the supraclavicular cannulation of the subclavian vein are identical to those used for the infraclavicular approach, except that the skin puncture site is located in the angle between the lateral head of the sternocleidomastoid muscle and the clavicle (Fig. 6–7). At this point, a small

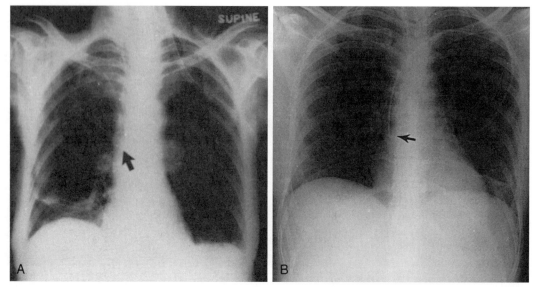

Figure 6–6. Following placement of a subclavian catheter, chest roentgenography is necessary to confirm its proper position in the superior vena cava and to rule out the presence of a pneumothorax. Arrows indicate the proper placement of a catheter inserted from the right subclavian vein *(A)* and from the left subclavian vein *(B)*.

wheal of local anesthetic is placed in the skin. The catheterization needle is inserted through this wheal of anesthetized skin, with the tip directed just behind the clavicle at a 45-degree angle to the sagittal plane and pointed 15 degrees forward of the coronal plane. Thus, as the needle is advanced, it is safely moving away from the structures of the subclavian artery and cupula of the lung. Gentle aspiration is intermittently applied to the syringe as the needle is advanced until the vein is entered just anterior to the

tubercle of the first rib. Once within the vein, the syringe is lowered toward the shoulder to align the needle with the vein. The guidewire is inserted, and the cannulation procedure is performed as for the infraclavicular approach.

With the supraclavicular approach, retrograde cannulation of the internal jugular vein is rarely encountered. However, the catheter can still go out the subclavian vein on the same side or on the opposite side, or it can pass into the mammary veins or other

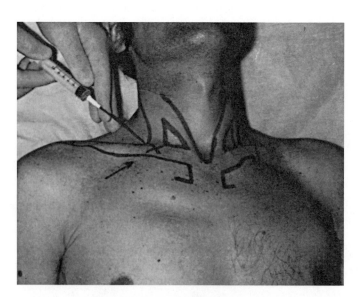

Figure 6–7. Landmarks used in the percutaneous placement of a subclavian catheter via the supraclavicular approach. The skin puncture site is located in the angle formed by the lateral head of the sternocleidomastoid muscle and the superior border of the clavicle. (From Grant JP: Handbook of Total Parenteral Nutrition, 2nd ed. Philadelphia WB Saunders, 1992, p 118.)

small tributaries. It is therefore important to check for the ease of blood flow by aspirating on the syringe and to check for proper catheter positioning with a postplacement chest roentgenogram. A sterile dressing should be applied, as discussed in a later section. Occasionally, it has been useful to tunnel the catheter over the anterior surface of the clavicle down to a point on the anterior chest wall to make the application of a sterile dressing easier and more comfortable for the patient, rather than placing the dressing in the more mobile, hair-bearing area of the neck.

Internal and External Jugular Vein Catheterization

The internal and external jugular veins for central venous access have found less use in long-term TPN than in short-term central venous pressure monitoring in the intensive care unit. Because of the higher positioning of the puncture site on the neck, difficulties in maintaining a sterile dressing limit their long-term use. In addition, the small size of the external jugular vein can result in thrombosis of this system, with tender thrombophlebitis extending distally from the puncture site and presenting a clinical problem for the patient. The use of these two access sites is not recommended for TPN, but in extenuating circumstances they can be used temporarily until more permanent access can be achieved.

Basilic Vein in the Antecubital Fossa

Experience with the use of polyvinyl chloride catheters through the basilic vein in the antecubital fossa has demonstrated a high incidence of thrombophlebitis that occurs within 4 to 10 days of catheter placement. This has seriously limited the use of the basilic vein for long-term TPN. The development and use of silicone elastomer and polyurethane catheters has improved the experience, with catheters being left in place for 4 to 6 weeks with few complications.[11] Skin preparation and dressing care are the same as those used in subclavian vein catheterization. Dressings should be changed routinely (as outlined later), and the system should be isolated for TPN. The catheters

do limit the mobility of the arm and are somewhat less comfortable than the subclavian catheters for long-term use.

Other Vascular Access Sites Useful in Extenuating Circumstances

As mentioned earlier, Duffy described the use of the femoral vein for cannulation of the inferior vena cava in 1949.[7] When no upper veins are available, for example, after thrombosis of both subclavian veins, the femoral approach has been used with variable success. The vein can be cannulated percutaneously, and a catheter can be inserted until the tip is just above the renal veins, as observed under fluoroscopy. The catheter should then be tunneled from the groin to just above the umbilicus to move it from the groin area. These patients must be monitored carefully for the development of phlebitis and particularly for possible pulmonary embolism. I have acquired experience with the use of Silastic catheters placed via the femoral system in five patients receiving home intravenous support. All patients have been maintained on low-dose anticoagulation therapy with sodium warfarin (Coumadin) to avoid potential complications of thrombosis.

On rare occasions when superior vena caval thrombosis is present and the risks of using the inferior vena cava are too high, catheters have been placed via a small anterior thoracotomy through the right atrial appendage into the right atrium. Experience with these catheters in thoracic surgery for monitoring pulmonary artery pressure has shown them to be safe in short-term use. A limited experience has proved that these catheters can be maintained for long-term intravenous feeding.

A few authors have suggested using an arteriovenous fistula or shunt for long-term vascular access in TPN.[12–14] When a shunt is employed, a small T is placed in the shunt, and access is achieved through the T, with infusion of the solution through the catheter while blood flow is maintained. When an arteriovenous fistula is used, a small-bore needle is placed into the access percutaneously, much as is done when dialysis is performed. The feeding solutions are infused either continuously or cyclically. Use of an arteriovenous fistula or shunt is associated with an increased risk of thrombosis of the vascular access. Fear of separation of the arteriovenous shunt and exsanguination limits its use to patients who are alert and cooperative.

The percutaneously placed subclavian catheters used in hemodialysis have also been used to supply hypertonic TPN solutions. Typically, one lumen of these two-lumen catheters is used when dialysis is not being performed. The solution is interrupted for the 2 to 6 hours of dialysis. Since these catheters are typically placed for short-term use only, their use is somewhat limited for TPN. A more permanent access must be established once the dialysis catheter is removed.

Finally, one of the portals of a Swan-Ganz catheter or a triple-lumen subclavian catheter has been used for TPN. The use of these catheters is likely associated with an increased risk of infection and is therefore limited to short-term use during acute illness.

Long-Term Vascular Access

Specially designed catheters are now available for long-term access to the central venous system. These catheters are particularly useful for patients receiving nutritional support at home, but they have also been used in the hospital for extended periods of care. Several designs are available, but in general they consist of a single or dual-lumen tubing with Luer-Lok caps on the end and a polyethylene terephthalate (Dacron) cuff positioned to be placed in the subcutaneous tissues to anchor the catheter in place. The catheters are composed of either silicone elastomer or polyurethane.

Initially, these catheters were all placed in the operating room by a small cutdown to the cephalic vein or external jugular vein and then advanced under fluoroscopic control into the right atrium.[15] The catheters were then advanced through a subcutaneous tunnel to exit at or just slightly below the nipple line. Subsequently, techniques have been modified so that these catheters are placed percutaneously.[16] Watters and I have described a method for the placement of these catheters using an electrocardiogram to position the catheter tip, avoiding the use of fluoroscopy.[17] Experience with these catheters has shown them to be very safe, with a low infectious complication rate.[18, 19] The

incidence of subclavian vein thrombosis may be as high as 3 to 5%. The catheters are of significant bore to allow easy passage of the TPN solutions, including fat emulsions. They come in sizes for use in infants, adolescents, and adults.

◆ SPECIAL CLINICAL CONSIDERATIONS IN VASCULAR ACCESS

After head and neck surgery or tracheostomy, patients have a higher incidence of subclavian vein catheter infection. This is likely caused by contamination of the area and the subsequent migration of bacteria along the course of the catheter into the subcutaneous tissues.

Patients who have suffered extensive burns of the shoulders, upper extremities, and head and neck area can be given intravenous nutritional support through the central veins of the neck if no other access is available. In general, if an adequate dressing cannot be maintained because of the burned area, it is suggested that the catheter be sutured in place and left uncovered by gauze. The skin around the catheter should be cleansed every 2 to 4 hours, and povidone-iodine ointment should be applied to cover the exit site. The catheter should be removed and placed at another site approximately every 48 to 72 hours.

Patients with clotting abnormalities or very low platelet counts present special risks for central vein cannulation. Little difficulty is encountered if the catheterization technique is uncomplicated. However, puncture of a major artery or arterial tributary can result in significant bleeding, which leads to hemothorax and hemomediastinum and possibly to cardiac tamponade and shock. If possible, before any cannulation, the clotting difficulty should be corrected by the administration of fresh-frozen plasma, platelets, or specific clotting factors. If heparin is being administered, it is suggested that the administration be interrupted and that the bleeding time or partial thromboplastin time be allowed to return to normal before cannulation. After uncomplicated placement of the catheter, heparin therapy can be resumed immediately.

Patients who are allergic to povidone-iodine solutions should undergo vigorous skin preparation with an antiseptic soap containing chlorhexidine or hexachlorophene and should undergo subsequent defatting with acetone, ether, or trichlorotrifluoroethane. Catheterization should then be accomplished with subsequent catheter dressing using a non–povidone-iodine ointment such as bacitracin or a polymyxin-bacitracin mixture. Many patients with a sensitivity to povidone-iodine solutions tolerate the placement of a povidone-iodine ointment and often the placement of a povidone-iodine solution when it is applied to the small area of the catheter exit site and dressing. A trial application should be undertaken before catheter care is compromised by nonapplication of the povidone-iodine solution.

REFERENCES

1. Aubaniac R: Une nouvelle voie d'injection ou de ponction veineuse: La voie sous-claviculaire. Semin Hop Paris 28:3445–3447, 1952.
2. Wilson JN, Grow JB, Demong CV, et al: Central venous pressure in optimal blood volume maintenance. Arch Surg 85:55–70, 1962.
3. Ashbaugh D, Thomson JWW: Subclavian-vein infusion. Lancet 2:1138–1139, 1963.
4. Estridge CE, Hughes FA, Prather JR, Clemmons EE: Use of central venous pressure in the management of circulatory failure: Review of indications and technique. Am Surg 32:121–125, 1966.
5. Dudrick SJ, Wilmore DW, Vars HM, Rhoads JE: Can intravenous feeding as the sole means of nutrition support growth in the child and restore weight loss in an adult? An affirmative answer. Ann Surg 169:974–984, 1969.
6. Yoffa D: Supraclavicular subclavian venipuncture and catheterization. Lancet 2:614–617, 1965.
7. Duffy BJ Jr: The clinical use of polyethylene tubing for intravenous therapy: A report on seventy-two cases. Ann Surg l30:929–936, 1949.
8. Wilson S, Sparks W, Williams V, Grant J: Modification of patient positioning for subclavian catheter insertion. JPEN J Parenter Enteral Nutr 14(Suppl 1):17s, 1990.
9. Bernard RW, Stahl WM: Subclavian vein catheterizations: A prospective study. Ann Surg 173:184–190, 1971.
10. Grant JP: Handbook of Total Parenteral Nutrition, 2nd ed. Philadelphia, WB Saunders, 1992.
11. Graham DR, Keldermans MM, Klemm LW, et al: Infectious complications among patients receiving home intravenous therapy with peripheral, central, or peripherally placed central venous catheters. Am J Med 91:95s–l00s, 1991.
12. Scribner BH, Cole JJ, Christopher TG, et al: Long-term total parenteral nutrition. JAMA 212:457–463, 1970.
13. Shils ME: Guidelines for total parenteral nutrition. JAMA 220:1721–1729, 1972.
14. Heizer WD, Orringer EP: Parenteral nutrition at home for 5 years via arteriovenous fistulae. Gastroenterology 72:527–532, 1977.
15. Heimbach DM, Ivey TD: Technique for placement of a permanent home hyperalimentation catheter. Surg Gynecol Obstet 143:634–636, 1976.
16. Vander Salm TJ, Fitzpatrick GF: New technique for placement of long-term venous catheters. JPEN J Parenter Enteral Nutr 5:326–327, 1981.
17. Watters VA, Grant JP: Use of electrocardiogram to position right atrial catheters during surgery. Ann Surg 225:165–171, 1997.
18. Pollack PF, Kadden BA, Byrne WJ, et al: 100 patient years' experience with the Broviac Silastic catheter for central venous nutrition. JPEN J Parenter Enteral Nutr 5:32–36, 1981.
19. Galandiuk S, O'Neill M, McDonald P, et al: A century of home parenteral nutrition for Crohn's disease. Am J Surg 159:540–545, 1990.

7

◆ Parenteral Formulas

Jay M. Mirtallo, M.S., R.Ph.

Since parenteral nutrition was introduced in the United States in the late 1960s, new challenges for providing optimal specialized nutritional support and drug therapy have arisen. As a result of expanded knowledge about the metabolic consequences of various illnesses, an increased demand for specialized parenteral nutrition solutions has resulted in the availability of myriad different types of solutions of amino acids, fat emulsions, carbohydrates, trace elements, vitamins, and electrolytes. Additionally, drug therapy has become more complex. Because patients who require parenteral nutrition often require intravenous drug therapy, drug-nutrient interactions and medication delivery options are important considerations in the management of these patients.

A thorough understanding of the scientific literature concerning the appropriate use of these products is necessary to optimize the clinical application of a parenteral nutrient formulation. The potential risks or favorable effects of concomitant medication and nutritional therapy should be considered. This chapter describes the individual components available for parenteral nutrition, solution admixture considerations, clinical application of parenteral nutrition solutions, and medication delivery issues.

◆ PARENTERAL NUTRITION COMPONENTS

Parenteral nutrition solutions are complex formulations that generally include energy supplied as dextrose and fat, as well as protein, electrolytes, trace elements, vitamins, and water. These components usually need to be individualized for patients according to their primary diagnosis, chronic diseases,

fluid and electrolyte balance, acid-base status, and specific goals of parenteral nutrition.

Energy (Macronutrients)

Dextrose

Dextrose is the primary source of parenteral carbohydrate. Dextrose is needed by the central nervous system, white blood cells, red blood cells, and renal medulla. Each gram of hydrated dextrose used in parenteral nutrition yields 3.4 kcal. Important to formulation design is the maximal rate of dextrose that is oxidized by the body: 5 mg/kg/min ($\cong$25 kcal/kg/day).[1] Formulations that infuse dextrose calories in excess of this amount cause hyperglycemia, even in patients with no predisposing conditions or illnesses[2]; excessive carbon dioxide production from fat synthesis; and hepatic steatosis. Commercial dextrose preparations are available in 2.5 to 70% concentrations. A 2.5% and a 70% dextrose concentration yield 2.5 and 70 g of dextrose per 100 ml of solution, respectively. The dextrose content of parenteral nutrition is a significant determinant of the formulation's osmolarity. Each 5% final concentration of dextrose is approximately 250 mOsm/L. The maximal osmolarity that can be tolerated by a peripheral vein is 900 mOsm/L. As such, parenteral nutrition solutions suitable for peripheral vein administration have dextrose concentrations of 10% or less. This method of parenteral nutrition administration is usually avoided because it depends on a patient's having satisfactory veins, tolerating large fluid volumes, having relatively normal nutritional needs, and requiring therapy for a short period (e.g., $\leq$1 week). Parenteral nutrition solutions with final concentrations of 10% or greater must be administered by a central vein because of the high osmolarity.

Fat

Intravenous fat emulsions are used in parenteral nutrition as an energy source and to

Portions of this chapter are derived from the chapter entitled "Parenteral Nutrition Solutions," written by Roland N. Dickerson, Rex Brown, and Kimberly G. White, in the second edition of this book. I extend my sincere appreciation to these authors.

provide essential fatty acids.[3] The first fat emulsion introduced in the United States in the early 1960s contained cottonseed oil, but it was removed from the market in 1965 as a result of severe adverse reactions. Today, the commercially available products in the United States are manufactured from soybean oil and safflower oil. These oils are predominantly made up of long-chain fatty acids having a high content of the polyunsaturated fatty acids linoleic and linolenic acid. They also differ somewhat in fatty acid composition but are similar in other characteristics important to maintaining the stability of the emulsion, for example, egg yolk, phosphatide emulsifier, pH, and osmolarity, resulting in a small particle size (Table 7–1). These characteristics are important in choosing products and formulating parenteral nutrition admixtures. It is essential to maintain a safe particle size of the emulsion. The metabolism of intravenous fat emulsions is similar to that of endogenous chylomicrons. In unstable emulsions, larger particle sizes develop and lead to symptoms of fat embolism when infused. Generally, acute reactions such as hypotension, pulmonary hypertension, and acidosis may result when a fat particle larger than 6 μm is infused. Additionally, the reticuloendothelial system in the lungs, liver, and spleen clears the larger particles more rapidly, limiting their usefulness as an energy source. Fat emulsion products having a high phospholipid-to-triglyceride ratio (the 10% product has a fourfold greater quantity of phospholipid than the 20% product) are more likely to produce high serum levels of phospholip-

ids, free cholesterol, and plasma triglycerides.[4]

Since fat emulsions contain predominantly long-chain fatty acids with a high content of essential fatty acids, their rate of hydrolysis and utilization by the body is not as efficient as that of emulsions containing smaller fatty acids such as those of medium-chain triglycerides. Combinations of long- and medium-chain triglycerides have been available in Europe for several years but are not available for commercial use in the United States.

Most clinicians provide intravenous fat daily during parenteral nutrition as an intermittent infusion, as a continuous infusion, or as a part of a total nutrient admixture (TNA). The latter two methods have gained considerable popularity because fewer fluctuations in serum triglyceride concentrations and improved fat oxidation occur when these products are given continuously in moderate doses.[5] The need for a test dose of intravenous fat is thus usually eliminated because the rate of administration during slow continuous infusion is less than the suggested test dose. Patients still need to be observed for fever, chills, headache, and back pain during the first dose of intravenous lipid. Absolute contraindications to the administration of intravenous fat emulsions include pathologic hyperlipidemia, lipoid nephrosis, severe egg allergy, and acute pancreatitis associated with hyperlipidemia. These products should be given cautiously to patients with severe liver disease, adult respiratory distress syndrome, or high metabolic stress. Although only approxi-

Table 7–1. Composition of Intravenous Fat Emulsions

Component or Characteristic	Intralipid (Clintec)	Liposyn II (Abbott) (10%, 20%)		Liposyn III (Abbott)
Oil (%)	Soybean (10, 20, 30)	Soybean (5, 10)	Safflower (5, 10)	Soybean (10, 20)
Egg yolk phosphatide (%)	1.2		1.2	1.2
Glycerin (%)	2.25		2.5	2.5
Fatty acids (%)				
Linoleic acid	50		65.8	54.5
Oleic acid	26		17.7	22.4
Palmitic acid	10		8.8	10.5
Linolenic acid	9		4.2	8.3
Stearic acid	3.5		3.4	4.2
Osmolarity (mOsm/L)	260–268		258–276	284–292
Approximate pH	8		8–8.3	8.3
Fat particle size (μm)	0.5		0.4	0.4

mately 2 to 4% of nonprotein calories are needed as fat to prevent essential fatty acid deficiency, most patients receive 10 to 40% (maximum, 60%) of their energy as intravenous lipid during parenteral nutrition. The usual daily adult dose of intravenous fat is 0.5 to 1 g/kg/day; the maximal dose is 2.5 g/kg/day. Most practitioners avoid the maximal dose of intravenous lipid because of reports that long-chain triglycerides may potentially be immunosuppressive.[6] It is currently recommended not to exceed 30% of calories as intravenous lipid since there is limited clinical benefit when this dose is exceeded.[7]

Intravenous fat emulsions are particularly beneficial as an energy source in patients or conditions that predispose to harmful effects of dextrose. These include diabetes, stress, and other hyperglycemic conditions; respiratory acidosis; and hepatic steatosis. When a substantial percentage of energy is administered as intravenous lipid (e.g., up to 30% of total calories), less dextrose needs to be given to meet energy requirements.

Glycerol

Dextrose requires insulin for transport into many cells for oxidation. Many clinical conditions impair the secretion and/or action of insulin. Therefore, other carbohydrate sources that are not dependent on insulin have been investigated for parenteral nutrition. Those that have received the most attention have been glycerol, xylitol, sorbitol, and fructose. Metabolism of these carbohydrates may require more energy or consume excessive quantities of essential nutrients such as phosphorus.[8] Of these carbohydrates, only glycerol is used commercially. Glycerol, which is a sugar alcohol that provides 4.3 kcal/g, is used in intravenous fat emulsions to provide tonicity so the product may be infused safely into a vein. It is also used as a nonprotein calorie source in the product ProcalAmine. This product contains 3% amino acids and 3% glycerol premixed in 1-L bottles. Glycerol is also called *glycerin*, and it appears to have a protein-sparing effect similar to that of an intravenous fat emulsion. ProcalAmine is marketed for short-term postoperative protein sparing, is nearly isotonic, and contains some electrolytes. Before this product is used, its costs and benefits compared with those of 5% dextrose in water should be assessed carefully. Additionally, the product has a standard electrolyte content, which may not be appropriate for some patients.

Protein

Initially, protein hydrolysates of naturally occurring proteins (e.g., fibrin and casein) were used as the protein source for parenteral nutrition. These were replaced with crystalline amino acid products, which were purer and had a consistent, known amino acid composition. Protein hydrolysates were avoided because of unfavorable microbial growth characteristics, the presence of preformed ammonia, and partial bioavailability (~85%) of the protein. In comparison, current amino acid products are of high biologic value, containing about 40 to 45% of their content as essential amino acids; have a known composition; and are associated with a lower incidence of metabolic acidosis. The incidence of metabolic acidosis was reduced further with reformulation of amino acid products to include acetate as a buffer for the chloride used to form soluble salts of some amino acids.

Amino acids provide 4 kcal/g when oxidized for energy. Generally, it is desired to provide enough total or nonprotein calories that the utilization of the amino acids for protein synthesis is optimized. The number of calories in relation to the nitrogen provided, termed the *calorie-to-nitrogen ratio*, sufficient to optimize amino acid utilization by the body is 120 to 150:1 for the healthy person, 200 to 220:1 for patients with renal or liver insufficiency, and 80 to 90:1 for acutely ill, stressed individuals.

Parenteral amino acid products can be conveniently divided into two groups: standard amino acid formulations and modified amino acid formulations. The standard amino acid products are used for patients with normal organ function and nutritional needs. These products have a high content of essential amino acids and have from 19% to 21% branched-chain amino acids. Although these products are commercially available in several concentrations ranging from 3% to 15%, many pharmacies stock only the 10% and 15% concentrations because any desired concentration less than this can be made by adding sterile water and using an automated compounder.

Modified amino acid products have been developed for patients with renal and liver

Table 7–2. Modified–Amino Acid Injection Products

Renal failure	Aminosyn-RF 5.2% (Abbott)	Essential amino acids only, plus histidine and arginine
	NephrAmine 5.4% (McGaw)	Essential amino acids only, plus histidine
	RenAmin 6.5% (Clintec)	Essential and nonessential amino acids with increased proportion of essential amino acids to 60% of total amount
	Aminess 5.2% (Clintec)	Essential amino acids only, plus histidine
Liver disease	HepatAmine 8% (McGaw)	Higher concentrations of branched-chain amino acids (BCAAs) and reduced content of aromatic amino acids
Stress or sepsis	Aminosyn-HBC 7% (Abbott)	Similar to standard amino acid products with higher content of BCAAs
	FreAmine HBC 6.9% (McGaw)	
	BranchAmin 4% (Clintec)	Only BCAAs for use as supplement to standard amino acid products
Pediatrics	Aminosyn-PF 7%, 10%	Similar to standard amino acid product with lower concentrations of methionine, phenylalanine, and glycine; also contains taurine, glutamate, and aspartate
	TrophAmine 6%, 10%	

Essential amino acids are those that the body is incapable of synthesizing in sufficient quantities to prevent deficiency symptoms in healthy individuals when exogenous sources of the amino acid are absent. These include isoleucine, leucine, lysine, methionine, phenylalanine, threonine, tryptophan, and valine. Histidine and arginine are considered conditionally essential in some clinical diseases such as renal or liver disease. BCAAs (leucine, isoleucine, valine) are used as an energy source by muscle and are the only class of amino acids not metabolized by the liver. They become a fuel source during acute illness, and decreased serum levels observed in liver disease may contribute to encephalopathic symptoms. The aromatic amino acids (phenylalanine, tyrosine, and tryptophan) accumulate in the serum of patients with hepatic insufficiency, creating an improper proportion of BCAAs to aromatic acids, the ratio of which has been shown to correlate with encephalopathic symptoms.

failure as well as stress and for neonates (Table 7–2). Even though these products have been shown to be effective protein sources, evidence of the superiority of these products to standard amino acid formulations is lacking. In a prospective, randomized double-blind trial, a modified amino acid product for renal patients provided no further benefit than a modified-dose standard amino acid product when administered in isocaloric, isonitrogenous doses.[9] In liver disease patients, the use of branched-chain amino acid–enriched and aromatic amino acid–reduced products has been questioned.[10] Munoz suggests that nutritional benefits for branched-chain amino acids reported so far are not clear.[10] Standard amino acids have been used safely in cirrhotic patients without inducing encephalopathy. Munoz proposes that protein therapy in liver disease ensures adequate doses (0.8 to 1 g dry weight per kilogram per day) to avoid negative nitrogen balance. Dietary protein restriction is required during periods of encephalopathy but at the highest tolerated dose.[10] Others, however, have considered the use of modified amino acid products for liver failure when patients experience an intolerance to the use of standard amino acid formulations. The modified amino acid product normalizes the abnormal amino acid serum profile observed in most patients with severe encephalopathy.

This has resulted in improvements in hepatic encephalopathy and a lower mortality in some patients.[11]

Many critically ill patients who require parenteral nutrition have marked fluid and sodium overload. In these patients, it is usually beneficial to provide this therapy in the smallest possible volume. A commercially available 15% standard amino acid solution admixed with 70% dextrose in water and administered with 20% lipid emulsion can be used to concentrate the parenteral nutrition formula in patients who are overhydrated or edematous. This maneuver can improve fluid balance in these patients when fluid intake from other sources is also minimized.[12]

Two parenteral protein products are marketed for neonatal and pediatric patients who require parenteral nutrition (Table 7–3). These products contain higher concentrations of histidine and tyrosine, which are considered essential for infants. In preterm neonates receiving parenteral nutrition with these particular amino acid products, growth and development have been similar to those in utero.[13] Clinical trials with these pediatric amino acid products have demonstrated superior nitrogen retention when compared with standard amino acid solutions.[14] Some preliminary evidence suggests that the incidence of cholestasis associated with parenteral nutrition is lower in neo-

Table 7–3. Neonatal and Pediatric Amino Acid Products

	TrophAmine 6% (McGaw)	Aminosyn-PF 7% (Abbott)
L-Amino acid content (g/100 ml)	6	7
Nitrogen (g/100 ml)	0.93	1.1
Essential Amino Acids (mg/100 ml)		
Isoleucine	490	534
Leucine	840	831
Lysine	490	475
Methionine	200	125
Phenylalanine	290	300
Threonine	250	360
Tryptophan	120	125
Valine	470	452
Nonessential Amino Acids (mg/100 ml)		
Alanine	320	490
Arginine	730	861
Histidine	290	220
Proline	410	570
Serine	230	347
Tyrosine	140	44
Glycine	220	270
Cysteine	<14	—
Electrolytes (mEq/100 ml)		
Sodium	5	3.4
Potassium	—	—
Magnesium	—	—
Chloride	<3	—
Acetate	56	33
Phosphorus (mM/L)	—	—
Osmolarity (mOsm/L)	525	586
Amount Supplied (ml)	500	250 and 500

nates who receive these modified amino acid formulations as part of parenteral nutrition.[14]

L-Cysteine hydrochloride is marketed as a single-entity amino acid for admixture with neonatal parenteral nutrition solutions. This amino acid is considered to be essential in neonates. Because cysteine can be converted to insoluble cystine, it should be added to the parenteral nutrition solution last and used within 24 hours of addition. The pa-renteral nutrition solution with cysteine should be refrigerated until used.

From a financial perspective, a significant cost of parenteral nutrition is the amino acid source. Modified amino acid products are more costly per gram of nitrogen infused.[15] Because the benefit of these amino acid products has not been clearly demonstrated, it is recommended to select a standard amino acid product having an amino acid profile that is consistent with that used in

Table 7–4. Composition of 10% Amino Acid Injection Products

Amino Acid Injection Product	Aminosyn II (Abbott)	FreAmine III (McGaw)	Travasol (Clintec)
Nitrogen content (g/dl)	1.53	1.53	1.65
Essential amino acid content (% of total amino acids)	43	46	45
Branched-chain amino acid content (% of total amino acids)	26	23	19
Aromatic amino acid content (% of total amino acids)	7	12	11
Glycine content (g/dl)	500	1400	1030

Table 7–5. Daily Electrolyte Requirements for Adults*

Electrolyte	Recommended Daily Supplementation	Conventional Dosing Range
Calcium	10 mEq	10–15 mEq
Magnesium	10 mEq	8–20 mEq
Phosphate	30 mmol	20–40 mmol
Sodium	Variable	1–2 mEq/kg + replacement
Potassium	Variable	1–2 mEq/kg
Acetate	Variable	As needed to maintain acid-base balance
Chloride	Variable	As needed to maintain acid-base balance

*Assuming patients have normal organ function.

renal, liver, and critical illness. For this, it is useful to create a table of products under consideration that allows comparison of essential with nonessential and branched-chain with aromatic amino acid content (Table 7–4).

Electrolytes, Vitamins, and Trace Elements (Micronutrients)

Electrolytes

Electrolytes in maintenance or therapeutic doses (Table 7–5) need to be added daily to the parenteral nutrition solution to preserve electrolyte homeostasis. Commercially available electrolyte products that may be added to the parenteral nutrition solution are listed in Table 7–6. Each patient's requirements for individual electrolytes depend on the primary disease state, renal function, hepatic function, pharmacotherapy, past intake, renal or extrarenal losses, and nutritional status. Extrarenal electrolyte losses may include those from diarrhea, ostomies, vomiting, fistulas, or nasogastric suctioning. Patients with large amounts of extrarenal losses may be candidates for electrolyte replacement with intravenous fluids

Table 7–6. Commercially Available Electrolyte Formulations

Sodium chloride	Calcium gluconate*
Sodium acetate	Calcium chloride
Sodium phosphate	Calcium gluceptate
Potassium chloride	Magnesium sulfate*
Potassium acetate	Magnesium chloride
Potassium phosphate	

*Preferred salt for parenteral nutrition.

administered separate from parenteral nutrition (Table 7–7).

Electrolytes may be added to parenteral nutrition solutions using single- or multiple-entity products. The multiple-electrolyte formulations may be used for patients who have normal organ function and normal serum concentrations of electrolytes. These products usually lack calcium or phosphorus, or both, so these must be added at the time of preparation. The obligate electrolyte content of the amino acid product should also be considered. Most amino acid products contain substantial amounts of chloride and acetate salts. Some amino acid products are formulated with maintenance electrolytes. During a pharmacy's compounding process, inadequate consideration of the phosphorus content of a manufacturer's amino acid product resulted in calcium phosphate precipitation.[16] This led to two deaths and two injuries when the formulation was infused into patients.

Vitamins

Vitamins are an essential component of a patient's daily parenteral nutrition regimen because they are necessary for normal metabolism and cellular function of the body. The Nutrition Advisory Group of the American Medical Association has established guidelines for the 13 essential vitamins (four fat-soluble vitamins and nine water-soluble vitamins) in adult and pediatric patients.[17, 18] Multiple-entity products that contain 12 (for adult use) or 13 (for pediatric use) vitamins are used (Table 7–8). Adult formulations do not contain vitamin K in order to avoid interaction in patients receiving oral anticoagulants. In adults, vitamin K supplementa-

Table 7–7. Source and Amount (mEq/L) of Electrolyte Loss

Source	Sodium	Hydrogen	Potassium	Chloride	Bicarbonate
Gastric	40–65	90	10	100–140	0
Pancreatic	135–150		5–10	60–75	70–90
Bile	128–160		4–12	90–120	30
Intestinal (jejunum)	95–120		5–15	80–130	10–20
Intestinal (ileum)	110–130		10–20	90–110	20–30
Diarrhea	90–120		5–10	75–120	5–40

tion of 2 to 4 mg/wk is recommended in patients not being anticoagulated with warfarin. Problems in the commercial availability of multiple-vitamin products occurred in 1988[19] and 1997.[20] Refractory lactic acidosis leading to three patient deaths resulted from thiamine deficiency when parenteral nutrition was provided without vitamins. Folic acid deficiency has also been reported.[21] During periods of multivitamin shortage because of production problems, it is recommended to ration vitamins by administering a dose with parenteral nutrition three times a week along with the daily addition of thiamine and folic acid. Individual parenteral vitamins are recommended when the multivitamin products are not available. Vitamins that are marketed as single-entity parenteral formulations include vitamins A, D, E, K, B_1 (thiamine), B_2 (riboflavin), B_3 (niacin), B_6 (pyridoxine), B_9 (folic acid), B_{12} (cyanocobalamin), and C (ascorbic acid). During vitamin shortages, oral multiple vitamins may also be used provided that the patient is able to absorb adequate amounts orally.

Trace Elements

Trace elements are essential micronutrients that are metabolic cofactors essential for the proper functioning of several enzyme systems. Most practitioners add these nutrients to the parenteral nutrition solution daily. The Nutrition Advisory Group of the American Medical Association has also published guidelines for four trace elements known to be important to human nutrition.[22] The suggested amounts of zinc, copper, manganese, and chromium for adults are listed in Table 7–9. Since the original recommendations, substantial evidence for the essentiality of selenium has accumulated.[23] Zinc requirements are increased in metabolic stress secondary to increased urinary losses and in gastrointestinal disease secondary to ostomy or diarrheal losses. Manganese and

Table 7–8. Suggested Composition for Parenteral Multivitamin Products

Vitamin	Units of Measurement	Infants and Children <11 yr	Adults
A	RE (IU)	690 (2300)	990 (3300)
D	μg* (IU)	10 (400)	5 (200)
E	mg† (IU)	4.7 (7)	6.7 (10)
K	μg	200	—
B_1 (thiamine)	mg	1.2	3.0
B_2 (riboflavin)	mg	1.4	3.6
Niacin	mg	17	40
Folic acid	μg	140	400
B_6 (pyridoxine)	mg	1.0	4.0
Pantothenic acid	mg	5.0	15.0
Biotin	μg	20	60
B_{12} (cyanocobalamin)	μg	1.0	5.0
C (ascorbic acid)	mg	80	100

RE, retinol equivalents; IU, international units.
*As cholecalciferol.
†As dl-α-tocopherol.

Table 7–9. Suggested Intakes for Parenteral Trace Elements

Trace Element	Adults	Children (µg/kg/day)	Neonates (µg/kg/day)
Zinc	2.5–4 mg/day	100	300
Copper	0.5–1.5 mg/day	20	20
Manganese	150–800 µg/day	2–10	2–10
Chromium	10–15 µg/day	0.14–0.2	0.14–0.2
Selenium	40–80 µg/day	2–3	2–3

copper are excreted through the biliary tract, whereas zinc, chromium, and selenium are excreted renally. Therefore, copper and manganese should be used with caution in patients with cholestatic liver disease. Further, evidence suggests that the amount of manganese in multiple–trace element formulations is too high, resulting in elevated serum levels that may lead to neurologic symptoms.[24]

Selenium stores have been shown to be depleted in patients receiving long-term parenteral nutrition[23] or in those with thermal injury,[25] acquired immunodeficiency syndrome,[26] or liver failure.[27] Therefore, selenium should be added initially to the parenteral nutrition solution for patients with these disease states or conditions. The trace elements are available as both single- or multiple-entity products. Parenteral guidelines for molybdenum and iodine have not been established; however, these trace elements are available commercially.

◆ FORMULATION DESIGN

Parenteral nutrition formulations are designed to provide nutrients in doses sufficient to meet the patient's daily requirements. Because parenteral nutrition is an extremely complex admixture containing amino acids, dextrose, lipids, water, electrolytes, trace elements, and vitamins—40 or more components—errors in their formulation and compounding have led to serious and lethal complications.[16] As a result, parenteral nutrition formulation design must consider the stability, compatibility, and sterility of the final admixture, which in some cases limits one's ability to individualize nutrient doses. Safety issues related to parenteral nutrition formulations have led to the development of guidelines for safe practices.[28] These guidelines were organized into five sections: labeling, compounding, formulas, stability, and filtering. Specific guidelines are highlighted in this section as infection control, nutrient stability, and compatibility are discussed.

The two major types of parenteral nutrient solutions are the traditional dextrose–amino acid solution and the TNA. The TNA system involves the addition of dextrose, amino acids, and lipid emulsion (with electrolytes, vitamins, trace minerals, and other additives) into a single container. TNA formulations are used frequently because of the convenience of only one infusion for parenteral nutrition purposes and the improved tolerance and oxidation of intravenous fatty acids. The stability of these formulations is a concern, however, because of the destabilization of the emulsion in the presence of an acidic pH and because of exposure to extremes of temperature. For parenteral nutrition, these concerns limit the doses of some nutrients such as divalent cations, zinc, and iron as well as amino acids.

The most cost-effective method of designing parenteral nutrition formulas is to use concentrated sources of amino acids, dextrose, intravenous fat emulsions, and water to compound, using automated methods, admixture volumes sufficient to last for a 24-hour period (once-a-day nutrient admixtures).[29] Accurate dispensing of each amount of macronutrient and water usually necessitates the use of an automated compounding device that is interfaced with a computer to provide rapid and accurate compounding of the admixture (Fig. 7–1). Concentrated sources of dextrose, amino acids, and intravenous fat emulsions can be admixed with one another and sterile water to make lower concentrations of macronutrients appropriate for infusion into the vein. As such, parenteral nutrition formulas for normal renal and liver function, stress, fluid restriction, and renal and liver impairment may be developed while providing the flexibility to individualize the formula further for conditions of intolerance. Intolerance to dextrose occurs in some critically ill patients, whereas intravenous fat emulsions should be used with caution in patients with moderately elevated serum triglyceride levels. In this manner, formulas may be designed to provide 30 to 33 kcal/kg/day, 1 to 1.5 g of protein per kilogram per day, and intravenous fat doses not to exceed 30% of calories.

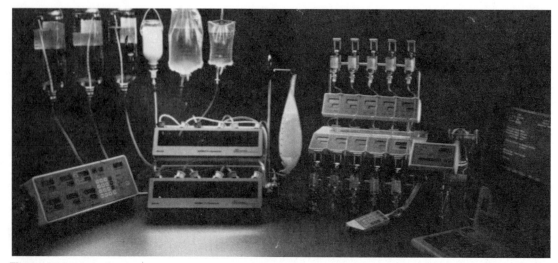

Figure 7–1. Example of an automated compounding system. The items in the photograph from left to right are the Automix 3 + 3 compounder, Micromix compounder, and computer for the multitask operating system software. (Courtesy of the Clintec Nutrition Company, Deerfield, Ill.)

To foster safe practices, guidelines for parenteral nutrition labels require the ingredients be listed as a quantity per day: grams for macronutrients, milliequivalents for electrolytes, millimoles for phosphorus, and appropriate units for other additives.[28] The patient's dosing weight is also required so that the adequacy of the nutrient dose may be assessed and to ensure a balanced formula. *Balanced* refers to the proper proportion of calories, protein, electrolytes, trace elements, and vitamins that allows adequate use and assimilation into the body. Serious harm and two patient deaths have occurred when the improper amount of dextrose was admixed into parenteral nutrition for pediatric patients. An infant was overdosed with dextrose when the parenteral nutrition solution was admixed with twice the amount of dextrose that was prescribed.[30] In another case, an infant suffered irreversible brain damage when parenteral nutrition without dextrose was administered.[31]

Infection Control

Catheter-related sepsis may be caused by the use of contaminated infusion fluid.[32–41] The infusion of contaminated fluid can be attributed to either a lack of aseptic technique in the preparation process or contamination that occurs during the manipulation of intravenous lines. Growth of microorganisms depends on the type of nutrient fluid infused.

Conventional (dextrose-based) parenteral nutrition solutions support microbial growth dependent on the protein sources present in the fluid. Original formulations using protein hydrolysates showed rapid proliferation of both bacteria and fungi, whereas no change was noted or a decreased concentration of inoculated bacteria was observed in parenteral solutions containing crystalline amino acids.[35, 42–50] The ability of protein hydrolysates to promote bacterial and fungal growth was attributed to the presence of peptides or preformed ammonia that the bacteria may use for growth. Similarly, it was found that by adding a large protein, such as albumin, the proliferation of microbial contaminants was increased.[47] The investigators suggested that adding albumin to crystalline amino acids provides the peptides necessary for the growth of organisms. Because of the hypertonicity and acidity of conventional crystalline amino acid–glucose admixtures, bacterial growth is suppressed.[42, 43] Fungi (e.g., *Candida albicans*), however, continue to proliferate in conventional admixtures from 7 to 10 days.[42] Refrigeration at 4°C or freezing at −20°C suppresses microbial growth, including the growth of *C. albicans*.[42, 48–50] Although one report suggests that pharmacy-prepared conventional glucose–amino acid solutions can be stored at room temperature for as long as 7 days without increased infectious risk to patients,[50] it is recommended that all parenteral nutrition admixtures be stored in a refrigerator at 2 to 8°C until the time of use. After removal from refrigeration, the solution should be used within 24 hours.[51] Storage should be in an adequately temperature-controlled refrigerator away from food.

Intravenous lipid emulsions, in contrast to glucose–crystalline amino acid mixtures, support the growth of both gram-positive and gram-negative bacteria, as well as fungi.[34, 40, 52–61] The growth of organisms reached high levels without any detectable changes in appearance or odor of the emulsion. Fungal strains appear to grow more slowly than bacteria but reached concentrations comparable to those in the bacteria-contaminated emulsions by 24 hours.[55] When admixed in TNAs, lipid emulsion fosters the growth of bacteria and fungi to a greater extent than conventional parenteral nutrition fluids but to a lesser extent than fat emulsion alone.[52–54, 62, 63] Dilute parenteral nutrition regimens used in neonatal patients had microbial growth patterns similar to those of adult solution counterparts, suggesting that slight dilution did not change the growth support characteristics of the study solutions.

There is some disparity in the results of microbial growth studies for TNAs. This may be explained by differences in the inocula used in studies or to the difficulty in doing microbial growth studies in lipid media. These data led the Centers for Disease Control and Prevention to limit the hanging time for intravenous fat emulsions.[64] Infusion of lipid-containing fluids (e.g., TNA) should be completed within 24 hours of hanging the fluid. Lipid emulsions given alone should be completely infused within 12 hours of hanging of the emulsion. Additionally, tubing used to administer lipids is to be replaced within 24 hours of initiating the infusion.[64] In contrast, an earlier report by Ebbert and coworkers found similar in-use contamination of intravenous lipids when administered for either 12 or 24 hours.[65] Of 103 consecutive patients, 45% of whom received lipid emulsion for 12.5 to 24 hours and 55% of whom received lipids for 5 to 12 hours, 92% were not contaminated. Of the eight contaminated samples, there were four each in the periods administered up to 12 hours and from 12 to 24 hours. It was observed by the investigators that the contamination may represent less stringent care of peripheral lines because all

contaminations occurred during the administration of peripheral parenteral nutrition. Ebbert and coworkers support the practice of administering lipid emulsions for 12 to 24 hours rather than limiting the infusion to 12 hours as the Centers for Disease Control and Prevention recommends.

Because of the widespread practice of sound aseptic techniques during the preparation and administration of parenteral nutrition, contamination of parenteral nutrition solutions has rarely been reported as a cause of sepsis in patients.[38–40] However, intravenous fat emulsion has been associated with *Malassezia furfur* sepsis in infants.[66–68] Because of its growth dependence on exogenous fatty acids, *M. furfur* grows readily in sebaceous glands and surrounding skin. It is among the normal flora of most adults as well as some premature infants in the neonatal intensive care unit. Sepsis was not from the lipid infusate but rather most likely from the skin by contamination of the catheter at the time of placement, and perhaps the fat emulsion provided the necessary environment for fungal growth.[66]

Nutrient Stability and Compatibility

Parenteral Nutrition Stability

Stability refers to the degradation of nutritional components over time. The compounding of parenteral nutrition admixtures accelerates the rate of physicochemical destabilization, resulting in the recommendation to administer parenteral nutrition as soon after its preparation as possible. Certain amino acids, lipids, and multivitamins are most susceptible to instability.

The Maillard reaction (the *browning reaction*) involves the reaction of carbohydrate with certain amino acids (e.g., glycine), causing the carbohydrate to decompose. This reaction is enhanced by the high temperatures used in sterilization. Thus, dextrose and amino acids combined in the same container are not available commercially but must be prepared by a pharmacist. Once prepared, dextrose–amino acid solutions without vitamins are chemically stable for 1 to 2 months if stored in a refrigerator (4°C) and protected from light.[49] At room temperature, concentrations of tryptophan, arginine, and methionine decrease significantly.[49, 69] Tryptophan is the least stable of the amino acids when admixed with dextrose,[69] and its degradation can be initiated by prolonged exposure to light[70] or the addition of hydrochloric acid.[71] The photoreduction of tryptophan leads to degradation products that result in an indigo blue discoloration. The clinical significance of tryptophan degradation products is controversial. Grant and coworkers suggest that these products may function as hepatotoxins.[72] Therefore, the discoloration should be prevented by avoiding exposure to extremes of light and temperature.

Characteristics of intravenous fat emulsions are very important to the stability, bioavailability, and metabolism of the fatty acids. The emulsifier egg yolk phosphatide maintains a physical barrier and produces electronegative repulsive charges (zeta potential) to stabilize the oil-in-water dispersion at a particle size of about 0.3 to 0.05 μm. The pH of the fluid significantly influences the particle size of the emulsion. Fat emulsions are more stable at an alkaline pH and are buffered to a pH range of from 8 to 8.3. When the fat emulsion is admixed with dextrose and amino acids, the final pH of the TNA is mostly dependent on the pH of the amino acid product used and usually ranges from 5.3 to 6.1. This effect is due to the amphoteric nature of amino acids, which act as a natural buffer. Problems with TNA stability were observed with the use of Aminosyn 7%, having a lower pH than other comparable amino acid formulations.[73] More recent information has demonstrated safe admixture of this manufacturer's amino acids in TNAs in a variety of combinations of dextrose, fat, and electrolytes.[74] Several other studies on TNA stability have been performed,[75–81] and considerable data have been generated by manufacturers. Because of differences in the pH of commercial amino acid products, the phospholipid content of fat emulsion, and parenteral nutrition preparation, distribution, storage, and administration, it is recommended that manufacturers be consulted for available stability guidelines.[28] Brown and coworkers provide an in-depth explanation of the physical chemistry of lipid emulsions, emulsion stabilization, electrostatic forces, individual parenteral nutrition component effects, compounding recommendations, and other important considerations in the understanding of the complex pharmaceutical chemistry of TNAs.[82] In general, final concentrations of TNA should be composed of about 2 to 6.7% lipids, 1.75 to 5% crystalline amino acids, and 3.3 to 35% dextrose.[83] Parenteral nutrition solution components outside this range may also be stable, but this information must be determined for the specific admixture and not be extrapolated from the literature.

Vitamin stability in parenteral nutrition solutions is influenced by many factors, including solution pH; temperature; the presence of other vitamins, minerals, preservatives (e.g., bisulfite), and macronutrients; storage time; the type of nutrient delivery equipment; the flow rate to the patient; and light exposure.[84–87] Under normal conditions of light and temperature, most vitamins should maintain their potency for up to 24 hours from the time of parenteral nutrition admixture. Despite their degradation, very few vitamin deficiencies have been reported in the acute care setting. Patients who have marginal body stores and who are dependent on long-term parenteral nutrition support are most likely to be affected by the short-term stability of vitamins. One case of night blindness was reported to be the result of vitamin A loss when a hospital pharmacy admixed weekly batches of parenteral nutrition for a home patient. Adding the vitamins to the parenteral nutrition formulation just before administration resolved the problem.[88] Similarly, ascorbic acid added in batch fashion to parenteral nutrition degraded and resulted in calcium oxalate precipitation.[89] Because of these short-term stability considerations, it is suggested that vitamins be added to parenteral nutrition formulations shortly before their administration. Parenteral nutrition with vitamins added should be given an expiration date and time of approximately 24 hours.

Parenteral Nutrition Compatibility

Parenteral nutrition is considered to be compatible when all the individual components remain in a form that may be safely administered to a patient. Combinations that form precipitates are considered to be incompatible. Precipitates can be solid and liquid. The most common solid precipitate in parenteral nutrition is calcium phosphate. Because both calcium and phosphorus are essential to ensure the proper assimilation of nutrients into the body, it is desirable to have both included in the parenteral nutrition formulation. Calcium salts, however, are reactive compounds and readily form insoluble products with several substances, for example, phosphorus, oxalate, and bicarbonate. Many factors influence the solubility of calcium and phosphorus in parenteral nutrition. Precipitation is more likely in the presence of high calcium and phosphorus concentrations, decreased amino acid concentrations, increased environmental temperature, increased solution pH, or prolonged hanging time beyond 24 hours.[84] This interaction is prevalent in neonatal parenteral nutrition solutions since this population requires large doses of calcium and phosphorus, yet fluid intakes are restricted and amino acid doses are low.[90, 91] Conventional dextrose–amino acid mixtures rarely pose an incompatibility problem if calcium gluconate concentrations are 10 mEq/L or less and the phosphorus content is 30 mmol/L or less at room temperature.[92] However, more ionized calcium is available for forming insoluble complexes with phosphate when the parenteral nutrition solution is warmed, as in infusion of the solution into the patient. Precipitation can occur in a solution at room temperature even if an identical cold solution is clear.[93, 94] The effect of body heat on the clinical significance of calcium phosphate solubility is evident by reports of venous catheter occlusions in parenteral nutrition solutions at the borderline limits of compatibility.[95, 96] As the pH of parenteral nutrition rises, the more soluble monobasic phosphate salt is converted to dibasic phosphate, which is more likely to bind with calcium and precipitate. It has been suggested that manipulation of the acidification of the solution by adding cysteine hydrochloride can improve solubility.[97]

The following guidelines have been suggested to avoid calcium phosphate precipitation in parenteral nutrition fluids. Calcium gluconate is the preferred salt since it is the least reactive form of calcium. Parenteral nutrition should be compounded in the proper sequence such that calcium and phosphorus are added separately and diluted well before mixing together in the final container. Maximal amounts of calcium and phosphorus doses must not be exceeded, and "borderline" doses should be avoided by considering separate infusion when higher-than-normal doses are required. When a base precursor is indicated, only acetate salts should be used; sodium bicarbonate should not be used. Sodium bicarbonate combines with calcium to form the water-insoluble salt calcium carbonate. Finally, stability should be ensured by using the most recent, up-to date information possible, or the information should be verified with the manufacturer before dispensing the formula to the patient.

Phase separation with the liberation of free oil in TNA formulations constitutes a liquid precipitate. This can occur when an excess of cation is added to a given admixture. The higher the cation valence, the greater the destabilizing effect on the emulsion. Monovalent cations such as sodium and potassium have little effect unless present in very high amounts.[98] Divalent cations, however, can create a bridge when binding with the anionic component of the emulsifier on two different emulsified fat particles. This neutralizes the zeta potential, creating repulsive charges, and keeps the particles near each other. These factors eventually cause the particles to join together to form larger particles and produce phase separation, the various phases of which are known as *aggregation, coalescence, flocculation* and *separation,* or *"oiling out."*[82] In the terminal stage of emulsion destabilization, small lipid particles form large droplets that may vary from 5 to 50 μm or more yet may escape visual detection. As the process continues, coalesced lipid particles in TNA may be seen as yellow-brown oil droplets at or near the TNA surface. These lipid particles may be either as individual spheric droplets or as segmented (discontinuous) oil layers.[28] The presence of free oil in TNA is considered to mean that the formulation is unsafe for parenteral administration. The risk associated with the infusion of unstable lipid droplets is unclear; however, the existence of lipid particles greater than 5 μm in diameter comprising more than 0.4% of the total fat present has been shown to mean that the formulation is pharmaceutically unstable.[99] Such admixtures are unfit for parenteral administration. Finally, trivalent cations such as iron (from iron dextran) are more disruptive to the emulsifier than divalent cations. Driscoll and associates found that there was no safe concentration of iron dextran that could be admixed with TNA.[99]

Drug Stability and Compatibility

Because many patients receiving parenteral nutrition solutions also receive concomitant drug therapy, the question of the stability of drugs mixed with these solutions is important to the patient's optimal care. Parenteral nutrition–drug admixture compatibility considerations are minimized with the increased use of multiple-lumen catheters. Also, parenteral nutrition may be cycled over a 12- to 16-hour period rather than a continuous 24-hour period to allow for drug administration when parenteral nutrition is not infusing. However, it is recommended that the catheter or port designated for parenteral nutrition be used solely for parenteral nutrition whenever possible. In patients with limited venous access, medication administration with parenteral nutrition is unavoidable. In these situations, compatibility considerations are relevant. One technique would be the direct admixture of the medication with the parenteral nutrition fluid. But parenteral nutrition is generally not used as a "drug-delivery vehicle" because of limited or unreliable compatibility information, especially with TNAs. Also, adequate assessment of specific pharmacotherapeutic criteria for the direct admixture of drugs with parenteral nutrition is required.[100] Specific criteria for drug admixture with parenteral nutrition are as follows:[100]

1. Stability and compatibility of the drug with the specific parenteral admixture over a 24-hour period must be determined before adding the medication.
2. The medication must have appropriate pharmacokinetics and proven efficacy for continuous infusion.
3. The medication dose must have remained constant throughout the previous 24-hour period before admixture in parenteral nutrition.
4. There should be a stable parenteral nutrition infusion rate for at least 24 hours before the medication is added.
5. Parenteral nutrition should include appropriate labeling to avoid pharmacotherapeutic problems associated with abrupt discontinuation of parenteral nutrition.

Usually, H_2 antagonists and insulin are the only medications that are admixed in TNA. These medications may also be added to conventional dextrose–amino acid solutions. Other medications that have been shown to be stable and efficacious in con-

ventional parenteral nutrition are heparin, aminophylline, hydromorphone, hydrochloric acid (maximal concentration of 100 mEq/L), and iron dextran.[92]

Medications are most often administered as piggyback admixtures given in the Y site along with parenteral nutrition. For Y-site administration, the drug is administered via piggyback, intravenous push, or other intravenous methods at the Y-site injection port or other access port between the parenteral nutrition admixture and the venous catheter. During simulated studies of compatibility, a 1:1 volume ratio of drug mixture with parenteral nutrition is used. For example, 1 ml of drug solution is combined with 1 ml of test parenteral nutrition admixture for a period of time consistent with that usually observed in practice. In adults, the time of medication exposure to parenteral nutrition is usually short because of the rapid infusion rate of both medication and parenteral nutrition. In pediatric patients, the time of exposure is longer because of slower rates of infusion (with smaller infusion volumes). Trissel and coworkers have studied 106 medications for compatibility in conventional dextrose-amino acid solutions[101] and TNAs.[102] This new information along with past reviews provides the compatibility data for Tables 7–10 through 7–13, which list drugs that have been found to be physically or chemically compatible or incompatible with parenteral nutrition. Caution should be used with aminophylline, ampicillin, and cephradine, because these medications raise the pH of the parenteral nutrition solution sufficiently to cause a calcium phosphate precipitate.[103, 104] Lists of medication compatibility are frequently made as a matter of convenience, but because of the nature of parenteral nutrition, the clinician should consult the original research reports regarding experimental conditions and assay determination methods. Study results of compatibility may vary depending on the methodology used and may not be applicable to the conditions for use at a specific institution.

Compounding Considerations for Parenteral Nutrition

Because of the complexity of parenteral nutrition products, safe preparation is a complicated task. The quality of the final prod-

Table 7–10. Drugs Compatible with Parenteral Dextrose–Amino Acid Solutions

Albumin	Cyclophosphamide	Isoproterenol	Oxacillin
Amikacin	Dexamethasone	Kanamycin	Oxytocin
Aminophylline	Digoxin	Leucovorin	Paclitaxel
Ampicillin	Diphenhydramine	Levorphanol	Penicillin G
Ampicillin-sulbactam	Dipyridamole	Lidocaine	Pentobarbital
Aztreonam	Dobutamine	Lorazepam	Phenobarbital
Azlocillin	Dopamine	Magnesium sulfate	Phytonadione
Bumetanide	Doxycycline	Meperidine	Piperacillin
Buprenorphine	Droperidol	Mesna	Piperacillin-tazobactam
Butorphanol	Enalaprilat	Metaraminol	Polymyxin B
Caffeine	Erythromcyin	Methicillin	Potassium chloride
Calcium gluconate	Famotidine	Methyldopa	Prochlorperazine
Carbenicillin	Fentanyl	Methylprednisolone	Propofol
Carboplatin	Fluconazole	Metronidazole	Ranitidine
Cefepime	Gallium nitrate	Mezlocillin	Sargramostim
Cefoperazone	Gentamicin	Miconazole	Sulfamethoxazole-trimethoprim
Cefonicid	Granisetron	Morphine	Tacrolimus
Cefotaxime	Haloperidol	Moxalactam	Tetracycline
Cefoxitin	Heparin	Nafcillin	Ticarcillin
Ceftazidime	Hydralazine	Nalbuphine	Ticarcillin-clavulanate
Ceftizoxime	Hydrochloric acid	Neostigmine	Tobramycin
Ceftriaxone	Hydrocortisone	Netilmicin	Urokinase
Cefuroxime	Hydromorphone	Nitroglycerin	Vancomycin
Cephalothin	Hydroxyzine	Nitroprusside	Vitamin A
Chloramphenicol	Ifosfamide	Norepinephrine	Vitamin C
Chlorpromazine	Imipenem-cilastatin	Octreotide	Zidovudine
Cimetidine	Insulin, regular	Ofloxacin	
Clindamycin	Iron dextran	Ondansetron	

Data from references 84, 92, and 101.

Table 7–11. Drugs Incompatible with Parenteral Dextrose–Amino Acid Solutions

Acyclovir	Cytarabine	Mannitol	Penicillin G
Amphotericin	Doxorubicin	Methotrexate	Phenytoin
Cefazolin	Fluorouracil	Metoclopramide	Potassium phosphate
Cephradine	Furosemide	Midazolam	Promethazine
Cisplatin	Ganciclovir	Minocycline	Sodium bicarbonate
Cyclosporine	Immune globulin	Mitoxantrone	Sodium phosphate

Data from references 84, 92, and 101.

Table 7–12. Drugs Incompatible with Parenteral Total Nutrient Admixtures

Acyclovir	Erythromycin	Iron dextran	Nalbuphine
Amphotericin	Fluorouracil	Levorphanol	Ondansetron
Cyclosporine	Ganciclovir	Lorazepam	Pentobarbital
Dopamine	Haloperidol	Magnesium sulfate	Phenobarbital
Doxorubicin	Heparin	Midazolam	Phenytoin
Doxycycline	Hydrochloric acid	Minocycline	Potassium phosphate
Droperidol	Hydromorphone	Morphine*	Sodium phosphate

*Morphine sulfate incompatible at concentration of 15 mg/ml but compatible at a concentration of 1 mg/ml.[102]
Data from references 83, 84, 92, and 102.

Table 7–13. Drugs Compatible with Parenteral Total Nutrient Admixtures

Albumin	Cimetidine	Kanamycin	Penicillin G
Amikacin	Cisplatin	Leucovorin	Phytonadione
Aminophylline	Clindamycin	Lidocaine	Piperacillin
Ampicillin	Cyclophosphamide	Meperidine	Piperacillin-tazobactam
Ampicillin-sulbactam	Cytarabine	Mesna	Polymyxin B
Aztreonam	Dexamethasone	Methicillin	Potassium chloride
Bumetanide	Digoxin	Methotrexate	Prochlorperazine
Buprenorphine	Diphenhydramine	Methyldopa	Promethazine
Butorphanol	Dobutamine	Methylprednisolone	Ranitidine
Calcium gluconate	Enalaprilat	Metronidazole	Sodium bicarbonate
Carboplatin	Famotidine	Mezlocillin	Nitroprusside
Cefoperazone	Fentanyl	Morphine*	Sulfamethoxazole-trimethoprim
Cefonicid	Fluconazole	Nafcillin	Tacrolimus
Cefotaxime	Furosemide	Netilmicin	Ticarcillin-clavulanate
Cefotetan	Gallium nitrate	Nitroglycerin	Tobramycin
Cefoxitin	Gentamicin	Nizatidine	Vancomycin
Ceftazidime	Hydrocortisone	Norepinephrine	Vitamin A
Ceftizoxime	Hydroxyzine	Octreotide	Vitamin C
Ceftriaxone	Ifosfamide	Ofloxacin	Zidovudine
Cefuroxime	Imipenem-cilastatin	Oxacillin	
Cephapirin	Insulin, regular	Paclitaxel	
Chlorpromazine	Isoproterenol		

*Morphine sulfate incompatible at concentration of 15 mg/ml but compatible at a concentration of 1 mg/ml.[102]
Data from references 83, 84, 92, and 102.

uct depends on the facilities, resources, personnel training, and products used in preparation. Since the inception of parenteral nutrition, pharmacists have developed policies and procedures for parenteral nutrition compounding based on their training and interpretation of the literature. As a result, inconsistent practices in parenteral nutrition preparation exist. This has led to some serious patient injuries.[28] Publications address these practices and provide evidence-based guidelines for parenteral nutrition admixture.[28, 51, 105, 106] A summary of the most recent parenteral nutrition guidelines for compounding, quality assurance, and stability and compatibility is provided in Table 7–14.[28] When applying these guidelines, one must remember that the order of mixing is critical. The order is specific so that conditionally compatible ingredients are diluted (e.g., calcium and phosphorus) or buffered (e.g., lipids with amino acids before dextrose is added) before their mixture together in the final container.[51]

Compounding methods include manual and automated. Manual compounding depends on the gravity transfer of nutrient components from a large source container to an empty plastic bag or glass bottle. One method of manual compounding is the use of a dual-compartment bag in which amino acids and dextrose are in separate compo-

nents of the same bag and mixed together by the release of a plug within the container just before administration. The manual method of admixture is slow, is prone to inaccuracies, and requires multiple manipulations, thereby increasing the likelihood of contamination. Automated compounding devices are faster and more accurate than the manual method. They also allow more versatility in formula design to be more specific to patient needs. Also, alerts for incompatible combinations of ingredients may be programmed in the machine's software, which flashes a warning on the screen when the nutrient and its dose are input into the computer.

Even with this advanced technology, problems continue to be reported concerning automated compounder use. Some examples of alerts received by the U.S. Pharmacopoeia are the incorrect placement of nutrient bottles, improper assembly of nutrient products, incorrect dosage programmed into the computer, inadequate flushing between the addition of incompatible substances, and machine malfunction.[51]

Parenteral nutrition is considered a high-risk sterile product.[105, 106] Its compounding includes complex and/or numerous aseptic manipulations.[105] Specific guidelines for aseptic processing include media fill validations of both the process and the personnel

Table 7–14. Guidelines for Parenteral Nutrition Compounding, Quality Assurance, and Sterility and Compatibility

Parenteral Nutrition	Practice Guidelines
Compounding	The additive sequence in compounding should be optimized and validated as a safe and efficacious method.
	The manual compounding method should be reviewed periodically or when the manufacturer's brand of nutrient products is about to change. This review should include the most current literature as well as consultation with the manufacturer when necessary.
	Manufacturers of automated compounding devices should provide an additive sequence that ensures safe parenteral nutrition (PN) compounding. This sequence should also be reviewed by the manufacturer of the nutrient products being used in preparing the PN product.
	Splitting PN contracts should be avoided unless there is specific stabilty data concerning the admixture of different brands of amino acids, dextrose, and fat.
	Each PN product prepared should be visually inspected.
Quality assurance	Gravimetric analysis is suggested as an indirect assessment of the accuracy for PN preparation. Attention should be focused on the most dangerous additives such as potassium chloride.
	Chemical analysis of the dextrose content may also be used to determine the accuracy of compounding.
	Refractometric analysis is an alternative as an indirect measurement of the dextrose concentration. This method is limited to PN formulations that do not contain lipids (e.g., neonatal formulations).
	In-process and end-product testing is recommended daily.
	Guidelines for aseptic preparation should be followed.[107]
Stability and compatibility	All methods used for PN (e.g., dose, admixture, packaging, delivery, storage, and administration) ensure a stable and compatible product.
	Medication administration in or with PN is safe, stable, and compatible.
	Stability and compatibility decisions are made with the most reliable information available from the literature or manufacturer.
	Because of limited stability information, the use of conventional dextrose-amino acid formulas with separate administration of fat is recommended for neonatal and infant patients.

Adapted from the National Advisory Group on Standards and Practice Guidelines for Parenteral Nutrition: Safe practices for parenteral nutrition formulations. JPEN J Parenter Enteral Nutr 22:49–66, 1998. American Society for Parenteral and Enteral Nutrition (A.S.P.E.N.) does not endorse this material in any form other than its entirety.

carrying out the process.[105] In addition, there are specific requirements for facilities, space, and environmental control similar to those of a Class 100 clean-room environment.[105] The sterile product release checks require visual inspection against a lighted white and black background for evidence of visible particulates or other foreign matter. In addition, compounding accuracy checks of the addition of all drug products or ingredients used to prepare the parenteral nutrition product are ensured by validating the volume and quantity used in admixture. Sterility testing should be done according to American Society of Health-System Pharmacists guidelines.[106] Presterilized disposable membrane filtration devices (e.g., Addi-Chek, Ivex-2), which are sensitive in detecting low levels of contamination[107, 108] and easy to use, are commercially available. The time frame from the preparation of the compound until sterility testing is important.[107, 108] It is recommended that the solution be tested within 60 minutes after preparation, because the chance of false-negative findings increases when the sample processing is delayed for a longer time after inoculation.[109]

◆ CLINICAL APPLICATION OF PARENTERAL NUTRITION

The previously mentioned concepts are useful in designing a parenteral nutrition program. A simple and cost-effective method is to develop standard parenteral nutrition formulas of known composition, stability, and compatibility. Seltzer and associates found standard formulas to be useful in 80% of their patient population at a savings of 25% over traditional parenteral nutrition

Table 7–15. Dosage Guidelines for Parenteral Nutrition

	Normal Range	Minimum Dose	Maximum Dose
Calories (kcal/kg/day)	30–33	20	40
Protein (g/kg/day)	1–1.5	0.8	2
Glucose (mg/kg/min)	2–3.5	1	4–5
Fat (% calories)	<30	4–6	30
(g/kg/day)			2.5

systems.[110] Table 7–15 provides some general dosage guidelines for macronutrients that may be useful in establishing formulas for patients with standard or individual requirements. In this manner, parenteral nutrition formulas for normal renal and liver function, stress, fluid restriction, and renal and liver impairment may be developed while providing the flexibility to individualize the formula for conditions of intolerance. For instance, most patients require 30 to 33 kcal/kg of actual body weight per day. For obese patients, 21 kcal/kg of actual body weight is used for individuals from 130 to 165% of their ideal body weight,[111] and patients greater than 165% of ideal body weight receive 2 g of protein per kilogram of ideal body weight while energy is derived using a fixed energy-to-protein ratio (kilocalories to gram of nitrogen) of 75:1.[112] Protein doses are modified based on renal and liver function and their treatments from a usual range of 1 to 1.5 g/kg/day to 0.8 to 1.2 g/kg/day, depending on the dose that is tolerated by the patient. Dextrose doses may also have to be modified when significant quantities of dextrose or carbohydrate are administered (e.g., dialysis solutions containing dextrose in differing concentrations). Also, the dose of intravenous fat should be decreased in patients being sedated with propofol continuous infusions because the vehicle for the drug is a 10% soybean oil emulsion. Formulas including dextrose, amino acids, and fat along with their nutrient composition are provided in Table 7–16. The level of any of these ingredients may be modified based on individual patient tolerances and needs. For example, more protein may be provided by the renal formula by increasing the amino acid dose to 50 g/L. Infusion of 30 to 33 kcal/kg/day usually provides 1.2 g of protein per kilogram per day. Contrarily, decreasing the amino acid dose to 30 g/L provides 0.8 g of protein per kilogram per day.

Table 7–17 outlines electrolyte additives for parenteral nutrition along with suggestions for modifying these doses based on individual tolerance and need. Increased requirements for sodium occur when excess losses through the urine, ostomy site, or fistula are not replaced. In cases of renal or liver impairment, it is prudent to restrict or withhold sodium. Potassium and phosphorus are required in order to incorporate nitrogen into the lean body mass. Potassium should be used with caution in patients with renal disease but still may be required to support anabolic processes despite significant impairments in renal function. Hypophosphatemia is often seen in malnourished patients and should be recognized and corrected before initiating parenteral nutrition. Because phosphorus is conditionally compatible with calcium in parenteral nutrition, the dose required to replenish body deficits may have to be administered separate from the parenteral nutrition fluid. Acetate is a precursor to bicarbonate in the body and is useful in correcting deficits caused by diarrhea or urinary bicarbonate losses. Increased requirements for magnesium and zinc are the result of excessive losses in diarrheal fluid. There are limits on the dosage of calcium, magnesium, and zinc that can be added to TNAs because the emulsion can be disrupted at high doses of these cations. Parenteral multivitamins added each day to parenteral nutrition maintain adequate vitamin stores in normal patients, but individual vitamin replacement is necessary for those patients diagnosed with vitamin deficiencies. Tables 7–18 and 7–19 illustrate adult parenteral nutrition formulas in the standard label format.[28] The formula in Table 7–18 is useful in patients with normal renal and liver function, and the formula in Table 7–19 is indicated in renal failure patients with fluid restriction. Note that some ingredients are provided as quantity per day so that each ingredient may be reviewed for its daily nutrient dose. The quantity per liter is provided for some additives so that the dose may be compared with the parenteral nutrition order or in a manner that is easier to interpret by the clinician, as well as quantity per day and according to the manner it was ordered or perceived by the clinician.

Table 7–16. Parenteral Nutrition Formulas

	Patient Condition			
	Normal	*Stress*	*Renal or Liver Failure*	*Obesity*
Formula (g/L of dextrose–amino acid–fat)	150-40-30	150-50-30	210-40-40	75-60-20
Nutrient Composition				
Calories (kcal/ml)	0.97	1.01	1.27	0.70
Nitrogen (g/L)†	6.6	8.25	6.6	9.9
Percentage total calories as fat	30	30	30	29
Nonprotein calorie/N ratio	123:1	98:1	135:1	50:1
Caloric dose (kcal/kg/day)	30–33	30–33	30–33	20–22*
Protein dose infused with usual caloric dose (g/kg/day)	1.2	1.5	1.0	2.0*

*Dose based on ideal body weight.
†The grams of nitrogen provided per liter of parenteral nutrition is dependent on the amino acid injection product used in its admixture and varies between manufacturers.

Table 7–17. Parenteral Nutrition Electrolyte Additives

Additive	Usual Dose	Modified Dose	Clinical Condition Requiring Modification
NaCl (mEq/L)	60–80	30–40	Renal or liver failure
		0	$Na_s > 150$ mEq/L
		120–140	Sodium deficit due to diarrhea or chloride deficit due to gastric fluid losses
Potassium (mEq/L)	40	10–20	Renal failure, hyperkalemia
Chloride salt	20	0	$K_s > 5.7$ mEq/L
		60–120	Excess loss due to diuresis or amphotericin B, deficit caused by malnutrition
Phosphate salt (mEq/L)	20		Equivalent to 13.6 mmol of phosphorus
Acetate	20–40	100–120	Use sodium salt for most metabolic acidosis conditions, but potassium salt may be preferred for bicarbonate losses caused by diarrhea since the potassium content of this fluid is high.
Phosphorus (mmol/L)	10–20	30–40	Malnutrition; dose may be limited because of compatibility concerns with calcium
		0–5	Renal failure, hyperphosphatemia
Magnesium (mEq/day)	8–16	24–40	Deficit due to malnutrition or excess loss due to diarrhea
		0–8	Renal failure, hypermagnesemia
Calcium (mEq/day)	4.5–9	0	Hypercalcemia
		13.5	Low ionized calcium levels

Table 7–18. Parenteral Nutrition Formula for an Adult Patient with Normal Nutritional Requirements

Institution or Pharmacy Name and Address, and Pharmacy Telephone Number: _____

Name _____ Dosing Weight 65 kg   Patient location _____
Administration date and time _____   Expiration date and time _____

Base Formula	*Amount/Day*	*(Amount/L)*
Dextrose	324 g	(150 g/L)
Amino acids*	86.4 g	(40 g/L)
Lipid*	64.8 g	(30 g/L)
Electrolytes		
Sodium chloride	173 mEq	(80 mEq/L)
Potassium acetate	43.2 mEq	(20 mEq/L)
Potassium phosphate	21.6 mmol of P	(10 mmol/L)
	(31.7 mEq of K)	(14.7 mEq/L)
Calcium gluconate	4.5 mEq	
Magnesium sulfate	8.0 mEq	
Vitamins, Trace Elements, and Medications		
Multiple vitamins*	10 ml	
Multiple trace elements*	2 ml	
Infuse at a rate of 90 ml/h	Volume 2160 ml	Infuse over 24 h

Admixture contains 2160 ml plus 100 ml overfill
Central line use only

*Specify product name.
Adapted from the National Advisory Group on Standards and Practice Guidelines for Parenteral Nutrition: Safe practices for parenteral nutrition formulations. JPEN J Parenter Enteral Nutr 22:49–66, 1998. American Society for Parenteral and Enteral Nutrition (A.S.P.E.N.) does not endorse this material in any form other than its entirety.

Table 7–19. Parenteral Nutrition Formula for an Adult Patient with Diabetes, Renal Failure, and Fluid Restriction

Institution or Pharmacy Name and Address, and Pharmacy Telephone Number: _____

Name _____ Dosing Weight 65 kg   Patient location _____
Administration date and time _____   Expiration date and time _____

Base Formula	*Amount/Day*	*(Amount/L)*
Dextrose	328 g	(210 g/L)
Amino acids*	62.4 g	(40 g/L)
Lipid*	62.4 g	(40 g/L)
Electrolytes		
Sodium chloride	31 mEq	(20 mEq/L)
Potassium acetate	31 mEq	(20 mEq/L)
Potassium phosphate	3.9 mmol of P	(2.5 mmol/L)
	(5.7 mEq of K)	(3.7 mEq/L)
Calcium gluconate	4.5 mEq	
Magnesium sulfate	4.0 mEq	
Vitamins, Trace Elements, and Medications		
Multiple vitamins*	10 ml	
Multiple trace elements*	2 ml	
Insulin	39 units	(25 units/L)
Infuse at a rate of 65 ml/h	Volume 1560 ml	Infuse over 24 h

Admixture contains 1560 ml plus 100 ml overfill
Central line use only

*Specify brand name.
Adapted from the National Advisory Group on Standards and Practice Guidelines for Parenteral Nutrition: Safe practices for parenteral nutrition formulations. JPEN J Parenter Enteral Nutr 22:49–66, 1998. American Society for Parenteral and Enteral Nutrition (A.S.P.E.N.) does not endorse this material in any form other than its entirety.

REFERENCES

1. Burke JF, Wolfe RR, Mullany CJ, et al: Glucose requirements following burn injury. Parameters of optimal glucose infusion and possible hepatic and respiratory abnormalities following excessive glucose intake. Ann Surg 190:274–283, 1979.
2. Rosmarin DK, Wardlaw GM, Mirtallo J: Hyperglycemia associated with high, continuous infusion rates of total parenteral nutrition dextrose. Nutr Clin Pract 11:151–156, 1996.
3. Roesner M, Grant JP: Intravenous lipid emulsions. Nutr Clin Pract 2:96–107, 1987.
4. Wolfe BM, Ney DM: Lipid metabolism in parenteral nutrition. In Rombeau JL, Caldwell MD (eds): Clinical Nutrition. Vol 2: Parenteral Nutrition. Philadelphia, WB Saunders, 1986, pp 72–99.
5. Abbott WC, Grakaukas AM, Bistrian BR, et al: Metabolic and respiratory effects of continuous and discontinuous lipid infusions. Arch Surg 119:1367–1371, 1984.
6. Siedner DL, Mascioli EA, Istfan NW, et al: Effects of long-chain triglyceride emulsions on reticuloendothelial system function in humans. JPEN J Parenter Enteral Nutr 13:614–619, 1989.
7. Delafosse B, Viale JP, Tissot S, et al: Effects of glucose-to-lipid ratio and type of lipid on substrate oxidation rate in patients. Am J Physiol 267:E775–E780, 1994.
8. Van den Berghe G, Hers HG: Dangers of intravenous fructose and sorbitol. Acta Pediatr Belg 31:115–119, 1978.
9. Mirtallo JM, Schneider PJ, Mavko K, et al: A comparison of essential and general amino acid infusions in the nutritional support of patients with compromised renal function. JPEN J Parenter Enteral Nutr 6:109–113, 1982.
10. Munoz SJ: Nutritional therapies in liver disease. Semin Liver Dis 11:278–291, 1991.
11. Cerra FB, Cheung NK, Fischer JE, et al: Disease-specific amino acid infusion (F080) in hepatic encephalopathy. A prospective, randomized, double-blind controlled trial. JPEN J Parenter Enteral Nutr 9:288–295, 1985.
12. Broyles JE, Brown RO, Vehe KL, et al: Pharmacist interventions improve fluid balance in fluid-restricted patients requiring parenteral nutrition. Ann Pharmacother 25:119–122, 1991.
13. Heird WC, Hay W, Helms RA, et al: Pediatric parenteral amino acid mixture in low birth weight infants. Pediatrics 81:503–510, 1990.
14. Helms RA, Christensen ML, Mauer EC, et al: Comparison of pediatric versus standard amino acid formulations in preterm neonates requiring parenteral nutrition. J Pediatr 110:466–470, 1987.
15. Melnik G: Value of specialty intravenous amino acid solutions. Am J Health Syst Pharm 53:671–674, 1996.
16. Food and Drug Administration Safety Alert: Hazards of precipitation associated with parenteral nutrition. Am J Hosp Pharm 51:1427–1428, 1994.
17. Multivitamin preparations for parenteral use. A statement by the Nutrition Advisory Group. JPEN J Parenter Enteral Nutr 3:258–262, 1979.
18. Green HL, Hambridge KN, Schanler R, et al: Guidelines for the use of vitamins, trace elements, calcium, magnesium, and phosphorus in infants and children receiving total parenteral nutrition. Report of the Subcommittee on Pediatric Parenteral Nutrient Requirements from the Committee on Clinical Practice Issues of the American Society for Clinical Nutrition. Am J Clin Nutr 48:1324–1342, 1988.
19. Anonymous: Death associated with thiamine deficient total parenteral nutrition. MMWR 38:38–43, 1987.
20. Alliou M, Ehrinpreis MN: Shortage of intravenous multivitamin solution in the United States [Letter]. N Engl J Med 337:54–55, 1997.
21. American Society for Parenteral and Enteral Nutrition: IV multivitamin shortage—Update 23, March 20, 1998. Management of chronic shortage of IV multivitamins. http://www.clinnutr.org/mvi.htm.
22. Guidelines for essential trace element preparations for parenteral use: A statement by the Nutrition Advisory Group. JPEN J Parenter Enteral Nutr 3:263–267, 1979.
23. Baptista RJ, Bistrian BR, Blackburn GL, et al: Utilizing selenious acid to reverse selenium deficiency in total parenteral nutrition patients. Am J Clin Nutr 39:816–820, 1984.
24. Ono J, Harada K, Kodaka R, et al: Manganese deposition in the brain during long-term total parenteral nutrition. JPEN J Parenter Enteral Nutr 19:310–312, 1995.
25. Hunt Dr, Lane HW, Beesinger D, et al: Selenium depletion in burn patients. JPEN J Parenter Enteral Nutr 8:695–699, 1984.
26. Dworkin BM, Rosenthal WS, Wormser GP, et al: Selenium deficiency in the acquired immunodeficiency syndrome. JPEN J Parenter Enteral Nutr 10:405–407, 1986.
27. Dworkin B, Rosenthal WS, Jankowski RH, et al: Low blood selenium levels in alcoholics with and without advanced liver disease. Dig Dis Sci 30:838–844, 1985.
28. National Advisory Group on Standards and Practice Guidelines for Parenteral Nutrition: Safe practices for parenteral nutrition formulations. JPEN J Parenter Enteral Nutr 22:49–66, 1998.
29. Mirtallo JM, Jozefczyck KG, Hale KM, et al: Providing 24-hour nutrient infusions to critically ill patients. Am J Hosp Pharm 43:2205–2208, 1986.
30. Cobel MR: Compounding pediatric dextrose solutions. Medication error alert. ASHP Newsletter August:3, 1995.
31. Gebbart F: Test hyperal solutions? Florida mom says yes. Hosp Pharm Rep February:35, 1992.
32. Bozzetti F, Bonfanti G, Regalia E et al: Catheter sepsis from infusate contamination. Nutr Clin Pract 5:156–159, 1990.
33. Williams WW: Infection control during parenteral nutrition therapy. JPEN J Parenter Enteral Nutr 9:735–746, 1985.
34. Miller SJ: Catheter related sepsis during parenteral nutrition. Hosp Pharm 23:991–996, 1988.
35. Herruzo-Bareara R, Garcia-Caballero J, Vera-Cortes L, et al: Growth of microorganisms in parenteral nutrient solutions. Am J Hosp Pharm 41:1178–1180, 1984.
36. Maki DG, Goldman DA, Rhame FS: Infection control in intravenous therapy. Ann Intern Med 79:867–887, 1973.
37. Maki DG, Rhame FS, Mackel DC, Bennet JV: Nationwide epidemic of septicemia caused by contaminated intravenous products. Am J Med 60:471–485, 1976.
38. Pouffe JF, Brown DG, Silva J Jr, et al: Nosocomial outbreak of Candida parapsilosis fungemia re-

lated intravenous infusions. Arch Intern Med 137:1686–1689, 1977.

39. Solomon SL, Khabbaz RF, Parker RH, et al: *Candida parapsilosis* bloodstream infections in patients receiving parenteral nutrition: Report of an outbreak. J Infect Dis 149:98–102, 1984.

40. McKee KT, Melly MA, Greene HL, et al: Gram-negative bacillary sepsis associated with the use of lipid emulsion in parenteral nutrition. Am J Dis Child 133:649–650, 1979.

41. Two children die after receiving infected TPN solutions. Pharm J August:3, 1994.

42. Goldman DA, Martin WT, Worthington JW: Growth of bacteria and fungi in total parenteral nutrition solutions. Am J Surg 126:314–318, 1971.

43. Wilkinson WR, Flores LL, Pagones JN: Growth of microorganisms in parenteral nutritional fluids. Drug Intell Clin Pharm 7:226–231, 1973.

44. Brennan MF, O'Connel RC, Rosol JA, et al: The growth of *Candida albicans* in nutritive solutions given parenterally. Arch Surg 103:705–708, 1971.

45. Deeb EN, Natsios GA: Contamination of intravenous fluids by bacteria and fungi during preparation and administration. Am J Hosp Pharm 28:764–767, 1971.

46. Gelbart SM, Reinhardt GF, Greenlee HB: Multiplication of nosocomial pathogens in intravenous feeding solutions. Appl Microbiol 106:874–879, 1973.

47. Mirtallo JM, Caryer K, Schneider PJ, et al: Growth of bacteria and fungi in parenteral nutrition solutions containing albumin. Am J Hosp Pharm 38:1907–1910, 1981.

48. Murray KM, Murri N, Schumann L, et al: Bacterial and fungal growth after freezing or refrigerating parenteral nutrient solutions. Am J Hosp Pharm 44:121–124, 1987.

49. Parr MD, Bertch KE, Rapp RP: Amino acid stability and microbial growth in total parenteral nutrient solutions. Am J Hosp Pharm 42:2688–2691, 1985.

50. Tagaki J, Khalidi N, Wolk RA, et al: Sterility of total parenteral nutrient solutions stored at room temperature for seven days. Am J Hosp Pharm 46:973–977, 1989.

51. Total Parenteral Nutrition/Total Nutrient Admixtures. USP DI Text, Vols I and II. Rockville, Md, United States Pharmacopeial Convention, 1996, pp 66–71.

52. Mershon J, Nogami W, Williams JM, et al: Bacterial/fungal growth in a combined parenteral nutrition solution. JPEN J Parenter Enteral Nutr 10:498–502, 1986.

53. D'Angio R, Quercia RA, Treiber NK, et al: The growth of microorganisms in total parenteral nutrition admixtures. JPEN J Parenter Enteral Nutr 11:394–397, 1987.

54. Gilbert M, Gallagher SC, Eads M, et al: Microbial growth patterns in a total parenteral nutrition formulation containing lipid emulsion. JPEN J Parenter Enteral Nutr 10:494–497, 1986.

55. Kim CH, Lewis DE, Kumar A: Bacterial and fungal growth in intravenous fat emulsions. Am J Hosp Pharm 40:2159–2161, 1983.

56. Keammerer D, Mayhall CG, Hall GO, et al: Microbial growth patterns in intravenous fat emulsions. Am J Hosp Pharm 40:1650–1653, 1983.

57. Deitel M, Kaminsky MV, Fuksa M: Growth of common bacteria and *Candida albicans* in 10% soybean oil emulsion. Can J Surg 18:531–535, 1975.

58. Melly MA, Meng HC, Schaffner W: Microbial growth in lipid emulsions used in parenteral nutrition. Arch Surg 110:1470–1481, 1975.

59. Jarvis WR, Highsmith AK, Aller Jr, et al: Polymicrobial bacteremia associated with lipid emulsion in a neonatal intensive care unit. Pediatr Infect Dis 2:203–208, 1983.

60. Vasilakis A, Apelgren KN: Answering the fat emulsion contamination question: Three in one admixtures vs conventional total parenteral nutrition in a clinical setting. JPEN J Parenter Enteral Nutr 12:356–359, 1988.

61. Crocker KL, Noga R, Filibeck DJ, et al: Microbial growth comparison of five commercial parenteral lipid emulsions. JPEN J Parenter Enteral Nutr 8:391–395, 1984.

62. Rowe CE, Fukuyama TT, Martinoff JT: Growth of microorganisms in total nutrient admixtures. Drug Intell Clin Pharm 21:633–638, 1987.

63. Scheckelhoff DJ, Mirtallo JM, Ayers LW, Visconti JA: Growth of bacteria and fungi in total nutrient admixtures. Am J Hosp Pharm 43:73–77, 1986.

64. Pearson ML, Hospital Infection Control Practices Advisory Committee: Guideline for prevention of intravascular device-related infections. Infect Control Hosp Epidemiol 17:438–473, 1996.

65. Ebbert ML, Farraj M, Hwang LT: The incidence and clinical significance of intravenous fat emulsion contamination during infusion. JPEN J Parenter Enteral Nutr 11:42–45, 1987.

66. Powell DA, August J, Snedden S, et al: Broviac catheter–related *Malassezia furfur* sepsis in five infants receiving intravenous fat emulsions. J Pediatr 105:987–990, 1984.

67. Redline RW, Dahms BB: *Malassezia* pulmonary vasculitis in an infant on long-term Intralipid therapy. N Engl J Med 305:1395–1398, 1981.

68. Long JG, Keyserling HL: Catheter-related infection in infants due to an unusual lipophilic yeast—*Malassezia furfur*. Pediatrics 76:896–900, 1985.

69. Jurgens RW, Henry RS, Welco A: Amino acid stability in a mixed parenteral nutrition solution. Am J Hosp Pharm 38:1358–1359, 1981.

70. Bhatia J, Stegink LD, Ziegler EE: Riboflavin enhances photo-oxidation of amino acids under simulated clinical conditions. JPEN J Parenter Enteral Nutr 7:277–279, 1983.

71. Mirtallo JM, Rogers KR, Johnson JA, et al: Stability of amino acids and the availability of acid in total parenteral nutrition solutions containing hydrochloric acid. Am J Hosp Pharm 38:1729–1731, 1981.

72. Grant JP, Cox CE, Kleinman LM, et al: Serum hepatic enzyme and bilirubin elevations during parenteral nutrition. Surg Gynecol Obstet 145:573–580, 1970.

73. Trissel LA: Amino acid injection. *In* Handbook on Injectable Drugs, 8th ed. Bethesda, Md, American Society for Health Systems Pharmacists, p 44.

74. Tripp MG, Menon SK, Mikrut BA: Stability of total nutrient admixtures in a dual-chamber flexible container. Am J Hosp Pharm 47:2496–2503, 1990.

75. Harrie KR, Jacob M, McCormick D, et al: Comparisons of total nutrient admixture stability using two intravenous fat emulsions. Soyacal and Intralipid 20%. JPEN J Parenter Enteral Nutr 10:381–387, 1986.

76. Sayeed FA, Tripp M, Sukumaran KB, et al: Stability of total nutrient admixtures using various in-

travenous fat emulsions. Am J Hosp Pharm 33:2271–2280, 1987.

77. Bettner FS, Stennett DJ: Effects of pH, temperature, concentration, and time on particle counts in lipid-containing total parenteral nutrition admixtures. JPEN J Parenter Enteral Nutr 10:375–380, 1986.

78. Barat AC, Harrie K, Jacob M, et al: Effect of amino acid solutions on total nutrient admixture stability. JPEN J Parenter Enteral Nutr 11:384–388, 1987.

79. Ang SD, Canhan JE, Daly JM: Parenteral infusion with an admixture of amino acids, dextrose, and fat emulsion solution. Compatibility and clinical safety. JPEN J Parenter Enteral Nutr 11:23–27, 1987.

80. Parry VA, Harrie KB, McIntosh-Lowe NL: Effect of various nutrient ratios on the emulsion stability of total nutrient admixtures. Am J Hosp Pharm 43:3017–3022, 1986.

81. Tripp MG, Menon SK, Mikrut BA: Stability of total nutrient admixtures in a dual-chamber flexible container. Am J Hosp Pharm 47:2496–2593, 1990.

82. Brown R, Quercia RA, Sigman R: Total nutrient admixture: A review. JPEN J Parenter Enteral Nutr 10:650–658, 1986.

83. 3-in-1 Reference Manual: Stability Data for Typical 3-in-1 TPN Formulations. Abbott Park, Ill, Abbott Laboratories, 1990.

84. Niemiec PW, Vanderveen TW: Compatibility considerations in parenteral nutrient solutions. Am J Hosp Pharm 41:893–911, 1984.

85. Riggle MA, Brandt RB: Decrease of available vitamin A in parenteral nutrition solutions. JPEN J Parenter Enteral Nutr 10:388–392, 1991.

86. Gutcher GR, Lax AA, Farrell PM: Vitamin losses to plastic intravenous infusion devices and an improved method of delivery. Am J Clin Nutr 40:8–13, 1984.

87. Smith JL, Canham JE, Wells PA: Effect of phototherapy light, sodium bisulfite, and pH on vitamin stability in total parenteral nutrition admixtures. JPEN J Parenter Enteral Nutr 12:394–402, 1988.

88. Howard L, Chu R, Feman S, et al: Vitamin A deficiency from long-term parenteral nutrition. Ann Intern Med 93:576–577, 1988.

89. Gupta VD: Stability of vitamins in total parenteral nutrient solutions. Am J Hosp Pharm 43:2132, 1986.

90. Eggert LD, Rusho WJ, MacKay MW, et al: Calcium and phosphorus compatibility in parenteral nutrition admixtures. Am J Hosp Pharm 39:49–53, 1982.

91. Lenz GT, Mikrut BA: Calcium and phosphate solubility in neonatal parenteral nutrient solutions containing Aminosyn-PF or TrophAmine. Am J Hosp Pharm 45:2367–2371, 1988.

92. Trissel LA: Handbook on Injectable Drugs, 6th ed. Bethesda, Md, American Society of Hospital Pharmacists, 1990.

93. Henry RS, Jurgens RW, Sturgeon R, et al: Compatibility of calcium chloride and calcium gluconate with sodium phosphate in a mixed TPN solution. Am J Hosp Pharm 37:673–674, 1980.

94. Knowles JB, Casson G, Smith M, et al: Pulmonary deposition of calcium phosphate crystals as a complication of home total parenteral nutrition. JPEN J Parenter Enteral Nutr 13:209–213, 1989.

95. Robinson LA, Wright BT: Central venous catheter occlusion caused by body-heat mediated calcium phosphate precipitation. Am J Hosp Pharm 39:120–121, 1982.

96. Stennett DJ, Gerwick WH, Egging PK, et al: Precipitate analysis from an indwelling total parenteral nutrition catheter. JPEN J Parenter Enteral Nutr 12:88–92, 1988.

97. Schmidt GL, Baumgartner TG, Fischlishweiger W, et al: Cost containment using cysteine HCl acidification to increase calcium/phosphate solubility in hyperalimentation. JPEN J Parenter Enter Nutr 10:203–207, 1986.

98. Black CD, Popovich NF: A study of intravenous emulsion compatibility: Effects of dextrose, amino acid, and selected electrolytes. Drug Intell Clin Pharm 15:184–193, 1981.

99. Driscoll DF, Bhargara HW, Li L, et al: Physicochemical stability of total nutrient admixtures. Am J Hosp Pharm 52:23–634, 1995.

100. Driscoll DF, Baptista RJ, Mitrano FP, et al: Parenteral nutrient admixtures as drug vehicles. Theory and practice in the critical care setting. Ann Pharmacother 25:276–283, 1991.

101. Trissel LA, Gilbert DL, Martinez JF: Compatibility of parenteral nutrient solutions with selected drugs during simulated Y-site administration. Am J Health Syst Pharm 54:1295–1300, 1997.

102. Trissel LA, Martinez JF, Gilbert DL, et al: Compatibility of medications with 3-in-1 parenteral nutrition admixtures. JPEN J Parenter Enteral Nutr 23:67–74, 1999.

103. Kirkpatrick AE, Holcombe BJ, Sawyer WT: Effect of retrograde aminophylline administration on calcium and phosphate solubility in neonatal total parenteral nutrient solutions. Am J Hosp Pharm 46:2496–2500, 1989.

104. Watson D: Techniques, materials, and devices: Piggyback compatibility of antibiotics with pediatric parenteral nutrition solutions. JPEN J Parenter Enteral Nutr 9:220–224, 1985.

105. Sterile Drug Products for Home Use (1206). UPS 23/NF18. Rockville, Md, United States Pharmacopeial Convention, 1995, pp 1963–1975.

106. ASHP Technical Assistance Bulletin on quality assurance for pharmacy-prepared sterile products. Am J Hosp Pharm 50:2386–2398, 1993.

107. Miller CM, Furtado D, Smith FM, et al: Evaluation of three methods for detecting low-level bacterial contamination in intravenous solutions. Am J Hosp Pharm 39:1302–1304, 1982.

108. Hoffman KH, Smith FM, Godwin HN, et al: Evaluation of three methods for detecting bacterial contamination in intravenous solutions. Am J Hosp Pharm 39:1299–1302, 1982.

109. DeChant RL, Furtado D, Smith FM, et al: Determining a time frame for sterility testing of intravenous admixtures. Am J Hosp Pharm 39:1305–1308, 1982.

110. Seltzer MH, Assaado M, Coao ET, et al: Use of a simplified standardized hyperalimentation formula. J Parenter Enteral Nutr 2:28–30, 1978.

111. Ireton-Jones C, Francis C: Obesity: Nutrition support practice and application to critical care. Nutr Clin Pract 10:144–149, 1995.

112. Choban PS, Burge JC, Scales D, Flancbaum L: Hypoenergetic nutrition support in hospitalized obese patients: A simplified method of clinical application. Am J Clin Nutr 66:546–550, 1997.

8

◆ Hepatobiliary Complications of Parenteral Nutrition

Karen E. Shattuck, M.D.
Gordon L. Klein, M.D.

◆ INTRODUCTION AND EPIDEMIOLOGY

Because of the development of parenteral nutrition (PN) three decades ago, countless patients who are unable to tolerate food because of gastrointestinal disease or immaturity have survived and recovered.[1, 2] Few medical advancements are free from complications; accordingly, hepatobiliary dysfunction associated with PN accounts for appreciable morbidity and occasional mortality.[3–7] The focus of this chapter is the clinical features, pathologic changes, proposed causes, and suggested management of the hepatobiliary dysfunction and cholestasis associated with PN administration. Particular attention is given to special patients such as preterm infants and to current investigations related to the etiology of PN-associated hepatic dysfunction.

Although PN-associated hepatic dysfunction occurs in patients of all ages, the majority of cases are found in preterm infants.[1–7] In fact, the first report of PN-associated liver disease was described in a 1000-g infant.[8] The infant, managed on PN without feeding because of severe apnea of prematurity, had clinical evidence of cholestasis beginning with hepatomegaly on day 18 of PN. When he died at 10 weeks of age, liver histologic examination demonstrated bile duct proliferation and early cirrhosis.

Subsequently, PN-associated liver disease has been documented in adults, children, and infants. Fortunately PN-associated liver disease is usually self-limiting, but it may progress to liver failure in a minority of patients, particularly preterm infants.[1–3, 5, 9] Although developments in PN solutions have been associated with apparent decreases in the incidence of liver disease,[2, 3] direct comparisons across time are difficult because of differences in the populations studied. The reported incidences of liver disease range from 7.4 to 84% of patients receiving PN (reviewed in references 1 through 7).

The incidence of cholestasis in the first reported series of 62 infants was 23%, with an incidence of 50% in infants with birth weight under 1000 g; 18% in those from 1000 to 1499 g; and 7% in those from 1500 to 2000 g.[9] In the neonatal intensive care unit at the University of Texas Medical Branch hospitals, the incidence of PN-associated cholestasis is defined as an elevation in levels of serum conjugated bilirubin to greater than 2 mg/dl. Over the past 10 years, cholestasis has been diagnosed in approximately 8% (range, 5 to 15%) of the infants receiving PN for more than 1 week (Fig. 8–1) (n = 1736). In agreement with previous studies,[1, 4, 6–7, 10] cholestasis associated with PN in our population is more common in extremely low birth weight infants (less than 1000 g), with an incidence of approximately 14% during the same time period. Between 1988 and 1993, the frequency of PN administration for more than 1 week steadily increased from 23% to 42% of total admissions and remains at that level, reflecting the universal use of PN in infants less than 1500 g birth weight. However, progressive or fatal liver disease in these preterm infants was extremely rare and always associated with additional complications.

Hepatic dysfunction has been reported in 40 to 60% of children on long-term PN, usually after months on PN.[6] The typical pediatric patient on PN has short bowel syndrome due to surgical intervention for neonatal necrotizing enterocolitis or bowel obstruction.

In adults, PN-associated elevations in serum transaminase or bilirubin levels are reported in 20 to 93% of patients. After a PN duration of 2 to 5 years, 15% of adults develop progressive liver disease, and 5% have severe or fatal disease.[2, 11] The typical adult patient on PN has chronic bowel dis-

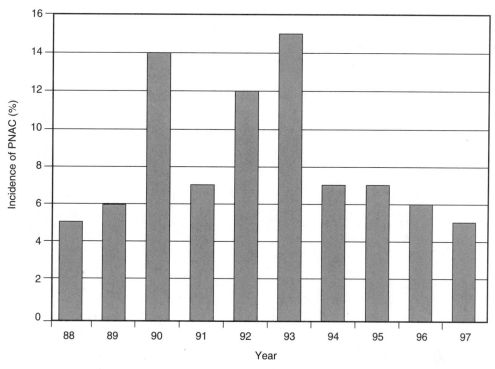

Figure 8–1. Incidence of parenteral nutrition–associated cholestasis (PNAC) in the neonatal intensive care unit at the University of Texas Medical Branch, Galveston, 1988–1997. Incidence represents the percentage of infants admitted who received parenteral nutrition for more than 1 week.

ease such as Crohn's disease, infarction, obstruction, or fistula, and most are on home PN for years.

◆ PATHOLOGY

No histologic finding that is pathognomonic of PN-associated liver injury has been identified; in fact, the histologic changes are nonspecific and vary considerably among patients.[1, 12–16] It is well recognized that the histologic features associated with PN are different in infants and adults, particularly in the early stages of hepatic dysfunction. In infants, cholestasis is prominent, and changes characteristic of neonatal hepatitis and biliary obstruction are observed. Biliary sludge and cholelithiasis may occur in any age group, although cholelithiasis is less common in infants.[7, 12, 15] PN-associated liver dysfunction in adults is more likely to present with hepatomegaly and histologic evidence of steatosis.[2, 12]

Liver biopsies are rarely obtained in infants with suspected PN-associated liver disease.[1, 7] Thus, much of the available information has been obtained from advanced cases or from autopsies. Canalicular and cytoplasmic cholestasis is a major feature, with accumulation of bile pigment in the cytoplasm. Hepatocytes may undergo feathery degeneration, possibly due to toxicity of hydrophobic bile acids such as lithocholate. In the Kupffer cells, consistent findings are hyperplasia and pigmentation with lipofuscin, indicating peroxidation of cell membranes. The hepatocytes in zone 3 (perivenular) appear particularly vulnerable. These changes have been noted within 10 days of PN introduction (Fig. 8–2).[1]

Hepatocellular changes of steatosis, extramedullary hematopoiesis, and giant cell transformation may be observed later in the course of PN cholestasis. Inflammatory changes and proliferation of bile ducts and bile plugs are characteristic after 3 weeks of PN. Canalicular microvilli may be diminished in number or they may form edematous blebs.[13, 15]

Portal or sinusoidal fibrosis does not usually develop until approximately 3 months of PN. These changes may persist even after PN is discontinued.[3, 14] Cirrhosis may de-

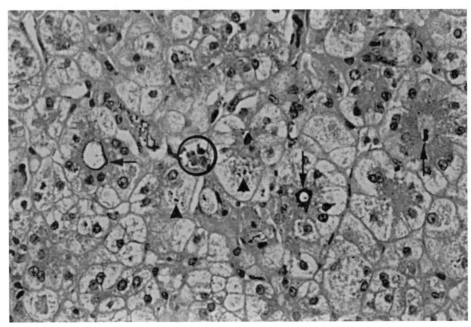

Figure 8–2. High-power view of liver parenchyma in a biopsy from a 3-month-old boy with parenteral nutrition–associated cholestasis. Hepatocytes are forming rosettes and have rarified cytoplasm. Bilirubinostasis is evident in canaliculi within the rosettes *(arrows)*, in hepatocyte cytoplasm *(arrowheads)*, and in Kupffer cells *(circle)*. Hematoxylin and eosin; original magnification ×400. (Courtesy of A. Brian West, Department of Pathology, University of Texas Medical Branch, Galveston.)

velop after 5 to 6 months and may progress to liver failure and death.[11, 17] Fatal liver malignancy has been described in a child who had required long-term PN because of necrotizing enterocolitis as a neonate.[18] Periportal fibrosis and cholestasis were documented at 13 months of age, and the PN was discontinued. One year later, the child died of hepatocellular carcinoma, considered to be a consequence of PN-associated cirrhosis, because hepatocellular carcinoma is not the typical liver malignancy in children.

In adults, hepatocellular changes predominate. Steatosis is the most common early finding, with intrahepatic cholestasis and triaditis also noted.[2, 12, 19] These changes may be found within a few weeks of PN initiation. After long-term PN, steatonecrosis and cirrhosis have been reported.[2, 11] When advanced liver disease is found in patients on PN, severe medical conditions such as pre-existing liver disease, sepsis, and renal failure are almost invariably associated.[19]

◆ CLINICAL FEATURES AND ASSOCIATED CONDITIONS
Clinical Features

As with the histopathologic features, there are no clinical findings specific for PN-asso-

ciated liver disease. Moreover, the pathologic and clinical features do not correlate in a predictable manner.[1–7, 14] The diagnosis of PN-associated cholestasis is therefore a diagnosis of exclusion, and other disorders should be considered, especially in neonates and infants[20–22] (Table 8–1).

PN cholestasis is usually suspected be-

Table 8–1. Examples of Typical Causes of Conjugated Hyperbilirubinemia to Consider in Neonates and Infants Receiving Parenteral Nutrition.*

Infectious hepatitis, i.e., hepatitis A, B, or C; cytomegalovirus; herpes simplex; coxsackie
Inborn metabolic disorders
    Galactosemia or other carbohydrate disorders
    Tyrosinemia or other amino acid disorders
    Wolman's disease or other lipid disorders
    α_1-Antitrypsin deficiency
Extrahepatic biliary obstruction, i.e., choledochal cyst, biliary atresia
Intrahepatic biliary obstruction, i.e., idiopathic neonatal hepatitis
Hypothyroidism or other endocrinologic disorders
Shock
Bowel obstruction

*These diagnoses are among those that should be excluded before cholestasis is attributed to parenteral nutrition.[20–22] This is not an exhaustive list.

cause of a rise in conjugated bilirubin levels within 2 weeks of starting PN.[6] The biochemical definition of PN-associated liver disease used most commonly is an elevation in serum conjugated bilirubin levels to greater than 2 mg/dl, but some studies select 1.5 mg/dl as the lower limit or include other serum markers in their definitions. These differences in definitions should be considered when comparing studies.[3] Early abnormalities in serum biochemistry results may be of uncertain significance because the patient may have no new symptoms or may present with only mild hepatomegaly.[3]

In all age groups, elevations in serum bile acid concentrations,[3, 23–25] 5' nucleotidase,[26] or γ-glutamyltransferase[26] may occur as early as 7 to 10 days after beginning PN, consistent with possible canalicular injury.[26] Within 4 to 6 weeks, an elevation in alkaline phosphatase and aminotransferase levels may be observed,[3–6] considered indicative of cholestasis and steatosis, respectively. The elevations in serum markers may persist for several weeks after the cessation of PN but usually normalize without apparent sequelae. In a small percentage of patients, PN-associated cholestasis progresses to hepatic failure.[27]

Therefore, monitoring serum markers of cholestasis is indicated in all patients on PN,[10] especially if PN is required for more than 1 week, and general guidelines have been published.[28] In our neonatal intensive care unit, baseline laboratory studies are obtained at the beginning of PN, after 4 weeks, and then every other week if the patient remains on PN or has evidence of cholestasis. Tests for levels of serum bilirubin (conjugated and unconjugated), albumin, transaminases, and γ-glutamyltransferase are included. The guidelines for monitoring pediatric patients at our institution are similar to these general guidelines.

Associated Conditions

A number of clinical conditions are associated with an increased risk of PN liver dysfunction and progressive liver disease in patients of all ages. The most notable risk factors are enteral fasting, infection, and a long duration of PN (summarized in Fig. 8–3). Small bowel resection presents an additional risk and often coexists with other conditions.

Enteral fasting has multiple effects on the gastrointestinal system that predispose the patient to cholestasis. Because substrate is absent, the normal pattern of interdigestive migrating motor complexes is not maintained, and intestinal motility is slowed. The secretion of the hormones cholecystokinin (CCK) and secretin is decreased, resulting in reductions in intestinal peristalsis and gallbladder contractility.[3, 29] Bile acid secretion by the liver is decreased because bile acid absorption from the intestine is reduced. The decreased rate of bile flow allows more opportunity for other solutes in bile, such as bilirubin, to undergo spontaneous or enzymatic deconjugation.[29–31] Unconjugated bilirubin may form concentrations of calcium bilirubinate, clinically significant as gallstones or biliary sludge.[29]

Because food substrate is needed to maintain the integrity of the small intestinal mucosa, fasting leads to atrophy of the enterocytes.[3, 5] In a miniswine model, the marked ileal atrophy while the miniswine were fasting on PN was associated with a 70% decrease in ileal absorption of the primary bile salt taurocholate, which could lead to a reduction in the bile acid pool.[32] The authors speculated that the decreased absorption of primary bile acids from the gut also resulted in increased deconjugation and dehydroxylation of bile acids by enteric flora to form the increased concentrations of cholestatic secondary bile acids that were observed.[32] Indeed, alterations in biliary bile acid composition have been documented in adults on PN because of inflammatory bowel disease, including an increase in lithocholic acid and its metabolites,[33] secondary bile acids that are known to cause cholestasis.[34–37] Lithocholate accounted for 7 to 15% of biliary bile salts after approximately 2 weeks of PN in patients with elevated serum aminotransferase activities compared with less than 1% of bile salts in patients without liver dysfunction.[33] The presence of lithocholate sulfate in serum is a sensitive marker of cholestasis.[38] Moreover, PN-associated cholestasis and lithocholate-induced cholestasis have similar histologic features.[15, 39]

Sepsis, especially associated with abdominal surgery or intestinal dysmotility, greatly increases the risk of PN cholestasis.[10, 19, 23, 40–42] In children on PN because of small bowel resection in the neonatal period, the risk is greatest when sepsis occurs within

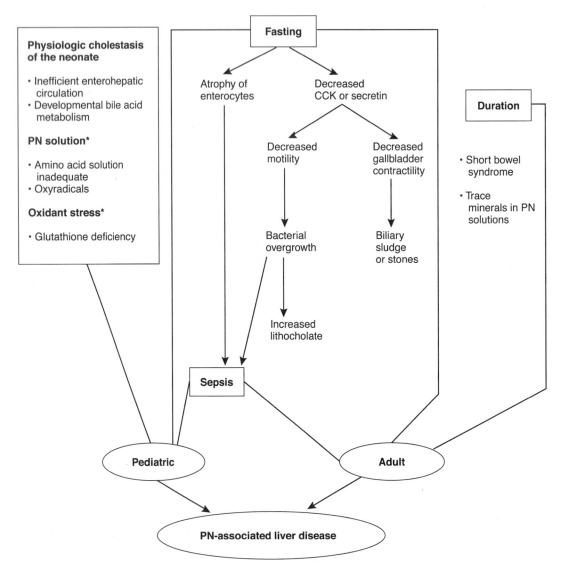

Figure 8–3. Major risk factors for parenteral nutrition–associated liver disease in pediatric and adult patients. Fasting and sepsis are important in all age groups. The duration of parenteral nutrition and developmental immaturity are important in the adult and pediatric groups, respectively. Asterisk (*) indicates an area under study or speculative. CCK, cholecystokinin.

only weeks of beginning PN.[40] In one series including infants on short-term PN, without bowel surgery, the incidence of cholestasis was 26% in those with infection, and it did not occur in those without infection.[41] Endotoxin, produced by gram-negative bacteria, mediates the hepatic dysfunction associated with sepsis by stimulating cytokine release.[43–45] Studies in rats and perfused rat livers have shown that tumor necrosis factor-α and interleukin 1 are released by the Kupffer cells in response to bacterial endotoxins, causing inflammation and fibro-

sis.[46] Cytokines also have direct effects on hepatic amino acid metabolism,[47, 48] including increases in biliary concentrations of branched-chain and gluconeogenetic amino acids[49] similar to changes observed during oxidant stress,[50] which is discussed later.

In adults, progressive liver disease is definitely related to *the duration of PN*.[51–53] Although the relation between PN duration and cholestasis appears to be weaker in infants, most studies support an association between the duration of PN and cholestasis.[54–56] In one early study of preterm infants, cholestasis developed in 10% of preterm infants on PN for 10 days but in 90% of those on PN for 90 days; the mean duration of PN until the onset of cholestasis was 42 days.[9] Other studies have demonstrated correlations between the duration of PN and the severity of cholestasis; correlations between surgery and the incidence of cholestasis were also identified.[55, 57]

Small bowel resection is associated with a fivefold increase in cholestasis in adults receiving PN.[58] In one series in which the entire small bowel was resected, 25% of patients developed cholestasis 46 to 88 months after PN was initiated.[52] Infants with bowel perforation due to necrotizing enterocolitis are subsequently at increased risk for cholestasis on PN; moreover, series have reported that up to 75% of infants with PN-associated cholestasis had necrotizing enterocolitis.[42, 59–61]

Additional Predisposing Conditions in Neonates and Infants

In the neonate, physiologic hepatic immaturity is a condition predisposing to the development of cholestasis if PN is administered.[21] This physiologic cholestasis is most commonly manifested as jaundice due to unconjugated hyperbilirubinemia. Less commonly appreciated is the developmental immaturity of bile acid metabolism that accompanies the jaundice.[62, 63] The severity of physiologic cholestasis is inversely related to the gestational age.[21]

To review the enterohepatic circulation of the normal adult, bile acids are synthesized from cholesterol, secreted into bile, resorbed from the intestine, efficiently extracted by the hepatocyte from the systemic circulation, and again secreted into bile.[64] In addition to bile acids, organic anions such as glutathione and amino acids are important constituents of bile flow.[65] Gallbladder storage of bile acids between meals and emptying during meals regulates the delivery of bile acids to the duodenum.[29] The rate of bile secretion and the plasma level of bile acids increase during meals, as intestinal absorption of bile salt–triglyceride products increases.[29] Bile acids also induce bile flow by stimulating the release of somatostatin[66, 67] and the secretion of biliary lipids.[29] The hepatic biosynthesis of bile acids is balanced with fecal loss.[29, 67]

In neonates of any gestational age, the relative size of the total bile acid pool is reduced and multiple steps of the enterohepatic circulation are less efficient compared with those of the normal adult (reviewed in Hofmann[29]). The hepatocellular uptake of bile acids from the plasma and the rate of intestinal conservation of bile acids are reduced. Enterohepatic circulation of bile acids is slow, in part due to reduced gastrointestinal motility rates.[29] In this environment, as previously discussed, bacterial overgrowth is enhanced so that the primary bile salts cholate and chenodeoxycholate are more likely to be metabolized to cholestatic secondary bile salts.[3, 14, 29, 34]

The developmental immaturity of bile acid metabolism also may contribute to PN cholestasis.[68] Neonates preferentially conjugate bile acids with taurine rather than glycine so that taurocholate rather than glycocholate is the main bile acid of infants.[62] Taurine deficiency has been documented in preterm neonates[69] and children,[70, 71] including three children who died of PN-associated hepatic failure.[71] Moreover, the glycine conjugate of lithocholic acid is more cholestatic than taurolithocholate,[34, 35] which is relevant if lithocholic acid concentrations are increased because of bacterial overgrowth.

◆ PROPOSED CAUSES
Amino Acid Solutions, Dextrose, and Lipids

Not surprisingly, the major nutritional components of PN are prominent on the long list of suspected contributors to PN-associated hepatic dysfunction. The clinical and laboratory evidence support a role for some PN components in liver dysfunction, but additional insults appear to be required for the development of progressive liver disease.[51–61]

The amino acid solution used for PN may have a direct effect on the canalicular membrane of the neonatal liver.[6, 26] The administration of amino acid solutions is associated with cholestasis in experimental animals, including the rat and the rabbit.[72, 73] In the isolated perfused rat liver, the administration of amino acid solution induces an acute reduction in bile flow[74–76] that is reversible, dose related, and ameliorated by taurocholate.[77]

Early studies demonstrated that the development of cholestatic jaundice in infants was related to the quantity of amino acids infused.[7] However, these studies were performed using adult formulations of amino acid solutions, so the direct relevance to the current clinical setting is uncertain. Guidelines for amino acid requirements are available.[28, 78]

The specific amino acids included in PN solutions are now considered to be of more importance, particularly in the neonate, in whom a number of metabolic pathways are immature.[79, 80] The trans-sulfuration pathway has received particular attention with regard to the liver because an adequate supply of taurine is necessary for neonatal bile acid metabolism.[62, 63] Because the enzyme cystathionase is found in inadequate quantities in the neonate, products of the trans-sulfuration pathway including taurine and cysteine may be deficient if methionine is the only precursor provided (reviewed in Rassin[80]).[81] These considerations contributed to the development of solutions formulated to reproduce the plasma amino acid profile of breast-fed infants.[55, 82, 83] The decrease in PN-associated liver disease in children and infants since their implementation suggests that pediatric amino acid solutions have reduced the incidence of PN-associated cholestasis, although there is little direct supporting evidence. Amino acid solutions are no longer implicated in PN-associated hepatic disease in adults.

Dextrose administration in amounts large enough to overwhelm the hepatic glucose-oxidizing capacity may result in steatosis and excess glycogen deposition in the liver; it is conceivable that this could cause hepatocellular enlargement sufficient to compress the canaliculi and obstruct bile flow.[84-86] In the adult rat, the infusion of glucose (~20%) at 139 kcal/kg/day for 5 days resulted in significant decreases in bile flow and bile acid output compared with chow-fed controls, with histologic abnormalities of the hepatocytes including fine lipid droplets.[87] However, during the infusion of a solution containing amino acids, vitamins, and glucose, conditions more similar to those of the patient receiving PN, the bile flow and bile acid output were reduced to a lesser degree than during the infusion of glucose alone.[87]

The infusion of hypertonic solutions of glucose reduces bile flow,[88] but the cholestatic effect of hypertonic solutions is not limited to those containing glucose. Hyperosmolar solutions of sodium, sucrose, and mannitol induce a similar response, at least in the isolated rat liver (Shattuck, unpublished observations). However, hyperosmolarity is not mandatory for hyperglycemia-induced cholestasis; decreased bile flow occurs in the isolated rat liver when glucose concentrations are greater than 15 to 20 mmol/L and insulin is absent.[89] Taken together, these observations suggest that glucose is not a major factor in the etiology of hepatic dysfunction under normoglycemic conditions, when infused as a component of PN, although the serum glucose level may affect bile flow in other clinical situations.

The original descriptions of PN cholestasis predated the inclusion of lipid emulsions in PN solutions,[1-7] and there is little evidence to support a direct role for nutrient lipids as a major factor in the etiology of PN-associated liver disease.[60] However, the role of potentially toxic by-products formed in lipid emulsions continues to be an open question. Lipid hydroperoxides have been measured in high concentrations in lipid emulsions;[90] this may be related to the histologic evidence of peroxidation of cell membranes in neonates with PN cholestasis.[90, 91] Clayton and colleagues have proposed that the plant sterols that contaminate lipid emulsions are not efficiently metabolized by the liver and may accumulate within hepatocytes.[92] Elevated concentrations of phytosterol were documented in children with cholestasis. In animal models, the daily injection of phytosterols resulted in their progressive accumulation in serum, liver, and bile, which was associated with significant increases in serum bile acid levels and inhibition of secretory function in hepatocyte couplets.[93] Further study is needed to confirm the clinical importance of these intriguing observations.

Trace Minerals and Contaminants

There is evidence that other components of PN, including trace minerals and contaminants, particularly aluminum, may contribute to liver disease. Small-volume additives to PN, such as heparin and calcium and/or phosphate salts, are contaminated with aluminum, which accumulates in the liver.[94-96] The hepatic aluminum concentration is known to be elevated in children on PN.[97] In animal models, reported effects include cholestasis, decreased bile flow, and biochemical abnormalities, such as decreased levels of hepatic mixed-function oxidases and increased levels of nonactivated glucuronyltransferase.[96, 98, 99] Moreover, aluminum-treated chow-fed rats with elevated serum bile acid concentrations and reduced bile flow have a reduction in the taurine conjugation of bile acids.[100] This change results in an increased glycine-to-taurine ratio that correlates with the duration of exposure to aluminum and the serum bile acid concentration. Additionally, there has been a single report that the intraperitoneal administration of aluminum over 7 to 14 days resulted in portal inflammation and a dose-related elevation in the levels of serum bile acids.[101] The increased biliary transferrin excretion in rats after parenteral aluminum loading may represent an attempt by the hepatocyte to reduce the toxicity of aluminum to the liver.[102]

Since the inclusion of trace minerals such as manganese, copper, and chromium in PN was recommended,[28, 78] occasional toxicity has been reported. Long-term PN is associated with increased chromium levels in children, although chromium toxicity has not been related to liver disease.[103] Chromium should be withheld from PN in patients with severe renal failure.[28] Because manganese and copper are excreted in bile,[104, 105] patients with pre-existing hepatic dysfunction are at particular risk for toxicity. It is uncertain whether high serum levels lead to cholestasis or are the result of decreased mineral secretion in bile.[6, 14] The accumulation of manganese and copper in the liver and basal ganglia associated with high blood concentrations has been documented in adults and children on long-term PN.[6, 106] Therefore, in patients with liver failure, copper and manganese should be withheld from PN,[28] or supplementation may be decreased and serum levels monitored.[28, 105, 107]

Metabolic Enzymes

In addition to the adverse effects of aluminum on the hepatic mixed-function oxidase system, PN solutions have been shown to reduce cytochrome P450 isoenzymes in the rat.[108] Thus, PN therapy itself may alter hepatic metabolism of P450-dependent intermediates of drugs or normal biochemical substances in order to produce hepatotoxic substances.

Oxidant Stress

Much attention has been directed toward oxidant stress as a potential risk factor in PN cholestasis, particularly in the neonate. The sick neonate is frequently subjected to oxidant stress because of fluctuations in blood oxygenation associated with respiratory distress, apnea of prematurity, and sepsis.[109] One of the histologic findings of cholestasis peculiar to the neonatal patient is Kupffer cell accumulation of lipofuscin pigment,[1, 7] a product of peroxidized cell membrane lipids.

During early sepsis, endotoxin stimulates the hepatic release of glutathione, which may protect from reactive oxygen species generated by the activated Kupffer cells.[41, 110] Depletion of hepatic glutathione is known to exacerbate hepatic reperfusion injury.[111, 112] Moreover, the neonate is relatively deficient in antioxidant defenses; in particular, erythrocyte concentrations of glutathione are known to be low in neonates with respiratory distress syndrome.[113] Thus, two sources of potential oxidant stress have been investigated—*glutathione depletion* and the *infusion of oxygen free radicals or lipid hydroperoxides*, which may be formed in photo-oxidized amino acid solutions and lipid emulsions.[89–91, 114]

The liver is a major site of synthesis and storage of the tripeptide glutathione (γ-glutamylcysteinylglycine).[115, 116] Glutathione functions as a cofactor for the enzyme glutathione peroxidase, which neutralizes reactive oxygen radicals, such as hydrogen peroxide and lipid hydroperoxides. In addition to this key role as an antioxidant, glutathione is a major stimulant of bile flow.[117, 118] In animal models, prolonged fasting[119] and a low-protein diet[120] are known to deplete glutathione stores.

Biliary glutathione concentrations were increased acutely during perfusion of the isolated rat liver with commercial amino acid solution,[77] possibly as an adaptive mechanism to preserve bile flow because amino acid solution decreases bile flow.[74–76] In the same model, oxygen exposure for 48 hours or the experimental inhibition of glutathione synthesis resulted in significant decreases in hepatic and biliary glutathione concentrations.[50] Decreased bile flow and increased biliary oxidized glutathione levels were observed in conditions of the most marked glutathione depletion. When glutathione stores are depleted, the biliary secretion of selected amino acids and taurine is increased.[50] Moreover, in fasted weanling rats, hepatic glutathione levels decreased to 16% of those of controls after 5 days of PN; after 8 days, elevated serum concentrations of alanine aminotransferase and glycocholate, and mitochondrial lipid peroxidation in the liver were observed.[121] Taken together, these studies suggest that in the glutathione-depleted liver, decreased biliary glutathione levels and increased biliary amino acid secretion may be factors in the development of cholestasis.

The other line of investigation related to antioxidant defense has examined the role of reactive oxygen species generated from two sources: the photo-oxidation of amino acids and the formation of lipid hydroperoxides by lipid emulsions. During storage, lipid emulsion undergoes peroxidation that causes in vitro hemolysis of erythrocytes,[90] and a 10-fold increase in expired pentane in neonates infused with lipid emulsion has been documented.[90-91]

The amino acid–vitamin solution used in PN has been shown to form toxic products when exposed to light. In particular, the riboflavin in the multivitamin solution used in PN has been implicated in the photo-oxidation of tryptophan,[114] methionine, histidine, tyrosine, and cysteine.[122-124] The oxidation of tryptophan also occurs enzymatically in the dark.[125] Products lethal to mammalian cells in culture are produced by the irradiation of tryptophan and tyrosine in the presence of riboflavin.[126, 127] In neonatal gerbils who received tryptophan intraperitoneally for 4 or 7 days, serum γ-glutamyltransferase activity, an indicator of hepatic canalicular membrane function and integrity, was increased compared with controls, and the increase was greatest in the gerbils receiving light-exposed tryptophan.[124] Chromatographic studies of these solutions revealed numerous photoadduct compounds of tryptophan and riboflavin after exposure to light.[128] Moreover, the infusion of PN irradiated with light is associated with alterations in hepatobiliary function and histologic appearance in rats infused with PN for 5, 7, and 10 days.[129, 130] Other abnormalities associated with light-exposed PN solution included decreased concentrations of biliary glutathione and hepatic amino acids and increased activity of biliary γ-glutamyltransferase.[131, 132] Finally, in the isolated rat liver, the infusion of a light-exposed amino acid–vitamin solution results in decreased bile flow and an increased biliary concentration of oxidized glutathione, a marker of oxidant stress, compared with the infusion of a light-protected solution.[133] These studies in animal models provide strong evidence that products of photo-oxidation could contribute to PN-associated liver dysfunction, but clinical data are not available.

◆ PREVENTION AND TREATMENT

There is no definitive medical therapy for PN-associated hepatic dysfunction. Fortunately, liver disease due to PN is reversible when PN is discontinued, unless severe fibrosis or cirrhosis has developed.[6, 16] Many strategies may be used for both prevention and treatment (Table 8–2).

Because sepsis is a major risk factor for cholestasis, preventing infections of the central venous catheter used for PN administration is of paramount importance.[6] The initiation of enteral feeding even in hypocaloric quantities should be attempted to prevent hepatic dysfunction and to treat established cholestasis,[6, 14, 15, 134] as discussed previously. In patients who require continued PN despite the development of cholestasis, cycling of PN may be useful.[7, 135] Antibiotics,[2, 3, 59, 136] to prevent bacterial overgrowth in the intestine, and phenobarbital[137-139] have been used with some success.

Table 8–2. Medical Therapy Used for the Prevention and Treatment of Parenteral Nutrition–Associated Liver Disease*

Use hypocaloric enteral feeding
Cycle parenteral nutrition (PN) and eliminate trace minerals
Discontinue PN (treatment only)
Aggressively treat sepsis and prevent central catheter infection
Administer phenobarbital or antibiotics (treatment only)
Administer ursodeoxycholic acid (investigational)
Administer cholecystokinin (investigational)

The decreased gastrointestinal motility that accompanies enteral fasting may result in bacterial overgrowth, which is undesirable because of the potential enhancement of the production of endotoxin and hepatotoxic secondary bile acids. Therefore, the administration of oral antibiotics has been used to prevent bacterial overgrowth. Metronidazole was shown in one study to prevent cholestasis in adults with Crohn's disease[136] and has also been recommended as treatment for cholestasis.[2, 3] Oral gentamicin has been associated with a possible protective effect against cholestasis in the very low birth weight preterm neonate,[59] although this study was not specifically designed to study the effect of prophylactic oral gentamicin on cholestasis. Thus, antibiotics may be useful in high-risk infants and adults as prevention or treatment for PN-associated cholestasis.

Phenobarbital has been used as a choleretic agent in the management of biliary atresia,[138] but its role in the treatment of PN-associated cholestasis remains unclear. Phenobarbital is thought to increase Na^+,K^+-ATPase activity in the hepatocyte, thereby increasing intrahepatic bile flow.[139] Although phenobarbital has not been proved to be effective, anecdotal cases of impending liver failure have been successfully treated with phenobarbital (5 mg/kg/day) with rapid decreases in serum alkaline phosphatase and bilirubin levels.[137] No study advocates the use of phenobarbital as prophylaxis to avoid PN-associated cholestasis.

Newer Therapies to Promote Bile Flow

Two medications that have attracted interest are ursodeoxycholic acid (UDCA) to increase bile flow and CCK to stimulate gallbladder emptying.

The choleretic bile acid UDCA (3α-hydroxy-7β-cholanoic acid), the 7β-epimer of chenodeoxycholic acid, is currently the recommended therapy for primary biliary cirrhosis.[140, 141] Although cholic acid, chenodeoxycholic acid, and deoxycholic acid constitute more than 90% of all biliary bile acids in healthy adults, UDCA accounts for less than 5% of the bile acid pool[29, 142] and is thought to be formed in the distal intestine. Oral supplementation with UDCA may

be of therapeutic benefit in cystic fibrosis and cholestasis in pregnancy[143] but probably not in primary sclerosing cholangitis.[144] The mechanism by which UDCA promotes bile flow is unclear, but possibilities include increasing the secretion of hydrophilic non-hepatotoxic bile acids into bile or having a direct cytoprotective effect.[29]

No controlled trials of UDCA in treating PN-associated liver disease are available, but preliminary studies are encouraging. In a single case report, UDCA was found to be effective in treating PN-associated liver disease in an adult.[145] In a small group of children on long-term PN for intractable diarrhea, the oral administration of UDCA at a dosage of 30 mg/kg/day was associated with the disappearance of jaundice and hepatomegaly within 1 to 2 weeks. Levels of serum transaminases, γ-glutamyltransferase, and bilirubin normalized within 6 to 8 weeks of UDCA administration in most children.[146] In a preliminary report, UDCA treatment (15 to 45 mg/kg/day) of infants on PN for more than 4 weeks prevented gallstones, cholangitis, and surgical intervention; of the 12 infants who did not receive UDCA, 9 developed one of these complications.[147]

Side effects of UDCA appear to be uncommon and include back pain, diarrhea, vomiting, and alopecia.[148] Unlike the other major bile acids, UDCA is not cytotoxic and is absorbed rapidly and passively.[29, 149, 150] One problem with its administration is noteworthy: the intestinal absorption of UDCA is incomplete even in healthy subjects because of the poor solubility of the compound below pH 8.[29] This problem could be overcome by the development of pH-sensitive microcapsules such as those used for pancreatic enzymes,[151] or the infusion of a solution of sodium UDCA into the small intestine.[29, 149, 150]

Intrahepatic bile flow and gallbladder contraction are stimulated by the release of CCK, which remains at very low levels during periods of fasting.[55] Prophylactic CCK has been shown to prevent the formation of biliary sludge in adults on long-term PN.[152] In one cohort of infants at high risk for PN-associated cholestasis, the prophylactic administration of CCK appeared to reduce the incidence of severe cholestasis (direct bilirubin levels >5 mg/dl) and was associated with lower direct bilirubin values than observed in the retrospective control group.[153] No side effects were observed at the dosages used in this study (0.02 to 0.04 µg/kg/dose two to three times daily). CCK has also been shown to decrease conjugated hyperbilirubinemia in neonates with established PN-associated cholestasis.[154] However, CCK was not effective in neonates with advanced liver failure. Side effects included feeding intolerance and apparent abdominal cramping due to pylorospasm when high doses were given (up to 0.32 µg/kg daily).[154]

Improvement in Parenteral Nutrition Formulations

Because amino acid solutions are generally agreed to contribute to cholestasis in the pediatric population, further refinement of these solutions could be beneficial in the prevention of PN-associated liver disease.

In this regard, the use of glutamine has received much attention. Amino acid solutions used for PN do not include glutamine because of its instability in solution when stored for long periods, and ready metabolism to ammonia and glutamate, both of which are both potentially toxic.[79–80] Glutamine, a gluconeogenetic amino acid that is released by skeletal muscle and liver during stress, is the major metabolic fuel of the enterocyte.[155] Moreover, deficiency of glutamine is thought to be one cause of the intestinal villous hypoplasia and decreased mucosal weight that occur within days of PN initiation.[156, 157] Enrichment of PN solution with glutamine has been shown to ameliorate these changes, at least in rats.[155] Glutamine may also prevent the depletion of immunoglobulin A in the gut that has been associated with PN.[158]

In addition, glutamine enrichment of PN may protect from the hepatic steatosis associated with the administration of hypercaloric PN, which is required for growth in infants. Steatosis, commonly observed in association with PN administration, may occur because of an imbalance of insulin and glucagon levels in the portal vein.[159] The gluconeogenetic amino acids (nonessential), such as glutamine, stimulate the secretion of glucagon, which causes the hepatic release of free fatty acids.[145] In contrast, essential amino acids have greater insulinogenic potential, which leads to the uptake of carbohydrate and the formation of triacylglycerols.[159] The protective effect of glutamine against hepatic steatosis in rats appears to be mediated by its ability to stimulate glucagon secretion, releasing fatty acids; the investigators commented that other gluconeogenetic amino acids might well have a similar effect.[159]

Glutamine is known to be well tolerated by adult volunteers and patients with malignancy, and no accumulation of ammonia or glutamate in serum was observed.[160] In a single case of a child on PN and an elemental diet, glutamine administration was associated with weight gain and decreased stool losses of fat and carbohydrate, indicating improved intestinal absorption.[161] In a randomized controlled trial, preterm infants receiving glutamine supplementation required fewer days on PN, a shorter length of time to full feedings, and fewer ventilator days.[162] Differences between control and study groups were significant only in the cohort under 800 g birth weight. Although serum ammonia, blood urea nitrogen, and glutamate levels were higher in infants treated with glutamine, the levels remained within normal limits. Additional studies are needed to confirm these promising results.

Because cysteine may be deficient in neonates,[80, 81] cysteine in the form of L-cysteine hydrochloride has been added to PN solutions administered in neonates.[82, 83] Thus far, the usefulness of cysteine hydrochloride supplementation in preventing glutathione depletion or PN-associated cholestasis has not been demonstrated. In rat models, the administration of cysteine in the form of N-acetylcysteine has been shown to prevent the glutathione depletion associated with oxidant stress[163] and to ameliorate the decrease in bile flow during the infusion of amino acid solution.[164] Clinical studies are needed.

If progressive liver disease is not responsive to medical management, laparotomy and surgical irrigation of the biliary tree may be successful, but this would be considered only in severe cases.[165, 166] In some centers,[167] isolated intestinal transplantation to avoid long-term PN in patients with short bowel syndrome or combined liver-bowel transplantations in patients with associated liver failure may be an option.[167]

◆ CHOLELITHIASIS AND BILIARY SLUDGE

Biliary sludge, acalculous cholecystitis, and gallstones have been reported in association with PN in all age groups.[1-3] The duration of PN is clearly related to the development of biliary sludge and gallstones. Biliary sludge has been reported in 44% of neonates receiving PN for a mean of 10 days[168] and may be as high as 100% after 6 to 13 weeks.[169] Gallstone formation, common (~30%) in adults and children after 2 to 3 years on PN,[3] is being reported with increasing frequency in children and infants.[170, 171] In adults, cholecystitis and cholangitis may complicate cholelithiasis, but pancreatitis is more common in children.[170] Moreover, unlike the situation in adults, PN-associated cholelithiasis is one of the principal causes of gallstones in pediatric patients.[170, 171] In addition to PN duration, clinical conditions that predispose to the development of gallstones include resection of the distal ileum or ileocecal valve, short bowel syndrome, multiple laparotomies, PN cholestasis, necrotizing enterocolitis, and enteral fasting.[1, 3]

The pathogenesis of PN-associated biliary tract disease is incompletely understood, but risk factors are similar to those for liver disease. In particular, enteral fasting is associated with increased biliary stasis, which encourages the formation of calcium bilirubinate stones.[1, 3] Treatment with ursodeoxycholic acid or CCK may be considered.[3] Biliary sludge usually resolves after PN is discontinued, but cholecystectomy may be necessary to treat cholelithiasis if medical management is unsuccessful.[170, 171]

SUMMARY

Hepatobiliary disease associated with PN administration remains a diagnostic and management challenge for the clinician and fortunately is usually self-limiting. PN-associated liver disease occurs most commonly in patients who are not being enterally fed, because fasting causes decreased intestinal motility, a reduction in the secretion of hormones such as CCK, atrophy of enterocytes, bacterial overgrowth, and overproduction of cholestatic bile acids. Sepsis and the duration of PN are also strongly related to the risk of PN-associated cholestasis. Patients who have extensive small bowel resection may be at the highest risk for progressive liver disease. Determining whether hepatic disease is due to PN or to these associated conditions is frequently impossible. Infants are especially vulnerable, probably because

of physiologic cholestasis, immature antioxidant defenses, and the constituents of the PN solutions.

The prevention and treatment of PN-associated liver disease may include enteral feedings, cycling of PN, and phenobarbital or prophylactic antibiotics. Future advances in the treatment of PN-associated hepatobiliary disease are likely to include more widespread use of ursodeoxycholic acid, hypocaloric feeding, and further improvements in the formulations of pediatric amino acid solutions.

REFERENCES

1. Balistreri WF, Bove KE: Hepatobiliary consequences of parenteral alimentation. *In* Popper H, Schaffner F (eds): Progress in Liver Disease, Vol 9. Philadelphia, WB Saunders, 1990, pp 567–601.
2. Fisher FL: Hepatobiliary abnormalities associated with total parenteral nutrition. Gastroenterol Clin North Am 18:645–666, 1989.
3. Quigley EMM, Marsh MN, Shaffer JL, Markin RS: Hepatobiliary complications of total parenteral nutrition. Gastroenterology 104:286–301, 1993.
4. Whitington PF: Cholestasis associated with total parenteral nutrition in infants. Hepatology 5:693–696, 1985.
5. Sax HC, Bower RH: Hepatic complications of total parenteral nutrition. JPEN J Parenter Enteral Nutr 12:615–618, 1988.
6. Kelly DA: Liver complications of pediatric parenteral nutrition—Epidemiology. Nutrition 14:153–157, 1998.
7. Farrell MK, Balistreri WF: Parenteral nutrition and hepatobiliary dysfunction. Clin Perinatol 13:197–212, 1986.
8. Peden VH, Witzleben CL, Skelton MA: Total parenteral nutrition [Letter]. J Pediatr 78:180–181, 1971.
9. Beale EF, Nelson RM, Bucciarell RL, et al: Intrahepatic cholestasis associated with parenteral nutrition in premature infants. Pediatrics 64:342–347, 1979.
10. Pereira GR, Sherman MS, DiGiacomo J, et al: Hyperalimentation-induced cholestasis: Increased incidence and severity in premature infants. Am J Dis Child 135:842–845, 1981.
11. Bowyer BA, Fleming CR, Ludwig J, et al: Does long-term home parenteral nutrition in adult patients cause chronic liver disease? JPEN J Parenter Enteral Nutr 9:11–17, 1985.
12. Briones ER, Iber FL: Liver and biliary tract changes and injury associated with total parenteral nutrition: Pathogenesis and prevention. J Am Coll Nutr 14:219–228, 1995.
13. Cohen C, Olsen MM: Pediatric total parenteral nutrition—Liver histopathology. Arch Pathol Lab Med 105:152–156, 1981.
14. Benjamin DR: Hepatobiliary dysfunction in infants and children associated with long-term total parenteral nutrition: A clinico-pathologic study. Am J Clin Pathol 76:276–283, 1981.
15. Hodes JE, Grosfeld JL, Weber TR, et al: Hepatic

failure in infants on total parenteral nutrition (TPN): Clinical and histopathologic observations. J Pediatr Surg 17:463–468, 1982.

16. Dahms BB, Halpin TC: Serial liver biopsies in parenteral nutrition associated cholestasis in early infancy. Gastroenterology 81:136–144, 1981.

17. Postuma R, Trevenen CL: Liver disease in infants receiving total parenteral nutrition. Pediatrics 63:110–115, 1979.

18. Vileisis RA, Sorenson K, Gonzales-Crussi F, Hunt CE: Liver malignancy after parenteral nutrition. J Pediatr 100:88–90, 1982.

19. Wolfe BM, Walker BK, Shaul DB, et al: Effect of total parenteral nutrition on hepatic histology. Arch Surg 123:1084–1090, 1988.

20. Davis AM: Initiation, monitoring and complications of pediatric parenteral nutrition. In Baker RD, Baker SS, Davis AM (eds): Pediatric Parenteral Nutrition. New York, Chapman & Hall, 1997, pp 228–237.

21. Balistreri WF: Neonatal cholestasis. J Pediatr 106:171–184, 1985.

22. Hughes CA, Talbot IC, Ducker DA, Harran MJ: Total parenteral nutrition in infancy: Effect on the liver and suggested pathogenesis. Gut 24:241–248, 1983.

23. Manginello FP, Javitt NB: Parenteral nutrition and neonatal cholestasis. J Pediatr 94:296–298, 1979.

24. Javitt NB: Cholestasis in infancy: Status report and conceptual approach. Gastroenterology 70:1172–1181, 1976.

25. Deleze G, Paumgartner G: Bile acids in serum and bile of infants with cholestatic syndromes. Helv Paediatr Acta 32:29–38, 1977.

26. Black DD, Sutle EA, Whitington PF, et al: The effect of short term total parenteral nutrition on hepatic function in the human neonate; a prospective randomized study demonstrating alteration of hepatic canalicular function. J Pediatr 99:445–449, 1981.

27. Rodgers BM, Hollenbeck JI, Donnelly WH, Talbert JL: Intrahepatic cholestasis with parenteral alimentation. Am J Surg 131:149–155, 1976.

28. ASPEN Board of Directors: Guidelines for the use of parenteral nutrition in adults and pediatric patients. JPEN J Parenter Enteral Nutr 17(Suppl): 275A–525A, 1993.

29. Hofmann AF: Defective biliary secretion during total parenteral nutrition: Probable mechanisms and possible solutions. J Pediatr Gastroenterol Nutr 20:376–390, 1995.

30. Spivak W, DiVenuto D, Yuey W: Non-enzymatic hydrolysis of bilirubin mono- and diglucuronide to unconjugated bilirubin in model and native bile systems—Potential role in the formation of gallstones. Biochem J 242:323–329, 1987.

31. Ho KJ: Human β glucuronidase—Studies on the effects of pH and bile acids in regard to its role in the pathogenesis of cholelithiasis. Biochim Biophys Acta 827:197–206, 1985.

32. Matsumura JS, Greiner MA, Nahrwold DL, Dawes LG: Reduced ileal taurocholate absorption with total parenteral nutrition. J Surg Res 54:517–522, 1993.

33. Fouin-Fortunet H, Quernec LL, Erlinger S, et al: Hepatic alterations during total parenteral nutrition in patients with inflammatory bowel disease: A possible consequence of lithocholate toxicity. Gastroenterology 82:932–937, 1982.

34. Little JM, Zimniak P, Shattuck KE, et al: Metabolism of lithocholic acid in the rat: Formation of lithocholic acid 3-O-glucuronide in vivo. J Lipid Res 31:615–622, 1990.

35. Yousef IM, Tuchweber B, Vonk RJ, et al: Lithocholate cholestasis-sulfated glycolithocholate-induced intrahepatic cholestasis in rats. Gastroenterology 80:233–241, 1981.

36. Kakis G, Yousef IM: Pathogenesis of lithocholate- and taurolithocholate-induced intrahepatic cholestasis in rats. Gastroenterology 75:595–607, 1978.

37. Oelberg DG, Chari MV, Little JM, et al: Lithocholate glucuronide is a cholestatic agent. J Clin Invest 73:1507–1514, 1984.

38. Farrell MK, Balistreri WF, Suchy FJ: Serum sulfated lithocholate as an indicator of cholestasis during parenteral nutrition in infants and children. JPEN J Parenter Enteral Nutr 6:30–33, 1982.

39. Miyai K, Price VM, Fisher MM: Bile acid metabolism in mammals: Ultrastructural studies on the intrahepatic cholestasis induced by lithocholate and chenodeoxycholic acids in the rat. Lab Invest 24:292–302, 1971.

40. Sondheimer JM, Asturiase E, Cadnapaphornchai M: Infection and cholestasis in neonates with intestinal resection and long-term parenteral nutrition. J Pediatr Gastroenterol Nutr 27:131–137, 1998.

41. Wolf A, Pohlandt F: Bacterial infection: The main cause of acute cholestasis in newborn infants receiving short term parenteral nutrition. J Pediatr Gastroenterol Nutr 8:297–303, 1989.

42. Moss RL, Das JB, Raffensperger JG: Necrotizing enterocolitis and total parenteral nutrition–associated cholestasis. Nutrition 12:340–343, 1996.

43. Nolan JP: Intestinal endotoxins as mediators of hepatic injury—An idea whose time has come again. Hepatology 10:887–891, 1989.

44. Tracey KJ, Beutler B, Lowry SF, et al: Shock and tissue injury induced by recombinant human cachectin. Science 234:470–474, 1986.

45. Dinarello CA, Cannon JG, Wolff SM, et al: Tumor necrosis factor (cachectin) is an endogenous pyrogen and induces production of interleukin-1. J Exp Med 163:1433–1450, 1986.

46. Lichtman SN, Wang J, Schwab JH, Lemasters JJ: Comparison of peptidoglycan-polysaccharide and lipopolysaccharide stimulation of Kupffer cells to produce tumor necrosis factor and interleukin-1. Hepatology 19:1013–1022, 1994.

47. Argiles JM, Lopez-Soriano FJ: The effects of tumor necrosis factor-α (cachectin) and tumor growth on hepatic amino acid utilization in the rat. Biochem J 266:123–126, 1990.

48. Argiles JM, Lopez-Soriano FJ, Wiggins D, Williamson DH: Comparative effects of tumor necrosis factor-α (cachectin), interleukin-1 and tumor growth on amino acid metabolism in the rat in vivo. Biochem J 261:357–362, 1989.

49. Shattuck KE, Grinnell CD, Goldman AS, Rassin DK: The acute effects of TNF-α on the isolated perfused rat liver. J Investig Med 44:64–69, 1996.

50. Shattuck KE, Grinnell CD, Keeney SE, et al: Hyperoxia and glutathione depletion in the isolated perfused rat liver. J Investig Med 45:576–583, 1997.

51. Touloukin RJ, Downing SE: Cholestasis associated with long-term parenteral nutrition. Arch Surg 106:58–62, 1973.

52. Ito Y, Shils ME: Liver dysfunction associated with long-term total parenteral nutrition in patients with massive bowel resection. JPEN J Parenter Enteral Nutr 15:271–276, 1991.

53. Stanko RT, Nathan FG, Mendelow H, Adibi SA: Development of hepatic cholestasis and fibrosis in patients with massive loss of intestine supported by prolonged parenteral nutrition. Gastroenterology 92:197–202, 1987.

54. Merritt RJ: Cholestasis associated with total parenteral nutrition. J Pediatr Gastroenterol Nutr 5:9–22, 1986.

55. Drongowski RA, Coran AG: An analysis of factors contributing to the development of total parenteral nutrition–induced cholestasis. JPEN J Parenter Enteral Nutr 13:586–589, 1989.

56. Forchielli ML, Gura KM, Sandler R, Lo C: Aminosyn PF or TrophAmine: Which provides more protection from cholestasis associated with total parenteral nutrition? J Pediatr Gastroenterol Nutr 21:374–382, 1995.

57. Benya R, Brasco J, McGreen T, et al: Intrahepatic cholestasis, bile excretory function and hyperbilirubinemia. Curr Hepatol 11:199–229, 1991.

58. Messing B, Zarka Y, Lemann M, et al: Chronic cholestasis associated with long-term parenteral nutrition. Transplant Proc 26:1438–1439, 1994.

59. Spurr SG, Grylack LJ, Mehta NR: Hyperalimentation associated neonatal cholestasis: Effect of oral gentamicin. JPEN J Parenter Enteral Nutr 13:633–636, 1989.

60. Moss RL, Das JB, Raffensperger JG: Total parenteral nutrition associated cholestasis: Clinical and histopathologic correlation. J Pediatr Surg 28:1270–1275, 1993.

61. Beath SV, Davies P, Papadopoulou A, et al: Parenteral nutrition–related cholestasis in postsurgical neonates: Multivariate analysis of risk factors. J Pediatr Surg 31:604–606, 1996.

62. Lester R, St Pyrek J, Little JM, Adcock EW: Diversity of bile acids in the fetus and newborn infant. J Pediatr Gastroenterol Nutr 2:355–364, 1983.

63. Lester R: Bile acid metabolism in the newborn. J Pediatr Gastroenterol Nutr 2:335-336, 1983.

64. Carey MC, Cahalane MJ: Enterohepatic circulation. In Arias IM, Jacoby WB, Popper H, et al (eds): The Liver: Biology and Pathobiology. New York, Raven Press, 1988, pp 573–615.

65. Erlinger S: Bile flow. In Arias IM, Jacoby WB, Popper H, et al (eds): The Liver: Biology and Pathobiology. New York, Raven Press, 1988, pp 643–661.

66. Riepl PL, Fiedler F, Teufel J, Lehnert P: Effect of intraduodenal bile and tauro-deoxycholate on exocrine pancreatic secretion and on plasma levels of vasoactive intestinal polypeptide and somatostatin in man. Pancreas 9:109–116, 1994.

67. Lin HC, Kwok G, Zhao XT, Gu YG: Bile acid–dependent inhibition of gallbladder emptying. Am J Physiol 269:G988–G993, 1995.

68. Watkins JB, Szczepanik P, Gould JB, et al: Bile salt metabolism in the human premature infant. Gastroenterology 69:706–713, 1975.

69. Malloy MH, Rassin DK, Richardson CJ: Total parenteral nutrition in sick preterm infants: Effects of cysteine supplementation with nitrogen intakes of 240 and 400 mg/kg/day. J Pediatr Gastroenterol Nutr 3:239–244, 1984.

70. Vinton NE, Laidlaw SA, Ament ME, Kopple JD: Taurine concentrations in plasma, blood cells and urine of children undergoing long-term total parenteral nutrition. Pediatr Res 21:399–403, 1987.

71. Cooper A, Betts JM, Pereira GR, Ziegler MM: Taurine deficiency in the severe hepatic dysfunction complicating total parenteral nutrition. J Pediatr Surg 19:462–466, 1984.

72. Zahavi I, Shaffer EA, Gall DG: Total parenteral nutrition associated cholestasis: Acute studies in infant and adult rabbits. J Pediatr Gastroenterol Nutr 4:622–627, 1985.

73. Belli DE, Fournier LA, Lepage G, et al: Total parenteral nutrition–associated cholestasis in rats: Comparison of different amino acid mixtures. JPEN J Parenter Enteral Nutr 11:67–73, 1987.

74. Graham MF, Tavill AS, Halpin TC, Louis LN: Inhibition of bile flow in the isolated perfused rat liver by a synthetic parenteral amino acid mixture: Associated net amino acid fluxes. Hepatology 4:69–73, 1984.

75. Shattuck KE, Grinnell CD, Rassin DK: Amino acid infusions induce reversible, dose-related decreases in bile flow in the isolated rat liver. JPEN J Parenter Enteral Nutr 17:171–176, 1993.

76. Perea A, Tuchweber B, Yousef IM, et al: Studies on effect of synthetic amino acid mixtures on bile secretion in the isolated perfused rat liver. Nutr Res 7:89–99, 1987.

77. Shattuck KE, Grinnell CD, Rassin DK: Biliary amino acid and glutathione secretion in response to amino acid infusion in the isolated rat liver. JPEN J Parenter Enteral Nutr 18:119–127, 1994.

78. Committee on Clinical Practice Issues of the American Society for Clinical Nutrition: Guidelines for pediatric parenteral nutrition. Am J Clin Nutr 48:1324–1342, 1988.

79. Rassin DK: Amino acid metabolism in total parenteral nutrition during development. In Friedman M (ed): Absorption and Utilization of Amino Acids, Vol 2. Boca Raton, Fla, CRC Press, 1989, pp 71–85.

80. Rassin DK: Amino acid requirements and profiles in total parenteral nutrition. In Lebenthal E (ed): Total Parenteral Nutrition: Indications, Utilization, Complications, and Pathophysiological Considerations. New York, Raven Press, 1986, pp 5–15.

81. Sturman JA, Gaull G, Raiha NC: Absence of cystathionase in human fetal liver: Is cysteine essential? Science 169:74–76, 1970.

82. Heird WC, Dell RB, Helms RA, et al: Amino acid mixture designed to maintain normal plasma amino acid patterns in infants and children requiring parenteral nutrition. Pediatrics 80:401–408, 1987.

83. Adamkin DH, McClead RE, Desai NS, et al: Comparison of two neonatal intravenous amino acid formulations in preterm infants: A multicenter study. J Perinatol 11:375–382, 1991.

84. Machytka B, Hoos I, Forster H: Fatty liver in rats following parenteral hyperalimentation with glucose or glucose substitutes. Nutr Metals 21:110–112, 1977.

85. Hirai Y, Sanada Y, Fujiwara T, et al: High calorie infusion–induced hepatic impairments in infants. JPEN J Parenter Enteral Nutr 3:146–150, 1979.

86. Chang S, Silvis SE: Fatty liver produced by hyperalimentation of rats. Am J Gastroenterol 62:410–418, 1974.

87. Rivera A Jr, Bhatia J, Rassin DK, et al: In vitro biliary function in the adult rat: The effect of parenteral glucose and amino acids. JPEN J Parenter Enteral Nutr 13:240–245, 1989.

88. Rutishauser SCB, Millward SE: The effects of hypertonic glucose solutions on hepatic bile formation. J Hepatol 11:22–28, 1990.

89. Marin JJG, Bravo P, Barriocanal FP, et al: Hyperglycemia-induced cholestasis in the isolated perfused rat liver. Hepatology 14:184–191, 1991.

90. Pitkanen O, Hallman M, Andersson S: Generation of free radicals in lipid emulsion used in parenteral nutrition. Pediatr Res 29:56–59, 1991.

91. Wispe JR, Bell EF, Roberts RJ: Assessment of lipid peroxidation in newborn infants and rabbits by measurements of expired ethane and pentane: Influence of parenteral lipid infusion. Pediatr Res 19:374–379, 1985.

92. Clayton PT, Bowron A, Mills KA, et al: Phytosterolemia in children with parenteral nutrition-associated cholestatic liver disease. Gastroenterology 105:1806–1813, 1993.

93. Iyer KR, Spitz L, Clayton P: New insight into mechanisms of parenteral nutrition–associated cholestasis: Role of plant sterols. J Pediatr Surg 33:1–6, 1998.

94. Milliner DS, Shinaberger JH, Shuman P, Coburn JW: Inadvertent aluminum administration during plasma exchange due to aluminum contamination of albumin-replacement solutions. N Engl J Med 312:165–167, 1985.

95. Sedman AB, Klein GL, Merritt RJ, et al: Evidence of aluminum loading in infants receiving intravenous therapy. N Engl J Med 312:1337–1343, 1985.

96. Klein GL, Heyman MB, Lee TC, et al: Aluminum-associated hepatobiliary dysfunction in rats: Relationships to dosage and duration of exposure. Pediatr Res 23:275–278, 1988.

97. Klein GL, Berquist WE, Ament ME, et al: Hepatic aluminum accumulation in children on total parenteral nutrition. J Pediatr Gastroenterol Nutr 3:740–743, 1984.

98. Bidlack WR, Brown RC, Meskin MS, et al: Effects of aluminum on the hepatic mixed function oxidase and drug metabolism. Drug Nutr Interact 5:33–42, 1987.

99. Klein GL, Sedman AB, Heyman MB, et al: Hepatic abnormalities associated with aluminum loading in piglets. JPEN J Parenter Enteral Nutr 11:293–297, 1987.

100. Klein GL, Lee TC, Heyman MB, Rassin DK: Altered glycine and taurine conjugation of bile acids following aluminum administration to rats. J Pediatr Gastroenterol Nutr 9:361–364, 1989.

101. Demircan M, Ergun O, Coker C, et al: Aluminum in total parenteral nutrition solutions produces portal inflammation in rats. J Pediatr Gastroenterol Nutr 26:274–278, 1998.

102. Klein GL, Goldblum RM, Moslen MT, et al: Increased biliary transferrin excretion following parenteral aluminum administration to rats. Pharmacol Toxicol 72:373–376, 1993.

103. Bougle D, Bureau F, Deschrevel G, et al: Chromium and parenteral nutrition in children. J Pediatr Gastroenterol Nutr 17:72–74, 1993.

104. Reynolds AP, Kiely E, Meadows N: Manganese in long term paediatric parenteral nutrition. Arch Dis Child 71:527–528, 1994.

105. Fell JME, Reynolds AP, Meadows N, et al: Manganese toxicity in children receiving long-term parenteral nutrition. Lancet 347:1218–1221, 1996.

106. Shike M, Roulet M, Kurian R, et al: Copper metabolism in total parenteral nutrition. Gastroenterology 81:290–297, 1981.

107. Plaa GL, DeLamirande E, Lewittes M, Yousef IM: Liver cell plasma lipids in manganese-bilirubin induced intrahepatic cholestasis. Biochem Pharmacol 31:3698–3701, 1982.

108. Knodell RG, Steele NM, Cerra FB, et al: Effects of parenteral and enteral alimentation on hepatic drug metabolism in the rat. J Pharmacol Exp Ther 229:589–597, 1984.

109. Dosi P, Raul AJ, Chelliah BP, et al: Perinatal factors underlying neonatal cholestasis. J Pediatr 106:471–474, 1985.

110. Toth CA, Thomas P: Liver endocytosis and Kupffer cells. Hepatology 16:255–266, 1992.

111. Jaeschke H: Vascular oxidant stress and hepatic ischemia-reperfusion injury. Free Radic Res Commun 12-13:737–743, 1991.

112. Jaeschke H: Enhanced sinusoidal glutathione efflux during endotoxin-induced oxidant stress in vivo. Am J Physiol 263:G60–G68, 1992.

113. Smith CV, Hansen TN, Martin NE, et al: Oxidant stress responses in premature infants during exposure to hyperoxia. Pediatr Res 34:360–365, 1993.

114. Kanner JD, Fennema OJ: Photooxidation of tryptophan in the presence of riboflavin. Agric Food Chem 35:71–76, 1987.

115. Meister A, Anderson ME: Glutathione. Annu Rev Biochem 52:711–760, 1983.

116. Kaplowitz N, Aw TY, Ookhtens M: The regulation of hepatic glutathione. Annu Rev Pharmacol Toxicol 25:715–744, 1985.

117. Ballatori N, Truong AT: Glutathione as a primary osmotic driving force in hepatic bile formation. Am J Physiol 263:G617–G624, 1992.

118. Ballatori N, Truong AT: Relation between biliary glutathione excretion and bile acid–independent bile flow. Am J Physiol 256:G22–G30, 1989.

119. Pessayre D, Dolder A, Artigou JY, et al: Effect of fasting on metabolite-mediated hepatotoxicity in the rat. Gastroenterology 77:264–271, 1979.

120. Leaf G, Neuberger A: The effect of diet on the glutathione content of the liver. Biochem J 41:280–287, 1947.

121. Sokol RJ, Taylor SF, Devereaux MW, et al: Hepatic oxidant injury and glutathione depletion during total parenteral nutrition in weanling rats. Am J Physiol 270:G691–G700, 1996.

122. Brawley V, Bhatia J, Karp WB: Hydrogen peroxide generation in a model pediatric parenteral amino acid solution. Clin Sci 85:709–712, 1993.

123. Bhatia J, Mims LC, Roesel RA: The effect of phototherapy on amino acid solutions containing multivitamins. J Pediatr 96:284–286, 1980.

124. Bhatia J, Rassin DK: Photosensitized oxidation of tryptophan and hepatic dysfunction in neonatal gerbils. JPEN J Parenter Enteral Nutr 9:491–495, 1985.

125. Rojas J, Silva E: Photochemical-like behavior of riboflavin in the dark promoted by enzyme-generated triplet acetone. Photochem Photobiol 47:467–470, 1988.

126. Wang R: Lethal effect of "daylight" fluorescent light on human cells in tissue culture medium. Photochem Photobiol 21:373–375, 1975.

127. Nixon TB, Wang RJ: Formation of photoproducts

lethal for human cells in culture by daylight fluorescent light and bilirubin light. Photochem Photobiol 26:589–591, 1977.

128. Bhatia J, Rassin DK, McAdoo DJ: Photosensitized oxidation of tryptophan: Effect on liver and brain tryptophan. JPEN J Parenter Enteral Nutr 15:637–641, 1991.

129. Bhatia J, Moslen MT, Hague AK, et al: Total parenteral nutrition–associated alterations in hepatobiliary function and histology in rats: Is light exposure a clue? Pediatr Res 33:487–492, 1993.

130. Grant JP, Cox CE, Kleinman LM, et al: Serum hepatic enzyme and bilirubin elevations during parenteral nutrition. Surg Gynecol Obstet 145:573–580, 1977.

131. Bhatia J, Rivera A, Moslen MT, et al: Hepatic function during short-term total parenteral nutrition: Effect of exposure of parenteral nutrients to light. Res Commun Chem Pathol Pharmacol 78:321–340, 1992.

132. Bhatia J, Moslen MT, Kaphalia L, Rassin DK: Glutathione and tissue amino acid responses to light-exposed parenteral nutrients. Toxicol Lett 63:79–89, 1992.

133. Shattuck KE, Bhatia J, Grinnell C, Rassin DK: The effects of light exposure on the in vitro hepatic response to an amino acid–vitamin solution. JPEN J Parenter Enteral Nutr 19:398–402, 1995.

134. Colomb V, Goulet O, Rambaud C, et al: Long-term parenteral nutrition in children; liver and gallbladder disease. Transplant Proc 24:1054–1055, 1992.

135. Collier S, Crouch J, Hendricks K, Caballero B: Use of cyclic parenteral nutrition in infants less than 6 months of age. Nutr Clin Pract 9:65–68, 1994.

136. Capron JP, Herve MA, Gineston JL, Braillon A: Metronidazole in prevention of cholestasis associated with total parenteral nutrition. Lancet 1:446–447, 1993.

137. South M, King A: Parenteral nutrition–associated cholestasis: Recovery following phenobarbitone. JPEN J Parenter Enteral Nutr 11:208–209, 1987.

138. Thaler MM: Effect of phenobarbital on hepatic transport and excretion of ^{131}I–Rose Bengal in children with cholestasis. Pediatr Res 6:100–110, 1972.

139. Palmer RH, Hruban Z: Production of bile duct hyperplasia and gallstones by lithocholic acid. J Clin Invest 45:1255–1267, 1964.

140. Poupon PE, Lindor KD, Cauch-Dudek K, et al: Combined analysis of randomized controlled trials of ursodeoxycholic acid in primary biliary cirrhosis. Gastroenterology 113:884–890, 1997.

141. Trauner M, Meier PJ, Boyer JL: Molecular pathogenesis of cholestasis. N Engl J Med 339:1217–1227, 1998.

142. Hofmann AF, Grundy SM, Lachin JM, et al: Pretreatment biliary lipid composition in white patients with radiolucent gallstones in the National Cooperative Gallstone Study. Gastroenterology 83:738–752, 1982.

143. Poupon R, Poupon RE: Ursodeoxycholic acid therapy of chronic cholestatic conditions in adults and children. Pharmacol Ther 66:1–15, 1995.

144. Lindor KD: Ursodiol for primary sclerosing cholangitis. N Engl J Med 336:691–695, 1997.

145. Lindor KD, Burnes J: Ursodeoxycholic acid for the treatment of home parenteral nutrition–associated cholestasis. A case report. Gastroenterology 101:250–253, 1991.

146. Spagnuolo MI, Iorio R, Vegnente A, Guarino G: Ursodeoxycholic acid for treatment of cholestasis in children on long-term total parenteral nutrition: A pilot study. Gastroenterology 111:716–719, 1996.

147. Cocjin J, Watanabe F, Sehgal S, et al: Does ursodeoxycholic acid (UDCA) alter the course of total parenteral nutrition–associated cholestasis (TPNAC) in the neonate [Abstract]? Pediatr Res 35:126A, 1994.

148. United States Pharmacopeial Convention Inc: USP DI Drug Information for the Health Care Professional, 18th ed. Rockville, Md, United States Pharmacopeial Convention, 1998, p 2921.

149. Ota M, Minami Y, Hoshita T: Intestinal absorption of ursodeoxycholic, glycoursodeoxycholic and tauroursodeoxycholic acids in rats. J Pharmacobiodyn 8:114–8, 1985.

150. Walker S, Stiehl A, Raedsch R, et al: Absorption of urso- and chenodeoxycholic acid and their taurine and glycine conjugates in rat jejunum, ileum and colon. Digestion 35:47–52, 1985.

151. Mundlos S, Kuhnelt P, Adler G: Monitoring enzyme replacement treatment in exocrine pancreatic insufficiency using the cholesteryl octanoate breath test. Gut 31:1324–1328, 1990.

152. Sitzmann JV, Pitt HA, Steinhorn PA, et al: Cholecystokinin prevents parenteral nutrition induced biliary sludge in humans. Surg Gynecol Obstet 170:25–31, 1990.

153. Teitelbaum DH, Han-Markey T, Drongowski RA, et al: Use of cholecystokinin to prevent the development of parenteral nutrition–associated cholestasis. JPEN J Parenter Enteral Nutr 21:100–103, 1997.

154. Teitelbaum DH, Han-Markey T, Schumacher RE: Treatment of parenteral nutrition–associated cholestasis with cholecystokinin-octapeptide. J Pediatr Surg 30:1082–1085, 1995.

155. Grant JP, Snyder PJ: Use of L-glutamine in total parenteral nutrition. J Surg Res 44:506–513, 1988.

156. Hughes CA, Dowling RH: Speed of onset of adaptive mucosal hypoplasia and hypofunction in the intestine of parenterally fed rats. Clin Sci 59:317–327, 1980.

157. Lo CW, Walker WA: Changes in the gastrointestinal tract during enteral or parenteral feeding. Nutr Rev 47:193–198, 1989.

158. Alverdy JA, Aoys E, Weiss-Carrington P, Burke DA: The effect of glutamine-enriched TPN on gut immune cellularity. J Surg Res 52:34–38, 1992.

159. Li S, Nussbaum MS, McFadden DW, et al: Addition of L-glutamine to total parenteral nutrition and its effects on portal insulin and glucagon and the development of hepatic steatosis in rats. J Surg Res 48:421–427, 1990.

160. Ziegler TR, Benfell K, Smith RJ, et al: Safety and metabolic effects of L-glutamine administration in humans. JPEN J Parenter Enteral Nutr 14(Suppl):137–146, 1990.

161. Allen SJ, Pierro A, Cope L, et al: Glutamine-supplemented parenteral nutrition in a child with short bowel syndrome. J Pediatr Gastroenterol Nutr 17:329–332, 1993.

162. Lacey JM, Crouch JB, Benfell K, et al: The effects of glutamine-supplemented parenteral nutrition in premature infants. JPEN J Parenter Enteral Nutr 20:74–80, 1996.

163. Shattuck KE, Rassin DK, Grinnell CD: N-Acetyl-

cysteine protects from glutathione depletion in rats exposed to hyperoxia. JPEN J Parenter Enteral Nutr 22:228–233, 1998.

164. Shattuck KE, Rassin DK, Grinnell CD: N-Acetyl-cysteine protects bile flow during amino acid infusion [Abstract]. Pediatr Res 45:117A, 1999.

165. Cooper A, Ross AJ, O'Neill JA Jr, et al: Resolution of intractable cholestasis associated with total parenteral nutrition following biliary irrigation. J Pediatr Surg 20:772–774, 1985.

166. Rintala R, Lindahl H, Pohjavuori M, et al: Surgical treatment of intractable cholestasis associated with total parenteral nutrition in premature infants. J Pediatr Surg 28:716–719, 1993.

167. Langnas AN, Shaw BW, Antonson DL, et al: Preliminary experience with intestinal transplantation in infants and children. Pediatrics 97:443–448, 1996.

168. Matos C, Avni EF, Van Gansbeke D, et al: Total parenteral nutrition (TPN) and gallbladder disease in neonates. Sonographic assessment. J Ultrasound Med 6:243–248, 1987.

169. Heubi JE, Soloway RD, Balistreri WF: Biliary lipid composition in healthy and diseased infants, children and young adults. Gastroenterology 82:1295–1299, 1982.

170. Reif S, Sloven DG, Lebenthal E: Gallstones in children. Characterization by age, etiology and outcome. Am J Dis Child 145:105–108, 1991.

171. Jonas A, Yahav J, Fradkin A, et al: Cholecholithiasis in infants: Diagnostic and therapeutic problems. J Pediatr Gastroenterol Nutr 11:513–517, 1990.

9

◆ Metabolic Bone Disease

Edward W. Lipkin, M.D., Ph.D.

The skeletal system serves several purposes: it is a structural framework for the body cell mass; it provides a reservoir of essential calcium, phosphate, and magnesium; and it constitutes one of the largest sources of bicarbonate buffering capacity for neutralization of acid. The skeletal system is dynamic, continuously undergoing a process of new bone formation, remodeling of existing bone, and bone resorption. A variety of disease processes, both intrinsic to bone and secondarily affecting bone, result in poor bone health and clinically in pain and fracture.

◆ OSTEOPOROSIS

Definition and Epidemiology

Osteoporosis is a state of reduced bone mass per unit volume with a normal ratio of mineral to matrix that results in increased bone fragility and fracture with minimal or no trauma, especially in the distal radius, the vertebrae, and the proximal femur. With advances in the technology, the current definition rests on the assessment of bone density. Thus, osteoporosis is defined as a bone density lower than 2.5 SDs below the mean for a young sex-matched healthy person. *Established osteoporosis* is osteoporosis and an established fracture. *Osteopenia* is considered a bone density lower than 1 SD below that of a young sex-matched healthy person.

More than 20 million women in the United States are affected by osteoporosis. From 25 to 30% of white women older than 65 years have symptomatic osteoporosis with fracture, pain, or a loss in height. There are 1.5 million fractures per year due to osteoporosis, at an annual health care cost of $8 to $10 billion per year.[1] Although osteoporosis primarily affects women, men have one seventh of all vertebral fractures and one quarter of all hip fractures resulting from osteoporosis. Men have a lesser incidence and prevalence of osteoporosis be-cause they have greater peak bone mass, a shorter life expectancy, and no menopause equivalent.[2, 3]

Major morbidity and mortality result from fractures due to osteoporosis. There are 350,000 hip fractures alone per year in North America.[4] A hip fracture occurs in 30% of women older than 80 years.[5] The average hip fracture results in hospitalization for 3 weeks and is associated with 12 to 30% mortality in the first year after hip fracture.[6] Of patients who sustain a hip fracture, 15 to 25% are discharged to a nursing home for at least 1 year and 25 to 35% are discharged to home but are dependent on other people or devices for mobility.[7, 8] Vertebral fractures are more prevalent (650,000 vertebral fractures per year) than hip fractures and occur in 25 to 30% of women older than 60 years.[9] Although mortality related to vertebral fractures is less than that of hip fractures, vertebral fractures may result in permanent deformity and chronic pain.[10] The third type of fracture, which is common in osteoporosis, is a Colles' fracture of the forearm. Over 200,000 Colles' fractures occur per year, and they are the most common fracture in adults younger than 75 years, at which age fractures of the hip become more common. [11] Colles' fractures may cause significant functional morbidity.

Pathophysiology and Risk Factors

Osteoporosis is a clinically heterogeneous disorder that results from a net resorption of bone greater than new bone formation. One factor influencing osteoporosis is the peak bone mass attained, typically in the third decade. The higher one's peak bone mass, the lesser the incidence of osteoporosis once bone loss occurs. Risk factors for decreased peak bone mass include thinness, weight loss, short stature, white race, a family history of osteoporosis, and low calcium intake. Insufficient accumulation of peak bone mass predisposes to later fractures.[12]

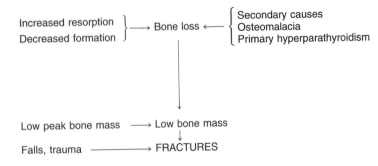

Figure 9–1. Development of osteoporosis.

The characteristics of bone loss differ for men and women.[13, 14] A slow phase of bone loss occurs throughout life in men. In women, there is an accelerated phase of exponential bone loss from estrogen deficiency lasting 5 to 10 years after menopause, followed by the slow phase of age-related bone loss. After the age of 40 years, women lose 50% of trabecular and 35% of cortical bone mass. Men lose two thirds of this amount. The attainment of peak bone mass is followed by age-related bone loss caused by an uncoupling of resorption and formation, resulting in a relative disproportionate increase of bone resorption.[15] Over the years, there is a slow increase in the fracture rate of the hip, humerus, tibia, and pelvis reflecting slow bone loss and impaired coordination, slowed reflexes, failing vision, increased medication use, and neuromuscular disease resulting in increased falls.

Researchers have identified a variety of risk factors for the development of osteoporosis that may be of clinical significance in any given individual. Of primary importance as a risk factor for the development of osteoporosis is estrogen deficiency, due to menopause, surgical ovariectomy, extreme exercise, or weight loss.[16] Estrogen deficiency results in increased sensitivity of bone to the resorptive effect of parathyroid hormone (PTH) and in decreased calcium absorption.[17, 18] With aging, the conversion of 25-hydroxyvitamin D to 1,25-dihydroxyvitamin D is reduced and parallels a decline in calcium absorption by the gut.[19, 20] In postmenopausal women, very low calcium intake (less than 500 mg/day, recommended dietary allowance = 800 mg/day) is associated with an increased incidence of osteoporosis,[21] and deficient calcium intake during adolescence results in decreased maximal bone mass[22] and predisposes to osteoporosis in later life. The intake of vitamin D may also be insufficient in elderly persons.[23] Body morphology is a major determinant of peak bone mass. Thus, individuals with a slender body build have less peak bone mass and less estrogen production than non-thin individuals of equivalent stature.[24] Obesity is protective against bone loss because of skeletal loading from weight bearing and stresses from muscle that stimulate osteoblast formation. Obese individuals also have increased conversion of androgens to estrogens in fat tissue. Genetic factors may influence the peak bone mass, and a family history of osteoporosis is a risk factor.[25, 26] Excessive intake of caffeine and protein may cause bone loss. Motor incoordination and weakness may lead to instability and falls that contribute to the risk of fracture.[27]

A simplified schema for how osteoporosis develops is presented in Figure 9–1.

Types

Osteoporosis can be considered to be either primary, due to a defect in the skeletal system, or secondary, due to a variety of factors and medical conditions.

Primary Osteoporisis

Primary osteoporosis results both from the aging process (senile osteoporosis) and from the loss of gonadal function (postmenopausal osteoporosis).[1] The differing clinical syndromes of primary osteoporosis and their causes are summarized in Table 9–1.

Secondary Osteoporosis

Secondary osteoporosis is due to a variety of endocrine diseases, malignancy, drugs, immobilization, liver disease, genetic defects in collagen, and nutritional deficiency.

Table 9–1. Primary Osteoporosis Syndromes

	Type 1 Postmenopausal*	Type 2 Senile†
Age (yr)	50–75	>75
Sex ratio (F/M)	6:1	2:1
Type of bone loss	Trabecular	Trabecular and cortical
Rate of bone loss	Accelerated (increased bone resorption)	Slow (decreased bone formation)
Fracture site	Distal radius	Vertebrae
	Vertebrae	Proximal femur
PTH	Decreased (secondary to estrogen deficiency)	Increased (secondary to decreased calcium absorption)
Calcium absorption	Decreased	Decreased
25-OH-D to 1,25-(OH)$_2$-D conversion	Decreased secondary to decreased PTH	Primary decrease in vitamin D conversion
Main cause	Estrogen deficiency	Aging

*Type 1: Not all postmenopausal women with the same lower estrogen level develop osteoporosis. Other factors must be responsible such as a higher sensitivity to PTH or the elaboration of interleukin-6, known to increase resorption.
†Type 2: Women develop type 2 twice as frequently as men older than 70 years. It is due to decreased osteoblastic function and calcium absorption, estrogen deficiency, a negative calcium balance, and a variety of environmental and genetic factors.
25-OH,D, 25-hydroxyvitamin D; 25-(OH)$_2$-D, 25, dihydroxyvitamin D; PTH, parathyroid hormone.

The endocrine diseases that need to be considered as causes of secondary osteoporosis include Cushing's disease (glucocorticoid excess), thyrotoxicosis, hypogonadism (e.g., secondary to a pituitary tumor), diabetes mellitus, primary hyperparathyroidism, and amenorrhea. Glucocorticoid excess, whether due to a pituitary tumor, an adrenal tumor, or medication, impairs calcium absorption,[28] increases calcium losses in the urine,[29] and inhibits bone formation.[30] Thyrotoxicosis increases bone turnover.[31] Muscle weakness can be a part of thyrotoxicosis and can aggravate bone loss and falls. Fractures are rare with thyroid over-replacement. Hypogonadism can result from a variety of pituitary tumors.[32] Diabetes mellitus type 1 is associated with osteoporosis, but osteoporotic fractures are rare.[33] Primary hyperparathyroidism increases bone turnover and can be a cause of osteoporosis.[34] Amenorrhea induces osteoporosis.[35] Paradoxically, exercise favors bone formation, but women who exercise to the point of amenorrhea experience bone loss.[36]

Malignant disease is another secondary cause of osteoporosis that is not necessarily due to direct lytic destruction of bone. The malignancies that are associated with osteoporosis include multiple myeloma, leukemia, lymphoma, mastocytosis, and disseminated carcinomatosis.[37]

A variety of drugs (see Drug-Induced Osteoporosis, below) should also be considered secondary causes of osteoporosis, including alcohol, which inhibits the function

and number of osteoblasts;[38] heparin, which induces a release of collagenase and other enzymes from lysozymes;[39] steroids;[40] and cigarettes, which increase sex steroid catabolism.[41]

Additional secondary causes of osteoporosis include immobilization,[42] liver disease such as primary biliary cirrhosis,[43] and a variety of genetic defects of bone collagen including osteogenesis imperfecta, Ehlers-Danlos syndrome, Marfan's syndrome, and homocystinuria.[44] Osteoporosis can be seen in scurvy (vitamin C deficiency)[45] and in severe malnutrition including conditions requiring total parenteral nutrition.[46]

Clinical Presentation and Diagnosis

The clinical presentation of osteoporosis is bone fracture with minimal or no trauma (50% associated with falls). Vertebral fractures are most common, typically fractures of the lower thoracic and upper lumbar area. Sharp back pain is often experienced, along with paravertebral muscle spasm and percussion tenderness. Many fractures, however, are asymptomatic. Complications from vertebral collapse such as nerve root or spinal cord compression are uncommon.[47] The compression fracture results in a loss of height, dorsal kyphosis (dowager's hump), and chronic back pain. Marked spine deformity results in abdominal discomfort, restrictive pulmonary disease, and painful rubbing of the ribs on the iliac crest. Additional sites of bone fractures in osteoporosis include the proximal femur, distal radius, humerus, and pelvis. Although a fracture is a common presenting complaint in osteoporosis, often the patient is asymptomatic, and osteopenia is discovered coincidentally.

The assessment of bone mass by standard radiography is inaccurate. On standard radiography, 30% of bone mineral or more may be lost before osteopenia is apparent.[48] Radiologically, vertebrae show a loss of horizontal trabeculations, localized herniation of the nucleus pulposus into the vertebral body (Schmorl's node), anterior wedge fractures, biconcavity resulting from ballooning of the intervertebral disks (codfish vertebrae), and complete compression fractures. Posterior wedging suggests a destructive lesion such as infection or a blood-borne tumor and not osteoporosis.

Osteoporosis is currently diagnosed from direct assessment of bone mineral, usually by dual-energy x-ray absorptiometry. The current technology for the noninvasive assessment of bone mineral is summarized in Table 9–2. To consider the patient to have primary osteoporosis, secondary causes should be excluded by history (drugs, menstrual) and physical examination, combined with thyroid function tests. A complete blood count, serum and urine protein electrophoresis, liver function tests, a general chemistry battery, and gonadal function tests (testosterone or estradiol, luteinizing hormone, and follicle-stimulating hormone) should be done. Primary hyperparathyroidism may be excluded by a normal serum calcium and PTH measurement.

A variety of other tests are used to assess the dynamics of bone remodeling. Serum alkaline phosphatase levels are increased in Paget's disease, fracture, hyperparathyroidism, and growth before puberty. Because alkaline phosphatase is released from bone, liver, and the gut, in bone disease it is useful to measure the bone-specific activity, which then is a very direct assessment of osteoblastic activity and indirectly of bone formation.[49] Serum osteocalcin is another measure of osteoblastic activity but correlates poorly with bone formation under a variety of conditions.[50] The rate of bone resorption is difficult to assess, but the current best measure is the concentration of cross-linked collagen-Pyridium relative to creatinine, which are excreted in the urine.[51] Most attempts to model the therapy of osteoporosis based on serum measurements of bone formation and resorption have not been fruitful.[52] The architecture of bone—and with tetracycline labeling, the rate of bone formation—can be very accurately assessed from a bone biopsy.[53] It is the most accurate means of diagnosing a mineralization defect in bone and establishing the diagnosis of osteomalacia. Bone biopsy may also be critical in establishing the diagnosis of aluminum bone disease, Paget's disease, or osteogenesis imperfecta.

The issue of population screening for osteoporosis remains controversial. Predicting osteoporosis risk is difficult despite a knowledge of individual risk factors. The problem is that we do not know any risk combination that can predict low bone mass. There is no single inexpensive test

Table 9–2. Noninvasive Assessment of Bone Mineral Content

Technique	Site	Precision* (%)	Accuracy† (%)	Exam Time (min)	Absorbed Dose of Radiation‡ (mrem)	Cost ($)
Single-photon absorptiometry	Proximal and distal radius, calcaneus	1–3	5	15	10–20	75
Dual-energy photon absorptiometry	Spine, hip, total body	2–4	4–10	20–40	5	1–150
Dual-energy x-ray absorptiometry	Spine, hip, total body	0.5–2	3–5	3–7	1–3	75–150
Quantitative computed tomography	Spine	2–5	5–20	10–15	100–1000	100–200

*Precision is the coefficient of variation (standard deviation divided by the mean) for repeated measurements over a short period of time in young healthy persons.

†Accuracy is the coefficient of variation for a measurement in a specimen whose mineral content has been determined by other means (e.g., measurement of ashed weight).

‡To convert millirems to millijoules per kilogram of body weight, multiply by 0.01.

that is reliable and precisely reflects the response to therapy. Densitometry remains the single most important tool for diagnosing osteoporosis and establishing the risk of fracture. As a practical strategy, it is wise to assume that all postmenopausal patients will develop osteoporosis if precautions are not taken. In general, for each patient, the more risk factors present and the longer the duration of their presence, the greater the risk of future problems. This approach can be used in two ways:

1. To sensitize the patient and the physician to the likelihood of osteoporosis
2. To address those risk factors that are amenable to alteration

Treatment

The drugs approved by the Food and Drug Administration (FDA) for the treatment of postmenopausal osteoporosis are estrogen, calcitonin, and bisphosphonates.[54] Osteoporosis is not an approved indication for calcitriol. Oral calcium and sodium fluoride are not subject to FDA regulations.

Studies suggest that calcium supplementation in perimenopausal females does decrease the rate of bone loss when administered in doses of 1000 to 1500 mg/day.[55] Note that five tablets of calcium carbonate (Tums) are equivalent to 3 cups of milk, which is equivalent to 1 g of elemental calcium. The majority of elderly women have inadequate calcium intake, and age-matched osteoporotic women have lower calcium intake than nonosteoporotic women. Calcium supplementation is more effective in type 2 (low bone formation) osteoporosis. The adequacy of calcium intake in patients requiring total parenteral nutrition may be especially problematic.[56]

Sodium fluoride was widely used for the treatment of osteoporosis but has fallen out of favor. Fluoride in doses between 50 and 75 mg/day increases spinal bone density an impressive 8% per year, twice that seen with estrogen, calcitonin, or bisphosphonates. However, the incidence of hip fractures may increase, and fluoridic bone is more brittle.[57] There is also a high incidence of side effects (40%) from fluoride at this dosage, including gastrointestinal upset, tendinitis, fasciitis, and synovitis. Its use cannot be recommended.

Studies using vitamin D_2 (ergocalciferol) have yielded equivocal results in reducing the vertebral fracture rate in postmenopausal osteoporosis.[54] There is inadequate vitamin D intake, however, in a significant proportion of the elderly population, and it is currently suggested that elderly persons ensure an intake of 400 IU of ergocalciferol, in pill form if necessary. The data on the use of 1,25-dihydroxyvitamin D (calcitriol) to reduce fracture rates in postmenopausal osteoporosis is controversial. However, intestinal calcium absorption is increased by calcitriol, often resulting in hypercalciuria and/or hypercalcemia.[58] The serum and urinary excretion of calcium should be monitored in patients taking calcitriol every 6 to 8 weeks as the signs of hypercalcemia and hypercalciuria are subtle and not clinically evident until irreversible renal damage has occurred.

Diphosphonates, potent inhibitors of bone resorption, can be of efficacy in the treatment of osteoporosis, and some have been shown to reduce fracture rates. Etidronate has been used in several trials and has been shown to reduce vertebral fracture rates.[59, 60] The treatment regimen for etidronate is 400 mg twice daily orally for 2 weeks followed by a 10- to 12-week etidronate-free period, with a repeat of this 3-month cycle for 3 years. Oral calcium is given concomitantly. With etidronate use there is a 2 to 3% increase in bone mass, and some studies have shown a 50% reduction in vertebral fractures. The main short-term side effect is nausea. Large doses can cause osteomalacia by inhibiting mineralization, but the bisphosphonates available in Europe do not have this side effect. The newer bisphosphonate, alendronate (Fosamax), has also been demonstrated to reduce fracture rates in clinical trials and does not cause osteomalacia.[61] Alendronate is taken as 5 to 20 mg once a day orally. With alendronate treatment, bone mass increases 5 to 7%. One major side effect is esophagitis, which may require discontinuing treatment.

Calcitonin has been used and is currently FDA approved for the treatment of postmenopausal osteoporosis.[62] Calcitonin directly inhibits osteoclasts and is useful in both osteoporosis and other metabolic bone diseases. It is available as the salmon hormone both as a subcutaneous injection and as a nasal spray.[63] The human recombinant product is available solely in injectable form. Salmon calcitonin is administered as 100 U/day. Antibodies may develop, limiting its usefulness. It has inherent analgesic properties and is used in the early postfracture period for this effect.[64]

Androgens and anabolic steroids have been used for the treatment of osteoporosis. For men with hypogonadism, a reasonable starting dose of testosterone is 200 mg intramuscularly every 10 to 14 days.[2] In the past, the anabolic steroid stanozolol was used for the treatment of osteoporosis but is not currently recommended because of liver toxicity.

Estrogen supplementation of the postmenopausal or ovariectomized woman remains the first-line treatment of choice for osteoporosis.[54] Estrogen inhibits the frequency of activation of the bone-remodeling cycle. Thus, estrogen is most efficient when turnover is increased, as in the first 5 to 10 years of menopause. In this period, fractures are decreased by 50% at the hip and wrist and by 75% at vertebrae.[65] Ten years after menopause, there is less, but still some, measurable impact of estrogen supplementation on reducing the rate of fracture even up to the eighth decade of age. The earlier therapy is begun, the more likely bone mass will be preserved. When treatment is stopped, bone loss occurs at a rate comparable to that after ovariectomy.[66] The usual dose is 0.625 mg of conjugated equine estrogen or 1 mg of estradiol orally, or transdermal estradiol delivered at a rate of 50 to 100 μg/day. The latter has ease of administration and no first-pass metabolism in the liver and so produces no alterations in blood-clotting factors or binding proteins. There are side effects of estrogen supplementation that require monitoring. One such side effect is endometrial cancer, the risk of which increases fourfold to 13-fold with the use of estrogens. This effect is negated with progestin therapy without impairing the response of bone to estrogen.[67]

If the patient has a uterus, medroxyprogesterone acetate (Provera) 10 mg/day on days 16 to 25 post-menses with yearly pelvic examinations and Pap smear with endometrial biopsy if abnormal menstrual bleeding occurs are obligatory parts of treatment. In order to avoid unacceptable discomfort, bleeding is sometimes induced with progesterone only every 3 months instead of monthly or the patient is prescribed 2.5 mg of medroxyprogesterone orally per day. Continuous estrogen-progestin combinations (2 mg of estradiol plus 1 mg of norethisterone acetate) avoid vaginal bleeding in 80% of patients, but endometrial safety has been documented to only a limited extent.[68]

Another more controversial side effect of estrogens is breast cancer. The long-term (>15 years) use of estrogens increases the relative risk of developing breast cancer 1.2- to 1.3-fold. The risk of mortality from breast cancer with increased estrogen exposure is less, however, than with no exposure, although the mechanism of this effect is not understood.[69] Another risk of estrogen use is pulmonary embolism, the incidence of which is increased two- to threefold.[70] There are several positive effects of estrogen use besides a reduction in the risk of postmenopausal fractures. The incidence of cardiovascular disease is decreased 50%, although it is unclear whether this is negated by intermittent progestin administration.[71] A prospective trial of estrogen-progesterone treatment for the secondary treatment of coronary artery disease failed to demonstrate a decrease in cardiovascular morbidity and mortality.[72] Estrogen also relieves the vasomotor instability (hot flashes) and vaginal atrophy characteristic of the menopause.

Drug-Induced Osteoporosis

Medications are the most common cause of secondary osteoporosis and also osteopenia.[73]

Glucocorticoids

Glucocorticoids are the most common offending medication. Chronic treatment with pharmacologic doses of glucocorticoids frequently produces severe osteopenia that clinically resembles age-related osteoporosis.[74] Bone loss is more severe in trabecular than in cortical bone. Thus, fractures are especially common in the ribs, vertebrae, and ends of long bones. Current data indicate a rapid loss of bone in the early weeks of steroid therapy, with perhaps 12 to 15% loss of trabecular mass over the first 12 to 18 months followed by a less marked rate of loss thereafter.[75] The primary risk factors for glucocorticoid-induced osteopenia are a high total cumulative dose of glucocorticoid, an age younger than 15 or older than 50 years, and a loss of gonadal function.

Other factors that contribute to this syndrome include a long duration of glucocorticoid therapy; disorders associated with increased interleukin-1, interleukin-6, or tumor necrosis factor production (e.g., rheumatoid arthritis); and all the general osteoporosis risk factors. The disorder results from multiple effects of glucocorticoids including the direct suppression of osteoblast function, inhibition of intestinal calcium absorption leading to secondary hyperparathyroidism, and increased bone resorption. The effect of glucocorticoids on intestinal calcium absorption is thought to be a direct inhibitory effect on the intestinal mucosa, independent of vitamin D. The biochemical changes are generally not striking. Serum alkaline phosphatase and osteocalcin levels decline progressively but usually remain within the normal range. Urinary calcium excretion is increased in the first several years and then declines. The diagnosis of glucocorticoid-induced osteopenia is made on the basis of the clinical situation and the exclusion of other causes of osteopenia. Radiography shows both a horizontal and a vertical loss of trabeculations and shows callus formation at the site of stress fractures. Aseptic necrosis can be detected early with a bone scan or magnetic resonance imaging.

Treatment of glucocorticoid-induced osteopenia involves minimizing exposure to steroids as much as possible.[76] A striking illustration of the impact of reducing the detrimental impact of steroids on bone is provided by the observation that after adrenalectomy in patients with Cushing's disease, there is a rebound increase in bone mass. This also occurs after the cessation of steroid therapy from asthma or rheumatic diseases. However, the bone mass is not restored to previous levels. Maintenance of the lowest effective dose of steroid is vital, but significant osteopenia has been seen with doses as low as 7.5 to 10 mg of prednisone a day. Deflazacort may have less deleterious effects on bone mass, but its effect on the fracture rate has not been studied. Exercise and weight bearing directly stimulate bone formation but have obvious limitations. Sodium fluoride and nandrolone decanoate have shown a stimulatory effect on bone density in postmenopausal women on steroids. However, this does not necessarily equate with decreased fractures. Reduced testosterone levels occur frequently in men on steroids because of the suppression of adrenal androgens. Testosterone helps bone mass in this instance. Vitamin D_2 produces a suppression of PTH levels, an increase in bone mass, and an improved histologic appearance of bone. With vitamin D_2 treatment, however, there is a significant risk of hypercalciuria and hypercalcemia. This may be treated with hydrochlorothiazide. Calcitonin has shown significant benefit in short-term studies. Oral pamidronate produced an initial increase in appendicular and cortical bone density followed by stabilization over 18 months. Alendronate has similar effects.

Anticonvulsants

Anticonvulsants are another class of medications capable of producing osteopenia and secondary osteoporosis.[73] The risk factors for this syndrome include high doses, multiple drug regimens, a long duration of therapy, low vitamin D intake and limited sunlight exposure, a reduced level of physical activity, the use of adjuvant regimens such as acetazolamide or a ketogenic diet, and the use of hepatic enzyme-inducing drugs such as glutethimide or rifampin. The diagnosis is based on the history and the risk factors described. Decreased fasting serum calcium and phosphate levels and elevated alkaline phosphatase activity are usually present. A reduced serum 25-hydroxyvitamin D_2 level, mildly increased serum PTH level, and quantitative osteopenia complete the picture. Up to 50% of institutionalized patients on anticonvulsant drugs have osteomalacia, but decreased sunlight and dietary vitamin D play a role. The prophylaxis against anticonvulsant-induced osteopenia includes maintaining an intake of 800 U of vitamin D plus 800 mg of calcium per day, maintaining physical activity as much as possible, and avoiding adjuvant regimens and hepatic enzyme–inducing drugs when possible. If the patient already has established osteopenia, other causes of osteopenia should be sought. Vitamin D_2 (50,000 IU [or 25-hydroxyvitamin D 50 μg]) one to three times per week plus calcium (1000 mg/day) should be given for 6 to 24 months until biochemical parameters are normalized and bone mass is stabilized; physical activity should be maintained, but there is no need to discontinue the anticonvulsant drug.

◆ OSTEOMALACIA

Osteomalacia is a metabolic bone disease characterized by defective mineralization of bone matrix.[77] In adults, it causes pain, fractures, osteopenia, and osteoporosis. In children, it affects the bone and the cartilage matrix of the growth plate, altering the columnar architecture such that the growth plate increases in size. This syndrome is specifically referred to as *rickets*.

Pathophysiology

Vitamin D Deficiency. The most common cause of osteomalacia is vitamin D deficiency. Dietary vitamin D (carried by chylomicrons and its absorption aided by bile salts) and skin vitamin D (carried by α_1-globulin) are transferred to the liver for hydroxylation via the cytochrome P450 system. Next, this compound is transferred to the kidney for further hydroxylation to become calcitriol, the active form of vitamin D. Vitamin D increases the intestinal absorption of calcium and phosphate, allows PTH to mobilize calcium and phosphate from bone, promotes mineralization of bone matrix, increases renal absorption of phosphate, and decreases the secretion of PTH. Phosphate is essential for adequate mineralization. Hypophosphatemia alone can cause osteomalacia.

Vitamin D deficiency can be due to inadequate ultraviolet light exposure, inadequate dietary intake, and fat malabsorption and is most often seen in persons living in developing countries, in elderly persons, and in food faddists.[78] Osteomalacia due to inadequate sunlight exposure or inadequate vitamin D intake is reversible within weeks to months with 100 IU a day of vitamin D_2.

Fat malabsorption can also cause osteomalacia. Vitamin D is absorbed in the proximal small bowel, undergoes enterohepatic circulation, and is 25-hydroxylated in the liver. Poor absorption results from a loss of bowel surface area as seen in short bowel syndrome, celiac disease, inflammatory bowel disease, and ileojejunal bypass. Absorption of vitamin D occurs in chylomicrons, so diseases of fat emulsification such as chronic biliary obstruction can lead to vitamin D deficiency. Treatment of malabsorption-related osteomalacia requires larger doses of 25-hydroxyvitamin D_2 and calcium. Liver disease (particularly cholestatic) can also cause osteomalacia.

Poor production of 25-hydroxyvitamin D_2 can result from end-stage liver disease, but more important is disruption of bile acid secretion and inadequate fat absorption. Renal failure and nephrotic syndrome can cause osteomalacia due to absent 1,25-dihydroxyvitamin D production.

Rarely, inborn errors of vitamin D_2 metabolism result in rickets. Vitamin D–dependent rickets (VDDR) is characterized by all the classic features of vitamin D deficiency without a therapeutic response to accepted vitamin D replacement therapy.[79] Two types exist, VDDR-1 and VDDR-2. Both are autosomal recessive, with type VDDR-2 affecting children more severely than adults. The biochemical findings in these disorders are noted in Table 9–3. The bone lesions of VDDR-1 heal with 1 µg of 1,25-dihydroxyvitamin D. In VDDR-2 there is hypocalcemia, early rickets, normal vitamin D levels, secondary hyperparathyroidism, and alopecia. Some get benefit from high-dose 1,25-dihydroxyvitamin D therapy.

Anticonvulsant medication can also cause a mineralization defect in bone, as can mesenchymal tumors and prostate cancer from a renal phosphate leak. Hypophostatemia may itself lead to osteomalacia because of a failure of mineralization of the bone matrix and the passive egress of calcium from bone. In hypophosphatemia, vitamin D levels are normal, and secondary hyperparathyroidism is not a feature because serum calcium levels are normal.

Table 9–3. Biochemical Findings in Vitamin D–Dependent Rickets

	Calcium	25-OH-D	1,25(OH)$_2$-D	iPTH	Presumed Defect
VDDR-1	↓	N- ↑	↓ ↓	↓	Renal 25-OH-D hydroxylase
VDDR-2	↓	N- ↑	N- ↑	↓	Intracellular 1,25-(OH)$_2$-D receptor

25-OH-D, 25-hydroxyvitamin D; 1,25-(OH)$_2$-D, 1,25-dihydroxyvitamin D; N, normal; iPTH, intact parathyroid hormone; VDDR, vitamin D–dependent rickets.

Renal Tubular Dysfunction. Renal tubular defects are capable of causing osteomalacia.[80] These defects are both inherited (X-linked) and acquired. The Fanconi syndrome describes a general defect in proximal tubular transport of phosphate and other molecules. Therapy involves phosphate repletion. Vitamin D or its metabolites are added depending on the disease.

Types I, II, and IV renal tubular acidosis can cause osteomalacia by a mechanism not primarily involving hypophosphatemia. Rather, osteomalacia results from the release of calcium from bone as a buffer to the chronic metabolic acidosis.

Malabsorption Syndromes and Other Causes. Malabsorption syndromes, sometimes due to phosphate-binding antacids, are a relatively rare cause of osteomalacia. Treatment includes phosphate and calcium supplementation and stopping the antacid therapy. Chronic dialysis[81] and total parenteral nutrition[82] are rare causes of mineralization defects and may cause osteomalacia. In these disorders, aluminum, either from calcium binders or as a contaminant of parenteral solutions, may contribute to defective mineralization in bone.[83] Common causes of hypophosphatemia are usually acute and seldom lead to osteomalacia. They include respiratory alkalosis, acute insulin administration, recovery from hypothermia, and leukemic blast crisis.

Tumors. Tumors are also capable of producing osteomalacia and rickets.[84] Since 1959, there have been reports of approximately 79 patients in whom rickets or osteomalacia has been associated with various tumors. There is usually remission after resection of the tumor. Symptoms of bone and muscle pain, weakness, and fractures occur an average of 4 years before diagnosis. The age at diagnosis is generally the fourth decade, with 10% younger than 18 years at presentation. Hypophosphatemia and an abnormally low renal tubular maximum for the reabsorption of phosphorus characterize this disorder. Most tumors are of mesenchymal origin, but breast cancer, prostate cancer, multiple myeloma, and chronic lymphocytic leukemia have been described. Regardless of the cell type responsible for the syndrome, the tumors at fault are often small, are difficult to locate, and present in obscure areas. Many have been located in a relatively inaccessible area within bone such as within the femur or tibia, sinuses, or nasopharynx. The pathogenesis is likely the tumor's production of a humoral factor that affects the proximal renal tubule, particularly phosphate reabsorption. Abnormal vitamin D metabolism may also contribute. However, osteomalacia secondary to hematologic malignancy has different features. In these patients, the nephropathy associated with light-chain proteinuria results in the decreased renal tubular reabsorption of phosphate characteristic of the disease.

Primary treatment is complete resection of the tumor. However, this is not always possible. Administration of 1,25-dihydroxyvitamin D alone or in combination with phosphorus supplementation has been effective with evidence of bone healing by bone biopsy when pharmacologic doses are employed. The doses used increase the possibility of nephrolithiasis, nephrocalcinosis, and hypercalcemia. Thus, careful assessment of parathyroid function, serum and urinary calcium levels, and renal function is essential.

Diagnosis

The incidence of osteomalacia is difficult to assess because of the nonspecific symptoms and laboratory values. Some report an incidence of 3.7 to 25% in geriatric inpatients.[85] It may coexist with osteoporosis and not be recognized. The clinical features of osteomalacia in children consist of the "rachitic rosary"—a prominence of the costochondral junction; saber shins due to discordant growth at the growth plate; bowing deformity of the long bones; kyphosis and lordosis plus limb bowing causing a waddling gait; an increased number of fractures; generalized muscle weakness and atonia in the skull; parietal flattening and frontal bossing; and in the teeth, delayed eruption of permanent teeth and enamel defects. The clinical features of osteomalacia in adults are more nonspecific and include diffuse skeletal pain and bony tenderness, especially with weight bearing; femoral and vertebral fractures; and proximal muscle weakness with normal muscle electrophysiology.

The radiographic features of rickets include osteopenia and growth retardation, decreased density and blurring of the trabecular pattern in the epiphysis, bowing of the arms and legs, and craniotabes of the skull. The radiologic features of osteomalacia include thinning of the cortex and rarefaction of the shaft of long bones, and radiolucent bands perpendicular to bone surface called *Looser's lines* or *pseudofractures*. Pseudofractures are pathognomonic for osteomalacia.[86]

◆ PAGET'S DISEASE

Paget's disease of bone is a not-uncommon cause of bone pain and fractures. Paget's disease of bone is a localized disorder of bone remodeling.[87] The process is initiated by increases in osteoclast-mediated bone resorption and has a strong genetic predilection.[88] There is a subsequent increase in new bone formation that is a disordered mosaic. This produces bone that is expanded in size, less compact, more vascular, and more susceptible to fracture or deformity than normal bone. Most patients are asymptomatic and are diagnosed coincidentally because of elevated serum alkaline phosphatase activity. From 15 to 30% of patients with Paget's disease have a family history of this disorder. The data suggest that the cumulative incidence to the age of 90 years is about 2% but increases to over 9% if one or more first-degree relatives are affected.[89] The highest incidence of this disease is in England, but it is also common in Europe, North America, and Australia, with white predominance. The data also support a viral cause of Paget's disease because inclusions that resemble viral nucleocapsids have been described in pagetic sites.

The putative virus is a paramyxovirus, possibly measles, canine distemper, or respiratory syncytial virus. A current "unifying" hypothesis of the evolution of Paget's disease is that a common viral infection occurring perhaps early in life in a genetically susceptible host predisposes to an osteoclast lesion that is manifested in adulthood (fifth or sixth decade) as Paget's disease. A characteristic of the pathology of Paget's disease is that osteoclasts are more numerous and contain up to 100 nuclei per cell. In the early stages, increased resorption dominates, causing an advancing lytic wedge or "blade-of-grass" lesion in a long bone or osteoporosis circumscripta in the skull. After this, there is tightly coupled new bone formation that is abnormal, with a high-turn-over mosaic pattern of woven bone. The bone marrow becomes infiltrated with fibrous tissue and increased blood vessels. In the final stages of Paget's disease, the hypercellularity may diminish, leaving a sclerotic, pagetic mosaic. This is "burned-out" Paget's disease. Typically, all stages can be seen at the same time at different sites.

The biochemical hallmark of Paget's disease is an increase in the urinary excretion of collagen N-telopeptides, reflecting bone resorption.[90] Elevated levels of alkaline phosphatase reflect increased osteoblast activity. In untreated patients, these rise in proportion, demonstrating preserved coupling of resorption and formation. The degree of elevation reflects the extent or severity. The highest elevations (10 times normal) imply that the skull is involved. These laboratory parameters allow the disorder to be monitored over time and the effects of treatment to be observed. Generally, approved therapies reduce these measures by about 50% in up to two thirds of patients. Typically, the serum calcium level is normal; however, it can be raised if a patient with extensive Paget's disease is immobilized, with a resultant loss of weight-bearing stimulus to new bone formation and dehydration or, coincidentally, primary hyperparathyroidism.

The epidemiologic features of Paget's disease include a slight male preponderance. Most cases occur in persons older than 40 years, with an average of 58 years.[89] The most common sites of bony involvement are the pelvis, femur, spine, skull, and tibia. Most patients are asymptomatic, and an elevated alkaline phosphatase level or abnormal radiograph taken for another reason diagnoses the disease. Clinical observation suggests that sites affected by Paget's disease are the only ones that will progress over time. Other clinical features of this disease are bone pain or warmth; a bowing appearance of the femur or tibia with secondary arthritis and gait disorder; back pain; kyphosis; and spinal cord compression with motor and sensory changes. The latter has been known to occur in Paget's disease as a result of a vascular steal syndrome.[91] Skull involvement leads to headache and cranial nerve palsies, especially hearing (cranial nerve VIII). Brain stem compression, obstructive hydrocephalus, and airway narrowing occur rarely. Fractures occur, especially in the femoral shaft in the subtrochanteric area. There may be substantial blood loss, and there is an increased rate of nonunion. The development of frank carcinoma (sarcomas) in bone occurs with Paget's disease but is rare (<1%).[92] The most common sites are the pelvis, femur, and humerus. These manifest as new pain at a pagetic site. Changes in bone pain should be examined by radiography because this carcinoma is curable surgically if detected early. Benign giant cell tumors also result from Paget's disease and are usually sensitive to glucocorticoids.[93] High-output cardiac failure occurs.

Paget's disease usually presents with characteristic radiographic and clinical features, eliminating problems with differential diagnosis. However, an older patient may present with severe bone pain, elevations of alkaline phosphatase and urinary collagen N-telopeptide levels, a positive bone scan, and equivocal radiologic findings. In such cases, the possibility of metastatic disease to bone or some other form of metabolic bone disease must be considered. Old radiographs and laboratory studies are very helpful. A similar problem occurs when someone with established Paget's disease develops multiple painful new sites. Bone biopsy for tissue diagnosis may be indicated.[94]

There are several agents that reduce the bone pain and biochemical activity of Paget's disease. It has not been proved that a reduction in elevated pagetic indices will prevent future complications. However, the consensus is that moderately active disease (alkaline phosphatase activity three to four times the upper limit of normal) in weight-bearing areas is an indication for treatment. This is especially true with young patients and when elective surgery is planned on the bone to reduce the amount of blood loss. The agents available for the treatment of Paget's disease include calcitonin and the bisphosphonates etidronate, pamidronate, and alendronate. Plicamycin (mithramycin) and gallium have also been used.

◆ HYPERPARATHYROIDISM

Parathyroid disease also causes metabolic bone disease.

Primary Hyperparathyroidism

Primary hyperparathyroidism is a primary disorder of the parathyroid glands. Primary hyperparathyroidism most commonly presents as inappropriately high plasma PTH levels in the presence of raised plasma calcium levels on routine biochemical screening.[95] If the patient is symptomatic, then bone disease, fractures, renal stones, constipation, duodenal ulcer, pancreatitis, nonspecific abdominal pain, and depression are the most common clinical features. Rarely, primary hyperparathyroidism is seen in multiple endocrine neoplasia.[96] One multiple endocrine neoplasia syndrome (type I) is hyperparathyroidism with a pancreatic islet cell tumor and pituitary adenoma. Another multiple endocrine neoplasia syndrome (type II) is hyperparathyroidism with a medullary carcinoma of the thyroid and pheochromocytoma. The most common cause of primary hyperparathyroidism is a single benign adenoma (90%); occasionally it is caused by multiple adenomas; and rarely, it is caused by hyperplasia or carcinoma.[95]

The diagnosis of primary hyperparathyroidism depends on the finding of an elevated serum calcium level and a decreased phosphate level. There is phosphaturia, and a normal serum phosphate level may signal impending renal failure. Mild hypercalciuria is evident, as is a mildly increased alkaline phosphatase level, hyperchloremic metabolic acidosis with alkaline urine, and an increased plasma PTH level. A normal PTH level does not exclude the diagnosis of primary hyperparathyroidism but may be abnormal for the degree of hypercalcemia, whereas undetectable levels of PTH do exclude this diagnosis. Measurement of intact PTH is the current assay of choice, although historically, other assays have been used. An elevated nephrogenous cyclic AMP level that is not suppressible with an oral calcium tolerance test has also been used. Radiographs show osteitis fibrosa cystica (brown tumors) and subperiosteal resorption (especially on hand radiographs). Skull radiography shows a pepper-pot skull.

The treatment of choice for primary hyperparathyroidism is surgical removal of the involved parathyroids. Neck exploration with removal of adenoma, if present, or removal of $3\frac{1}{2}$ glands if hyperplasia is documented by frozen section in the operating room, is the approach of choice. The remaining tissue may be buried in a more accessible site. Venous sampling or ultrasonography may be used to locate the source of PTH if initial surgery is unsuccessful.

There is a potential for postoperative hypocalcemia.

Secondary Hyperparathyroidism

Secondary hyperparathyroidism results from low serum calcium levels that stimulate an appropriate rise in PTH levels. The causes of secondary hyperparathyroidism include chronic renal failure and dietary deficiency of vitamin D.[97]

Uremic Osteodystrophy

In renal osteodystrophy, there are numerous contributing causes. As nephrons drop off, PTH levels rise and calcitriol levels drop. Mineralization remains intact until the glomerular filtration rate is less than 40%. Further falls in the glomerular filtration rate cause phosphate retention, which lowers the serum calcium levels and further stimulates PTH release. Anorexia, heparin usage, and aluminum usage also contribute.

The skeletal lesions seen with renal failure may be of several types.[97] High-turnover hyperparathyroid bone disease occurs in 5 to 30% of patients on dialysis. Numerous remodeling sites, irregular trabeculae, and overproduction of collagen leading to woven osteoid and marrow fibrosis (osteitis fibrosa) characterize this syndrome. Fragile bone susceptible to fracture results. Low-turnover uremic osteodystrophy occurs in 5 to 30% of patients on dialysis. Aluminum toxicity is the main cause of low-turnover uremic osteodystrophy, but parathyroidectomy, anticonvulsant therapy, and diabetes mellitus may contribute. The picture is one of osteomalacia. This type is becoming less common with the reduced use of aluminum phosphate binders.

Depending on its definition, mixed uremic osteodystrophy occurs in 5 to 80% of patients on dialysis. This disorder is usually seen in patients with established osteitis fibrosa who develop aluminum-related bone disease or in patients with aluminum accumulation who develop increased bone remodeling with deferoxamine treatment. β2-Microglobulin disease is a disorder in which this protein is retained in renal failure and deposits in bone and soft tissue. An algorithm for differentiating the diagnosis of these disorders is as follows:

PTH	>200–400 pg/ml	Hyperparathyroid bone disease, severe if >400
	<200 pg/ml	Usually low-turnover bone disease
Aluminum	>200 μg/L	Aluminum bone toxicity
	<80 μg/L	No aluminum bone disease

Radiographic changes appear late. Changes are nonspecific and can be a confusing combination of cortical erosions and a rugger-jersey appearance of the spine typically seen in osteitis fibrosa, and pseudofractures and typical rib and/or hip fractures and vertebral compression fractures seen in osteomalacia. A bone biopsy with double tetracycline labeling is helpful if noninvasive testing is equivocal.[98]

There is no single means of treatment for uremic osteodystrophy. Initiating prophylactic treatment early in renal failure, however, may prevent secondary hyperparathyroidism. A suggested approach is as follows:

1. Control of calcium via manipulation of the dialysate calcium concentration. No calcium supplements are given until the phosphate level is less than 6.5 mg/dl.
2. Control of phosphate. Dietary restriction and phosphate binders are indicated, but note the potential for aluminum toxicity. Calcium salts (acetate) are less potent and decrease the risk of hypercalcemia and extraosseous calcification, especially with vitamin D therapy.
3. Removal of aluminum. Deferoxamine, a chelator, works but can increase the infectious risk. There is a need to follow serum aluminum levels until they drop consistently and to confirm improvement of bone formation with a bone biopsy. Muscle and bone pain relief are signs of improvement.
4. Supplementation with 1,25-dihydroxyvitamin D. This has been shown to prevent renal bone disease and decrease bone pain in adults and increase growth velocity in children. It is not effective in the osteomalacia type of renal bone disease due to aluminum toxicity and can cause

hypercalcemia and hypercalciuria. Pulse therapy and intravenous administration have fewer side effects.

5. Parathyroidectomy. This is a last-resort treatment. Indications are sustained hypercalcemia, intractable pruritus, severe skeletal pain, and refractory calciphylaxis unresponsive to other measures. There is a higher risk of aluminum toxicity after the surgery.

Uremic hyperparathyroidism occasionally is associated with an autonomously functioning parathyroid adenoma in the setting of long-standing secondary hyperparathyroidism. In this disorder, there is continued secretion of large amounts of PTH after prolonged secondary hyperparathyroidism despite adequate dialysis. The original cause of the secondary hyperparathyroidism may have been removed, but the parathyroids act autonomously and cause hypercalcemia. Treatment is as for primary hyperparathyroidism.[99]

REFERENCES

1. Riggs BL: Overview of osteoporosis. West J Med 154:63–77, 1991.
2. Orwall ES, Klein RF: Osteoporosis in men. Endocr Rev 16:87–116, 1995.
3. Jackson JA: Osteoporosis in men In Favus MJ (ed): Primer on Metabolic Bone Diseases and Disorders of Mineral Metabolism, 13th ed. Philadelphia, Lippincott-Raven, 1996, pp 283–286.
4. Cooper C, Campion G, Melton J III: Hip fractures in the elderly: A world-wide perspective. Osteoporos Int 2:285–289, 1992.
5. Keene GS, Parker MJ, Pryor GA: Morbidity and mortality after hip fractures. BMJ 307:1248–1250, 1989.
6. Ray WA, Griffin MR, Baugh DK: Mortality following hip fracture before and after implementation of the prospective payment system. Arch Intern Med 150:2109–2114, 1990.
7. Palmer RM: The impact of the prospective payment system on the treatment of hip fractures in the elderly. Arch Intern Med 149:2237–2241, 1989.
8. Chrischilles EA, Butler CD, Davis CS, Wallace RB: A model of lifetime osteoporosis impact. Arch Intern Med 151:2026–2032, 1991.
9. Melton LJ III: Epidemiology of vertebral fractures in women. Am J Epidemiol 129:1000–1011, 1989.
10. Barrett-Connor E: The economics and human costs of osteoporotic fracture. Am J Med 98:3–8, 1995.
11. Wasnich RD: Epidemiology of osteoporosis In Favus MJ (ed): Primer on Metabolic Bone Diseases and Disorders of Mineral Metabolism, 13th ed. Philadelphia, Lippincott-Raven, 1996, pp 249–251.
12. Hui SL, Slemeda CW, Johnson CC Jr: Baseline

13. measurement of bone mass predicts fracture in white women. Ann Intern Med 111:355–361, 1989.
13. Riggs BL, Wahner HW, Dunn WL, et al: Differential changes in bone mineral density of the appendicular and axial skeleton with aging: Relationship to spinal osteoporosis. J Clin Invest 67:328–335, 1981.
14. Hannon MT, Felton DT, Anderson JL: Bone mineral density in elderly men and women: Results from the Framingham Osteoporosis Study. J Bone Miner Res 7:547–552, 1992.
15. Parfitt AM: Bone remodeling: Relationship to the amount and structure of bone, and the pathogenesis and prevention of fractures In Riggs BL, Melton LJ III (eds): Osteoporosis: Etiology, Diagnosis, and Management. New York, Raven Press, 1988, pp 45–93.
16. Marcus R: Understanding osteoporosis. West J Med 155:53–60, 1991.
17. Sallagher JC, Riggs BL, DeLuca HF: Effect of estrogen on calcium absorption and serum vitamin D metabolites in postmenopausal osteoporosis. J Clin Endocrinol Metab 51:1359–1364, 1980.
18. Cheema C, Grant BF, Marcus R: Effects of estrogen on "free" and total 1,25-dihydroxyvitamin D and the parathyroid–vitamin D axis in postmenopausal women. J Clin Invest 83:537–542, 1989.
19. Bullamore JR, Gallagher JC, Wilkinson R, et al: Effect of age on calcium absorption. Lancet 2:353–537, 1970.
20. Heaney RP, Gallagher JC, Johnson CC, et al: Calcium nutrition and bone health in the elderly. Am J Clin Nutr 36:986–1013, 1982.
21. Heaney RP: Nutrition and risk for osteoporosis In Marcus R, Feldman D, Kelsey J (eds): Osteoporosis. San Diego, Academic Press, 1996, pp 483–505.
22. Chan GM, Hess M, Hollis J, Brooks LS: Bone mineral status in childhood accidental fractures. Am J Dis Child 138:569–570, 1984.
23. Holick MF, Matsouka LY, Wortman J: Age, vitamin D, and solar ultraviolet radiation. Lancet 4:1104–1105, 1989.
24. Chen Z, Lohman TG, Stini WA, et al: Fat or lean mass: Which one is the major determinant of bone mineral mass in healthy postmenopausal women? J Bone Miner Res 12:144–151, 1997.
25. Seeman E, Hopper JL, Bach LA, et al: Reduced bone mass in daughters of women with osteoporosis. N Engl J Med 320:554–558, 1989.
26. Cummings SR, Nevitt MC, Browner WS, et al: Risk factors for hip fracture in white women. Study of Osteoporotic Fractures Research Group. N Engl J Med 332:767–773, 1995.
27. Cummings SR, Kelsey JL, Nevitt MC, O'Dowd KJ: Epidemiology of osteoporosis and osteoporotic fractures. Epidemiol Rev 7:178–208, 1985.
28. Lukert BP, Stanbury SW, Mawer EB: Vitamin D and the intestinal transport of calcium: Effects of prednisolone. Endocrinology 93:718–727, 1973.
29. Suzuki Y, Ichikawa Y, Saito E, Homma M: Importance of increased urinary calcium excretion in the development of secondary hyperparathyroidism of patients under glucocorticoid therapy. Metabolism 32:151–156, 1983.
30. Dempster DW: Bone histomorphometry in glucocorticoid-induced osteoporosis. J Bone Miner Res 4:137–141, 1989.
31. Rosen HN, Moses AC, Grundberg C, et al: Therapy with parenteral pamidronate prevents thyroid hor-

mone–induced bone turnover in humans. J Clin Endocrinol Metab 77:664–669, 1993.

32. Greenspan GL, Oppenheim DS, Klibanski A: Importance of gonadal steroids to bone mass in men with hyperprolactinemic hypogonadism. Ann Intern Med 110:526–531, 1989.

33. Levin ME, Bosseau VC, Avioli LV: Effects of diabetes mellitus on bone mass in juvenile and adult-onset diabetes. N Engl J Med 294:241–245, 1976.

34. Silverberg SL, Shane E, de la Cruz L, et al: Skeletal disease in primary hyperparathyroidism. J Bone Miner Res 4:283–291, 1989.

35. Schlechte J, Simerman B, Martin R: Bone density in amenorrheic women with and without hyperprolactinemia. J Clin Endocrinol Metab 56:1120–1123, 1983.

36. Drinkwater BL, Wilson K, Chesnut C III, et al: Bone mineral content of amenorrheic and eumenorrheic athletes. N Engl J Med 311:277–281, 1984.

37. Whyte MP: Skeletal neoplasms. In Favus MJ (ed): Primer on Metabolic Bone Diseases and Disorders of Mineral Metabolism, 13th ed. Philadelphia, Lippincott-Raven, 1996, pp 391–399.

38. Diamon T, Stiel D, Lunzer M, et al: Ethanol reduces bone formation and may cause osteoporosis. Am J Med 86:282–288, 1989.

39. Avioli LV: Heparin-induced osteopenia: An appraisal. Adv Exp Biol Med 52:375–387, 1975.

40. Hahn TJ: Corticosteroid-induced osteopenia. Arch Intern Med 138:882–885, 1978.

41. Slemenda CW, Hui SL, Longscope C, Johnston CC Jr: Cigarette smoking, obesity, and bone mass. J Bone Miner Res 4:737–741, 1989.

42. Leblanc AD, Schneider VS, Evans HJ, et al: Bone mineral loss and recovery after 17 weeks of bed rest. J Bone Miner Res 5:843–850, 1990.

43. Lipkin EW: Metabolic bone diseases in gut diseases. Gastroenterol Clin North Am 27:513–523, 1998.

44. Pinnell SR, Murad S: Disorders of collagen. In Stanbury JB, Wyngaarden JB, Fredrickson DS, et al (eds): The Metabolic Basis of Inherited Disease, 5th ed. New York, McGraw-Hill, 1983, pp 1425–1449.

45. Shamash R, Laufer D, Tulchinsky V: Scurvy—A disease not only of historical interest. Br J Oral Maxillofac Surg 26:258–260, 1988.

46. Lipkin EW, Ott SM, Klein GL: Heterogeneity of bone histology in parenteral nutrition patients. Am J Clin Nutr 11:586–589, 1987.

47. Einhorn TA: Orthopedic complications of osteoporosis In Favus MJ (ed): Primer on Metabolic Bone Diseases and Disorders of Mineral Metabolism, 13th ed. Philadelphia, Lippincott-Raven, 1996, pp 293–299.

48. Steiner E, Jergas M, Genant HK: Radiology of osteoporosis In Marcus R, Feldman D, Kelsey J (eds): Osteoporosis. San Diego, Academic Press, 1996, pp 1019–1054.

49. Baumann AA, Scheffer PG, Ooms ME, et al: Two bone alkaline phosphatase assays compared with osteocalcin as a marker of bone formation in healthy elderly women. Clin Chem 41:196–199, 1995.

50. Diaz-Diego EM, Diaz-Martin MA, de la Piedra C, Rapado A: Lack of correlation between levels of osteocalcin and bone alkaline phosphatase in healthy control and post-menopausal osteoporotic women. Horm Metab Res 27:151–154, 1995.

51. Hanson DA, Weiss M-AE, Bollen A-M, et al: A specific radioimmunoassay for monitoring human bone resorption. Quantitation of type I collagen cross-linked N-telopeptide in urine. J Bone Miner Res 7:1251–1258, 1992.

52. Eriksen EF, Brixen K, Charles P: New markers of bone metabolism: Clinical use in metabolic bone disease. Eur J Endocrinol 132:251–263, 1995.

53. Recker RR (ed): Bone Histomorphometry: Techniques, and Interpretation. Boca Raton, Fla, Academic Press, 1983.

54. Eastell R: Treatment of postmenopausal osteoporosis. N Engl J Med 338:736–746, 1998.

55. Ott SM: Calcium and vitamin D in the pathogenesis and treatment of osteoporosis In Marcus R (ed): Osteoporosis. Oxford, Scientific, 1994, pp 227–287.

56. Lipkin EW, Ott SM, Chesnut C III, Chait A: Mineral loss in the long-term parenteral nutrition patient. Am J Clin Nutr 47:515–523, 1988.

57. Riggs BL, Hodgson SF, O'Fallon WM, et al: Effect of fluoride treatment on the fracture rate in postmenopausal women with osteoporosis. N Engl J Med 322:802–809, 1990.

58. Ott SM, Chesnut CH III: Calcitriol treatment is not effective in postmenopausal osteoporosis. Ann Intern Med 110:267–274, 1989.

59. Storm T, Thamsborg G, Steiniche T, et al: Effect of intermittent cyclic etidronate therapy on bone mass and fracture rate in women with postmenopausal osteoporosis. N Engl J Med 322:1265–1271, 1990.

60. Watts NB, Harris ST, Genant HK, et al: Intermittent cyclic etidronate treatment of postmenopausal osteoporosis. N Engl J Med 323:73–79, 1990.

61. Liberman VA, Weiss SR, Brull J, et al: Effect of oral alendronate on bone mineral density and the incidence of fractures in postmenopausal osteoporosis. The phase II Osteoporosis Treatment Study Group. N Engl J Med 333:1437–1443, 1995.

62. Rico H, Revilla M, Hernandez ER, et al: Total and regional bone mineral content and fracture rate in postmenopausal osteoporosis treated with salmon calcitonin: A prospective study. Calcif Tissue Int 56:181–185, 1995.

63. Overgaard K, Hansen MA, Jensen SB, Chirstiansen C: Effect of salcatonin given intranasally on bone mass and fracture rates in established osteoporosis: A dose response study. BMJ 305:556–561, 1992.

64. Gennari C, Agnuspei D, Camporeale A: Use of calcitonin in the treatment of bone pain associated with osteoporosis. Calcif Tissue Int 49(Suppl 2):s9–s13, 1991.

65. Maxim P, Ettinger B, Spitalny GM: Fracture prevention by long-term estrogen treatment. Osteoporos Int 5:23–29, 1995.

66. Cauley JA, Seeley DG, Ensrud K, et al: Estrogen replacement therapy and fractures in older women: Study of Osteoporotic Fractures Research Group. Ann Intern Med 122:12–16, 1995.

67. Beresford SAA, Weiss NS, Voigt LF, McKnight B: Risk of endometrial cancer in relation to the use of oestrogen combined with cyclic progestogen therapy in postmenopausal women. Lancet 349:458–461, 1997.

68. Piegsa K, Calder A, Davis JA, et al: Endometrial status in post-menopausal women on long-term continuous combined hormone replacement therapy (Kliofem). A comparative study of endometrial biopsy, outpatient hysteroscopy and transvaginal ultrasound. Eur J Obstet Gynecol Reprod Biol 72:175–180, 1997.

69. Colditz GA, Hankinson SE, Hunter DJ, et al: The use of estrogens and progestins and the risk of breast cancer in postmenopausal women. N Engl J Med 332:1589–1593, 1995.

70. Grodstein F, Stamfer MJ, Goldhaber SZ, et al: Prospective study of exogenous hormones and risk of pulmonary embolism in women. Lancet 348:983–987, 1996.

71. Grodstein F, Stamfer MJ, Mason JE, et al: Postmenopausal estrogen and progesterone use and the risk of cardiovascular disease. N Engl J Med 335:453–461, 1996.

72. Hulley S, Grady D, Bush T, et al: Randomized trial of estrogen plus progestin for secondary prevention of coronary heart disease in postmenopausal women. Heart and Estrogen/Progestin Replacement Study (HERS) Research Group. N Engl J Med 280:605–613, 1998.

73. Lukert BP: Glucocorticoid and drug-induced osteoporosis. In Favus MJ (ed): Primer on Metabolic Bone Diseases and Disorders of Mineral Metabolism, 13th ed. Philadelphia, Lippincott-Raven, 1996, pp 278–282.

74. Arger RA, Rosen CJ: Glucocorticoids and osteoporosis. Endocrinol Metab Clin North Am 23:641–654, 1994.

75. Olbright T, Benker G: Glucocorticoid-induced osteoporosis: Pathogenesis, prevention, and treatment with special regard to the rheumatic diseases. J Intern Med 234:737–744, 1993.

76. American College of Rheumatology Task Force on Osteoporosis Guidelines: Recommendations for the prevention and treatment of glucocorticoid-induced osteoporosis. Arthritis Rheum 39:1791–1801, 1996.

77. Parfitt AM: Otseomalacia and related disorders. In Avioli LV, Krane SM (eds): Metabolic Bone Disease and Clinically Related Disorders, 2nd ed. Philadelphia, WB Saunders, 1990, pp 329–396.

78. Holick MF: Vitamin D: Photobiology, metabolism, and clinical applications. In DeGroot L, Besser H, Burger HG, et al (eds): Endocrinology, 3rd ed. Philadelphia, WB Saunders, 1995, pp 990–1013.

79. Liberman UA, Marx SJ: Vitamin D–dependent rickets. In Favus MJ (ed): Primer on Metabolic Bone Diseases and Disorders of Mineral Metabolism, 13th ed. Philadelphia, Lippincott-Raven, 1996, pp 311–319.

80. Chesney RW, Jones DP: Renal tubular disorders. In Gonick HC (ed): Current Nephrology, Vol 19. Chicago, Mosby–Year Book, 1995.

81. Goodman WG–Coburn JW, Slatopolsky E, Salusky IB: Renal osteodystrophy in adults and children. In Favus MJ (ed): Primer on Metabolic Bone Diseases and Disorders of Mineral Metabolism, 13th ed. Philadelphia, Lippincott-Raven, 1996, pp 341–360.

82. Lipkin EW: Metabolic bone disease in the long-term parenteral nutrition patient. Clin Nutr 14(Suppl 1):65–69, 1995.

83. Ott SM, Maloney NA, Klein GA, et al: Aluminum is associated with low bone formation in patients receiving chronic parenteral nutrition. Ann Intern Med 98:910–914, 1983.

84. Drezner MK: Tumor-associated rickets and osteomalacia. In Favus MJ (ed): Primer on Metabolic Bone Diseases and Disorders of Mineral Metabolism, 13th ed. Philadelphia, Lippincott-Raven, 1996, pp 319–325.

85. Thomas MK, Lloyd Jones DM, Thadhani RI, et al: Hypovitaminosis in medical inpatients. N Engl J Med 338:777–783, 1998.

86. Pitt MJ: Rachitic and osteomalacic syndromes. Radiol Clin North Am 19:581–599, 1981.

87. Rebel A, Basle M, Pouplard A, et al: Bone tissue in Paget's disease of bone. Ultrastructure and immunology. Arthritis Rheum 23:1004–1014, 1980.

88. Siris ES, Ottman R, Flaster E, Kelsey JL: Familial aggregation of Paget's disease of bone. J Bone Miner Res 6:495–500, 1991.

89. Siris ES: Paget's disease of bone. In Favus MJ (ed): Primer on Metabolic Bone Diseases and Disorders of Mineral Metabolism, 13th ed. Philadelphia, Lippincott-Raven, 1996, pp 409–419.

90. Vebelhart D, Ginetys E, Chapoy MC, Delmas PD: Urinary excretion of Pyridium crosslinks. A new marker of bone resorption in metabolic bone disease. Arthritis Rheum 8:87–96, 1990.

91. Herzberg L, Bayliss E: Spinal cord syndrome due to non-compressive Paget's disease of bone: A spinal artery steal phenomenon reversible with calcitonin. Lancet 2:13–15, 1980.

92. Wick MR, Siegel GP, Unni KK, et al: Sarcomas of bone complicating osteitis deformans (Paget's disease). Am J Surg 5:47–59, 1981.

93. Upchurch KS, Simon LS, Schiller AL, et al: Giant cell reparative granuloma of Paget's disease of bone: A unique clinical entity. Ann Intern Med 98:35–40, 1983.

94. Meunier PJ, Coindre JM, Edouard CM, Arlot ME: Bone histomorphometry in Paget's disease: Quantitative and dynamic analysis of pagetic and non-pagetic bone tissue. Arthritis Rheum 23:1095–1103, 1980.

95. Strewler GJ, Rosenblatt M: Mineral metabolism. In Felig P, Baxter JD, Frohman LA (eds): Endocrinology and Metabolism, 13th ed. New York, McGraw-Hill, 1995, pp 1452–1467.

96. Heath H III, Hobbs MR: Familial hyperparathyroid syndromes in bone. In Favus MJ (ed): Primer on Metabolic Bone Diseases and Disorders of Mineral Metabolism, 13th ed. Philadelphia, Lippincott-Raven, 1996, pp 187–189.

97. Coburn JW, Slatopolsky E: Vitamin D, parathyroid hormone, and the renal osteodystrophies. In Brenner B, Rector F (eds): The Kidney, 4th ed. Philadelphia, WB Saunders, 1990, pp 2036–2120.

98. Sherrard DJ: Renal osteodystrophy. Semin Nephrol 6:56–67, 1986.

99. Llach F: Parathyroidectomy in chronic renal failure: Indications, surgical approach, and calcitriol. Kidney Int 38(Suppl 29):s62–s68, 1990.

10

◆ Perioperative Nutritional Support

Manoj K. Maloo
R. Armour Forse

> Thy food shall be thy remedy   (nay it be thy poison)
> *Hippocrates c. 400* B.C.   *MM/AF 2000* A.D.

Cuthbertsons' work[1] outlining the catabolic response and Whipple's work[2] demonstrating protein breakdown and negative nitrogen balance in patients with injury and infection were the early landmarks in the field of surgical nutrition. Over 60 years ago, Studley[3] appreciated that malnutrition is a key factor negatively influencing a desired surgical outcome. Associating this malnutrition with increased stress on the body and increased infectious complications led Rhoads and Alexander to the idea of postoperative nutritional therapy.[4, 5] Although there was little enthusiasm for the introduction of total parenteral nutrition (TPN) in Sweden in the early 1960s, Aubaniac's description of subclavian vein catheterization[6] provided an efficient means of delivery of the hypertonic solutions. In 1968, Wilmore and Dudrick showed that parenteral nutrition could be used as a sole source of nutrition.[7]

◆ MALNUTRITION IN THE SURGICAL PATIENT

Over 25 years ago, Bistrian and colleagues documented that malnutrition was a problem in hospitalized patients.[8, 9] Malnutrition continues to be a widespread problem in the hospitalized patient population, with an approximate prevalence of 50%. The incidence tends to increase over the course of the hospitalization.[10, 11] Despite advances in patient care in all fields of medicine, evaluations continue to reflect a widespread prevalence of malnutrition, with a 40% incidence of malnutrition in British hospitals, and 54% in Norwegian institutions.[12]

Surveys of surgical patients have suggested that malnutrition may be quite rampant, existing in up to 70% of surgical candidates.[8, 13–15] Forty to 70% of patients undergoing surgery for benign and malig-

nant gastrointestinal tract disease are malnourished preoperatively and of these, over 60% with esophageal, gastric, and pancreatic malignancies suffer from malnutrition.[13–16] Patients with gastrointestinal fistulas also have a high incidence of malnutrition, varying with the fistula location. The incidence is up to 53% in patients with gastric or duodenal fistulas, 74% in those with jejunal or ileal fistulas, and 20% in those with fistulas involving the large intestine.[17] A prospective study found that 50% of patients undergoing reduction pneumoplasty for emphysema had a deficient nutritional status as judged by body mass index. This was associated with increased postoperative morbidity as measured by an increased length of time on a ventilator, a greater number of postoperative infections, and a longer length of stay in the intensive care unit and hospital.[18]

One problem is that malnutrition and its potential debilitating and life-threatening consequences can be generally difficult to appreciate when the observer is untrained.[19, 20] A poor nutritional state is associated with a reduction in muscle function, respiratory function, and immune function; impaired wound healing; and an impaired quality of life[12] as well as numerous complications as outlined in Table 10–1. It is obvious that these medical problems will add to both the morbidity and the mortality of any surgical procedure.

Current investigations into the biology of malnutrition are further demonstrating cellular dysfunction particularly in the peritoneal macrophage, where there is a reduction in ubiquitous nuclear factor κ-B (NF-κB) activation and increased apoptosis, a biologic response that would increase the risk of postoperative infection.[21–23] These observations only increase the need for the awareness that nutrition is important in the overall management of the surgical patient.

Table 10–1. Complications in the Malnourished Surgical Patient

Impaired organ function
  Skeletal muscle: Loss of bulk and strength secondary to proteolysis[24]
  Gastrointestinal tract: Delay in resumption of postoperative function[24]
  Cardiac muscle: Decreased mass, force of contractility, and rate[19, 25, 26]
  Respiratory: Decreased respiratory muscle function[18]
    Impaired hypoxic ventilatory response[19, 27]
  Kidney: Decreased function secondary to hypovolemia
  Liver: Global reduction in synthetic and metabolic functions
  Skin: Atrophy, decubitus ulcer, and susceptibility to infections[19]
  Bone: Reduced callus formation[28]
  Generalized dysfunction secondary to tissue edema of hypoalbuminemic state
Impaired host defense and wound healing[19]
Longer recovery period[19]
Anemia
Hypothermia
Decreased basal metabolic rate[19]
Impaired coordination[28]
Accelerated age-dependent bone loss inducing osteoporosis[29]
Psychologic: apathy and loss of motivation[24]

Types of Malnutrition in the Surgical Patient

Surgical patients are susceptible to all forms of malnutrition, resulting from their preoperative clinical condition as well as their postoperative care. Marasmus, or protein-calorie malnutrition, is often seen in the elderly and the emaciated surgical candidate who has been chronically ill. Manifesting as weight loss, depleted fat stores, weakness, bradycardia, and being prone to hypothermia, it is often easily recognized. This type of malnutrition usually develops over time and requires time to completely correct.

Kwashiorkor, or protein malnutrition, on the other hand, may be difficult to recognize. There is concern that protein depletion exists in a number of elderly persons because of the "tea and toast diet" that they can often exist on. Using the patient's dietary history and measuring the patient's serum albumin level can indicate this malnutrition.

The degree of protein depletion that is acceptable in the surgical patient is an area of debate. Protein depletion is an independent risk factor for a significant increase in the frequency and severity of complications in hospitalized patients.[19] The marked protein depletion results in not only impaired immunocompetence with its poor consequences, but also anemia, edema, muscle wasting, and delayed wound healing.

Most authors linking preoperative protein malnutrition to poor surgical outcomes mention losses of protein stores of up to 5 to 7% to be acceptable without incurring a significant increase in complications.[24] Vernon and Hill have suggested that the negative impact of hypoproteinemia occurs when the degree of protein depletion has resulted in a decrease in muscle function.[30] This may be too great a degree of protein depletion to accept, as the threshold at which muscle function is affected is a protein loss of 20% of that of the healthy state. In the postoperative recovery phase when parenteral nutritional support is provided, restoration of muscle function is appreciably earlier than changes in body composition, which remain delayed for several weeks.[31] Acceptable levels of protein depletion in surgical patients probably exist somewhere between these limits.

Markers of Nutritional Status in the Perioperative Patient

A number of nutritional parameters have individually correlated with outcomes, but none have been able to accurately predict malnutrition. The use of markers in predicting clinical outcomes is difficult because of the intertwined nature of malnutrition and other clinical factors that influence outcomes. Different objective and subjective parameters including clinical judgment, physical parameters, biochemical analysis, immunologic determination, and nutritional indices are outlined.

Judgment

Baker and Detsky and associates demonstrated clinical acumen alone to be superior to nutritional indices in determining post-surgical results.[32, 33] The Subjective Global Assessment is based on a thorough history and physical evaluation to predict medical complications. Blinded observers demonstrated an 80% reproducibility with the same patients in one study, and another study found the preoperative Subjective

Global Assessment to have a better predictive value of postoperative infections than anthropometrics, serum albumin levels, transferrin levels, delayed cutaneous hypersensitivity, the creatinine-height index, and the prognostic nutritional index.[34] General physical features applied in the subjective analysis of an individual's status often include appearance, the prominence of malar eminencies, and signs of temporal, digital, or gluteal muscle wasting. Gait and affect as measured by a subjective psychological profile may also be employed but can be influenced by non-nutritional factors.

Traditional Physical Parameters Including Anthropometrics

Evidence of recent weight loss has played a pivotal role in the nutritional assessment of the surgical patient. Recent weight loss greater than 10% (within 6 months) indicates moderate protein-calorie malnutrition and has been shown repeatedly to be predictive of an increased mortality rate after surgery,[13, 35] whereas greater than 20% indicates severe protein-calorie malnutrition and even further morbidity and mortality.[36]

Numerous disease processes (i.e., congestive heart failure, chronic renal insufficiency, liver failure, an underlying disease requiring steroid use) may confound the accuracy of serum albumin measurements because of larger-than-normal interstitial volume loads inherent in these conditions. Changes in water distribution, which generally occur rather slowly unless precipitated by acute illness or stress, greatly influence this parameter, and the use of this information in caring for patients must be tempered by the knowledge of fluid dynamic characteristics in health and illness, tailoring treatment appropriately.

Two parameters, the triceps skinfold thickness and the midarm muscle circumference have been the traditional anthropometric measurements. The triceps skinfold thickness in the nondominant arm has been used as an indicator of fat reserves, with values less than the 5th to 10th percentiles associated with significant malnutrition and poor surgical results. Midarm muscle circumference values of less than the 10th percentile reflect a greater than 30% loss of lean tissue and severe protein-calorie malnutrition.[37] Despite a poor experimental correlation with accurate objective tools of measurement of lean body mass (LBM), midarm muscle circumference is used as a rapid adjunct to confirm a suspected state of protein depletion with a significant weight loss. Although these are simple, quick, and easily done at the bedside, low sensitivity in individual patients with mild to moderate malnutrition have limited the use of anthropometrics to confirming severe malnutrition.

Biochemical Parameters

Various serum protein determinations and the resulting formulas have been used to attempt to correlate nutritional parameters and outcomes. The serum albumin level is often included and heavily relied on as an important marker of nutritional assessment. The association of low serum albumin levels and poor surgical outcomes is well recognized.[8, 38–41] A multicenter trial of over 54,000 patients at Veteran Affairs (VA) hospitals looking at 62 perioperative parameters found a preoperative serum albumin level to have about a 70% accuracy in predicting postoperative mortality.[42]

Early measures of postoperative serum albumin levels are not only unnecessary but also misleading as a measure of the postoperative nutritional state. This is mainly because of a reduction in the synthesis of albumin as a result of the postoperative release of the cytokines interleukin 1, tumor necrosis factor, and interleukin 6 and a concomitant increase in protein catabolism. A redirection of hepatic and intestinal mucosal protein synthesis toward acute-phase proteins[23, 43] combined with the increase in interstitial accumulation of albumin because of capillary leak account for the low serum albumin levels seen in the early postoperative period. The normal rate of albumin exchange between intravascular and extravascular compartments is greater than 10 times the rate of albumin synthesis or degradation, and this accounts for the quickest changes in serum albumin concentrations. In septic patients, there is a threefold albumin loss from intravascular to extravascular spaces.[44] Hyaluronan helps to maintain albumin exclusion from the extracellular matrix; however, the postoperative washout of interstitial hyaluronan because of increased hydrostatic pressure is an additional factor leading to the hypoalbuminemic state of postoperative patients.[45–47]

Using the serum albumin level as an index has provided some general information and guidelines. Brennan and colleagues have demonstrated no benefit with preoperative nutritional support in patients with albumin levels over 4 g/dL,[48] whereas Daly and associates demonstrated that if the preoperative albumin level was less than 3 g/dL, nutritional supplementation of postoperative cancer patients was associated with a reduced incidence of wound infection and dehiscence.[49, 50]

Other biochemical markers (prealbumin, transferrin, retinal binding protein, insulin-like growth factor) have not been reliable as nutritional markers in the postoperative period because of factors similar to those responsible for the low serum albumin levels.

Immunologic Determinants

Although the immune system is altered on a number of levels by malnutrition, the routine use of immune parameters to assess the nutritional state has not been successful. Blackburn and his colleagues demonstrated that a lymphocyte count less than 3000/mm^3 with malnutrition reflects an immune deficiency.[10] However, the total lymphocyte count was a poor measure of the patient's nutritional state when compared with an isotope measurement of the body cell mass.[51] Redmond and colleagues have done extensive work demonstrating that various immunosuppressive mechanisms are at work in protein-calorie malnutrition.[52–54] A major component of the immune dysfunction is the macrophage defects, including macrophage microbicidal function with decreased phagocytosis and impaired respiratory burst activity (superoxide anion generation). The cause of this appears to be depletion of critical membrane phospholipids, resulting in altered prostaglandin levels, nitric oxide production, signal transduction, and cytokine (interleukin 1, interleukin 6) production. As an extension of this work, they demonstrated that malnutrition-induced depressed host responses predispose to *Candida albicans* sepsis.[55] Despite the new descriptions of the mechanisms, there is still no reliable clinical assessment of the immune defects as a reflection of the degree of malnutrition. Skin testing of recall antigens can be used to define anergy, or a clinical state of immunosuppression. The state

of anergy is associated with higher rates of postoperative morbidity and mortality.[56, 57] Copeland and his colleagues were able to show an improved outcome with the use of parenteral nutrition (PN) to reverse the state of anergy.[58] When 257 patients were evaluated, a significant relationship between the nutritional status and immunocompetance as defined by anergy was described. Forty-three percent of anergic patients who demonstrated anergy converted with aggressive and appropriate TPN therapy; however, other patients who had an improved nutritional status remained anergic.[59] These data as well as others indicate that anergy is not a reliable indicator of the surgical patient's nutritional state.

Body Composition Studies

The body can be described as a number of compartments, with the principal ones being the fat mass, the extracellular mass, and the body cell mass. These compartments can be directly and indirectly measured by determining the total body potassium, sodium, or nitrogen levels. Successful measurements have been made with the use of isotope dilution principles and isotopes that were either radioactive or heavy. Still other systems took advantage of naturally occurring isotopes and their ratios. Although in many instances the data were a good reflection of the nutritional state, the systems are not easily applied and the detection systems not universally applicable. Isotopes of water such as deuterium can be used to measure the total body water (TBW). The TBW is a reflection of the LBM, and the body weight minus the LBM gives the body fat mass. Body cell mass can be measured using potassium scanning or through direct and indirect isotope dilution techniques. The total body nitrogen and thus indirectly the body protein can be measured by neutron activation measurement.[60, 61] Although these techniques have been successfully used in surgical patients to help answer research questions, there is no reliable system that can be used clinically in surgical patients. In addition, the fluid and electrolyte changes that occur with surgical stress can make the interpretation of the data difficult.

Bioelectric Impedance Analysis

Bioelectric impedance analysis (BIA) is a more practical system in terms of clinical application. BIA detects subtle changes in body composition such as the increased extracellular mass–to–body cell mass ratio, which is an early sign of malnutrition.[61, 62] TBW and thus the LBM and the total body fat can be predicted using the BIA measurements. The basis of the measurements is the resistance of the whole body to a low-voltage electric current. In diseases with either malnutrition or other causes of water and electrolyte abnormalities, the BIA measurements are abnormal. This of course includes the electrolyte and fluid changes seen in surgical stress. Studies by Jacobs and associates using BIA in the surgical patient raise concerns about its ability to measure malnutrition, and its precision and clinical utility remain limited.[63, 64]

Muscle Function

As previously mentioned, Vernon and Hill have shown that postoperative outcomes are poor in patients with preoperative muscle impairment.[25] There are some data to suggest that testing of muscle function is more specific and sensitive than traditional nutritional markers in preoperatively predicting postoperative complications.[65, 66] Means of measuring muscle strength include measuring the grip strength, respiratory muscle strength, and response of specific muscles to electric stimulation. The latter is an attempt to be more precise and to eliminate subjective aspects of the test. However, the adductor pollicis stimulation studies suggest that the results are measuring functional improvements as a result of energy repletion and that the improvements occur before changes in body composition, including the amounts of nitrogen, protein, or muscle.[67, 68] This type of testing ranges from uncomfortable to painful and is affected by a number of drugs. Its regular clinical use is thus very limited.

Comorbidities

Renal failure, cirrhosis, congestive heart failure, chronic pulmonary disease, chronic diarrhea, infection, and systemic inflammatory response syndrome (SIRS) are among many common chronic or acute comorbidities that may concomitantly plague the surgical patient. Surgery not uncommonly unmasks underlying clinically quiescent conditions, revealing a patient's nutritional status to be more deficient than expected. Although some of these conditions may have existed for years, a few are of an acute nature, and all negatively influence patient outcomes.

Various metabolic and nutritional conditions characteristic of different disease processes exist in patients with end-organ failure. For example, the changes related to kidney disease are well recognized. The metabolic acidosis of renal insufficiency stimulates the irreversible degradation of essential branched-chain amino acids and muscle protein. The ability to reduce the oxidation of the amino acids in malnutrition is impaired by the metabolic acidosis of renal failure, and, associated with the anorexia of renal failure, the LBM loss is increased.[69]

The presence and degree of the inflammatory response as a function of the severity of ongoing SIRS in the critically ill postoperative patient deserves special mention, as the development of malnutrition is accelerated. Loss of up to 40 g of nitrogen per day in these patients makes significant malnutrition occur much earlier than in the usual postoperative patient. This type of patient will require earlier provision of adjuvant nutritional support.

In summary, there is no single parameter that can help identify all the surgical patients at risk for malnutrition. The Subjective Global Assessment done by a trained observer is perhaps the best clinical tool for identifying the preoperative patient who would benefit from nutritional support and thus have an improved clinical outcome. Despite the existence of a number of highly accurate research tools, evidence of recent preoperative weight loss and measuring a preoperative albumin level remain the best, simple, and fairly correct objective markers of preoperative malnutrition. The consensus statement issued by the National Institutes of Health (NIH), American Society for Parenteral and Enteral Nutrition (ASPEN), and American Society for Clinical Nutrition (ASCN)[44] supports this. More recent patient series have further confirmed these preoperative markers to correlate with the hospital length of stay.[70]

◆ PERIOPERATIVE ENTERAL NUTRITION VERSUS PARENTERAL NUTRITION

Once the malnourished patient is identified and a decision is made to provide nutritional support, the route of delivery must be decided. The enteral route remains the route of choice for the surgical patient, with the parenteral route reserved for those who cannot, should not, or will not eat. Malnourished patients who are not compromised and at risk for complications should have their nutritional needs immediately dealt with. If the enteral route is available, then enteral nutrition (EN) is started, but it is often necessary to simultaneously start TPN.

Though the evidence is often anecdotal, most clinicians have maintained that EN is always better than PN. Lower cost, greater safety, a more physiologic nature, the prevention of bacterial translocation in the gut, and most of all an improved outcome have all been associated with an enteral route of delivery of nutrients.

In a broad review of the subject based on current literature, Lipman compared both means of nutritional delivery, examining these widely held beliefs.[71] As both pre- and postoperative nutrition are often intertwined, both are discussed here, and the cited studies are limited primarily to prospective randomized controlled trials (PRCTs).

With the exception of the increased number of infectious complications in patients with abdominal trauma and the cost of PN, no differences have been found between EN and PN. The infectious complications are predominantly line-related; however, many of the PN patients were suffering from hyperglycemia, a confounding risk factor with infections. The cost has not been reevaluated and with the cost of PN delivery being decreased to a fraction of earlier prices, the cost comparison merits reanalysis.

Both TPN and starvation are associated with changes in gut function and architecture, and although this is well recognized in small rodents, the same has not been demonstrated in humans.[72] Changes in intestinal permeability are well known to occur in humans after upper gastrointestinal surgery for malignancies, major vascular surgery, after multiple trauma, and in severe burns.[73–76] A few studies have gone further to demonstrate the association of increased gut permeability with the development of sepsis and SIRS.[76–79]

With the use of physiologic parameters such as nitrogen balance and protein, metabolic, and immune markers, the "improved physiology" of nonvolitional EN was compared with PN in eight PRCTs of perioperative patients. With the exception of an increase in serum protein levels in groups with abdominal or head trauma, other evidence of EN's being more physiologic than PN could not be demonstrated.[80–88] In two groups with esophageal cancer, each consisting of 12 patients receiving either EN or PN, Lim and coworkers found early increases in nitrogen balance in the TPN group, whereas no overall differences in the postoperative wound infection rate, morbidity, or mortality were noted between the two groups.[89]

It remains important to bear in mind the important maintenance role of EN. Luminal feeding promotes enteral flow, obviates stasis, and stimulates biliary kinetics, resulting in improved enterohepatic circulation, thus preventing TPN-associated cholestasis along with a reduction in the incidence of calculous and acalculous cholecystitis.[90–92]

Evaluating intestinal absorption and/or permeability, four PRCTs found no differences in either gut function or morphology when EN and PN were compared.[71, 77, 80, 93, 94] In a PRCT of postoperative patients who had undergone esophageal, gastric, or pancreatic surgery, Rowlands and colleagues found no significant difference in intestinal permeability, or levels of serum albumin, C-reactive protein, or various immunoglobulins.[82] Of a total of 203 surgical patients, in the 28 patients who received at least 10 days of preoperative TPN, Sedman and colleagues found no increase in intestinal atrophy when compared with enterally fed controls.[95] Interestingly, in eight healthy volunteers, Buchman and associates noted intestinal immune function not to be affected after 2 weeks of PN.[96]

Despite what appears to be adequate EN, pre-existing abnormalities of intestinal structure and function have remained with EN. Cummins and coworkers demonstrated that even 2 to 3 months of EN was unable to reverse pre-existing villous atrophy and abnormal permeability.[97] These studies show that the changes in intestinal permeability associated with major surgery are not completely treated by luminal nutrition administration. Though not conclusive, a number of studies have shown that, depending on the disease and degree of illness, PN does not adversely affect intestinal morphology or function, whereas EN does not completely correct the pre-existing intestinal disease.[73–76]

Although bacterial translocation is known to occur in humans, its clinical significance remains unclear. In two studies, Sedman and associates were unable to correlate subsequent bacterial translocation with preoperative TPN delivery.[95]

A PRCT reported by Sako and coworkers in head and neck cancer surgery patients who were randomized to TPN or nasogastric feeding after surgery found no difference in wound healing, complications (septic and nonseptic), or short-term outcomes.[98] In a similar patient population and study type, Iovinelli and associates also found no difference in nutritional outcomes or surgical complications, though the length of stay in the hospital appeared to be longer by over a week in the group receiving TPN.[99]

Von Meyenfeldt and colleagues compared 50 patients receiving EN with 50 patients receiving TPN along with two control groups of a similar size receiving no form of nutritional support and found no differences in the number of complications (septic or nonseptic), length of stay, or mortality in the two study groups.[100] Both study groups and one of the two control groups were considered to be "depleted" before nutritional therapy, whereas the other control group was labeled well nourished.

Few data exist to compare the safety of PN with that of EN. Moore and associates reported a larger number of complications with EN related to gastrostomy and jejunostomy placement and/or migration; this study was limited to abdominal trauma patients.[101] Baigrie and coworkers randomized 97 patients after esophagogastric surgery to EN or TPN, finding 21 catheter-related complications in 18 of 47 patients randomized to TPN and 20 jejunal catheter problems in 20 of 50 patients in the EN group.[102] There were also 15 compared with 9 life-threatening complications and 6 compared with 4 deaths in the TPN group compared with the EN group, though these differences were not statistically significant.

With the significantly larger patient population receiving EN and not PN, which is reflective of general nutritional support delivery in the United States, naturally more complications would be expected in the EN group. In 10 years of Lipman's own retrospective analysis of a VA center's experience, no death was directly attributable to TPN, whereas deaths due to EN were sec-

ondary to improper catheter placement and migration, resulting in nasopulmonary intubation, pneumothorax, feeding into the pleural space, and ileal placement of surgical jejunostomy tubes, leading to lethal small bowel obstruction.[71] Aspiration, epistaxis, nasoalar necrosis, sinusitis, otitis, nasopharyngeal perforation, cranial insertion, carotid artery blowout, esophageal strictures, and esophageal and intestinal perforations have been not uncommonly described.[103–106] Without overstressing the self-evident, both routes of nutritional delivery need to be cautiously administered and monitored.

Poor nutritional intake status is a prescription for a poor outcome in the complicated surgical patient. An important outlook toward nutritional support should include a complementary, not competitive, approach of parenteral and enteral routes of delivery. This is most importantly reflected in the critically ill patient. A middle ground with protein-calorie delivery as the top aim is possible and may be achieved in the large majority of surgical patients. Metabolic and nutritional support can be begun parenterally when EN is not initially practical, transitioning to enteral feedings as bowel function returns, weaning the patient from TPN. Using a combination of PN and EN, using variations in the proportion of each, tailored to the clinical situation, and ultimately making the transition to EN, allows a majority of postoperative patients to receive complete metabolic, immune, and nutritional support.

Finally, small study sizes and inconsistencies in outcomes cannot allow enteral perioperative nutrition to be labeled better than perioperative TPN. And except for a questionable cost benefit of EN and a reduction in septic morbidity after abdominal and head trauma, no significant differences in EN and PN have yet been demonstrated.

◆ DELETERIOUS EFFECTS OF HYPERGLYCEMIA

The insulin resistance induced by stress is of both central and peripheral types and results in the decreased capacity for insulin to inhibit gluconeogenesis through increased secretion of catecholamines, cortisol, glucagon, growth hormone, and cytokines; combined, all these factors result in hyperglycemia. Peripheral insulin resistance results in a reduced facilitation of glucose transport into peripheral cells, and although hepato-cellular uptake is insulin independent, he-patocellular metabolism of glucose is insulin dependent. Increased amino acid mobilization and gluconeogenesis, and the increased mobilization of free fatty acids without significant ketogenesis, results in further amplification of the hyperglycemia.

The consequences of TPN-associated hyperglycemia have been well elucidated by Bistrian.[107] The widespread glycosylation of various proteins results in their dysfunction. Immunoglobulin glycosylation results in poor immune function, and collagen glycosylation is associated with poor wound healing. Hyperglycemia is known to result in the expression of a glucose-inducible protein by *Candida*; the protein aids in *Candida's* adherence to tissues and in eluding host defenses by being disguised structurally and functionally as a complement receptor fragment.[108]

Acute elevations in blood sugar levels are known to enhance proteolysis in normal humans.[109] Hyperglycemia is one of several deleterious effects of overfeeding (Table 10–2) and is responsible at least in part for other complications such as decreased immune function, poor wound healing, and increased infections. Pomposelli and associates have demonstrated a definite correlation between poor blood sugar control and an increased rate of nosocomial infections in the diabetic postoperative patient population,[110] whereas enhanced glycemic regulation has been demonstrated to correlate with improved adherence, chemotaxis, phagocytosis, and antibacterial activity of neutrophils.[111–114]

Table 10–2. Deleterious Effects of Overfeeding in Surgical Patients

Hyperglycemia
Depressed white blood cell function (i.e., adherence, chemotaxis, bactericidal activity)
Depressed immunoglobulin and macrophage function (secondary to glycosylation)
Collagen glycosylation → poor wound healing
Increased CO_2 production → increased minute ventilation and work of breathing,[18, 27] leading to difficulty in weaning off ventilator
Impaired amino acid mobilization
Hepatic steatosis
Lipogenesis
Increased rate of nosocomial and wound infections[110]
Increased proteolysis
Expression of unique mechanism of virulence in *Candida* in hyperglycemic environment.[10]

Further, iatrogenic hyperinsulinemia created by efforts to control elevations in blood sugar levels can itself result in impaired amino acid mobilization and an increased incidence of fatty liver.

◆ PREOPERATIVE NUTRITION

Goals

Preoperative nutritional therapy goals vary depending on the patient's clinical status, energy requirements, and volume limitations, but need to remain focused toward attempts to correct the effects of the malnourished state that occurred as a result of earlier therapies or the disease state. Only with therapy directed at an impaired immune response, widespread latent organ dysfunction, and various biochemical abnormalities evident on repletion efforts will nutritional support translate into improvements in clinical outcomes or at the least attenuate poor clinical results.

Preoperative enteral tube feeding has been less well studied, with two PRCTs demonstrating fewer postoperative complications with preoperative feeding than with controls.[100, 115]

Nutritional repletion aims at achieving a positive nitrogen and energy balance, which coupled with glycogen loading of tissues helps to provide the patient the nutritional wherewithal to cope with the stress of surgery and the obligatory postoperative catabolic period. Despite unappreciable changes in LBM from such nutritional therapy, the improvements in outcomes appear to be reflective of some yet-unidentified processes. These changes appear to be on the cellular and subcellular level and may range from immunologic enhancement to an improved cellular energy and biochemical state as described by Russel and associates.[31]

At the cellular level, the objectives of preoperative TPN include an increase in glycogen stores and intracellular ATP and ions, while decreasing inorganic phosphate and ADP levels and thus biochemically optimizing the energy stores in the preoperative patient.[116–119] The ability to attenuate postoperative insulin resistance with preoperative glucose loading as discussed later is another desirable goal.

Practical guidelines for nutritional intervention in the perioperative surgical patient should include evidence of weight loss of greater than 10% of usual body weight over the previous few months. In the euvolemic, preoperative state, an albumin level of less than 3.3 g/dL is noted by Rombeau, Kudsk, and colleagues also to be an indication for nutritional support.[120]

In patients who will benefit from presurgical nutritive repletion, the past practice of a 7- to 10-day in-hospital stay solely for preoperative nutritional therapy in the absence of comorbidities is no longer practical in the present cost-containment environment of managed care. Central venous line or feeding tube placement and 24 to 48 hours of monitoring usually necessitates an initial brief admission, whereas the remaining preoperative period can be spent in a subacute care or rehabilitation facility or even in the patients' homes, depending on the patients' and families' ability and willingness to undertake care, with appropriate visiting health care workers for monitoring.

Monitoring most importantly relates specifically to the severely malnourished group in whom the development of the refeeding syndrome is a distinct possibility.[121] The anabolic effects of insulin as a necessary response to a dextrose infusion result in a burst of cellular ion uptake leading to potentially life-threatening hypokalemia or hypophosphatemia or magnesium derangement. Recognition of such problems by initial daily evaluation of electrolyte levels and adequate parenteral correction by supplementation are crucial to appropriate clinical care.

As a state of relative extracellular water (ECW) overload is inherent to the chronic malnourished state,[47] fluid and sodium delivery must be rigidly controlled. This is even more important in the severely malnourished group, as these patients may also manifest an element of nutritional cardiomyopathy.[25] Historically, overenthusiastic repletion has on occasion had fatal consequences.[122, 123] The rapid weight gain accounted for by increases in ECW in many patients receiving preoperative TPN has long been associated with an impaired clinical outcome, including increased postoperative respiratory complication rates[47, 124, 125] and heart failure.[25, 122, 123]

Zimmer and associates demonstrated the fluid-retentive effects of a low-protein high-carbohydrate diet, showing that when starved prisoners of war were refed diets high in glucose, they had a tendency to retain sodium along with other fluid and electrolyte abnormalities.[126] Rudman and colleagues[127] demonstrated that up to 50% of the weight gain noted after high-glucose-loaded TPN was due to ECW expansion, preventable with the elimination of sodium from the TPN. Trials with different preoperative TPN formulations aimed at reducing TPN-induced preoperative ECW expansion have concluded that the use of high-lipid, low-sodium TPN may be of benefit.[128]

Calorie and Protein Requirements

Glucose metabolism is significantly altered in ill nondiabetic hospitalized patients. Important differences in glucose metabolism are seen between mildly hypermetabolic patients (uncomplicated postoperative patients) and those more severely stressed (trauma, sepsis, burns). Studies have demonstrated the rate of hepatic gluconeogenesis to be in the range of 2 mg/kg/min in normal fasted volunteers. In any moderately stressed patient the rate increases to 4 mg/kg/min. Infusions of dextrose in the control or the surgical patient in whom the surgical stress has resolved will suppress hepatic gluconeogenesis.[129] The critically ill patient or the patient who has undergone major surgery will have increased rates of hepatic gluconeogeneis that are not suppressible. Catabolic phenomena secondary to the stress response result in an obligatory protein breakdown along the ubiquitin-proteosome pathway, beginning at surgery and continuing well into the postoperative period. This has been shown to be not amenable to any currently known repletion efforts including supplying dextrose at up to maximal oxidation rates (4 mg/kg/min). Carbohydrates delivered in excess of this amount have a larger proportion used by way of nonoxidative pathways without further improvements in the energy balance[23] and a respiratory quotient (RQ) greater than 1, signifying net lipogenesis, a futile metabolic event in a malnourished hypermetabolic patient whose priorities do not include fat synthesis. Therefore, one of the keys to TPN is to provide sufficient exogenous glucose to meet metabolic needs without the development of glucose intolerance. The glucose infusion in TPN in most patients should not in any event exceed 4 mg/kg/min.

Although a daily protein intake of 0.8 g/kg of the patient's usual body weight is an accepted adequate intake for 95% of the healthy population,[130] hospitalized patients, and specifically perioperative surgical patients, require protein intakes of at least 1.2 g/kg/day when accompanied by adequate caloric intake to obviate the features of malnutrition. Historically, in attempts to provide patients with adequate calories, protein delivery has often been suboptimal because of limitations of the volume to use for nutritional delivery due to the fluid overload of the perioperative period or the volume restriction due to the patient's underlying disease. As expected, marked losses in LBM are noted in such cases. When energy delivery is inadequate, referred to as hypocaloric feeding (often necessitated by volume restriction or the need for glycemic control), greater amounts of protein, up to 1.5 g/kg/day, are required to achieve protein sparing.[131, 132]

A large step in achieving an adequate provision of proteins has been to unlink the historically combined protein intake with that of caloric delivery. Generally, this is not necessary with a majority of preoperative surgical patients, but a small number along with most postoperative patients are not tolerant of the volume and/or dextrose load inherent to total caloric delivery because of fluid constraints or hyperglycemia engendered by their disease or hypervolemic state. Therefore, rather than provide less nitrogen and thus fewer calories, we believe it is imperative to break the linkage between protein and calories, dispensing protein at a rate of at least 1.2 mg/kg/day, ideally at 1.5 mg/kg/day and if possible 22 to 25 kcal/kg/day to meet the energy expenditure of the LBM.[133]

Shaw and associates have shown a reduction in net protein breakdown with different rates of amino acid infusion from 1.1 to 1.5 g/kg/day, whereas an increase in net protein breakdown was noted with a further rate increase to 2.2 g/kg/day.[134] Using isotope tracer methodology, Wolfe and Shaw and associates demonstrated in burn and septic patients that the optimal balance between protein synthesis and breakdown was attained with protein delivery at 1.5 g/kg/day.[135, 136] During periods of maximal catabolism, for example, in patients ranging from ongoing SIRS patients to burn patients, when the resting energy expenditure is increased from 1.5 to 2 times normal, maximal protein sparing is achieved with the delivery of protein at a rate of 1.5 g/kg/day. Although nutritional support cannot suppress protein catabolism despite delivery at this level, maximal sparing does occur.

The prevalence of hyperglycemia is markedly increased when attempts to meet the patient's energy balance are made in trauma and sepsis patients.[8, 136] Underfeeding modestly while providing higher amounts of protein is one way to avoid this problem.

Lipids are another source of nonprotein calories, also allowing smaller volumes to be infused. Because of their calorically dense nature, they allow a reduction in the amount of carbon dioxide generated, thus aiding in obviating a potentially increased respiratory load and also in protein sparing when administered with sufficient protein.

Overfeeding of patients receiving PN is a widespread phenomenon common to academic medical centers in the United States. In a survey of one university system and its associate partners, using two hypothetical patient types, 25% of practitioners were found to be providing their patients with glucose at a rate of greater than 4.5 mg/kg/min, with nearly 50% using a 25% dextrose formula. Conclusions reached by Schloerb and colleagues were that over 25% of these centers were using dextrose in amounts resulting in an RQ of greater than 1.[137]

In summary, based on current knowledge, we recommend the provision of protein at 1.2 to 1.5 g/kg/day, 22 to 25 kcal/kg/day of calories of which dextrose is administered not in excess of 4 mg/kg/min with the balance made up by lipids. These guidelines are in accordance with the recommendations of a number of nutritional specialists.

We would be remiss in not mentioning the crucial role that adequate vitamins, minerals, and trace elements play. As vital components of most metabolic processes and biochemical reactions ranging from enzyme function enhancement to all aspects of a sustained immune response, they are a critical component in the nutritional repletion of any patient.

The previously mentioned precautions concerning the refeeding syndrome should be kept in mind when these orders are written; the orders may include low volume, low sodium, and adequate amounts of potassium, phosphorus, and magnesium.

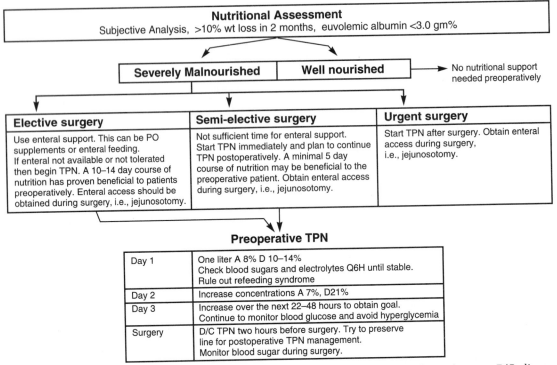

Figure 10–1. Algorithm for the use of preoperative hyperalimentation. A, amino acids; D, dextrose; D/C, discontinue; TPN, total parenteral nutrition. INC, increase.

Benefits

Preoperative nutritional therapy is not for every surgical patient. When nutrition is used as an adjunct to complete patient support, patient selection is critical in enhancing recovery and minimizing morbidity. Candidates for preoperative hyperalimentation are outlined in Figure 10–1.

The objective is multifold: by the provision of adequate protein and calories, patients benefit at the cellular level, and this is reflected in improved organ system function, translating to improved outcomes. Preoperative nutritional therapy aims to optimize each and every aspect of body function; a few of the beneficial effects are discussed.

Glycogen, electrolyte, and protein repletion improve muscle substrate and the cellular energy and kinetics with improved muscle function not only in cardiomyocytes but throughout the body. This has a wide-ranging effect with positive inotropy for cardiac tissue and glycogen loading of skeletal tissue, providing more strength and a better energy state and resulting in increased activity and better respiratory muscle function.

Enhanced immune function with amino acid provision has been shown as demonstrated by anergy conversion.[58, 59] The gastrointestinal tract, the largest immune organ, is also supported by an improved nutritional state. Substrate delivery in the form of amino acids helps to maintain mucosal integrity and boost immunity through Peyer's patches of the gut-associated lymphoid tissue (GALT) system. This substrate availability allows optimal immunoglobulin A (IgA) production, which then provides protection against mucosal invasion. A similar role for IgA in the respiratory mucosal epithelium has been proposed.

Another area of interest is the fixed reduction in insulin sensitivity (IS) seen postoperatively. A dose-response relationship to trauma severity has been noted and seems to be independent of numerous variables. Its attenuation by preoperative glucose infusion appears to correlate with enhanced outcomes. The role of modifying this fixed reduction in IS in the perioperative period promises to be an exciting new area of research with potential applicability and is discussed in detail later.[138]

Evaluation of Clinical Data
(Table 10–3)

In 1983, using linear regression analysis in a large group of patients undergoing gastrointestinal surgery, Meguid and associates[139] were among the first to recognize the importance of appropriate patient selection in achieving some of the beneficial effects of TPN instead of practicing the universal delivery of TPN to perioperative patients without regard to their nutritional status. Three distinct groups based on the nutritional status, diagnosis, age, and period of inadequate oral intake were retrospectively identified. The first group included high-risk malnourished patients of any age with a gastrointestinal cancer, who they recommended should receive perioperative TPN. The second group consisted of patients younger than 40 years with a primary carcinoma at any site in whom perioperative TPN was not recommended, and the third group consisted of well-nourished patients older than 40 years or malnourished patients of any age with genitourinary, gynecologic, or lymphoproliferative disease. This third group was followed carefully, and TPN was recommended if an adequate oral intake had not been established by day 10. If a complication developed in either of groups 2 or 3, TPN was instituted immediately. Refinement of these criteria over the ensuing years has resulted in inclusion and later exclusion of various criteria improving the utilization of TPN by being more specific in patient selection.

Evaluating only PRCTs, a consensus statement issued by NIH, ASPEN, and ASCN described preoperatively moderate to severely malnourished candidates identified in various trials based on weight loss, plasma protein levels, and prognostic indices as the groups in whom 7 days of preoperative TPN provided a clear benefit in surgical outcomes.[44]

Moghissi and colleagues in a PRCT of patients with esophageal cancer and preoperative weight loss of 4 to 13 kg allocated patients in one group to 5 to 7 days of preoperative TPN and another to an oral diet plus

Table 10–3. Prospective Randomized Controlled Trials Evaluating Preoperative Total Parenteral Nutrition

Reference	First Authors	Nonprotein Calories (kcal/kg/day) [% of goal]	Nitrogen (g/kg/day) [% of goal]	Lipids (kcal/kg/day)	End-Point	Complications Control (%)	TPN (%)	Mortality Control (%)	TPN (%)
140	Fan	Goal: 19 [100] >40 [>211]	Goal: 0.24 [100] 0.25 [104]	NR	Any complication	75.0	85.0	30.0	30.0
141	Thompson	40–50 [211–263]	0.30 [125]	NR	Any complication	11.1	16.7	0.0	0.0
142	Muller	32–46 [168–242]	0.24 [100]	13.5	Major complication	32.0	37.0	18.6	21.7
143	VA	45 [237]	0.30 [125]	5.3	Any complication	24.6	25.5	10.5	13.4
144	Bellantone	30 [158]	0.20 [83]	9	Sepsis	35.3	30.0	3.9	2.5
145	Muller	40 [211]	0.24 [100]	0	Major complication	32.2	16.7	18.6	4.5
142	Muller	32–45 [168–237]	0.24 [100]	0	Major complication	30.9	13.8	20.0	6.9
146	Smith	50–60 [263–316]	0.25–0.30 [104–125]	0	Any complication	35.3	17.6	17.6	5.9
147	Heatley	40 [211]	0.20 [83]	0	Anastomotic leak	44.4	23.7	22.2	15.7
148	Fan	30]158]	0.24 [100]	15	Any complication	55.0	34.0	15.0	7.8
149	Meguid	35 [184]	0.16 [67]	NR	Any complication	56.0	31.3	0.0	3.0
150	Bellantone	30 [158]	0.20 (83)	9	Sepsis	7.8	14.8	2.2	1.8
151	Moghissi	34–36 [179–189]	0.18–0.20 [75–83]	7	Delayed healing	80.0	0.0	0.0	0.0
100	Von Meyenfeldt	35–40 [184–211]	0.16–0.20 [67–83]	4	Major complication	14.0	12.0	4.0	4.0

NR, not reported; TPN, total parenteral nutrition; [ ], Numbers in brackets reflect the percentage of current recommendations fed to patients.

dextrose, intravenous fluids, and electro-lytes without additional protein.[151] Patients in the group receiving TPN established posi-tive nitrogen balance preoperatively and re-mained in positive balance postoperatively, demonstrating better wound healing, whereas the other group remained in nega-tive nitrogen balance throughout the periop-erative course. In a prospective randomized trial involving 100 patients undergoing ma-jor gastrointestinal surgical procedures, Bel-lantone and coworkers found that patients randomized to receive 7 days of preopera-tive TPN showed a 21% rate of sepsis com-pared with 53% in those receiving a stan-dard hospital diet.[144] Postoperative mortality was also lower in the TPN group but not significantly. In a similar trial of 125 patients with gastrointestinal cancers, Muller and as-sociates randomized one group to 10 days of preoperative TPN and the other to a hospital diet, noting both a reduction in major com-plications (17% vs. 32%) and in mortality (5% vs. 18%) in the TPN group.[145] Campos and coworkers showed a statistically sig-nificant reduction in major postoperative complications (i.e., anastomotic leakage, wound infection, and other infections) and a reduction in mortality with 7 to 10 days of preoperative TPN.[152]

The conclusions reached at the consensus conference[39] echo the results of 13 PRCTs involving over 1250 patients, that TPN for 5 to 7 days may positively influence the even-tual outcome, whereas 7 to 10 days of preop-erative TPN do result in an overall reduction of postoperative complications from 40% to 30%.

Nine of 13 PRCTs demonstrated a clear benefit of preoperative TPN in severely mal-nourished patients.[100, 140, 144–149, 151] The mildly to moderately malnourished patients receiving TPN had a higher complication rate than those not receiving TPN.[147] How-ever, retrospective analysis revealed that these patients receiving TPN were inappro-priately overfed with calories in the range of 150 to 316% of the what is currently acceptable (see Table 10–3). This would greatly increase the incidence of hyperglyce-mia as well as the other complications of overfeeding.

The hazards of this overfeeding include, but are not limited to, hyperglycemia and associated hepatic steatosis, fat production, immune impairment, respiratory dysfunc-tion, and derangements in fluid distribution. Each one of these changes results in system

dysfunction and has numerous associated pathologic results as outlined throughout this chapter, and all correlate with poor out-comes in the postoperative patient.

The question then remains: Could those in the preoperative groups studied retro-spectively have shown a greater reduction in postoperative complications? If so, it would be expected that future PRCTs may demonstrate an even greater reduction in postoperative complications in those receiv-ing nutrition at levels consistent with cur-rently acceptable goals.

◆ POSTOPERATIVE NUTRITION

In the severely catabolic postoperative pa-tient, energy balance and lean tissue reple-tion should not be the primary aims. The goals are to provide adequate protein and calories, to support the immune response, and to provide metabolic support including the pH and electrolyte corrections. Equally important is the avoidance of nutritional therapy–induced complications, which re-sulted from overfeeding. This was the conse-quence of aggressive TPN or "hyperalimen-tation," an approach that gave TPN a poor reputation.[143]

Two key assets to improving the nitrogen balance in the surgical patient are immuno-competence and wound healing. These can be obtained by providing an adequate amount of protein, which can be achieved with modest levels of energy delivery. By maximizing the protein intake and avoiding the problems of overfeeding, including hyperglycemia, Daly and his associates demonstrated that postoperative nutritional support reduced wound infections and de-hiscence in cancer patients with a preopera-tive albumin level of 3.0 g/dL.[49, 50]

The endocrine response to both intravas-cular depletion and postoperative pain fa-vors salt and water retention as a result of aldosterone and antidiuretic hormone re-lease. When this endocrine response is ac-companied by often-necessary aggressive re-hydration therapy in the early postoperative period, a state of fluid overload rapidly de-velops. As mentioned earlier, expansion of cellular water is an index of sickness, whereas subsequent recovery correlates well with changes in the distribution of TBW,[153] and restoration of the exchangeable sodium ratio appears to be one of the best predictors of outcomes.[154]

Enough emphasis cannot be placed on the need for daily weighing of postoperative patients. When done with the same zeroed scale and at the same time daily, weighing will reflect the acute changes in the TBW over a short period of time.[47]

Activation of the stress response and a resultant increase in the counterregulatory hormones and cytokines including cortisol, catecholamines, glucagon, growth hormone, tumor necrosis factor, and interleukin 1 result in an obligatory proteolysis not obviated from even the protein-sparing effects of nutritional support. Activation of the ubiquitin-proteosome system is the principal mechanism of this proteolysis. This requisite protein catabolism appears to be phylogenetically mandated, ensuring adequate substrate availability necessary for protein synthesis and gluconeogenesis (and thus providing the building blocks for an adequate immune response and wound healing). This primarily glucocorticoid-activated and insulinopenic-driven signal[155, 156] in an acidotic state demonstrates the body's attempt to satisfy primal protein and energy demands as in a state of survival mode at the expense of incurring obligatory skeletal muscle loss.

Further, the effects of surgical stress increase glucose turnover two to four times the normal levels, with a major portion of the glucose from skeletal muscle protein–derived gluconeogenesis. A 50% increase in energy expenditure may increase proteolysis two to four times secondary to the disproportionate increase in glucose turnover. With the severity of injury proportional to the intensity of nitrogen loss, it should be readily apparent how, for example, a postoperative patient with a wound infection can become markedly catabolic and quickly lose a large amount of body cell mass.[157, 158] The starved patient loses approximately 75 g of protein per day, whereas the stressed patient's losses are proportional to the degree of stress encountered. Major surgery is correlated with a 20% increase in metabolism, sepsis with 50%, and burns with up to 100%, as outlined by Elwyn and colleagues.[159] In such a scenario, nitrogen excretion can increase up to 40 g/day, or 250 g of muscle protein per day, equating to approximately 1000 g of muscle mass lost per day.[160, 161] In a 1998 study by Plank and associates, a loss of 13% of total body protein over a 3-week period was noted in a series of 12 patients with severe sepsis secondary to perforation of an abdominal viscus despite the provision of adequate nutritional support.[162] These data highlight the inability of exogenous protein to block the catabolic state and emphasize the importance of trying to match the protein loss estimated with nitrogen balance.

EN, which often takes a minimum of several days to reach protein-calorie goal rates, is commonly erratic and unpredictable in tolerance, whereas TPN provides not only rapid metabolic support to the critically ill but nearly always ensures goal protein, if not calorie, delivery in a predictable and timely fashion in most patients unless limited by volume or difficult glycemic management issues.

EN is usually begun with an isotonic full-strength formula. It may then be advanced 10 to 20 mL every 12 hours to goal. Caveats to administration include the following: (1) Tolerance as reflected by diarrhea (one must rule out colonic overgrowth, multiple antibiotic use, and prokinetics first), distention, high residuals in the case of gastric feeding (>100 mL/4 h), and nausea or vomiting must be monitored. Assessment includes clinical examination and, as needed, abdominal films to check for colonic distention and the location of the tube. (2) Feeding into the small bowel (beyond the ligament of Treitz) is better tolerated and remains the "gold standard" in difficult-to-feed patients along with being associated with decreased infectious complications.[163] A crucial concern in the enterally fed postoperative patient is hemodynamic stability, which should be a prerequisite to enteral feeding. Poor perfusion of the splanchnic bed as reflected in a low urine output, the presence of acidosis, vasopressor use (other than low-dose dopamine therapy), or hypovolemic shock should be absolute contraindications to small bowel feeding.

Despite disadvantages associated with PN and EN, protein-calorie delivery can still be satisfactorily achieved in a majority of patients when both routes are simultaneously used in a balanced fashion when the use of either exclusively is not tolerated. This common ground of combined delivery allows an earlier reduction in obligatory protein losses; the postoperative scenario is often conducive to PN and the gut is often "not ready." Although PN may not provide the optimal calorie delivery, it can provide

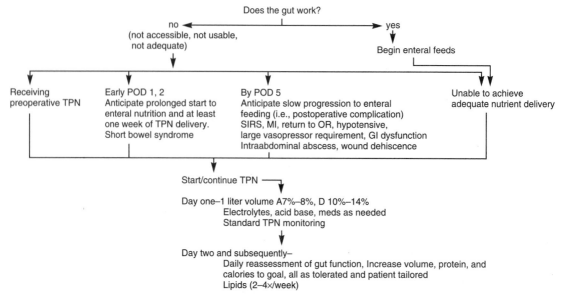

Figure 10–2. Algorithm for the Initiation of Postoperative Nutritional/Metabolic Therapy. Corollary: In preoperative and intraoperative decision making, consider if this patient would benefit from a surgical feeding tube (e.g., trauma, burns, esophageal or gastric resection, gastric bypass surgery, débridement of necrotic pancreatitis). A, amino acids; D, dextrose; GI, gastrointestinal; MI, myocardial infarction; OR, operating room; POD, postoperative day; SIRS, systemic inflammatory response syndrome; TPN, total parenteral nutrition.

70 to 80 g of amino acids per day, or more, enough to allow a reduction in obligatory proteolysis. Its delivery is then either increased daily or the clinical picture changes to allow the start of EN, paving the path for a smooth transition to luminal nutrition. Thus, a well-planned combination of protein-calorie delivery involving PN and EN can effectively be complementary, aiding in postsurgical recovery. This is currently a preferred mode of nutritional delivery for most clinicians. Data in trauma and burn patients also advocate the importance of early luminal nutrition.[19, 101, 164, 165]

Candidates

In patients with good nutritional balance preoperatively, studies have shown the body's ability to withstand starvation for 5 to 7[34] days without the untoward effects of poor wound healing and increasing difficulty in weaning from the ventilator. At around 1 week postoperatively without nutritional support, wound healing and recovery become adversely affected, and an increase in the rate of postoperative infections is noted.[17] Thus, for patients undergoing major surgery, nutritional support should be instituted if oral feeding is not resumed by

postoperative day 5 (Fig. 10–2), this finding often heralding the development of a postoperative complication. The time threshold toward the initiation of PN is reduced in proportion to the severity of the illness (i.e., infection, ileus, systemic inflammatory response syndrome, inability to wean off mechanical ventilation)[166] and the onset of complications. Starvation beyond 7 to 10 days will result in complications related to protein malnutrition.

A significant increase in morbidity in the postoperative patient is seen when associated with preoperative weight loss. As previously mentioned, this also bears a strong association with increased postoperative and 1-year mortality rates.[167]

Evaluation of Clinical Data

Evaluation of nine PRCTs involving over 700 general surgery and cardiac postoperative patients to whom TPN was routinely given regardless of nutritional status showed that this practice increased the overall risk of complications by 10% without statistical differences in mortality. In the assessment of this statement, it is imperative to recognize that the TPN delivered to each of these patients was not only not optimal in both calories and protein administered but also far in excess of needs based on present understanding of nutritional requirements in terms of calories.[44] These complications of hyperglycemia and overfeeding distracted from the potential benefits that could have been provided had its use involved current discretions. Patients received calories in the range 132 to 263% of their actual needs while the protein delivery was often below (46 to 100%) currently accepted levels of repletion in five of nine groups (Table 10–4).

In a different subset of patients, those with gastrointestinal fistulas, before the use of TPN, mortality was commonly secondary to electrolyte and fluid losses, malnutrition, and peritonitis.[168] Though the efficacy of TPN has not been established with PRCTs, one retrospective study of patients with small bowel fistulas noted higher rates of spontaneous and surgical closure and lower mortality rates[169] with its use.

Four PRCTs evaluating early postoperative jejunostomy tube feeding in patients with gastrointestinal carcinoma demonstrated no major differences in postoperative morbidity and mortality in comparison to regular diets.[116, 170–172] One PRCT using glutamine dipeptide–enriched TPN postoperatively in patients undergoing elective abdominal surgery demonstrated significantly better nitrogen balance and a 6.2-day-shorter stay than in the control group.[173]

Various amino acids are used for specific roles in aiding patients' recovery. When provided to a group of patients undergoing major elective surgery,[49] formulations enriched with arginine, ribonucleic acid (in the form of uracil), and n-3 fatty acids have resulted in fewer infections, fewer wound complications, and a decreased length of stay in the hospital in comparison with a standard formula. When n-3 fatty acids were used in perioperative cancer patients, an improvement in renal and hepatic function along with a low incidence of infections was noted.[174] Branched-chain amino acids have been shown to improve nitrogen balance, and in patients with compromised renal function, a reduction in ureageneis is seen. Arginine has an immunostimulatory role and appears to be involved in aiding immunocyte stimulation through second messenger nitric oxide.[49, 175] A clinical trial evaluating arginine's role in abetting an improved outcome is awaited. Uracil itself is known to aid in the proliferation of intestinal crypt cells, lymphocytic proliferation, and cellular RNA and DNA synthesis. Glutamine, the most widely found amino acid in the body, appears to have a host of functions including the maintenance of enterocyte and immunocyte function and is discussed later.

In the orthopedic population two studies merit mention. Based on anthropometric measurements on admission, 122 of 744 patients who were classified as more than 1

Table 10–4. Prospective Randomized Controlled Trials Evaluating Preoperative Total Parenteral Nutrition

Reference	First Authors	Nonprotein Calories (kcal/kg/day) [% of goal]	Nitrogen (g/kg/day) [% of goal]	Lipids (kcal/kg/day)	End-Point	Complications Control (%)	Complications TPN (%)	Mortality Control (%)	Mortality TPN (%)
		Goal: 19 [100]	Goal: 0.24 [100]						
176	Abel	16–25 [84–132]	0.11 [46]	0	Total complications	29.2	80.0	12.5	20.0
48	Brennan	30–35 [158–184]	0.15 [63]	10	Major complications	22.8	45.0	1.8	6.7
177	Preshaw	40 [211]	0.16 [67]	6.4	Anastomosis leak	17.4	33.0	0.0	0.0
178	Sandstrom	29 [153]	0.27 [113]	8.6	Sepsis	16.0	27.3	6.7	8.0
179	Woolfson	35 [184]	0.20 [83]	4	Anastomosis leak	6.7	9.7	13.3	12.0
14	Holter	30 [158]	0.20 [83]	0	Major complication	19.2	13.3	7.6	6.6
180	Jensen	40–50 [211–263]	0.24–32 [100–133]	0	Major complication	40.0	10.0	0.0	0.0
181	Collins	37 [195]	0.23 [96]	0	Slow healing	90.0	20.0	0.0	0.0
182	Reily	35 [184]	0.24 [100]	6.2	ICU stay	NR	NR	20.0	5.6

ICU, intensive care unit; NR, not reported; TPN, total parenteral nutrition; [ ], Numbers in brackets reflect percentage of current recommended nutrients fed to patients.

standard deviation below mean weight, were randomized to receive a regular diet and 1000 kcal plus 28 g of protein by nocturnal nasogastric feeding or regular diet alone, and demonstrated a shorter time to rehabilitation and a reduction in the time to independent mobility as well as decreased lengths of stay in the hospital along with a reduction in mortality. The second study demonstrated a decreased length of stay in the hospital and fewer short- and long-term complications in elderly women with femoral neck fractures provided once-a-day nutritional supplementation with meals compared with hospital meals alone.[183, 184]

Other specific subsets of postoperative patients require tailoring of formulas to their unique requirements, as described in the following sections.

Critically Ill Postoperative Patients

In the critically ill postoperative patient, even more important than addressing protein support, it is often necessary to address a deranged metabolic state in which astute TPN management can play a critical and very successful role. With progressively sophisticated means and a better understanding of managing the critically ill, appropriate patient care entrusts the caregivers to practice nutritional and metabolic support judiciously.

Initially developed for the delivery of protein and calories, hyperalimentation has evolved into a powerful multifaceted metabolic corrective tool, playing a crucial role in the early postoperative care of critically ill patients with severe metabolic derangements. A single 1-L or even smaller volume bag of PN can provide necessary electrolytes for homeostasis, protons or buffers for acid-base balance, and compatible medications, which combined can uniquely aid in strict fluid control while helping to minimize the catabolic effect of stress.

Nutritional support in the critically ill patient should aim at achieving a nitrogen balance that is less negative, rather than overtly positive. Placing a critically ill patient into positive nitrogen balance is often not feasible or possible and should not necessarily be the goal of TPN in the intensive care unit setting. The efforts of metabolic and nutritional support at this point should be to aid in achieving metabolic control and correcting the immediate problems of vol-

ume overload, hyponatremia, hypocalcemia, hypoalbuminemia secondary to redistributive phenomena, severe acid-base disturbances (including alkalosis associated with aggressive diuretic therapy), and the insulin resistance of stress. Babineau and coworkers concluded that PN in fact often becomes necessary to correct these metabolic abnormalities in patients with postoperative complications after cardiopulmonary bypass.[185] A minimal-volume bag of PN can have a maximal impact, correcting severe acid-base disturbances while simultaneously providing a baseline tissue-sparing protein delivery mechanism and minimizing LBM catabolism and consequential severe negative nitrogen balance (Table 10–5).

Surgical patients necessarily burdened with excess fluid not uncommonly require pharmacologic diuresis, which can result in severe metabolic alkalosis. Large bowel di-

Table 10–5. Minimal Volume–Maximal Impact: 1 L of A7–8%, D14–21%

Protein: 70–80 g
Carbohydrates: 140–210 g
Maintenance electrolytes: usually low sodium but always patient specific
Maintenance multivitamins and minerals
Acid-base homeostasis
  Acidoses: bicarbonate delivery as sodium or potassium acetate
  Alkalosis: HCl delivery*

pH	HCl (mEq/L)
7.50–7.51	50
7.52–7.53	75–100
>7.54	100–125

Compatible medications
  Insulin
  Antacid prophylaxis: H$_2$-receptor blockers
  DVT prophylaxis: low-dose heparin
  Steroids
  Aminophylline
  Pharmacologic doses of micronutrients
    Thiamine
    Folic acid
    Zinc

Vitamin K, 10 mg, should be given once a week subcutaneously.

*HCl delivery requires closely monitored setting (usually in the ICU) with frequent blood gas analysis (maybe venous).

HCl amount required may also be calculated in terms of base excess, using the following formula: [body weight (kg) × 0.6] × [serum HCO$_3$ − 24] (0.5 is used for females).

Two important issues regarding HCl infusion merit attention.

HCl delivery >150 meq/L has been demonstrated to result in catheter damage.

Lipids and HCl do not mix. The combination results in cracking of the emulsion and potentially lethal fat embolization).

DVT, deep venous thrombosis; ICU, intensive care unit.

arrhea, large nasogastric losses, or large volume blood transfusions with a massive citrate burden are other well-known conditions that may also result in a similar change. Progressive metabolic alkalosis that does not respond to the first-line treatment of chloride replacement as normal saline usually requiring large volumes warrants the use of hydrochloric acid. A pH above 7.5 is physiologically unacceptable, and as a potentially lethal entity with the increased risk of therapy-resistant ventricular tachyarrthymmias, it demands that corrective measures be instituted.

Acidosis can just as commonly upset the internal milieu and can be caused by a host of factors, many resulting in reduced tissue perfusion. The first line of therapy for this acidosis is fluid resuscitation; effective tissue perfusion often requires pharmacologic approaches. If these are unsuccessful in controlling pH, acetate can be added to the TPN bag. Of primary importance is determination of the cause of the pH disturbance, which must be meticulously sought and an attempt made to rectify it before giving exogenous aid.

Metabolic acidosis is known to favor proteolysis, stimulating essential branched-chain amino acid and muscle protein degradation in the presence of glucocorticoids. Glucocorticoids are responsible for the increase in messenger RNA's encoding ubiquitin and proteosome subunits. The ubiquitin-proteosome mechanism of protein breakdown is how this muscle proteolysis is carried out.[186–189]

The purpose of exogenous protein is to provide amino acids for the synthesis of acute-phase proteins and other components of the stress-immune response. Protein calories should be included in the total caloric delivery formula, as the amino acids delivered are not used for net protein synthesis in the early postoperative period, even if adequate nonprotein calories are provided in the form of carbohydrate and lipid. During this early stage of stress, protein is shunted toward caloric utilization, and as often occurs in the recovery phase, only a small fraction of the administered amino acids are used for net protein synthesis.[24] Some of the metabolic abnormalities common to the postoperative period, including insulin glucose resistance and decreased utilization of fat as a calorie source, help to explain the excess protein degradation

noted during stress, that is, amino acids are used as a source of energy.[190]

Several investigators have demonstrated tolerance of and unimpaired metabolism with lipid administration in the critically ill.[191–193] A significant reduction in arterial oxygen tension and increases in mean pulmonary artery pressures have been noted during fat emulsion infusions in patients with acute respiratory distress syndrome, warranting caution in patients experiencing marginal respiratory function.[191] Though this is transient and levels return to preinfusion numbers, adequate tissue oxygenation should be ensured. Lipids should to be used as a source of additional calories to help meet energy requirements, allowing a reduction in the dextrose load with concomitantly less concern for hyperglycemia. The maximal rate of lipid infusion tolerated is usually under 0.11 mg/kg/h without the deleterious effects of impaired reticuloendothelial system dysfunction and subsequent potential increases in infection rates.[192, 193]

As part of the metabolic and immune support provided by nutritional delivery in the postoperative setting, monitoring of its efficacy and the adequacy of delivery is necessary. Lack of early improvement in the critically ill patient also demands scrutiny of each aspect of patient care. At this point, assessment of the resting energy expenditure becomes necessary. The added burden of abetting the difficult-to-wean ventilator-dependent patient by overfeeding must be recognized early and corrective steps to optimize nutritional delivery taken, obviating further dietary-provoked exacerbations of respiratory dysfunction.

Historically, the Harris-Benedict equation has been used to determine the energy expenditure of a patient, although even when a stress factor is added into the equation, the values obtained have remained overestimates, often resulting in overfeeding of the critically ill. Makk and coworkers have demonstrated poor correlation between values obtained by metabolic cart and calculations from the Harris-Benedict equation.[194]

Energy requirements may be measured by indirect calorimetry or by calculations using the cardiac output (measured by thermodilution) and the arterial–mixed venous oxygen difference using the reverse-Fick technique.[195] Metabolic cart measurements of oxygen consumption and carbon dioxide production by indirect calorimetry provide the most accurate determinations of energy expenditure as well as the RQ determination, based on the modified Weir formula, whereas the thermodilution technique lacks accuracy. An RQ greater than 1 is indicative of carbohydrate excess in nutritional delivery, necessitating a reduction in the dextrose load. Appropriate formulations delivering mixed fuels correlate with an ideal RQ of 0.82 to 0.83. Limiting carbohydrate delivery to 4 mg/kg/min precludes increased carbon dioxide production with the accompanying increased minute ventilation and work of breathing. Very large or very small patients, those with a marked increase in ECW (TBW overloaded), or ventilator-dependent patients also make ideal candidates for the metabolic cart.

Twenty-four-hour measurements of urinary nitrogen loss allow calculation of a patient's nitrogen balance and aid as a guide toward improved protein delivery, preventing underestimation of protein requirements.

Interestingly, the plasma amino acid pattern of sepsis is similar to that in liver failure. Although aromatic amino acid levels are elevated, the branched chain amino acid levels are low to normal (decreased in liver failure).[196] Whether manipulation of these ratios through basic alterations in catabolic cycles is one of the keys to potentially influencing outcomes through specialized nutritive delivery needs to be studied. Knowledge of the mechanisms of the catabolic processes in stress including manipulation of fixed reductions in IS along with changes in fluid dynamics and nutrient distributions as well as losses may in the future allow interceding before activation of this cascade.

In summary, the central strategy remains unchanged, with the aims of providing a minimal volume–maximal impact PN bag that will effect a metabolic balance through an exacting pH and electrolyte management strategy while simultaneously reducing the obligatory nitrogen loss with protein-calorie delivery.

Recent trends toward early enteral feeding in the intensive care unit population with specialized enteral formulations aimed at attenuating the inflammatory response have been seen, based on studies demonstrating a reduction in postoperative complications.[197] Variations in fat emulsions have evolved with newer formulations incorporating medium-chain triglycerides and n-3 fatty acids. Sufficiently strong data exist demonstrating improved outcomes with use of both lipids in the critically ill postoperative patient population. The n-3 lipids' immunomodulatory role altering prostanoid and leukotriene production to less inflammatory products has been well elucidated. Their rapid substitution for arachidonic acid in cellular membranes resulting in production of the 3-prostanoids and the 5-leukotriene product lines has demonstrated a significant improvement in septic postoperative patients.[49, 174] EN supplemented with fish oil has reduced the complications and length of stay in burn patients, while the use of fish oil with arginine and nucleotides decreased infections and the hospital length of stay in GI oncology patients.[49, 198] A multicenter trial of similar EN preparations in critically ill patients provided further evidence of beneficial effects with a reduced length of stay in the hospital.[199] Once multiorgan failure is established, enteral feeding makes no difference in the outcomes, and in fact Raina and associates have demonstrated increased damage and mucosal permeability in rats infused with tumor necrosis factor[197] and given early EN. Babineau and colleagues hypothesize that hyperlipasemia may be a better marker for intolerance to early enteral feeding in patients after cardiopulmonary bypass when compared with hyperamylasemia.[200]

Maintenance of the integrity of the gut mucosal barrier is an important aspect of the well state, and breakdowns in this barrier during critical illness are felt to be involved in the pathogenesis and continued exacerbation of SIRS. The enterocyte uses both luminal substrates (short-chain fatty acids in the colon) and glutamine systemically to support its function. Studies in bone marrow patients receiving glutamine-supplemented TPN have demonstrated improved outcomes as mentioned later.[201]

Diabetes

Strict blood sugar control is important for reasons previously detailed. Pomposelli and associates[114] demonstrated a clear reduction in nosocomial infections in diabetic patients able to maintain blood sugar levels less than 220 mg/dL[202] in the immediate postoperative period. Values over this are associated with immunologic suppression including poor granulocyte function. In a study by

Rady and colleagues, early postoperative hyperglycemia in patients older than 75 years undergoing cardiac surgery was a significant predictor of early postoperative mortality.[203] Patients who died in the early postoperative period demonstrated a 39% rate of nosocomial infections compared with 5% in survivors. In a retrospective study of over 8900 patients undergoing cardiac surgery, Zarr and coworkers demonstrated a 1.7% versus 0.4% rate of deep wound infections in diabetic (18% of total) versus nondiabetic patients.[204] This rate was six times higher in patients who on postoperative day 1 had blood glucose levels over 250 mg/dL as opposed to those maintained between 100 and 150 mg/dL. Interestingly, with maintenance of strict glycemic control over the last 3 years of the study, the rate of deep wound infections was impressively reduced from 2.8% (5 years before change) to 0.74%, whereas no change was observed in the nondiabetic group over the same period (0.4% vs. 0.38%). A review by Khaodhiar and colleagues examining the current studies concludes that hyperglycemia in the early postoperative period is clearly associated with a rate of infection considerably higher than in those patients remaining euglycemic during the same period.[205] Likening healing areas of myocardial infarct to surgical wounds with respect to immune function, the Diabetes Insulin-Glucose in Acute Myocardial Infarction study involved patients with acute myocardial infarctions (AMIs) who were randomly assigned to strict blood sugar control versus usual therapy. Marked reductions in 1-year mortality by 30% and sustained reductions to 11% over long-term follow-up in the group with fastidious control of their blood sugar were found.[206]

Sometimes the brittle diabetic patient and the occasional postoperative diabetic patient make adequate control of blood sugar with sliding scale insulin ineffectual, necessitating either a reduction in the dextrose load, which then becomes difficult without reducing the protein delivery in the TPN, or the initiation of a continuous intravenous insulin infusion until blood sugar levels are well controlled. When this happens, at the time of preparation of the next bag of hyperalimentation, two thirds of the previous 24-hours' total amount of administered insulin may be added to the new preparation. Initial hourly monitoring of blood sugar levels and appropriate titration of the insulin infusion

is required until satisfactory euglycemic control is attained.

Simultaneously, it is important to ascertain that poor glucose control is not due to a hypovolemic state or poor peripheral circulation, common in postoperative patients, impeding the absorption of subcutaneously administered regular insulin.

Perioperative Insulin Sensitivity and Implications

Using the hyperinsulinemic clamp technique, Thorell and colleagues have shown that IS shows a marked variation in the healthy nondiabetic individual.[138, 206a] More importantly, the relative reduction in IS after a given operation is quite reproducible with a coefficient of variation down to 12.3% or less. With moderate operative trauma, a reduction in IS occurs by postoperative day 1, lasting until day 5 and taking up to 3 weeks to return to normal.

Three other observations that may permanently change the perioperative management of the surgical patient include the following:

1. The postoperative reduction in IS demonstrates a dose-response relationship to the degree of trauma and is not related to the age, body weight, length of the procedure, or known preoperative sensitivity.
2. Ljungqvist and colleagues[138] found that in patients undergoing hip replacement, a continuous glucose-insulin infusion intraoperatively abolished the usually reproducibly expected postoperative reduction in IS.
3. Significant correlation with the decrease in IS seen on postoperative day 1 can be made with the length of the hospital stay.

This finding of a reduction in the expected postoperative IS with preoperative glucose infusion provides further supporting evidence, along with the inotropic effect of glucose-insulin-potassium (GIK) infusion in perioperative cardiac surgery patients, for a crucial role of insulin in the perioperative period. Somehow, insulin seems to attenuate the characteristic obligatory postoperative catabolic response of the surgical patient.

Reduced IS, fixed and predictable after a defined procedure, and the means to abolish this expected fall and therefore a reduction in postoperative complications by preoperative glucose loading, are being re-examined under different conditions, including surgery in abdominal and cardiac surgery patients. If this understanding stands up to strict clinical scrutiny, then its applicability may have a far-reaching impact and widespread implications for the care of the surgical patient.

Cardiac Surgical Patients

Sodi-Pollares over 35 years ago first reported the beneficial "membrane-stabilizing" effects of a GIK infusion on limiting electrocardiographic changes in patients with AMI.[207] Conflicting data later discouraged its widespread use with the biochemical reasoning that glucose may be cytotoxic if NADH reoxidation does not occur.

Since then, work investigating these solutions has demonstrated the reduction of inhouse mortality from AMIs and enhanced recovery and decreased mortality after various elective and urgent aortocoronary bypass procedures, including cases of pump (left ventricular) failure.[116, 117, 208–211] GIK has also been utilized for recurrent chest pain in chronic angina pectoris[212] and improvement in decreased left ventricular function in acute ischemia.

There are several studies, including the meta-analysis of Fath-Ordoubadi and Beatt, outlining the benefits of GIK infusion in AMI with mortality reductions ranging from 28% to 48%.[208–210] Demonstrating a dose-response relationship, high doses (Rackley regimen[213]) of the GIK formula appear to correlate with the greater mortality reduction of 48%. This appears to be in concordance with the recognized effect of maximal suppression of circulating free fatty acid (FFA) levels and suppression of myocardial FFA uptake with high-dose GIK. Recognized as toxic to the ischemic myocardium and associated with an increased incidence of arrhythmias, FFAs depress cardiac function. A landmark PRCT further reiterated the benefits of GIK in AMI, demonstrating a 66% relative reduction of in-house mortality when used in conjunction with thrombolytic therapy.[211]

In similar fashion as infusing GIK, glycogen loading of the heart before hypothermic ischemic arrest has been found to improve tolerance to ischemia.[118, 122] Prospective randomized trials with the control group receiving a standard protocol have shown improvement in cardiac parameters (40% increase in cardiac index), a shorter time of ventilator support, less weight gain and inotrope use, a reduced incidence of arrhythmias, and shorter intensive care unit and hospital stays in patients after urgent coronary bypass surgery.[116] Patients with traditionally high mortality from refractory left ventricular failure after cardiopulmonary bypass have similarly demonstrated significant improvement in cardiac parameters and required less inotropic support with use of the GIK solution.[117]

The low-flow (as opposed to the long-held notion of no-flow) ischemia demonstrated in perfusion studies of patients with an AMI have revealed residual perfusion adequate to maintain substrate delivery and to wash out lactate from the myocardium. With critical circulation available, the GIK can be effective in delivering an increased glycolytic flux and thus increased intracellular ATP to the cardiac myocyte. The consequence of this is the preservation of moiety-conserved cycles due to the protection of efficient energy transfer cycles usually lost with ischemia. The use of the large amounts of insulin to overcome the stress-induced insulin resistance with the large doses of glucose is the reason for the effectiveness of GIK therapy and its resulting improved outcomes. This is of particular value in the maintenance of critical membrane function including calcium and sodium homeostasis, adding an element of myocyte protection to the toxic effects of the elevations in intracellular calcium found during hypoxic states. This substrate enhancement with a glucose-potassium solution appears to have a significant role in limiting myocardial necrosis.

Current thought advocates a cardioprotective role for insulin in ischemia and reperfusion injury, responsible for an earlier return to aerobic metabolism via increased pyruvate dehydrogenase activity. In vitro studies with human myocytes support this avenue of thought. Notably, glucose alone has been found to result in greater cellular injury.[119]

In our own preliminary (unpublished) experience with metabolic modulation in postoperative coronary artery bypass graft patients, low-dose glucose, potassium, and 70 g of protein appears to achieve insulin levels similar to those seen with GIK infusion. Preliminary data show increases in the cardiac output and index from 20% to 60% within 4 to 12 hours of beginning TPN.

The use of amino acids in cardiac surgery has been based on their salutary effects on the arrested heart intraoperatively, and thus aspartate and glutamate are used in enriched blood cardioplegic solutions.[214–221] Krebs cycle intermediates lost during ischemia are replenished primarily by amino acid or carbohydrate substrates. With the systemic neuroendocrine stress response activated and causing insulin resistance, glucose uptake is impeded. With the rapid utilization of the next available substrate, amino acid levels are subsequently found to be diminished,[222, 223] and therefore it would be logical for amino acids to have an important role in the recovery of myocardial oxidative metabolism. The addition of amino acids to a GIK-type of solution, then, would potentially provide gluconeogenetic precursors, and thus their benefit may in fact be synergistic to the recognized effects of GIK alone. Their role in protein synthesis may prove to be of less importance, and the real utility of amino acids appears to be as important metabolic intermediates in the Krebs cycle. Glutamate, aspartate, arginine, and ornithine are the main Krebs cycle amino acids because of their close association with the malate-aspartate shuttle and the transport of reducing equivalents across the mitochondria.

Based on the above basic science, amino acids appear to play a role in the recovery of oxidative metabolism after ischemia,[224, 225] this idea being strengthened by the finding of a relative shortage of glutamate after cardiac surgery.[222, 223] In agreement with this concept, postoperative glutamate infusion has been shown to improve the metabolic and functional state of the heart after routine coronary artery bypass grafting and also in postoperative heart failure.[227]

Interestingly, in another study, patients with postoperative refractory heart failure after hypothermic ischemic arrest treated with GIK demonstrated a reduction of in-house mortality from 26.6% to 17.6% compared with controls, and a third group treated with GIK plus amino acids had an even lower in-house mortality of 13.9%. Svedjeholm and associates have gone further to advocate metabolic support as a more efficacious mode of therapy in the treatment of postoperative heart failure in the place of current treatments utilizing inotropes and mechanical assistive devices.[228]

Babineau and colleagues retrospectively reviewed over 4000 patients who had undergone cardiopulmonary bypass, of which approximately 5% developed complications, necessitating the institution of TPN support. These patients were found to be older, with a higher prevalence of diabetes and multiple metabolic derangements including volume overload, hyperglycemia, hyponatremia, alkalosis, and uremia, compounded by marked hypotension requiring pharmacologic support in the early postoperative period.[185]

In regard to enteral feedings after bypass surgery, hyperlipasemia has been found to be a marker of intolerance to EN, as discussed by Babineau and coworkers.[200] This syndrome appears to be distinct from the postpump pancreatitis seen after cardiopulmonary bypass. Bowel infarction secondary to low-flow states after bypass in patients on pressor therapy is another dreaded complication of enteral feeding in this subset.

It remains to be seen if substrate enhancement may be extended to other surgical subgroups to achieve similar positive outcomes.

Hepatic and Renal Disease

Nutritional and other therapy in hepatic failure is often a play for time until regeneration allows a return of normal function. Fulminant hepatic failure, usually viral or secondary to toxic hepatitis, may benefit from nutritional support before transplantation, as such support may reduce protein depletion, allowing an improved immune status after transplantation.

In patients with hypermetabolism such as liver failure and kidney failure, branched-chain amino acids decrease postinjury catabolism and muscle amino acid mobilization and oxidation, and increase hepatic protein synthesis in a dose-dependent fashion.[213] In patients with acute renal failure, branched-chain amino acids have shown an inhibitory effect on ureagenesis. The acidotic milieu responsible for the irreversible breakdown of branched-chain amino acids in patients with renal failure is glucocorticoid-dependent and proceeds through the ubiquitin-proteosome proteolytic pathway.

Improved outcomes with the use of branched-chain amino acids in patients with end-stage liver disease developing hepatic encephalopathy have been through a significant reduction in "wake-up time" compared with other regimens, noted in a 1989 meta-analysis.[229] In a prospective study of 124 patients undergoing partial hepatectomy for hepatocellular carcinoma, Fan and associates randomized 64 patients to receive PN in addition to an oral diet for a 14-day perioperative period while a control group of 60 patients received a hospital diet.[148] The parenteral solution consisted of a 35% branched-chain amino acid–enriched and aromatic amino acid–deficient solution. An overall decrease in postoperative morbidity (34% vs. 55%) in the PN group was found and noted to be statistically significant largely because of fewer septic complications (17% vs. 37%), while mortality was also reduced (5 patients vs. 9 patients). A reduction in diuretic use, weight loss, and hepatic enzymes in the group provided with PN was also observed. Both a U.S. multicenter trial and an Italian trial demonstrated statistical differences in survival with branched-chain amino acid–enriched solutions when compared with neomycin and lactulose therapy, respectively, in critically ill patients with hepatic encephalopathy.[230, 231]

Solid Organ Transplantation

The nutritional status of patients with end-organ failure awaiting transplantation is an important issue. Patients awaiting kidney transplantation may be on the waiting list for months to years before an organ is available. In the ensuing period, marked metabolic and nutritional changes resulting from poor intake and increased catabolic processes are noted.

Most liver transplantation patients suffer from malnutrition.[232–234] This appears to translate to a direct increase in morbidity and mortality after transplantation.[235] Pikul and colleagues retrospectively evaluated 68 liver transplantation recipients, finding a 79% incidence of malnutrition that correlated with an increase in the number of days on the ventilator and in the intensive care unit and hospital.[236] Another review of 500 transplantation patients found an overall malnutrition incidence of 70%.[237] Though liver transplantation patients are not hypermetabolic, studies have shown large urinary nitrogen losses to continue well into the post-transplantation period, and despite gradual nutritional and clinical improvements, the patients continue to have negative balance when they have been measured.[238, 239]

The problems of end-stage organ disease are compounded by the associated cachexia. For example, cardiac cachexia is a well-known entity in candidates awaiting heart transplantation. The anorexia of uremia associated with end-stage renal disease is also a commonly recognized entity. Often oral intake is limited, engendered by the nature of the disease. Early satiety, anorexia, nausea, vomiting, and diarrhea may be a result of restrictions imposed by the disease process. In transplantation with these problems and consequently, inadequate oral intake, enteral feeding is the preferred route, with PN used in patients with intestinal intolerance.

Wicks and colleagues[94] have shown early enteral feeding to be as effective as TPN after transplantation and along with Hasse and associates[240] found it to be well tolerated. Highlighting the immunomodulatory effects of n-3 fatty acids, animal models have demonstrated the increased survival time of kidney and heart transplants after infusion or luminal feeding of these preparations. After kidney transplantation, human studies have demonstrated increased graft vascularity and function with a reduction in cyclosporine nephrotoxicity as well as a reduced rate of rejection with fish oil supplementation.[241–244] In a prospective randomized trial with the control group receiving a standard hospital diet, Reilly and colleagues have shown that the metabolic support provided by TPN may decrease morbidity and shorten the length of stay in the intensive care unit in liver transplantation recipients.[182]

Patients receiving bone marrow transplants deserve mention. When assessed for transplantation, these patients are generally well nourished, but complications from chemotherapy and radiotherapy toxicity; graft-versus-host disease; and infections result in severe catabolism, marked by negative nitrogen balance, hyperglycemia, and hypertriglyceridemia. Especially in this population, the gut may play a significant role as a portal for bacterial entry into the blood, and with the severe gastrointestinal side effects of therapy, EN is often not an early consideration. At the time of transplantation, these patients require PN, and though the effect is not repeatedly reproducible, glutamine supplementation may provide improved mucosal integrity.[201]

Overall short-term nutritional complications remain similar to those of the nontransplanted surgical population. Long-term nutritional and metabolic issues after transplantation, including hyperlipidemia, hypertension, obesity, osteoporosis, diabetes, and accelerated heart and atherosclerotic disease, are only now coming to the forefront with appreciable improvements in survival because of refinements in immunosuppressive regimens. With research and advancements (in metabolism and nutrition) directed at making immunosuppressor regimens more efficacious, improvements in patient metabolic and long-term nutritional status and decreased morbidity can be expected.

Trauma

In now-classic studies, Moore and Kudsk and coworkers[101, 164, 165] have shown that early EN provided to patients with abdominal trauma is associated with significantly fewer septic complications than in patients receiving PN. Trice and associates reiterated this in their own meta-analysis, similarly comparing patients receiving TPN or EN.[245]

A recent PRCT evaluating glutamine-enriched EN versus a nonsupplemented enteral feeding in patients with multiple trauma demonstrated far fewer episodes of pneumonia (17% vs. 45%), bacteremia (7% vs. 42%), and sepsis (3% vs. 26%) in the patients on the supplemented regimen, though the length of hospital stay and the number of days on a ventilator did not differ significantly.[246] Developments in immune-modulating diets appear to be demonstrating reproducible benefits. Better immune function, a decreased rate of septic complications, and a reduced length of stay in the hospital, including the time in the intensive care unit have all been demonstrated, whereas withholding EN is clearly associated with the highest rates of infection.

The immunologic basis for the association of EN with the lower rate of infection appears to be the mucosal immunity conferred by the Peyer's patches of the GALT. Sensitized to intraluminal antigens, B and T lymphocytes multiply in the mesenteric lymph nodes, followed by systemic dissemination, including into the lamina propria of the intestine. The resulting area-specific IgA production provides protection against mucosal invasion.

It is here that immune-enhancing TPN may have a role with the addition of glutamine to the TPN. Attenuation of TPN-induced GALT atrophy and improved respiratory tract immunity have been shown with glutamine supplementation.[247] Whether this correlates with clinical improvement and improves patient outcomes remains to be seen. Widespread use will need peer-reviewed evaluation through prospective randomized controlled studies.

◆ IMMUNO AND METABOLIC MODULATORS

Glutamine

Glutamine and growth hormone (GH) are both known to enhance skeletal muscle protein synthesis, upregulate the immune system, and enhance enterocyte proliferation in the gastrointestinal tract. Glutamine is essential as an enterocyte and immune cell metabolic substrate, and studies appear to categorize it as a conditionally essential amino acid in the stressed catabolic state. It is recognized to play a fundamental role in the metabolic adaptation to injury, and it is important as fuel for all rapidly dividing cells, serving as a precursor for glutathione, pyrimidine, and purine synthesis. Glutamine is also used as an aid in bowel adaptation, especially in the premature infant.

A glutamine source, ornithine α-ketoglutarate, has been demonstrated to improve gut morphology and function, reduce trauma-induced immunosuppression, and have an antiproteolytic effect on catabolism while maintaining a potent sparing effect on endogenous glutamine pools. In animal studies, oral α-ketoglutarate has demonstrated a protective effect on intestinal function in orthotopic bowel transplantation, and those subjected to abdominal irradiation showed both an increased protein synthesis rate and a significant reduction in bacterial translocation.

In clinical studies there is evidence that glutamine-supplemented nutrition may be beneficial to injured and postoperative patients. Bone marrow transplantation patients have been the only group in which there has been consistently demonstrated improved clinical outcome such as decreased infections and decreased hospital length of stay.[201]

Growth Hormone

With the frustrating realization that nutritional support alone will not maintain LBM in the early postoperative period, attention turned to pharmacologic adjuncts, most prominent of which included GH and insulin-like growth factor I (IGF-I). IGF-I mediates the metabolic and anabolic effects of GH, the clinically most important of which is the increased rate of protein synthesis. GH also enhances the mobilization of fat stores for energy during periods of stress, and IGF-I promotes amino acid incorporation and cellular proliferation and attenuates proteolysis in skeletal muscle and liver.

It is clear that GH, IGF-I, insulin, and glucocorticoids have a complex interplay acting with and by means of the proinflammatory cytokines tumor necrosis factor, interleukin 1, and interleukin 6 in the complex catabolic show of proteolysis after surgery, after trauma, and with sepsis. These cytokines affect IGF-I production by the liver by attenuating the ability of GH to stimulate IGF-I production.[248, 249] Nutritional status appears to have a critical role in how this is regulated (i.e., IGF-I synthesis is reduced by nutrient restriction and stimulated by refeeding) through transcription and post-transcriptional changes in IGF-I gene expression.

Initial studies in healthy volunteers provided hypocaloric diets demonstrated nitrogen retention and weight gain with GH administration. This efficacy waned with time and appeared to be inversely proportional to the degree of caloric restriction, thus showing that the maximal benefit of GH in trauma and septic patients must include complete nutritional support.[250]

Mean baseline GH concentrations are clearly elevated in critically ill fasted patients, but unlike healthy individuals, who show a reduction in GH levels after the administration of TPN, the GH levels remain elevated in critically ill patients.[251] What was originally felt to be partial GH resistance, initially described in septic patients in whom exogenous GH failed to elevate serum IGF-I levels, now appears to be characterized as a down-regulation of GH receptor messenger RNA expression, in both liver and skeletal muscle as noted in the trauma of surgery.[252, 253] Postreceptor resistance to IGF-I inhibition of protein breakdown, a mechanism similar to that of insulin resistance, is noted in rat muscle in sepsis.[254] Current ongoing research is aimed at identifying the specific mechanisms of IGF-I resistance in sepsis-stimulated muscle catabolism and potential similarities with the insulin resistance of stress.

In a PRCT, the postoperative use of GH for 8 days demonstrated improved nitrogen balance, enhanced humoral and cellular immunity, and a reduction in wound infections and the length of the hospital stay.[255] A similar trial in septic surgical patients on TPN receiving GH demonstrated a reduction in net protein catabolism compared with a similar group receiving only TPN.[256]

In the pediatric population with over 40% burns, Herndon and associates have shown that through an increase in IGF-I receptors in the wound, GH in fact accelerated donor site healing and wound closure time, increased muscle strength, and decreased hospital costs by 25%.[257, 258] Similar though less dramatic results have been obtained in the adult burn population.[259]

Jauck has suggested a reduction in the time to recovery for the postoperative elderly (>80 years) population after operative procedures for hip fractures with the use of GH compared with those given placebos.[260]

More recently, speculation that the administration of GH may limit endogenous skeletal muscle glutamine availability during critical illness has been met with concern.[261] Two randomized placebo-controlled trials in a large European multicenter setting in which critically ill postoperative patients were administered GH demonstrated a twofold increase in mortality compared with the placebo group. Whether limiting glutamine availability or in fact other mechanisms were responsible for the deleterious effects in septic patients remains to be seen.[262]

Among certain design flaws noted in the study, two appear to be the most important. First, the GH dosage administered was 0.08 mg/kg/day instead of the more common dose of 0.03 mg/kg/day (the latter a commonly used pharmacologic dose). Second, the timing of administration was felt to be early in the course of the illness when GH is known to have deleterious effects on splanchnic blood flow.[263, 264]

Other undesirable effects of GH administration include fluid retention, hyperglycemia, and hypercalcemia, and there are constant concerns about stimulating preexisting or new neoplasms.

Inappropriately written preoperative hyperalimentation prescriptions often result in artificial disturbances in water and salt metabolism, correlating with a greater incidence of postoperative complications.[47, 124, 125] The use of GH as an aid to prevent against ECW expansion continues with conflicting results, some studies demonstrating benefit[265, 266] and others not.[267, 268]

Although previous clinical trials with GH and IGF-I have suggested clinical utility in enhancing protein metabolism, Wilmore advocates that to obtain the optimal effect of these anabolic agents one must have peak delivery of all substrates including amino acids, calories, and micronutrients while ensuring adequate tissue oxygenation, preventing organ dysfunction.[261]

Intravenous infusion of IGF-I has also been shown to improve nitrogen balance in malnourished persons, and its administration in burned or septic rats appears to improve the gut barrier by preventing atrophy,[250, 269] though no clinical trials in critically ill humans are available.

It appears that GH and IGF-I certainly may have benefits in some patient populations, but their dynamics appear to be broad and not well understood. Prior to general use in perioperative patients, large strides in elucidating their specific biochemical spectrum of activity must be made.

Designer or Structured Lipids

Medium-chain triglycerides (MCTs) have numerous desirable qualities including not requiring micellar formation for absorption from the gut lumen, being rapidly hydrolyzed, and not requiring the presence of bile or pancreatic lipase for digestion or absorption. They rapidly enter the portal vein bound to albumin and, without a need for carnitine, are readily transported into mitochondria for rapid oxidation. Most importantly, they do not promote eicosanoid synthesis or serve as precursors for oxygen free radical production, and they have nitrogen-sparing effects owing to their efficacy as a fuel. Because they are not significantly stored in adipose tissue or accumulated in the liver, their use avoids the pitfalls of cholestasis, steatosis, and fatty liver. Combinations of MCTs and long-chain triglycerides (LCTs) are metabolized faster than LCTs alone, and their combination is cleared faster than LCTs because of faster hydrolysis by lipoprotein lipase and rapid removal of remnant particles.[270] Together they provide a better source of fat by meeting energy and essential fatty acid needs while simultaneously improving clearance and oxidation of fatty acids without inciting the inflammatory system to the extent of LCTs alone. A prospective trial in patients undergoing liver resection in which an MCT-LCT emulsion was provided with TPN demonstrated a reduction in septic complications, improvement in hepatic function, a reduction in diuretics required, and weight loss.[148]

The fatty acids at the sn-2 position of the triglyceride molecule are the preferentially preserved components at absorption and the ones ultimately incorporated into cellular membranes.[271] This makes the placement of specific fatty acids, be they n-3 fatty acids with their anti-inflammatory and antithrombogenic effects or MCTs or other modulating fatty acids, into this position uniquely able to effect a clinical change. The development of a structured triglyceride emulsion with various combinations of MCT-LCTs may ideally allow tailoring of nutritional and metabolic support to meet the demands of specific disease states.

Rapid (<4 days) incorporation of n-3 fatty acids into membrane phospholipids of the rat lung alveolar macrophages and hepatic Kupffer and endothelial cells with short-term continuous enteral feeding has been demonstrated by Palombo and colleagues.[272, 273]

These rapid cellular effects with the n-3 enriched diets are associated with alterations in the eicosanoids. Displacement of arachidonic acid with blunting of the arachidonic acid eicosanoids by n-3 polyunsaturated fatty acid (PUFA) decrease neutrophil aggregation, thrombosis, immunosuppression, and tissue injury. This is secondary to a shift in production to the fourth series of prostaglandins (less inflammatory and less vasoconstrictive) and the fifth series of leukotrienes (less inflammatory).[272–275] As a result of these biological effects a number of n-3 products have been designed for patients with acute respiratory distress syndrome, burns, oncology surgery, and transplants.

In animal studies of endotoxemia, n-3 PUFA enteral delivery has been shown to reduce lactic acidosis and maintain or improve tissue perfusion and microcirculation in the heart, brain, lung, and gut.[276–280] Clinically, the success of the n-3 PUFA with organ transplantation is thought to be a result of improvement in the grafted organs' microcirculation along with a protection against a marked inflammatory response.[241–244]

The hyperexcitable ischemic myocardium (because of decreased Na^+,K^+-ATPase pump function) is readily arrhythmogenic because of a lower excitatory threshold. Work by Leaf and colleagues points to inhibition of Na^+ and Ca^{2+} currents along with other PUFA-infusion–related inducible changes in the electrophysiology of the cardiomyocytes as the mechanism of the potent antiarrhythmic effects of these PUFAs.[281] They further found that

- The n-3 and n-6 fatty acids except arachidonic acid appear to have antiarrhythmic effects.
- It is the free PUFA partitioning into membrane phospholipids that is responsible, with the site of action at the carboxyl end.
- The electrophysiology specifically involved is
  1. Slight hyperpolarization of the resting membrane potential
  2. An increased threshold voltage for Na^+ channel opening
  3. A threefold increase in the relative refractory period

For the cardiac surgery patient, the potential combination of GIK, amino acids, and n-3 oils may provide a solution combining glycogen loading, protein sparing, and antiarrhythmic protection as an all-in-one combination.

Nonperioperative patients with injury or diseases such as cancer, trauma, burns, critical illness, IgA nephropathy, ulcerative colitis, and regional enteritis who had nutritional supplementation with n-3 PUFA had significant improvement in their clinical outcome parameters. Enterally delivered n-3 PUFA provides a basis for enteral immunomodulation, with clinical evidence of remissions with regional enteritis and reduced disease activity and reduced rate of early relapses with ulcerative colitis.[282–288]

Ongoing trials will determine the true efficacy of perioperative TPN in reducing the rate of postoperative complications. Some have even suggested that the preoperative use of TPN may have a role in reducing the amount of intestine removed at surgery.[44]

◆ FUTURE DIRECTIONS

The intricate biochemical changes activated by surgery are only beginning to be understood. Stimulation of enzyme activities as well as large-scale gene transcription appears to be involved. With a better understanding of these processes, there can be a more specific therapeutic approach to the metabolic and nutritional changes that accompany surgery. An example is the protein catabolism that is consistently present with surgery. Through the understanding of the regulation of the ATP-dependent ubiquitin-proteosome mechanism of proteolysis, a common pathway of protein breakdown with surgery, the protein catabolism may be truncated, and the need for exogenous protein decreased. Future advancements in the nutritional and metabolic management of the critically ill postoperative patient may routinely involve the use of immunonutrition with various additives including glutamine, arginine, and n-3 fatty acids. Rapid, accurate evaluation and correction of protein-energy requirements with continual metabolic cart and bedside body composition studies aiding in the evaluation of fluid and electrolyte changes along with limiting preoperative sodium and fluid through strict delivery criteria and the use of other potential aids (i.e., growth hormone, which blocks ECW expansion when administered in a well-timed fashion) may further positively impact postoperative patient outcomes.

The potential benefits and roles of specific pharmacologically dosed amino acids including arginine and glutamine, nucleotides and nucleosides, and antioxidants, each acting in different capacities from immunomodulators to aids in gut adaptation, still remain to be better delineated. Metabolic support and thus protection will remain one of the keys to early recovery and will often be as important as eradication of the inciting pathologic agent in promoting a more rapid recovery.

◆ NEW NUTRITIONAL MARKERS

Newer means to evaluate body composition (i.e., bedside neutron activation measurement) are necessary to aid in accurate assessment and thus the appropriate delivery of protein-calorie nutrition in the difficult-to-evaluate critically ill postoperative patient.

Painless, rapid, simple bedside evaluation of muscle function is needed to identify preoperatively those at risk of postoperative complications and thus correctly institute preoperative TPN support in those most likely to benefit.

◆ DISCUSSION

Traditional definitions of successful patient outcomes have encompassed declines in morbidity and mortality rates and improvements in symptomatology and patient comfort. Although these definitions are still applicable, in today's cost-containment, algorithm-driven, result-oriented health care system, those parameters constituting a successful outcome have been molded to include a reduced length of stay in the intensive care unit and hospital and diagnosis-related cost reductions. Thus on many an occasion practitioners are coerced into choosing a less desirable therapeutic option among the many available, based on lower cost, and therefore not uncommonly not serving the patients' best interests.[289]

Much remains to be done in identifying the specific patient subsets in whom preoperative TPN would be beneficial. Data from previous studies are for the most part not applicable to today's practice in light of the inappropriate feeding regimens used at the time and based on current understanding of patients' preoperative and postoperative nutritional and metabolic needs. Present and future studies must be tailored to current thought in regard to not only protein and calorie provision but also fluid, electrolyte, and micronutrient composition, thus optimizing patients' chances for a more desirable outcome. As our understanding of critical illness continues to improve, metabolic support has become increasingly entwined in and an integral part of nutritional delivery.

As medical resources become more limited, preoperative TPN administration must be delivered in the nonacute medical center or even at home. This is important as the length of time for preoperative repletion of minerals and vitamins, as well as calories and high-energy phosphates and possibly some protein is estimated as 10 to 14 days or more.

It is expected that the current and future trials based on current protein-calorie delivery recommendations will reaffirm the necessity of TPN for certain perioperative patient subsets, but it is hoped that these criteria may be further expanded, thus benefiting other groups that have been excluded based on historical misgivings.

REFERENCES

1. Cuthbertsons DP: Further observation on the disturbance of metabolism caused by injury, with particular reference to the dietary requirements of fracture cases. Br J Surg 23:505, 1936.
2. Whipple GH: Protein production exchange in the body including hemoglobin, plasma protein, and cell protein. Am J Med Sci 196:609, 1938.
3. Studley HO: Percentage of weight loss. A basic indicator of surgical risk in patients with chronic peptic ulcer. JAMA 106:458–460, 1936.
4. Rhoads JE: Memoir of a surgical nutritionist. JAMA 28:968, 1994.
5. Rhoads JE, Alexander CE: Nutritional problems of surgical patients. Ann N Y Acad Sci 63:268, 1955.
6. Aubaniac R: L'injection intraveineuse sous-claviculaire: Advantages et technique. Presse Med 60:1456, 1952.
7. Wilmore DW, Dudrick SJ: Growth and development of an infant receiving all nutrients exclusively by vein. JAMA 203:860, 1968.
8. Bistrian BR, Blackburn GL, Hallowell E, et al: Protein status of general surgery patients. JAMA 230:858, 1974.
9. Vitale J, Cochran D, Nagfar J: Prevalence of protein-calorie malnutrition in general medical patients. JAMA 235:1976.
10. Blackburn GL, Bistrian BR, Maini BS, et al: Nutritional and metabolic assessment of the hospitalized patient. JPEN J Parenter Enteral Nutr 1:11–22, 1977.
11. Bistrian BR, Blackburn GL, Vitale J, et al: Prevalence of malnutrition in general medical patients. JAMA 235:1567–1570, 1976.
12. Bruun LI, Bosaeus I, Bergstad I, et al: Prevalence of malnutrition in surgical patients: Evaluation of nutritional support and documentation. Clin Nutr 18:141–147, 1999.
13. Mughal MM, Meguid MM: The effect of nutritional status on morbidity after elective surgery for benign gastrointestinal disease. JPEN J Parenter Enteral Nutr 11:140–143, 1987.
14. Holter AR, Fischer JE: The effects of perioperative hyperalimentation on complications in patients with carcinoma and weight loss. J Surg Res 23:31–37, 1977.
15. Meguid MM, Campos AC, Hammond WG: Nutritional support in surgical practice, I. Am J Surg 159:345–358, 1990.

16. Moore EE, Jones TN: Nutritional assessment and preliminary report on early support of the trauma patient. J Am Coll Nutr 2:45–54, 1983.

17. American Society for Parenteral and Enteral Nutrition Board of Directors: Guidelines for the use of parenteral and enteral nutrition in adult and pediatric patients. JPEN J Parenter Enteral Nutr 17(Suppl):1SA–52SA, 1993.

18. Mazolewski P, Turner JF, Baker M, et al: The impact of nutritional status on the outcome of lung volume reduction surgery. A prospective study. Chest 116:693–696, 1999.

19. Bistrian BR: Nutritional assessment of the hospitalized patients; a practical approach. In Wright RA, Heymsfield S, McManus CB III (eds): Nutritional Assessment. Boston, Blackwell, 1984, pp 183–205.

20. Babineau TJ, Borlase BC, Blackburn GL: Applied total parenteral nutrition in the critically ill. In Rippe JM, Irwin LS, Alpert JS, Fink MP (eds): Intensive Care Medicine. Boston, Little, Brown, 1991, pp 1675–1691.

21. Rivadeneira DE, Grobmyer SR, Naama HA, et al: Protein-calorie malnutrition increases apoptosis in peritoneal macrophages. Surg Forum 49:62–64, 1998.

22. Barry L, Mestre J, McCarter M, et al: Protein-calorie malnutrition attenuates NF-κB activation in peritoneal macrophages. Surg Forum 49:117–119, 1998.

23. Hasselgren PO: Burns and metabolism. J Am Coll Surg 188:98–103, 1999.

24. Bistrian BR: Apex: The Preceptorship for Excellence in Parenteral Nutrition Support. Health Management Solutions, Inc. South Norwalk, CT, 1996, pp 2–7.

25. Keys A, Henchel A, Taylor HL: The size and function of the human heart at rest in semi-starvation and in subsequent rehabilitation. Am J Physiol 50:153, 1947.

26. Gibbons GN, Blackburn GL, Harken DE, et al: Pre- and postoperative hyperalimentation in the treatment of cardiac cachexia. J Surg Res 20:439–444, 1976.

27. Askanazi J, Weissman C, La Sala PA, et al: Effect of protein intake on ventilatory drive. Anesthesiology 60:106–110, 1984.

28. Baston MD, Rawlings J, Allison SP: Undernutrition, hypothermia, and injury in elderly women with fractured femur an injury response to altered metabolism? Lancet 1:143–146, 1983.

29. Parsons V, Symulker G, Brown SJ: Fracturing osteoporosis in young women with anorexia nervosa. Calcif Tissue Int 35 (Suppl):2, 1983.

30. Vernon DR, Hill GL: The relationship between tissue loss and function: Recent developments. Curr Opin Clin Nutr Metab Care 1:5–8, 1998.

31. Russel DM, Prendergast PJ, Darby PL, et al: A comparison between muscle function and body composition in anorexia nervosa: The effect of refeeding. Am J Clin Nutr 38:229–237, 1983.

32. Baker JP, Detsky AS, Wesson DE, et al: Nutritional assessment: A comparison of clinical judgment and objective measurements. N Engl J Med 306:969–972, 1982.

33. Detsky AS, Baker JP, Mendelson RA, et al: Evaluation of accuracy of nutritional assessment techniques applied to hospitalized patients: Methodology and comparisons. JPEN J Parenter Enteral Nutr 8:153–159, 1984.

34. Buzby GP, Mullen JP, Matthews DC: Prognostic nutritional index in gastrointestinal surgery. Am J Surg 139:160, 1980.

35. Seltzer MH, Slocum BA, Cataldi-Betcher EL, et al: Instant assessment: Absolute weight loss and surgical mortality. JPEN J Parenter Enteral Nutr 6:218–221, 1982.

36. McMahon MM, Bistrian BR: The physiology of nutritional assessment in protein-calorie malnutrition. Dis Mon 36:373–417, 1990.

37. Bishop CW, Bowe PE, Ritchey SJ: Norms for the nutritional assessment of American adults by upper arm anthropometrics. Am J Clin Nutr 34:2530–2539, 1981.

38. Reinhardt GF, Mycofski JW, Wilkens DB, et al: Incidence and mortality of hypoalbuminemic patients and hospitalized veterans. JPEN J Parenter Enteral Nutr 4:357–359, 1980.

39. Seltzer MH, Bastidas JA, Cooper DM, et al: Instant nutritional assessment. JPEN J Parenter Enteral Nutr 3:157–159, 1979.

40. Rady MY, Ryan T, Starr NJ: Clinical characteristics of preoperative hypoalbuminemia predict outcome of cardiovascular surgery. JPEN J Parenter Enteral Nutr 21:81–90, 1997.

41. Friedenberg F, Jensen G, Gujral N, et al: Serum albumin as predictive of 30-day survival after percutaneous endoscopic gastrostomy. JPEN J Parenter Enteral Nutr 21:72–74, 1997.

42. Gibbs J, Cull W, Henderson W, et al: Preoperative serum albumin level as a predictor of operative mortality and morbidity: Results from the national VA surgical risk study. Arch Surg 134:36–42, 1999.

43. Hill AG, Hill GL: Metabolic response to severe injury. Br J Surg 85:884–890, 1998.

44. Nutrition support in clinical practice: Review of published data and recommendations for future research directions. JPEN J Parenter Enteral Nutr 21:133–156, 1997.

45. Lebel L, Smith L, Risberg B, et al: Effect of increased hydrostatic pressure on lymphatic elimination of hyaluronan from sheep lung. J Appl Physiol 64:1327–1332, 1988.

46. Townsley MI, Reed RK, Ishibashi M, et al: Hyaluronan efflux from canine lung with increased hydrostatic pressure and saline loading. Am J Respir Crit Care Med 150:1605–1610, 1994.

47. Sitges-Serra A, Franch-Arcas G: Fluid and sodium problems in perioperative feeding: What further studies need to be done? Curr Opin Clin Metab Care 1:9–14, 1998.

48. Brennan MF, Pisters PWT, Posner M, et al: A prospective randomized trial of total parenteral nutrition after major pancreatic resection for malignancy. Ann Surg 220:436–444, 1994.

49. Daly JM, Lieberman MD, Goldfine J, et al: Enteral nutrition with supplemental arginine, RNA, and omega-3 fatty acids in patients after operation: Immunologic, metabolic and clinical outcome. Surgery 112:56–67, 1992.

50. Daly JM, Weintraub FN, Shou J, et al: Enteral nutrition during multimodality therapy in upper gastrointestinal cancer patients. Ann Surg 221:327–338, 1995.

51. Forse RA, Rompre C, Crosilla P, et al: Reliability of the total lymphocyte count as a parameter of nutrition. Can J Surg 28:216–219, 1985.

52. Redmond HP, Leon P, Leiberman MD, et al: Im-

paired macrophage function in severe protein energy malnutrition. Arch Surg 126:192–196, 1991.

53. Redmond HP, Gallagher HJ, Shou J, Daly JM: Antigen presentation in protein-energy malnutrition. Cell Immunol 163:80–87, 1995.

54. Redmond HP, Shou J, Kelly CJ, et al: Immunosuppressive mechanisms in protein-calorie malnutrition. Surgery 110:311–317, 1991.

55. Redmond HP, Shou J, Kelly CJ, et al: Protein-calorie malnutrition impairs host defense against *Candida albicans.* J Surg Res 50:552–559, 1991.

56. Harvey KB, Moldawer LL, Bistrian BR, Blackburn GL: Biological measures for the formulation of a hospital prognostic index. Am J Clin Nutr 34:2013–2022, 1981.

57. Christou NV, Meakins JL: Neutrophil function in anergic surgical patients: Neutrophil adherence and chemotaxis. Ann Surg 190:557–564, 1979.

58. Copeland EM, MacFadyen BV, Dudrick SJ: Effect of intravenous hyperalimentation on established delayed hypersensitivity in the cancer patient. Ann Surg 184:60–64, 1979.

59. Forse RA, Christou N, Meakins JL, et al: Reliability of skin testing as a measure of nutritional state. Arch Surg 116:1284–1288, 1981.

60. Ishibashi N, Plank LD, Sando K, Hill GL: Optimal protein requirements during the first 2 weeks after the onset of critical illness. Crit Care Med 26:1529–1535, 1998.

61. Forse RA, Shizgal HM: The assessment of malnutrition. Surgery 88:17–24, 1980.

62. Bell SJ, Bistrian BR, Connolly CA, et al: Body composition changes in patients with human immunodeficiency virus infection. Nutrition 13:629–632, 1997.

63. Jacobs DO: Use of bioelectrical impedance analysis measurements in the clinical management of critical illness. Am J Clin Nutr 64(3 Suppl):498S–502S, 1996.

64. Scheltinga MR, Jacobs DO, Kimbrough TD, Wilmore DW: Identifying body fluid distribution by measuring electrical impedance. J Trauma 33:665–670, 1992.

65. Zeiderman MR, McMahon MJ: The role of objective measurement of skeletal muscle function in the preoperative patient. Clin Nutr 8:161, 1989.

66. Windsor JA, Hill GL: Weight loss with physiologic impairment: A basic indicator of surgical risk. Ann Surg 207:290, 1988.

67. Russell D, Leiter LA, Whitwell J, et al: Skeletal muscle function during hypocaloric diets and fasting: A comparison with standard nutritional assessment parameters. Am J Clin Nutr 37:133, 1983.

68. Meguid MM, Certas S, Chen M, Nole E: Adductor pollicis muscle tests to detect and correct subclinical malnutrition in preoperative cancer patients [Abstract]. Am J Clin Nutr 45:843, 1987.

69. Mitch WE: Mechanisms causing loss of lean body mass in kidney disease. Am J Clin Nutr 67:359–366, 1998.

70. King BK, Blackwell AP, Minard G, Kudsk KA: Predicting patient outcome using preoperative nutritional markers. Surg Forum 48:592–595, 1997.

71. Lipman TO: Grains or veins: Is enteral nutrition really better than parenteral nutrition? A look at the evidence. JPEN J Parenter Enteral Nutr 22:167–182, 1998.

72. Levine GM, Deren JJ, Steiger E, et al: Role of oral intake in maintenance of gut mass and disaccharide activity. Gastroenterology 67:975–982, 1974.

73. Deitz EA: Intestinal permeability is increased in burn patients shortly after injury. Surgery 102:411–412, 1990.

74. LeVoyer T, Cioffi WG, Pratt L, et al: Alterations in intestinal permeability after thermal injury. Arch Surg 127:26–29, 1992.

75. O'Dwyer SJ, Michie HR, Zeigler TR, et al: A single dose of endotoxin increases intestinal permeability in healthy humans. Arch Surg 123:1459–1464, 1988.

76. Roumen RM, van der Vliet JA, Wevers RA, et al: Intestinal permeability is increased after major vascular surgery. J Vasc Surg 17:734–737, 1993.

77. Reynolds JV, Kanwar S, Welsh FKS, et al: Does the route of feeding modify gut barrier function and clinical outcome in patients after major upper gastrointestinal surgery? JPEN J Parenter Enteral Nutr 21:196–201, 1997.

78. Page HC, Dwenger A, Regl G, et al: Increased gut permeability after multiple trauma. Br J Surg 81:850–852, 1994.

79. Zeigler TR, Smith RJ, O'Dwyer ST, et al: Increased intestinal permeability associated with infection in burn patients. Arch Surg 123:1313–1339, 1988.

80. Suchner U, Senftleben U, Eckart T, et al: Enteral versus parenteral nutrition: Effects on gastrointestinal function and metabolism. Nutrition 12:13–22, 1996.

81. Hindmarsh JT, Clark RG: The effects of intravenous and intraduodenal feeding on nitrogen balance after surgery. Br J Surg 60:589–594, 1973.

82. Rowlands BJ, Giddings AEB, Johnston AOB, et al: Nitrogen-sparing effect of different feeding regimes in patients after operation. Br J Anaesth 49:781–787, 1977.

83. Peterson VM, Moore EE, Jones TN, et al: Total enteral nutrition versus total parenteral nutrition after major torso injury: Attenuation of hepatic protein reprioritization. Surgery 104:199–207, 1988.

84. Kudsk KA, Minard G, Wojtysiak SL, et al: Visceral protein response to enteral versus parenteral nutrition and sepsis in patients with trauma. Surgery 116:516–523, 1994.

85. Pearlstone DB, Lee JI, Alexander RH, et al: Effect of enteral and parenteral nutrition on amino acid levels in cancer patients. JPEN J Parenter Enteral Nutr 19:204–208, 1995.

86. Braga M, Vignali A, Gianotti L, et al: Immune and nutritional effects of early enteral nutrition after major abdominal operations. Eur J Surg 162:105–112, 1996.

87. Fish J, Sporay G, Beyer K, et al: A prospective randomized study of glutamine-enriched parenteral compared with enteral feeding in postoperative patients. Am J Clin Nutr 65:977–983, 1997.

88. Shirabe K, Matsumata T, Shimada M, et al: A comparison of parenteral hyperalimentation and early enteral feeding regarding systemic immunity after major hepatic resection—The results of a randomized prospective study. Hepatogastroenterology 44:205–209, 1997.

89. Lim STK, Choa RG, Lam KH, et al: Total parenteral nutrition versus gastrostomy in the preoperative preparation of patients with carcinoma of the oesophagus. Br J Surg 68:69–72, 1981.

90. Merritt R: Cholestasis associated with total paren-

teral nutrition. J Pediatr Gastroenterol Nutr 5:9–22, 1986.

91. Drongowski RA, Coran AG: Analysis of factors contributing to the development of total parental nutrition–induced cholestasis. JPEN J Parenter Enteral Nutr 13:586–589, 1989.

92. Pitt HA, King WI II, Mann LL, et al: Increased risk of cholelithiasis with prolonged total parenteral nutrition. Am J Surg 145:106–112, 1983.

93. Hadfield RJ, Sinclair DG, Houldsworth PE, et al: Effects of enteral versus parenteral nutrition on gut mucosal permeability in the critically ill. Am J Respir Crit Care Med 152:1545–1548, 1995.

94. Wicks C, Somasundaram S, Bjarnason I, et al: Comparison of enteral feeding and total parenteral nutrition after liver transplantation. Lancet 344:837–840, 1994.

95. Sedman PC, Macfie J, Palmer MD, et al: Preoperative total parenteral nutrition is not associated with mucosal atrophy or bacterial translocation in humans. Br J Surg 82:1663–1667, 1995.

96. Buchman AL, Mestecky J, Moukarzel A, et al: Intestinal immune function is unaffected by parenteral nutrition in man. J Am Coll Nutr 14:656–661, 1995.

97. Cummins A, Chu G, Faust L, et al: Malabsorption and villous atrophy in patients receiving enteral feeding. JPEN J Parenter Enteral Nutr 19:193–198, 1995.

98. Sako K, Lore JM, Kaufman S, et al: Parenteral hyperalimentation in surgical patients with head and neck cancer: A randomized study. J Surg Oncol 16:392–402, 1981.

99. Iovenelli G, Marsili I, Varrassi G: Nutrition support after total laryngectomy. JPEN J Parenter Enteral Nutr 17:445–448, 1993.

100. Von Meyenfeldt MF, Meijerink W, Rouflart M, et al: Perioperative nutritional support: A randomized clinical trial. Clin Nutr 11:180–186, 1992.

101. Moore FA, Feliciano DV, Andrassy RJ, et al: Early enteral feeding, compared with parenteral, reduces postoperative septic complications. The result of a meta-analysis. Ann Surg 216:172–183, 1992.

102. Baigrie RJ, Devitt PG, Watkin DS: Enteral versus parenteral nutrition after oesophagogastric surgery: A prospective randomized comparison. Aust N Z Surg 66:668–670, 1996.

103. Bohnker BK, Artman LE, Hoskins WJ: Narrow bore nasogastric feeding tube complication: A literature review. Nutr Clin Pract 2:203–209, 1987.

104. Care E, Gussul MA: Complications of enteral feeding. Nutrition 9:1–9, 1992.

105. Benya R, Mobarahn S: Enteral alimentation: Administration and complications. J Am Coll Nutr 10:209–219, 1991.

106. Ciocon JO, Silverstone FA, Graver LM, et al: Tube feedings in elderly patients: Indications, benefits and complications. Arch Intern Med 148:429–433, 1988.

107. Bistrian BR: Interactions of metabolic and infectious complications in total parenteral nutrition. Presented at the 20th Clinical Congress of the American Society of Parenteral and Enteral Nutrition Washington, DC, January 14, 1996.

108. Hostetter M: Handicaps to host defense: Effects of hyperglycemia on C3 and *Candida albicans.* Diabetes 39:271–275, 1990.

109. Flakoll PJ, Hill JO, Abumrad NN: Acute hyperglycemia enhances proteolysis in normal man. Am J Physiol 265:E715–E721, 1993.

110. Pomposelli J, Baxter JK, Babineau TJ, et al: Early postoperative glucose control predicts nosocomial infection rate in diabetic patients. JPEN J Parenter Enteral Nutr 22:77–81, 1998.

111. Jones R, Peterson C: Hematologic alterations in diabetes mellitus. Am J Med 70:339–352, 1981.

112. Mowat A, Baum J: Chemotaxis of polymorphonuclear leukocytes from patients with diabetes mellitus. N Engl J Med 284:621–627, 1971.

113. Bagdade J, Neilson K, Bulger R: Reversible abnormalities in phagocytic function in poorly controlled diabetic patients. Am J Med Sci 263:451–456, 1972.

114. Nolan C, Beatty H, Bagdade J: Impaired granulocyte bactericidal function in patients with poorly controlled diabetes. Diabetes 27:889–894, 1978.

115. Shukla HS, Rao RR, Banu, et al: Enteral hyperalimentation in malnourished surgical patients. Indian J Med Res 80:339–346, 1984.

116. Lazar HL, Philippides G, Fitzgerald C, et al: Glucose-insulin-potassium solutions enhance recovery after urgent coronary artery bypass grafting. J Thorac Cardiovasc Surg 113:354–362, 1997.

117. Coleman GM, Gradinac S, Taegtmeyer H, et al: Efficacy of metabolic support with glucose-insulin-potassium for left ventricular pump failure after aortocoronary bypass surgery. Circulation (Suppl I):80(3 Pt. 1):I91–I96, 1989.

118. McElroy DD, Taegtmeyer H, Walker WE: Effects of glycogen on function and energy metabolism of the isolated rabbit heart after hypothermic ischemic arrest [Abstract]. Clin Res 35:304A, 1987.

119. Rao V, Merante F, Weisel R, et al: Insulin stimulates pyruvate dehydrogenase and protects human ventricular cardiomyocytes from simulated ischemia. J Thorac Cardiovasc Surg 116:485–494, 1998.

120. Symposium: Nutritional support for surgical patients. Contemp Surg 55:96–108, 1999.

121. Apovian CM, McMahon MM, Bistrian BR: Guidelines for refeeding the marasmic patient. Crit Care Med 18:1030, 1990.

122. Foxx Orenstein A, Jensen GL: Overzealous resuscitation of an extremely malnourished patient with nutritional cardiomyopathy. Nutr Rev 48:406–411, 1990.

123. Weinsier RL, Krumdock CL: Death resulting from overzealous total parenteral nutrition: The refeeding syndrome revisited. Am J Clin Nutr 34:393–399, 1981.

124. Starker PM, Lasala PA, Askanazi J, et al: The response to TPN. A form of nutritional assessment. Ann Surg 198:720–724, 1983.

125. Starker PM, Lasala PA, Forse RA, et al: Response to total parenteral nutrition in the extremely malnourished patient. JPEN J Parenter Enteral Nutr 9:300–302, 1985.

126. Zimmer R, Weill J, Dubois M: The nutritional situation in the camps of the unoccupied zone of France in 1941 and 1942 and its consequences. N Engl J Med 230:303–314, 1944.

127. Rudman D, Millikan WJ, Richardson TJ, et al: Elemental balances during intravenous hyperalimentation of underweight adult subjects. J Clin Invest 55:94–104, 1975.

128. Gill MJ, Franch-Arcas G, Guirao X, et al: Response of severely malnourished patients to preoperative parenteral nutrition: A randomized trial of water and sodium restriction. Nutrition 13:26–31, 1997.

129. Tappy L, Schwarz J-M, Schneiter P, et al: Effects of isoenergetic glucose-based or lipid-based parenteral nutrition on glucose metabolism, de novo lipogenesis, and respiratory gas exchanges in critically ill patients. Crit Care Med 26:860–867, 1998.

130. Recommended Dietary Allowances, 10th ed. Washington, DC, National Academy Press, 1989, p 285.

131. Hoffer LJ, Bistrian BR, Young VR, et al: Metabolic effects of very low calorie weight reduction diets. J Clin Invest 73:750–758, 1984.

132. Munro HW, Crim MC: The proteins and amino acids. *In* Goodhart R, Shils M (eds): Modern Nutrition in Health and Disease, 6th ed. Philadelphia, Lea Febiger, 1980, p 78.

133. Bistrian BR, Babineau TJ: Optimal protein intake in critical illness? Crit Care Med 26:1476–1477, 1998.

134. Shaw JHF, Wilbore M, Wolfe RR: Whole body protein kinetics in severely septic patients. Ann Surg 205:288–294, 1987.

135. Shaw JHF, Wolfe RR, Goodenough RD, et al: Response of protein and urea kinetics in burn patients to different levels of protein intake. Ann Surg 197:163–171, 1983.

136. Shaw J, Wolfe RR: An integrated analysis of glucose, fat, and protein metabolism in severely traumatized patients: Studies in the basal state and the response to total parenteral nutrition. Ann Surg 209:63–72, 1989.

137. Schloerb PR, Henning JF: Patterns and problems of adult total parenteral nutrition use in US academic medical centers. Arch Surg 133:7–12, 1998.

138. Ljungqvist O, Thorell A, Gutniak, et al: Glucose infusion instead of preoperative fasting reduces postoperative insulin resistance. J Am Coll Surg 178:329–336, 1994.

139. Meguid MM, Campos ACL, Meguid V, et al: IONIP: A criterion of surgical outcome and patient selection for perioperative nutritional support. Br J Clin Pract 42:8–14, 1988.

140. Fan S, Lau W, Wong K, et al: Preoperative parenteral nutrition in patients with oesophageal cancer: A prospective, randomised clinical trial. Clin Nutr 8:23–27, 1989.

141. Thompson B, Julian T, Stremple J: Perioperative total parenteral nutrition in patients with gastrointestinal cancer. J Surg Res 30:497–450, 1981.

142. Muller J, Keller H, Brenner U, et al: Indications and effects of preoperative parenteral nutrition. World J Surg 10:53–63, 1986.

143. The VA TPN Cooperative Study Group: Perioperative total parenteral nutrition in surgical patients. N Engl J Med 325:525–532, 1991.

144. Bellantone R, Doglietto G, Bossola M, et al: Preoperative parenteral nutrition in the high risk surgical patients. JPEN J Parenter Enteral Nutr 12:195–197, 1988.

145. Muller J, Brenner U, Dienst C, et al: Preoperative parenteral feeding in patients with gastrointestinal carcinoma. Lancet 1:68–71, 1982.

146. Smith R, Hartemick R: Improvement of nutritional measures during preoperative parenteral nutrition in patients selected by the prognostic nutritional index: A randomized controlled trial. JPEN J Parenter Enteral Nutr 12:587–591, 1988.

147. Heatley RV, Williams RHP, Lewis MH: Preoperative intravenous feeding: A controlled trial. Postgrad Med J 55:541–545, 1979.

148. Fan S, Lo C, Lai E, et al: Perioperative nutritional support in patients undergoing hepatectomy for hepatocellular carcinoma. N Engl J Med 331:1547–1552, 1994.

149. Meguid M, Curtas M, Meguid V, et al: Effects of preoperative TPN on surgical risk—preliminary status report. Br J Clin Pract 42(Suppl):53–58, 1988.

150. Bellantone R, Doglietto G, Bossola M, et al: Preoperative parenteral nutrition of malnourished patients. Acta Chir Scand 22:249–251, 1988.

151. Moghissi K, Hornshaw J, Teasdale PR, Dawes EA: Parenteral nutrition in carcinoma of the esophagus treated by surgery: Nitrogen balance and clinical studies. Br J Surg 64:125–128, 1977.

152. Campos ACL, Meguid MM: A critical appraisal of the usefulness of perioperative nutritional support. Am J Clin Nutr 55:117–130, 1992.

153. Carlson RG, Miller SF, Finley RR, et al: Fluid retention and burn survival. J Trauma 27:127–135, 1987.

154. Tellado JM, Garcia-Sabrido JL, Hanley JA, et al: Predicting mortality based on body composition analysis. Ann Surg 209:81–87, 1989.

155. Price SR, Mitch WE: Mechanisms stimulating protein degradation to cause muscle atrophy. Curr Opin Clin Nutr Metab Care 1:79–83, 1998.

156. Price SR, Bailey JL, Wang X, et al: Muscle wasting in insulinopenic rats results from activation of the ATP-dependent, ubiquitin proteosome proteolytic pathway by a mechanism including gene transcription. J Clin Invest 98:1703–1708, 1996.

157. Wilmore DW: The metabolic management of the critically ill. New York, Plenum Press, 1977, p 149.

158. Clifton GL, Robertson CS, Grossman RG, et al: The metabolic response to severe head injury. J Neurosurg 60:687–696, 1984.

159. Elwyn DH, Kinney JM, Askanazi J: Energy expenditure in surgical patients. Surg Clin North Am 61:545–556, 1981.

160. Van Way CW III: Nutritional support in the injured patient. Surg Clin North Am 71:537–548, 1991.

161. Shaw JMF, Wolfe RR: An integrated analysis of glucose, fat, and protein metabolism in severely injured patients. Ann Surg 209:63–72, 1989.

162. Plank LD, Connolly AB, Hill GL: Sequential changes in the metabolic response in severely septic patients during the first 23 days after the onset of peritonitis. Ann Surg 228:146–158, 1998.

163. Grahm TW, Zadrozny DB, Harrington T: The benefits of early jejunal hyperalimentation in the head-injured patient. Neurosurgery 19:367–373, 1986.

164. Kudsk KA, Croce MA, Fabian TC, et al: Enteral vs. parenteral feeding: Effects on septic morbidity following blunt and penetrating abdominal trauma. Ann Surg 215:503–513, 1992.

165. Moore FA, Moore EE, Jones TN, et al: TEN vs TPN following major abdominal trauma—Reduced septic morbidity. J Trauma 29:916–923, 1989.

166. Meguid MM, Muscaritoli M: Current uses of total parenteral nutrition. Am Fam Physician 47:383–394, 1993.

167. Stack JA, Babineau TJ, Bistrian BR: Assessment of nutritional status in clinical practice. Gastroenterologist 4(Suppl I):S8–S15, 1996.

168. Edmunds LH Jr, Williams GM, Welch CE: External fistulas arising from the gastrointestinal tract. Ann Surg 152:445, 1960.

169. Himal HS, Allard JR, Nadeau JE, et al: The importance of adequate nutrition in closure of small intestinal fistulas. Br J Surg 61:724, 1974.

170. Sagar S, Harland P, Shields R: Early postoperative feeding with elemental diet. BMJ 1:293–295, 1979.

171. Ryan JA, Page CP, Babcock L: Early postoperative jejunal feeding of elemental diet in gastrointestinal surgery. Ann Surg 47:393–403, 1981.

172. Smith RC, Hartemink RJ, Hollinshead JW, et al: Fine bore jejunostomy feeding following major abdominal surgery: A controlled randomized clinical trial. Br J Surg 72:458–461, 1985.

173. Morlion BJ, Stehle P, Wachtler P et al: Total parenteral nutrition with glutamine dipeptide after major abdominal surgery: A randomized, double-blind, controlled study. Ann Surg 227:302–308, 1998.

174. Kenler AS, Swails WS, Driscoll DF, et al: Early enteral feeding in postsurgical cancer patients: Fish oil structured lipid-based polymeric formula. Ann Surg 223:316–333, 1996.

175. Daly JM, Reynolds J, Thom A, et al: Immune and metabolic effects of arginine in the surgical patient. Ann Surg 208:512–523, 1988.

176. Abel R, Fischer J, Buckley M, et al: Malnutrition in cardiac surgical patients: Results of a prospective randomized evaluation of early postoperative parenteral nutrition. Arch Surg 111:45–50, 1976.

177. Preshaw R, Attisha R, Hollingworth W: Randomized sequential trial of parenteral nutrition in healing of colonic anastomoses in man. Can J Surg 22:437–439, 1979.

178. Sandstrom R, Drott C, Hyltander A, et al: The effect of postoperative intravenous feeding (TPN) on outcome following major surgery evaluated in a randomized study. Ann Surg 217:185–195, 1993.

179. Woolfson A, Smith J: Elective nutritional support after major surgery: A prospective randomized trial. Clin Nutr 8:15, 1989.

180. Jensen S: Clinical effects of enteral and parenteral nutrition preceding cancer surgery. Med Oncol 2:225–229, 1985.

181. Collins J, Oxby C, Hill G: Intravenous amino acids and intravenous hyperalimentation as protein-sparing therapy after major surgery: A controlled clinical trial. Lancet 1:778–791, 1978.

182. Reilly J, Mehta R, Teperman L, et al: Nutritional support after liver transplantation: A randomized prospective study. JPEN J Parenter Enteral Nutr 14:386–391, 1990.

183. Bastow MD, Rawlings J, Allison S: Benefits of supplementary tube feeding after fractured neck of the femur: A randomized controlled trial. BMJ 187:1589–1592, 1983.

184. Delmi M, Rapin CH, Bengoa JM, et al: Dietary supplementation in elderly patients with fractured neck of the femur. Lancet 335:1013–1016, 1990.

185. Babineau TJ, Bollinger WS, Forse RA, Bistrian BR: Nutritional support for patients after cardiopulmonary bypass. Ann Surg 228:701–706, 1998.

186. Wing SS, Goldberg AL: Glucocorticoids activate the ATP-ubiquitin–dependent proteolytic system in skeletal muscle during fasting. Am J Physiol 264:E668–E676, 1993.

187. Mitch WE, Medina R, Greiber S, et al: Metabolic acidosis stimulates muscle protein degradation by activating the ATP-dependent pathway involving ubiquitin and proteosomes. J Clin Invest 93:2127–2133, 1994.

188. May RC, Kelly RA, Mitch WE: Metabolic acidosis stimulates protein degradation in rat muscle by a glucocorticoid-dependent mechanism. J Clin Invest 77:614–621, 1986.

189. Price SR, England BK, Bailey JL, et al: Acidosis and glucocorticoids concomitantly increase ubiquitin and proteosome subunit mRNAs in rat muscle. Am J Physiol 267:C955–C960, 1994.

190. Fischer JE, Tiao GM: Nutritional support in hepatic failure. *In* Fischer JE (ed): Nutrition and metabolism in the surgical patient, 2nd ed. Boston, Little, Brown, p 647.

191. Venus B, Smith RA, Patel C, et al: Hemodynamic and gas exchange alterations during intralipid infusion in patients with adult respiratory distress syndrome. Chest 95:1278–1281, 1989.

192. Klein S, Miles JM: Metabolic effects of long chain and medium-chain triglyceride emulsions in humans [Editorial Comment]. JPEN J Parenter Enteral Nutr 18:396–397, 1994.

193. Hamawy KJ, Moldawer LL, Georgieff M, et al: The Henry M Vars Award. The effect of lipid emulsion on reticuloendothelial system function in the injured animal. JPEN J Parenter Enteral Nutr 9:559–565, 1985.

194. Makk LJ, McClave SA, Creech PW, et al: Clinical application of the metabolic cart to the delivery of TPN. Crit Care Med 18:1320, 1990.

195. Stock MC, Ryan ME: Oxygen consumption calculated from the Fick equation has limited utility. Crit Care Med 24:86–95, 1996.

196. Freund H, Ryan JA, Fischer JE: Amino acid derangements in patients with sepsis treated with branch chain amino acid enriched infusions. Ann Surg 188:423, 1978.

197. Raina N, Cameron RG, Jeejeebhoy KN: Gastrointestinal, hepatic and metabolic effects of enteral and parenteral nutrition in rats infused with tumor necrosis factor. JPEN J Parenter Enteral Nutr 21:7–13, 1997.

198. Gottschlich MM, Jenkins M, Warden GD, et al: Differential effects of the three enteral dietary regimens on selected outcome variables in burn patients. JPEN J Parenter Enteral Nutr 14:225–236, 1990.

199. Bower RG, Cerra FB, Bershadsky B, et al: Early enteral administration of a formula (Impact) supplemented with arginine, nucleotides, and fish oil in intensive care unit patients: Results of a multicenter, prospective, randomised, clinical trial. Crit Care Med 23:436–449, 1995.

200. Babineau TJ, Hernandez E, Forse RA, Bistrian BR: Symptomatic hyperlipasemia after cardiopulmonary bypass: Implications for enteral nutritional support. Nutrition 9:237–239, 1993.

201. Schloerb PR, Amare M: Total parenteral nutrition with glutamine in bone marrow transplantation and other clinical applications (a randomized double blind study). JPEN J Parenter Enter Nutr 17:407–413, 1993.

202. Baxter RK, Babineau TJ, Apovian CM, et al: Perioperative glucose control predicts increased nosocomial infection in diabetics. Crit Care Med 18:S207, 1990.

203. Rady M, Ryan T, Starr N: Perioperative determinants of morbidity and mortality in elderly patients undergoing cardiac surgery. Crit Care Med 6:225–235, 1998.

204. Zarr K, Furnary A, Grunkemier G, et al: Glucose

control lowers the risk of wound infection in diabetics after open heart operation. Ann Thorac Surg 63:356–361, 1997.

205. Khaodhiar L, McCowen K, Bistrian BR: Perioperative hyperglycemia, infection or risk? Curr Opin Clin Nutr Metab Care 2:79–82, 1999.

206. Malmberg K, Ryden L, Hamsten A, et al: Effects of insulin treatment on cause-specific one-year mortality and morbidity in diabetic patients with acute myocardial infarction: DIGAMI study group: Diabetes Insulin-Glucose in Acute Myocardial Infarction. Eur Heart J 17:1337–1344, 1996.

206a. Thorell A, Nygren J, Ljungqvist O: Insulin resistance: A marker of surgical stress. Cur Opin Clin Nutr Metab Care 2:69–78, 1999.

207. Sodi-Pollares D, Testelli M, Fishleder F: Effects of an intravenous infusion of a potassium-insulin-glucose solution on the electrocardiographic signs of myocardial infarction. Am J Cardiol 9:166–181, 1962.

208. Apstein CS, Taegtmeyer H: Glucose-insulin-potassium in acute myocardial infarction: The time has come for a large, prospective trial. Circulation 96:1074–1077, 1997.

209. Fath-Ordoubadi F, Beat KJ: Glucose-insulin-potassium therapy for treatment of acute myocardial infarction: An overview of randomized placebo-controlled trials. Circulation 96:1152–1156, 1997.

210. Apstein CS: Glucose-insulin-potassium for acute myocardial infarction: Remarkable results from a new prospective, randomized trial. Circulation 98:2223–2226, 1998.

211. Diaz R, Paolasso EC, Piegas LS, et al: Metabolic modulation of acute myocardial infarction: The ECLA Glucose-Insulin-Potassium Pilot Trial. Circulation 98:2227–2234, 1998.

212. Smith KS: Insulin and glucose in the treatment of heart disease with specific reference to angina pectoris. BMJ 1:693–696, 1933.

213. Rogers WJ, Stanley AW, Breinig JB, et al: Reduction of hospital mortality rate of acute myocardial infarction with glucose-insulin-potassium infusion. Am Heart J 92:441–454, 1976.

214. Taegtmeyer H, Goodwin GW, Doenst T, et al: Substrate metabolism as a determinant for post-ischemic functional recovery of the heart. Am J Cardiol 80:3A–10A, 1997.

215. Taegtmeyer H: Metabolic responses to hypoxia: Increased production of succinate by rabbit papillary muscles. Circ Res 43:808–815, 1978.

216. Sanborn T, Gavin W, Berkowitz S, et al: Augmented conversion of aspartate and glutamate to succinate during anoxia in rabbit heart. Am J Physiol 237:H535–H541, 1979.

217. Rau E, Shine KI, Gervais A, et al: Enhanced mechanical recovery of anoxic and ischemic myocardium by amino acid perfusion. Am J Physiol 236:H873–H879, 1979.

218. Haas GS, DeBoer LWV, O'Keefe DD, et al: Reduction of postischemic myocardial dysfunction by substrate repletion during reperfusion. Circulation 70(Suppl 1):65–74, 1984.

219. Lazar HL, Buckberg GD, Manganaro AJ, et al: Myocardial energy replenishment and reversal of ischemic damage by substrate enhancement of secondary blood cardioplegia with amino acids during reperfusion. J Thorac Cardiovasc Surg 80:350–359, 1980.

220. Weldner PW, Myers JL, Miller CA, et al: Improved recovery of immature myocardium with L-glutamate blood cardioplegia. Ann Thorac Surg 55:102–105, 1993.

221. Engelman RM, Dobbs WA, Rousou JH, et al: Myocardial high-energy phosphate replenishment during ischemic arrest: Aerobic versus anaerobic metabolism. Ann Thorac Surg 33:453–458, 1982.

222. Svedjeholm R, Svensson SE, Ekroth R, et al: Trauma metabolism and the heart: Studies of heart and leg amino acid flux after cardiac surgery. Thorac Cardiovasc Surg 38:1–5, 1990.

223. Svedjeholm R, Ekroth R, Joachimsson PO, et al: Myocardial uptake of amino acids and other substrates in relation to myocardial oxygen consumption four hours after cardiac surgery. J Thorac Cardiovasc Surg 101:688–694, 1991.

224. Lazar HL, Buckberg GD, Manganaro AJ, et al: Reversal of ischemic damage with amino acid substrate enhancement during reperfusion. Surgery 80:702–709, 1980.

225. Burns AH, Reddy WJ: Amino acid stimulation of oxygen and substrate utilization by cardiac myocytes. Am J Physiol 235:E461–E466, 1978.

226. Vanhanen I, Huljebrant I, Hakanson E, et al: Glutamate infusion stimulates oxidative metabolism of the heart early after coronary surgery [Abstract 64]. Presented at the Forty-first Annual Meeting of the Scandinavian Association for Thoracic and Cardiovascular Surgery, Tromso, Norway, Aug 20–23, 1992.

227. Pisarenko OI, Lepilin MG, Ivanov VE: Cardiac metabolism and performance during L-glutamic acid infusion in postoperative cardiac failure. Clin Sci 70:7–12, 1986.

228. Svedjeholm R, Heljebrant I, Hakanson E, et al: Glutamate and high-dose glucose-insulin-potassium (GIK) in the treatment of severe cardiac failure after cardiac operations. Ann Thorac Surg 59:S23–S30, 1995.

229. Naylor CD, et al: Parenteral nutrition with branch chain amino acids in hepatic encephalopathy: A meta-analysis. Gastroenterology 97:1033, 1989.

230. Cerra FB, et al: Disease specific amino acid infusion in hepatic encephalopathy: A prospective randomised double-blind control study. JPEN J Parenter Enteral Nutr 9:288, 1985.

231. Fiaccadori F, et al: Branch chain amino acid enriched solutions in the treatment of hepatic encephalopathy: A controlled trial. In Capocaccia L, Fischer JE, Rossi-Fanelli F (eds): Hepatic Encephalopathy in Chronic Liver Failure. New York, Plenum Press, 1984, p 333.

232. Hehir DJ, Jenkins RL, Bistrian BR, et al: Nutrition in patients undergoing orthotopic liver transplant. JPEN J Parenter Enteral Nutr 9:695–700, 1985.

233. DiCecco S, Wieners EJ, Weisner RH, et al: Assessment of nutritional status of patients with end-stage liver disease. Mayo Clin Proc 64:95–102, 1989.

234. Porayko MK, DiCecco S, O'Keefe SJD: Impact of malnutrition and its therapy on liver transplantation. Semin Liver Dis 11:305–314, 1991.

235. Shaw BW, Wood RP, Gordon RD, et al: Influence of selected patient variables and operative blood loss on six-month survival following liver transplantation. Semin Liver Dis 5:385–393, 1985.

236. Pikul J, Sharpe MD, Lowndes R, et al: Degree of properative malnutrition is predictive of postoperative morbidity and mortality in liver transplant recipients. Transplantation 57:469–472, 1994.

237. Hasse JM, Blue LS, Crippin LS, et al: The effect of nutritional status on length of stay and clinical outcomes following liver transplantation [Abstract]. J Am Diet Assoc 94(Suppl):A38, 1994.

238. Shanbhogue RLK, Bistrian BR, Jenkins RL, et al: Increased protein catabolism without hypermetabolism after human orthotopic liver transplantation. Surgery 101:146–149, 1987.

239. Plevak DJ, DiCecco SR, Wiesner RH, et al: Nutritional support for liver transplantation: Identifying caloric and protein requirements. Mayo Clinic Proceedings 69:225–230, 1994.

240. Hasse JM, Blue LS, Liepa GU, et al: Early enteral nutrition support in patients undergoing liver transplantation. JPEN J Parenter Enteral Nutr 19:437–443, 1995.

241. Berthoux FC, Guerin C, Bertoux P, et al: One-year randomized controlled trial with omega-3 fatty acid–rich fish oil in clinical renal transplant. Transplant Proc 24:2578–2582, 1992.

242. Homan van der Heide JJ, Bilo HJG, Donker JM, et al: Effect of dietary fish oil on renal function and rejection in cyclosporine-treated recipients of renal transplants. N Engl J Med 329:769–773, 1993.

243. Maachi K, Berthoux P, Burgard G, et al: Results of a 1-year randomized controlled trial with omega-3 fatty acid fish oil in renal transplantation under triple immunosuppressive therapy. Transplant Proc 27:846–849, 1995.

244. Bennett WM, Carpenter CB, Shapiro ME, et al: Delayed omega-3 fatty acid supplements in renal transplantation. Transplantation 59:352–356, 1995.

245. Trice S, Melnik G, Page CP: Complications and costs of early postoperative parenteral versus enteral nutrition in trauma patients. Nutr Clin Pract 12:114–119, 1997.

246. Houdijk AP, Rijnsburger ER, Jansen J, et al: Randomised trial of glutamine-enriched enteral nutrition on infectious morbidity in patients with multiple trauma. Lancet 352:772–776, 1998.

247. Li J, Kudsk KA, Janu P, Renegar KB: Effect of glutamine-enriched total parenteral nutrition on small intestinal gut-associated lymphoid tissue and upper respiratory tract immunity. Surgery 121:542–549, 1997.

248. Thissen JP, Verniers J: Inhibition by interleukin-1Beta and tumor necrosis factor alpha of the insulin-like growth factor-1 messenger ribonucleic acid response to growth hormone in rat hepatocyte primary culture. Endocrinology 138:1078–1084, 1997.

249. Wolf M, Bohm S, Brand M, et al: Proinflammatory cytokines interleukin-1Beta and tumor necrosis factor alpha inhibit growth hormone stimulation of insulin-like growth factor-1 synthesis and growth hormone receptor mRNA levels in cultured rat liver cells. Eur J Endocrinol 135:729–737, 1996.

250. Clemmons DR: Use of growth hormone and insulin-like growth factor-1 in catabolism that is induced by negative energy balance. Horm Res 40:62–67, 1993.

251. Ross, R, Miell J, Freeman E, et al: Critically ill patients have high basal growth hormone levels with attenuated oscillatory activity associated with low levels of insulin-like growth factor-1. Clin Endocrinol 35:47–54, 1991.

252. Dahn MS, Lange MP, Jacobs LA: Insulin-like growth factor-1 production is inhibited in human sepsis. Arch Surg 123:1409–1414, 1988.

253. Hermansson M, Wickelgren RB, Hammaqvist F, et al: Measurement of human growth hormone receptor messenger ribonucleic acid by a quantitative polymerase chain reaction–based assay: Demonstration of reduced expression after elective surgery. J Clin Endocrinol Metab 82:421–428, 1997.

254. Hobler SD, Williams AB, Fischer JE, et al: IGF-1 stimulates protein synthesis but does not inhibit protein breakdown in muscle from septic rats. Am J Physiol 274:R571–R576, 1998.

255. Vara-Thorbeck R, Ruiz-Requena E, Guerrero-Fernandez JA: Effects of human growth hormone on the catabolic state after surgical trauma. Horm Res 45:55–60, 1996.

256. Koea JB, Breier BH, Douglas RG, et al: Anabolic and cardiovascular effects of recombinant human growth hormone in surgical patients with sepsis. Br J Surg 83:196–202, 1996.

257. Herndon DN, Hawkins HK, Nguyen TT, et al: Characterization of growth hormone enhanced donor-site healing in patients with large cutaneous burns. Ann Surg 221:649–659, 1995.

258. Herndon DN, Barrow RE, Kunkel KR, et al: Effects of recombinant human growth hormone on donor-site healing in severly burned children. Ann Surg 212:424–429, 1990.

259. Frost RA, Lang CH: Growth factors in critical illness: Regulation and therapeutic aspects. Curr Opin Clin Nutr Metab Care 1:195–204, 1998.

260. Jauck KW: Growth hormone interventions in the postsurgical patients. Presented at International Workshop on Cellular and Molecular Mechanisms in Surgery and Critical Care, Bonn, Germany, March 5, 1998.

261. Wilmore DW: Deterrents to the successful clinical use of growth factors that enhance protein anabolism. Curr Opin Clin Nutr Metab Care 2:15–21, 1999.

262. Pharmacia and Upjohn: Important Drug Warning 10–11, 1997, USA.

263. Unneberg K, Balteskard L, Mjaaland M, et al: Growth hormone increases and IGF-1 reduces the response to *Escherichia coli* infusion in injured pigs. Eur J Surg 163:779–788, 1997.

264. Dahn MS, Lange MP: Systemic and splanchnic metabolic response to exogenous human growth hormone. Surgery 123:528–538, 1998.

265. Gatzen C, Scheltinga MR, Kimbrough TD, et al: Growth hormone attenuates the abnormal distribution of body water in critically ill surgical patients. Surgery 112:181–187, 1992.

266. Byrne TA, Morrissey TB, Gatzen C, et al: Anabolic therapy with growth hormone accelerates protein gain in surgical patients requiring nutritional rehabilitation. Ann Surg 218:400–418, 1993.

267. Hoffman DM, Crampton L, Sernia C, et al: Short term growth hormone (GH) treatment of GH-deficient adults increases body sodium and extracellular water, but not blood pressure. J Clin Endocrinol Metab 81:1123–1128, 1996.

268. Ho KK, O'Sullivan AJ, Hoffman DM: Metabolic actions of growth hormone in man. Endocrinol 42:S57–S63, 1996.

269. Chen K, Okuma T, Okumura K, et al: Insulin-like growth factor-1 prevents gut atrophy and maintains intestinal integrity in septic rats. JPEN J Parenter Enteral Nutr 19:119–124, 1995.

270. Chan S, McCowen KC, Bistrian BR: Medium-chain triglyceride and n-3 polyunsaturated fatty acid–containing emulsions in intravenous nutrition. Curr Opin Clin Nutr Metab Care 1:163–169, 1998.

271. Bell SJ, Bradley D, Forse RA, Bistrian BR: The new dietary fats in health and disease. J Am Diet Assoc 97:280–286, 1997.

272. Palombo JD, Lydon EE, Chen PL, et al: Fatty acid composition of lung, macrophage and surfactant phospholipids after short-term enteral feeding with omega-3 lipids. Lipids 29:643–649, 1994.

273. Palombo JD, DeMichele SJ, Lydon EE, et al: Rapid modulation of lung and liver macrophage phospholipid fatty acids in endotoxemic rats by continuous enteral feeding with omega-3 and gamma-linolenic fatty acids. Am J Clin Nutr 63:208–219, 1996.

274. Palombo JD, Bistrian BR, Fechner KD, et al: Rapid incorporation of fish or olive oil fatty acids into rat hepatic sinusoidal cell phospholipids after continuous enteral feeding during endotoxemia. Am J Clin Nutr 57:643–649, 1993.

275. Utsunomiya T, Chavali SR, Zhong WW, Forse RA: Effects of continuous tube feeding of dietary fat emulsions on eicosanoid production and on fatty acid composition during an acute septic shock in rats. Biochim Biophy Acta 1214:333–339, 1994.

276. Pomposelli JJ, Flores E, Blackburn GL, et al: Diets enriched with n-3 fatty acids ameliorate lactic acidosis by improving endotoxin-induced tissue hypoperfusion in guinea pigs. Am Surg 213:166–176, 1991.

277. Pomposelli JJ, Flores E, Hirschberg Y, et al: Short term TPN containing n-3 fatty acids ameliorate lactic acidosis induced by endotoxin in guinea pigs. Am J Clin Nutr 52:548–552, 1990.

278. Pscheidl EM, Wan JM, Blackburn GL, et al: Influence of omega-3 fatty acids on splanchnic blood flow and lactate metabolism in an endotoxemic rat model. Metab Clin Exp 41:698–705, 1992.

279. Ellis EF, Police RJ, Dodson LY, et al: Effect of dietary n-3 fatty acids on cerebral microcirculation. Am J Physiol 262:H1379–H1386, 1992.

280. Murray MJ, Svingen BA, Holman, et al: Effects of a fish oil diet on pigs' cardiopulmonary response to bacteremia. JPEN J Parenter Enteral Nutr 15:152–158, 1991.

281. Leaf A, Kang JX, Xiao Y, Billman GE: Dietary n-3 fatty acids in the prevention of cardiac arrhythmias. Curr Opin Clin Nutr Metab Care 1:225–228, 1998.

282. Lornz-Meyer H, Bauer P, Nicolay C, et al: Omega-3 fatty acids and low carbohydrate diet for the maintenance of remission in Crohn's disease. Scand J Gastroenterol 31:778–785, 1996.

283. Asian A, Triadafilopoulos G: Fish oil fatty acid supplementation in active ulcerative colitis: A double-blind, placebo-controlled, cross-over study. Am J Gastroenterol 87:432–437, 1992.

284. Lorenz R, Weber PC, Szimnau P, et al: Supplementation with n-3 fatty acids from fish oil in chronic inflammatory bowel disease—A randomized, placebo-controlled, double-blind cross-over trial. J Intern Med 225:225–232, 1989.

285. Hawthorne AB, Daneshmend TK, Hawkey CJ, et al: Treatment of ulcerative colitis with fish oil supplementation: A prospective 12 month randomized controlled trial. Gut 33:922–928, 1992.

286. Stenson WF, Cort D, Rodgers J, et al: Dietary supplementation with fish oils in ulcerative colitis. Ann Intern Med 116:609–614, 1992.

287. Koeschke K, Ueberschaer B, Pietsch A, et al: n-3 fatty acids only delay early relapse of ulcerative colitis in remission. Dig Dis Sci 41:2087–2094, 1996.

288. Belluzi A, Brignola C, Campieri M, et al: Effect of an enteric-coated fish oil preparation on relapses in Crohn's disease. N Engl J Med 334:1557–1560, 1996.

289. Maloo MC, Maloo MK: Privatize the profits and socialize the risks: Are health maintenance organizations tangling with doctors, hospital and cash flows? [Abstract] Page No. 1678 Volume No.3 Presented at the 29th Annual Meeting of the Decision Sciences Institute. Las Vegas, Nevada. Nov 21–24, 1998.

11

◆ Parenteral Nutrition in Inflammatory Bowel Disease

Michael E. Kupferman, M.D.
John L. Rombeau, M.D.

Inflammatory bowel disease (IBD), including Crohn's disease (CD) and ulcerative colitis (UC), results in some degree of malnutrition in the majority of patients. Treating the nutritional deficiencies by either oral or enteral feeding is complicated by the diseased gastrointestinal tract; thus, total parenteral nutrition (TPN) is often needed to meet nutritional needs and correct pre-existing deficits. This chapter reviews the etiology of malnutrition and the ensuing metabolic and physiologic alterations, the evaluation of the malnourished patient, and the indications for TPN in both CD and UC.

◆ ETIOLOGY OF MALNUTRITION IN INFLAMMATORY BOWEL DISEASE

The malnutritive sequelae of IBD are protean, resulting in severe metabolic disturbances in both adults and children. Approximately two thirds of patients hospitalized for IBD are malnourished, as evidenced by weight loss, anemia, hypoalbuminemia, and vitamin deficiencies.[1] These deficiencies are the result of four processes: (1) decreased oral intake, (2) nutrient losses from the intestines, (3) increased metabolic demand, and (4) drug-nutrient interaction.

Decreased Oral Intake

Decreased oral intake results from anorexia, abdominal symptoms, and dietary restriction. The active inflammatory process in the intestine is accompanied by the release of numerous cytokines, such as interleukin 6 and tumor necrosis factor, which cause anorexia.[2] Symptoms experienced by patients with either UC or CD are similar. These include bloating, early satiety, altered taste, diarrhea, and abdominal cramping, all re-

sulting in decreased food intake. Additionally, the postprandial abdominal pain often leads to an avoidance of food. Other factors contributing to decreased nutrient intake include physician-ordered dietary restriction and selective restriction of trigger foods. In an observational study, patients with CD who experienced weight loss had lower protein and caloric intake, less enjoyment from eating, and less hunger.[3] Decreased nutrient intake has been recognized as being the primary cause of malnutrition in patients with CD.[4]

Nutrient Losses from the Intestine

IBD-induced malabsorption leads to a loss of vital nutrients and minerals in the stool. The inflammatory process causes rapid transit, a decreased absorptive area, a loss of brush-border colonocytes, decreased nutrient absorption, and excess intestinal secretions. Histologic abnormalities in radiographically and grossly normal bowel have also been demonstrated. Multiple intestinal resections are often required in patients with CD and contribute to a decreased absorptive area. Bacterial overgrowth in the small and large intestine prevents normal epithelial absorptive function. Inflammation leads to shedding of the brush-border epithelium and digestive enzymes, contributing not only to the malabsorption but also to the protein-losing enteropathy of IBD.[5] Protein loss can be as high as 80 to 90 g/day in patients with CD.[6] Excess intestinal mucus secretion and inflammatory-induced bleeding exacerbate the loss of proteins and minerals. Impaired recycling of bile salts by the terminal ileum leads to steatorrhea and decreased lipid and lipid-soluble vitamin absorption. Diarrhea results in not only fluid loss but also electrolyte imbalance.

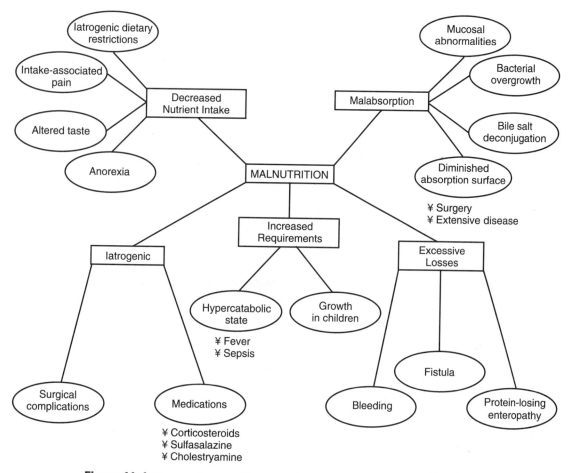

Figure 11–1. Causes of malnutrition in patients with inflammatory bowel disease.

Increased Metabolic Demand

The chronic inflammatory process presumably leads to an increased resting energy requirement in patients with IBD, which in turn exacerbates the underlying weight loss and malnutrition. Fever, sepsis, and operative treatment increase the patient's fat, protein, and carbohydrate requirement to enhance healing. The resting energy expenditure (REE) is increased in sepsis, and every degree Celsius rise increases the REE by 13%.[7] The increased cell turnover in the colon and treatment with corticosteroids induce a catabolic state that contributes to increased metabolic demand in patients with IBD.[8]

However, recent studies have shown that REE levels are equal to or even less than those predicted by the Harris-Benedict equation, suggesting that REE in IBD patients is the same as that in normal individuals.[9, 10]

Further, it has been shown that as disease activity increases, the active energy expenditure decreases, maintaining a constant level of total REE.[11] In a study of patients with CD who had evidence of weight loss (63 patients) and those who did not (30 patients), no difference was seen in regard to REE and fecal energy losses.[12] Weight loss occurred in the patients with lower protein and energy intake and more food restrictions. Nonetheless, metabolic demands seem to play a role in the development of malnutrition.

In the pediatric population, nutrient requirements are increased to allow normal growth and development.[13] However, the nutritional intake is often inadequate, leading to growth retardation or failure in a significant number of patients.[14] These findings support the aggressive use of nutritional therapy in children with IBD.

Drug-Nutrient Interaction

Pharmacologic therapy for IBD can itself contribute to the development of malnutrition. Calcium metabolism is altered by corticosteroids and can lead to a decrease in intestinal absorption and an increase in urinary excretion.[15] Corticosteroids deplete body stores by increasing albumin metabolism.[16] Immunomodulators, such as cyclosporine, methotrexate, and azathioprine, can induce a plethora of gastrointestinal side effects, including nausea, vomiting, diarrhea, stomatitis, and esophagitis, all leading to increased loss or decreased intake of nutrients.[17–20] Folate absorption is impaired with the coadministration of sulfasalazine.[3]

◆ NUTRITIONAL DEFICIENCIES IN PATIENTS WITH INFLAMMATORY BOWEL DISEASE (Table 11–1)

Hypoalbuminemia

Serum albumin levels reflect the nutritional status in patients over prolonged periods and have been used to measure chronic protein malnutrition. One group reported the

Table 11–1. Reported Prevalence of Nutritional Deficiencies in Inflammatory Bowel Disease

Deficiency	Prevalence (%)	
	Crohn's Disease	Ulcerative Colitis
Weight loss	65–75	18–62
Hypoalbuminemia	25–80	25–50
Intestinal protein loss	75	ND
Negative nitrogen balance	69	ND
Anemia	25–85	66
Low iron	39	81
Low vitamin B_{12}	48	5
Low folic acid	67	30–40
Low calcium	13	ND
Low magnesium	14–33	ND
Low potassium	5–20	ND
Low vitamin A	11	NR
Low vitamin C	ND	NR
Low vitamin D	75	35
Low vitamin K	ND	NR
Low zinc	50	ND
Low copper	ND	

Adapted from Dieleman LA, Heizer WD: Nutritional issues in inflammatory bowel disease. Gastroenterol Clin North Am 27:435–451, 1998.

ND, reported but incidence not described; NR, not reported.

presence of hypoalbuminemia in 25 to 80% of patients with CD and in 25 to 50% with UC, reflecting the chronicity of malnutrition in a significant number of patients with IBD.[5] In children, 59% with CD and 33% with UC were found to have abnormally decreased albumin levels.[21] Other researchers found a mean serum albumin level of 2.9 ± 13 g/dL in a 10-year review of 74 adults with IBD.[22] Hypoalbuminemia has been correlated with disease activity in a study of 46 patients with "severe" attacks of UC, in whom the mean serum albumin level was 3.34 g/dL.[23] However, single measurements of serum albumin levels do not accurately reflect disease activity and acute or recent malnutrition in CD.[24]

Vitamin Deficiencies

The vitamin deficiencies seen in IBD, and CD in particular, are protean. Decreased levels of vitamins A, E, B_6, B_1, riboflavin, and folate were found in patients with CD when compared with controls.[25] Similarly, when compared with controls, patients with CD in remission had decreased levels of vitamins A, C, and E and β-carotene. Metabolic bone disease has been associated with CD,[26] with concomitant low serum levels of vitamin D that have been correlated with disease activity.[27] Vitamin deficiencies are exacerbated by the use of sulfasalazine and corticosteroids. Patients with IBD are at increased risk of developing osteopenia and osteoporosis, particularly from the effects of steroids and inflammation.[3, 28] A study failed to show any benefit or increase in bone density in IBD patients after 1 year of therapy with vitamin D and calcium supplementation.[29] Deficiencies in other vitamins, including niacin and ascorbic acid, have also been described.[17]

Mineral Deficiencies

In addition to depleted sodium and potassium stores from diarrhea and malabsorption,[30, 31] numerous other mineral deficiencies are present in IBD. The clinical importance of trace elements has gained wide acceptance, and recognizing these deficiencies in patients with IBD is imperative. Zinc deficiency is the most common trace mineral deficiency in IBD.[32] One study reported significant decreases in serum concentrations of zinc and magnesium in patients with CD in remission.[33] Deficiencies of copper, chromium, molybdenum, selenium, and manganese in patients with IBD have been described.[34, 36] Patients on long-term TPN treatment are at increased risk for developing trace element deficiencies. Patients on long-term home TPN were found to have severely depleted body stores of selenium[37] due to reduced absorption, excessive endogenous intestinal loss, and decreased intake.[38] Selenium deficiency can predispose to cardiomyopathy.[39]

◆ NUTRIENT-RELATED CLINICAL ABNORMALITIES IN PATIENTS WITH INFLAMMATORY BOWEL DISEASE

Body Weight Loss

Significant weight loss in patients with both CD and UC has been extensively documented and is accompanied by alterations in other anthropomorphic measurements.[40, 41] Clinically relevant weight loss occurs in 65 to 75% of patients with CD and in 18 to 62% of patients with UC.[32, 42] Weight loss has been reported to be above 80% in children with CD.[43]

Anemia

There is a high incidence of anemia in IBD, with reports of 60 to 80% in CD and 66% in UC.[21, 42] Iron deficiency anemia is found in 81% of patients with UC and in 39% with CD. Iron absorption is maintained;[44] however, mucosal hemorrhage, intestinal ulceration, and subsequent fecal blood loss account for the iron deficiency anemia seen in UC. Low iron stores, which occur in approximately 60 to 80% of patients with UC,[5] can be confirmed with a bone marrow smear or with a serum ferritin test, which correlates well with bone marrow stores.[45] Release of inflammatory mediators from diseased colonic mucosa can cause an anemia of chronic disease and exacerbate the iron deficiency anemia of IBD.[2] Anemia in CD is complicated by disease involving the entire gastrointestinal tract. Sulfasalazine, one of the mainstays of treatment in CD, decreases the absorption of folate in the proximal

small bowel.[46] One study found an association between low red blood cell folate levels and the development of dysplasia and cancer in UC. Supplementing folate in this patient population resulted in a decreased incidence of cancer.[47]

The anemia in CD can often be megaloblastic, due to decreased folate and vitamin B_{12} absorption. Although folate deficiency has been well documented in patients with CD,[21, 42] no study has linked disease in the proximal bowel, the site of folate absorption, to folate malabsorption.[48] It has been postulated that the ongoing inflammatory process that is characteristic of the disease leads to greater cell turnover and subsequent folate depletion when the intake is insufficient.[49] Steatorrhea, bacterial overgrowth, and involvement or resection of the terminal ileum results in impaired vitamin B_{12} absorption, leading to a megaloblastic anemia.[8, 48]

Growth Retardation

IBD in children is particularly devastating, as the disease chronicity and nutritional deficiencies lead to growth failure or growth retardation. Approximately 30% of children with CD and 5 to 10% with UC have growth failure.[50] Body height, weight, and growth velocity are all substandard in this group of patients.[14] Delay in the onset of puberty, skeletal maturation, and the development of secondary sex characteristics is common in children with IBD.[51] Intestinal symptoms may not develop until growth failure has been apparent for years,[52] and as few as 14% and as many as 88% of children may have subnormal growth before IBD is diagnosed.[53, 54]

The etiology of growth failure in pediatric IBD is multifactorial and shares similarities with the malnutrition of adult IBD. Decreased oral intake; malabsorption; increased metabolic demand; steroid therapy; and growth hormone deficiency all contribute to growth failure, but inadequate nutrient intake plays the largest role.[52, 55–57] Children with CD have an intake of 2760 kcal/day compared with the average requirements for chronologic age of 3180 kcal/day.[13] The growth failure syndrome seen in CD is clinically similar to the well-characterized *nutritional dwarfing*.[58] It has been noted that children with CD have similar rates of protein synthesis and breakdown and net protein retention when compared with controls,[59] providing further evidence that nutrient intake plays a primary role in the development of growth failure in these patients.

Although surgical resection of the diseased intestine, as well as conventional medical treatment, contributes to improved growth development,[21] nutritional management is the primary means to promote growth. Nutritional therapy must be started as soon as the diagnosis of Crohn's disease–induced growth arrest is established. Bone maturation, when advanced, may make it difficult if not impossible to achieve normal height at the adult age. An assessment of the development of permanent growth failure in children and adolescents with IBD showed that 19 to 35% of children and adolescents who suffer from IBD have permanent growth failure in adulthood and are noticeably shorter in stature than the general population.[60] Restoration of normal body composition and reversal of growth failure can be accomplished with the administration of nutritional support but will be successful only if it is initiated before the completion of skeletal growth.[61]

◆ NUTRITIONAL ASSESSMENT IN PATIENTS WITH INFLAMMATORY BOWEL DISEASE

It is imperative that all patients with IBD undergo nutritional assessment. A number of clinical and biochemical parameters have been proposed to diagnose malnutrition accurately; however, many of the measurements and indices have inherent inadequacies and alone would be insufficient for assessing nutritional status. Malnutrition is most accurately defined by a method that predicts nutrition-associated complications and prognosis, thus providing the physician with a predication of the clinical outcome.[62] A precise nutritional assessment of the patient with IBD includes taking a thorough medical history, performing a comprehensive physical examination, and conducting selected laboratory tests. Components of nutritional assessment include the following:

1. *Body composition analyses.* Although the technology exists to perform accurate measurements of all body components, these techniques are not readily available, and no single body component measurement predicts the outcome of malnourished patients.[63]

2. *Weight loss.* Body weight and weight loss can be assessed by determining the patient's ideal body weight and comparing that with the usual weight or by determining a patient's body mass index (kg/m²). These measurements can be confounded by errors of recall,[64] body habitus, and hydration status. Despite these limitations, body weight loss is still the most important predictor of adverse clinical outcome in most hospitalized patients.

3. *Anthropometry.* Muscle mass and the body fat index are determined by measuring the midarm muscle circumference and triceps skinfold thickness, respectively. Although the oft-employed published standards used to assess anthropomorphic data have their limitations in comparative studies, there is a consensus that abnormal values below the fifth percentile are indicative of malnutrition and bode poorly for clinical outcomes.[64]

4. *Serum proteins.* Although serum albumin levels are depressed in a number of chronic disease processes and correlate with increased medical complications, they are not adequate indicators of acute protein malnutrition.[65–68] Protein malnutrition does suppress the hepatic synthesis of albumin, but because of albumin's long half-life and large circulating pool, albumin levels do not change significantly in an acutely malnourished patient. Multiple studies have shown that a protein-deficient diet, although resulting in weight loss and decreased lean body mass, does not lead to decreased serum albumin levels.[69, 70] Levels of prealbumin, another serum protein, are suppressed in malnourished patients and are used as markers of acute malnutrition, mainly due to its short half-life. Additionally, reduced prealbumin levels can be reversed with refeeding.[71] However, the serum concentration of this transport protein can be affected by other physiologic factors, and thus it is not a reliable indicator of malnutrition.

5. *Discriminant analyses.* Various indices have been developed to quantitatively assess the nutritional status in malnourished patients and to predict outcomes. Buzby and colleagues proposed the Prognostic Nutritional Index, using serum al-

bumin and prealbumin concentrations, triceps skinfold thickness, and immune competence, to predict clinical outcomes in malnourished patients.[72] Similarly, the Nutrition Risk Index utilizes serum albumin levels and body weight changes as variables to stratify malnourished surgical patients.[73-75]

The Subjective Global Assessment is based on nutritionally relevant features of the patient's medical history and physical examination.[76, 77] It is the most frequently used composite index of nutritional status. The assessment allows the physician to identify malnourished patients who have an increased risk for medical complications and who would obtain significant clinical improvement from nutritional therapy. The patient is analyzed for restriction of nutrient intake, for physiologic alterations due to malnutrition, and for the influence of disease on nutrient requirements. The medical history emphasizes: (1) weight loss, (2) food intake, (3) gastrointestinal symptoms, (4) functional capacity, and (5) disease type and catabolic effects.

The physical examination focuses on body habitus and alterations in body composition: (1) loss of subcutaneous fat in the triceps and mid–axillary line area, (2) temporalis, deltoid, and quadriceps muscle wasting, (3) edema, and (4) mucosal and cutaneous lesions. These measurements are graded as normal, mild, moderate, or severe.

On the basis of the data obtained from the medical history and physical examination, the patient's nutritional status is categorized as well nourished, moderately malnourished, or severely malnourished.

Geering and colleagues assessed the nutritional status of patients with Crohn's disease in remission using four parameters: (1) body composition, (2) dietary intake, (3) biochemical indices, and (4) muscle strength (Table 11–2).[33] The investigators found that compared with control subjects, men with CD had statistically significant lower levels of percentage body fat ($P < .05$, $P < .01$) and total body bone mineral content ($P < .05$). Among women, only the bone mineral content was different from control levels ($P < .025$). Except for amounts of fiber, phosphorus, and vitamin A, the nutritional intake among the control and CD groups was not significantly different. A number of serum biochemical indices were markedly lower in the CD group compared with con-

Table 11–2. Indicators of Nutritional Status in Patients with Crohn's Disease in Remission

Indicator	Crohn's Disease	Control
Body fat (%), male	18.2	24.7
Bone mineral content (kg)	2.4	2.6
Fiber intake (g/MJ)	1.5	1.9
Phosphorus intake (g)	1.4	1.7
Serum albumin (g/L)	37.7	42.5
Serum β-carotene (μmol/L)	0.98	2.33
Serum vitamin C (μmol/L)	35.3	57.8
Serum vitamin E (μmol/L)	29.2	34.8
Serum mgnesium (mmol/L)	0.79	0.85
Serum selenium (μmol/L)	0.86	1.03
Serum zinc (μmol/L)	12.0	13.4
Serum glutathione peroxidase (U/mmol HgB)	768	967
Serum cholesterol (mmol/L)	4.3	5.7
Serum lipids (g/L)	1.16	1.37

HgB, hemoglobin
Adapted from Geerping BJ, Badart-Smook A, Stockbrugger RW, Brummer RJ: Comprehensive nutritional status in patients with long-standing Crohn disease currently in remission. Am J Clin Nutr 67:919–926, 1998.

trols. These included albumin, β-carotene, vitamins C and E, magnesium, selenium, zinc, cholesterol, and total lipid levels. Various measures of muscle strength, using an isokinetic dynamometer, revealed significant differences between the CD and the control group. The authors conclude that a comprehensive nutritional assessment will better detect nutritional deficiencies than using a single dimension of nutritional status.

The Subjective Global Assessment is indeed subjective; as a consequence, there are no absolute values for measurement. It is effective in predicting complications in general surgical patients,[78] dialysis patients,[79] and liver transplantation patients.[80, 81] To our knowledge, there are no reports confirming its accuracy in malnourished IBD patients. However, it is our preferred method of assessing nutritional status in patients with IBD. Consideration of the complete clinical picture and the physician's common sense and judgment determine the value of this assessment.

◆ NUTRITIONAL REQUIREMENTS AND INFLAMMATORY BOWEL DISEASE

After the common nutritional deficiencies are determined and the nutritional status of a patient with IBD is assessed, it is important to determine the patient's energy and protein requirements. Energy requirements are calculated from the patient's weight, height, age, and gender. The basis for this calculation is the Harris-Benedict equation for determining resting metabolic expenditure:

$$\text{Male RME (kcal/day)} = 66 + (13.7 \times W) + (5 \times H) - (6.8 \times A)$$
$$\text{Female RME (kcal/day)} = 655 + (9.6 \times W) + (1.7 \times H) - (4.7 \times A)$$

where RME is resting metabolic expenditure, W is body weight in kilograms, H is height in centimeters, A is age in years.

After determination of the resting metabolic expenditure, total energy requirements are adjusted according to the patient's disease or clinical status.

Indirect calorimetry is a more accurate yet more complicated and expensive method for determining energy requirements. This method is based on the oxidation of organic fuels, measuring oxygen consumption and carbon dioxide production, and determining energy expenditure from a metabolic equation. Using indirect calorimetry, one group determined the energy requirements in 35 patients with nonseptic IBD.[82] They found that the predicted basal energy expenditure as calculated by the Harris-Benedict formula was equivalent to the measured REE. When patients had body weights greater than 90% of ideal body weight, their measured REEs did not differ from those of control subjects. Patients whose body weights were less than 90% of ideal body weight had significantly higher measured energy expenditure per kilogram of body weight than either control subjects or patients whose body weights were 90% or more of ideal body weight ($P < .001$). However, this increase could also be predicted by using the Harris-Benedict formula for these patients. The authors concluded that the Harris-Benedict equation can be used to determine caloric requirements of patients with IBD in the absence of significant weight loss or sepsis. In general, calorie requirements for nonseptic, fairly weight-stable patients are 1.5 times the basal energy expenditure. However, in situations in which multiple stress factors are combined with acute changes in nutritional status, techniques that measure the actual energy expenditure, such as indirect calorimetry, may be preferable.

In active IBD, protein is lost into the intestinal lumen and excreted as fecal nitrogen.[83] In addition, patients with CD have reduced pancreatic enzymatic output; therefore, their rate of proteolytic digestion may be impaired by as much as 30%.[84] There is also a poorly understood effect of the inflammatory process per se on protein metabolism, which is similar to that occurring in infectious diseases. Intestinal mucosal disease may interfere with peptide and amino acid absorption, and bacterial overgrowth can interfere with protein homeostasis.[85] Because of these pathologic changes, patients with IBD may present with severe protein deficiency, and their protein requirements may be greater than anticipated, especially when diarrhea, steatorrhea, hematochezia, or melena is present.

As a general rule, the amount of protein needed to meet the daily requirement of patients with IBD ranges from 0.75 to 2 g/kg body weight per day. This amount is higher in the hypercatabolic patient and lower in the patient with liver disease or renal failure.

As previously stated, vitamin, mineral, and trace element deficiencies are common in patients with IBD. Adequate daily supplies of these nutrients must be provided for patients with IBD who are receiving TPN.

◆ PARENTERAL NUTRITION AND INFLAMMATORY BOWEL DISEASE

The three indications for the use of TPN in patients with IBD are perioperative support, nutritional replacement, and primary therapy.

The use of TPN for nutritional replacement in IBD does not differ from its use in other diseases. The clinician must be aware, however, of the specific nutritional deficits occurring in patients with IBD and must keep in mind that in the presence of sepsis, energy requirements increase above the normal needs.

The use of TPN as perioperative support is controversial because of its expense and questionable efficacy in the few clinical trials.

Another possible indication for TPN in IBD is primary therapy. When conventional medical treatment fails, the alternative is to start the patient on "bowel rest" with TPN. The availability of TPN makes the use of bowel rest nutritionally feasible and has prompted the combined use of TPN, bowel rest, and anti-inflammatory medications as the primary therapy for IBD, especially for CD. The rationale for using bowel rest as a therapeutic maneuver is to avoid oral intake because of the presence of symptoms of obstruction or in the hope that patients will have symptomatic improvement as a result of the decreased mechanical, physical, and chemical activities of the bowel. It should be noted that the clinical practice of bowel rest is undergoing vigorous scientific scrutiny, mainly because of its adverse effects of decreasing intestinal absorptive surface area and reducing enzymatic activity of the gut.[86-89] Furthermore, bowel rest may aid in promoting bacterial translocation and transmigration of endotoxin, especially in conditions such as IBD, in which disruption of the intestinal epithelium occurs.[90-93]

When the reported effects of TPN in patients with IBD are analyzed, there are some noteworthy considerations. Both CD and UC are frequently reported together as IBD, without adequate differentiation between the two diseases. Although the diseases share several pathologic features, the overall prognosis, surgical success, and long-term sequelae are different for each condition. Therefore, it is essential that the two diseases be analyzed separately. Another problem is the lack of uniform long-term follow-up. In published reports, follow-ups vary from weeks to years; therefore, comparative reports must be evaluated very cautiously. Further problems include the lack of uniformity in defining the terms *remission* and *relapse*. Finally, no consensus exists as to what constitutes medical failure. In most "nutritional" studies, adjuvant medical treatment was continued during the period of nutritional therapy, further confounding the interpretation of results.

In the following section, we review the published trials of TPN and IBD that have addressed (1) TPN as primary therapy for CD, (2) TPN as primary therapy for UC, (3) preoperative TPN and CD, and (4) TPN and fistulous CD.

◆ TOTAL PARENTERAL NUTRITION AS PRIMARY THERAPY FOR CROHN'S DISEASE

Tables 11–3 and 11–4 summarize the reported series of the use of TPN as primary

therapy for patients with CD. Among the 17 retrospective studies shown in Table 11–3, the mean hospital remission rate was 55.5%. Long-term remission rates were lower, and in many cases the time of follow-up was not reported. Only a few prospective studies have been reported (see Table 11–4).

Elson and colleagues reported on 20 patients with CD who were treated with TPN for 36 days.[96] They achieved a 75% remission rate during hospitalization, which decreased to 44% after 20 to 48 months of follow-up. They also reported five partial remissions that were controlled with medication.

Müller and associates reported on a pilot project to obtain reliable data for a clinical trial comparing TPN with intestinal resection in patients with CD.[97] Thirty patients entered the study. All of them were hospitalized for surgery because they either had failed to respond to medical therapy or had developed complications such as enterocutaneous fistulas, intermittent ileus, or bleeding. During the trial, all medications were discontinued. TPN was started in the hospital and continued for as long as 12 weeks at home. Twenty-five patients responded promptly to TPN. Surgery was avoided in these patients, and they were discharged within 11 to 23 days after beginning TPN. In five patients, TPN did not control the active disease, and surgery was performed. During the first 12 months of follow-up, 8 of the 25 patients who were early in remission had to be hospitalized because of a recurrence of the disease. In the following 12 to 48 months, relapses occurred in another nine patients, one of whom died. The remaining eight patients were in remission after 48 months, without evidence of active disease. The authors compared the results of their series with the results in historical control patients from the same hospital who underwent surgery. The cumulative recurrence rate after 4 years of follow-up was about four times higher in the group receiving TPN than in the surgical control group.

Lerebours and colleagues reported an evaluation of TPN in the management of steroid-dependent and steroid-resistant patients with CD.[98] Twenty patients with severe CD, defined by the Best index[99] as higher than 150, were investigated. Steroid therapy during TPN was conducted without protocol according to the overall course of the disease. The clinical response was judged to be positive if a marked diminution

Table 11–3. Crohn's Disease and Total Parenteral Nutrition as Primary Therapy: Retrospective Studies

Study	No. of Patients	Duration of TPN (days)	Hospital Remissions	Long-Term Remissions	Length of Follow-up (mo)	Remarks
Anderson and Boyce (1973)[94a]	4	30	4 (100%)	1 (25%)	3	
Fischer et al. (1973)[106]	7	NR	3 (43%)	NR	NR	Additional medical therapy
Vogel et al. (1974)[95]	8	9–50	8 (100%)	4 (50%)	4–36	Additional medical therapy
Eisenberg et al. (1974)[120]	9	21	5 (55%)	NR	NR	
Fazio et al. (1976)[108] and Harford and Fazio (1979)[109]	18	20	11 (61%)	4 (22%)	27	
Reilly et al. (1976)[107]	23	33	14 (61%)	12 (52%)	42	Additional steroids
Dean et al. (1976)[110]	11	14	4 (36%)	NR	NR	Additional medical therapy
Mullen et al. (1978)[22]	50	26	19 (38%)	10 (20%)	120	Additional medical therapy
Bos and Westerman (1980)[95a]	86	41.1	24 (28%)	NR	NR	
Holm (1981)[95b]	8	79	7 (87.5)	4 (57%)	42	
Shiloni and Freund (1983)[95c]	16	53	9 (56%)	6 (37%)	3–36	
Ostro et al. (1985)[122]	100	NR	77 (77%)	68 (69%) 50 (54%)	3 12	49% receiving steroids
Kushner et al. (1986)[95d]	10	124	3 (30%)	0 (0%)	18.6	Partial remissions with prednisone
Shiloni et al. (1989)[104]	49	30	22 (45%)	25 (50%)	1.5–29.3	Medications used in some instances
Sitzmann et al. (1990)[95e]	16	35.6	15 (94%)	11 (73.3%)	30.6	Additional medical therapy
Cravo et al. (1991)[95f]	24	NR	18 (75%)	Partial: 12 (52%) Total: 7 (31%)	21.1	Additional medical therapy

NR, not reported; TPN, total parenteral nutrition.

or cessation of symptoms was observed, with the Best index shifting below 150, and if steroid therapy could be discontinued or decreased without causing relapse. A long-term remission was defined as the absence of symptoms and the discontinuation of all medications, according to the classification of Elson and colleagues.[96] A positive clinical response to TPN was obtained in 19 patients. The results were not significantly different between the steroid-resistant and the steroid-dependent groups. After a mean 25 months of follow-up, 3 of the 19 patients who had had positive responses were symptom-free without any medications. The remaining 16 patients had relapses, which either were uncontrolled (four patients) or were controlled with steroids or other medical therapy.

To our knowledge, the trial described in the 1980 paper by Dickinson and colleagues was the first prospective controlled trial of TPN and CD.[86] Nineteen patients with acute Crohn's colitis were divided into two groups. The control group (receiving a normal hospital diet) consisted of 3 patients, and the group receiving TPN comprised 16 individuals. All patients were treated with bed rest and prednisone at 40 mg/day. The long-term follow-up, for a minimum of 15 months, revealed that all control patients had relapsed, and only one patient remained free of symptoms in the group receiving TPN.

McIntyre and colleagues reported a multicenter controlled trial of bowel rest in the treatment of acute colitis in 16 patients with CD.[87] The patients were randomly assigned to receive either TPN and only water by mouth (the bowel rest group) or an oral diet consisting of hospital meals. After a median length of 43 months of follow-up, 11 of the 16 patients with CD had relapsed (5 in the group on oral diet and 6 in the group on TPN).

In 1987, Alun Jones reported the results of a controlled trial to determine the relative efficacy of TPN and an elemental diet in the induction of remission of CD. The long-term outcome was not reported. Twenty-nine patients were assigned to one of two groups: TPN (n = 16) and elemental diet (n = 13). Two patients in each group failed to achieve remission after 14 days of therapy.[88]

Greenberg and coworkers reported a controlled trial of bowel rest and nutritional support in 51 patients with active CD that was unresponsive to other medical treatments.[89] The patients were randomly assigned to one of three nutritional support groups designed to be administered in the hospital for 21 days. The groups were TPN and nothing by mouth (n = 17), defined-formula enteral diet (n = 19), and partial parenteral nutrition and oral food (n = 15). All medications were discontinued, with the exception of prednisone. A full clinical remission included a Crohn's Disease Activity Index (CDAI)[100] of less than 150 by the 21st day of therapy and the maintenance of a full oral diet without an increase in the index score, medication, or surgery. A relapse included the CDAI's rising to greater than 250; complications requiring an increase in the prednisone dosage, TPN, or surgery; or other medical reasons (drug toxicity) that made continuous therapy hazardous. Remission rates after the 3 weeks of nutritional support were 71% for the group receiving TPN, 58% for the group receiving a defined enteral diet, and 60% for the third group (partial parenteral nutrition and oral diet). After 12 months of follow-up, the remission rates were equivalent among the three groups and were not influenced by the type of nutritional support initially administered. The authors concluded that nutritional support without bowel rest induced a clinical remission in the majority of patients with active CD who had not responded to medical management. The outcome with defined-formula enteral diets was equivalent to that of TPN.

Wright and Adler conducted a prospective randomized trial to evaluate the relative efficacy of peripheral parenteral nutrition and an elemental diet in patients with acute exacerbations of CD.[101] Eleven patients were randomly assigned to receive either the TPN (n = 5) or elemental diet (n = 6). Patients were treated with either TPN or total enteral nutrition (TEN) for 7 to 14 days. The endpoints were defined as a CDAI of less than 150 or 14 days of treatment. The patients' response to treatment was assessed by both clinical and biochemical parameters, including the CDAI, serum transferrin levels, retinol-binding protein levels, the lympho-

Table 11–4. Crohn's Disease and Total Parenteral Nutrition as Primary Therapy: Prospective Studies

Study	No. of Patients	Duration of TPN (days)	Hospital Remissions	Long-Term Remissions	Length of Follow-up (mo)	Remarks
Prospective Studies						
Greenberg et al. (1976)[121]	43	25	33 (77%)	29 (67%)	24	
Elson et al. (1980)[96]	20	36	13 (65%)	3 (15%)	20–48	Partial remissions with medication
Müller et al. (1983)[97]	30	84	25 (83.3%)	8 (27%)	48	
Lerebours et al. (1986)[98]	20	42	19 (95%)	3 (15%)	25	Prednisone
Prospective Randomized Controlled Studies						
Dickinson et al. (1980)[86]	3 C 6 TPN	24 19	3 (100%) 4 (67%)	0 (0%) 1 (17%)	16–48	Prednisone
McIntyre et al. (1986)[87]	9 TPN 7 OD	7	9 (100%) 5 (71.4%)	3 (33%) 2 (28.6%)	27–64	Prednisone, 20 mg/8 h
Alun Jones (1987)[88]	16 TPN 14 ED	7–14	14 (87.5%) 11 (85%)	NR	NR	No medications, no bed rest
Greenberg et al. (1988)[89]	17 TPN 19 ED 15 PPN	21	12 (71%) 11 (58%) 9 (60%)	5 (29%) 6 (32%) 5 (33%)	12	Prednisone
Wright and Adler (1990)[101]	5 TPN 6 ED	7–14	5 (100%) 6 (100%)	NR	NR	Remission based on CDAI

C, control group; CDAL, Crohn's Disease Activity Index; ED, element diet; NR, not reported; OD, oral diet; PPN, partial parenteral nutrition; TPN, total parenteral nutrition.

cyte count, and anthropomorphic data. In both groups, the CDAI improved significantly after nutritional therapy was instituted ($P < .05$), but changes in weight did not correlate with clinical subjective improvement of disease. Among the group receiving TEN, the serum transferrin level improved significantly ($P < .05$), but it did not in the TPN group. Similarly, the total lymphocyte count increased among the patients receiving TEN but did not change significantly in the patients receiving TPN. Additionally, the group receiving enteral nutrition had an increased caloric intake compared with the TPN group. This was attributed to the limitations in the method of administering TPN. The authors conclude that the mode of nutritional therapy in acute exacerbations of CD does not significantly affect the clinical outcome or the short-term outcome, as assessed by the CDAI. Because the alterations in biochemical and anthropometric data did not correlate with clinical disease improvement, enteral nutrition does not appear to be superior to TPN.

Christie and Hill analyzed the effect of TPN on protein metabolism and muscle physiology in patients with acute attacks of CD and UC.[102] Nineteen patients were admitted to the hospital for IBD that was unresponsive to outpatient medical therapy for at least 3 weeks. Fifteen patients had CD and four had UC. Inclusion criteria included a weight loss greater than 10% over a 3-month period, skinfold testing, exercise intolerance, a serum albumin level less than 32 g/L, and other physiologic impairments. Patients were age-, gender- and height-matched to a group of normal healthy volunteers. Before the onset of TPN, patients were evaluated for total body protein, plasma proteins, respiratory muscle function, and skeletal muscle function, and they were evaluated again at 7 and 14 days after the initiation of TPN. Long-term data were obtained on an outpatient basis at an average of 200 days after therapy. TPN was administered for 14 days, along with 40 mg of prednisone per day. Initially, patients had lost 27% ($P < .001$) of their body weight, 35% of their protein ($P < .0001$), and 32% of their fat ($P < .01$), compared with the control group. Patients demonstrated impairments in both skeletal and respiratory muscle function. However, respiratory and skeletal muscle function improved rapidly within 7 days of the initiation of therapy

and continued to improve during the study. The total body protein did not improve significantly during the TPN-treatment phase but did improve over the course of the convalescent phase. The authors concluded that the initiation of TPN in acute exacerbations of IBD significantly improved skeletal and respiratory muscle function early in treatment, with concomitant prevention of continued protein loss and eventual repletion of total protein levels.

Although TPN has been shown to improve the clinical outcome of patients with acute flares of CD, the role of luminal contents in the progression of disease and in bowel integrity is becoming more apparent with clinical studies. Payne-James and Silk recommend that TPN be used only for nutritional support and not as a primary therapeutic modality.[103] Additional data from Shiloni and colleagues have confirmed this observation, reporting that the use of TPN in severe exacerbations of CD will only delay the need for eventual surgery, with a higher cost and greater risk to the patient.[104]

It has become apparent, based on more recent studies, that the traditional therapy of bowel rest and TPN in the management of acute CD is as efficacious as enteral nutrition. TPN does induce remission during acute attacks of CD. The increased costs of TPN and the increased incidence of complications associated with TPN are making TPN less attractive in acute exacerbations of CD. Because enteral nutrition with an elemental diet can achieve equivalent remissions, without the increased cost and risk, TPN should be implemented as primary therapy only in select situations of acute CD. These include patients with (1) a failure to respond to enteral diets, (2) a condition in which the enteral route is not feasible, (3) intestinal obstruction, (4) short bowel syndrome, (5) symptomatic fistulas, and (6) associated severe malnutrition failing to respond to medical therapy (Table 11–5).

◆ TOTAL PARENTERAL NUTRITION AS PRIMARY THERAPY FOR ULCERATIVE COLITIS

Fewer studies have examined the effect of TPN in UC, and their results are less encouraging (Table 11–6). UC is a disease restricted to the colon with minimal or no small bowel

Table 11–5. Indications for the Use of Total Parenteral Nutrition as Primary Therapy in Crohn's Disease

Failure of enteral diet
Enteral route not feasible
Intestinal obstruction
Short bowel syndrome
Symptomatic fistula
Intractable severe malnutrition

involvement, which may explain the decreased response to bowel rest. Patients with UC tend to have less severe nutritional deficits, further indicating a reduced need for nutritional support. Additionally, TPN does not reduce the inflammation of UC, unlike its effect in CD.[105]

In 1973, Fischer and colleagues reported on four patients with UC who were treated with TPN as a means of achieving clinical remission.[106] After one course of TPN, they achieved one remission, defined as the avoidance of surgery. After 6 months of follow-up, these patients remained in remission.

Reilly and coworkers in 1976 reported on a series of 11 patients with UC.[107] After 29 days of TPN, surgery was avoided in only one patient. The authors retrospectively compared this group with a control group of 16 patients who underwent colectomy before the introduction of TPN at their hospital and found a significantly higher rate of postsurgical complications among the patients who did not receive TPN.

Fazio and colleagues in 1976[108] and Harford and Fazio in 1978[109] reported on their series of 14 patients with UC who were treated with TPN. Among them, five patients were given TPN as primary therapy for an average period of 20 days. They achieved four remissions, defined as a return of the patient's health to the premorbid state and the maintenance of this state for 3 months or more. After a follow-up of 20 to 41 months, three of the patients who had initially responded had not relapsed.

In 1976, Dean and colleagues reported on five patients with UC.[110] After 14 days of TPN, four of them avoided surgery. No data regarding long-term follow-up were provided in the report.

Mullen and colleagues reported in 1978 their experience with 24 patients with UC who received TPN as primary therapy.[22] After an average time on TPN of 26 ± 3.7 days, they achieved nine remissions (surgery was avoided). After 6 to 120 months of follow-up, only four remained free of symptoms.

Table 11–6. Ulcerative Colitis and Total Parenteral Nutrition as Primary Therapy

Study	No. of Patients	Duration of TPN (days)	Hospital Remissions	Long-Term Remissions	Length of Follow-up (mo)	Remarks
Retrospective Studies						
Fischer et al. (1973)[106]	4	NR	1 (25%)	1 (25%)	6	Medical therapy
Fazio et al. (1976)[108] and Harford and Fazio (1978)[109]	5	20	4 (80%)	3 (60%)	20–41	
Reilly et al. (1976)[107]	11	29	1 (9%)	NR	NR	Steroids
Dean et al. (1976)[110]	5	14	4 (80%)	NR	NR	Medical therapy
Mullen et al. (1978)[22]	24	26	9 (37.5)	4 (16.6%)	6–120	Medical therapy
Hanauer et al. (1984)[111]	38	22	17 (44.7%)	13 (34.2%)	27	Prednisone
Sitzmann et al. (1990)[95e]	22	21.4	6 (27%)	3 (13.6%)	39 (mean)	Steroids, azathioprine
Prospective Nonrandomized Studies						
Elson et al. (1980)[94]	10	21	4 (40%)	1 (10%)	44	
Prospective Randomized Controlled Studies						
Dickinson et al. (1980)[99]	16 C 13 TPN	NR	8 (50%) 6 (46%)	3 (18.7%) 1 (7.7%)	16–48	Prednisone
McIntyre et al. (1986)[87]	12 OD 15 TPN	7	7 (58.3%) 6 (40%)	3 (25%) 2 (13.3%)	27–64	Prednisone
Gonzalez-Huix et al. (1993)[112]	22 TEN 20 TPN	16	12 (55%) 10 (50%)	NR	Prednisone	

C, control group; NR, not reported; OD, oral diet; TEN, total enteral nutrition; TPN, total parenteral nutrition.

Hanauer and coworkers reported on 38 patients with UC who were treated with TPN.[111] After 22 days of TPN, 17 patients achieved remission and were discharged on medical therapy. After 27 months of follow-up, there were four relapses among the initial responders. All patients in that series were given prednisone. The authors found that continued blood loss, as manifested by transfusion requirements, was a singular prognostic indicator of a poor response to TPN.

In 1980, Elson and colleagues reported on their prospective nonrandomized trial of TPN in 10 patients with UC.[96] After 21 days of TPN, four patients were discharged with improved conditions and could thus avoid colectomy. Of these, one was readmitted for colectomy one month after discharge. Two continued to have their active disease controlled with medication 5 and 43 months, respectively, after discharge. Only one was symptom-free and off all medication 44 months after discharge.

Dickinson and colleagues reported in 1980 on their prospective controlled trial of TPN and bowel rest as an adjunct therapy for acute colitis.[86] They divided 29 patients with UC into two groups: 16 control patients and 13 patients treated with TPN. All patients received prednisone at 40 mg/day. During the hospitalization period, eight remissions occurred among the control patients and six occurred in the group receiving TPN. Remission was defined as the avoidance of surgery. After a long-term follow-up of 16 to 48 months, three control patients remained in remission, and only one of the patients receiving TPN did.

McIntyre and colleagues reported in 1986 a controlled trial of bowel rest in the treatment of severe acute colitis.[87] Among 47 patients who made up the trial, 27 had UC. They were divided into two groups: 12 received an oral diet, and 15 received TPN and bowel rest. Both groups were given 60 mg/day of prednisone. After 7 days of study, remission was achieved in six patients on TPN and in seven patients on the oral diet. After 27 to 64 months of follow-up, two patients on TPN and three on the oral diet remained free of symptoms.

In 1993, Gonzalez-Huix and colleagues published their results from a prospective randomized trial that compared the use of TPN with TEN as an adjunct to steroid therapy in hospitalized patients with acute exacerbations of UC.[112] Forty-two patients with moderate and severe disease, as determined by the criteria of Truelove and Witts[113] and by abdominal leukocyte scintigraphy,[114] were randomized to either TPN (n = 20) or TEN (n = 22) treatment when the severity of disease remained moderate or severe after 48 hours of intravenous steroid therapy (1 mg/kg/day). The end-points were defined as either colectomy or mild or inactive disease stabilized on less than 30 mg of steroids per day. Assessment of the nutritional status was performed at the onset and at the end of the study. Differences among the various clinical and nutritional parameters were not significant between the two groups at the onset of the study. After 16 days of therapy, 10 patients (50%) on TPN and 12 (55%) on TEN achieved remission in the hospital. The amount of time spent on either TEN (16.5 days) or TPN (16.0 days) was not significantly different between the two groups. Anthropometric parameters were unchanged at the end of the study in both groups. Serum albumin levels rose significantly in the TEN group but not in the TPN group ($P = 0.028$). Ten patients in each group required a colectomy, but those on TPN had a higher rate of postoperative complications when compared with those in the TEN group who required colectomy ($P = 0.028$). The treatment-related complication rate was significantly higher ($P = 0.046$) among patients on TPN (35%) than among those treated with TEN (9%). Additionally, major complications, including subclavian vein thrombosis and catheter sepsis, occurred only in the TPN-treated group. Long-term remission rates were not reported. The authors conclude that TEN is as effective as TPN therapy in acute UC when used in conjunction with steroids and results in fewer and less severe complications. Therefore, the authors state, TPN should not play a primary role in the management of acute exacerbations of UC.

Currently, the American Society for Parenteral and Enteral Nutrition practice guidelines recommend TPN for malnourished patients with acute exacerbations of UC when the patient is being considered for surgery. Also, when enteral nutrition administration is impossible or does not adequately preserve lean body mass and functional capacity, TPN should be used. However, it must be recognized that disease activity is not influenced by TPN in severe acute exacerbations of UC.[115]

In conclusion, a positive nutritional response has been found in most of the studies, but a positive clinical response occurred less often. Overall, the average response rate to short-course TPN therapy is 41%. On a long-term basis, this rate falls to 22%. Response rates in individual studies vary greatly, from as high as 80% to as low as 9% when short courses of TPN treatment are analyzed. Similarly, long-term response rates vary from 8% to 60%. Differences in study design, treatment regimens, patient populations, and end-point determination are only some of the factors that prevent accurate comparisons for overall treatment recommendations.

In summary, TPN is not indicated in fulminant UC when surgery is the first choice or in cases of elective colectomy in the absence of nutritional depletion. Between these extremes, the possible benefits must be carefully evaluated against the expense and the inherent risks.

◆ PREOPERATIVE TOTAL PARENTERAL NUTRITION AND CROHN'S DISEASE

Preoperative TPN has been advocated to increase tissue integrity, simplify surgical dissection, shift the patient to an anabolic state, and limit bowel resection by decreasing the extent of disease.[116] Most of the reports of preoperative TPN in CD (Table 11–7) are either retrospective or uncontrolled. How-

ever, a few investigators have tested the value of preoperative TPN in a controlled setting.

Additionally, many studies of preoperative and perioperative nutrition analyze the use of TPN preoperatively in pooled patient populations with a variety of surgical problems. One such study was the Veterans Affairs Total Parenteral Nutrition Cooperative Study, which sought to determine whether perioperative TPN would decrease the incidence of complications in malnourished patients.[74] The authors noted that patients receiving TPN had more infectious complications than controls (14.1% vs. 6.4%, $P = .01$). In a post hoc subset analysis, patients who were severely malnourished preoperatively had significantly fewer complications than the control group (5% vs. 43%, $P = .03$). Some investigators prescribe TPN preoperatively for 1 week to 10 days before surgery in severely malnourished patients who cannot tolerate enteral feeding.[17]

In 1989, Lashner and colleagues reported on 103 preoperative patients with CD, 49 of whom received TPN and 54 of whom did not.[117] The patients were divided into three groups according to the site of resection: colonic, segmental small bowel, or ileocolectomy. Preoperative TPN benefited patients undergoing small bowel resection by reducing the length of small bowel that needed removal ($P < .001$ in ileocolectomy patients). This effect was independent of the length of diseased bowel determined preoperatively. For patients undergoing co-

Table 11–7. Preoperative Total Parenteral Nutrition in Crohn's Disease

Study	No. of Patients	Duration of Preoperative TPN (days)	No. of Complications	Remarks
Vogel et al. (1974)[95]	6	14	1	
Eisenberg et al. (1974)[120]	25	21	2	
Fazio et al. (1976)[108]	48	20	NR	30 patients had improved postoperative courses; 12 patients avoided surgery
Allardyce (1978)[116a]	7	49.5	NR	Nutritional improvement
Bos and Westerman (1980)[95a]	25	41	2	
				Two deaths
Rombeau et al. (1982)[119]	30	<5 (10 patients)	5	
		>5 (20 patients)	1	
Gouma et al. (1988)[123]	15	33	5	
Lashner et al. (1989)[117]	49 TPN	NR	NR	Significant reduction of resected small bowel in TPN group
	54 no TPN		NR	

NR, not reported; TPN, total parenteral nutrition.
From Lashner BA, Evans AA, Hanauer SB: Preoperative total parenteral nutrition for bowel resection in Crohn's disease. Dig Dis Sci 34:741–746, 1989.

lectomy, there was little benefit from preoperative TPN. There were no significant differences in the postoperative complication rates. A longer hospital stay was reported in the patients receiving TPN ($P < .001$) in both the ileocolectomy and the colonic resection groups.

In 1992, Steffes and Fromm reported on 46 patients undergoing right-sided ileocolectomy for ileal CD who were not treated with preoperative TPN.[118] During the perioperative period, all patients were administered antibiotics, and those who had received prednisone within the previous 12 months (n = 44) were given 250 to 300 mg of hydrocortisone every 24 hours postoperatively for 2 days, then tapered. The patients were followed for 1 to 10 years. Twenty-four of the patients received an elemental diet 1 to 2 days before surgery, and none received preoperative parenteral nutrition or postoperative TPN. Enterocutaneous fistula was the primary indication for surgery in seven patients. Long-term follow-up was obtained from all patients. No patients developed an abscess or fistula within the first year, nor did any require reoperation. The reported incidence of perioperative complications was 2.2%, and the incidence of late complications was 6.5%. Although 93.5% of the patients had serum albumin levels of less than 35 g/L, and 80.4% had a loss of body weight greater than 15% (markers of malnutrition that warrant preoperative TPN, according to one report),[119] the authors were unable to identify a group of patients in their population who would benefit from preoperative TPN.

From the analysis of the cited reports, some conclusions can be made. Almost every report showed positive changes in nutritional parameters with preoperative TPN; however, these changes were not accompanied by reduced postoperative complications. Predictably, there was a substantial increase in the cost of therapy and in the number of hospitalization days for the TPN-treated patients when compared with non-treated patients. It is concluded that 5 to 10 days of preoperative TPN in CD should be restricted to patients who are severely malnourished and who are not candidates for enteral nutrition.

◆ TOTAL PARENTERAL NUTRITION AND FISTULOUS CROHN'S DISEASE

Patients with CD who have fistulas deserve a separate review, because the nutritional therapy is not as efficacious when compared with those with nonfistulous disease. A comprehensive review of the effects of TPN on fistulous disease is provided in Chapter 13. Like other studies of TPN and CD, most of these reports (Table 11–8) are either retrospective or uncontrolled. Furthermore, in some reports it is difficult to discern whether the fistula was due to the intrinsic disease or anastomotic breakdown.

Eisenberg and colleagues reported on 18 patients who had Crohn's fistulas.[120] In their series, fistula closure with TPN was achieved in five patients. After 3 months of follow-up, there was one recurrence. Greenberg and colleagues reported on 14 patients with Crohn's fistulas who were treated with TPN alone (n = 7) or with TPN plus prednisone (n = 7).[121] Closure was achieved in one patient in the group receiving TPN

Table 11–8. Crohn's Disease Fistulas and Total Parenteral Nutrition

Study	No. of Patients	Duration of TPN (days)	Short-Term Closures	Long-Term Closures	Length of Follow-up (mo)
Eisenberg et al. (1974)[120]	18	NR	5 (27%)	4 (22%)	3
Greenberg et al. (1976)[121]	7 TPN	21	1 (14%)		NR
	7 TPN + prednisone		6 (85%)	NR	
Mullen et al. (1978)[22]	20	26	12 (60%)	10 (50%)	120
Driscoll et al. (1978)[5]	6	NR	0 (0%)	NR	NR
Elson et al. (1980)[96]	4	36	1 (25%)	NR	NR
Holm (1981)[95b]	3	71	3 (100%)	3 (100%)	60
Müller et al. (1983)[97]	3	84	2 (66%)	NR	NR
Ostro et al. (1985)[122]	24	NR	15 (62%)	8 (33%)	12
Gouma et al. (1988)[123]	22	33	13 (59%)	NR	NR

NR, not reported; TPN, total parenteral nutrition.

and in six patients in the group receiving TPN plus prednisone. The long-term outcome was not reported. Mullen and associates reported on 20 patients with CD who had a total of 37 fistulas.[22] After a course of TPN, closure was achieved in 12 fistulas. After a follow-up of 120 months, two fistulas recurred. Ostro and colleagues reported on 24 patients with Crohn's fistulas.[122] After a course of TPN, closure was obtained in 15. After a year of follow-up, only eight remained closed. In 1988, Gouma and colleagues reported on 22 patients with Crohn's fistulas who were treated for a mean of 33 days with TPN and bowel rest.[123] They obtained 13 closures, 5 failures, and 4 improvements, defined as a diminution of the number of fistulous tracts present in the same patient.

When the cited reports are analyzed as a group, there is a 38% average fistula closure rate after TPN (see Table 11–8). This rate is less than that reported with TPN as primary therapy for patients with CD taken as a whole (see Tables 11–2 and 11–4). Of particular concern is the absence of a non-TPN control group and the absence of long-term follow-up in most studies. We conclude that TPN, although useful in patients with postoperative anastomotic fistulas or in those who are prohibitive surgical risks, does not lead to a definitive closure in most instances, and surgery is usually needed. We also believe that the factors influencing spontaneous closure of enteric fistulas,[124] as well as the general principles of treatment (fluid and electrolyte replacement and the evaluation of sepsis, if present), must be considered in the management of these patients.

◆ HOME NUTRITIONAL SUPPORT

The development of improved devices and systems for home nutritional support, including home parenteral nutrition (HPN), has made the use of this technique feasible, allowing patients with IBD, especially those with CD, to receive TPN for long periods at home, thus reducing the length of hospitalization. A comprehensive review of home TPN in children and adults is provided in Chapters 25 and 26.

In patients with IBD who do not require an acute care setting, there are three major indications for the use of HPN: (1) patients with short bowel syndrome; (2) treatment and nutritional support in the presence of enteric fistulas; and (3) malnourished patients who do not tolerate enteral feeding. Special care must be taken to reduce sepsis, which is by far the most frequent complication of HPN. Appropriate training of the patient in using the delivery system and in recognizing the onset of complications is mandatory. An experienced nutritional support team or nurse is also needed.

Howard and Hassan have set forth the following criteria in determining the propriety of HPN in each individual patient:[125]

1. The bowel dysfunction will persist for a prolonged time.
2. Oral or tube enteral feeding does not provide sufficient nutrition to the patient.
3. The therapy will restore and maintain the patient at a normal nutritional status.
4. The therapy will restore or maintain the patient at a partial or complete functional capacity.
5. Support at home for the patient is available to manage the therapy and prevent complications.

In 1988, Stokes and Irving reported a study of 89 patients with CD in the United Kingdom and Ireland who had HPN.[126] These patients underwent 100 courses of HPN during 10 years. Indications for starting therapy were short bowel syndrome in 60 cases, enteric fistulas in 29, and exacerbations of the disease in 41. Thirty patients had more than one indication. At the end of the 10th year of follow-up, nine patients had died and eight had stopped HPN because of treatment complications. The complication rate per patient per year was 28%, with a sepsis rate of 13% per patient per year. Fifty-two patients had no HPN-associated complications. Patients with short bowel syndrome spent a significantly longer time on HPN than patients with CD who did not have short bowel syndrome. Half of the patients with short bowel syndrome were still receiving HPN, and only one quarter had resumed enteral feeding. Among the patients without short bowel syndrome, 57.5% had successfully resumed enteral feeding and only 27.5% were still receiving HPN.

In 1990, Galandiuk and colleagues published a retrospective study involving 41 patients with CD who were receiving HPN.[127]

The end-points of their study were the effects on the numbers of surgical procedures, the intensity of medical therapy, the nutritional state, and the quality of life. The patients were followed for up to 11 years. Fifty-nine percent of the patients underwent surgery for CD during the course of HPN. There was no significant difference in the number of surgical procedures when compared with that for the pre-HPN period. Twenty-nine percent of the patients were taking prednisone while receiving HPN, compared with 54% of the patients during the pre-HPN period. No significant change in body weight was noted; however, both the serum albumin and transferrin levels increased during HPN. The quality of life was assessed by a quality-of-life score, a social activity score, and a psychologic well-being score. These scores showed a significant improvement during the HPN period compared with the pre-HPN period. Fifty-six percent of the patients had complications related to HPN: catheter sepsis in 19 patients, a blocked or damaged catheter in 15 patients, electrolyte imbalance in 5 patients, and hyperglycemia in 1 patient. The authors conclude that although HPN is indispensable for patients with CD and short bowel syndrome or a high-output stoma, it is associated with a definitive morbidity and mortality and does not provide protection against surgery for CD. It does, however, provide the patient with an increased sense of well-being, an improved nutritional status, a reduction in other medical therapy, and an improved quality of life.

Howard and colleagues published the results of HPN in the United States in a series of 497 patients with CD in whom data were collected between 1984 and 1987.[128] A total of 298 patients began therapy while in the national HPN registry. In this group, a mortality rate of 5% per year was noted, although none of the 12 patient deaths were attributable to HPN. In this group, 38% resumed oral nutrition after 1 year, 47% remained on HPN, and 11% switched to home enteral therapy. Complete rehabilitation was achieved in 75% of patients in their first year, 73% in their second year, and 60% in their third year. Although the remainder experienced partial rehabilitation, less than 5% obtained little benefit from the HPN. The complication rate was 2.8 per year, of which 1.1 hospitalizations were HPN-related. Sepsis was suspected or confirmed in

54% of HPN complications. The distribution of HPN-related complications was notable for its predilection for a small group of patients. Within the first year of HPN, 77% of 231 patients had no complications, 51% of 37 had none through the second year, and 43% of 30 had none through the third and fourth year. Thus, a small group of patients suffered from multiple complications, and in fact 1% had more than four HPN-related complications within the first year. A total of 199 patients were enrolled in the HPN registry having already been on HPN for an average of 70 months. The mortality rate in this group was 2% per year. After the first year of follow-up, 87% of 135 patients were still on HPN, and only 7% had resumed oral nutrition. In this group of long-term HPN patients, the complication rate was significantly lower than in the other group: the hospitalization rate was 1.2 per year, with only half of hospitalizations related to the HPN therapy. In a previous report, the authors stated that in 1986 more than $600 million was spent on HPN and home enteral nutrition in the United States.[129] Only 14% of the 131,000 persons on home nutritional support were on parenteral nutrition, but they accounted for 55% of the total dollars spent.

Howard and colleagues examined the usage of HPN in the United States over a 7-year period, from 1985 to 1992.[130, 131] By analyzing data from the North American Home Parenteral and Enteral Nutrition Patient Registry, the investigators assessed the disease distribution and therapy outcomes in patients using HPN. Four parameters were used to assess the clinical outcome of patients on HPN therapy: (1) the survival rate, determined by 36 months of follow-up data; (2) the therapy status, determined by the nutritional status at 1 year; (3) the rehabilitation status, determined by a global assessment of function over 1 year; and (4) the complication rate. From a total of 5357 patients on HPN, 562 (10.5%) suffered from CD, with a mean age of 36 years. The annual survival rate was 96%. After 1 year of treatment, 70% had resumed a full oral diet, 25% continued on the HPN, and 2% died. Sixty percent of patients achieved a complete rehabilitation status, 38% had achieved a partial rehabilitation, and 2% had minimal rehabilitation. There were 2 complications per patient per year, one half related to HPN therapy. The authors also evaluated the impact of the patients' age on the outcome using pooled clinical data on patients with CD and ischemic bowel and motility disorders. The survival rates in the pediatric (ages zero to 18 years), middle (35 to 55 years), and geriatric (65 years and older) groups were 92, 90, and 67%, respectively. Pediatric and adult patients were more likely to resume an oral diet (62 and 48%, vs. 34% in the geriatric patients) and achieved a complete rehabilitation status (63 and 62% vs. 38%). However, adult and geriatric patients had fewer complications (0.9/yr, 0.9/yr) compared with pediatric patients (1.8/yr). The authors concluded that the use of HPN in CD is an effective and safe therapy, with favorable survival rehabilitation rates. Additionally, patients with CD on HPN, regardless of age, had good clinical outcomes. Thus, age should not be an exclusionary criteria when determining the role of HPN in the management of a patient with CD.

In conclusion, HPN is an important advance in the treatment of patients with CD who require long-term nutritional therapy. Although complication rates in the reported series vary, complications are always present, and care must be taken to avoid them, especially access-related sepsis, which accounts for approximately one half of HPN-related complications. The high cost of this therapy warrants careful selection of patients and close supervision and training by a multidisciplinary nutritional support team. However, this treatment modality is a lifesaving therapy, especially when severe short bowel syndrome is present, and when it is well utilized, it provides the patient with an improved nutritional status and quality of life, in addition to a reduction in other medical therapy.

◆ FUTURE DIRECTIONS

Greater understanding of the etiology and pathogenesis of IBD and the inflammatory process has led to a new understanding of nutritional support. The recognition that luminal antigens, from both bacteria and foods, play a role in the progression of IBD has important implications for nutritional therapy.[132] The role of local factors such as cytokine production and immunoregulatory cells in the disease process continues to be elucidated.[133, 134] Directing medical therapy

at tempering the immune response and altering the intestinal microenvironment may prove beneficial to patients with IBD and malnutrition. By varying the lipid formulation of TPN, researchers have shown an improvement in disease activity in a rat model, presumably by suppressing the formation of proinflammatory mediators such as leukotrienes and prostaglandins.[135] Similarly, colitis activity was reported to be decreased when intravenous fish oil was administered to a patient with severe UC.[136] The function of butyrate and antioxidants in colonocyte viability and the disease process has demonstrated the importance of using them in managing IBD. Further investigation in these areas is warranted.

SUMMARY

The etiology of malnutrition in IBD is multifactorial and manifests itself in a variety of clinical conditions and syndromes. Patients often suffer from coexisting protein, vitamin, and mineral deficiencies that severely affect their disease. Malnutrition is particularly devastating in children and can lead to growth retardation, growth failure, and delayed sexual maturity. It is imperative that the physician recognize the malnutritive state early in its appearance and institute appropriate nutritional therapy immediately to prevent and reverse underlying deficiencies.

Although a number of indices and methods are available to assess the patient's nutritional status, the Subjective Global Assessment does so accurately, accounting for historical, physical, and biochemical data. The Harris-Benedict formula can be used with acceptable accuracy to calculate energy requirements. When the patient is severely stressed, or when the nutritional status changes acutely, indirect calorimetry can be used to assess energy requirements, albeit a more complicated and expensive process.

The reported trials of TPN and IBD must be interpreted cautiously, because most authors do not separate patients with CD from those with UC. Despite several shared characteristics, the clinical courses and prognoses of CD and UC are different, as are their impacts on nutritional status.

In acute attacks of CD, TPN can be used effectively as a primary therapy to induce remission. However, the same results can be achieved with TEN without the complications associated with TPN. In the perioperative setting, TPN should be reserved for those patients with CD who have severe nutritional deficiencies. Clinical data do not support the supposition that TPN therapy can lead to fistula closure in patients with CD. For patients with acute exacerbations of UC in whom enteral feeding is impossible, TPN should be instituted to restore and to preserve lean body mass and functional capacity. Additionally, it may be used to improve the nutritional status of malnourished patients in whom surgery can be delayed. It is not indicated in situations of fulminant UC when emergent surgery is needed or when elective colectomy is needed in the absence of nutritional depletion.

Home nutritional therapy is recognized as an important advance in the outpatient management of severely malnourished patients and of those with short bowel syndrome as a result of IBD. It has offered patients an improved quality of life, improved nutritional status, and decreased hospitalization, with good results and low mortality.

REFERENCES

1. Wall AJ, Kirsner JB: Ulcerative colitis and Crohn's disease of the colon: Symptoms, signs and laboratory aspects. *In* Kirsner JB, Shorter RG (eds): Inflammatory Bowel Disease. Philadelphia, Lea & Febiger, 1975, pp 101–108.
2. Sartor RB: Current concepts of the etiology and pathogenesis of ulcerative colitis and Crohn's disease. Gastroenterol Clin North Am 24:475–507, 1995.
3. Husain A, Korzenik JR: Nutritional issues and therapy in inflammatory bowel disease. Semin Gastrointest Dis 9:21–30, 1998.
4. Rigaud D, Angel A, Cerf M, et al: Mechanisms of decreased food intake during weight loss in adult Crohn's disease patients without obvious malabsorption. Am J Clin Nutr 60:775–781, 1994.
5. Driscoll RH, Rosenberg IH: Total parenteral nutrition in inflammatory bowel disease. Med Clin North Am 62:185–201, 1978.
6. Fischer JE: Inflammatory bowel disease. *In* Fischer JE (ed): Total Parenteral Nutrition, 2nd ed. Boston, Little, Brown, 1991, pp 239–251.
7. Blackburn GL, Bistrian BR, Maini BS, et al: Nutritional and metabolic assessment of the hospitalized patient. JPEN J Parenter Enteral Nutr 1:11–22, 1977.
8. Dudrick SJ, Latifi R, Schrager R: Nutritional management of inflammatory bowel disease. Surg Clin North Am 71:609–623, 1991.
9. Chan AT, Fleming R, O'Fallon WM, Huizenga KA: Estimated versus measured basal energy requirements in patients with Crohn's disease. Gastroenterology 91:75–78, 1986.
10. Kushner RF, Schoeller DA: Resting and total energy expenditure in patients with inflammatory bowel disease. Am J Clin Nutr 53:161–165, 1991.
11. Stokes MA, Hill GL: Total energy expenditure in patients with Crohn's disease: Measurement by the combined body scan technique. JPEN J Parenter Enteral Nutr 17:3–7, 1993.
12. Rigaud D, Cerf M, Angel Alberto L, et al: Increase in resting energy expenditure during flare-ups in Crohn's disease. Gastroenterol Clin Biol 17:932–937, 1993.
13. Motil KJ, Grand RJ: Nutritional management of inflammatory bowel disease. Pediatr Clin North Am 32:447–469, 1985.
14. Motil KJ, Grand RJ, Davis-Kraft L, et al: Growth failure in children with inflammatory bowel disease: A prospective study. Gastroenterology 105:681–691, 1993.
15. Reid IR: Pathogenesis and treatment of steroid osteoporosis. Clin Endocrinol 30:83–103, 1989.
16. O'Keefe SJD, Ogden J, Rund J, Potter P: Steroids and bowel rest versus elemental diet in the treatment of patients with Crohn's disease: The effect on protein metabolism and immune function. JPEN J Parenter Enteral Nutr 13:455–460, 1989.
17. Zurita VF, Rawls DE, Dyck WP: Nutritional support in inflammatory bowel disease. Dig Dis 13:92–107, 1995.
18. Elton E, Hanauer SB: Review article: The medical management of Crohn's disease. Aliment Pharmacol Ther 10:1–22, 1996.
19. Sandborn WJ, Tremaine WJ: Cyclosporin treatment of inflammatory bowel disease. Mayo Clin Proc 67:981–990, 1992.
20. Kozarek PA, Patterson DJ, Gelfand MD, et al: Methotrexate induces clinical and histologic remission in patients with refractory inflammatory bowel disease. Ann Intern Med 110:353–356, 1989.
21. Seidman EG: Nutritional management of inflammatory bowel disease. Gastroenterol Clin North Am 17:129–155, 1989.
22. Mullen JL, Hargrove WC, Dudrick SJ, et al: Ten years experience with intravenous hyperalimentation and inflammatory bowel disease. Ann Surg 187:523–529, 1978.
23. DeDombal FT: Prognostic value of the serum protein during severe attacks of ulcerative colitis. Gut 9:144–149, 1968.
24. Novacek G, Vogelsang H, Schmidt B, et al: Are single measurements of pseudocholinesterase and albumin markers for inflammatory activity or nutritional status in Crohn's disease? Wien Klin Wochenschr 105:111–115, 1993.
25. Kukori F, Iida M, Tominaga M, et al: Multiple vitamin status in Crohn's disease. Correlation with disease activity. Dig Dis Sci 38:1614–1618, 1993.
26. Driscoll RH, Meredith SC, Sitrin MD, et al: Vitamin D deficiency and bone disease in patients with Crohn's disease. Gastroenterology 83:1252–1258, 1982.
27. Harries AD, Brown R, Heatly RV, et al: Vitamin D status in Crohn's disease: Association with nutrition and disease activity. Gut 26:1197–1203, 1985.
28. Bischoff SC, Hermann A, Goke M, et al: Altered bone metabolism in inflammatory bowel disease. Am J Gastroenterol 92:1157–1163, 1997.
29. Bernstein CN, Seeger LL, Anton PA, et al: A randomized, placebo-controlled trial of calcium supplementation for decreased bone density in corticosteroid-using patients with inflammatory bowel

disease: A pilot study. Aliment Pharmacol Ther 10:777–786, 1996.

30. Atwell JD, Duthie HL: The absorption of water, sodium and potassium from the serum of humans showing the effects of regional enteritis. Gastroenterology 46:16–22, 1964.

31. Lehr L, Schober O, Hundeshagen H, et al: Total body potassium depletion and the need for preoperative nutritional support in Crohn's disease. Ann Surg 196:709–714, 1982.

32. Dieleman LA, Heizer WD: Nutritional issues in inflammatory bowel disease. Gastroenterol Clin North Am 27:435–451, 1998.

33. Geerling BJ, Badart-Smook A, Stockbrugger RW, Brummer RJM: Comprehensive nutritional status in patients with long-standing Crohn's disease currently in remission. Am J Clin Nutr 67:919–926, 1998.

34. Rannem T, Ladefoged K, Hylander E, et al: Selenium status in patients with Crohn's disease. Am J Clin Nutr 56:933–937, 1992.

35. Goldschmid S, Graham M: Trace element deficiencies in inflammatory bowel disease. Gastroenterol Clin North Am 18:579–587, 1989.

36. Hinks LJ, Inwards KD, Lloyd B, et al: Reduced concentrations of selenium in mild Crohn's disease. J Clin Pathol 41:198–201, 1988.

37. Rannem T, Ladefoged K, Hylander E, et al: The effect of selenium supplementation in skeletal and cardiac muscle in selenium-depleted patients. JPEN J Parenter Enteral Nutr 19:351–355, 1995.

38. Rannem T, Hylander E, Ladefoged K, et al: The metabolism of [^{75}Se]selenite in patients with short bowel syndrome. JPEN J Parenter Enteral Nutr 20:412–416, 1996.

39. Johnson RA, Baker SS, Fallon JT, et al: An occidental case of cardiomyopathy and selenium deficiency. N Engl J Med 304:1210–1212, 1981.

40. Crohn BB, Ginzburg L, Oppenheimer GD: Regional ileitis, a pathologic and clinical entity. JAMA 99:1323–1329, 1932.

41. Mekhjian HS, Switz DM, Melnyk CS, et al: Clinical features and natural history of Crohn's disease. Gastroenterology 77:898–906, 1979.

42. Kelley DG, Fleming CR: Nutritional considerations in inflammatory bowel disease. Gastroenterol Clin North Am 24:597–611, 1995.

43. Kirschner BS: Inflammatory bowel disease. Pediatr Clin North Am 35:189–208, 1988.

44. Bartels U, Strandberg Pedersen N, Jarnum S: Iron absorption and serum ferritin in chronic inflammatory bowel disease. Scand J Gastroenterol 13:649–656, 1978.

45. Thomson AIR, Brust R, Ali MAM, et al: Iron deficiency in inflammatory bowel disease. Diagnostic efficacy of serum ferritin. Am J Dig Dis 23:705–709, 1978.

46. Franklin JL, Rosenberg IH: Impaired folic acid absorption in inflammatory bowel disease: Effects of salicylazosulfapyridine. Gastroenterology 64:517–525, 1973.

47. Lashner BA: Red blood cell folate is associated with development of dysplasia and cancer in ulcerative colitis. J Cancer Res Clin Oncol 119:549–554, 1993.

48. Dyer HH, Child JA, Mollin DL: Anemia in Crohn's disease. QJM 41:419–436, 1972.

49. Dyer NH, Dawson AM: Malnutrition and malabsorption in Crohn's disease with reference to the effect of surgery. Br J Surg 60:134–140, 1973.

50. Rosenthal SR, Snyder JD, Hendricks KM, et al: Growth failure and inflammatory bowel disease: Approach to the treatment of a complicated adolescent problem. Pediatrics 72:481–490, 1983.

51. Grand RJ, Homer DR: Approaches to inflammatory bowel disease in childhood and adolescence. Pediatr Clin North Am 22:835–850, 1975.

52. Grand RJ, Ramakrishna J, Calenda KA: Inflammatory bowel disease in the pediatric patient. Gastroenterol Clin North Am 24:613–632, 1995.

53. Kirschner BS, Voinchet O, Rosenberg IH: Growth retardation in inflammatory bowel disease. Gastroenterology 75:505–511, 1978.

54. Kanoff ME, Lake AM, Bayless TM: Decreased height velocity in children and adolescents before the diagnosis of Crohn's disease. Gastroenterology 95:1523–1527, 1988.

55. Belli DC, Seidman E, Bouthillier L, et al: Chronic intermittent elemental diet improves growth failure in children with Crohn's disease. Gastroenterology 94:603–610, 1988.

56. Kirschner BS, Klich JR, Kalman SS, et al: Reversal of growth retardation in Crohn's disease with therapy emphasizing oral nutritional restitution. Gastroenterology 80:10–15, 1981.

57. Kirschner BS: Ulcerative colitis and Crohn's disease in children: Diagnosis and management. Gastroenterol Clin North Am 24:99–117, 1995.

58. Afonso JJ, Rombeau JL: Nutritional care for patients with Crohn's disease. Hepatogastroenterology 37:32–41, 1990.

59. Motil KJ, Grand RJ, Maletskos CJ, et al: The effect of disease, drugs and diet on whole body protein metabolism in adolescents with Crohn's disease and growth failure. Pediatrics 101:345–351, 1982.

60. Markowitz J, Grancher K, Rose J, et al: Growth failure in pediatric inflammatory bowel disease. J Pediatr Gastroenterol Nutr 16:373–380, 1993.

61. Oliva MM, Lake AM: Nutritional considerations and management of the child with inflammatory bowel disease. Nutrition 12:151–158, 1996.

62. Jeejeebhoy KN: Nutritional assessment. Gastroenterol Clin North Am 27:347–369, 1998.

63. Klein S, Kinney J, Jeejeebhoy K, et al: Nutrition support in clinical practice: Review of published data and recommendations for future research directions. JPEN J Parenter Enteral Nutr 21:133–156, 1997.

64. Morgan DB, Hill GL, Burkinshaw L: The assessment of weight loss from a single measurement of body weight: The problems and limitations. Am J Clin Nutr 33:2101–2105, 1980.

65. Reinhardt GF, Myscofski JW, Wilkens DB, et al: Incidence and mortality of hypoalbuminemic patients in hospitalized veterans. JPEN J Parenter Enteral Nutr 4:357–359, 1980.

66. Anderson CF, Wochos DN: The utility of serum albumin values in the nutritional assessment of hospitalized patients. Mayo Clin Proc 57:181–184, 1982.

67. Apelgren KN, Rombeau JL, Twomey PL, et al: Comparison of nutritional indices and outcome in critically ill patients. Crit Care Med 10:305–307, 1982.

68. Klein S: The myth of serum albumin as a measure of nutritional status. Gastroenterology 99:1845–1846, 1990.

69. Castenada C, Charnley JM, Evans WJ, et al: Elderly women accommodate to a low-protein diet with losses of body cell mass, muscle function, and immune response. Am J Clin Nutr 62:30–39, 1995.

70. Halmi KA, Struss AL, Owen WP, et al: Plasma and erythrocyte amino acid concentrations in anorexia nervosa. JPEN J Parenter Enteral Nutr 11:458–464, 1987.

71. Prealbumin in Nutritional Care Consensus Group: Measurement of visceral protein status in assessing protein and energy malnutrition: Standards of care. Nutrition 11:169–171, 1995.

72. Buzby GP, Mullen JP, Matthew DC: Prognostic Nutritional Index in gastrointestinal surgery. Am J Surg 139:160–167, 1980.

73. Buzby GP, Williford WO, Peterson OL, et al: A randomized clinical trial of total parenteral nutrition in malnourished surgical patients: The rationale and impact of previous clinical trials and pilot study on protocol design. Am J Clin Nutr 47:357–365, 1988.

74. Veterans Affairs Total Parenteral Nutrition Cooperative Study Group: Perioperative total parenteral nutrition in surgical patients. N Engl J Med 325:525–532, 1991.

75. Duerksen DR, Nehra V, Bistrian BR, Blackburn GL: Appropriate nutritional support in acute and complicated Crohn's disease. Nutrition 14:462–465, 1998.

76. Baker JP, Detsky AS, Wesson DE, et al: Nutritional assessment: A comparison of clinical judgement and objective measurements. N Engl J Med 306:969–972, 1982.

77. Detsky AS, McLaughlin JR, Baker JP, et al: What is subjective global assessment of nutritional status? JPEN J Parenter Enteral Nutr 11:8–13, 1987.

78. Hirsch S, de Obldia N, Petermann M, et al: Subjective global assessment of nutritional status: Further validation. Nutrition 7:35–37, 1991.

79. Enia G, Sicuso C, Alati G, et al: Subjective global assessment of nutrition in dialysis patients. Nephrol Dial Transplant 8:1094–1098, 1993.

80. Hasse J, Strong S, Gorman MA, et al: Subjective global assessment: Alternative nutrition-assessment technique for liver-transplant candidates. Nutrition 9:339–343, 1993.

81. Pikul J, Sharpe MD, Lowndes R, et al: Degree of preoperative malnutrition is predictive of postoperative morbidity and mortality in liver transplant recipients. Transplantation 57:469–472, 1994.

82. Barot LR, Rombeau JL, Feurer ID, Mullen JL: Caloric requirements in patients with inflammatory bowel disease. Ann Surg 195:214–218, 1982.

83. Welch CS, Adams M, Wakefield EG: Metabolic studies in ulcerative colitis. J Clin Invest 16:161–168, 1937.

84. Worming H, Mullertz S, Thaysen EH, Rang HO: pH concentration of pancreatic enzymes in aspirates from the human duodenum during ingestion of a standard meal in patients with intestinal disorders. Scand J Gastroenterol 2:81–89, 1967.

85. Rutgerts P, Ghoos Y, Vantrappen G, Eyssen H: Ileal dysfunction and bacterial overgrowth in patients with Crohn's disease. Eur J Clin Invest 11:199–206, 1981.

86. Dickinson RJ, Ashton MG, Axton ATR, et al: Controlled trial of intravenous hyperalimentation and total bowel rest as an adjunct to the routine therapy of acute colitis. Gastroenterology 79:1199–1204, 1980.

87. McIntyre PB, Powell-Tuck J, Wood SR, et al: Controlled trial of bowel rest in the treatment of severe acute colitis. Gut 27:481–485, 1986.

88. Alun Jones V: Comparison of total parenteral nutrition and elemental diet in induction of remission of Crohn's disease: Long-term maintenance of remission by personalized food exclusion diets. Dig Dis Sci 32(Suppl):100S–107S, 1987.

89. Greenberg GR, Fleming CR, Jeejeebhoy KN, et al: Controlled trial of bowel rest and nutritional support in the management of Crohn's disease. Gut 29:1309–1315, 1988.

90. Ambrose NS, Johnson M, Burdon DW, Keighley MRB: Incidence of pathogenic bacteria from mesenteric lymph nodes and ileal serosa during Crohn's disease surgery. Br J Surg 71:623–625, 1984.

91. Deitch EA, Maejima K, Berg R: Effect of oral antibiotics and bacterial overgrowth on the translocation of the GI tract microflora in burned rats. J Trauma 25:385–392, 1985.

92. Wellman W, Fink PC, Schmidt FW: Whole-gut irrigation as anti-endotoxinaemic therapy in inflammatory bowel disease. Hepato-gastroenterology 31:91–93, 1984.

93. Keller GA, West MA, Cerra FB, et al: Multiple systems organ failure: Modulation of hepatocyte protein synthesis by endotoxin activated Kupffer cells. Ann Surg 201:87–95, 1985.

94. Anderson DL, Boyce HW: Use of parenteral nutrition in the treatment of advanced regional enteritis. Am J Dig Dis 18:633–640, 1973.

95. Vogel CM, Corwin TR, Bave AE: Intravenous hyperalimentation in the treatment of inflammatory diseases of the bowel. Arch Surg 108:460–467, 1974.

95a. Bos LP, Westerman I: Total parenteral nutrition in Crohn's disease. World J Surg 4:163–166, 1980.

95b. Holm I: Benefits of total parenteral nutrition (TPN) in the treatment of Crohn's disease and ulcerative colitis. Acta Chir Scand 147:271–276, 1983.

95c. Shiloni E, Freund HR: Total parenteral nutrition in Crohn's disease: Is it a primary or supportive mode of therapy? Dis Colon Rectum 26:275–278, 1983.

95d. Kushner RF, Shapir J, Sitrin MD: Endoscopic, radiographic and clinical response to prolonged bowel rest and home parenteral nutrition in Crohn's disease. JPEN J Parenter Enteral Nutr 10:568–573, 1986.

95e. Sitzmann JV, Converse RL, Bayless TM: Favorable response to parenteral nutrition and medical therapy in Crohn's colitis. Gastroenterology 99:1647–1652, 1990.

95f. Cravo M, Camilo ME, Correia JP: Nutritional support in Crohn's disease: Which route? Am J Gastroenterology 86:317–321, 1991.

96. Elson CO, Layden TJ, Nemchausky BA, et al: An evaluation of total parenteral nutrition in the management of inflammatory bowel disease. Dig Dis Sci 25:42–48, 1980.

97. Müller JM, Keller HW, Erasmi H, Pichlmaier H: Total parenteral nutrition as the sole therapy in Crohn's disease: A prospective study. Br J Surg 70:40–43, 1983.

98. Lerebours E, Messing B, Chevalier B, et al: An evaluation of total parenteral nutrition in the management of steroid-dependant and steroid-resistant patients with Crohn's disease. JPEN J Parenter Enteral Nutr 10:274–278, 1986.

99. Best WR, Bectel JM, Singelton JW, et al: Development of a Crohn's disease activity index. Gastroenterology 70:439–444, 1976.

100. Summers RW, Switz DM, Sessions JT, et al: National cooperative Crohn's disease study: Results

of drug treatment. Gastroenterology 77:847–869, 1979.

101. Wright RA, Adler EC: Peripheral parenteral nutrition is no better than enteral nutrition in acute exacerbation of Crohn's disease: A prospective trial. J Clin Gastroenterol 12:396–399, 1990.

102. Christie PM, Hill GL: Effect of intravenous nutrition on nutrition and function in acute attacks of inflammatory bowel disease. Gastroenterology 99:730–736, 1990.

103. Payne-James JJ, Silk DBA: Total parenteral nutrition as primary treatment in Crohn's disease—RIP? Gut 29:1304–1308, 1988.

104. Shiloni E, Coronado E, Freund HR: Role of total parenteral nutrition in the treatment of Crohn's disease. Am J Surg 157:180–185, 1989.

105. Hanauer SB: Inflammatory bowel disease. N Engl J Med 334:841–848, 1996.

106. Fischer JE, Foster GS, Abel RM, et al: Hyperalimentation as primary therapy for inflammatory bowel disease. Am J Surg 125:165–175, 1973.

107. Reilly J, Ryan JA, Strole W, Fischer JE: Hyperalimentation in inflammatory bowel disease. Am J Surg 131:192–200, 1976.

108. Fazio VW, Kodner I, Jagelman DG, et al: Inflammatory disease of the bowel. Dis Colon Rectum 19:574–578, 1976.

109. Harford FJ, Fazio VW: Total parenteral nutrition as primary therapy for inflammatory disease of the bowel. Dis Colon Rectum 21:555–557, 1978.

110. Dean RE, Campos MM, Barret B: Hyperalimentation in the management of chronic inflammatory intestinal disease. Dis Colon Rectum 19:601–604, 1976.

111. Hanauer SB, Evans AA, Newcomb SA, Kirsner JB: Can response of ulcerative colitis to total parenteral nutrition (TPN) be predicted [Abstract]? Gastroenterology 86:1106, 1984.

112. Gonzalez-Huix F, Fernandez-Banares F, Esteve-Comas M, et al: Enteral versus parenteral nutrition as adjunct therapy in acute ulcerative colitis. Am J Gastroenterol 88:227–232, 1993.

113. Truelove SC, Witts LJ: Cortisone in ulcerative colitis. Final report on a therapeutic trial. BMJ 2:1041–1048, 1955.

114. Giné JJ, Villa R, Martin-Comin J, et al: The value of ^{111}In-labeled autologous leukocyte scan in attacks of inflammatory bowel disease. J Clin Nutr Gastroenterol 1:37–44, 1986.

115. ASPEN Board of Directors: Practice guidelines: Inflammatory bowel disease. JPEN J Parenter Enteral Nutr 17:1–52SA, 1993.

116. Jacobs DO, Rolandelli R, Fried R, Rombeau JL: Malnutrition and inflammatory bowel disease: Indications for and complications of parenteral nutritional support. *In* Rombeau JL, Caldwell MD (eds): Clinical Nutrition. Vol II: Parenteral Nutrition. Philadelphia, WB Saunders, 1984, pp 380–400.

116a. Allardyce DB: Preoperative parenteral feeding in Crohn's disease: Preoperatively, to induce remission, and at home. Am Surg 44:510–516, 1978.

117. Lashner BA, Evans AA, Hanauer SB: Preoperative total parenteral nutrition for bowel resection in Crohn's disease. Dig Dis Sci 34:741–746, 1989.

118. Steffes C, Fromm D: Is preoperative parenteral nutrition necessary for patients with predominantly ileal Crohn's disease? Arch Surg 127:1210–1212, 1992.

119. Rombeau JL, Barot LR, Williamson CE, Mullen JL: Preoperative total parenteral nutrition and surgical outcome in patients with inflammatory bowel disease. Am J Surg 143:139–143, 1982.

120. Eisenberg HW, Turnbull RB, Weakley FL: Hyperalimentation as preparation for surgery in transmural colitis (Crohn's disease). Dis Colon Rectum 17:469–475, 1974.

121. Greenberg GL, Haber GB, Jeejeebhoy KN: Total parenteral nutrition (TPN) and bowel rest in the management of Crohn's disease [Abstract]. Gut 17:828, 1976.

122. Ostro MJ, Greenberg GR, Jeejeebhoy KN: Total parenteral nutrition and complete bowel rest in the management of Crohn's disease. JPEN J Parenter Enteral Nutr 9:280–287, 1985.

123. Gouma DJ, Meyenfeldt MF, Rouflart M, Soeters PB: Preoperative total parenteral nutrition (TPN) in severe Crohn's disease. Surgery 103:648–652, 1988.

124. Rombeau JL, Rolandelli R: Enteral and parenteral nutrition in patients with enteric fistulas and short bowel syndrome. Surg Clin North Am 67:551–571, 1987.

125. Howard L, Hassan N: Home parenteral nutrition: 25 years later. Gastroenterol Clin North Am 27:481–512, 1998.

126. Stokes MA, Irving MH: How do patients with Crohn's disease fare on home parenteral nutrition? Dis Colon Rectum 31:454–458, 1988.

127. Galandiuk S, O'Neill M, McDonald P, et al: A century of home parenteral nutrition for Crohn's disease. Am J Surg 159:540–544, 1990.

128. Howard L, Heaphey L, Fleming CR, et al: Four years of North American registry home parenteral nutrition outcome data and their implications for patient management. JPEN J Parenter Enteral Nutr 15:384–393, 1991.

129. Howard L, Claunch C, Fleming R, et al: The outcome of Crohn's patients on home parenteral nutrition as shown in 3 years of national registry data. Paper presented at Digestive Disease Week, 90th annual meeting of the American Gastroenterological Association, Washington, DC, 1989.

130. Howard L, Ament M, Fleming CR, et al: Current use and clinical outcome of home parenteral and enteral nutrition therapies in the United States. Gastroenterology 109:355–365, 1995.

131. Howard L, Malone M: Current status of home parenteral nutrition in the United States. Transplant Proc 28:2691–2695, 1996.

132. Burke A, Lichtenstein GR, Rombeau JL: Nutrition and ulcerative colitis. Ballieres Clin Gastroenterol 11:153–174, 1997.

133. Sartor RB: Current concepts of the etiology and pathogenesis of ulcerative colitis and Crohn's disease. Gastroenterol Clin North Am 24:475–507, 1995.

134. Rogler G, Andus T: Cytokines in inflammatory bowel disease. World J Surg 22:382–389, 1998.

135. Inui K, Kukuta Y, Ikeda A, et al: The nutritional effect of alpha-linolenic acid–rich emulsion with total parenteral nutrition in a rat model with inflammatory bowel disease. Ann Nutr Metab 40:227–233, 1996.

136. Grimminger F, Fuehrer D, Papavassilis C, et al: Influence of intravenous n-3 lipid supplementation on fatty acid profiles and lipid mediator generation in a patient with severe ulcerative colitis. Eur J Clin Invest 23:706–715, 1993.

12

◆ Intravenous Nutrition in Patients with Acute Pancreatitis

Catherine McIsaac, M.S., R.D.
W. Scott Helton, M.D.

This chapter discusses the use of intravenous nutrition in clinical pancreatitis. The clinical indications and therapeutic goals of intravenous nutrition and specific nutritional needs of patients with pancreatitis are addressed. In addition, the safety, clinical efficacy, and risks of intravenous nutrition in the care of patients with pancreatitis and its complications are reviewed. Controversies about the use of lipid emulsions and enteral feedings during pancreatitis are addressed. The last part of this chapter provides readers with a rational treatment algorithm for the use of total parenteral nutrition (TPN) in patients with pancreatitis and outlines important areas for future investigation. The etiology, pathophysiology, and medical and surgical management of pancreatitis are not discussed in detail. Several excellent reviews of these topics are provided for readers' reference.[1-6] Several comprehensive reviews of intravenous nutrition in patients with pancreatitis are listed as additional references on the subject.[7-10]

◆ BACKGROUND

Pancreatitis represents a wide spectrum of inflammatory pancreatic diseases of variable intensity, ranging from mild edema to partial or generalized pancreatic necrosis. Because the severity of pancreatitis often dictates the therapy and prognosis, it is clinically useful to classify pancreatitis into several types. Patients with pancreatitis usually have one of three variations: mild edematous pancreatitis, relapsing acute or chronic pancreatitis, or acute hemorrhagic and necrotizing pancreatitis.

The vast majority of patients with acute pancreatitis have a self-limiting mild edematous form that resolves quickly with several days of conservative medical management.[1, 11] These patients are usually able to eat within 5 to 7 days[12] and thus are in little need of vigorous nutritional support.

Patients who have chronic relapsing pancreatitis, particularly that related to alcohol intake, may be malnourished on admission to the hospital.[13] These patients may have chronic pancreatic exocrine or endocrine insufficiency resulting in malabsorption, steatorrhea, diabetes, and vitamin and mineral deficiencies. In addition, these patients may be undernourished because of alcohol abuse or chronically decreased dietary intake in an attempt to avoid postprandial pancreatic pain. Although episodes of recurrent chronic pancreatitis usually respond promptly to conservative treatment and patients usually are in the hospital for less than 1 week, the cumulative effects of repeated attacks of pancreatitis may eventually result in an acute or chronic malnourished state requiring acute nutritional support. In such situations, prompt administration of intravenous nutrition for short periods may be of some clinical benefit.

In 5 to 15% of patients with pancreatitis, a moderate to severe necrotizing process develops and results in local and systemic life-threatening complications.[2, 14] This form of pancreatitis is often complicated by intra-abdominal sepsis.[2, 15] Patients need intensive medical support for weeks to months[3, 4] and often require one or more operations.[2, 16] Severe necrotizing pancreatitis has a mortality between 5 and 20%.[2, 11, 13, 14] Unlike patients with mild, self-limited edematous pancreatitis or recurrent relapsing chronic pancreatitis, patients with severe necrotizing pancreatitis are highly catabolic and predisposed to malnutrition. The necrotizing retroperitoneal inflammatory process leads to severe postprandial pain, nausea, vomiting, gastric stasis, and duodenal ileus, all of which preclude oral, gastric, or duodenal feeding. A lack of intensive nutritional support in these patients can result in rapid wasting, which can potentially contribute significantly to subsequent morbidity and mortality.[13, 17–19]

◆ HISTORICAL USE OF TOTAL PARENTERAL NUTRITION IN PANCREATITIS

Severe acute pancreatitis produces a hypercatabolic state similar to the metabolic effects of sepsis, burns, and trauma[20–25] and results in rapid loss of body weight, fat, and protein.[13, 26, 27] Soon after parenteral nutrition was introduced in 1968 by the University of Pennsylvania group of Dudrick and colleagues,[28] parenteral nutrition was used in patients with pancreatitis.[26] The inability to feed patients with severe pancreatitis enterally because of gastric and duodenal ileus, combined with physicians' increased awareness of these patients' nutritional risks, led to the common use of TPN in patients afflicted with severe forms of the disease.[16–19, 26, 29, 30] The initial experience with intravenous feeding in patients with severe pancreatitis reported improved survival,[13, 26] thus further encouraging the use of TPN in pancreatitis.

A standardized approach to operating on patients with severe necrotizing pancreatitis, which included gastrostomy for decompression of gastric and duodenal ileus, cholecystostomy for biliary diversion, and jejunostomy for alimentation,[17, 31] was practiced in the early 1970s, when intravenous nutrition was gaining wide acceptance. Many of the patients included in the reports of severe necrotizing pancreatitis were therefore being given both jejunal and intravenous feeding.[13, 17, 18] The simultaneous emergence of these two clinical approaches to this disease was associated with a decrease in mortality that was most likely related to improved nutritional support.[13, 17–19, 26]

A historical review of the literature describing the use of TPN in pancreatitis demonstrates no decrease in mortality in patients with severe disease between 1974[26] and 1991.[29] In fact, the literature shows that the first three major reports on the use of TPN and pancreatitis by Feller and associates,[26] White and Heimbach,[17] and Blackburn and coworkers[13] included a much higher proportion of patients with severe pancreatitis than later studies.[19, 29, 32] The outcome for patients in the earlier series was as good as, if not better than, that for patients in more recent reports[16, 19, 29] who had pancreatitis of similar severity (Table 12–1).

Predating the clinical reports on the successful use of TPN in severe pancreatitis were descriptions of the successful use of jejunal feeding of elemental diets to patients with severe pancreatitis. In 1970, Lawson and associates reported a mortality of 26% in a group of patients who had severe pancreatitis and were fed exclusively by jejunostomy tube.[31] In fact, the first reports of TPN in pancreatitis by Feller and colleagues[26] and White and Heimbach[17] described the administration of TPN early in the course of severe pancreatitis, followed by jejunal feedings as soon as the gut could tolerate them.

The improvement in the outcome of patients with severe pancreatitis observed in the early 1970s was believed to be partly related to vigorous nutritional support and not to any specific effect of TPN. This belief led Goodgame and Fischer to proclaim that "hyperalimentation should be seen as a method of support and not primary therapy" and that in "patients with acute pancreatitis who require laparotomy for diagnosis or therapy, jejunostomy should be performed as a potential means of long-term nutritional management."[18] Similar recommendations for jejunostomy tube feedings have been made by other investigators.[33–35]

Several explanations have been offered for the lack of a demonstrable clinical effect of TPN on pancreatitis. The variability in the severity and etiology of the disease makes it very difficult to conduct studies in which sufficient numbers of patients are stratified according to the etiology, severity, nutritional status at the onset of disease, and associated medical conditions in order to achieve the necessary statistical power to show a treatment effect. Most of the studies to date have included insufficient numbers of patients, so that the probability of a type II statistical error (an inability to demonstrate an effect when an effect may be present) is great. These factors contribute to the fact that no medical treatment to date, including TPN, has been shown to significantly influence the clinical course and final outcome of pancreatitis.[1, 4, 9]

Although any improvement in the outcome of this disease during the past 20 years cannot be attributed directly to nutritional support, there are reasons why TPN is po-

Table 12–1. Trials of Intravenous Nutrition in Patients with Pancreatitis

Study	No. of Patients	Type of Study	Ranson Score	Mortality (%)	Diet Information	Observations and Conclusions
Feller et al., 1974[26]	83	R		14	Early TPN + jejunal feeds (Flexical)	Nut met, mortality 22–14%
White and Heimbach, 1976[17]	30	R	100% necrotizing pancreatitis	20	TPN + jejunal feeds	WT, Nut met
Blackburn et al., 1976[13]	13	R	100% operated 100% > 5 RS	15	TPN + oral Precision LR 4.25% FreAmine 25% glucose	WR, NE
Goodgame, and Fischer, 1977[18]	46	R	78% operated	20	FreAmine + glucose	WT, NE, Nut met, ↑CS
Motton et al., 1982[97]	68	P, NR	NA	19	NA	TPN mortality
Silberman et al., 1982[36]	11	P, NR	Mild	NA	Peripheral TPN Intralipid + 10% glucose + 5.9% amino acids	NE, WT, lipid safe
Grant et al., 1984[19]	73	R	38% > 3 RS	20	Calories = 1.7–1.9 × BEE Protein = 1.5–2.5 g/kg/day + 10% Intralipid Peripheral TPN	WT, ↑CS, 82% required insulin
Hyde and Floch, 1984[37, 178]	21	PR	NA	NA	Glucose 1.7 g/kg/24 h or Glucose + protein 1 g/kg/24 h, or Glucose, protein + 10% lipid	WT, NE, lipid safe
Durr et al., 1985[96]	31	PR	Mild	NA	IV lipid vs. NPO 1.5 g fat/kg/day	NE, lipid safe
Sax et al., 1987[12]	54	PR	Mild 0.8–1.4 RS	1.8	TPN vs. nothing 25% glucose, 4.25% amino acids 10% lipid 2 ×/wk	NE, WT

Study	No.	Design	Severity	Nutritional regimen	Results
Gossum et al., 1988[16]	18	R	5.6 RS	55	10% Aminosyn 1 g protein/kg/day 30 kcal nonprotein/kg/day Lipid—55% nonprotein calories	Triglyceride + glucose intolerance predicted poor outcome
Sitzmann et al., 1989[30]	73	P, NR	50% > 3 RS	11 (42% operated)	1.65 × BEE Glucose + lipid 2 ×/wk, or lipid daily, or no lipid + glucose 7 mg/kg/min	81% ↑ Nut status after TPN, WT Lipid safe Negative N balance associated with 10× ↑ mortality
Steininger et al., 1989[79]	4	P, NR	NA	NA	Glucose-to-fat ratio of 2:1 35 kcal/kg/day	↓Plasma glutamine Glutamine dipeptide safe, and muscle and plasma glutamine ↓ WT, lipid safe
Robin et al., 1990[32]	156	R	29% > 3 RS	4	Lipid 1 ×/wk 85% only glucose	
Kalfarentzos et al., 1991[29]	67	P, NR	3.8 RS	24	1.5–2.5 g protein/kg/day 20–30% of calories as fat	NE, lipid safe, WT, 88% of patients needed insulin ↑ CS
De Beaux et al., 1994[39]	14	PR	Severe (Glasgow score)	0	TPN provided 29.4 kcal/kg/day; 1.5 g protein/kg/day Glutamine supplementation: 0.22 g glutamine/kg/day for 7 days	↓ Proinflammatory cytokine interleukin 8 in glutamine-supplemented group
Braunschweig et al., 1997[100]	44	PR	NA	0	Standard TPN provided 21 patients randomized to receive 30 mg zinc/day (in TPN) for 3 days	Zinc-supplemented group had ↑ febrile response, suggesting exaggerated acute-phase response

BEE, basal energy expenditure; CS, catheter sepsis; IV, intravenous; NA, not available; NE, no effect on clinical course; NPO, nothing per mouth; NR, nonrandomized; Nut met, nutritional needs met; P, prospective; PR, prospective randomized; R, retrospective; RS, Ranson score; TPN, total parenteral nutrition; WT, well tolerated.

tentially beneficial to patients with the more severe forms of pancreatitis. First, the incidence of malnutrition is high in patients suffering from acute pancreatitis.[13, 26, 36] Second, patients with pancreatic necrosis frequently require multiple abdominal operations,[2, 4, 5] which result in extended periods of gastric and intestinal ileus and an inability to eat or be fed by the proximal gut. Third, these patients usually are initially unable to have their high caloric needs completely satisfied by the oral or enteral route because of ileus and the time it takes to adapt to full-strength enteral feeding.

◆ RATIONALE FOR USING TOTAL PARENTERAL NUTRITION IN PANCREATITIS: INDICATIONS AND NUTRITIONAL OBJECTIVES

The major objectives of nutritional support are to meet the metabolic and nutritional needs of patients and to replete patients who may have underlying malnutrition. In this respect, both intravenous and enteral feeding have been shown to be effective in supporting the nutritional needs of patients with pancreatitis. Early reports of enteral support suggested that enteral feeding via the jejunum was safe and well tolerated in pancreatitis,[37–40] although the literature was limited to case reports and small series of patients (Table 12–2). More recently, there have been several prospective randomized clinical trials that illustrate that total enteral nutrition (TEN) is the preferred route of nutritional support in patients with pancreatitis (Table 12–3).

McClave and coworkers conducted a prospective trial to compare the use of early TEN with the use of early TPN in mild pancreatitis.[41] Thirty patients were studied over 32 admissions, randomized to receive TEN[16] or TPN.[16] Nutritional support was initiated within 48 hours of hospital admission. Both groups received isocaloric, isonitrogenous feedings to provide a goal of 25 kcal/kg and 1.2 g of protein per kilogram. TPN was administered through a central or peripheral catheter, TEN was administered as a semielemental formulation (Peptamen, Clintec/Nestle Clinical Nutrition) through an endoscopically placed nasojejunal tube. By the fourth day of hospitalization, typically feeding day 4, the TEN group had reached an average of 72% of goal feedings, which was not significantly different from the 81% of goal feedings achieved by the TPN group. The TEN group tended to have a shorter length of hospitalization at 9.7 ± 1.3 days compared with the TPN group, at 11.9 ± 2.6 days. In addition, the patients receiving TEN tended to have fewer days to normal amylase levels (4.8 ± 0.6 days vs. 6.8 ± 1.5 days) and diet by mouth (5.6 ± 0.8 days vs. 7.1 ± 1.1 days), although these differences were not significant. In addition, there were no differences in serial pain scores, serum albumin levels, nosocomial infections, or mortality. The average cost of nutritional support, based on charges to the patient, was four times greater in the TPN group than in the TEN group. The results suggest that TEN may promote a more rapid resolution to the episode of pancreatitis and the associated stress response. The authors concluded that TEN is as safe and effective, but far less costly, than TPN in mild acute pancreatitis, and the jejunal route should be used preferentially.

Kalfarentzos and associates, compared the use of TEN with TPN in 38 patients with severe necrotizing pancreatitis.[42] TEN was provided as a peptide-base formula (Reabilan HN, Roussel Uclaf Nutrition, France) through a nasoenteric feeding tube placed under fluoroscopy distal to the ligament of Treitz. TPN was provided as a three-in-one solution administered through a subclavian line over 24 hours. Both the TEN and the TPN were well tolerated, and average intakes were comparable between the two groups: approximately 24 kcal/kg/day and 1.4 g of protein. The length of nutritional support was similar in the two groups; the average was 34.8 days for the TEN group and 32.8 days for the TPN group. Hyperglycemia was the most frequently occurring metabolic complication of the nutritional support, occurring in 78% of patients in the TEN group and 90% in the TPN group, although patients with severe hyperglycemia requiring insulin (blood glucose >200 mg/dL) occurred twice as often in the TPN group (50%) as in the TEN group (22%). The TPN group had a significantly greater number of patients with complications, including septic complications, which occurred in 50% of the patients receiving TPN compared with 28% of the TEN group. In this study of patients, the risk of developing metabolic, infectious, and pancreatitis-

Table 12–2. Early Experiences with Total Enteral Support in Pancreatitis

Study	No. of Patients	Severity of Pancreatitis	Route of Nutritional Support	Diet Information	Length of Nutritional Support	Observations
Kudsk et al., 1990[37]	11	Severe, complicated, required exploratory laparotomy Hemorrhagic: 4 Abscess: 5 Pseudocyst: 2	Surgical feeding jejunostomy, with gastrostomy, cholecystostomy	Full-strength Vital HN via feeding jejunostomy	31 ± 6.8 days	Mortality: 2 (18%) Diarrhea/loose stools common TEN well tolerated
Bodoky et al., 1991[38]	12	Chronic pancreatitis, pancreatoduodenectomy	Needle-catheter jejunostomy, pancreatic secretions collected by nasopancreatic tube	TEN: semielemental Peptisorb 2000 kcal, 90 g protein TPN (central line) 2025 kcal, 100 g protein	Experimental period: 7 days	Exocrine pancreas stimulation in jejunostomy feeding similar to that with TPN
De Beaux et al., 1994[39]	1	Severe Glasgow score: 5	Feeding jejunostomy with gastrostomy, TPN	TEN product not reported TPN: 2540 kcal/day; 84 g protein	104 days	Combination of TPN and TEN effective in reducing protein losses
Simpson and Centes, 1995[40]	5	Mild Ranson score: 1.8 (0–3)	Endoscopically placed nasojejunostomy	Standard formulas: Osmolite (2) Elemental: Vital HN and Vivonex (3)	Average: 28 days (10–59 days)	TEN well tolerated TEN did not worsen pancreatitis Nutritional needs met

TEN, total enteral nutrition; TPN, total parenteral nutrition.

Table 12-3. Prospective Randomized Trials Comparing Total Parenteral Nutrition and Total Enteral Nutrition

Study	Patients (no.)		Pancreatitis Severity Score		Patients With Catheter-Related Infections (%)		Patients With Complications (%)		Average Length of Hospitalization (days)		Estimated Cost of Nutritional Support ($/day)	
	TPN	TEN	TPN	TEN	TPN	TEN	TPN	TEN	TPN	TEN	TPN	TEN
McClave et al., 1997[41]	16	16	Mild RS: 1.3	Mild RS: 1.3	12.5	0	31.25*	25	Mean: 11.9	Mean: 9.7	464§	135
Kalfarentzos et al., 1997[42]	20	18	35% severe 65% mild	22% severe 78% mild	10	0	75†	44	Mean: 39	Mean: 40	150	45
Windsor et al., 1998[43]	18	16 TF: 6 PO: 10	38.8% severe (GS)	37.5% severe (GS)	0	0	44‡	6.25	Median: 12.5	Median: 15	115	8

*Complication reported was hyperglycemia requiring insulin.

†Complications reported were hyperglycemia, infections, pneumonia, sepsis, pancreatic pseudocyst, fistula, abscess, and necrosis.

‡Complications reported were sepsis, multiorgan failure, operative interventions.

§Cost of nutritional support per day: average charge for nutritional support based on charges to the patient divided by the average length of nutritional support, 7.1±1.1 days for TPN; 5.6±0.8 days for TEN.

BC, severity assessed by Balthazar's criteria; GS, severity assessed by Glasgow criteria; NR, not reported; PO, by mouth; RS, severity assessed by Ranson score criteria; TEN, total enteral nutrition; TF, tube feeding; TPN, total parenteral nutrition.

related complications in patients receiving TPN was 3.47 times greater than that of patients receiving TEN. The authors concluded that the enteral route should be used preferably for patients with acute severe pancreatitis.

Windsor and colleagues investigated the effects of TPN compared with TEN and oral feedings on the acute-phase response and disease severity in both mild and acute pancreatitis, with the clinical end-point being the incidence of systemic inflammatory response syndrome (SIRS).[43] On admission to the hospital, the severity of pancreatitis was determined by the Glasgow score. Patients were stratified according to disease severity and then randomized to receive either TPN or TEN. The standard TPN solution was formulated to provide 2500 mL 2084 kcal, 57 g of protein, and 110 g of lipid (55% of nonprotein calories). In patients with severe disease (n = 7), TPN was delivered through a central venous catheter, and in mild or moderate disease (n = 11), it was administered through a peripherally inserted catheter. In patients with severe disease (n = 6), TEN was delivered through an endoscopically placed nasojejunal feeding tube as a standard intact protein formula (Osmolite, Ross) to provide 2000 mL, 2018 kcal, 75 g of protein, and 69 g of lipid (36% of nonprotein calories). For patients with mild or moderate pancreatitis (n = 12), TEN was administered as oral supplements in addition to a clear liquid diet. Within the first 48 hours of hospitalization, the patients were evaluated for etiology of pancreatitis, Glasgow and Acute Physiology and Chronic Health Evaluation (APACHE) II scores, levels of serum C-reactive protein, immunoglobulin M (IgM) anti–core endotoxin antibodies, and total antioxidant potential, as well as having a contrast-enhanced computed tomography (CT) scan. The patients received their nutritional support regimen as determined by randomization for 7 days, after which the patients were re-evaluated as outlined previously. Patients continued to be monitored until discharged, and nutritional support was continued as determined by the attending physician.

After 7 days of nutritional support, there was a significant reduction in APACHE II scores and C-reactive protein in the TEN group, whereas there were no changes in the TPN group. Serum IgM anticore endotoxin antibodies increased in the TPN group and

remained stable in the TEN group. The total antioxidant potential decreased by 27% in the TPN group, whereas it increased by 33% in the TEN group. No changes were noted in the serial CT scans in either group. Clinical outcome measures were all improved in the TEN group compared with the TPN group. In the group receiving TEN, SIRS was present in 69% of patients at the onset of nutritional support; this number was reduced to 13% after 7 days. In the TPN group, however, SIRS was initially present in 67% of patients, and the incidence was not significantly reduced over the course of nutritional support, being present in 56% of the group at the end of the seventh day. In addition, sepsis and multiorgan failure occurred only in the patients receiving TPN.

Although the study was limited in the small number of patients with severe acute pancreatitis,[13] the results suggest that enteral feeding is not only feasible and desirable, but that it appears to improve the severity and outcome of disease by modifying the acute-phase response in acute pancreatitis.

Sax and colleagues conducted a randomized prospective study comparing nothing by mouth versus early administration of TPN in patients with pancreatitis.[12] This well-designed and superbly executed study deserves discussion. In this study, TPN had no effect on the clinical course and resolution of pancreatitis or on the incidence of pancreatitis-related complications. Patients receiving TPN tended to have a prolonged time to initiation of oral diet ($P < .09$) and time to reach full oral caloric intake ($P < .06$) when compared with the group. The duration of hospital stay and total hospital costs were also greater in the TPN group. Patients in the TPN group also had a significantly higher incidence of catheter infection than did patients with central lines who did not have pancreatitis ($P < .003$). Because the patients in this trial had mild pancreatitis as judged by Ranson's criteria (Table 12–4) (average Ranson scores were 1.1 and 0.9 in the two groups),[44] the conclusions reached from this trial cannot be generalized to patients with more severe pancreatitis (Ranson score >2). The study by Sax and coworkers demonstrates that patients with mild pancreatitis have early resolution of disease and little need for vigorous nutritional support. Sax's group concluded that the routine use of TPN in patients with mild pancreatitis is not warranted and perhaps is

Table 12–4. Ranson's Prognostic Criteria in Pancreatitis

At admission
  Age > 55 yr
  Glucose > 200 mg/dL
  White blood cell count > 16,000 mm³
  Serum lactic dehydrogenase > 700 IU
  Serum aspartate aminotransferase > 250 Sigma
    Frankel units (U/L)
Within first 48 h
  Hematocrit drop > 10%
  Serum calcium < 8 mg/dL
  Base deficit > 4 mEq/L
  Blood urea nitrogen increase > 5 mg/dL
  Fluid sequestration > 6 L
  Arterial Po₂ < 60 mm Hg
Three or more positive prognostic criteria are
  indicative of severe pancreatitis.

From Ranson JHC, Rifland KM, Roses DF, et al: Prognostic signs and the role of operative management in acute pancreatitis. Surg Gynecol Obstet 139:69–81, 1974. By permission of Surgery, Gynecology, and Obstetrics.

contraindicated. The higher costs of TPN, risks associated with central venous access, and high incidence of line sepsis in patients with pancreatitis (Table 12–5) argue against the use of TPN in these patients.[12]

The absence of any proven clinical benefit of TPN in mild pancreatitis should not preclude the use of intravenous feeding in individual patients who cannot tolerate either TEN or oral feeding. When patients' nutritional needs cannot be met by the oral or enteral route after 5 days of hospitalization for any reason, they should be fed intravenously. The published American Society of Parenteral and Enteral Nutrition (ASPEN) guidelines state: "Enteral feeding should be used to prevent nutritional deficits in patients with acute pancreatitis when abdominal pain, ascites, or an increase in serum amylase does not restrict the use of the gastrointestinal tract. TPN should be used when enteral feeding exacerbated abdominal pain, ascites, or fistulous output in patients with pancreatitis and limited oral intake."[45] The Patient Care Committee of the American Gastroenterology Association lists pancreatitis as a clinical condition that is potentially benefited by intravenous nutrition and states that "regardless of the effect on the underlying disease process, the decision to institute TPN should be made on the basis of (1) the degree of malnutrition, (2) the anticipated length of disability, and (3) the state of metabolic stress."[46]

If the ASPEN and American Gastroenterological Association (AGA) guidelines are followed, then the routine use of intravenous nutritional support in all patients with pancreatitis is not indicated. Patients with mild pancreatitis (e.g., with an APACHE II score <9 [see Fig. 12–1] or Ranson's score <2) who have an expected low complication rate and can usually eat within 5 days do not need nutritional support.[44, 47] The report by

Table 12–5. Total Parenteral Nutrition Catheter Infection Rate in Patients With and Without Pancreatitis

Study	No. of Pancreatitis Patients Infected	Organisms Isolated	Nonpancreatitis Catheter Infection Rate (%)	P Value*
Goodgame and Fischer, 1977[18]	8 of 46 patients (17%) 8 of 99 catheters (8%)	5 Staphylococcus aureus 2 Staphylococcus epidermidis 1 Enterococcus	3.0	
Grant et al., 1984[19]	10 of 121 patients (8.2%)	6 Coagulase-negative staphylococci 2 Candida albicans 4 Gram-negative rods	2.3	<.0005
Sax et al., 1987[12]	3 of 28 catheters (10.7%)	3 Staphylococcus aureus	1.5	<.003
Kalfarentzos et al., 1991[29]	6 of 67 patients (8.9%)	2 Staphylococcus epidermidis 1 Staphylococcus aureus 2 Enterobacter cloacae 1 Candida	2.9	<.01
Jackson et al., 1993[123]	11 of 43 patients (25.6%)	5 Candida spp. 2 Staphylococcus epidermidis 4 Culture-negative "sepsis syndrome" organisms	Not reported	

*Comparison between total parenteral nutrition line infection rates in patients with pancreatitis and in those without pancreatitis at the same institution.

Sax and colleagues suggests that routine use of TPN in patients with mild pancreatitis may be contraindicated from a cost-effective and risk-benefit point of view.[12] On the other hand, patients with severe pancreatitis. (>9 APACHE II score[47] and >2 Ranson score[44]) are catabolic and have a high probability of developing complications, needing one or more operations, and having significantly prolonged periods of gastric and duodenal ileus. The ASPEN and AGA guidelines clearly support the early implementation and use of nutritional support in these patients.

◆ NUTRITIONAL SUPPORT ALGORITHM FOR PATIENTS WITH PANCREATITIS

The following proposal for the use of intravenous nutrition in patients with pancreatitis is not intended to be dogmatic but rather to serve as a guideline. It is based on a comprehensive review of the world literature. An outline for this algorithm is illustrated in Figure 12–1, and proposed energy and fuel requirements are outlined in Table 12–6.

Mild Pancreatitis

The first step in evaluating any patient for intravenous nutritional support should be

Table 12–6. Suggested Energy and Fuel Requirements for Total Parenteral Nutrition During Acute Severe Pancreatitis

Energy: Estimate by	
1. Indirect calorimetry	
2. 2 × basal energy expenditure by Harris-Benedict equation for uninfected; 2.5 × basal energy expenditure for infected necrosis	
Fraction of total daily caloric load	
Glucose	50–60 or <4.0 mg/kg/min
Protein	15–20% or 2–2.5 g/kg/day
Lipid	20–30%
Nonprotein calorie/ nitrogen	100 kcal/g of protein

Data from Nordenstrom J, Carpenter AY, Askanzi J, et al: Free fatty acid mobilization and oxidation during total parenteral nutrition in trauma and infection. Ann Surg 198:725–735, 1983; Long CL: Fuel preferences in the septic patient: Glucose or lipid? J Parenter Enteral Nutr 11:333–335, 1987; and Long CL. Schaffel N, Geiger JW, et al: Metabolic response to injury and illness: Estimation of energy and protein needs from indirect calorimetry and nitrogen balance. JPEN J Parenter Enteral Nutr 3:452–456, 1979.

based on the patient's nutritional status. Patients with malnutrition, which often accompanies chronic alcoholism and chronic pancreatitis, should be started on intravenous nutrition as soon as they are admitted to the hospital. In the absence of underlying malnutrition, patients with mild pancreatitis (Ranson score <2 or an APACHE II score <9) should receive nothing by mouth and should be treated conservatively with fluid and electrolytes and analgesia while a search for the underlying cause of the pancreatitis is sought. When gastrointestinal symptoms and abdominal pain resolve, these patients can be fed orally with a diet low in fat. Experience has shown that patients treated in such a fashion usually are able to tolerate a complete oral diet within 7 days of admission to the hospital.[12] If abdominal pain, nausea and vomiting, and persistent or progressive hyperamylasemia persist beyond 5 days, however, intravenous nutritional support should probably be initiated because the time to resolution of the underlying disease is less predictable and a patient's risk of developing malnutrition increases daily.

Severe Pancreatitis

Patients who arrive at the hospital with severe pancreatitis (Ranson score >2 or APACHE II score >9) should have immediate and vigorous resuscitation in an intensive care setting, and dynamic CT should be performed to further assess the severity of the disease. These patients have a high probability of prolonged gastric and duodenal ileus, as well as a risk of retroperitoneal necrosis, sepsis, and the need for one or more operations. These patients should receive enteral nutritional support by nasojejunal feeding tube within 48 hours of admission to the hospital. If TEN is not tolerated as evidenced by an increase in abdominal pain, vomiting, or amylase levels, then intravenous nutritional support should be initiated. The intravenous line used for TPN should have a single lumen and a silver- or iodine-impregnated cuff in order to minimize the risk of catheter infection.

Initial intravenous diets should consist of glucose and amino acids until serum triglyceride and lipid levels can be determined. Total daily energy requirements should be

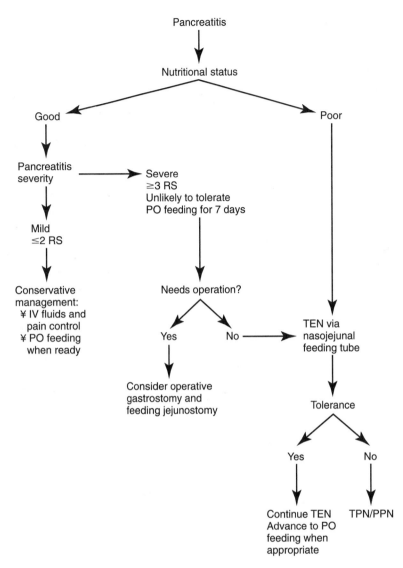

Figure 12–1. Algorithm for nutritional support for patients with pancreatitis. IV, intravenous; PO oral; PPN, peripheral parenteral nutrition; RS, Ranson criteria score; TEN, total enteral nutrition; TPN, total parenteral nutrition.

determined by indirect calorimetry. Alternatively, requirements can be estimated by using the Harris-Benedict equation (see Table 12–8) with appropriate stress qualifiers.[8, 48] Total nonprotein calories, as estimated by indirect calorimetry, usually are less than 2500 kcal/day. The calorie-to-nitrogen ratio should be approximately 100:1, and hence the total protein supplied should be between 2 and 2.5 g/kg/day. Serum glucose levels should be closely monitored, particularly at the beginning of TPN, and a peripheral insulin infusion begun in order to maintain serum glucose levels at less than 200 mg/dL. After several days, when a patient's insulin needs become more stable and predictable, insulin can be added to the TPN solution bag.

Indirect calorimetry should be used when and if available in order to predict a patient's caloric needs accurately and to avoid over- and underfeeding. Serum triglycerides should be measured in all patients before intravenous lipids are administered. If the triglyceride level is normal, intravenous lipids should then be added to the intravenous feeding regimen to supply between 20 and 30% of total nonprotein calories. Total lipids should probably not exceed 1.5 g/kg/day. Patients with hypertriglyceridemia should not be given lipids until their plasma lipid profile normalizes. Plasma triglyceride levels should be monitored in all patients after lipids are included in the TPN in order to demonstrate an adequate capacity to clear lipids.

Consideration should be given to placing a nasojejunal transpyloric feeding tube in all patients for transition to enteral feeding. If abdominal surgery is performed, needle catheter jejunostomy should be performed and the patient should be started on enteral elemental feeding postoperatively. Parenteral nutrition can be decreased as enteral nutrient delivery is increased and tolerated.

Enteral Feeding in Severe Pancreatitis

Intravenous nutrition is not without complications; therefore, it is appropriate to briefly discuss alternative methods of nutritional support—namely, enteral feeding—in patients with pancreatitis. There is no controversy about the fact that patients with severe pancreatitis require intensive nutritional support. For reasons stated earlier, current practice is to feed these patients intravenously even though reports in the literature have demonstrated that patients with severe pancreatitis can have their nutritional needs adequately and safely met by the enteral route when the diet is instilled into the jejunum.[31, 33, 34, 49] Enteral feeding should always be considered as an alternative or supplemental method of nutritional support in patients with pancreatitis because it poses fewer risks, is less invasive, is generally less expensive, affords greater comfort, eases nursing care, and may support gastrointestinal barrier function and integrity. Furthermore research illustrates that enteral feeding is the preferred route of nutritional support in severe pancreatitis (see Table 12–3), as it was associated with fewer complications[42] and improved disease severity and moderation of the acute-phase response.[43]

Infusion of an enteral diet directly into the stomach or duodenum is not recommended because of gastric and duodenal ileus. Although pancreatic rest has yet to be demonstrated to be a clinically meaningful end-point in the treatment of pancreatitis,[9] most authorities still recommend that enteral feedings be given into the jejunum.[33, 34, 49] They should be low in fat,[50] high in carbohydrate,[51] and high in osmolality[49] to reduce pancreatic exocrine secretion.

The decision to use the enteral rather than the parenteral route of feeding should take into consideration not only the effectiveness of both methods but also the costs, the risks, and patients' comfort. The lower costs and avoidance of central line complications should make the use of enteral feedings the preferable method of nutritional support in patients with pancreatitis, provided a patient's gut tolerates being fed and nutritional requirements can be met. Surgeons are often hesitant to place feeding jejunostomies in patients who have pancreatitis and are very ill and require operation for débridement of necrotic or infected tissue because of the fear of potential complications resulting from a leaking jejunostomy. A number of reports, however, have demonstrated that, when placed with a Witzel tunnel, feeding jejunostomies are safe and efficacious methods of feeding patients with pancreatitis.[17, 31, 33] Some clinicians advocate the placement of a feeding jejunostomy in all patients who undergo operation for pancreatitis.[18, 33, 35] Kudsk and colleagues placed jejunal feeding tubes in 11 patients who had severe necrotizing pancreatitis and required operations.[33] Five of these patients were operated on within 48 hours of the onset of pancreatitis and were fed immediately after surgery without any adverse effect on the clinical course of the pancreatitis.

◆ PANCREATIC REST AS A THERAPEUTIC GOAL

Most physicians do not base the decision to use TPN in patients with pancreatitis on the stated guidelines of the ASPEN or the AGA but rather on the theory that *pancreatic rest* is important in the treatment of pancreatitis.[52, 53] The therapeutic rationale for pancreatic rest during pancreatitis is based on the hypothesis that reduced pancreatic protein synthesis and secretion alleviate pancreatic inflammation, minimize complications, and thus accelerate the rate of recovery from pancreatitis. Blackburn and colleagues stated that nutritional depletion must be corrected without stimulation of the pancreas and its attendant exacerbation of the pancreatitis.[13] Ranson and Spencer also advocated that oral feeding be avoided in patients with pancreatitis and claimed that premature oral feeding of patients not fully recovered from pancreatitis exacerbated the disease and led to an increased incidence of subsequent complications.[53] These reports contributed to the overzealous use of TPN in patients with pancreatitis.

Because most physicians believe in therapeutic approaches that promote pancreatic rest for the treatment of acute pancreatitis, feeding patients with pancreatitis without stimulating pancreatic exocrine secretion has become an important objective despite the absence of any clinical or scientific evidence to support this approach. Contrary to popular belief, pancreatic rest by avoiding pancreatic exocrine secretion has not made any impact on the clinical outcome of pancreatitis.[4–9] Furthermore, there is no conclusive evidence to date that any medical treatment intended to decrease pancreatic exocrine secretion has any clinical benefit, other than the avoidance of pain, on the course of the disease.[4, 9, 54] These observations are not surprising when one considers the fact that pancreatic exocrine secretion is severely impaired in an inflamed pancreas.[55–57] If the pancreas is unable to respond to secretory stimuli, it makes perfect sense that therapeutic maneuvers to avoid pancreatic exocrine stimulation will have no bearing on the disease process.

If pancreatic rest is eventually demonstrated to be beneficial to patients with pancreatitis, it will then be relevant to know what the effects of individual nutrients on pancreatic exocrine secretion are. The effects of individual nutrients and the route of feeding on pancreatic exocrine secretion have been thoroughly discussed elsewhere[8–10] and therefore are only briefly reviewed here.

Clinical and experimental experience has demonstrated that none of the individual components of TPN stimulate pancreatic exocrine secretion.[58–64] A singular report by Konturek and colleagues at one time cast some doubt on this fact.[65] These researchers reported that intravenous fat infusion stimulated pancreatic exocrine secretion in dogs. Subsequent studies, performed in both dogs[60, 63, 64, 66] and humans,[62, 67] did not confirm these findings and demonstrated that intravenous fat did not stimulate pancreatic exocrine secretion. TPN has consistently been shown to decrease pancreatic exocrine secretion in experimental animals and humans.[58–61] Among the various components of TPN, hypertonic glucose has a profound suppressant effect on the exocrine pancreas, and amino acids do not stimulate pancreatic enzyme secretion above basal levels.[60] The results of these studies added more support to the use of TPN in pancreatitis and led to its wide use in almost all patients with the disease, despite the lack of any proven clinical benefit from controlled, randomized trials.

◆ METABOLIC CHANGES IN PATIENTS WITH PANCREATITIS

In order to recommend appropriate feeding, it is important to know the changes in intermediary metabolism and substrate needs of patients with pancreatitis. Patients with severe acute pancreatitis undergo a hyperdynamic catabolic state that is characterized by the same metabolic, cardiovascular, and hemodynamic features observed in stressed, postoperative, and septic patients.[20, 24, 68–71] These physiologic changes are initiated and sustained by injured, dead, and ischemic tissues, as well as by invading bacteria. The hypermetabolism of pancreatitis has been well described[8, 22, 25, 72, 73] and is summarized in Table 12–7. The hormonal and metabolic derangements in these patients lead to changes in carbohydrate, protein, and lipid metabolism, which in turn lead to increased resting energy expenditure (REE), peripheral insulin resistance and lipolysis, hyperglycemia and hypertriglyceridemia, decreased glucose oxidation, and increased circulating levels of catecholamines, insulin, and glucagon.

Table 12–7. Metabolic Changes During Acute Pancreatitis

Hormonal changes
  ↑ Insulin and glucagon, ↓ insulin-to-glucagon ratio
  ↑ Catecholamines
Substrate changes
  ↑ Serum glucose, urea, and triglycerides
  ↑ Aromatic amino acids
  ↓ Plasma total amino acids, BCAAs, and glutamine
  ↓ Gluconeogenic amino acids: alanine, threonine, and serine
  ↓ Glucose oxidation, ↑ peripheral lipolysis
Energy utilization
  Mild pancreatitis
    ↑ Resting energy expenditure
    ↑ Oxygen consumption
  Severe pancreatitis
    ↑ Arteriovenous shunting
    ↓ Oxygen consumption
    ↓ Energy utilization
  Skeletal muscle changes
    ↓ Total free amino acids, glutamine, and BCAAs
    ↑ Water content and fat

BCAAs, branched-chain amino acids.

Caloric Needs

Patients with pancreatitis are extremely hypermetabolic and can have profoundly increased energy requirements. Because optimal nutritional support requires knowledge of a patient's energy requirements and provision of appropriate amounts of calories, it is important to determine a patient's energy expenditure. Caloric needs of patients with pancreatitis vary and are determined by the severity of the disease, the presence of infection, and a patient's age, height, weight, and temperature.[23, 73, 74]

Basal energy expenditure (BEE) in critically ill patients is usually assessed by one of two methods. BEE is most often estimated by using the Harris-Benedict formula (Table 12–8)[75] modified by stress factors to account for the severity of illness.[26, 48, 76] Studies have now demonstrated that the modified Harris-Benedict formula is not a reliable estimator of BEE in patients with pancreatitis.[8, 23, 73, 74] The most accurate way of assessing caloric requirements in patients with pancreatitis is by estimating the REE by indirect calorimetry.[76] When comparing REE measured by indirect calorimetry with predicted energy expenditure (PEE) by the modified Harris-Benedict formula, Mann and coworkers demonstrated that this formula significantly overestimated the caloric needs of patients with acute pancreatitis.[23] Using indirect calorimetry, Dickerson and colleagues reported a wide distribution of REE in hospitalized patients with pancreatitis.[74] 10% of patients with pancreatitis were hypometabolic (<90% of PEE), 38% were normometabolic (90 to 110% of PEE), and 52% were hypermetabolic (>110% of PEE). In these patients, REE varied from 77 to 139% of PEE. Boufard and associates demonstrated that patients with more severe pancreatitis

(those with a Ranson score >5) had a mean energy expenditure, assessed by indirect calorimetry, that was 1.49 times the PEE measured by the Harris-Benedict formula.[73] Additional research in patients with chronic pancreatitis and pancreatic abscess further underscores the difficulty in estimating energy needs. In patients with stable alcoholic chronic pancreatitis, it was found that measured energy expenditure was significantly higher than PEE in those patients who were underweight, that is, approximately 60% of these patients were hypermetabolic.[77] In patients with pancreatic abscess, Arouni and colleagues found that energy expenditure as determined by indirect calorimetry did not correlate with Harris-Benedict calculations, covering a wide range (22.4 to 46.8 kcal/kg/day).[78] This research further illustrates the need to use indirect calorimetry for careful determination of caloric requirements in this population of patients, who tend to be undernourished as well as hypermetabolic during episodes of acute pancreatitis.

These studies illustrate that the nutritional needs of patients with pancreatitis cannot be accurately estimated by using modifications of the Harris-Benedict formula and suggest that critically ill patients with pancreatitis should have their caloric needs calculated by indirect calorimetry.[23] Another important reason for accurately assessing the total energy expenditure is to avoid administering calories in excess of metabolic needs, because overfeeding has deleterious consequences in critically ill patients.[76]

Protein and Amino Acid Metabolism

Acute pancreatitis is attended by accelerated skeletal muscle proteolysis and amino acid release[79] coupled with increased consumption of circulating amino acids, resulting in amino acid depletion,[22] increased ureagenesis,[72] and nitrogen excretion[16] that can reach 20 to 40 g/day.[13] Roth and colleagues described the changes in amino acid concentrations in plasma and skeletal muscle in patients with acute hemorrhagic necrotizing pancreatitis.[80] They demonstrated that total amino acid concentrations in the plasma of these patients were lower than those in healthy control subjects. Particularly low were concentrations of amino

Table 12–8. Harris-Benedict Equation

Male basal energy expenditure = 66 + (13.7 × weight in kg) + (5 × height in cm) − (6.8 × age)
Female basal energy expenditure = 655 + (9.6 × weight in kg) + (1.7 × height in cm) − (4.7 × age)

From Harris JA, Benedict FG: A Biometric Study of Basal Metabolism in Man, Vol 2. Washington, DC, Carnegie Institution of Washington, 1919, p 227; and Roza AM, Shizgas HM: The Harris Benedict equation reevaluated: Resting energy requirements and the body cell mass. Am J Clin Nutr 40:168–182, 1984.

acids used for gluconeogenesis in the liver: alanine, threonine, and serine. The level of glutamine the most abundant amino acid in plasma, was only 55% of normal. This depression in glutamine and alanine levels occurred despite a significant release of both amino acids from skeletal muscle.[79]

The changes in skeletal muscle protein metabolism and amino acid concentrations in patients with pancreatitis are similar to those observed in patients after operations,[81] during sepsis,[21] and with multiple organ failure.[20, 24] The total free amino acid pool decreases to 40% of normal, and intracellular skeletal muscle glutamine, the most abundant free amino acid in skeletal muscle, diminishes to levels as low as 15% of normal.[80] Simultaneous increases occur in the concentrations of the branched-chain amino acids, phenylalanine, tyrosine, methionine, and taurine.[21, 25, 80]

The specific changes of amino acid metabolism in patients with pancreatitis suggest that the administration of amino acid solutions rich in branched-chain amino acids or in glutamine may support the underlying metabolism and therefore be clinically beneficial to patients with severe forms of pancreatitis. Intravenous administration of glutamine dipeptides to patients with severe pancreatitis attenuates the decrement in intracellular levels of glutamine in skeletal muscle, as well as the reduction in plasma concentrations of glutamine.[79] Compared with conventional TPN, glutamine dipeptide–supplemented TPN was found to reduce the release of the proinflammatory cytokine interleukin 8 from peripheral blood mononuclear cells from patients with severe acute pancreatitis.[82] The clinical effects of providing intravenous glutamine to patients with pancreatitis have not been reported, however. Also, no clinical studies have demonstrated that administration of branched-chain amino acid preparations has a beneficial effect on the outcome of severe pancreatitis.

Carbohydrate Metabolism

Increased circulating plasma cortisol and catecholamine levels, peripheral insulin resistance, a decreased insulin-to-glucagon ratio, and a decreased clearance rate and oxidation of glucose result in hyperglycemia in patients with pancreatitis.[80] Patients with pancreatitis tend to develop significant hyperglycemia with the administration of hypertonic dextrose solutions and usually require supplemental insulin administration. Grant and colleagues[19] and Kalforentzos and associates[29] reported that 80 to 88% of patients with pancreatitis required between 46 and 85 U of insulin per day while receiving glucose-based TPN. Gossum and colleagues found that severe glucose intolerance and high insulin requirements (>3 U/h) were associated with a fatal outcome.[16] It should be noted that the high insulin requirements reported in these studies are associated with predominantly glucose-based diets and not with constant lipid infusion as a three-in-one mixture. The latter would be anticipated to result in less glucose intolerance and lower insulin requirements.[83]

Intravenous glucose should never be administered in excess of the maximal endogenous capacity to oxidize glucose (5 mg/kg/min in normal adults). In seriously ill patients with pancreatitis, glucose clearance and oxidation may be severely impaired and lower than the maximal capacity. If glucose is provided in an amount exceeding the glucose oxidation rate, hepatic steatosis develops.[16] Hence, glucose should provide no more than 60% of a patient's total caloric needs. In a 70-kg man with a BEE of 2500 kcal/day, this would equate with a glucose infusion rate of less than 5.0 mg/kg/min.[24] Several studies have demonstrated that the respiratory quotient for patients with acute pancreatitis ranges between 0.78 and 0.91 reflecting a mixed-fuel oxidation.[23, 73, 74]

Fat

The use of lipid emulsions in patients with pancreatitis continues to be controversial because of the etiologic association of hyperlipidemia and pancreatitis.[84–90] The literature convincingly demonstrates, however, that no controversy should exist over the use of lipid in patients with pancreatitis. All physicians need to know the important considerations and facts about the use of lipid in patients with pancreatitis.

The package insert from the manufacturers of lipid emulsions cautions against their use in patients with dyslipoproteinemias and acute pancreatitis because of a number of reports in the literature. Cameron and colleagues, in a series of studies on pancreatitis and hypertriglyceridemia, concluded that increased serum triglycerides can initiate acute pancreatitis.[85-87] Additional evidence to support a relationship between hypertriglyceridemia and pancreatitis comes from the observations of (1) increased susceptibility to recurrent pancreatitis in patients with types I and V hyperlipoproteinemia,[84, 91] (2) the association between hypertriglyceridemia after ingestion of large amounts of alcohol and acute pancreatitis,[87] (3) the association of hyperlipidemia and pancreatitis with oral contraceptive therapy,[89] and (4) the development of pancreatitis in children who have inflammatory bowel disease and are receiving steroids and intravenous fat.[88, 90] These associations between lipid infusion and pancreatitis have resulted in the current standard of care for all patients initially presenting with acute pancreatitis—their triglyceride level is measured. If the triglyceride level is elevated, lipids should not be administered until the level returns to normal.

Certain patients may have a previously unrecognized lipid disorder or impaired ability to metabolize lipids.[92] Hence, administration of lipid emulsions to patients with pancreatitis requires careful observation. Patients with previous episodes of pancreatitis may have an impaired ability to clear circulating lipid[92] and therefore may be susceptible to the development of hyperlipidemia while receiving lipid infusion. Hence, in patients with pancreatitis, it is important to check not only the serum lipid level before infusion but also the postinfusion level to demonstrate adequate clearance capacity. If the serum triglyceride level is normal, a 100-mL test dose of 20% lipid should be infused. If this test dose is well tolerated, up to 30% of nonprotein calories can be provided as fat, and the serum triglyceride level should be evaluated weekly.

Numerous clinical trials have demonstrated the safety of administering lipids intravenously to patients who have acute pancreatitis and in whom hypertriglyceridemia was not an etiologic factor for their disease (see Table 12–1). Tanimura and colleagues first reported on the use of intravenous lipid in patients with pancreatitis in Japan.[93] They observed that acute pancreatitis in a group of patients with essential fatty acid deficiency abated when an infusion of fat was started. Kawaura and coworkers subsequently administered fat-supplemented TPN to four patients with favorable results and claimed that "the most important thing in intravenous nutritional support of patients with pancreatitis is to give fat emulsion intravenously."[94] Lochs, from Vienna, infused fat intravenously into 10 patients with acute pancreatitis and observed that triglycerides were eliminated from the plasma at a rate only slightly slower than that observed in healthy control subjects.[95] Significant hyperlipidemia was not observed during the lipid infusions, and pancreatitis was not exacerbated. Durr and coworkers performed the first controlled randomized study of the use of intravenous fat in patients with acute pancreatitis.[96] Sixteen patients received fat intravenously (1.5 g/kg/day), and 15 patients received only standard conservative management with no nutritional support. Fat infusion caused no apparent benefit or detriment. Surprisingly, the plasma triglyceride levels were similar between the two groups, thus demonstrating that patients with pancreatitis tolerate fat infusion without difficulty. Motton and associates[97] and Silberman and colleagues[36] administered lipid emulsions intravenously to patients with acute pancreatitis in amounts ranging from 60 to 350 g/day without any untoward effects.

In addition to the fact that intravenous administration of fat is safe during pancreatitis, several physiologic reasons exist to support its use. First, the altered metabolism of pancreatitis is characterized by a decreased capacity to oxidize glucose, peripheral insulin resistance, and hyperglycemia. Reliance on glucose as the sole nonprotein calorie source increases the risk of hyperglycemia and hepatic steatosis, whereas adding fat to TPN solutions decreases hyperglycemia and reduces hepatic steatosis. Second, the addition of lipid to intravenous glucose infusions improves nitrogen balance[98] in patients on TPN, including those patients with pancreatitis.[30] Third, patients with pancreatitis have respiratory quotients between 0.76 and 0.91, demonstrating a mixed-fuel utilization. These patients metabolize their own fat stores; hence, daily administration of lipid is not absolutely necessary provided a patient has reasonable body fat. In such patients, lipid emulsions should be provided at least twice a week to prevent essential fatty acid deficiency.

Lipid emulsions are ideally administered

continuously along with amino acids and glucose in a three-in-one mix. This method offers the advantage of simple administration and fewer metabolic complications than bolus infusions of lipid alone over 8 hours.[99] MacFie and colleagues have shown that the substrate and hormone profiles during continuous lipid infusion approximates, those of the normal postabsorptive state, whereas wide fluctuations in substrate levels, persistent hyperinsulinemia, and impaired oxidation of exogenous fat occur during intermittent lipid infusion.[99]

Electrolytes, Minerals, and Vitamins

Patients with severe acute pancreatitis have significant fluid sequestration early in the course of their disease and require aggressive fluid and electrolyte resuscitation in an intensive care unit setting.[1, 2] It is common to delay the initiation of TPN in these patients until after the initial resuscitation, when the patient's metabolic milieu is more stable. There is no reason, however, that severely ill patients with pancreatitis cannot have TPN administered within 24 hours of illness. When TPN is begun early, additional intravenous lines are necessary so that other fluids, electrolytes, and drugs can be administered independently of the nutrient solution. No attempt should be made to correct initial abnormalities in the patient's electrolyte, glucose, or acid-base status through the administration of the parenteral nutrient solution. If supplemental insulin is required, as is usual, it too should be administered through a separate intravenous line. Once the initial resuscitation phase is complete and a patient's metabolic status is more stable, then daily insulin requirements and maintenance or replacement amounts of fluids and electrolytes can be administered through the parenteral nutrient solution.

Hypocalcemia is the most common mineral abnormality in acute pancreatitis and may require intravenous supplementation.[44] This should not be via the TPN solution. Hypomagnesemia commonly occurs during acute pancreatitis, particularly in alcoholic patients, and may initially require large amounts of replacement.[19] This is also best administered separately and not in the TPN solution. Alcoholic patients are particularly likely to have depleted total body magnesium levels. In addition, they are also likely to have depleted total body zinc levels. Serum zinc levels further decline by 10 to 69% during the acute-phase response. Brunschweig and coworkers conducted a prospective randomized trial of parenteral zinc supplementation in a group of patients with pancreatitis or catheter-related sepsis previously receiving home TPN.[100] It was found that 30 mg per day of elemental zinc sulfate administered in TPN increased serum zinc levels by 50%, whereas levels in the control group, receiving unsupplemented TPN, remained unchanged. However, during the first 3 days of nutritional support, the zinc-supplemented group had a significantly higher febrile response, evidence of an exaggerated acute-phase response. There was a significant correlation between serum interleukin b levels and body temperatures. It appears that excessive supplementation (30 mg/day) of parenteral zinc may exaggerate the acute-phase response, suggesting that overzealous zinc supplementation to correct depleted plasma zinc levels be avoided in acute pancreatitis. Repletion of total body stores of these and other micronutrients can be progressively achieved by daily administration of minerals in the TPN solution.

All patients receiving TPN should be given the recommended daily allowance of vitamins in their TPN. Alcoholic patients should receive supplemental thiamine and folate at the initiation of TPN, and these supplements can be administered in the TPN bag.[12] In addition, patients with acute pancreatitis have been found to have significantly decreased levels of total vitamin C and its bioactive component, ascorbic acid, compared with a groups of healthy controls and patients with acute intra-abdominal crisis.[101] Levels of plasma ascorbic acid were undetectable in 14 of 25 patients with acute pancreatitis. Researchers advocate the intravenous administration of 500 mg of ascorbic acid daily to accelerate recovery.

Although the pathophysiology of pancreatitis is not yet understood, evidence is increasing to support the role of oxidative damage in the development of pancreatic inflammation. Increased oxidative stress as measured by increased lipid peroxidation and decreased antioxidant defenses occurs in a number of experimental models of pancreatitis. Evidence of oxidative stress has also been identified in studies of human patients with both acute and chronic pancre-

Table 12–9. Antioxidant Nutrient Levels in Patients with Pancreatitis

Study	Total No. of Subjects	Types of Pancreatitis (no. of patients of total number of subjects)	Antioxidant Levels in Pancreatitis Group Compared with Control Group (%)			
			Vit A	Vit C	Vit E	Se
DeWaele et al., 1992[173]	60	Gallstones/biliary (20)	85.7	77.4		N/A
		Acute alcoholic (20)	73.1*	52.4*	77.3*	N/A
Scott et al., 1993[101]	86	Acute (29) Gallstones/alcoholism/ idiopathic	N/A	18.7*	N/A	N/A
Uden et al., 1992[103]	60	Recurrent pancreatitis (20)	35.4*†	N/A	79.1*	72.6*
Braganza et al., 1995[174]	94	Acute (42) Gallstones/alcoholism/ idiopathic	27.8*†	13.8‡	78.4*	66.2*
Van Gossum et al., 1996[175]	49	Chronic alcoholism (35)	61.2*	N/A	50*	62.1*

*Statistical significance between pancreatic patient levels and control levels (number of patients is the residual number from total number of subjects and equals the number of controls).

†Vitamin A is β-carotene.

‡Vitamin C is ascorbic acid.

NA, not available.

atitis. In addition, decreased levels of antioxidant nutrients have been found in patients with pancreatitis of various causes (Table 12–9). Uncontrolled clinical experiences suggest that the administration of antioxidants ameliorates many of the consequences of pancreatitis. Since 1990, clinicians in Germany have treated patients with acute pancreatitis with intravenous sodium selenite producing dramatic reductions in complications, the need for operations, and mortality.[102] In a double-blind crossover trial of oral antioxidant supplementation in patients with recurrent nongallstone pancreatitis, there were significantly fewer attacks of pancreatitis during the treatment phase and a decrease in background pain.[103] These studies suggest that there may be therapeutic potential for antioxidants in the management of patients with pancreatitis.

◆ IS TOTAL PARENTERAL NUTRITION BENEFICIAL AND SAFE DURING PANCREATITIS?

Before trials of enteral support in acute pancreatitis in the late 1990s, there had been unanimous support in the medical and surgical literature for the use of TPN in the treatment of pancreatitis. Table 12–1 lists a number of clinical reports in which intravenous nutrition was used in patients with pancreatitis. The majority of the investigators in these trials strongly endorsed the use of TPN during pancreatitis, predominantly because of the ability of intravenous nutrition to meet the nutritional needs of patients with pancreatitis. A prospective randomized trial of TPN in the care of patients with pancreatitis, conducted by Sax and colleagues and discussed earlier, did not demonstrate any clinical benefit of TPN.[12] The prospective randomized trials comparing TPN and TEN (see Table 12–3) illustrate that TEN is the preferred route of nutritional support in acute pancreatitis, as it is associated with fewer complications, improvement in disease severity, and lower cost.[41–43] However, in accordance with ASPEN guidelines, TPN should be used in pancreatitis when TEN "exacerbates abdominal pain, ascites, or fistulous output in patients with pancreatitis."[45]

Several conclusions, can be made from a review of the reported worldwide clinical experience with the use of TPN during pancreatitis. First and most important, the administration of TPN to patients with acute pancreatitis is generally safe and well tolerated, meets patients' nutritional needs, and corrects underlying malnutrition. Second, intravenous lipid is safe, does not cause or exacerbate pancreatitis in nonhyperlipidemic individuals, and should constitute approximately 25 to 30% of nonprotein calories. Third, TPN does not alter the course of pancreatitis or influence mortality. Fourth, TPN suppresses pancreatic secretion and is useful in the treatment of pancreatic duct fistulas. Fifth, the incidence of central intravenous catheter infection is significantly greater in patients with pancreatitis than in TPN-fed patients without pancreatitis.

◆ RISKS, BENEFITS, AND COST OF TOTAL PARENTERAL NUTRITION DURING PANCREATITIS

In the absence of any proven clinical benefit, it is imperative that the risks and potential side effects of any form of therapy be carefully evaluated. The inherent risks of TPN administration include catheter sepsis, pneumothorax and hemothorax, major venous thrombosis, air embolism, and a number of potential metabolic complications. Catheter infection is the major concern in patients who have pancreatitis and are given TPN through a central line. Four studies have demonstrated that the TPN catheter infection rate in patients with pancreatitis is significantly greater than that in patients receiving TPN for other medical reasons (see Table 12–5). This high incidence of line infection warrants scrupulous attention to central venous catheter care in patients with pancreatitis and argues against the use of triple-lumen catheters for TPN administration because they are more often infected than single-lumen catheters. Careful consideration should be given to the preferential use of catheters with silver-impregnated cuffs,[104, 105] which have a documented decreased infection rate. The reason why patients with pancreatitis have an increased susceptibility to line infection is not entirely clear but may be related to impaired opsonization, phagocytosis, and bacterial killing by mononuclear cells.[106–108]

Because TPN has not been shown to change the course of the disease and because the catheter infection rate in patients with acute pancreatitis appears to be significantly increased (see Table 12–5), the administration of TPN to patients with pancreatitis should not be undertaken lightly and should be based on sound reasoning and proper indications. Furthermore, because the vast majority of patients with pancreatitis (>80%) have a mild, quickly resolving form of the disease that allows an early return of gut function, the routine administration of TPN to all patients with pancreatitis is neither justified nor indicated.

The time-limiting factors in the number of days that patients with pancreatitis spend in the hospital (which equate directly to hospital costs) are related primarily to the time it takes to tolerate oral feeding and to alleviate pain.[12] It is standard practice not to feed patients by the oral route until their abdominal pain and tenderness resolve. Ranson and Spencer claimed that premature oral feeding may prevent complete resolution of pancreatitis, result in an early return of pain, and cause the development of pseudocyst.[53] No clinical trials have substantiated this claim, although one experimental study performed in rats demonstrated that increased oral intake during mild pancreatitis increased mortality.[109] No published evidence to date suggests that jejunal enteral feeding adversely affects the course of pancreatitis. In fact, reports have demonstrated that patients with severe pancreatitis can be safely and effectively fed by jejunal feedings.[33, 34]

It is generally assumed that enteral feeding is substantially less expensive than intravenous feeding, although costs vary by institution. At the University of Illinois Medical Center in Chicago, the cost of administering nasojejunal feedings (approximately $850/w) is substantially less than the cost of TPN (approximately $4200/w). These cost estimates are based on the charges to the patient for the formula alone, either 2000 mL of Peptamen VHP (semielemental diet) or TPN. They do not include the additional costs including line or feeding tube placement, diet delivery, or nutritional assessment and monitoring. The higher cost of TPN, however, should not be an argument for its avoidance in patients with pancreatitis who are unable to tolerate enteral nutrition.

The rapid increase in health care costs has led to therapeutic treatment plans designed to discharge patients earlier from the hospital. These socioeconomic forces unfortunately result in premature feeding and discharge of patients who have pancreatitis but are not yet ready to be fed. Ironically, such clinical strategies may actually prolong patients' illnesses by resulting in their readmission to the hospital with pancreatitis. These patients are often labeled as having chronic relapsing or recurrent pancreatitis when, in effect, the original bout of pancreatitis may never have resolved. Despite the forces being mounted against physicians by hospital administrators, cost-containment policy, and third-party reimbursement, it is my opinion that patients should demonstrate complete resolution of pancreatitis before being fed orally and discharged from the hospital. Complete resolution of pancreatitis is defined as complete resolution of pain and abdominal tenderness, normal serum amylase levels, and the ability to tolerate oral alimentation without nausea and vomiting. In patients in whom mild pancreatitis has not resolved after 5 days of conservative therapy, nutritional support should be implemented in the form of either jejunal feeding or TPN.

Ideally, the decision to use TPN in patients with pancreatitis should be based on cost-effectiveness and risk-benefit analysis derived from controlled clinical trials. Current research suggests that enteral nutrition is the preferred route of nutritional support; however, intravenous feedings are indicated when patients are unable to tolerate tube feedings because of increased pain, vomiting, or increased amylase levels. A physician's decision to use TPN in a patient with pancreatitis should be based on his or her personal experience, the condition of the patient, and the guidelines set forth by the ASPEN and AGA committees, not by hospital cost-containment policy or third-party reimbursement.

◆ TOTAL PARENTERAL NUTRITION FOR COMPLICATIONS OF PANCREATITIS

The use of TPN in patients with pancreatitis may be most strongly indicated and clinically effective in those who develop complications of the disease, such as intestinal and pancreatic fistulas, pancreatic ascites, pseudocysts, and pancreatic abscesses. Many of these complications preclude feeding by the oral, gastric, or small intestinal route.

Pancreatic Fistulas

Patients with severe acute necrotizing pancreatitis can develop both enterocutaneous and pancreaticocutaneous fistulas. Thomas and Ross first reported the closure of a pancreatic fistula by intravenous support using dextrose and amino acid solutions.[110] Dudrick and colleagues subsequently described the use of TPN to successfully close a traumatic pancreaticoduodenal fistula.[111] The clinical efficacy of TPN in facilitating the closure of pancreatic fistulas has subsequently been demonstrated by many others.[67, 112–114] The rationale for using TPN in patients with pancreatic fistulas is based on the fact that intravenous nutrition causes less pancreatic secretion than do enteral feedings[66, 115] and is related to the inhibitory effect of hypertonic glucose infusion on pancreatic exocrine secretion.[60] Pancreatic fistulas heal faster when the volume of the fistula output is decreased by the use of TPN. Concern was at one time expressed that intravenous lipid might stimulate pancreatic exocrine secretion,[65] but clinical and experimental data demonstrate that this is not the case.[62, 63, 66, 67, 116] Therefore, there is no contraindication to the use of intravenous lipids in patients with pancreatic fistulas. Studies have also demonstrated that decreasing pancreatic fistula output by the combination of TPN and somatostatin accelerates healing even more quickly than does the use of TPN alone.[117, 118] If octreotide is used concomitantly with TPN in patients with acute or chronic pancreatitis, there may be greater glucose intolerance and need for insulin.

Pancreatic Ascites

Spontaneous rupture of pancreatic pseudocysts can result in massive ascites secondary to an internal pancreatic duct leak. Treating internal pancreatic fistulas only by oral dietary restriction and parenteral nutrition results in closure of the fistulas less than 50% of the time.[118, 119] Sanfey and Cameron advocate that surgery be performed if internal fistulas do not heal after 2 to 3 weeks of medical therapy.[120] It would be reasonable, however, to try other nonsurgical approaches aimed at decreasing pancreatic secretion, such as somatostatin, terbutaline, or exogenous pancreatic enzyme ingestion, before resorting to surgery.[121, 122]

Pseudocysts

Pancreatic pseudocysts commonly develop in patients after severe pancreatitis and are secondary to disruption of the pancreatic ductule system and extravasation of pancreatic juice into the peripancreatic tissues. If the development of pancreatic pseudocysts is dependent on the accumulation of pancreatic exocrine secretions outside the pancreatic ductule system, then TPN should theoretically decrease pancreatic pseudocyst evolution by inhibiting pancreatic exocrine secretion. There are no published clinical trials demonstrating that administration of TPN to patients with pancreatitis decreases the subsequent development of pancreatic pseudocysts. Jackson and associates demonstrated clinical and radiographic improvement in a retrospective study of the use of TPN in 40 patients with pancreatic pseudocyst.[123] After an average of 32.5 days on TPN, there was complete (13.9%) or partial (53.5%) regression of the pseudocyst based on serial CT or ultrasonography. Twelve patients (27.9%) underwent drainage of the pseudocyst. Of note, however, was the high rate (34.9%) of catheter-related complications, including catheter-related infection, that occurred in 25.6% of these patients. Further controlled clinical trials comparing TPN to TEN are needed to determine if the route of nutritional support alters the course of the disease, as well as the most beneficial and cost-effect route.

Chronic pancreatic pseudocysts often have a communication with the pancreatic duct. In such cases, when the pseudocyst is drained externally by a percutaneous catheter, a pancreatic duct fistula is created by way of the pseudocyst. In this setting, the use of TPN with or without somatostatin will have the same beneficial effects reported in the healing of pancreatic fistulas, provided that a patient has no proximal pancreatic duct obstruction.[124]

Abscesses

Pancreatic abscesses usually develop from superinfection of a pancreatic pseudocyst. If the abscess is localized, it can often be drained percutaneously. The anatomic location of the abscess often causes localized colonic, gastric, or duodenal ileus, as well as nausea and vomiting. In such a setting, nutritional support can be achieved by the use of TPN until the abscess is drained and gastrointestinal function returns. There are

no published clinical data on the ability of TPN during acute pancreatitis to decrease the incidence of retroperitoneal infection or pancreatic infections after a severe episode of pancreatitis.

◆ FUTURE RESEARCH

Designing Clinical Trials for Total Parenteral Nutrition in Patients with Pancreatitis

The lack of any proven clinical effect of TPN on the outcome of pancreatitis is possibly related to the heterogeneity of the disease, the lack of prospective clinical trials in which patients have been randomly assigned to treatment arms based on disease severity, and the failure to initiate TPN early in the course of the disease. In order to conduct studies that control for these factors, it will be necessary to identify immediately on their hospital admission patients who are most likely to benefit from the early institution of TPN and to use a reliable method of stratification based on the severity of disease.

A number of methods can quantitate the severity of pancreatitis and can be useful for predicting the likelihood that the patient will experience organ failure, complications, and death. The most popular and widely used method for quantitating the severity of pancreatitis, described by Ranson and colleagues (see Table 12–4), consists of 11 signs.[44] An inherent problem with Ranson's scoring system is that it can be calculated only after a patient has been in the hospital for 48 hours. Hence, the Ranson score cannot be used to rapidly stratify patients to treatment groups at the time of admission to the hospital. The APACHE II score,[125] which is weighted average score based on a patient's health and physiologic status, has been shown to be a better predictor of subsequent complications and death in patients with severe pancreatitis.[47] A score is used to stratify patients into those with severe (score >9) and mild (score <9) pancreatitis. The APACHE II score has the advantage of being calculated within 24 hours of admission to the hospital, allowing patients to be stratified according to severity on their initial presentation to the hospital. Abdominal CT with intravenous contrast material, referred to as *dynamic CT scanning*, is a useful way of ascertaining the presence of infarcted and necrotic pancreatic and peripancreatic tissues. Dynamic CT scanning is useful in predicting the risk of developing pancreatic pseudocyst or abscess and the need for operative débridement.[126-128]

The power of a staging system such as the Ranson score or APACHE II score for predicting the development of later complications can be enhanced by combining it with the results of dynamic CT scanning, as illustrated by the study by Clavien and colleagues.[129] Because early randomization and assignment to different treatment groups is necessary to test whether or not intravenous nutrition instituted early in the course of a patient's illness will have significant clinical impact, future attempts to stratify patients should use APACHE II, or a similar physiologic scoring system, combined with dynamic CT scanning.

The design of clinical trials should include the use of power analysis to determine the number of patients needed to be studied in order to reach significant conclusions about specific treatment effects. Clinical evidence suggests that TPN will be cost-effective and clinically efficacious only in patients with severe disease, and only 5 to 10% of all patients with pancreatitis develop a severe form of the disease. For example, a prospective trial attempting to demonstrate a 50% reduction in mortality (e.g., from 20% to 10%) for acute severe pancreatitis with a power of 0.8 would require approximately 400 paients randomly assigned to one of two treatment arms. Assuming a 10% incidence of severe pancreatitis in the general population, such a trial would require approximately 4000 initially evaluated patients. The accruement of such large numbers of patients obviously requires that multi-institutional studies be performed. Larger treatment effects on end-points other than mortality, such as the time to resolution of disease; infection; pseudocyst; the time in the intensive care unit; and the hospital cost, may of course require much smaller numbers of patients.

In addition to early stratification, multi-institutional trials will require all participating centers and physicians to have a standardized treatment algorithm, such as the one described by Beger,[2] if the treatment effect of early TPN on the clinical course of acute pancreatitis is to be evaluated.

Potential Role of Specific Nutrients in Modulating the Inflammatory, Hepatic, and Immunologic Response in Patients with Pancreatitis

The lack of any demonstrable clinical benefit of TPN on pancreatitis, other than the ability to support patients' nutritional needs and corretct their underlying malnutrition, may be related to the fact that current intravenous formulations are deficient in nutrients that are critically important to the maintenance of specific organ and physiologic functions.[130] Three areas of currently active research in nutritional support have potential for improving the clinical outcome of patients with severe pancreatitis. They are the study of the effects that specific nutrients have on (1) immune and reticuloendothelial function, (2) intestinal barrier function, and (3) the catabolic response to injury and infection.

Immunity and Reticuloendothelial Cell Function

The ability to modulate the immune system nutritionally[131-133] has tremendous potential for improving the outcome of pancreatitis in patients who have deficits in reticuloendothelial cell and macrophage function and are at increased risk for developing infection.[105-107]

The contribution of altered macrophage function to host morbidity and mortality during severe pancreatitis is illustrated by several experimental and clinical observations. First, macrophages from rodents with experimentally induced pancreatitis have impaired phagocytic and killing capacity for bacteria.[134] Second, there is an upregulation of proinflammatory cytokine release (tumor necrosis factor and interleukins 6 and 8) from peripheral-blood mononuclear cells from patients with acute pancreatitis.[135] Third, increased cytokine elaboration in patients with severe pancreatitis is more likely to occur in those who develop systemic complications suggesting a causal relationship.[136] Finally, stimulation of macrophages by exogenously administered glucan significantly decreases mortality in experimental pancreatitis.[137] Studies have demonstrated that lymphocyte,[138, 139] polymorphonuclear neutrophil,[140] and macrophage[141–144] functions can be altered by specific amino acids and fats and by the route of nutrient delivery.[133, 145, 146]

The proinflammatory cytokines (tumor necrosis factor and interleukins 1, 6, and 8) are known to play important pathophysiologic roles in the development and morbid consequences of severe pancreatitis.[136, 147] It is also known that a number of nutrients (e.g., glutamine, arginine, and fish oil) and vitamins (vitamin E) can modulate the production of cytokines as well as the host's reponse to infection.[148a] This link between nutrients, cytokine biology, and pancreatitis provides a potential new route of modulating the course of pancreatitis. The use of modified structured lipids, high in ω-3 and low in ω-6 fatty acids, has not been reported in animals or in patients with pancreatitis and may have significant beneficial effects on the clinical course of pancreatitis by altering a number of biologic responses. Modified lipid emulsions may alter the cellular response in the pancreas by changing the responsiveness of acinar cells to external stimuli or the stability of acinar cell zymogen granules and lysosomes.[148] In addition, the use of specialized lipid formulations may modulate the catabolic host response to pancreatitis.[132, 142]

One of a host's major defense mechanisms against pancreatitis is clearance of activated proteases from the circulation by Kupffer cells of the liver.[107, 108] α_2-Macroglobulin, an acute-phase protein made by the liver, binds to circulating trypsins. The trypsin–α_2-macroglobulin complex is cleared from the circulation by Kupffer cells. This clearance is dependent on the presence of fibronectin. Patients with pancreatitis have a relative deficiency of fibronectin as well as alterations in hepatic Kupffer cell function,[107, 108, 149] which together result in decreased phagocytosis by Kupffer cells. This deficit may partly explain the increased susceptibility of patients with pancreatitis to infection. The effect of intravenous diets enriched with specific amino acids such as glutamine and arginine or fats high in ω-3 fatty acids, which influence cell function,[141, 150, 151] should be investigated in terms of the incidence of infection or the host response to infection. In a prospective randomized double-blind clinical trial the addition of glutamine to parenteral nutrition was found to significantly decrease peripheral mononuclear cell production of interleukin 8 but did not affect the production of interleukin 6 or tumor necrosis factor α.[82] Two commercial enteral diets high in glutamine, arginine, and ω-3 fatty acids (Impact, Sandoz Nutritionals; Immun-Aid, McGaw) are now commercially available and are specifically designed to preserve or restore immune function. The effects of these diets should be carefully studied prospectively before wide generalized use because the effect of their individual dietary components on immune function and the inflammatory resonse are poorly understood. One report demonstrated that high doses of arginine can induce pancreatitis.[152]

Supporting the Gut Barrier

The most common cause of death in patients with severe necrotizing pancreatitis is sepsis.[153] Up to 60% of pancreatic phlegmons and peripancreatic fluid collections in patients with severe acute pancreatitis are colonized with gram-negative bacteria.[154] It is believed, although not proved in humans, that the high incidence of infection of the peripancreatic and retroperitoneal spaces is a result of microorganisms transported into the area of necrosis via lymphatic channels between the transverse colon and the pancreas[155, 156] and through microperforations of the large bowel.[157] Experimental evidence supports this hypothesis, because rats with chemically induced pancreatitis develop bacterial contamination of inflamed peripancreatic tissues.[155, 158, 159] Additional experimental evidence suggesting that bacterial translocation occurs during pancreatitis comes from the observation that intestinal decontamination in rats with pancreatitis decreases the incidence of bacterial colonization of mesenteric lymph nodes and death.[158] Intestinal decontamination by oral antibiotics has also been reported to reduce the incidence of severe infections and sepsis in patients with severe pancreatitis.[156]

Currently available commercial parenteral formulations do not contain many of the important fuels for the intestinal mucosa, including glutamine and short-chain fatty acids.[160] The addition of glutamine[161] or short-chain fatty acids[162, 163] to parenteral diets or the administration of gut trophic peptides such as cholecystokinin,[164] bombesin,[165] and neurotensin[166–168] stimulates gut growth and may preserve gut barrier function.[168, 169] The potential for enteral feeding in very small amounts during parenteral feeding to prevent gut barrier dysfunction and the hypercatabolic response to injury[170-172] is great and needs to be tested. Whether nutritional strategies of preserving intestinal barrier integrity and/or immunity will influence the outcome of severe acute pancreatitis is unknown and needs to be tested in prospective clinical trials.

In summary, future nutritional and clinical strategies should be designed to meet not only the overall nutritional needs of patients but also the specific nutritional needs of the gut, liver, and immune system. Additional research should be directed at investigating the effects of enteral feeding on the host catabolic response and the incidence of retroperitoneal infection.

REFERENCES

1. Levelle-Jones M, Neoptolemos JP: Recent advances in the treatment of acute pancreatitis. Surg Annu 22:235–261, 1990.
2. Beger HG: Surgical management of necrotizing pancreatitis. Surg Clin North Am 69:529–549, 1989.
3. Creutzfeldt W, Lankisch PG: Intensive medical treatment of severe acute pancreatitis. World J Surg 5:341–350, 1981.
4. Ranson JHC: Acute pancreatitis: Pathogenesis, outcome and treatment. Clin Gastroenterol 13:843–863, 1984.
5. Ranson JHC: The role of surgery in the management of acute pancreatitis. Ann Surg 211:382–393, 1990.
6. Durr GHK: Enteral and parenteral nutrition in acute pancreatitis. *In* Beger HG, Buchler M (eds): Acute Pancreatitis. Berlin, Springer-Verlag, 1987, pp 285–288.
7. Grant JP: Nutritional support in acute pancreatitis. Aspen Update 3(3):1, 10, 1981.
8. Havala T, Shronts E, Cerra F: Nutritional support in acute pancreatitis. Gastroenterol Clin North Am 18:525–542, 1989.
9. Kirby DF, Craig RM: The value of intensive nutritional support in pancreatitis. JPEN J Parenter Enteral Nutr 9:353–357, 1985.
10. McMahon MJ: Diseases of the exocrine pancreas. *In* Kinney JM, Jeejeebhoy KN, Hill GL, Owens OE (eds): Nutrition and Metabolism in Patient Care. Philadelphia, WB Saunders, 1988, pp 386–404.
11. Dammann HG, Dreyer M, Walter TA, et al: Prognostic indicators in acute pancreatitis: Clinical experience and limitations. *In* Beger HG, Buchler M (eds): Acute Pancreatitis. Berlin, Springer-Verlag, 1987, pp 25–31.
12. Sax HC, Warner BW, Talamini MA, et al: Early total parenteral nutrition in acute pancreatitis: Lack of beneficial effects. Am J Surg 153:117–124, 1987.
13. Blackburn GL, Williams LF, Bistrian BR, et al: New approaches to the management of severe acute pancreatitis. Am J Surg 131:114–124, 1976.
14. Allardyce DB: Incidence of necrotizing pancreatitis and factors related to mortality. Am J Surg 154:295–299, 1987.
15. Gerzoff SG, Banks PA, Robbins AH, et al: Early diagnosis of pancreatic infection by computed tomography–guided aspiration. Gastroenterology 93:1315–1320, 1987.
16. Gossum AV, Memoyne M, Greig OD, Jeejeebhoy KN: Lipid-associated total parenteral nutrition in patients with severe acute pancreatitis. JPEN J Parenter Enteral Nutr 12:250–255, 1988.
17. White TT, Heimbach DM: Sequestrectomy and hyperalimentation in the treatment of haemorrhagic pancreatitis. Am J Surg 132:270–275, 1976.
18. Goodgame JT, Fischer JE: Parenteral nutrition in the treatment of acute pancreatitis: Effect on complications and mortality. Ann Surg 186:651–658, 1977.
19. Grant JP, James S, Grabowski V, Trexler KM: Total parenteral nutrition in pancreatic disease. Ann Surg 200:627–631, 1984.
20. Roth E, Funovics J, Muhlbacher F, et al: Metabolic disorders in severe abdominal sepsis: Glutamine deficiency in skeletal muscle. Clin Nutr 1:25–41, 1982.
21. Freund H, Ryan JA, Fischer JE: Amino acid derangements in patients with sepsis: Treatment with branched-chain amino acid rich infusions. Ann Surg 188:423–430, 1978.
22. Holbling N, Funovics J, Roth E, et al: Amino acid metabolism in acute necrotising pancreatitis: Aspects of parenteral nutrition. *In* Hollender LF (ed): Controversies in Acute Pancreatitis. Berlin, Springer-Verlag, 1982, pp 297–301.
23. Mann S. Westernkow DR, Houtchens BA: Measured and predicted caloric expenditure in the acutely ill. Crit Care Med 13:173–177, 1985.
24. Cerra FB: Hypermetabolism, organ failure, and metabolic support. Surgery 101:1–14, 1987.
25. Di Carlo V, Nespoli A, Chiesa R, et al: Hemodynamic and metabolic impairment in acute pancreatitis. World J Surg 5:329–339, 1981.
26. Feller JH, Brown RA, Toussant GPM, Thompson AG: Changing methods in the treatment of severe pancreatitis. Am J Surg 127:196–201, 1974.
27. Voitk A, Brown RA, Echave V, et al: Use of an elemental diet in the treatment of complicated pancreatitis. Am J Surg 125:223–227, 1973.
28. Dudrick SJ, Wilmore DW, Vars HM, Rhoads JE: Can intravenous feeding as the sole means of nutrition support in the child and restore weight loss in an adult? An affirmative answer. Ann surg 169:974–984, 1969.
29. Kalfarentzos FE, Daravias DD, Karatzas TM, et al: Total parenteral nutrition in severe acute pancreatitis. J Am Coll Nutr 10:156–162, 1991.
30. Sitzmann JV, Steinborn PA, Zinner MJ, Cameron JL: Total parenteral nutrition and alternate energy substrates in treatment of severe acute pancreatitis. Surg Gynecol Obstet 168:311–317, 1989.
31. Lawson DW, Daggertt WM, Civetta JM, et al: Surgical treatment of acute necrotizing pancreatitis. Ann Surg 172:605–617, 1970.
32. Robin AP, Campbell R, Palani CK, et al: Total parenteral nutrition during acute pancreatitis: Clinical experience with 156 patients. World J Surg 14:572–579, 1990.
33. Kudsk KA, Campbell SM, O'Brien T, Fuller R: Postoperative jejunal feedings following complicated pancreatitis. Nutr Clin Pract 5:14–17, 1990.

34. Baulieux J, Boulex J, Peix JL, Donee R: La nutrition entérale par jejunostomie d'alimentation au cour des pancreatities aigues graves. Chirurgie 107:59–63, 1981.

35. Choudhuri G, Tandon RK: Nutritional support in acute pancreatitis. J Gastroenterol Hepatol 3:483–488, 1988.

36. Silberman M, Dixon NP, Gisenberg D: The safety and efficacy of a lipid-based system of parenteral nutrition in acute pancreatitis. Am J Gastroenterol 77:494–497, 1982.

37. Kudsk KA, O'Brien T, Fuller R: Postoperative jejunal feedings following complicated pancreatitis. Nutr Clin Pract 5:14–17, 1990.

38. Bodoky G, Harsanyi L, Pap A, et al: Effect of enteral nutrition on exocrine pancreatic function. Am J Surg 161:144–147, 1991.

39. De Beaux AC, Plester C, Fearon KC: Fexible approach to nutrition support in severe acute pancreatitis. Nutrition 10:246–249, 1994.

40. Simpson WG, Marsano L, Gates L: Enteral nutritional support in acute alcoholic pancreatitis. J Am Coll Nutr 14:662–665, 1995.

41. McClave SA, Greene LM, Snider HL, et al: Comparison of the safety of early enteral vs parenteral nutrition in mild acute pancreatitis. JPEN J Parenter Enteral Nutr 21:14–21, 1997.

42. Kalfarentzos F, Kehagras J, Mead N, et al: Enteral nutrition is superior to parenteral nutrition in severe acute pancreatitis: Results of a randomized prospective trial. B J Surg 84:1665–1669, 1997.

43. Windsor AC, Kanwar S, Li AG, et al: Compared with parenteral nutrition, enteral feeding attenuates the acute phase response and improves severity in acute pancreatitis. Gut 42:431–435, 1988.

44. Ranson JHC, Rifkind KM, Roses DF, et al: Prognostic signs and the role of operative management in acute pancreatitis. Surg Gynecol Obstet 139:69–81, 1974.

45. Shronts EP, Fish JA, Pesce-Hammond K: Nutrition Assessment. In Souba WW (ed): The ASPEN Nutrition Support Practice Manual. Silver Springs, MD, American Society of Parenteral and Enteral Nutrition, 1998, pp 1:1–1:4.

46. Sitzmann JV, Pitt HA: Statement on guidelines for total parenteral nutrition. The Patient Care Committee of the American Gastroenterological Association. Dig Dis Sci 34:489–496, 1989.

47. Larvin M, McMahon MJ: APACHE-II score for assessment and monitoring of acute pancreatitis. Lancet 2:201–204, 1989.

48. Roza AM, Shizgal HM: The Harris Benedict equation reevaluated: Resting energy requirements and the body cell mass. Am J Clin Nutr 40:168–182. 1984.

49. Keith RG: Effect of a low fat elemental diet on pancreatic secretion during pancreatitis. Surg Gynecol Obstet 151:337–343, 1980.

50. Stevens RV, Randall HT: Use of concentrated balanced, liquid elemental diet for nutritional management of catabolic states. Ann Surg 170:642–667, 1969.

51. Ragins H, Levenson SM, Signer R, et al: Intrajejunal administration of an elemental diet at neutral pH avoids pancreatic stimulation: Studies in dog and man. Am J Surg 126:606–614, 1973.

52. Ettien JT, Webster PD: The management of acute pancreatitis. Adv Intern Med 25:169–198, 1980.

53. Ranson JHC, Spencer FC: Prevention, diagnosis and treatment of pancreatic abscess. Surgery 82:99–106, 1977.

54. D'Amico D, Favia G, Biasiato R, et al: The use of somatostatin in acute pancreatitis—results of a multi-center trial. Hepatogastroenterology 37:92–98, 1990.

55. Evander A, Hederstrom E, Hultberg B, Ihse I: Exocrine pancreatic secretion in acute experimental pancreatitis. Digestion 24:159–167, 1982.

56. Mitchell CJ, Playforth MJ, Kelleher J, McMahon MJ: Functional recovery of the exocrine pancreas after acute pancreatitis. Scand J Gastroenterol 18:5–8, 1983.

57. Niederau C, Niederau M, Luthen R, et al: Pancreatic exocrine secretion in acute experimental pancreatitis. Gastroenterology 99:1120–1127, 1990.

58. Nakajima S, Magee DF: Inhibition of exocrine pancreatitis secretion by glucagon and D-glucose given intravenously. Can J Physiol Pharmacol 48:299–305, 1970.

59. Hamilton RF, Davis WC, Stephenson DV, Magee DF: Effects of parenteral hyperalimentation on upper gastrointestinal secretions. Arch Surg 102:348–352, 1971.

60. Towne JB, Hamilton RF, Stephenson DV: Mechanism of hyperalimentation in the suppression of upper gastrointestinal secretions. Am J Surg 126:714–716, 1973.

61. Kelly GA, Nahrwold DL: Pancreatic secretion in response to an elemental diet and intravenous hyperalimentation. Surg Gynecol Obstet 143:87–91, 1976.

62. Edelman K, Valenzuela JE: Effect of intravenous lipid on human pancreatic secretion. Gastroenterology 85:1063–1066, 1983.

63. Meyer JH, Jones RS: Canine pancreatic responses to intestinally perfused fat and products of fat digestion. Am J Physiol 226:1178–1187, 1974.

64. Fried GM, Ogden WE, Rhea A, et al: Pancreatic protein secretion and gastrointestinal hormone release in response to parenteral amino acids and lipid in dogs. Surgery 92:902–905, 1982.

65. Konturek SJ, Tasler J, Cieszkowski M, et al: Intravenous amino acids and fat stimulate pancreatic secretion. Am J Physiol 236:E676–E684, 1979.

66. Stabile BE, Debas HT: Intravenous versus intraduodenal amino acids, fats and glucose as stimulants of pancreatic secretion. Surg Forum 32:224–226, 1981.

67. Grundfest S, Steiger E, Selinkoff P, Fletcher J: The effect of intravenous fat emulsions in patients with pancreatic fistulas. JPEN J Parenter Enteral Nutr 4:27–31, 1980.

68. Ganong WF: Neuroendocrine responses to injury. In Little R, Frayn K (eds): The Scientific Basis for the Care of the Critically Ill. Manchester, UK, Manchester University Press, 1986, pp 45–60.

69. Bessey P, Watters J, Aoki T, Wilmore D: Combined hormonal infusion stimulates the metabolic response to injury. Ann Surg 200:264–281, 1984.

70. Woolfson AMM, Heatley RV, Allison SP: Insulin to inhibit protein catabolism after injury. N Engl J Med 300:14–17, 1979.

71. Duke JH Jr, Jorgensen BS, Browell JR, et al: Contribution of protein to caloric expenditure following injury. Surgery 78:168–174, 1970.

72. Shaw JH, Wolfe RR: Glucose, fatty acid, and urea kinetics in patients with severe pancreatitis: The response to substrate infusion and total parenteral nutrition. Ann Surg 204:665–672, 1986.

73. Bouffard YH, Delafosse BX, Annat GJ, et al: Energy expenditure during severe acute pancreatitis. JPEN J Parenter Enteral Nutr 13:26–29, 1989.

74. Dickerson RN, Vehe KL, Mullen JL, Feurer ID: Resting energy expenditure in patients with pancreatitis. Crit Care Med 19:484–490, 1991.

75. Harris JA, Benedict FG: A Biometric Study of Basal Metabolism in Man, Vol 2. Washington, DC, Carnegie Institution of Washington, 1919, p 227.

76. Rutten P, Blackburn GL, Flatt JP, et al: Determination of optimal hyperalimentation infusion rate. J Surg Res 18:477–483, 1975.

77. Hebuterne X, Hastier P, Peroux JL, et al: Resting energy expenditure in patients with alcoholic chronic pancreatitis. Dig Dis Sci 41:533–539, 1996.

78. Arouni MA, Fagan DR, Jasnowski J, et al: Nonprotein caloric requirement for patients with pancreatic abscess as measured by indirect calorimetry. Pancreas 5:95–98, 1990.

79. Steininger R, Karner J, Roth E, Langer K: Infusion of dipeptides as nutitional substrates for glutamine, tyrosine, and branched-chain amino acids in patients with acute pancreatitis. Metabolism 38(Suppl 1):78–81, 1989.

80. Roth E, Zoch G, Schulz F, et al: Amino acid concentrations in plasma and skeletal muscle of patients with acute hemorrhagic necrotizing pancreatitis. Clin Chem 31:1305–1309, 1985.

81. Vinnars E, Bergstrom J, Furst P: Influence of the postoperative state on the intracellular free amino acids in human muscle tissue. Ann Surg 182:665–671, 1975.

82. De Beaux AC, O'Riordain MG, Ross JA, et al: Glutamine-supplemented total parenteral nutrition reduces blood mononuclear cell interleukin-8 release in severe acute pancreatitis. Nutrition 14:261–265, 1998.

83. Blackburn GL: In search of the "preferred fuel." Nutr Clin Pract 4:3–5, 1989.

84. Greenberger NJ, Hatch F, Drummey G, Isselbacher KJ: Pancreatitis and hyperlipemia: A study of serum lipid alterations in 25 patients with acute pancreatitis. Medicine 45:161–174, 1966.

85. Cameron JL, Capuzzi DM, Zuidema GD, Margolis S: Acute pancreatitis with hyperlipemia: Evidence for a persistent defect in lipid metabolism. Am J Med 56:482–487, 1974.

86. Cameron JL, Capuzzi DM, Zuidema GD, Margolis S: Acute pancreatitis with hyperlipidemia: The incidence of lipid abnormalities in acute pancreatitis. Ann Surg 177:483–489, 1973.

87. Cameron JL, Zuidema GD, Margolis S: A pathogenesis for alcoholic pancreatitis. Surgery 77:754–763, 1975.

88. Noseworthy J, Colodny AH, Eraklis AJ: Pancreatitis and intravenous fat: An association in patients with inflammatory bowel disease. J Pediatr Surg 18:269–272, 1983.

89. Davidoff F, Tishler S, Rosoff C: Marked hyperlipidemia and pancreatitis associated with oral contraceptive therapy: N Engl J Med 289:552–555, 1973.

90. Lashner BA, Kirsner JB, Hanauer SB: Acute pancreatitis associated with high-concentration lipid emulsion during total parenteral nutrition therapy for Crohn's disease. Gastroenterology 90:1039–1041, 1986.

91. Frederickson DS, Lees RS: Familial hyperlipoproteinemia. In Stanbury JB, Wyngaarden JB, Frederickson DS (eds): The Metabolic Basis of Inherited Disease, 2nd ed. New York, McGraw-Hill, 1966, pp 429–485.

92. Guzman S, Nervi F, Llanos O, et al: Impaired lipid clearance in patients with previous acute pancreatitis. Gut 26:888–891, 1985.

93. Tanimura H, Takaneka M, Setoyama M, et al: Pathogenesis and treatment of pancreatitis due to essential fatty acid deficiency. Gastroenterol Jpn 12:483–489, 1977.

94. Kawaura Y, Sata H, Fukatani G, Iwa T: The therapy of acute pancreatitis through intravenous hyperalimentation with fat emulsions. Proceedings of the 5th Asian Pacific Congress of Gastroenterology, Singapore, 1976, pp 682–658.

95. Lochs H: Parenterale Ernährung bei akuter Pankreatitis. In Kleinberger G, Dölp R (eds): Basis der parenteralen und enteralen Ernährung. Klinische Ernährung, Vol 10. München, Zuckschwerdt, 1982, pp 180–185.

96. Durr GHK, Schaefers A, Maroske D, Bode JC: A controlled study on the use of intravenous fat in patients suffering from acute attacks of pancreatitis. Infusionsther Klin Ernahr 12:128–133, 1985.

97. Motton G, Pistorelli C, Fracastroro G, et al: Role of complete parenteral treatment nutrition in acute pancreatitis. In Hollender IF (ed): Controversies in Acute Pancreatitis. Berlin, Springer-Verlag, 1982, pp 293–296.

98. Long JM, Wilmore DW, Mason AD, Pruitt BA: Effect of carbohydrate and fat intake on nitrogen excretion during total intravenous feeding. Ann Surg 185:417–422, 1977.

99. MacFie J, Courtney DF, Brennan TG: Continuous versus intermittent infusion of fat emulsions during total parenteral nutrition. Clin Trial Nutr 7:163–168, 1991.

100. Braunschweig CL, Slowers M, Kovacevich DS, et al: Parenteral zinc supplementation in adult humans during the acute phase response increases the febrile response. J Nutr 127:70–74, 1997.

101. Scott P, Bruce C, Schofield D, et al: Vitamin C status in patients with acute pancreatitis. Br J Surg 80:750–754, 1993.

102. Kuklinski B, Zimmermann T, Schweder R: Decreasing mortality in acute pancreatitis with sodium selenite. Med Klin 90:36, 1995.

103. Uden S, Schofield D, Miller PF, et al: Antioxidant therapy for recurrent pancreatitis: Biochemical profiles in a placebo-controlled trial. Aliment Pharmacol Ther 6:229–240, 1992.

104. Maki DG, Cobb L, Garman JK, et al: An attachable silver-impregnated cuff for prevention of infection with central venous catheters: A prospective randomized multicenter trial. Am J Med 85:307–314, 1988.

105. Flowers RH, Schwenzer J, Kopel RF, et al: Efficacy of an attachable subcutaneous cuff for the prevention of intravascular catheter-related infection: A randomized, controlled trial. JAMA 261:878–883, 1989.

106. Ellenbogen S, Roberts NB, Day DW, et al: The effects of SMS 201-995 on reticuloendothelial system activity and pulmonary function in rats with acute pancreatitis. Br J Surg 75:606, 1988.

107. Adham NF, Song MK, Haberfeld GC: Relationship between the functional status of the reticuloendothelial system and the outcome of experimentally

induced pancreatitis in young mice. Gastroenterology 84:461–469, 1983.

108. Larvin M, Switala SF, McMahon MJ: Impaired clearance of circulating macromolecular enzyme inhibitor complexes in severe acute pancreatitis: An important aspect of pathogenesis? Br J Surg 74:1165, 1987.

109. Evander A, Lundquist I, Ihse I: Influence of gastrointestinal hormones on the course of acute experimental pancreatitis. Hepatogastroenterology 29:161–166, 1982.

110. Thomas PO, Ross CA: Effect of exclusive parenteral feeding on closure of pancreatic fistula: Study made after duodenopancreatic resection for carcinoma of ampulla of Vater. Arch Surg 57:104–112, 1948.

111. Dudrick SJ, Wilmore DW, Steiger E, et al: Spontaneous closure of traumatic pancreatoduodenal fistulas with total intravenous nutrition. J Trauma 10:542–552, 1970.

112. MacFadyen BV, Dudrick SJ, Ruberg RL: Management of gastrointestinal fistulas with parenteral hyperalimentation. Surgery 74:100–105, 1973.

113. Zinner MJ, Baker RR, Cameron JL: Pancreatic cutaneous fistulas. Surg Gynecol Obstet 138:710–712, 1974.

114. Pederzoli P, Bassi C, Falconi M, et al: Conservative treatment of external pancreatic fistulas with parenteral nutrition alone or in combination with continuous intravenous infusion of somatostatin, glucagon or calcitonin. Surg Gynecol Obstet 163:428–432, 1986.

115. Ertan A, Brooks FP, Ostrow JD, et al: Effect of jejunal amino acid perfusion and exogenous cholecystokinin on the exocrine pancreatic and biliary secretions in man. Gastroenterology 61:686–692, 1971.

116. Bivins BA, Bell RM, Rapp RP, Toedebusch WH: Pancreatic exocrine response to parenteral nutrition. JPEN J Parenter Enteral Nutr 8:34–36, 1984.

117. Prinz RA, Picleman J, Hoffman JP: Treatment of pancreatic cutaneous fistulas with a somatostatin analog. Am J Surg 155:36–42, 1988.

118. Variyam EP: Central vein hyperalimentation in pancreatic ascites. Am J Gastroenterol 78:178–181, 1983.

119. Barkin JS: Ascites as a complication of chronic pancreatic disease. Postgrad Med 64:195–200, 1978.

120. Sanfey H, Cameron JL: The management of internal pancreatic fistulas. Surg Rounds 7:26–37, 1984.

121. Gislason H, Gronbech JE, Soreide O: Pancreatic ascites: Treatment by continuous somatostatin infusion. Am J Gastroenterol 86:519–521, 1991.

122. Joehl RJ, Nahrwold DL: Inhibition of human pancreatic secretion by terbutaline as a potential agent for treating patients with pancreatic fistula. Surg Gynecol Obstet 160:109–114, 1985.

123. Jackson MW, Schuman BM, Bowden TA, et al: The limited role of total parenteral nutrition in the management of pancreatic pseudocyst. Am Surg 59: 736–739, 1993.

124. Morali GA, Braverman DZ, Shemesh D, et al: Successful treatment of pancreatic pseudocyst with a somatostatin analogue and catheter drainage. Am J Gastroenterol 86:515–518, 1991.

125. Knaus WA, Draper EA, Wagner DP, Zimmerman JE: APACHE II: A severity of disease classification system. Crit Care Med 13:818–829, 1985.

126. Kivisaari L, Somer K, Standertskjold-Nordenstam CG, et al: Early detection of acute fulminant pancreatitis by contrast-enhanced computed tomography. Scand J Gastroenterol 18:39–41, 1983.

127. Ranson JHC, Balthazar E, Caccavale R, Cooper M: Computed tomography and the prediction of pancreatic abscess in acute pancreatitis. Ann Surg 201:656–663, 1985.

128. Rotman N, Bonnet F, Larde D, Fagniez PL: Computerized tomography in the evaluation of the late complications of acute pancreatitis. Am J Surg 152:286, 1986.

129. Clavien PA, Hauser H, Meyer P, Rohner H: Value of contrast-enhanced computerized tomography in the early diagnosis and prognosis of acute pancreatitis: A prospective study of 202 patients. Am J Surg 155:457–466, 1988.

130. Wilmore DW, Smith RJ, O'Dwyer ST, et al: The gut: A central organ after surgical stress. Surgery 104:917–923, 1988.

131. Alexander JW, Peck MD: Future prospects for adjunctive therapy: Pharmacologic and nutritional approaches to immune system modulation. Crit Care Med 18:S159–S164, 1990.

132. Trocki O, Heyd TJ, Waymack JP, Alexander JW: Effects of fish oil on postburn metabolism and immunity. JPEN J Parenter Enteral Nutr 11:521–528, 1987.

133. Lowry SF: The route of feeding influences injury responses. J Trauma 30:S10–S15, 1990.

134. Wang X, Andersson R, Soltesz V, et al: But origin sepsis, macrophage function, and oxygen extraction associated with acute pancreatitis in the rat. World J Surg 20:299–308, 1996.

135. De Beaux AC, Ross JA, Maingay JP, et al: Proinflammatory cytokine release by peripheral blood mononuclear cells from patients with acute pancreatitis. B J Surg 83:1071–1075, 1996.

136. McKay C, Imrie CW, Baxter JN: Mononuclear phagocyte activation and acute pancreatitis. Scand J Gastroenterol 31(Suppl 2) 19:32–36, 1996.

137. Browder IW, Sherwood E, Williams D, et al: Protective effect of glucan-enhanced macrophage function in experimental pancreatitis. Am J Surg 153:25–33, 1987.

138. Daly JM, Reynolds J, Thom A, et al: Immune and metabolic effects of arginine in the surgical patient. Ann Surg 208:512–523, 1988.

139. Saito H, Trocki O, Wang SL, et al: Metabolic and immune effects of dietary arginine supplementation after burn. Arch Surg 122:784–789, 1987.

140. Ogle CK, Simon J, Ogle JD, Alexander JW: Enhancement of neutrophil function by glutamine. Paper presented at the 27th Annual Meeting of the Society for Leukocyte Biology, Heraklion, Greece, 1990.

141. Billiar TR, Bankey PE, Svingen BA, et al: Fatty acid intake and Kupffer cell function: Fish oil alters eicosanoid and monokine production to endotoxin stimulation. Surgery 104:343–349, 1988.

142. Mascioli EA, Leader L, Flores E, et al: Enhanced survival to endotoxin in guinea pigs fed IV fish oil emulsion. Lipids 23:623–625, 1988.

143. Wan JMF, Teo TT, Babayan VK, Blackburn GL: Invited comment: Lipids and the development of immune dysfunction and infection. JPEN J Parenter Enteral Nutr 12:43s, 1988.

144. Alexander JW, Saito H, Trocki O, Ogle CK: The importance of lipid type in the diet after burn injury. Ann Surg 204:1–8, 1986.

145. Myer J, Yurt RW, Duhaney R, et al: Differential neutrophil activation before and after endotoxin infusion in enterally versus parenterally fed volunteers. Surg Gynecol Obstet 167:501–509, 1988.

146. Saito H, Trocki O, Alexander JW, et al: The effect of route of nutrient administration on the nutritional state, catabolic hormone secretion and gut mucosal integrity after burn injury. JPEN J Parenter Enteral Nutr 11:1–7, 1987.

147. Denham W, Yang J, Norman J: Evidence for an unknown component of pancreatic ascites that induces adult respiratory distress syndrome through an interleukin-1 and tumor necrosis factor–dependent mechanism. Surgery 122:295–302, 1997.

148. Kinsella JE: Lipids, membrane receptors, and enzymes: Effects of dietary fatty acids. JPEN J Parenter Enteral Nutr 14:200s–217s, 1990.

148a. Bulger EM, Helton WS, Clinton CM, et al: Enteral vitamin E supplementation inhibits the cytokine response to endotoxin. Arch Surg 132:1337–1341, 1997.

149. Wilson C, Maharaj D, McCall F, et al: Can fibronectin predict outcome of acute pancreatitis? Br J Surg 75:607, 1988.

150. Hong RW, Robinson MK, Rounds JD, et al: Glutamine protects the liver following *C. parvum*/endotoxin induced hepatic necrosis. Surg Forum 42:1–3, 1991.

151. Spolarics Z, Lang CH, Bagby GJ, Spitzer JJ: Glutamine and fatty acid oxidation are the main sources of energy for Kupffer and endothelial cells. Am J Physiol 261:G185–G190, 1991.

152. Tani S, Tioh H, Okabayashi Y, et al: New model of acute necrotizing pancreatitis induced by excessive doses of arginine in rats. Dig Dis Sci 35:367–374, 1990.

153. Beger HG, Bittner R, Block S, Buchler M: Bacterial contamination of pancreatic necrosis: A prospective clinical study. Gastroenterology 91:433–438, 1986.

154. Gerzof SG, Banks PA, Robbins AH, et al: Early diagnosis of pancreatic infection by computed tomography–guided aspiration. Gastroenterology 93:1315–1320, 1987.

155. Hancke E, Marlein G: Bacterial contamination of the pancreas with intestinal germs: A cause of acute suppurative pancreatitis. *In* Beger HG (ed): Acute Pancreatitis. Berlin, Springer-Verlag, 1987, pp 87–89.

156. McClelland P, Murray A, Yaqoob M, et al: Prevention of bacterial infection and sepsis in acute severe pancreatitis. Ann R Coll Surg Eng 74:329–334, 1992.

157. Russel JC, Welch JP, Clark DG: Colonic complications of acute pancreatitis and pancreatic abscess. Am J Surg 146:558–564, 1983.

158. Lange JF, van Gool J, Tytgat GNJ: The protective effect of a reduction in intestinal flora on mortality of acute haemorrhagic pancreatitis in the rat. Hepatogastroenterology 34:28–30, 1987.

159. Gianotti L, Munda R, Alexander JW, et al: Bacterial translocation: A potential source for infection in acute pancreatitis. Pancreas 8: 551–558, 1993.

160. Windmeuller HG, Spaeth AE: Identification of ketone bodies and glutamine as the major respiratory fuels in vivo for postoperative rat small intestine. J Biol Chem 10:69–76, 1978.

161. O'Dwyer ST, Smith RJ, Hwang TL, Wilmore DW: Maintenance of small bowel mucosa with glutamine-enriched parenteral nutrition. JPEN J Parenter Enteral Nutr 13:579–585, 1989.

162. Koruda MJ, Rolandelli RH, Bliss DZ, et al: Parenteral nutrition supplemented with short-chain fatty acids: Effect on the small-bowel mucosa in normal rats. Am J Clin Nutr 51:685–689, 1990.

163. Kripke SA, Fox AD, Berman JM, et al: Inhibition of TPN-associated intestinal mucosal atrophy with monoacetoacetin. J Surg Res 44:436–444, 1988.

164. Weser E, Bell D, Tawil T: Effects of octapeptide-cholecystokinin, secretin, and glucagon on intestinal mucosal growth in parenterally nourished rats. Dig Dis Sci 26:409–416, 1981.

165. Coffey JA, Milhoan RA, Abdullah A, et al: Bombesin inhibits bacterial translocation from the gut in burned rats. Surg Forum 39:109–110, 1988.

166. Wood J, Hoang HD, Bussjaeger J, Solomon TE: Neurotensin stimulates growth of small intestine in rats. Am J Physiol 18:G813–G817, 1988.

167. Helton WS, Scheltinga M, Rounds J, et al: Exogenous neurotensin stimulates ileal but not jejunal mucosal growth during intravenous feeding in rats. JPEN J Parenter Enteral Nutr 14:9S, 1990.

168. Helton WS, Scheltinga M, Hong RW, et al: Neurotensin attenuates increased intestinal permeability during intravenous feeding in rats. Gastroenterology 100:A525, 1991.

169. Alverdy J, Chi HS, Sheldon GS: The effect of parenteral nutrition on gastrointestinal immunity: The importance of enteral stimulation. Ann Surg 202:681–685, 1985.

170. Grey VL, Garofalo C, Greenberg GR, Morein CL: The adaptation of the small intestine after resection in response to free fatty acids. Am J Clin Nutr 40:1235–1242, 1984.

171. Mochizuki H, Trocki O, Dominioni L, et al: Optimal lipid content for enteral diets following thermal injury. JPEN J Parenter Enteral Nutr 8:638–646, 1984.

172. Fong Y, Maran MA, Barber A, et al: Total parenteral nutrition and bowel rest modify the metabolic response to endotoxin in man. Ann Surg 210:449–457, 1989.

173. DeWaele B, Vierendeels T, Willems G: Vitamin status in patients with acute pancreatitis. Clin Nutr 11:83–86, 1992.

174. Braganza JM, Scott P, Bilton D, et al: Evidence for early oxidative stress in acute pancreatitis. Int J Pancreatol 17:69–81, 1995.

175. Van Gossum A, Closset P, Noel E, et al: Deficiency in antioxidant factors in patients with alcohol-related chronic pancreatitis. Dig Dis Sci 41:1225–1231, 1996.

176. Hyde D, Floch MG: The effect of peripheral nutritional support and nitrogen balance in acute pancreatitis. Gastroenterology 86:1119, 1984.

13

◆ Gastrointestinal Fistulas: Clinical and Nutritional Management

Humberto Arenas-Marquez, M.D.

Roberto Anaya-Prado, M.D.

Alejandro Gonzalez-Ojeda, M.D.

Jose L. Gutierrez de la Rosa, M.D.

Juan M. Palma-Vargas, M.D.

Luis M. Barrera-Zepeda, M.D.

Enrique Sánchez-Perez Verdia, M.D.

Fistula has been defined as an anomalous communication between two epithelial- or endothelial-lined surfaces. Fistulas may be internal or external. Internal fistulas are communications between one part of the gastrointestinal (GI) tract and either another part of the GI tract or an adjacent organ. External fistulas result in drainage of enteric contents onto the skin (gastrointestinal cutaneous fistula) or from the vagina.[1, 2] Most external fistulas arising from the GI tract occur as complications of surgical procedures, leading to increased costs and high morbidity and mortality rates, the latter ranging from 20 to 30%.[1] Because many surgeons lack sufficient experience in the management of fistulas, almost 20,000 patients per year with GI fistulas are referred to specialized centers for treatment.[3] University hospitals in Mexico to which patients are referred for specialized care receive an average of 70 patients per year with GI fistulas,[1] and their estimated frequency for all surgical interventions performed on the digestive tract varies between 2 and 5%.

◆ ETIOLOGY

Most GI fistulas occur either after surgical procedures in the abdominal cavity or after penetrating abdominal trauma. These two circumstances represent approximately 80 to 90% of all cases.[4–6] Spontaneous fistulas are secondary to either extension of bowel disease to adjacent structures or complications of the underlying disease affecting the bowel, such as Crohn's disease, diverticuli-

tis, cancer, appendicitis, ischemic bowel disease, or peptic ulcer.[7, 8] Many external fistulas appearing after abdominal surgery occur either because of failure of the surgical procedure (e.g., anastomosis leakage) or because of poor surgical skills (e.g., excessive cautery burning of bowel wall, extensive stoma devascularization, fixation of the intestines while suturing the abdominal wall). Patients undergoing bowel resections for Crohn's disease may develop internal or external fistulas early in the postoperative period, even with appropriate surgical procedures. Finally, a patient who has had previous surgery (e.g., open liver biopsy) may develop a spontaneous fistula secondary to another intra-abdominal process (e.g., diverticulitis complicated with enterocutaneous fistula). These fistulas are considered postoperative, clearly with no relation to the previous surgery.[9]

GI fistulas usually result from complications of surgical procedures performed for trauma, intestinal obstruction, cancer, infected pancreas necrosis, inflammatory bowel disease, extensive adhesions, or abdominal wall hernia repair with prosthetic mesh placement, and from an open abdominal wound approach to the treatment of specific pathologic lesions. Risk factors for GI fistulas can be divided into three categories: (1) general factors, which are factors related to the host, especially malnutrition and hypotension with poor tissue perfusion; (2) local factors, which are factors related to intrinsic tissue characteristics, such as a local inflammatory process, the presence or absence of infection, the type of suture material used, and excessive manipulation; and (3) iatrogenic, which are factors related to inappropriate surgical indications or techniques.

◆ CLASSIFICATION

GI fistulas have been classified in different ways. These descriptive classifications are helpful both in predicting the likelihood of spontaneous closure and in designing an initial management plan.[8, 10]

Etiologic Classification. Etiologic classification includes (1) congenital fistulas, those related to embryologic malformations; and (2) acquired fistulas, both spontaneous and postoperative.

Anatomic Classification. Depending on the site of drainage, these can be (1) external, when a hollow viscus is connected to the skin; and (2) internal, when an abnormal communication has been established between the GI tract and either another part of the GI tract or an adjacent organ.

Organic Classification. This classification describes the organ where the fistula first originated; the fistula can be esophageal, gastric, duodenal, small bowel (jejunal, ileal), colonic, pancreatic, or biliary.

Physiologic Classification. This is based on daily output: (1) high-output, greater than 500 mL/24 h; (2) moderate-output, 200 to 500 mL/24 h; (3) low-output, less than 200 mL/24 h. High-output fistulas tend to arise from the small bowel, whereas low-output fistulas are generally those that involve the colon. Although the fistula output is not predictive of spontaneous closure, malnutrition and water and electrolyte imbalances observed in high-output fistulas will have a great impact on morbidity and mortality. Thus, characterization of the fistula output is helpful in both treating and preventing metabolic, nutritional, and fluid losses.[2]

Epidemiologic Classification. First described by Sitges-Serra and colleagues,[11, 12] this considers the morbidity and mortality of a GI fistula according to its anatomy and physiology. This classification is recommended for epidemiologic and research purposes only. Type 1 includes those arising from the stomach, duodenum, pancreas, and small bowel. These can be either type 1a (output <1000 mL/48 h) or type 1b (output >1000 mL/48 h). Type 2 is those fistulas originating from colonic lesions and/or anastomosis leakage.

Finally, we must stress those factors that both have a direct impact on fistula outcome and significantly reduce the likelihood of spontaneous closure: (1) total or partial intestinal obstruction; (2) proximal-end fistulas; (3) the persistence of peritoneal inflammatory processes near the fistula tract; (4) neoplasms; (5) radiation damage; (6) inflammatory bowel disease; (7) foreign materials; (8) a short fistula tract; (9) an extremely large viscus defect; (10) epithelialization of the fistula tract; (11) multiple fistulas with abdominal wall destruction; and (12) an established high-output fistula and no signs of imminent closure after 4 to 5 weeks of nutritional support, without sepsis.[11]

◆ PATHOLOGIC PHYSIOLOGY

There is a common issue affecting every fistula patient after acute abdominal inflammation, which can be severe: the fistula tract must heal the same way an open contaminated wound does; that is, by inflammation, fibrosis, and contraction. Nevertheless, a fistula tract arising from the GI tract is somehow different from that of an open wound. Granulation tissue in the fistula tract does not have an even surface as does an infected surgical incision; instead, it is a three-dimensional structure formed by an irregular tube of continuous inner wall. This tube cannot be inspected, mechanically débrided, or cleansed by dressing changes, and its epithelial lining is always covered with intestinal contents, usually rich in bacteria. Finally, since the fistula tract usually communicates with its source organ through what is functionally an intervening abscess cavity, the dynamics of natural healing in the tract as well as in the cavity itself may be out of phase because the cavity's inner diameter frequently exceeds that of the distal tract.[9] Fluid and electrolyte imbalances, malnutrition, and sepsis are factors most frequently associated with major morbidity and mortality. The surgeon must deal with these in order to avoid the natural downward course toward multiple organ system failure and death.

Fluid and Electrolyte Imbalances. Primarily associated with high-output fistulas in the proximity of the ligament of Treitz that may drain up to 4 L/day, 2 L originating from the stomach and saliva and 2 L from pancreatic and biliary secretions, these lost fluids are rich in proteins, electrolytes, and other components. A critical feature is that these fluids are hypertonic to plasma, particularly in regard to sodium (Na^+), bicarbonate (HCO_3^-), and potassium (K^+), and a significant amount of energy is wasted to maintain this concentration gradient.

Malnutrition. There are three factors contributing to malnutrition: (1) a lack of adequate food intake (2) sepsis and its associated hypercatabolism; and (3) the loss of protein-rich, energy-containing fluids from the fistula.

Sepsis. This is the most common cause of death in patients with GI fistula. Organisms frequently involved tend to be those from the bowel (e.g., coliforms, *Bacteroides*, and enterococci). Staphylococci also play a role in abscess formation.

◆ CLINICAL PRESENTATION

Postoperative external fistulas are sometimes diagnosed in the period of hospital confinement after surgery, but an important number are diagnosed after the patient has been discharged. A common story is that of a patient not doing well and running a fever of 101 to 102° F (38.3 to 39.0° C). About the sixth postoperative day, purulent material is obtained through either an infected wound or a previously placed abdominal drainage tube, or through a drainage tract after drain removal. Twenty-four hours later, bowel contents drain in the form of feces or bile-tinged purulent material (Fig. 13–1). Signs and symptoms can be divided into (1) general, such as tachycardia; fever; abdominal pain and distention; abdominal tenderness; vomiting; and bowel obstruction; and (2) local, such as erythema and purulent or intestinal discharge through either the drainage site or the surgical wound, or both. Internal fistulas are commonly asymptomatic or produce minor recurrent infections if the bypassed segment is short and inflammation is not present. However, symptoms may appear if severe localized infection is present or long segments of bowel are bypassed. This leads to an intestinal short-circuit effect with malabsorption and fluid and electrolyte disturbances, which manifest as chronic diarrhea.

◆ ASSESSMENT AND INITIAL MANAGEMENT

The main goal in the management of patients with GI fistulas is to close the fistula

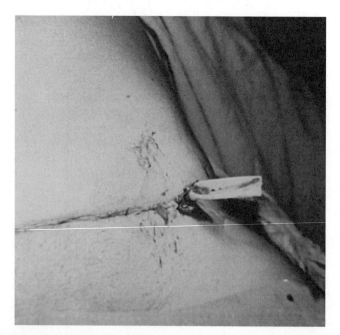

Figure 13–1. Fistulous drainage through site and an abdominal wound. An unrecognized lesion to the sigmoid colon during hysterectomy led to a colocutaneous fistula.

Table 13–1. Management of Fistulas

Stabilization
  Restore blood volume and begin correction of
    fluid and electrolyte imbalances
  Drain obvious abscesses surgically
  Control fistula and measure losses
  Protect skin
  Administer broad-spectrum antibiotics
  Begin nutritional support
  Begin treatment with H_2 antagonists
Investigation
  Delineate anatomy of fistula by radiographic
    studies
  Perform gastrointestinal endoscopy
Definitive Therapy
  Operate if fistula fails to close

and re-establish intestinal continuity, while restoring and maintaining an optimal nutritional state. To accomplish this, a systematic approach that combines diagnostic, supportive, and surgical procedures is essential. The therapeutic goals, essential for a successful resolution of the fistula, have been divided into three phases of care: (1) stabilization, (2) investigation, and (3) definitive therapy (Table 13–1).[2]

Stabilization

The stabilization phase must be carried out within 24 to 48 hours of recognition of the fistula. General tasks during the stabilization phase of gastric and duodenal fistulas that are generally applicable to the management of all GI fistulas are as follows:[13]

1. Give nothing by mouth; provide total bowel rest.
2. Place a nasogastric tube.
3. Begin treatment with H_2 antagonists.
4. Administer broad-spectrum antibiotics.
5. Correct fluid, electrolyte, and nutritional imbalances.
6. Protect the skin.
7. If diffuse peritonitis or localized abscess exists, drain surgically.

Giving the patient nothing by mouth and placing a nasogastric tube may be particularly helpful in fistulas of the esophagus, stomach, and duodenum, since oral intake increases protein and electrolyte losses by the upper GI tract through the fistula; but little evidence suggests that this helps distal fistulas or low-output fistulas. Many fistula patients are profoundly depleted of intravascular and interstitial volume, and replacement with isotonic saline solution takes first priority. Frequent assessment of vital signs and accurate measurements of fluid intake and losses, daily weight, central venous pressure, urine output, and skin turgor are needed in order to determine the patient's overall fluid balance. Blood is sent to the laboratory for measurement of the serum electrolyte concentration, arterial blood gasses, blood urea nitrogen, glucose, liver function, amylase levels, and red blood cell count. The latter indicates the status of anemia and confirms the presence of sepsis, whereas the other blood work determines the degree of hydration, electrolyte imbalances, acid-base abnormalities, liver condition, and whether inflammation of the pancreas exists. A clean sample of the fistula output must be obtained; its composition indicates the likely intra-abdominal injury that led to the fistula formation. Fistula drainage fluid must be collected not only to measure volume losses, but also to avoid excoriation of the skin (Fig. 13–2). Control of fistula drainage can be achieved by sump suction of the continuous fistula effluent. Once a satisfactory tract has been established, the sump drain should be replaced by progressively smaller suction drainage tubes until a tube is no longer needed.

A number of measures, including karaya powder and stoma adhesives, may be useful to protect the skin. When the skin is dry and intact, a collection bag can be applied to the edges of the fistula to protect the skin. If necessary, the sump tubes can be placed through the bag. If the abdominal wall surface is irregular, it may be difficult to create a flat area for adherence of the appliance. Under these circumstances, great skill and ingenuity are needed by the stoma therapist to tailor protection of the tissue around the fistula while collecting the fistula effluent (Fig. 13–3). H_2 antagonists and $H^+,-K^+$-ATPase inhibitors decrease gastric secretion and thus may decrease the volume of pancreatic and duodenal secretions, but, more importantly, they decrease the incidence of peptic ulcerations, which can occur in stressed patients taking nothing by mouth for extended periods of time. Sepsis has been found to be a major source of mortality and is associated with a decreased rate of healing of GI fistulas.[5] Thus, the recognition

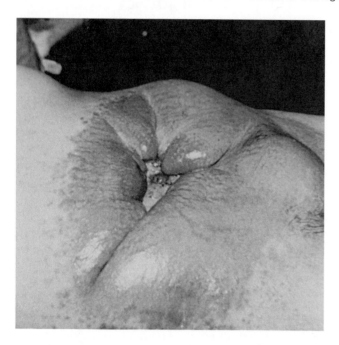

Figure 13–2. Epithelialized central fistula. The lack of appropriate skin protection produced skin excoriation and pain.

and control of sepsis are very important in fistula management. Abscesses should be drained as soon as they are diagnosed. Unfortunately, the source of sepsis is often obscure, and a continual diligent search for abscesses must be made by repeated physical examinations and radiologic studies until the infection is located and treated. Broad-spectrum antibiotics should be used when the fistula first appears and continued until the fistula is controlled and the patient's condition has stabilized. If an abscess is present, short courses of antibiotics should be used in conjunction with surgical drainage. However, blind therapy with broad-spectrum antibiotics is not a substitute for the drainage of abscesses. The appropriate use of antibiotics is also indicated in systemic sepsis, in cholangitis, and in preparation for operation.[14] If signs of ab-

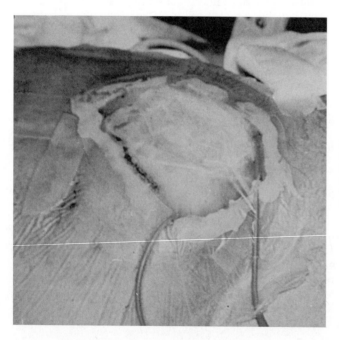

Figure 13–3. Skin protection and local control of fistula drainage. A cellulose plaque, stoma adhesives, sump suction of the continuous fistula effluent, and transparent dressing were used to achieve control of fistula drainage while protecting the skin.

dominal sepsis recur, intra-abdominal collections should be surgically drained. Nutritional support is a key element in the care of these patients; although total parenteral nutrition may be indicated, some have advocated the use of enteral feedings to preserve the gut mucosal barrier, which may prevent bacterial translocation.[15]

Investigation

Seven to 10 days after the patient's condition has stabilized, appropriate contrast studies may be undertaken to delineate the anatomy of the fistula, and gastroscopy may be useful in demonstrating gastrocolic or duodenocolic fistula. The purposes of these studies are to (1) identify the fistula site, (2) determine whether the bowel is in continuity with a lateral fistula or whether there is an end fistula with complete disruption, (3) determine whether any distal obstruction is present, (4) establish the condition of the bowel immediately adjacent to the fistula, and (5) determine the presence or absence of an intra-abdominal abscess either in conjunction with, immediately adjacent to, or remote from the site of the GI fistula.

Upright and supine plain radiographic views may demonstrate the presence of air or fluid levels below the diaphragm that are indicative of subphrenic abscess. The presence of gas within the biliary tree is a clear indication of an enterobiliary fistula. A fistulogram with contrast material (Hypaque) may outline the fistula tract and any associated cavities (Fig. 13–4). Computed tomography and ultrasonography are highly effective tools in diagnosing intra-abdominal abscesses. Gastroscopy may be useful in demonstrating gastrocolic or duodenocolic fistula. Endoscopic retrograde cholangiopancreatography is of prime value in demonstrating pancreatic and biliary fistulas. Both upper endoscopy and colonoscopy are helpful in detecting areas of abnormal mucosa in patients with Crohn's disease and in excluding cancer. These studies allow biopsy of mucosal lesions that can provide important histologic data. Colonoscopy is useful in determining the fistula opening in patients with colovaginal fistulas. The gathering and collection of all these data, integrated with the overall clinical picture, provide the basis for a clinical judgment of whether the fistula is likely to close spontaneously.

Definitive Therapy

The restoration of intestinal continuity is generally achieved most favorably by spontaneous closure. However, spontaneous closure in complicated fistulas occurs in only one third of patients. If they are going to heal spontaneously, fistulas usually close within a month after infection has been eradicated and nutritional support has been

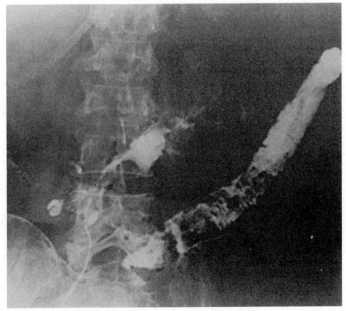

Figure 13–4. Fistulogram delineating the anatomy of a fistula tract to the transverse colon and an associated cavity.

instituted. Persistence of a fistula beyond a month indicates the need for surgical closure in most cases. The basic principles of thorough patient preparation, meticulous attention to operative detail, and supportive postoperative care are essential for successful surgical management. During surgery, the bowel should be freed from the ligament of Treitz to the rectum, because the presence of an occult abscess or distal obstruction will undo any attempts at successful surgical closure. The timing of the operation and the various surgical procedures are discussed elsewhere in this chapter.

◆ NUTRITIONAL ASSESSMENT

Evaluating nutritional status refers to identifying patients at increased risk for malnutrition. Patients with stress or hypermetabolism indicated by the fistula or surgical procedure may develop short-term malnutrition without adequate nutrient intake.[16] Alteration in nutritional status may occur because of inadequate intake (e.g., starvation) or because of alterations in the metabolism of substrates (e.g., sepsis). The aim of nutritional assessment and support is to prevent malnutrition from becoming a major cofactor in organ dysfunction and in morbidity and mortality. Historically, a complete nutritional assessment has consisted of a combination of subjective and objective parameters; however, no single parameter has been shown to be useful for all patients. Ideally, a nutritional assessment parameter should be highly sensitive and specific, be unaffected by cofactors unrelated to nutrition, and correlate with the response to nutritional therapy. Unfortunately, most nutritional parameters lack sensitivity and specificity; therefore, methods of identifying malnourished patients are not entirely satisfactory. Until improved methods for identifying malnutrition are developed, carefully selected objective parameters in combination with a thorough, nutritionally focused physical examination and other objective parameters are most reliable for identifying patients who are at most risk.

History and Physical Examination

The history and physical examination are the cornerstone of nutritional assessment. In most cases, the possibility of malnutrition is suggested by the underlying GI (fistula) disease affecting either oral intake, or absorption, or by a history of recent weight loss. The dietary history can give a good estimate of the patient's intake of proteins and calories. The extent of malnutrition can also be estimated from the physical findings. The amount of subcutaneous tissue on the extremities and buttocks and in the buccal fat pads reflects the status of caloric intake. Protein nutrition is evaluated from the bulk and strength of extremity muscles, visible evidence of temporal muscle wasting, and edema on the lower extremities. Vitamin malnutrition may be manifested by changes in the texture of the skin; the presence of follicular plugging or a skin rash; corneal vascularization; cracks at the corners of the mouth (cheilosis); hyperemia of the oral mucosa (glossitis); cardiac enlargement and murmurs; altered sensation in the hands and feet; the absence of vibration and position sense; and abnormal quality and texture of the hair. Trace metal deficiency produce abnormalities associated with those of vitamin deficiency (Fig. 13–5) plus changes in mental status. The presence of an enlarged or shrunken liver, skin telangiectasias, and perianal disease should also arouse suspicion of nutritional deficiency. With all these, weight loss is the main clinical sign of malnutrition. This is calculated in relation to the patient's usual body weight (Table 13–2). The greater the body weight loss, the greater the consequences for morbidity.[17] Ever since 1936, when Dr. Hiram Studley showed that a preoperative weight loss greater than 20% of total body weight was associated with a 33.3% mortality and that a body weight loss of less than 20% was associated with a 4% mortality, the estimation of weight loss has played a key role in the nutritional assessment of the surgical patient. A weight loss greater than 4.5 kg was reported by Seltzer and colleagues[14] and numerous other investigators, including Mughal and Meguid,[19] to be highly predictive.

Laboratory Measurements

Laboratory tests of value in detecting nutritional abnormalities are listed in Table 13–2. The complete blood cell count is affected by abnormal vitamin and trace element nutrition (e.g., microcytosis; iron deficiency, macrocytosis; folate and vitamin B_{12} deficiency, pancytopenia; copper deficiency). Abnor-

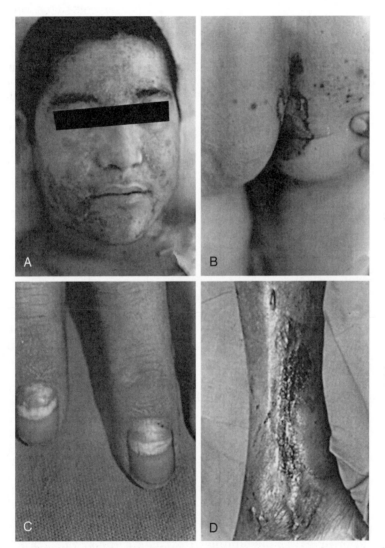

Figure 13–5. Trace metal deficiencies in severe cases of malnutrition and/or inadequate supply. *A*, Exfolitative dermatitis and loss of hair. *B*, Perianal dermatitis. *C*, Beau's lines. *D*, Skin ulcerations on the distal parts of the extremities.

Table 13–2. Basic Parameters for Nutritional Assessment

History
  Present illness

  $$\text{Absolute Weight Deficit} = \frac{\text{Actual Body Weight (100)}}{\text{Ideal Body Weight}}$$

  $$\text{Percentage Usual Body Weight} = \frac{\text{Actual Body Weight (100)}}{\text{Usual Body Weight}}$$

  Past illness predisposing to malnutrition

Physical examination
  Skin: quality, texture, rash, follicles, hyperkeratosis, nail deformities
  Eyes: keratoconjunctivitis, night blindness
  Mouth: cheilosis, glossitis, mucosal atrophy, dentition
  Hair: quality, texture, recent loss
  Heart: chamber enlargement, murmurs
  Abdomen: hepatomegaly, abdominal mass, ostomy, fistula
  Rectum: stool color, perineal fistula
  Neurologic: psychiatric, peripheral neuropathy, dorsolateral column deficit
  Extremities: muscle size and strength, pedal edema

Routine laboratory tests
  CBC: hemoglobin, hematocrit, red blood cell indices, white blood cell count, total lymphocyte count,* thrombocytopenia
  Electrolytes: sodium, potassium, chloride, calcium, phosphate, magnesium
  Liver function tests: AST, ALT, alkaline phosphatase, bilirubin, albumin,† prothrombin time
  Other tests: BUN, creatinine, triglycerides, cholesterol, free fatty acids, ketones, uric acid

---

*Normal = 2000–1500/μL; moderate malnutrition = 1500–1000/μL; severe malnutrition = <1000/μL.
†Normal = 4.5–3.5 g/dL; moderate malnutrition = 3.5–2.5 g/dL; severe malnutrition = <2.5 g/dL.
ALT, alanine aminotransferase; AST, aspastate aminotransferase; BUN, blood usea nitrogen; CBC, complete blood cell count.

---

malities in serum electrolyte concentrations may result from external losses (e.g., fistulas), decreased excretion (e.g., renal dysfunction), or overzealous treatment (e.g., cirrhosis). Liver function tests may be abnormal because of the primary disease, the administration of too many calories during total parenteral nutrition, or deficiencies of choline, carnitine, or essential fatty acids. The initial serum albumin level provides a general estimate of protein nutrition or liver function, but because the half-life of albumin is so long (18 days), other serum proteins such as transferrin, thyroxine-binding prealbumin, retinol-binding protein, and ceruloplasmin, which have half-lives of a few hours, may respond more quickly to changes in nutritional status. Unfortunately, the serum levels of these proteins are also influenced by changes in intravascular volume, and most are acute-phase reactants that rise nonspecifically during acute illness.

Special Measurements

Anthropometrics can be used to estimate the stores of body fat and protein (Table 13–3).

Body fat is approximated by the thickness of the triceps skin fold as measured with calipers. Protein, most of which resides in skeletal muscle, is estimated by correcting the midarm circumference to account for subcutaneous tissue, which gives the midarm muscle circumference. These data are compared with normal values for the patient's age and sex to determine the extent of depletion. However, a knowledge of energy requirements is often the first step in the process of nutritional assessment. These energy requirements are determined using the Harris-Benedict equation, nomograms, or indirect calorimetry.[20] With the Harris-Benedict equation, energy expenditure can be estimated as a function of height and weight, age, and sex. Nomograms relate basal metabolic requirements to age, sex, height, and weight. The Ireton-Jones equation was developed specifically for hospitalized patients and takes into account mechanical ventilation and measures energy expenditure by indirect calorimetry; the O_2 (V_{O_2}) and CO_2 (V_{CO_2}) production rates are calculated from the timed volumetric collection of expired O_2, CO_2, and urinary nitrogen (see Table 13–3).

Indirect calorimetry is based on the premise that all energy is produced as a result of fat, carbohydrate, and protein oxidation, and that the amount of consumed oxygen and produced carbon dioxide are constant and characteristic for every energy source. When indirect calorimetry is used, energy expenditure (heat production) is determined by the amount of consumed oxygen and the production of carbon dioxide during gas respiratory exchange. These two measurements provide the necessary information for energy expenditure estimates. The volume of both consumed oxygen and produced carbon dioxide are multiplied by a constant and then extrapolated for the 24-hour energy expenditure. The nonprotein respiratory quotation (RQ) indicates the percentage of carbohydrate and fat used for energy production. When the RQ is 1, pure carbohydrate is being oxidized, and when the RQ is 0.7, only fat is being oxidized. The nonprotein RQ is used to gauge the patient's metabolic response to nutritional therapy.

The synthesis and breakdown of protein can be determined by measuring the nitrogen balance (the difference between nitrogen intake and nitrogen excretion). The total nitrogen intake is the sum of nitrogen delivered from oral, intravenous, and tube feed-

Table 13–3. Special Measurements for Nutritional Assessment

Anthropometrics
  Triceps skin fold (TSF)
  Midarm circumference (MAC)

$$\text{Arm Muscle Circumference} = \frac{\text{MAC} - (\pi)\,(\text{TSF})}{10}$$

$$\text{Creatinine-Height Index} = \frac{\text{24-Hour Urine Creatinine Excretion}}{\text{Ideal Creatinine Excretion for Height}}$$

Energy
  Harris-Benedict equation

  Man = 66.5 + 13.8 (weight) + 5 (height) − 6.8 (age)
  Woman = 655.1 + 9.6 (weight) + 1.8 (height) − 4.7 (age)
  Ireton-Jones

  EEE(v) = 1784 − 11(A) + 5(W) + 244(S) + 239(T) + 804(B)
  EEE(s) = 629 − 11(A) + 25(W) − 609(O)
  where v is ventilator; s is spontaneous breath; A is age (yr); W is weight (kg); S is sex
  (male = 1, female = 0); T is trauma (present = 1, absent = 0); B is burns
  (present = 1, absent = 0); O is obesity (present = 1, absent = 0)

  Weir formula:

  (REE) (kcal/min) = 3.9 (V_{O_2}) + 1.1 (V_{CO_2}) − 2.2 (Urinary Nitrogen)*

$$\text{Nonprotein RQ} = \frac{V_{CO_2} - 4.8\,(\text{Urine N})}{V_{O_2} - 5.9\,(\text{Urine N})}$$

Protein

  Nitrogen Balance = Nitrogen Intake − Nitrogen Output
  Nitrogen Output = Urine Nitrogen + 4 g/day
  Urine Nitrogen = (Urinary Urea) (0.85)

  3-Methylhistidine urinary excretion
  Isotopic determination of protein turnover ([^{15}N]glycine, [^{15}N]lysine, [^{14}C] leucine infusion)
Body composition
  Total body water (TBW): [^{3}H] or [^{2}H]H_2O isotope dilution
  Extracellular water: ^{22}Na-isotope dilution
  Lean body mass TBW/0.73
  Body cell mass: (K_e)(0.083) or (TBN)(6.25)(4)
  Total body potassium: ^{42}K-isotope dilution, ^{40}K whole-body counting; K_e (exchangeable potassium)
  Total body nitrogen (TBN): Neutron activation
Immunologic testing
  Skin tests, lymphocyte blastogenesis, mixed lymphocyte response, immunoglobulin levels, complement
    levels, lymphokine production
Other important laboratory tests
  Transferrin; thyroxine-binding prealbumin; Retinol-binding protein

*V_{O_2} and V_{CO_2} are O_2 consumption and CO_2 production in milliliters per minute; urine nitrogen is grams per minute.
EEE, estimated energy expenditure; REE, resting energy expenditure; RQ, repirators quotient.

ings. The total nitrogen output is the sum of the nitrogen content of urine, fistulous output, diarrhea, and so forth. In most patients, only urea output needs to be measured directly. The urea or total nitrogen content is measured from a timed volumetric collection of urine, and a correction factor is added to account for nitrogen losses in stools and from skin exfoliation. The resulting value for nitrogen balance is not highly precise, however, because it represents a small difference between two large numbers. When large losses of nitrogen oc-

cur (e.g., GI fistulas), measurements of nitrogen balance are inaccurate because of the difficulties in collecting all the secretions. Nevertheless, nitrogen balance is easy to measure and should be a routine part of the process of assessing and monitoring of all candidates for nutritional therapy.

◆ NUTRITIONAL SUPPORT

Risk factors for morbidity and mortality in patients with GI fistulas are malnutrition, fluid and electrolyte imbalances, and sepsis. Malnutrition, defined as a loss of 10% or greater of usual body weight and hypoproteinemia, is present in most patients with GI fistulas and occurs because of decreased food intake, excessive losses of GI secretions, increased energy expenditure, and muscle proteolysis generated by sepsis.[21] Malnutrition has been shown to have an adverse effect on the morbidity and mortality of patients with GI fistulas. A review of 157 patients with GI fistulas demonstrated that malnutrition was responsible for the death of 61% of the patients.[19] In another series of 119 patients, Soeters and colleagues showed that 68 patients had moderate malnutrition and 36 were severely malnourished, whereas 86% had some degree of malnutrition that affected the final outcome.[5] Parenteral nutrition increases the spontaneous closure rate of GI fistula although both the underlying disease that led to fistula formation and the fistula output are also important in this regard. Improvement in mortality rates after the introduction of parenteral nutrition is multifactorial: the development of broad-spectrum antibiotics; advances in the management of fluids and electrolytes and in acid-base balance alterations; cardiopulmonary supportive care; and the surgical treatment of sepsis have all played a key role. Parenteral nutrition has been an important factor contributing to the decrease in mortality rates, although not necessarily the most important. In selected patients with good tolerance to enteral feedings, the mortality and spontaneous closure of fistulas are similar to those of patients with parenteral nutrition.[22, 23]

Parenteral Versus Enteral Nutrition

Nutritional support should be administered by the enteral route whenever possible. A length of at least 4 ft of functional bowel, both distal and proximal to the fistula, is needed for the delivery of enteral nutrition.[2] Nutritional requirements of patients with GI fistulas can be met with enteral feedings when tolerance is adequate.[24] When tolerance is partial, a combination of both parenteral and enteral nutrition must be used for a complete and adequate nutritional supply. Whenever enteral nutrition is not feasible, parenteral nutrition must be instituted immediately; even under these circumstances, low-dose (10–20 mL/h) enteral feedings must be pursued for bowel stimuli. Whether the nutritional support should be instituted by the enteral or the parenteral routes depends on the origin of the fistula, length of available functional bowel, fistula output, and tolerance to enteral feedings.

Parenteral Nutrition

Parenteral nutrition is indicated for patients with intolerance to enteral feedings; high-output small bowel fistulas; and esophageal, gastric, and duodenal fistulas.[22] Patients with GI fistulas often suffer from complex medical problems that mandate emergency surgical operations, either for drainage of abscesses or intestinal diversion. It is highly advisable that hemodynamic instability, fluid and electrolyte imbalances, and acid-base and metabolic alterations be corrected before intravenous nutrition is started. The central route facilitates the adaptation of formulas to the changing clinical conditions frequently encountered in these patients. Regular insulin must be added to the formula in those patients with glucose intolerance to maintain blood glucose levels below 200 mg/dL. Thus, all patients must be monitored with fingerstick blood sugar measurements, with sliding-scale insulin injected subcutaneously as needed, and two thirds of the insulin requirements of the previous day must be added to the parenteral nutrition admixture for the next 24-h delivery. This scheme must be continued until blood glucose levels are below 200 mg/dL. If necessary, the glucose supply is increased to meet the patient's energy requirements. For those patients with mechanical ventilation, a total calorie and glucose excess must be avoided in order not to increase CO_2 production, which prevents short-term weaning from mechanical ventilation. Fluid and protein restrictions in patients with renal failure depend on whether the patient is on hemodialysis. The use of special solutions containing high concentrations of branched-chain amino acids in patients with liver failure and encephalopathy is recommended if there is an initial good response to solutions containing standard amino acids.

The first step to begin adequate nutritional support is to determine the patient's energy requirements. These can be calculated using the Harris-Benedict equation and multiplying the result by a stress factor that defines the needs for the next 24 hours (see Table 13–3). A stress factor of 1.3 to 1.5 is recommended for most of the patients with GI fistulas, because of both the hypercatabolic state and the associated losses with the intestinal discharge. For patients without sepsis and with no excessive losses, a stress factor of 1.2 or less is appropriate.[2] Patients confined to the intensive care unit may develop fluid overload, overnutrition, hyperglycemia, an increase in energy expenditure, liver failure, azotemia, and respiratory distress with the use of Harris-Benedict equation corrected with a stress factor. In these types of patients, we recommend using the Harris-Benedict equation without a stress factor, or 22 kcal/kg of body weight at the beginning of nutritional support.[25] Attempts to acutely correct nutritional deficits must be avoided, since the excessive administration of nutrients produces an equally excessive production and retention of CO_2, liver steatosis, hyperglycemia, immunosuppression, and an increase in energy expenditure. Thus, weight gain must not be a priority in severely ill patients. Delivery systems must provide only the energy necessary to maintain body weight throughout a complicated clinical course. Once the acute process has been resolved, the hormonal environment is altered to favor anabolism. Furthermore, an increase in spontaneous activity and planned exercises stimulate lean body mass buildup.

Protein requirements have been estimated from the amount of protein and energy necessary to achieve a positive nitrogen balance. It must be emphasized that protein and energy intake are dominant factors, but this balance is achieved only with an adequate trace element supply. Protein needs are greater in patients with GI fistulas than in healthy individuals because of external losses and metabolic stress. Thus, we recommend a protein supply of 1.5 to 2.5 g/kg/ day. The calorie-to-nitrogen ratio is 100– 150:1 kcal/g of nitrogen. The protein supply can easily be assessed from the nitrogen intake and nitrogen excretion, which define what we usually know as nitrogen balance.

Fluid requirements can be estimated either from body weight (30 mL/kg) or by the square meter of body surface (1500 mL/m²). The resulting amount is either added to the formula in order to recover losses from the fistula or adjusted in patients with poor tolerance to large volume loads.[2] The baseline formula for parenteral nutrition has to be estimated on a daily basis: the calorie requirements can be met by glucose or fat. In most cases, 50 to 70% of calories are delivered as glucose, and 30 to 50% as lipids. The protein supply is given as 10% amino acid solution. The recommended electrolyte and trace metal contents are as follows: sodium, 60 to 100 mEq; potassium, 60 to 80 mEq; calcium, 10 to 15 mEq; magnesium, 8 to 20 mEq; phosphorus, 20 to 30 mmol; zinc, 5 mg; selenium, 100 μg; chromium, 20 μg; copper, 1 mg; manganese, 0.5 mg; multivitamins, 5 to 10 mL standard solution; heparin, 1 IU/mL. Fistula losses ought to be added to the recommended electrolyte and trace metal requirements. Patients with fistulas of the small bowel lose up to 12 mg of zinc and 10 mEq of magnesium for each liter of discharge. The vitamin C supply is 5 to 10 times that of the recommended daily allowance, water-soluble vitamins are two times the recommended daily allowance, and vitamin K is 10 mg intramuscularly once a week. The patient's daily progress dictates modifications to the formula. The parenteral nutrition admixture is prepared in a specialized center under the supervision of a pharmacist. In practice, these solutions combine 50 to 70% dextrose, 8.5 to 10% amino acids, and 10 to 20% lipid emulsion. Electrolytes, vitamins, and trace metals are added to the admixture. The composition is modified as fluid intolerance, nitrogen metabolism alterations, fluid and electrolyte imbalances, and excessive CO_2 production are demonstrated. The admixture is delivered in a 24-hour period. The central route through a central venous catheter inserted in the subclavian vein is preferred, with the tip of the catheter placed in the superior vena cava. This facilitates the care of the insertion site by specialized personnel, decreasing the risk of catheter sepsis. Catheter placement must always be verified with radiography before infusion is begun.

The administration of parenteral nutrition can produce serious life-threatening mechanical, septic, and metabolic complications. Thus, we recommend (1) catheter placement by an experienced physician with strict adherence to aseptic techniques; (2) catheter care by experienced nurses; and (3) metabolic monitoring to both prevent and treat complications as they occur. When parenteral or enteral nutrition is first begun, baseline determinations of electrolytes, calcium, magnesium, phosphorus, glucose, urea, creatinine, total proteins, albumin, aminotransferases, alkaline phosphatase, cholesterol, triglycerides, prothrombin clotting time, red blood cell count, and urine constituents must be obtained (see Table 13–2). For the first week, daily determinations of magnesium, phosphorus, glucose, urea, and creatinine levels are needed. Once the patient has stabilized, these are determined twice a week. The rest of the tests are performed once a week. The nitrogen balance is estimated once a week. Daily monitoring of the patient includes vital signs four times a day, fluid intake and output once a day, fingerstick blood sugar with sliding-scale insulin four times a day, weight once a day.

Enteral Nutrition

Enteral nutrition is indicated for patients with colocutaneous fistulas; low-output fistulas of the ileum; and high-output fistulas of the esophagus, stomach, duodenum, and jejunum, if distal access is possible. The benefits of enteral nutrition are digestive tract structural and functional preservation; better utilization of nutrients; decreased septic complication rates; and immune response preservation. Elemental diets have not demonstrated advantages over polymeric diets in patients with GI fistulas. Thus, we recommend polymeric diets as the first choice, although intolerance mandates changing to an elemental diet. Almost all colocutaneous fistulas can be treated with polymeric diets. Elemental diets delivered with continuous pump infusion for 24 hours are the most practical and well-tolerated means. Elemental diet infusion should initially be given at 20 mL/h, increasing by 10 to 20 mL/h every 8 hours until projected caloric requirements are met. For fistulas of the esophagus, stomach, duodenum, and small intestine, enteral nutrition should be delivered distal to the fistula; hence, adequate placement of the feeding tube is important. Quite often this is accomplished with the help of endoscopy and fluoroscopy. When surgery is indicated to close a fistula, gastric decompression through a gastrojejunal tube is advisable, and enteral feeding is begun early in the postoperative period. Jejunostomy tube placement is also advisable for those patients undergoing major GI surgery; if a fistula develops, nutrition can be started by the enteral route, thus decreasing the risk of complications related to intravenous nutrition. A multidisciplinary approach that uses intensive care resources, adequate nutritional support, and reasonable surgical criteria gives successful and satisfactory results both for the patients with GI fistulas and for the medical teams taking care of the patients.

◆ INTRA-ABDOMINAL INFECTION: DIAGNOSIS AND TREATMENT

Complications most frequently related to GI fistulas are infectious. These complications can be observed either in the abdominal wall (cellulitis, fasciitis), or within the abdominal cavity (abscess and/or primary peritonitis). The systemic repercussion of infection, known as sepsis, will be observed depending on the severity of complications.

Diagnosis

The past medical history, including information on previous operations and the details of the operative procedures preceding the presentation of the fistula, is of prime importance, especially in patients in whom primary anastomoses were made in the presence of either infection or hollow viscus perforation. It is also important to consider high-risk patients such as severely ill, immunosupressed (cancer, acquired immunodeficiency syndrome, renal failure), and malnourished patients, in whom healing of the suture line may fail, leading to leakage and fistula formation.

On physical examination, postoperative secondary peritonitis should be suspected when GI contents are obtained either through a infected wound or through a previously placed drainage tube early in the postoperative period (within the first 5 days). Low output through a drainage tube should not exclude the presence of intra-abdominal infection. In fact, peritoneal signs, once present, mandate immediate surgical exploration, although these findings are infrequent, since most of the patients are immunosupressed and on antibiotics and analgesic therapy. Laboratory confirmation of leukocytosis suggests the presence of uncontrolled intra-abdominal infection, although a great number of patients with GI fistulas show leukopenia. Hyperglycemia is frequently encountered in fistulous patients with associated infection. The clinical progress suggests the possibility of intra-abdominal infection. A collaborative effort between the surgeon and the radiologist early in the course is mandatory in order to identify intra-abdominal fluid collections. Only when these have been excluded is parenteral nutrition indicated. A multidisciplinary approach and follow-up by the surgical team are pivotal.[26–30]

Treatment

The therapeutic goals in the management of intra-abdominal infections should include a systematic approach that combines diagnostic, supportive, and surgical procedures aimed at aborting the source of infection. Broad-spectrum antibiotics, nutritional support, surgical treatment, and intervention radiology are all important in this regard.[31]

Broad-spectrum antibiotics, which include *Escherichia coli* and *Bacteroides* F. coverage, should be used empirically in community-acquired infections when the fistula first appears. Coverage should include *Pseudomonas* in hospital-acquired infections.[32] There is no evidence suggesting that results are improved when the established therapy is changed based on culture results. In fact, several retrospective studies have concluded that culturing samples from the first surgical procedure are not justified. The main reason for this is that there are a great number of potentially contaminating species within the GI tract, yet less than 5% of them are isolated in cultures.[33] The use of cultures is recommended to identify special organisms, such as fungi or resistant bacteria, than as a therapeutic guide. Some have advocated long-term antibiotic therapy base only on leukocytosis and fever.[34] However, studies have reported favorable results with shortened antibiotic regimens titrated according to the findings during surgery.[35] Thus, antibiotics are administered only for a week in severe cases of infection. Otherwise, the following recommendations are suggested: one-dose antibiotics for cases of either simple contamination or gastroduodenal perforation with an evolution of less than 12 hours; 24-hour antibiotic therapy for operable infections such as gangrenous appendicitis or bowel ischemia without perforation; and 2- to 5-day antibiotic therapy for cases of diffuse intra-abdominal contamination. As soon as the patient resumes oral intake, the oral administration of antibiotics is advisable.[36]

Only after intra-abdominal infection has been controlled and other sources of secondary infection have been excluded is tertiary peritonitis considered in the presence of persistent systemic and peritoneal inflammation. This clearly modifies the aim of therapy, since additional antibiotics and other surgical interventions may contribute not only to worsening of the patient's condition but to the possibility of overinfection. Thus, the goal should be to improve the host's immunologic state either with enteral nutrition or specific nutrients such as glutamine.[30, 37]

The goals of surgical management of intra-abdominal sepsis should be aimed at controlling the source of infection; adequate abdominal drainage; management of the compartment syndrome; and the prevention and management of persistent and recurrent infections. Thus, a planned, organized, and collaborative effort is important, paying special attention to keen surgical judgment and meticulous surgical technique, in order to prevent further complications (Figs. 13–6 and 13–7).[31, 38]

When the surgeon deals with a patient with intra-abdominal infection, the first thing to consider is whether the infection is under control; if not, mortality rates can far exceed 30 to 50%. A controlled intra-abdominal infection refers to the presence of contained abscesses within the peritoneal cavity (Fig. 13–8). These can be either simple (single unilocular collection) or multiple and can be best approached through either percutaneous drainage or open surgical drainage. Uncontrolled infection refers to active contamination and requires strict surgical control.[39] At celiotomy, a careful surgical approach of the peritoneal cavity is mandatory, and all necrotic material and bacterial contamination should be identified and dealt with. Furthermore, all suture lines should be examined and the rest of the bowel digitally inspected. In uncontrolled intra-abdominal infection associated with either hollow viscus perforation or suture line leakage, proximal diversion is the treat-

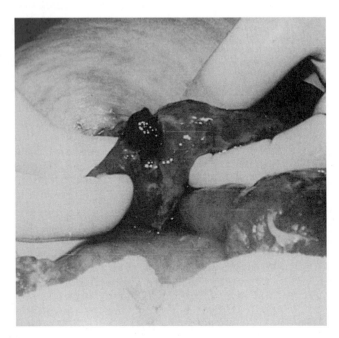

Figure 13–6. Partial dehiscence of small bowel anastomosis is identified and associated with generalized sepsis.

Figure 13–7. Performing anastomosis in the presence of severely inflamed peritoneal cavity should be avoided. A controlled fistula through functional ostomies, open abdomen management with a nonabsorbable mesh prosthesis anchored to the fascia, and covering the intestines with the omentum to prevent further fistula formation is recommended.

This patient underwent this type of approach. Three months after surgery, the functional ostomies and the wound's closing secondarily, over a mesh prosthesis, are shown.

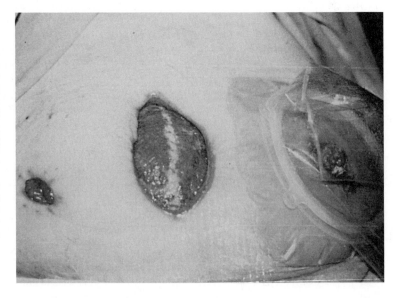

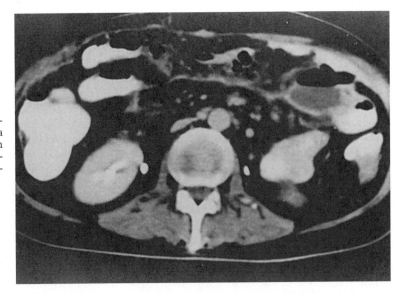

Figure 13–8. Computed tomographic scan demonstrating a small bowel fistula draining to an abscess cavity. Control of this abscess was achieved through percutaneous drainage.

ment of choice. As a general rule, the surgeon should avoid making new anastomoses in the presence of a severely inflamed peritoneal cavity. Proximal diversion is both safe and effective and achieves drainage control through an exposed fistula.[40]

The final decision in the surgical management depends on a planned reoperation based on the findings during surgery. This planned reoperation is indicated in cases of fecal peritonitis, pancreatic necrosis, and necrotizing fasciitis of the abdominal wall and is best performed no later than 5 days after the initial re-exploration. If performed after this period, adhesions will become firm and the chances of reperforation will be high. While the abdominal wall is sutured, a nonabsorbable mesh prosthesis is applied and anchored to the fascia, since a tensionless direct closure of the abdominal wall is not always possible under these circumstances. Thus, planned reoperation includes temporarily closing the abdominal wall after a thorough peritoneal cleansing has been achieved and all infectious material and any other source of contamination have been controlled.

Technical problems most frequently encountered when operating on patients with GI fistulas are iatrogenic in origin. Perforation of the GI tract may occur in the presence of an inflamed, friable bowel; especially in cases of infected open abdomen. New suture lines applied under these circumstances can either fail or become a new source of infection. Furthermore, trouble-

some bleeding coming from the mesentery may be difficult to control. Thus, careful surgical exploration is advised.[39–41]

Intra-abdominal abscess has been erroneously considered a synonym of peritonitis. Actually, an abscess appears as an effective host response to an infectious process.[37] At this point, the interventional radiologist plays a key role in both the detection and the treatment of postoperative intra-abdominal abscesses. Computed tomography has demonstrated advantages over ultrasonography as an investigative tool that is highly effective in diagnosing intra-abdominal abscesses and for successful percutaneous drainage in high-risk patients (see Fig. 13–8), as recommended by Butler and colleagues.[42] When the abscess is accessible and the computed tomographic characteristics suggest a simple abscess, radiologic percutaneous drainage is preferable because the results are comparable to those of operative therapy and morbidity is lower. In contrast, when multiple abscesses are identified, operative treatment is preferable, since treatment of the coexisting abnormalities must be addressed by surgery.[43]

◆ SURGICAL MANAGEMENT

Oropharyngeocutaneous and Esophageal Fistulas

Oropharyngeocutaneous and esophageal fistulas usually occur as a result of surgical operation performed on the neck for cancer, and from high-risk anastomosis after radiotherapy. Frequently, they have a sinuus tract. In order to obtain control of the fistula, it may be necessary to enlarge the tract, thus achieving local control of infection while preventing extension and exposure of vital structures such as the carotid artery. Any factor that prevents spontaneous closure of the fistula such as obstruction, a malignant tumor, or foreign materials should be treated accordingly. Substitutive therapy is required for those patients who develop iatrogenic hypothyroidism either after radiotherapy or because of thyroid resections.[2]

Chylous fistulas require conservative therapy with specific parenteral nutrition, possibly with enteral nutrition with either elemental lipids or medium-chain triglycerides.[44, 45] Definitive surgical correction is recommended for those patients with oropharyngeocutaneous fistulas in whom spontaneous closure has not occurred within 4 to 6 weeks. There are several techniques available for this purpose, such as primary closure; local and regional cutaneous flaps either with muscle or without it; esophageal resections with gastric and colonic interposition; or free jejunal grafts.[46]

Small oropharyngeocutaneous fistulas and small fistulas of the cervical esophagus can be closed primarily by separating mucosal and skin edges and closing each layer independently. Successful treatment reduces the time of spontaneous closure. Free cutaneous flaps are not recommended, both because they lack vascularity and because of poor perfusion on the receptor bed (e.g., radiated tissues). For larger fistulas, rotation of vascularized myocutaneous flaps is more convenient in order to transfer healthy tissues into the damaged area.[47, 48] Colonic or gastric interposition offers excellent results, although these procedures can be technically demanding.[49] Jejunal interposition is limited to the management of circumferential defects of the pharynx and the esophagus.[50]

Internal fistulas of the thoracic esophagus can involve one or two organs; thus, they are divided into esophagorespiratory and esophagocardiovascular fistulas. Both can be benign or malignant. Most cases of esophagorespiratory fistulas are secondary to either esophageal or lung cancer. Patients usually develop dysphagia and recurrent pulmonary infections. Surgical treatment includes esophageal diversion, resection, and bronchopulmonary resection with replacement. Ong and Kwong have proposed surgical resection,[51] and Kato and associates demonstrated good results on selected patients with small lesions and direct invasion to the lung.[52] The overall survival rate was 22.7%. Other treatment measures include organ diversion. Symbas and Burt and coworkers demonstrated better survival rates with esophageal exclusion and either gastrostomy or jejunostomy, as well as with cervical esophagostomy and distal closure of the esophagus.[53, 54] These measures do not decrease the risk of pulmonary infections. Stent placement for malignant stenosis has a mortality rate of 35%.[55]

The frequency of benign esophagorespiratory fistulas is lower. Although congenital fistulas are almost always found in a neonate patient, they can rarely present in adulthood. They can also occur after trauma (penetrating, orotracheal intubation), inflammatory disease states (chemical lesions, peptic ulcer, granulomatous disease, diverticula, and achalasia), and infectious diseases (tuberculosis, mycosis, syphilis, and infections associated with human immunodeficiency virus).[56] Definitive therapy should always include an approach by thoracotomy, with both fistula division and closure of the esophagorespiratory communication with pleural patch and muscular flap placement. Occasionally, organ resection may be necessary with esophageal replacement. Specific therapy may heal fistulas of infectious origin. Esophageal, aortic, and cardiac chamber fistulas may present as massive hemorrhage of the GI tract, usually so major that very few patients survive the event. Depending on the damage state of both the aorta and the esophagus, a left thoracotomy approach is indicated, with reconstruction in situ. Fistulas that communicate with pericardium have a high mortality rate because of purulent polymicrobial pericarditis. Surgical management should consist of organ bypass, proximal esophagostomy, gastrojejunostomy, closure of the fistula with a pleural or muscle flap, and even esophageal resection with replacement.[57] After an esophageal resection or transection has been performed, a partial or complete anastomotic dehiscence leads to either local or overt generalized sepsis. The surgical management is directed toward appropriate drainage (neck, thorax, abdomen) and to an adequate lung compliance.[58]

Gastroduodenal Fistulas

Ninety-five percent of duodenal fistulas occur after surgical operations and as a result of complete or partial suture line dehiscence. They are always associated with either abscess or local infection. Unlike some gastric fistulas, which appear after a period of time (after resection or gastroenteric diversion), duodenal fistulas appear early in the postoperative period.[13] Internal fistulas are rare; in fact, most internal fistulas reported in the literature are associated with Crohn's disease.[59] The surgical management of these fistulas is not straightforward. There is no specific rule indicating that a postoperative external fistula will fail to improve with medical treatment, thus requiring surgical management. Early surgical management should be considered for those patients who showing unfavorable factors that prevent spontaneous closure of the fistula (Table 13–4). Three surgical approaches have been devised for the management of these fistulas: exclusion, resection, and leakage closure.[60] Exclusion is reserved both for extremely ill patients and for severe sepsis that prevents establishing continuity of the GI tract. Exclusion consists of both resection of the fistula site and proximal and distal exteriorization of the affected segment. Exteriorization of the duodenum in generally achieved through a duodenostomy tube, thus converting an uncontrolled drainage tract to a controlled external fistula. The proximal segment can be exteriorized through a gastrostomy. Pyloric exclusion with gastrojejunostomy, or pyloric closure with gastrojejunostomy, is not recommended for duodenal fistulas. Resection of the fistulized segment with an end-to-end anastomosis is the treatment of choice. Primary closure of lateral fistulas is not indicated. A serosal patch with a Roux-en-Y diversion should be used in these cases.[61] Fistulas that appear after a gastroduodenostomy (Billroth I) are best approach by resection of the affected segment and a Roux-en-Y gastrojejunostomy reconstruction. A terminal duodenostomy tube should be placed when the duodenal stump is fibrotic and the closure is unsafe.

Biliary and Pancreatic Fistulas

Biliary and pancreatic fistulas can be internal or external. Biliary internal fistulas occur as a result of gallstone disease and recurrent episodes of inflammation. Organs most commonly affected are the colon and duodenum. Spontaneous cholecystocutaneous fistula is extremely rare. External fistulas are more frequent and usually occur after surgical procedures. The surgical treatment of internal fistulas includes cholecystectomy and closure of the communication to the affected organ. Endoscopic evaluation through retrograde cholangiography is generally required for external fistulas. The anatomic definition dictates the type of treatment. Special therapeutic maneuvers, such as endoscopic

Table 13–4. Predictive Factors for Spontaneous Closure of Gastrointestinal Fistulas

Factor	Favorable	Unfavorable
Anatomic location	Oropharyngeal, esophageal, duodenal stump, pancreatobiliary and jejunal	Gastric, lateral duodenal, ligament of Treitz, and ileal
Nutritional status	Well nourished	Malnourished
Sepsis	Absent	Present
Cause	Appendicitis, diverticulitis, postoperative	Crohn's disease, cancer, foreign body, radiation enteritis
Bowel condition	Healthy bowel, small leak, no abscess	Active disease, abscess, distal obstruction, total disruption
Miscellaneous	Tract >2 cm long Defect <1 cm²	Epithelialization, foreign body
Output		
Enteric fistula	<500 mL/day	>500 mL/day
Pancreatic fistula	<200 mL/day	>200 mL/day
Transferrin	>200 mg/dL	<200 mg/dL

sphincterotomy with residual stone extraction and stent placement, can be performed for fistulas originating in small bile ducts.[62] Surgical repair through an internal Roux-en-Y biliary diversion is required for fistulas that appear after a complete extrahepatic biliary transection has been produced.[63]

Pancreatic fistulas can be internal or external. Internal fistulas are always a consequence of an attack of pancreatitis or pancreatic trauma. The common clinical presentation includes pancreatic ascites, pleural effusion, or a pseudocyst.[64] Most external fistulas are secondary to surgical procedures on the gland. Fistula output greater than 200 mL/day is usually due to obstruction of the pancreatic duct. Diagnosis is established through amylase determinations on the fistula effluent. The anatomic delineation of the fistula tract is usually achieved through fistulography, retrograde pancreatography, and imaging studies such as computed tomography. The initial treatment for external pancreatic fistulas should consist of control of associated sepsis while good external drainage is ensured. Leaving the pancreas at rest is necessary and is generally achieved by the patient having nothing by mouth, nutritional support either parenteral or enteral distal to the pancreas, and the administration of somatostatin and its analogues. The placement of endostents through the ampulla of Vater can solve anomalous communications in cases of proximal obstruction of pancreatic duct. With all these measures, up to 80% of external pancreatic fistulas experience spontaneous closure. Initial surgical management should be considered for internal fistulas, since spontaneous closure occurs in less than 50% of the cases.[65] Accurate knowledge of the damaged duct anatomy is mandatory; thus, pancreatography may be required during surgery. Distal pancreatectomy should be performed for lesions on the body and tail of the pancreas, with a normal duct. However, fistulas arising in the head of the pancreas, and pseudocysts, should undergo some type of internal drainage. These can be constructed with stomach, duodenum, or a Roux-en-Y jejunal loop.[66]

Small Bowel Fistulas

Despite the technological advances of the last four decades, the average mortality rates for bowel fistulas vary between 15 and 25%. Fistulas can be classified according to their location into internal, external, or mixed. Internal fistulas represent only 25% of all cases.[2, 67] These are usually secondary to Crohn's disease (most common cause in Western countries), radiation, diverticular disease, ischemic bowel, and neoplasia. Enteroenteric fistulas between short segments of the small bowel can be overlooked unless a communication between largely separated segments has been established, such as a jejunoileal fistula, or jejunocolonic fistulas that result in diarrhea, electrolyte imbalances, and deficient intestinal absorption. Recurrent urinary infections prevail in cases of communication with the bladder. Small bowel follow-through and barium enema are necessary to establish the diagnosis of internal fistula. Computed tomography is helpful both in determining the presence of associated abscesses and for percutaneous drainage. Spontaneous closure is rarely observed. Thus, most of the patients require elective surgical operation, the main goal of which is to resect the affected segment or segments with a primary end-to-end anastomosis between healthy segments.

External fistulas represent 75% of all fistulas. The more proximal the fistula, the greater the output. Most of these fistulas are postoperative (complete or partial dehiscence of intestinal anastomosis, lesions to the bowel wall or to the vascular supply). Spontaneous closure rates can reach up to 70% of all cases (see Table 13–4). If the fistula persists despite conservative measures, surgical treatment must be considered aimed at re-establishing intestinal continuity and preserving as much small bowel as possible. It is also important to preserve the omentum, which is used to cover the intestines with vascularized tissue while avoiding contact with the abdominal wall, flaps, or prosthetic materials. Surgical operation should be performed 3 months after the resolution of sepsis, when adhesions are easily taken down and irrigation to inflamed tissues has improved. Care should be taken not to damage the remaining bowel, in order to avoid anastomosis dehiscence, perforation, or sepsis de novo. The abdominal cavity should be entered through areas not previously affected by sepsis or radiation. When intra-abdominal abscesses are found, these should be aspirated and drained through separate incisions. Special care should be paid to the reconstruction of the abdominal wall. Large wall defects may need myocutaneous flaps or the use of prosthetic mesh (Fig. 13–9).[68]

Colonic Fistulas

Most external colonic fistulas occur after surgical operations, as a consequence of complete or partial anastomotic dehiscence, or after a pericolic abscess has been drained. Internal fistulas are a direct consequence of diverticular disease, Crohn's disease, colon cancer, and radiation enteritis. External fistula output depends on the size of dehiscence and the clinical manifestations produced after fecal contamination and peritoneal inflammation. Spontaneous clo-

sure of low-output fistulas can be expected to occur in 80% of the patients, if they are adequately drained, no associated sepsis is found, and distal obstruction has been excluded.[69] Oral feeding, or a low-residue enteral diet can be used for these patients. Parenteral nutrition and the patients having nothing by mouth may be necessary for high-output fistulas. Surgical management should be considered for fistulas associated with severe sepsis and for those occurring after a total anastomotic dehiscence. Conventional treatment includes proximal-end colostomy and either a mucus fistula or a blind pouch (Hartmann's pouch) construction of the distal end. A proximal ostomy, preferably with distal ileum, can be used in cases of partial dehiscence with localized abscess formation, since a transverse colos-

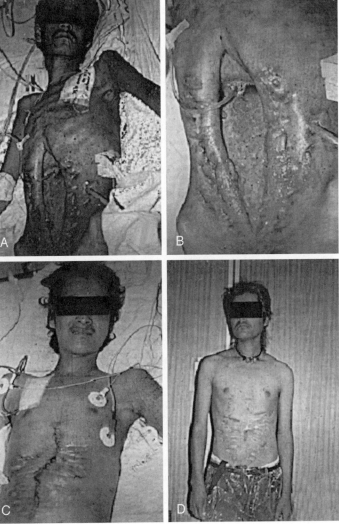

Figure 13–9. A 25-year-old multi-injured man who developed small bowel fistulas after multiple operations. *A* and *B*, Fistula tracts through the abdominal wall and severe malnutrition are appreciated. Performing surgery under these circumstances leads to a negligible surgical failure. Total parenteral nutrition support becomes a key element *(C)* and should be continued after surgery for a successful outcome *(D)*.

tomy may seriously endanger the vascular supply to the anastomosis. Ileostomy closure should be performed 3 to 4 months later, once fistula healing has been demonstrated and anastomosis stricture has been excluded. A new anastomosis and closure of the protecting ileostomy should be performed if stenosis is demonstrated during surgery.

Surgical treatment is always necessary for internal fistulas, before radiologic (intestinal follow-through, barium enema, intravenous pyelogram) and endoscopic (colonoscopy, cystoscopy) assessments. Up to 20% of the patients with diverticular disease develop coloenterovesical fistulas.[70] Resection of the affected colon with a primary anastomosis is the treatment of choice. Resection may also be necessary for fistulas to the small bowel. In fistulas that communicate with the bladder, the tract is dissected free and an indwelling catheter is left in place for 7 days. Identifying the communication to the bladder is not necessary, and if there is an inflammatory membrane or infection, this is just débrided without surgical closure. Wider resections of the affected organ or organs may be necessary in the presence of cancer. Fistulas associated with radiation represent a challenge for the surgeon. Trying to dismantle these fistulas resection of adjacent organs may be dangerous. Better results are obtained with the use of diverting ostomies of either proximal colon or distal ileum.[71]

◆ FUTURE PERSPECTIVES

Octreotide (Somatostatin)

The somatostatin synthetic analogue octreotide was initially approved by the Food and Drug Administration in 1988 for the treatment of VIPomas and carcinoid syndrome.[72] However, its pharmacologic properties have encountered several applications in the field of modern medicine such as adjuvant therapy for fistulas of the GI tract. The first reports were made by Heij and associates in 1986, when they described the use of octreotide in patients with external pancreatic fistulas.[73] Although results were not conclusive, a significant reduction in fistula output was observed. In 1987, Nubiola-Calonge and colleagues reported for the first time the use of octreotide as adjuvant therapy after con-

ventional treatment for small bowel fistulas.[74] In this preliminary report, octreotide significantly decreased fistula output and was capable of achieving spontaneous closure in 11 of 14 patients with fistulas 4 days after treatment. Since then, several reports have been published with the use of octreotide as adjuvant therapy in fistulas of the GI tract with promising results. These results include both a substantial reduction in hospital stays and a subsequent reduction in morbidity and mortality.[75–77] However, as Martineau and coworkers have pointed out,[78] further controlled studies with better methodology will be necessary in order to determine the actual roll of octreotide as adjuvant therapy in the management of GI tract fistulas.

Fibrin Sealant

Like octreotide, fibrin sealant (also known as fibrin tissue adhesive and fibrin glue; Omrix Biopharmaceuticals, Brussels, Belgium) has multiple therapeutic potentials (Fig. 13–10). Preliminary studies by Eleftheriadis and associates in 1990 report the use of fibrin in seven patients with enterocutaneous fistulas after gastric surgery.[79] In this study, fibrin was applied endoscopically in one or several sessions with no complications at all. The fistula output decreased rapidly, and closure was achieved in all cases. In 1992, Waclawiczek and colleagues proposed its use as a preventive measure in fistula formation after the Whipple operation.[80] In this study, the authors report a pancreatic fistula rate of zero in 67 procedures. After these preliminary reports, newer studies have been published reporting both its successful use in patients with pancreatic fistula secondary to pancreatitis[81] and as palliative therapy for patients with fistula secondary to malignancies, such as the gastrocolic fistula in a patient with Hodgkin's disease.[82] Because of its simplicity, it is expected that within the near future, fibrin use will expand and prospective studies will be able to determine its therapeutic potentials.

Collagen

Placenta-derived collagen has been reported experimentally in rats as a substitute for intestinal wall. In this study, the use of colla-

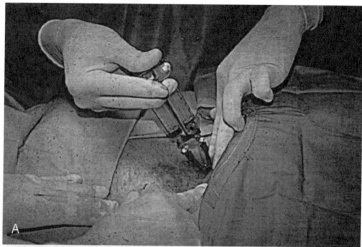

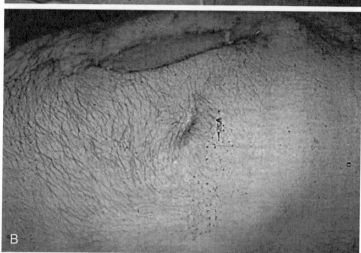

Figure 13–10. Gastrocutaneous fistula after gastrostomy tube removal. Fibrin sealant was applied *(A)*, and closure was achieved only 48 hours after its application *(B)*.

gen was compared with the use of fibrin after 25% of the anterior wall of the cecum was removed; results were similar in both groups. However, in another experiment, an 80% defect was created in the cecal wall, and neither primary repair nor the use fibrin were feasible, although a successful repair was achieved with the use of collagen.[83] The use of collagen as a substitute for bowel wall will probably be the aim of future studies.

Other Alternatives

There are several studies reporting the use of *n*-2-butylcyanocrylate in the management of GI fistulas.[84] A group from Japan has also reported the use of factor XIII as a treatment for GI fistulas occurring after surgery.[85] However, their contribution to the therapeutic armamentarium will have to be determined.

REFERENCES

1. Arenas-Marquez H, Anaya-Prado R, Hurtado H, et al: Mexican consensus on the integral management of digestive tract fistulas. Nutrition 15(3):1–4, 1999.
2. Berry SM, Fisher JE: Enterocutaneous fistula. Curr Probl Surg 31:469–576, 1994.
3. Frileux P, Attal E: Anastomotic dehiscence and external fistulas. In Schein M, Wise L (eds): Crucial Controversies in surgery. Brooklyn, NY, Karger Landes Systems, 1997, pp 257–269.
4. Schein M, Decker GA: Postoperative external alimentary tract fistulas. Am J Surg 161:435–438, 1991.
5. Soeters PB, Ebeid AM, Fisher JE: Review of 404 patients with gastrointestinal fistulas. Impact of parenteral nutrition. Ann Surg 190:189–202, 1979.
6. Hollender LF, Meyer C, Aven D, Zeyer B: Postoperative fistulas of the small intestine: Therapeutic principles. World J Surg 7:474–480, 1983.
7. Berry SM, Fisher JE: Classification and pathophysiology of enterocutaneous fistulae. Surg Clin North Am 76:1009–1018, 1996.
8. Michelassi F, Stella M, Balestracci T, et al: Incidence, diagnosis, and treatment of enteric and colo-

rectal fistulas in patients with Crohn's disease. Ann Surg 218:660–666, 1993.

9. James T, Lee JD Jr: Reoperative care of postoperative external fistulas: Stomach, pancreas, duodenum, small intestine. In McKuarrie DG, Humphrey EW (eds): Reoperations in General Surgery. New York, Mosby, 1992, pp 393–422.

10. Altomare DF, Serio G, Pannarale OC, et al: Prediction of mortality by logistic regression analysis in patients with postoperative enterocutaneous fistulae. Br J Surg 77:450–453, 1990.

11. Sancho JJ, DiConstanzo J, Nubiola P, et al: Randomized double-blind placebo-controlled trial of early octreotide in patients with postoperative enterocutaneous fistula. Br J Surg 82:638–641, 1995.

12. Sitges-Serra A, Jaurrieta E, Sitges-Creus: Management of postoperative enterocutaneous fistulas: The roles of parenteral nutrition and surgery. Br J Surg 69:147–150, 1982.

13. Tarzani R, Coutsoftides T, Steiger E, et al: Gastric and duodenal cutaneous fistulas. World J Surg 7:463–473, 1983.

14. Meguid MM, Campos ACL: Gastrointestinal fistulas: Clinical and nutritional management. In Rombeau JL, Caldwell MD (eds): Clinical Nutrition—Parenteral Nutrition. Philadelphia, WB Saunders, 2nd ed., 1993, pp. 462–497.

15. Rombeau JL, Takala J: Summary of round table conference; gut dysfunction in critical illness. Clin Nut 16:57–60, 1997.

16. ASPN Board of Directors: Section II. Rationale for adult nutrition support guidelines. JPEN J Parent Enteral Nutr 17 (Suppl 4):5SA–6SA, 1993.

17. Satyanarayana R, Klein S: Clinical efficacy of perioperative nutrition support. Curr Opin Clin Nutr Metab Care 1:51–58, 1998.

18. Studley HO: Percentage of weight loss: A basic indicator of surgical risk in patients with chronic peptic ulcer. JAMA 106:458–460, 1936.

19. Mughal MM, Meguid MM: The effect of nutritional status on morbidity after elective surgery for benign gastrointestinal disease. JPEN J Parenter Enteral Nutr 11:140–143, 1987.

20. Garrel DR, Jobin N, De Jonje LHM: Should we still use the Harris-Benedict equation? Nutr Clin Pract 11:99–103, 1996.

21. Rombeau JL, Rolandelli RH: Enteral and parenteral nutrition in patients with enteral fistulas and short bowel syndrome. Surg Clin North Am 67:551–570, 1987.

22. Fukuchi S, Seeburger J, Parquet G, Rolandelli RH: Nutritional support of patients with enterocutaneous fistulas. Nutr Clin Pract 13:59–65, 1998.

23. Eng K: Pitfalls in management of small bowel fistulas. Probl Gen Surg 3:64–69, 1986.

24. Levy PF, Cugnenc PH, Honiger J, Olliver JM: High-output external fistulas of the small bowel: Management with continuous enteral nutrition. Br J Surg 78:676–679, 1989.

25. Hunter DC, Lewis D, Benotti PN, et al: Resting energy expenditure in critically ill: Estimations versus measurement. Br J Surg 75:875–878, 1988.

26. Schein M: Intestinal fistulas and the open management of the septic abdomen. Arch Surg 125:1516–1517, 1990.

27. Sancho J, Hernandez R, Girvent M, Stieges-Serra A: Management of enterocutaneous fistulas. Dig Surg 14:483–491, 1997.

28. Gorbach SL: Intra-abdominal infections: State of the art clinical article. Clin Infect Dis 17:961–967, 1993.

29. Nystrom PO, Bax R, Delliger EP, et al: Proposed definition for diagnosis severity, scoring stratification and outcome for trials on intraabdominal infection. World J Surg 14:148–158, 1990.

30. Ronstein OD, Meakins JL: Diagnostic and therapeutic challenges of intraabdominal infections. World J Surg 14:159–166, 1990.

31. Wittman DH: Newer methods of operative therapy for peritonitis. In Nyhus LM, Baker RJ, Fischer JE (eds): Mastery of Surgery, 3rd ed. Boston, Little, Brown, 1996, p 146–152.

32. Montravers P, Gauzi R, Muller JP, Desmont JM: Emergence of antibiotic-resistant bacteria in cases of peritonitis after intraabdominal surgery affects the efficacy of empirical antimicrobial therapy. Clin Infect Dis 23:486–494, 1996.

33. Dougherty SH: Antimicrobial culture and susceptibility testing has little value for routine management of secondary bacterial peritonitis. Clin Infect Dis 25 (Suppl 2):S258–S261, 1997.

34. Lennard ES, Delliger EP, Minshew BH, et al: Implications of leukocytosis and fever at conclusion of antibiotic therapy for intraabdominal sepsis. Ann Surg 195:19–24, 1982.

35. Schein M, Assalia A, Bachus H: Minimal antibiotic therapy after emergency abdominal surgery: A prospective study. Br J Surg 81:989–991, 1994.

36. Witmann DH, Schein M: Let us shorten antibiotic prophylaxis and therapy in surgery. Am J Surg 172:S26–S32, 1996.

37. Witmann DH, Schein M, Condon RE: Management of secondary peritonitis. Ann Surg 224:10–18, 1996.

38. Wilson SE: A critical analysis of recent innovations in the treatment of intra-abdominal infections. Surg Gynecol Obstet 177:11–17, 1993.

39. Schein M, Hirshberg A, Hashnoan M: Correct surgical management of severe intraabdominal infections. Surgery 112:489–496, 1992.

40. Hirshberg A, Stein M, Adar R: Reoperation: Planned and unplanned. Surg Clin North Am 77:897–907, 1997.

41. Pennick FM, Kerremans RPS, Lauwers PM: Planned relaparotomies in the surgical treatment of severe generalized peritonitis from intestinal origin. World J Surg 7:762–768, 1983.

42. Butler JA, Huang J, Wilson SE: Repeated laparotomy for postoperative intraabdominal sepsis: An analysis of outcome predictors: Arch Surg 122:702–707, 1987.

43. Malagoni MA, Shumate CR, Thomas HA, et al: Factors influencing the treatment of intraabdominal abscesses. Am J Surg 159:167–171, 1990.

44. Al-Khayat M, Kenyon GS, Fawcett HV, et al: Nutritional support in patients with low volume chylous fistula following radical neck dissection. J Laryngol Otol 105:1952–1056, 1991.

45. Younus M, Chang RWC: Chyle fistula: Treatment with total parenteral nutrition. J Laryngol Otol 83:306–309, 1988.

46. Myer EN: The management of pharyngocutaneous fistula. Arch Otolaryngol 95:10–17, 1972.

47. Chen H, Tang Y, Noordhoff MS: Patch esophagoplasty with musculocutaneous flaps as treatment of complications after esophageal reconstruction. Ann Plast Surg 19:448–453, 1987.

48. Friedman M, Toriumi DM, Strorigl T, et al: The

sternocleidomastoid myoperiosteal flap for esophagopharyngeal reconstruction and fistula repair. Clinical and experimental study. Laryngoscope 98:1084–1091, 1988.

49. Watson TJ, Peters JH, DeMeester TR: Esophageal replacement for end-stage benign esophageal disease. Surg Clin North Am 77:1099–1113, 1997.

50. Jones NF, Eadie PA, Myers EN: Double lumen free jejunal transfer for reconstruction of the entire floor of the mouth, pharynx, and cervical esophagus. Br J Plast Surg 44:44–48, 1991.

51. Ong GB, Kwong KH: Management of malignant esophagobronchial fistula. Surgery 67:293–301, 1970.

52. Kato H, Tachimori Y, Watanabe H, et al: Surgical treatment of thoracoesophageal carcinoma directly invading the lung. Cancer 70:1457–1461, 1992.

53. Symbas PN, McKeown PP, Hatcher CR, et al: Tracheoesophageal fistula from carcinoma of the esophagus. Ann Thorac Surg 38:382–386, 1984.

54. Burt M, Diehl W, Martini N, et al: Malignant esophagorespiratory fistula: Management options and survival. Ann Thorac Surg 52:1222–1228, 1991.

55. Wong K, Goldstraw P: Role of covered esophageal stents in malignant esophagorespiratory fistula. Ann Thorac Surg 60:199–200, 1995.

56. Fernando CH, Benfield JR: Surgical management and treatment of esophageal fistula. Surg Clin North Am 76:1123–1135, 1996.

57. Miller WL, Osborn MJ, Sinak LJ, Westbrook BM: Pyopneumopericardium attributed to an esophagopericardial fistula: Report of a survivor and review of the literature. Mayo Clin Proc 66:1041–1045, 1991.

58. Alexander-Williams J, Irving M: Oesophageal fistulas. In Alexander-Williams J, Irving M (eds): Intestinal Fistulas. Wright PSG, Bristol, London, 1982, pp 115–127.

59. Pinchey LS, Fantry GT, Graham SM: Gastrocolic and gastroduodenal fistulas in Crohn's disease. J Clin Gastroenterol 15:205–211, 1992.

60. Chung MA, Wanebo HJ: Surgical management and treatment of gastric and duodenal fistulas. Surg Clin North Am 76:1137–1146, 1996.

61. Ujiki GT, Shields TW: Roux-en-Y operation in the management of postoperative fistula. Arch Surg 116:614–617, 1981.

62. Davids PHP, Rauws EAJ, Tytgat GNJ, et al: Postoperative bile leak: Endoscopic management. Gut 33:1118–1122, 1992.

63. Blumgart LH: Hiliar and intrahepatic biliary enteric anastomosis. Surg Clin North Am 74:845–863, 1994.

64. Lipsett PA, Cameron JL: Internal pancreatic fistula. Am J Surg 163:216–220, 1992.

65. Ihse I, Larson J, Lindstrom E: Surgical management of pure pancreatic fistulas. Hepatogastroenterology 41:271–275, 1994.

66. Ridgeway MG, Stabile BE: Surgical management and treatment of pancreatic fistulas. Surg Clin North Am 76:1159–1173, 1996.

67. Sansoni B, Irving M: Small bowel fistulas. World J Surg 9:897–903, 1985.

68. Tassiopoulos AK, Baum G, Halverson JD: Small bowel fistulas. Surg Clin North Am 76:1175–1190, 1996.

69. Lavery IC: Colonic fistulas. Surg Clin North Am 76:1183–1190, 1996.

70. Woods RJ, Lavery IC, Fazio VW, et al: Internal fistulas and diverticular disease. Dis Colon Rectum 51:591–596, 1988.

71. Saclarides TJ: Radiation injuries of the gastrointestinal tract. Surg Clin North Am 77:261–268, 1997.

72. Katz MD, Erstad BL: Octreotide: A new somatostatin analogue. Clin Pharm 8:255–273, 1989.

73. Heij HA, Bruining HA, Verschoor L: A comparison of the effects of two somatostatin analogues in a patient with an external pancreatic fistula. Pancreas 1:188–190, 1986.

74. Nubiola-Calonge P, Badia JM, Sanco J, et al: Blind evaluation of the effect of octreotide (SMS201–995), a somatostatin analogue, on small-bowel fistula output. Lancet 19:672–674, 1987.

75. Nubiola P, Badia JM, Martinez-Rodenas F, et al: Treatment of 27 postoperative enterocutaneous fistulas with the long half-life somatostatin analogue SMS 201–995, Ann Surg 210:56–58, 1989.

76. Miranda-Ruiz R, Castanon-Gonzalez J, Perez-Aldana C, et al: Effect of a synthetic somatostatin analogue with delayed action (SMS 201–995) on the biliary expenditure in a patient with an external biliary tract fistula. Rev Gastroenterol Mex 55:67–69, 1990.

77. Hernandez-Aranda JC, Gallo-Chico B, Flores-Ramirez LA, et al: Treatment of enterocutaneous fistula with or without octreotide and parenteral nutrition. Nutr Hosp 11:226–229, 1996.

78. Martineau P, Shwed JA, Denis R: Is octreotide a new hope for enterocutaneous and external pancreatic fistulas closure? Am J Surg 172:386–395, 1996.

79. Eleftheriadis E, Tzartinoglou E, Kotzampassi K, Aletras H: Early endoscopic fibril sealing of high-output postoperative enterocutaneous fistulas. Acta Chir Scand 156:625–628, 1990.

80. Waclawiczek HW, Heinerman M, Meiser G, et al: Prevention and treatment of postperative fistulae—New indications for fibrin gluing. Wien Klin Wochenschr 104:474–481, 1992.

81. Engler S, Dorlars D, Riemann JF: Endoscopic fibrin gluing of a pancreatic duct fistula following acute pancreatitis. Dtsch Med Wochenschr 121:1396–1400, 1996.

82. Shand A, Reading S, Ewing J, et al: Palliation of a malignant gastrocolic fistula by endoscopic human sealant injection. Eur J Gastroenterol Hepatol 9:1009–1011, 1997.

83. Alam H, Kim D, Brun E, et al: A placental-derived tissue matrix as a bowel wall substitute in rats. Preliminary study. Surgery 124:87–91, 1998.

84. Billi P, Alberani A, Baroncini D, et al: Management of gastrointestinal fistulas with n-2-butylcyanocrylate. Endoscopy 30:S69, 1998.

14

◆ Parenteral Nutrition in Short Bowel Syndrome

Steven Fukuchi, M.D.
Robin Bankhead, C.R.N.P., M.S., C.N.S.N.
Rolando H. Rolandelli, M.D.

◆ DEFINITION

The short bowel syndrome (SBS) is a constellation of signs and symptoms used to describe the metabolic and nutritional sequelae from a massive loss of the absorptive capacity of the small intestine. Although there can be a great variability among patients, SBS is characterized by malabsorption, severe diarrhea, dehydration, electrolyte disturbances, and malnutrition. Before the introduction of total parenteral nutrition (TPN), survival of patients with SBS was extremely rare.[1, 2] Today, with the use of home parenteral and enteral nutrition, it is estimated that nearly 275,000 patients are leading relatively normal and productive lives while receiving nutritional support at home.[3]

◆ INTESTINAL ANATOMY AND PHYSIOLOGY

The mucosa of the small intestine comprises *epithelium, lamina propria,* and *muscularis* layers. Absorptive, secretory, and barrier functions are regulated by the epithelial layer of the small intestine. This layer, one cell thick, lines the villi and their crypts and is responsible for the absorption of water, electrolytes, and nutrients. The crypt at the base of each villus is the source of epithelial cell renewal, exocrine and endocrine secretions, and water and ion secretion.[4] As epithelial cells mature, they are transported upward toward the tips of the villi, which are finger-shaped projections lining the small intestine, and are shed from the tips into the intestinal lumen. The turnover of epithelial cells is tightly regulated; normal human cells migrate from the crypt to the villus tip over a period of 5 to 6 days. Factors influencing cell turnover include the presence of luminal nutrients and digestive secretions, the nutritional state of the individual, the presence of infection and/or inflammation, and the administration of agents that impair cell replication (i.e., chemotherapy, radiation therapy). Impaired cell turnover results in villi that are blunted and flattened with diminished surface area.[5]

The process of absorption requires a large absorptive surface area. By the presence of villi and their microvilli, the intestinal surface area is multiplied to reach a size equivalent to that of a tennis court. The jejunum has a larger absorptive surface due to longer villi, whereas the ileum has shorter villi. The surface area of the intestine is further increased by the presence of 1-cm concentric folds every 5 cm of mucosa in the distal duodenum and proximal jejunum. Each villus is supplied by an arteriole and a lymphatic duct. Any disease that alters villous structure reduces the absorptive capacity.[6]

The small intestine extends from the pylorus to the ileocecal valve. Measurement of its length varies greatly, depending on the situation in which the measurement is taken (i.e., at laparotomy, radiographically, or at autopsy). Estimates range from 300 to 850 cm with a mean length of 620 cm in adults.[7] The duodenum (25 cm) extends from the pylorus to the ligament of Treitz. The jejunum (240 cm) and the ileum (360 cm) compose the proximal two fifths and the distal three fifths of the small intestine, respectively. The ileocecal valve functions as a barrier to prevent both the reflux of colonic contents into the small intestine and the rapid passage of contents through the ileum.[6]

◆ CAUSES AND SEVERITY OF SHORT BOWEL SYNDROME

In adults, the leading cause of SBS is massive small intestinal resection with or without a loss of colonic length as a result of mesenteric vascular disease, complications of Crohn's disease, or malignancy (Table 14–1). The reasons for massive resection of the small intestine in the pediatric population include necrotizing enterocolitis, midgut volvulus, and intestinal atresia. Additionally, children and adults may have a functional, rather than an anatomic, cause of SBS even though the small intestinal length is preserved. The functional impairment can be due to severe inflammatory bowel disease, intestinal pseudo-obstruction, or radiation enteritis.

The severity of the SBS is dependent on the length, location, and absorptive function of the remaining intestine as well as the physiologic process of intestinal adaptation.[8] In healthy adults, the absorptive and digestive surface area of the small intestine exceeds that required to maintain adequate nutrition. Therefore, limited resections of short segments of small intestine do not lead to clinical symptoms of SBS. The minimal length of intestine required for sufficient absorption is still controversial. This controversy arises from the wide variation in intestinal length as well as the difficulty in estimating the length of remaining intestine at the time of surgery. It is difficult to determine the length of the remaining intestine and to estimate the percentage of the total length of intestine this segment represents in a patient undergoing massive intestinal resection. Despite this difficulty, it is essential to obtain an estimate of the percentage of intestinal length remaining from the total length of intestine at the time of resection.

Table 14–1. Causes of Short Bowel Syndrome

Adult	Pediatric
Vascular (thrombosis, embolization, coagulopathy, chronic ischemia)	Necrotizing enterocolitis
	Intestinal atresia
	Intrauterine volvulus
Hypotension/low-flow state	Gastroschisis or omphalocele
Crohn's disease requiring resections	Extensive aganglionosis
Malignancy	Pseudo-obstruction
Abdominal trauma	
Strangulated hernia	
Small intestine volvulus	
Intestinal bypass for obesity	
Radiation enteritis	
Pseudo-obstruction	

Inflamed intestine can undergo either shortening or lengthening after surgery, which partially explains why the symptomatic outcome of massive small intestinal resection does not correlate well with the estimated length of resection.[9] However, resection of 75% or more of the small intestine usually leaves the patient with 70 to 100 cm (2 ft 4 in. to 3 ft 4 in.) of remaining intestine and is associated with severe metabolic sequelae that require intensive nutritional support.[8, 10–13]

The type and length of remaining intestine—that is, duodenum, jejunum, ileum, or a combination—determine the clinical symptoms of SBS. Complete duodenectomy or surgical bypass may result in anemia due to malabsorption of dietary iron and folate, as well as osteomalacia due to impaired calcium absorption.[14] Jejunectomy with preservation of the ileum produces no permanent defect in the absorption of protein, carbohydrates, and electrolytes.[15] The ileum can adapt to the increased absorptive requirements, but it cannot replace the jejunal secretion of enterohormones. Jejunal resection results in decreased secretion of cholecystokinin (CCK) and secretin, with resultant decreased gallbladder contraction and pancreatic secretion, respectively.[16] Decreased jejunal secretion of gastric inhibitory peptide and vasoactive intestinal polypeptide is associated with increased levels of gastrin release and gastric hypersecretion. The high solute load and the inactivation of digestive enzymes due to the low intraluminal pH are additional causes of diarrhea in SBS. Although resection of all or part of the jejunum is relatively well tolerated, extensive resection of the ileum has a profound effect on both small intestinal transit time and absorption.[14] Transit time through the ileum is longer than that through the duodenum and jejunum and, in addition, resection of the ileum effectively removes the "ileal brake," decreasing transit time in the remaining proximal intestine.[17] Absorption of conjugated bile salts through the enterohepatic circulation occurs exclusively in the ileum.[18] Resection of less than 100 cm of distal ileum with an intact colon results in watery choleretic diarrhea. Little or no steatorrhea occurs in this situation, because increased hepatic synthesis of bile salts compensates for their lower enterohepatic reabsorption. However, bile salts reaching the colon are deconjugated, stimulating water and ion secretion in the mucosa as well as colonic motility.[19, 20] If more than 100 cm of distal ileum are resected, increased hepatic synthesis of bile salts cannot match intestinal losses, and fat malabsorption occurs. Fatty acids reaching the colon stimulate motility and impair water and ion absorption, resulting in steatorrhea.

Colonic resection accompanying small intestinal resection also determines the severity of SBS. The colon is the major site of water and electrolyte absorption, and with increased volumes of ileal effluent, the colon can respond with three- to fivefold increments in absorptive capacity.[21] The colon also has a moderate capacity to absorb nutrients. Nonabsorbed carbohydrates reaching the colon undergo bacterial fermentation to yield short-chain fatty acids (SCFAs), principally acetate, propionate, and butyrate.[22] These SCFAs are efficiently absorbed by the colonic mucosa and enter the portal circulation to become a fuel source for the body.[23, 24] The normal human colon can absorb an estimated 500 kcal/day in the form of SCFAs.[25] Although the usual substrate for colonic fermentation is dietary fiber, malabsorbed starch polysaccharides also contribute to the production of SCFAs. Whenever SCFAs are produced in excess of the absorptive capacity of the colonic mucosa, diarrhea develops; this effect is exploited to rid the body of ammonia in patients with hepatic encephalopathy by administering lactulose, a highly fermentable nonstarch polysaccharide.

In patients with a segment of small intestine in continuity with all or part of the colon, the presence of the ileocecal valve can reduce the severity of diarrhea, increase nutrient absorption, and reduce the dependence on TPN. The physiologic role of the ileocecal valve is controversial; however, an intact ileocecal valve regulates the delivery of ileal contents into the colon and prevents the reflux of colonic bacteria into the ileum. Bacterial overgrowth in the remaining small intestine can lead to deconjugation of bile acids and subsequent diarrhea.

◆ SEQUELAE OF SHORT BOWEL SYNDROME

Gastric Hypersecretion

Gastric hypersecretion occurs in up to one third of patients with SBS.[26] Parietal cell hyperplasia and hypergastrinemia are common after massive intestinal resection.[9, 27] Fortunately, this acute hypersecretory state is usually transient, lasting only a few months. Gastric hypersecretion is greater after jejunal than after ileal resection. It is associated with high levels of serum gastrin and appears to result from the loss of inhibitory hormones such as gastric inhibitory peptide and vasoactive intestinal polypeptide secreted in the jejunum.[28]

In the patient with SBS, who already has a compromise in nutrient absorption because of the reduced small intestinal mucosal surface, the increased gastric acid load further impairs absorption by inactivating pancreatic lipase and deconjugating intraluminal bile salts. Gastric secretions can contribute to significant fluid losses and ostomy output, exacerbate diarrhea, and lead to peptic ulcer disease.[29] Medical management is generally successful in decreasing gastric hypersecretion in most of these patients.[30, 31] In patients who do not respond to medical management, complications of peptic ulcer disease such as obstruction, bleeding, and perforation may ensue.[32]

Cholelithiasis

The absorption of conjugated bile salts, as part of the enterohepatic circulation, occurs solely within the ileum; therefore, bypass or removal of this segment disrupts bile salt recirculation.[18] Cholelithiasis becomes a frequent problem in patients with SBS, particularly in those on long-term TPN.[33–36]

Despite the fact that the saturation of bile with cholesterol increases after ileectomy, 40% of these patients have radiopaque (calcium-rich) rather than radiolucent (cholesterol-rich) gallstones. Three possible reasons have been proposed to explain these phenomena.[14] First, excess unconjugated bile salts returning to the liver escape into the canaliculi and pass down into the ductules, where they are absorbed in exchange for bicarbonate, thus increasing the precipitation of calcium. Second, the low concentration of bile acids in the canaliculi induces passive diffusion of calcium through the leaky tight junctions of hepatocytes. Third, the deconjugation of bile salts by bacteria leads to excessive production of ursodeoxycholic acid, which produces bicarbonate secretion.

Increased operative morbidity and mortality in patients with SBS and the higher incidence of cholelithiasis have prompted some physicians to recommend prophylactic cholecystectomy before gallstone formation.[37, 38] This avoids the need for another surgical operation and also eliminates the diagnostic dilemma one often faces in patients with SBS who have already developed liver dysfunction. The first strategy in preventing cholelithiasis is early enteral feedings. If this is not feasible, intermittent administration of CCK may prevent bile stasis.[39] Cholecystectomy is often not possible at the time of massive small intestinal resection and should be considered at subsequent abdominal operations.

Liver Disease

Nearly all patients with SBS surviving on TPN develop some signs of liver dysfunction. The etiology of liver dysfunction in patients with SBS is multifactorial. Some of these factors relate to the loss of intestine, whereas others are secondary to the use of long-term TPN. Even the underlying cause of SBS may also have an independent influence on the development of liver dysfunction. With the loss of intestine, there is a proportional loss of portal blood flow. Since the liver receives most of its nourishment and oxygenation via the portal vein, this decrease in blood flow decreases the influx of trophic factors for the hepatic parenchyma. The subject of TPN-induced liver dysfunction is addressed in Chapter 8 of this book. The state of the remaining small intestine can also contribute to liver dysfunction. For instance, patients on long-term TPN for SBS secondary to Crohn's disease have a high incidence of liver dysfunction.

This dysfunction can be partially reversed by the concomitant administration of antibiotic agents by mouth, suggesting that bacterial overgrowth in the intestinal lumen plays a causative role in liver dysfunction.

Nephrolithiasis

Normally, dietary oxalate binds to intraluminal calcium to form an insoluble complex that is excreted in the stool. However, in patients with SBS, and colon in continuity, calcium preferentially binds to unabsorbed fatty acids, leaving oxalate free for absorption in the colon.[40] Additionally, bile salts reaching the colon increase oxalate absorption by increasing intestinal permeability.[19] Increased absorption of dietary oxalate eventually results in the development of calcium oxalate nephroureterolithiasis. Maintaining adequate hydration and a diet low in oxalate and administering oral calcium salts reduces the risk of this complication.[5]

◆ INTESTINAL ADAPTATION

After extensive small intestinal resection, the remaining intestine adapts to the loss of absorptive area. The adaptive response begins 12 to 24 hours after resection and continues for 1 to 2 years.[5] Increased nutrient and fluid absorption occurs through both structural and functional changes in the remaining intestine (Table 14–2). In general, the intestine dilates and elongates as the mucosal surface area increases owing to villus cell hyperplasia and increased crypt depth.[41] Functionally, fluid and nutrient absorption is enhanced by an increase in brush-border enzyme activity.[42, 43] The precise mechanisms of intestinal adaptation are

Table 14–2. Prognostic Indicators in Short Bowel Syndrome

Prognosis Indicator	Intestinal Adaptation	Long-Term Survival
Age	Negative correlation Younger always better	Infants and elderly have poor TPN tolerance
Remaining bowel	The longer the better Disease-free is better Ileum better than jejunum; colon preservation is better	The longer the better Disease-free is better Ileocecal valve preservation is better
Associated conditions	Ongoing sepsis or ischemia is worse	Organ dysfunction (cardiac, renal, pulmonary, or hepatic) is worse

TPN, total parenteral nutrition.

not completely understood, but known factors include luminal nutrients, biliopancreatic secretions, and intestinal hormones and peptide growth factors.

Exposure of the remaining intestine to luminal nutrients is essential for intestinal adaptation. Numerous animal studies have demonstrated that the absence of luminal nutrients causes mucosal atrophy.[44–47] Further evidence for the direct effect of luminal nutrients on epithelial cells is demonstrated by the decreasing gradient of villus height, nucleic acid content, and mucosal enzyme activities from the duodenum to the ileum.[48] Levy and colleagues showed that enteral feedings during the early phase of intestinal adaptation of patients with SBS decrease the likelihood of dependence on long-term TPN.[49] Although elemental feedings were thought to offer an advantage over polymeric diets, there does not appear to be a difference in absorption or tolerance.[50, 51] Additionally, elemental diets are known to induce colonic mucosal atrophy.[52]

Glutamine

Glutamine, a neutral gluconeogenetic amino acid, is considered a major fuel source for enterocytes and colonocytes.[53, 54] In addition to maintaining intestinal structure in normal and diseased states, glutamine appears to be of particular benefit after extensive intestinal resection.[55] Several studies have demonstrated beneficial effects ranging from postresectional enterocyte hyperplasia to enhanced fluid and electrolyte absorption.[56–59] Many of these effects are observed after enteral but not parenteral administration of glutamine, perhaps implicating its direct trophic effects. Likewise, oral glutamine has been shown to increase serum levels of growth hormone in humans, which is also considered to have trophic effects on the small intestine.[60]

Triglycerides and Fatty Acids

The superiority of long-chain triglycerides (LCTs) over proteins and polysaccharides on inducing intestinal adaptation has been demonstrated in several animal studies.[61] The relative saturation of LCTs also has an impact on the degree of intestinal adaptation. Menhaden oil, a highly unsaturated fat, increases the mucosal weight, DNA content, and intestinal protein content when compared with other sources of unsaturated fat.[62] In addition, medium-chain triglycerides (MCTs), which do not require pancreatic enzymes for digestion, do not increase intestinal adaptation as much as LCTs.[63] The essential fatty acids, linolenic and linoleic acid, appear to be as effective as LCTs alone in promoting intestinal adaptation. During intestinal adaptation, supplemental linoleic acid increases the intestinal adaptation mucosal protein content compared with minimal daily requirements of LCTs.[64]

Fiber and Short-Chain Fatty Acids

Dietary fiber and its by-products (SCFAs) have a variety of effects throughout the gastrointestinal (GI) tract, including effects on intestinal morphology, transit time, and nutrient absorption. Pectin, a water-soluble and fermentable fiber, promotes mucosal cell proliferation in both the small intestine and the colon of rats after massive small intestinal resection.[65] Fermentable fibers given during the intestinal adaptation phase can delay gastric emptying,[66] lengthen the small intestinal and colonic transit times,[67] and bind bile salts.[68] The viscous properties of pectin produce entrapment of water and solutes, thereby increasing the intestinal transit time. However, this effect may also limit the exposure of nutrients, water, minerals, and electrolytes to the intestinal epithelium and worsen diarrhea. As already mentioned, fermentable fibers and unabsorbed starch polysaccharides reaching the colon can contribute to the energy requirements of an individual with SBS.[69] It is estimated that the absorption of SCFAs from the colon provides 5 to 10% of daily energy requirements.[70] In addition to SCFAs' trophic effects on the intestine,[71] animals administered TPN supplemented with SCFAs had enhanced sodium and water absorption[72] and less mucosal atrophy after extensive intestinal resection.[73]

Enteric Hormones and Growth Factors

During intestinal adaptation, the delivery of nutrients to the small intestine produces direct trophic and functional changes and also stimulates enteric hormone and biliopancreatic secretion. It is well documented that hypergastrinemia, with accompanying mucosal hyperplasia, occurs after extensive small intestinal resection. However, this trophic effect is not seen in the distal small intestine.[74, 75] Biliopancreatic secretions diverted to the distal small intestine result in ileal mucosal hyperplasia.[76, 77] Because biliopancreatic secretions are stimulated in response to CCK and secretin, the direct effects of these two hormones on intestinal adaptation have been investigated. The administration of CCK to animals has rendered conflicting results. It appears that the potential beneficial effect of CCK on intestinal adaptation is related to the stimulation of biliopancreatic secretions, which in turn influence the release of other enteric hormones such as enteroglucagon.[5]

In animal models of intestinal resection, enteroglucagon is trophic to the small intestine.[78] The serum concentration of enteroglucagon increases after small intestinal resection primarily in response to the increased nutrient load entering the ileum.[79] The effects of enteric hormones on intestinal adaptation may be related to the production of polyamines (e.g., putrescine, spermidine, spermine, and cadaverine), which are trophic compounds whose production is regulated by the enzyme ornithine decarboxylase.[80] After intestinal resection in rats, the inhibition of ornithine decarboxylase activity resulted in the suppression of DNA synthesis and a complete absence of intestinal adaptation.[81] Forget and colleagues found higher levels of polyamines in the feces of children with malabsorption, including SBS, than in healthy control subjects.[82]

Epidermal growth factor (EGF), insulin-like growth factor I (IGF-I), and recombinant human growth hormone (rHGH) have shown the most promise in enhancing intestinal adaptation after extensive resection. EGF is secreted by the salivary glands and enteroendocrine glands of the proximal small intestine. EGF enhances cell replication, DNA and RNA synthesis, and polyamine levels, as well as ornithine decarboxylase activity in vitro.[83] In animal models of massive small intestinal resection, EGF increases nutrient absorption and intestinal regeneration.[84, 85] The trophic effects of EGF on intestinal cell proliferation require the presence of glutamine.[86]

The administration of exogenous rHGH promotes mucosal hyperplasia after extensive small intestinal resection.[87] The rHGH increases amino acid transport in the jejunum and ileum by increasing the number of functional carriers in the brush-border membrane.[88] It has also been shown to increase colonic mass and mechanical strength.[89] The administration of EGF and rHGH has been shown to accelerate intestinal adaptation as demonstrated by increased nutrient transport and villous hypertrophy.[90] IGF-I, which is regulated by growth hormone, enhances intestinal hyperplasia, hypertrophy, and nutrient absorption.[91] Like EGF, IGF-I induces ornithine decarboxylase activity, thereby increasing polyamine synthesis.[92] When glutamine is combined with IGF-I, protein accretion is significantly enhanced after extensive intestinal resection.[93] New peptides and cytokines (e.g., glucagon-like peptide 2 and interleukin 11) continue to be discovered and may eventually be described as the primary mediators of intestinal adaptation.[94, 95]

Clinical trials of rHGH in patients with SBS have shown mixed results. In a study by Byrne and coworkers, patients receiving rHGH, glutamine, and a modified diet improved nutrient absorption, decreased stool output, and decreased their dependence on TPN.[96] In contrast, Scolapio and colleagues reported modest improvements in electrolyte absorption and delayed gastric emptying, but no change in small intestinal morphology, stool losses, or macronutrient absorption.[7] An issue that is difficult to resolve is whether rHGH administration has its greatest effect on intestinal adaptation in the early postresectional period or if its administration months later to the time of injury will reinitiate the adaptive process. Furthermore, the long-lasting effects of short-term administration of rHGH on intestinal adaptation are unknown. Intestinal hormones and growth factors demonstrate a complex interrelationship of effects on the small intestinal mucosa; future research will, one hopes, elucidate the most important growth factor or combination of growth factors to enhance the process of intestinal adaptation.

◆ SURGICAL THERAPY

Surgical intervention in patients with SBS falls into two categories: (1) treatment required for the inciting event and (2) delayed surgery to improve intestinal function and, ideally, to provide autonomy from TPN. The goal of the initial surgery is to treat the primary illness and/or its complications while preserving as much small intestine as possible.[14] The surgical approach follows standard rules of surgery, such as intra-abdominal abscess drainage, proper management of enteric fistulas, and relief of intestinal obstruction. Abdominal reoperation is required in approximately 50% of patients with SBS.[32] The decision to perform delayed surgery to improve intestinal function is not as well defined as the decision to perform surgery after the inciting event.

Reoperations in patients with prior massive resections are extremely difficult. Peritoneal spaces collapse just from the loss of the small intestine, and the development of adhesions makes it extremely difficult to establish planes of dissection and expose the remaining small intestine. In the process of dissecting adhesions, the intestinal lumen is often entered (enterotomy), and this creates the risk of a further loss of intestine. In addition, the indication for surgery is usually not a life-or-death issue but a quality-of-life matter, which makes determination of a risk-to-benefit ratio very subjective. The benefit is usually not freedom from TPN but the ability to enjoy normal eating, that is, without pain, bloating, and an urgency to defecate. The importance of this physiologic activity can be appreciated only when one has cared for patients with SBS. In addition to an attempt to improve quality of life, surgery may become necessary in patients with SBS who enter a downward spiral of complications. These include recurrent catheter sepsis and thrombosis with a loss of venous access and hepatic failure.[97, 98] Mortality in the pediatric population has been reported as high as 20%.[99, 100]

Indications for surgical intervention in patients with SBS include the inability to advance enteral feeding in the presence of TPN-induced complications.[48] The procedures developed to improve intestinal function have not been uniformly successful, and most surgeons will not consider performing surgery until the intestine has reached maximal intestinal adaptation.

The goal of surgical therapy is to address the specific anatomic and physiologic abnormalities of the remaining small intestine. The abnormalities involve increased intestinal transit time, decreased mucosal surface

area, and ineffective peristalsis resulting in bacterial overgrowth of the intestine. Procedures designed to decrease the intestinal transit time include intestinal valves, reversed segments of intestine, colonic interposition, and intestinal pacing. Tapering enteroplasty, intestinal lengthening (Bianchi's procedure), and the growth of neomucosa are alternatives for the patient with insufficient mucosal surface area and poor peristalsis. Finally, improved immunosuppressive agents and insight into small intestinal immunology are making transplantation a realistic alternative for the patient with SBS.

Intestinal Valves

The importance of the ileocecal valve (ICV) in patients with SBS became evident in an early report of survival in SBS.[101] Infants with an ICV required a minimum of 15 cm of small intestine, compared with 40 cm in those without an ICV. The ICV slows intestinal transit, allowing increased nutrient contact with the mucosal surface, and prevents the reflux of stool from the colon into the small intestine, decreasing bacterial overgrowth. Preservation of the ICV is therefore a priority during any surgical procedure for SBS. Multiple techniques for creating artificial valves have been described, but clinically only a few cases have been reported. Ricotta and associates reported success with a 4-cm valve,[102] and Waddell and colleagues reported three patients with various lengths of small intestine who underwent creation of a 2-cm valve in the distal limb.[103] Two of the patients of Waddell and colleagues improved after the procedure, but the third patient developed an obstruction at the site of the valve, necessitating its removal. Elaborate valves have been designed in experimental models, but many potential problems, such as valve necrosis, intestinal obstruction, intussusception, and poor sphincter function, still exist.

Reversed Segments and Colonic Interposition

Successful outcomes with reversed intestinal segments in postvagotomy diarrhea (dumping syndrome) to slow peristalsis have prompted surgeons to apply this procedure to patients with SBS and rapid intestinal transit. Although most reports in the literature have been limited to case studies, two reviews of patients with SBS and reversed intestinal segments have shown some benefit.[104, 105] The reversed segment accomplishes two goals: it creates a functional valve, slowing peristalsis, and it disrupts the intrinsic nerve plexus, decreasing distal myoelectric activity.[106] The length of intestine to be reversed is important because a segment that is too short may be ineffective in slowing peristalsis, whereas a segment that is too long may create an intestinal obstruction.

Colonic interposition has been used in both the isoperistaltic and antiperistaltic directions in patients with rapid intestinal transit. The clinical experience with colonic interposition is even more limited than with reversed segments of small intestine. Glick and colleagues reported the results of six patients with colonic interposition, three of whom were eventually weaned from TPN.[107] The mechanism by which this procedure is effective is related to the intrinsic ability of the colon to absorb nutrients, water, and electrolytes and its slower peristaltic activity.[108, 109]

Intestinal Pacing

Under normal circumstances, small intestinal transit and motility are controlled by pacesetters initiating myoelectric impulses in the proximal duodenum.[110] Experimental models of intestinal pacing involve transection of the intrinsic nerve plexus in the proximal intestine with pacing of the distal small intestine.[111] Improvements in absorption have been demonstrated, but the safety and efficacy of this procedure have not yet met the criteria for clinical application.

Intestinal Tapering

Dilated small intestine is prone to bacterial overgrowth that can further aggravate malabsorption in the patient with SBS.[112] One of the options for improving intestinal function is intestinal tapering, that is, tapering enteroplasty. This procedure reduces the circumference of the intestine by either imbricating or excising the redundant intestinal wall along the antimesenteric border.[113] We-

ber and colleagues reported the efficacy of this procedure in 16 infants with SBS.[114]

Intestinal Lengthening

Bianchi has reported a procedure designed to improve peristalsis, increase mucosal surface area, and increase intestinal transit time while correcting dilatation.[115] The procedure is based on the anatomic feature of the intestinal vasculature, which bifurcates just before reaching the edge of the intestine, branching out independently to each side of its wall. This hemicircumferential segmental blood supply allows division of the intestine along its longitudinal axis into two tubes. The parallel tubes are closed off on the lateral aspect and then anastomosed at the ends, resulting in a narrower segment of intestine that is twice as long. The results of the Bianchi procedure and its modifications have been encouraging in infants and children with SBS, with investigators reporting reduced dependence on TPN and minimal operative morbidity.[116–119]

Other Experimental Procedures for Treating Short Bowel Syndrome

Tissue expanders and mechanical distraction have been used in animal models to increase the mucosal surface area.[120–122] The idea of neomucosa has evolved from growing mucosal cells on the serosal surface of intestine to creating artificial intestine on collagen scaffolds.[123, 124] Additionally, intestinal stem cell transplantation has been successful in experimental animals.[125]

Intestinal Transplantation

Intestinal transplantation is an alternative for a very select group of patients with SBS and life-threatening complications of TPN. Technically, small intestinal transplantation is not difficult. The first technically successful small intestinal transplant in an animal was performed in 1902 by Alexis Carrel. However, some inherent characteristics of the intestine have created major obstacles in expanding the clinical applications of small intestinal transplantation. These include the large amount of lymphoid tissue contained in the intestinal epithelium, the lamina propria, Peyer's patches, and mesenteric lymph nodes; the symbiotic presence of enteric bacteria; and the abundant expression of major histocompatibility complex class II molecules on the surface of mucosal cells.[126] These immunologic features of the intestine create the need for very potent doses of immunosuppressive agents to prevent and control rejection, and these agents can render the grafted intestine inefficient in dealing with luminal bacteria.

SBS is the most common indication for intestinal transplantation in children and adolescents and accounts for two thirds of the cases. Through February 1997, 273 intestinal transplants have been performed in 260 patients.[127] Approximately half of the patients were alive 2 years after transplantation, and 80% of them were free of TPN. The principal complications of intestinal transplantation are acute and chronic rejection, lymphoproliferative disorders, graft-versus-host disease, and infection. Previous efforts to prevent graft rejection too often resulted in lethal infection and death.[128]

The development of new immunosuppressive agents (tacrolimus) and the advances in immunomodulatory techniques (donor–bone marrow transplantation) have created new enthusiasm for intestinal and composite visceral transplantation. In the early 1990s, investigators discovered that hematopoietic cells of bone marrow origin, which are found in all organs, migrate and engraft peripherally after transplantation.[54, 129] This has evolved into the theory of chimerism: a dual immune reaction with allograft acceptance involving the responses of coexisting donor and recipient immune cells, each to the other causing reciprocal clonal expansion followed by peripheral clonal deletion. Improving graft tolerance through chimerism is the basis for concomitant bone marrow transplantation from the same donor.

In a review by the University of Pittsburgh, 80% of the 98 patients in their report had SBS as the cause of their intestinal failure.[130] Some patients received a combined liver–small intestinal transplant, whereas others received small intestine alone. The conditions necessitating transplantation in the "only small intestine" group included frequent catheter sepsis, vanishing central venous access, and early signs of hepatic dysfunction. Actuarial survival at 1 and 5 years was 72% and 48%, respectively, with over 90% of their patients independent of TPN. The researchers concluded that allograft acceptance is compatible with that of other solid organs, the liver is significantly but marginally protective of concomitantly engrafted intestine, and the morbidity and mortality of the procedure is still too high for widespread application. The long-term effects on graft tolerance after bone marrow augmentation will be of particular interest in years to come. Future advances in transplantation may involve ex vivo intestinal irradiation to deplete mature donor leukocytes in combination with bone marrow augmentation, as well as the use of closely matched live donors from whom only short segments are harvested. Through the development of new modalities for immunosuppression and the expansion and improvement of the donor pool, intestinal transplantation may become the preferred treatment option for patients with SBS.

◆ MANAGEMENT OF PATIENTS WITH SHORT BOWEL SYNDROME

The management of patients with SBS is based on optimizing nutrient assimilation and preventing the complications of TPN and the sequelae of chronic malabsorption. After a massive small intestinal resection, patients generally progress through three phases, and in each phase the management priorities are different (Table 14–3). These phases are (1) the early, or postoperative, phase; (2) the intermediate, or stabilization, phase; and (3) the late, long-term phase in which intestinal adaptation may be achieved or the patient may become dependent on TPN for life. Although there are some common sequelae and treatment modalities to all phases of SBS, the management must be individualized to each patient, taking into consideration the underlying illness and comorbidities and therefore the patient's prognosis.

Early Phase of Short Bowel Syndrome

In the early, or postoperative, phase (first month), the priorities of care are fluid and electrolyte repletion, preservation of the venous system, and salvage of as much intes-

Table 14–3. Phases of Short Bowel Syndrome

	Timing	Intermediate	Late
Timing	Resection–POD 30	POD 30–POD 90	POD 90–adaptation
Life threats	Sepsis, dehydration	Macronutrient deficits	Micronutrients deficits
	Comorbidities	Comorbidities	SBS sequelae
			TPN complications
Priorities	Gain IV access	Stabilize fluid and nutrients	Facilitate quality living
	Preserve gut length	Pharmacotherapy	Consider surgery
Nutritional intervention	Continuous TPN	Cycled TPN	Cycled TPN
	NPO	Enteral stimulation	Enteral vs. oral

IV, intravenous; NPO, nothing by mouth; POD, postoperative day; SPS, short bowel syndrome; TPN, total parenteral nutrition.

tine as possible. Fluid losses are common in all phases of recovery but are much greater in the early phase and can amount to several liters per day. If not appropriately replaced, these losses can result in hypovolemia, hypotension, and even more intestinal ischemia in patients with marginal splanchnic perfusion. Close monitoring of intakes, outputs, and hemodynamic parameters, even pulmonary pressures in some cases, is essential. Frequent measurement of serum and urine chemical constituents are also essential to gauge the adequacy of fluid and electrolyte replacement. Of all electrolytes, sodium is the one that deserves particular attention because losses in this phase are very high, ranging between 80 and 100 mEq/L of GI output (i.e., stool or ostomy effluent). Zinc is a trace element also lost in GI secretions and therefore is required in supranormal amounts by patients with SBS.

Pharmacologic treatment of diarrhea is initiated early to help reduce fluid and electrolyte losses. Octreotide is now used as the first line of treatment to control fluid and electrolyte losses during the early phase of SBS. This somatostatin analogue has a greater half-life than somatostatin and has proven efficacious in drastically reducing GI secretions, as well as reducing biliopancreatic fluid production. The major drawbacks of octreotide are the production of biliary sludge and even gallstones. Because both SBS and TPN administration are independent risk factors for gallstone formation, the use of octreotide can be risky if the patient has not undergone cholecystectomy. Another matter of concern with the use of octreotide is the risk of causing further intestinal ischemia. Octreotide has been successfully used to treat bleeding from esophageal varices in patients with portal hypertension because of its potent effect on decreasing

mesenteric blood flow. This can also be of concern in patients with marginal perfusion who underwent extensive suturing and/or anastomosing of the intestine because of the risk of poor wound healing and leakage. Octreotide was administered only subcutaneously, and because injections were painful, patients' acceptance and compliance were also a problem. Fortunately, it is now well accepted that octreotide is just as effective when mixed with TPN and administered intravenously. Finally, a side effect to keep in mind when using octreotide is the induction or worsening of hyperglycemia.

All patients who undergo massive intestinal resection must receive a gastric antisecretory agent, that is, H_2-receptor antagonists or proton pump inhibitors. This is necessary to treat the hypersecretory state induced by SBS and can also help reduce stool output. Other pharmacologic agents used in the early phase of SBS include opiates as antimotility agents, and cholestyramine as a bile salt binder. Cholestyramine is most effective in patients who have lost their ileum but maintained some colon in continuity. Although it may be very helpful in this early phase when the patient is consuming very little or no fat by mouth, it may also produce steatorrhea once the patient resumes oral intake of fat.

As stated, one important priority in the early phase of SBS is the preservation of the venous system. In patients who sustained a massive loss of intestine, the venous system becomes their "lifeline" because it is the main route for nutrition, hydration, and the delivery of medications. Misuse or abuse of superficial veins can lead to thrombosis that progresses into deep veins and, over time, to the loss of venous access, which will then preclude the administration of TPN, leading to the demise of the patient. Therefore, this must be communicated to all health care professionals caring for the patient, even by posting signs in the patient's room. Typical offenses in the category of vein abuse are pulmonary artery catheter introducers left in place for long periods of time. These introducers are large-bore, stiff catheters that should remain in place only during the 48 to 72 hours that a pulmonary artery catheter is used for central venous pressure monitoring. Once there is no longer a need for central venous pressure monitoring, the introducer must be removed; if that venous access is to be preserved, then the introducer is exchanged over a guidewire for a small-bore catheter. It should be clear to every caregiver in the intensive care unit that the recent addition of extra lumens to the pulmonary artery catheter (Swan-Ganz) is not a reason to maintain an introducer in place any longer than what is required for hemodynamic monitoring. Another avoidable cause of venous thrombosis is the use of peripheral parenteral nutrition. Although very effective in many other types of patients, peripheral parenteral nutrition is not used in patients with SBS owing to their high protein requirements as well as the long-term nature of the nutritional intervention.

The best way of preserving the venous system is to place a long-term catheter (i.e., made of silicone rubber) as early as the diagnosis of SBS is established. A more in-depth discussion on vascular access is presented later in this chapter. Whenever possible, all septic foci should be eliminated before the placement of a long-term catheter. In modern medicine, the old dictum of using a dedicated single-lumen line for TPN has become obsolete. Most patients now receive a double-lumen catheter in which one lumen may be dedicated to TPN and the other is used for medications and blood drawing. In patients with a single-lumen catheter or with a double-lumen catheter with one blocked lumen, the only lumen available is often used for more purposes than TPN administration.

Intermediate Phase of Short Bowel Syndrome

The intermediate, or stabilization, phase ranges from postoperative days 30 to 90.

Nowadays, patients in this phase of SBS are being discharged from the acute care facility and transferred to an extended care facility or rehabilitation center. During that transition, the nutritional support team is intimately involved with the entire discharge process, verifying the adequacy of all other therapies aside from TPN. Many patients with SBS are discharged from the acute care facility with one or more of the following problems and therapies: open wounds, a tracheostomy, drain tubes, ostomy appliances, dialysis, chronic intravenous (IV) antibiotic therapy, anticoagulation therapy, feeding tubes, dermal patches, and many other forms of medications. The care of patients with SBS can become so complex that many patients lose their primary physician and become patients of multiple specialists. Because of the natural experience of the nutritional support team with SBS patients, the responsibility of coordinating the entire care of these patients falls on this team. For instance, a careful review of all the therapies ordered for a patient often reveals contradicting or overlapping orders and even the continuation of therapies that are no longer needed.

The treatment priorities in the intermediate phase are the accurate assessment of nutrient and fluid requirements and the introduction of enteral nutrients. Before being discharged from the acute care facility, patients with SBS should have the best possible assessment of energy and nitrogen needs. Next to a loss of IV access, the second most common complication in patients with SBS is liver dysfunction. In order to minimize the risk of liver dysfunction, caloric requirements should be gauged as accurately as possible, and this is best done by indirect calorimetry. The total energy needs are estimated, and the mix of fuels is adjusted according to the respiratory quotient measured in each patient. Nitrogen needs are best determined by nitrogen balance, which can be done simply by the measurement of urinary urea or, more accurately, by a Kjeldahl test of urine as well as stool.

Although experimental data suggest that early stimulation to the GI tract would foster better intestinal adaptation, this is not very practical in the clinical setting. The early introduction of enteral nutrients is followed by increased GI losses; therefore, most patients with SBS are maintained with nothing by mouth until fluid losses can be accurately matched with fluid replacement and a positive balance is reached for all nutrients. Once the patient has reached a point of stabilization, enteral stimuli are introduced to the GI tract. Some patients with SBS reach this intermediate phase with some form of access to the GI tract, for example, gastrostomy, jejunostomy, or some type of tube in a fistula. When such an access to the GI tract is available, intestinal adaptation can be stimulated by the slow infusion of a diluted elemental diet (very low fat) or a semielemental diet (peptide based with MCTs). In patients without an access to the GI tract, liquid diets can be offered to the patient by mouth. Ideally, the diet should be lactose-free, high in protein, low in fat, and isotonic and include minerals and electrolytes in concentrations that favor intestinal absorption and reduce secretion. There are now ready-to-use commercially available diets that meet some of these criteria—for example, the World Health Organization rehydration solution and Pedialyte.

Late Phase of Short Bowel Syndrome

The late phase of SBS begins after the third month from the loss of intestine. It is during this phase when the ultimate fate of the remaining intestine will be decided, that is, whether intestinal adaptation is sufficient to fully compensate for the loss of intestine or whether instead the patient will become entirely or partially dependent on parenteral replacement of nutrients and fluids. The exact time at which intestinal adaptation occurs is highly variable and depends on the same factors that determine the severity of SBS. These include the length and level of remaining intestine, the presence or absence of intrinsic disease in the remaining intestine, and the presence or absence of the ileocecal valve and/or colon. Because all these factors occur in variable combinations among patients with SBS, there is no simple formula to predict the final outcome in an individual patient. However, it is widely accepted that if a patient has not reached intestinal adaptation by 2 years after a loss of the intestine, that person will be dependent on TPN for life.

Some patients may not require replacement of all nutrients parenterally, but only of those that cannot be supplemented orally in sufficient quantities. A typical example is the patient who can meet all nutrient and fluid requirements by the oral route except for essential fatty acids, magnesium, and calcium. This is a common scenario in patients who have lost their ileum to resections for radiation enteritis. High-dose pelvic radiation (without protection of the small intestine) has been a common therapeutic modality for women with gynecologic malignancies. Usually, the full damage to the ileum does not become evident until many years (e.g., 20 to 30) after the radiation treatment. These patients often achieve good intestinal adaptation, but they may require a monthly infusion of fat emulsions, magnesium, and calcium. The parenteral replacement of magnesium and calcium is also necessary because oral supplementation tends to worsen diarrhea and malabsorption.

Patients who become life-dependent on TPN are prone to certain complications. This predisposition may be simply due to the long-term nature of TPN in these patients (e.g., catheter-related complications); other complications may be precipitated by the combination of long-term TPN and long-term sequelae of SBS (e.g., hepatobiliary dysfunction and metabolic bone disease).

◆ TOTAL PARENTERAL NUTRITION (TPN) TO PATIENTS WITH SHORT BOWEL SYNDROME

Once the diagnosis of SBS is made, TPN is immediately begun. Establishing venous access with a multilumen catheter (a catheter with more than one access port) is essential for proper TPN administration while replacing the fluctuating fluid and electrolyte losses. Replacement of fluid and electrolytes through another access port prevents frequent reformulations of the TPN solution. Once fluid and electrolyte losses reach a steady state, all fluid and nutrient requirements are incorporated into the TPN formula. The challenge in this early phase is to meet all fluid and nutrient requirements without creating an intravascular volume overload. In particular, patients with underlying cardiac, pulmonary, or renal insufficiency are at risk of developing fluid overload.

Nutrient prescription is made based on the patient's age, body size, degree of metabolic stress, nutritional status, glucose tolerance, and comorbid conditions such as sepsis or renal or hepatic insufficiency. The amount of amino acids included in TPN formulas for patients with SBS is higher than that prescribed to patients with no loss of intestine. In the absence of renal or hepatic insufficiency, nitrogen prescription usually ranges between 1.5 and 2 g of amino acids per kilogram per day. Aside from the early hypercatabolism after surgery, patients with SBS continue to have increased protein losses by malabsorption of proteins secreted in the GI tract, such as digestive enzymes, and desquamated mucous and epithelial cells. Caloric requirements are usually within the range of nonstressed patients on long-term TPN, that is, 25 to 30 kcal/day. Most physicians who manage patients with SBS prescribe a mixed-fuel formula, that is, 60 to 70 percent of calories as carbohydrates and 30 to 40 percent of calories as fat. There are some concerns about the long-term use of lipid emulsions made exclusively with LCTs. These are discussed in Chapter 3 and include overloading of the reticuloendothelial system and possible immune compromise. Fortunately, new lipid emulsions, already commercially available in Europe, are made of a combination of LCTs and MCTs. This combination reduces the potential side effects of LCTs while providing MCTs, which are more easily oxidized.

Several micronutrients are prescribed to patients with SBS in larger amounts than the amounts normally included in TPN formulas. These include sodium, potassium, chloride, calcium, magnesium, zinc, copper, selenium, ascorbic acid, and vitamin D. The exact amounts are determined in the early phase of SBS by supplementation and monitoring of serum levels. Iron supplementation may also be required, and this can be done by a loading dose or by daily supplementation after adequate testing for allergic hypersensitivity responses, ranging from itching, urticaria, and bronchospasm to fatal reactions.

Before discharge, the TPN regimen is "compressed" into a fraction of hours to create cycles of infusion alternating with cycles of no infusion of TPN. The cycling of TPN makes a substantial difference in the quality of life of patients by "freeing" them from the formula infusion during the day so they can lead a productive and enjoyable life. In addition, there are physiologic ad-

vantages to the cycling of TPN by creating fluctuating levels of circulating insulin. This allows lipolysis and fat mobilization, thereby reducing the likelihood of fatty liver and possibly increasing protein synthesis.

Daily fluid and nutritional requirements need to be met at a steady state before beginning the compression process. Cardiac and pulmonary compromise, as well as glucose intolerance, are the main limiting factors in achieving cycling of the TPN formula. Cycling is preferably accomplished in the hospital over a 3- to 4-day period. The infusion period is progressively reduced to 20 hours the first day, 16 hours the second day, and 12 hours the third day, depending on the glucose and fluid tolerance. At each step of the compression, the rate is cut by half before discontinuing the infusion to prevent rebound hypoglycemia. For example, a patient who was requiring daily infusions of 2400 mL receives 120 mL/h over 20 hours the first day of compression, but the rate is tapered to 60 mL/h for 60 minutes before disconnecting the infusion. This hypothetical patient receives 150 ml/h over 16 hours the second day and 200 mL/h over 12 hours by the third day of compression with the rates decreasing to 75 and 100 ml/h over the last 60 minutes of infusion, respectively. After discharge, routine blood chemistry tests are performed weekly before renewing the prescription of the TPN formula.

◆ VENOUS ACCESS FOR LONG-TERM TOTAL PARENTERAL NUTRITION

Venous access devices (VADs) used for long-term TPN consist of single- or multilumen peripherally inserted central catheters (PICCs) and centrally inserted tunneled or implanted ports (Table 14–4). The tunneled catheter was designed originally by Broviac for use in home TPN and revised by Hickman to provide a larger lumen for blood withdrawal and the administration of chemotherapy. The selection among the different VADs is based on several factors. Some of these factors are a history of previous venous access or accesses, a history of prior surgery or surgeries in proximity to the access sites, the estimated length of therapy, the diagnosis, other uses of the VAD, the cognitive and motor function of the patient or caregiver, the patient's lifestyle, and body

Table 14–4. Long-Term Venous Access Devices

Catheter	Features	Advantages	Disadvantages
PICC	Silicone rubber (most common), also polyurethane and Aquavene Single and multilumen available Groshong type is available Subcutaneous port available Available with or without guidewire	Lower incidence of insertion complications Less trauma to superficial venous system Outpatient and bedside placement Easy to remove	Requires daily heparin flushing, except for Groshong Small bore size does not allow blood sampling and high-rate infusion Self-care can be difficult Arm movement is restricted Requires adequate vein Requires sterile dressings Breakage is common Body image is disturbed
Tunneled catheters	Silicone rubber (most common), also polyurethane Single and multilumen available Groshong is available Antimicrobial cuff available	Easier self-care Repair is possible Modified clean dressings Easier to remove than implanted ports More secure than PICC	Requires daily heparin flushing, except for Groshong Body image is disturbed
Implanted ports	Catheter and septum: silicone rubber (most common), also polyurethane; port: titanium, stainless steel, or plastic Single and multiport available Groshong is available	Reduced maintenance while not being accessed (no dressing and heparinization only every month) Body image is better preserved	Requires transdermic needle Greater procedure for insertion Greater procedure for removal Self-care can be difficult Needle dislodgment can occur

PICC, peripherally inserted central catheter.

image issues. PICCs have gained popularity for the simplicity with which they are inserted. Initially, PICCs were considered for therapies estimated to last a few months; however, their use has been extended for periods as long as 1 year. The drawbacks of PICCs are the difficulty of obtaining a superficial vein in the arm suitable for catheterization in patients who already had multiple venipunctures and the inconvenience of having a foreign body and a dressing in the arm. Also, the lumen of PICCs is significantly narrower than the lumen of tunneled catheters and implanted ports. This can become a problem in patients with SBS who require high-volume infusion to replace large fluid losses.

The purported advantage of implanted ports is the avoidance of an external catheter. For this reason, implanted ports are very convenient for chemotherapy, which is usually administered on an intermittent basis, weekly or monthly. In patients with SBS, however, the need for daily infusions demands either daily cutaneous punctures into the port or the maintenance of a needle through the port for extended periods of time. This second option is usually taken by patients with SBS, and that decision voids the only advantage of implanted ports over tunneled catheters. Melding patient and VAD selection criteria is essential.

Venous Access Device Placement

VADs are placed in the operating suite, in the interventional radiology suite, or even at the bedside. Anesthesia ranges from local infiltration with or without IV sedation to general anesthesia, depending on the type of VAD, the setting, and the preference of the patient and the physician. Prophylactic antibiotics are administered both pre- and postoperatively. Placement of a long-term VAD is contraindicated in patients with unexplained fevers to avoid seeding of the VAD with bacteria. Insertion is preferably performed with fluoroscopic guidance, and chest radiography is always obtained at the end of the procedure.

The antecubital veins such as the basilic, cephalic, and medial cubital veins are used for the placement of PICCs.[131] For tunneled catheters and for implanted ports, the usual access sites are, in order of preference, the subclavian vein, the internal jugular vein, the external jugular vein, and the cephalic vein at the deltopectoral groove. The optimal catheter tip location is the innominate vein or proximal superior vena cava, 3 to 5 cm proximal to the caval-atrial junction or proximal to the cardiac silhouette on chest radiography.[132]

PICCs can be placed at the patient's bedside or in the interventional radiology suite. Tunneled catheters are placed either in the interventional radiology suite or in the operating suite. Implanted ports are always placed in the operating suite. The placement of tunneled catheters can be done by either a percutaneous approach or an open technique. The catheter component of an implanted port can also be placed by a percutaneous approach, whereas the actual implantation of the port requires a skin incision.

During the course of long-term IV therapy, the more common sites for vascular access may become exhausted, and nontraditional approaches must be considered. The use of infraumbilical, translumbar, and transhepatic approaches to the inferior vena cava has been reported in both pediatric and adult patients.[133–135] Gorman and Buzby categorize these approaches as innovative superior vena cava through direct cutdown or via its tributaries; peripheral inferior vena cava via saphenous, inferior epigastric, or femoral veins; retroperitoneal (gonadal and lumbar veins); direct transthoracic (azygos vein, superior vena cava, right atrium); radiographic (translumbar and transhepatic approach); combined surgical-radiologic; and arteriovenous fistulas.[136] The combined surgical and radiologic approach has been described by Torosian and coworkers.[137] This approach consists of using venography to identify a patent peripheral vein and its tributaries; then a guidewire and a Dormier basket are advanced retrograde under fluoroscopic guidance through tributaries to a patent peripheral vein. A venotomy is then performed over the guidewire while the basket is used to pull the catheter into the appropriate position. Bennett reported on the use of the translumbar approach to the inferior vena cava in 29 patients who had obstruction, thrombosis, or local conditions preventing access to the jugular or subclavian vein.[138] Three insertion complications were encountered including inadvertent cannulation of the right renal artery, a small groin hematoma, and a retroperitoneal hematoma. The average catheter days in this series was 121 days with an infection rate of 2.8 per 1000 catheter days.

Venous Access Device Occlusion

A major complication of long-term TPN is VAD occlusion, that is, the inability of fluids to be flushed through the catheter or of blood to be withdrawn. The occlusion is the result of intraluminal, extraluminal, or mural thrombi. The formation of a fibrin sheath can also cause catheter occlusion. The fibrin sheath can originate either at the site of insertion or at the point at which the catheter tip touches the intima of the vein. The presence of the fibrin sheath does not always compromise catheter patency; however, if the sheath covers the tip of the catheter, causing a ball-valve effect, a withdrawal occlusion results. Precipitates from drugs, minerals, or lipid residue can also cause VAD occlusion.[139] Other causes of occlusion include catheter malposition, mechanical occlusion, and compression between the clavicle and the first rib.

Like catheter sepsis, catheter occlusion can jeopardize the life of the VAD and require hospitalization, VAD replacement, diagnostic testing, and the loss of venous access sites. Diagnosis of catheter-related venous thrombosis (CRVT) can be difficult, especially because it can be completely asymptomatic. Patients may present with VAD infection; ipsilateral pain and swelling of the arm, shoulder, and neck; an inability to infuse and/or withdraw fluids; or high infusion pressures. Duplex Doppler imaging,[140] computed axial tomography, and magnetic resonance imaging have all been used for the diagnosis of CRVT or occlusion. The definitive test to determine CRVT is venography performed through both the VAD and the respective extremity.

Factors that contribute to the incidence of CRVT include local trauma, the size of the catheter in relation to the vein, the length of catheterization, and the catheter material. Silicone elastomer and polyurethane produce less platelet aggregation than polyethylene and polyvinyl chloride catheters. One third of all patients with a temporary central venous catheter in place for at least 1 month have mural thrombosis.[141] Multiple cannulations of large veins often predispose to the development of thrombosis.[136] Therefore, the use of short-term polyvinyl chloride catheters, that is, triple-lumen catheters, should be avoided in patients with SBS to minimize the incidence of thrombotic complications and, thereby, the loss of venous access sites. Hyperosmolar, caustic, and extreme pH levels also contribute to thrombus formation. One issue still not fully understood is the relationship between catheter-related infection and thrombus formation, that is, does the presence of sepsis result in CRVT or does the thrombus or fibrin sheath become a target for colonization? In order to reduce the likelihood of CRVT, the prophylactic instillation of urokinase and the use of heparin-bonded catheters have been proposed, although their efficacy still remains unclear.

The prevention and treatment of CRVT include the use of thrombolytic agents, anticoagulation, and tissue plasminogen activator. Decisions regarding whether to remove or to "salvage" a VAD need to be made taking into consideration the availability of other access sites. Catheter occlusions resulting from a fibrin sheath or thrombosis are usually treated with an instillation of 1 mL of 5000 units of urokinase per milliliter (Abbokinase, Abbott Laboratories, Chicago) into the affected catheter lumen.* This procedure can be repeated up to three times and has replaced the use of streptokinase due to its lack of antigenicity, low incidence of side effects, and short half-life. The use of a short-term infusion of urokinase over either 12[142] or 6[143] hours has also been successful in clearing occluded catheters when patency could not be restored with a bolus injection. Precipitation of calcium salts and drugs can also cause catheter occlusion; thrombolytic agents are not effective in this situation. Shulman and associates report the use of 0.1 N hydrochloric acid (0.2 to 1 mL) to successfully restore catheter patency in the case of insolubility-induced precipitates.[144]

Catheter-Related Bloodstream Infection

Catheter-related bloodstream infection (CR-BSI) is the isolation of the same organism from a semiquantitative or quantitative culture of the catheter segment and from the blood (preferably drawn from a peripheral vein) of a patient with an accompanying clinical syndrome of sepsis and no other apparent source of infection. Although the experience with PICC lines is not as large as that with tunneled catheters and implanted ports, the rate of CR-BSI seems to be relatively low. In fact, Loughran and Borzatta report 0.8 infections per 1000 catheter days in their experience of 2506 days.[145] This is quite low when compared with the rate of CR-BSI of implanted ports, 0.21 per 1000 catheter days, and tunneled catheters, 2.77 infections per 1000 catheter days.[146]

The most common pathogens causing CR-BSI are *Staphylococcus epidermidis*, *Staphylococcus aureus*, enterococci, and *Candida albicans*.[146] Most CR-BSIs result from contamination at the cutaneous exit site of the VAD or at the catheter hub; hematogenous seeding from a distant focus of infection; or contaminated infusate.[147] Raad and coworkers describe the nature of intra- and extraluminal colonization of silicone catheters.[148] Extraluminal colonization originates from the skin and occurs within the first 10 days of catheterization. Intraluminal colonization originates from the hub and is seen after 30 days. In long-term VADs, the catheter hub has been shown to be the primary source of CR-BSI.[149] Overall, the incidence of catheter infection in long-term VADs is lower than in temporary catheters.

An alternative to VAD removal is the use of IV antibiotic therapy. The administration of high concentrations of antibiotic agents, instilled through the VAD lumen as an antibiotic lock[150] with the concomitant administration of urokinase,[151] is directed at clearing the biofilm that adheres to the surfaces of the catheter. The formation of this biofilm facilitates the adherence of microorganisms on catheter surfaces and protects them from antibiotics, antibodies, and host phagocytic activity. Jones and associates report successfully using urokinase to clear bacteremia and candidemia from 92% of infected right atrial catheters in children with long-term VADs.[152] Failure and recurrence (2%) occurred more frequently in infection caused by gram-positive organisms (Fig. 14–1).

◆ DRUG THERAPY IN PATIENTS WITH SHORT BOWEL SYNDROME

In patients with SBS, drug malabsorption becomes just as much of a problem as nutri-

---

*Urokinase is no longer commercially available; however, other agents such as recombinant tissue plasminogen activator (rTPA) are currently under investigation.

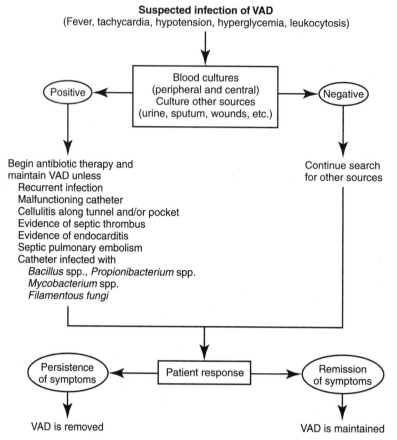

Suspected infection of VAD
(Fever, tachycardia, hypotension, hyperglycemia, leukocytosis)

Blood cultures
(peripheral and central)
Culture other sources
(urine, sputum, wounds, etc.)

Positive

Negative

Begin antibiotic therapy and
maintain VAD unless
   Recurrent infection
   Malfunctioning catheter
   Cellulitis along tunnel and/or pocket
   Evidence of septic thrombus
   Evidence of endocarditis
   Septic pulmonary embolism
   Catheter infected with
      Bacillus spp., *Propionibacterium* spp.
      Mycobacterium spp.
      Filamentous fungi

Continue search
for other sources

Persistence
of symptoms

Patient response

Remission
of symptoms

VAD is removed

VAD is maintained

Figure 14–1. Algorithm for management of vascular access device (VAD).

ent malabsorption. For some particular medications, the problem can be more serious than that of nutrient malabsorption because preparations for IV administration may not yet be available. Even when IV preparations do exist, they may not be compatible with TPN, which makes administration very difficult. Factors that influence drug absorption in SBS include the chemical and physical characteristics of the drug in relation to the level and surface area of the remaining intestine, the mesenteric blood flow, and intrinsic disease in the remaining intestine[153, 154] (Table 14–5).

Medications that are absorbed in the proximal GI tract have the best chance of being absorbed in SBS. The type of preparation of a medication also determines the possibility of absorption in SBS. The rapid transit in SBS prevents the dissolution of enteric coating and the activation of sustained-release mechanisms. Ehrenpreis and colleagues report poor absorption of digoxin in all forms (gels, tablets, and elixirs) in a patient with an end jejunostomy and 18 cm of remaining jejunum.[155] Aside from the IV route, the other routes particularly useful in patients with SBS are the rectal and the transdermal.

Suppositories and dermal patches are commercially available for a variety of medications. Even when not commercially avail-

Table 14–5. Factors Affecting Drug Absorption in Patients with Short Bowel Syndrome

Dependent on Patient's GI Tract	Dependent on Drug
Remaining absorptive surface	Preparation: tablet, elixir
Intrinsic disease	Release: enteric coating
Intestinal transit time	Solubility: aqueous vs. oil
Bacterial overgrowth	Absorption PK: acidic vs. alkaline
Microcurculation	Nutrient interaction

GI, gastrointestinal.

able, some drugs can be prepared for rectal or transdermal administration.[156] Other potential routes for drug delivery are buccal, sublingual, and pulmonary (inhalation of aerosolized drugs). In order to achieve the desired therapeutic effect, drugs may need to be administered to patients with SBS at higher than the recommended dosages. Whenever possible, drug levels in serum should be monitored periodically to take into account changes in absorption as the intestine adapts.

SUMMARY

The advent of TPN has enabled the survival of patients with SBS. This three-decade experience in maintaining patients with SBS alive has allowed a better understanding of the role of the gut in human physiology and redefined the essentiality of nutrients and their respective requirements. Bypassing the gut for nutrient administration with TPN is associated with liver dysfunction, gallstone formation, and metabolic bone disease, whereas the loss of small intestine per se can cause peptic ulcer disease and nephrolithiasis. Patients with SBS are also at risk of complications related to the placement and long-term maintenance of VADs. The nutritional support team has made an enormous difference in the quantity and quality of life for patients with SBS. The services provided by the nutritional support team extend beyond the provision of TPN to include pharmacotherapy and the coordination of all therapies in the ambulatory setting.

REFERENCES

1. Kinney JM, Goldwyn RM, Barr JS Jr, Moore FD: Loss of the entire jejunum and ileum and the ascending colon. JAMA 179:153–156, 1962.
2. Meyer HW: Sixteen-year survival following extensive resection of small and large intestine for thrombosis of superior mesenteric artery. Surgery 51:755–759, 1962.
3. Meguid MM, Campos AC, Hammond WG: Nutritional support in surgical practice, Part II. Am J Surg 159:427–444, 1990.
4. Madara JL, Trier JS: The functional morphology of the mucosa of the small intestine. In Johnson LR, Alpers DH, Christensen J, et al (eds): Physiology of the Gastrointestinal Tract, Vol 2. New York, Raven Press, 1994, pp 925–961.
5. Wilmore DW, Byrne TA, Persinger RL: Short bowel syndrome: New therapeutic approaches. Curr Probl Surg 34:389–444, 1997.
6. Thomson JS: Intestinal resection and the short bowel syndrome. In Quigley EM, Sorrell MF (eds): The Gastrointestinal Surgical Patient. Philadelphia, Williams & Wilkins, 1994, pp 327–352.
7. Scolapio JS, Camilleri M, Fleming CR, et al: Effect of growth hormone, glutamine, and diet on adaptation in short-bowel syndrome: A randomized, controlled study. Gastroenterology 113:1074–1081, 1997.
8. Rombeau JL, Rolandelli RH: Enteral and parenteral nutrition in patients with enteric fistulas and short bowel syndrome. Surg Clin North Am 67:551–571, 1987.
9. Tilson MD: Pathophysiology and treatment of short bowel syndrome. Surg Clin North Am 60:1273–1284, 1980.
10. Dudrick SJ, Latifi R, Fosnocht DE: Management of the short bowel syndrome. Surg Clin North Am 71:625–643, 1991.
11. Gouttebel MC, Aubert BS, Colette C, et al: Intestinal adaptation in patients with short bowel syndrome. Dig Dis Sci 34:709–715, 1989.
12. Koyama S, Hatakeyama K, Muto T: Nutritional management using elemental diet for adult patients with severe short bowel syndrome. Acta Med Biol 40:97–103, 1992.
13. Weser E, Fletcher JT, Urban E: Short bowel syndrome. Gastroenterology 77:572–579, 1979.
14. Hiyama DT, Rolandelli RH: Short bowel syndrome. In Rombeau JL, Caldwell MD (eds): Clinical nutrition: Parenteral nutrition. Philadelphia, WB Saunders, 1993, pp 498–511.
15. Wright HK, Tilson MD: Short gut syndrome, pathophysiology and treatment. Curr Probl Surg 8:1–51, 1971.
16. Hill GL, Mair WSJ, Goligher JC: Gallstones after ileostomy and ileal resection. Gut 16:932–936, 1975.
17. Nightingale JM, Kamm MA, van der Sijp JR, et al: Gastrointestinal hormones in short bowel syndrome. Peptide YY may be the "colonic brake" to gastric emptying. Gut 39:267–272, 1996.
18. Hofman AF: Bile secretion and the enterohepatic circulation of bile acids. In Feldman M, Sleisenger MH, Schorschmidt BF (eds): Sleisenger and Fordtran's Gastrointestinal and Liver Disease: Pathophysiology/Diagnosis/Management. Philadelphia, WB Saunders, 1998, pp 937–946.
19. Chadwick VS, Gaginella TS, Carlson GL, et al: Effect of molecular structure on bile acid–induced alterations in the absorptive function, permeability, and morphology in the perfused rabbit colon. J Lab Clin Med 94:661–674, 1979.
20. Mekhjian HS, Phillips SF, Hofmann AF: Colonic secretion of water and electrolytes induced by the bile acids: Perfusion studies in man. J Clin Invest 50:1569–1577, 1971.
21. Phillips SF, Giller J: The contribution of the colon to electrolyte and water conservation in man. J Lab Clin Med 81:733–746, 1973.
22. Bond JH, Currier BE, Buchwald H, Levitt MD: Colonic conservation of malabsorbed carbohydrates. Gastroenterology 78:445–447, 1980.
23. Haverstad T: Studies of short-chain fatty acid absorption in man. Scand J Gastroenterol 21:257–260, 1980.
24. Pomare EW, Branch WJ, Cummings JH: Carbohydrate fermentation in the human colon and its relation to blood acetate concentrations in venous blood. J Clin Invest 75:1148–1154, 1985.

25. Ruppin H, Barmier S, Sowrgel KH, et al: Absorption of short-chain fatty acids by the colon. Gastroenterology 78:1500–1507, 1980.

26. Carol A, Fleming R, Malagelada JR: Improved nutrient absorption after cimetidine in short bowel syndrome with gastric hypersecretion. N Engl J Med 300:79–80, 1979.

27. Williams NS, Evans P, King RF: Gastric acid secretion and gastrin production in the short bowel syndrome. Gut 26:914–919, 1985.

28. Strause E, Gerson E, Yalow RS: Hypersecretion of gastrin associated with the short bowel syndrome. Gastroenterology 66:175–180, 1974.

29. Thompson JS: Edgar J Poth Memorial Lecture. Surgical aspects of the short-bowel syndrome. Am J Surg 170:532–536, 1995.

30. Murphy JP, King DR, Dubois A: Treatment of gastric hypersecretion with cimetidine in the short bowel syndrome. N Engl J Med 300:80–81, 1979.

31. Nightingale JM, Walker ER, Farthing MJ, Lennard-Jones JE: Effect of omeprazole on intestinal output in the short bowel syndrome. Aliment Pharmacol Ther 5:405–412, 1991.

32. Thompson JS: Reoperation in patients with the short bowel syndrome. Am J Surg 164:453–457, 1992.

33. Manjo N, Bistrian BR, Mansioli EA, et al: Gallstone disease in patients with severe short bowel syndrome dependent on parenteral nutrition. J Parenter Enteral Nutr 12:461–464, 1989.

34. Nightingale JMD, Lennard-Jones JE, Gertner DJ, et al: Colonic preservation reduces need of parenteral therapy, increases incidence of renal stones, but does not change high prevalence of gallstones in patients with a short bowel. Gut 33:1493–1497, 1992.

35. Pitt HA, Lewinski MA, Moller EL, et al: Ileal resection induced gallstones: Altered bilirubin or cholesterol metabolism. Surgery 96:154–162, 1984.

36. Roslyn JJ, Pitt HA, Mann LL, et al: Gallbladder disease in patients on long term parenteral nutrition. Gastroenterology 84:148–154, 1983.

37. Roslyn JJ, Pitt HA, Mann LL, et al: Parenteral nutrition–induced gallbladder disease: A reason for early cholecystectomy. Am J Surg 148:58–63, 1984.

38. Thompson JS: The role of prophylactic cholecystectomy in the short-bowel syndrome. Arch Surg 131:556–559, 1996.

39. Sitzman JV, Pitt HA, Steinborn PA, et al: Cholecystokinin prevents parenteral nutrition induced biliary sludge in humans. Surg Gynecol Obstet 170:25–31, 1990.

40. Dobbins JW, Binder HJ: Importance of the colon in enteric hyperoxaluria. N Engl J Med 296:298–301, 1977.

41. Williamson RC: Intestinal adaptation: Structural, functional, and cytokinetic changes. N Engl J Med 298:1393–1402, 1978.

42. Chaves M, Smith M, Williamson RCN. Increased activity of digestive enzymes in ileal enterocytes adapting to proximal small bowel resection. Gut 28:981–987, 1987.

43. McCarthy DM, Kim YS: Changes in sucrase, enterokinase, and peptide hydrolase after intestinal resection: The association of cellular hyperplasia and adaptation. J Clin Invest 52:942–951, 1973.

44. Bury KD: Carbohydrate digestion and absorption after massive resection of the small intestine. Surg Gynecol Obstet 135:177–187, 1972.

45. Feldman EJ, Dowling RH, McNaughton J, et al: Effects of oral versus intravenous nutrition on intestinal adaptation after small bowel resection in the dog. Gastroenterology 70(pt 1):712–719, 1976.

46. Ford WDA, Boelhouwer RU, King WWK, et al: Total parenteral nutrition inhibits intestinal adaptive hyperplasia in young rats: Reversal by feeding. Surgery 96:527–534, 1983.

47. Hughes CA, Dowling RH: Speed of onset of adaptive mucosal hypoplasia and hypofunction in the intestine of parenterally fed rats. Clin Sci 59:317–327, 1980.

48. Warner BW, Ziegler MM: Management of the short bowel syndrome in the pediatric population. Pediatr Clin North Am 40:1335–1350, 1993.

49. Levy E, Frileux P, Sandrucci S, et al: Continuous enteral nutrition during the early adaptive stage of the short bowel syndrome. Br J Surg 75:549–553, 1988.

50. Lai HS, Chen WJ, Chen KM, Lee YN: Effects of monomeric and polymeric diets on small intestine following massive resection. Taiwan I Hsueh Hui Tsa Chih 88:982–988, 1989.

51. McIntyre PB, Fitchew M, Lennard-Jones JE: Patients with a high jejunostomy do not need a special diet. Gastroenterology 91:25–33, 1986.

52. Janne P, Carpentier Y, Willems G: Colonic mucosal atrophy induced by a liquid elemental diet in rats. Dig Dis 22:808–812, 1977.

53. Souba WW, Smith RJ, Wilmore DW: Glutamine metabolism by the intestinal tract. J Parenter Enteral Nutr 9:608–617, 1985.

54. Souba W, Klimberg S, Plumley D, et al: The role of glutamine in maintaining a healthy gut and supporting the metabolic response to injury and infection. J Surg Res 48:383–391, 1990.

55. Darmaun D, Messing B, Just B, et al: Glutamine metabolism after small intestinal resection in humans. Metabolism 40:42–44, 1991.

56. Gouttebel MC, Astre C, Briand D, et al: Influence of N-acetylglutamine or glutamine infusion on plasma amino acid concentrations during the early phase of small-bowel adaptation in the dog. J Parenter Enteral Nutr 16:117–121, 1992.

57. Kandil HM, Argenzio RA, Chen W, et al: L-glutamine and L-asparagine stimulates ODC activity and proliferation in a porcine jejunal enterocyte line. Am J Physiol 269:g591–g599, 1995.

58. Rhoads JM, Keku EO, Quinn J, et al: L-glutamine stimulates jejunal sodium and chloride absorption in pig rotavirus enteritis. Gastroenterology 100:683–691, 1991.

59. Tamada H, Nezu R, Matsuo Y, et al: Alanyl glutamine enriched total parenteral nutrition restores intestinal adaptation after either proximal or distal massive resection in rats. J Parenter Enteral Nutr 17:236–242, 1993.

60. Welbourne TC: Increased plasma bicarbonate and growth hormone after oral glutamine load. Am J Clin Nutr 61:1058–1061, 1995.

61. Grey VL, Garofalo C, Greenberg GR, Morin CL: The adaptation of the small intestine after resection in response to free fatty acids. Am J Clin Nutr 40:1235–1242, 1984.

62. Vanderhoof JA, Park JH, Herrington MK, Adrian TE: Effects of dietary menhaden oil on mucosal adaptation after small bowel resection in rats. J Parenter Enteral Nutr 106:94–99, 1994.

63. Chen WJ, Yang CL, Lai HS, Chen KM: Effects of lipids on intestinal adaptation following 60% resection in rats. J Surg Res 58:253–259, 1995.

64. Park JH, Grandjean CJ, Hart MH, et al: Effects of dietary linoleic acid on mucosal adaptation after small bowel resection. Digestion 44:57–65, 1989.

65. Koruda MJ, Rolandelli RH, Settle RG, et al: The effect of a pectin-supplemented elemental diet on intestinal adaptation to massive bowel resection. J Parenter Enteral Nutr 10:343–350, 1986.

66. Lawetz O, Blackburn AM, Bloom SR: Effect of pectin on gastric emptying and gut hormone release in the dumping syndrome. Scand J Gastroenterol 18:327–336, 1983.

67. Hillman L, Peters S, Fisher A, et al: Differing effects of pectin, cellulose and liquid on stool pH, transit time and weight. Br J Nutr 50:189–195, 1983.

68. Miettenen TA, Tarpila S: Effect of pectin on serum cholesterol, fecal-bile acids and biliary lipids in normolipemic and hyperlipemic individuals. Clin Chim Acta 79:471–477, 1977.

69. Rombeau JL, Kripke SA: Metabolic and intestinal effects of short-chain fatty acids. J Parenter Enteral Nutr 14(Suppl):181–185, 1990.

70. McNeil NI: The contribution of the large intestine to energy supplies in man. Am J Clin Nutr 39:338–342, 1984.

71. Kripke SA, Fox AD, Berman JM, et al: Stimulation of intestinal mucosal growth with intracolonic infusion of short-chain fatty acids. J Parenter Enteral Nutr 13:109–116, 1989.

72. Roediger WEW, Rae DA: Trophic effects of short chain fatty acids on mucosal handling of ions by the defunctioned colon. Br J Surg 69:23–25, 1982.

73. Koruda MJ, Rolandelli RH, Settle RG, et al: Effect of parenteral nutrition supplemented with short-chain fatty acids on adaptation to massive bowel resection. Gastroenterology 95:715–720, 1988.

74. Sagor GR, Al-Mukhtar MY, Ghatei MA, et al: The effect of altered luminal nutrition on cellular proliferation and plasma concentrations of enteroglucagon and gastrin after small bowel resection in the rat. Br J Surg 69:14–18, 1982.

75. Weser E: Nutritional aspects of malabsorption: Short gut adaptation. Clin Gastroenterol 12:443–456, 1983.

76. Altman GC: Influence of bile and pancreatic secretions on the size of the intestinal villi in the rat. Am J Anat 132:167–178, 1971.

77. Weser E, Heller R, Tawil T: Stimulation of mucosal growth in the rat ileum by bile and pancreatic secretions after jejunal resection. Gastroenterology 73:524–529, 1977.

78. Al-Mukhtar MY, Sagor GR, Ghatel MA, et al: The role of pancreatico-biliary secretions in intestinal adaptation after resection, and its relationship to plasma enteroglucagon. Br J Surg 70:398–400, 1983.

79. Bloom SR: Gut hormones in adaptation. Gut 28(Suppl):31–35, 1987.

80. Dowling RH: Polyamines in intestinal adaptation and disease. Digestion 2(Suppl 46):331–344, 1990.

81. Luk GD, Baylin SB: Inhibition of intestinal epithelial DNA synthesis and adaptive hyperplasia after jejunectomy in the rat by suppression of polyamine biosynthesis. J Clin Invest 74:698–704, 1984.

82. Forget P, Sinaasappel M, Bouquet J, et al: Fecal polyamine concentration in children with and without nutrient malabsorption. J Pediatr Gastroenterol Nutr 24:285–288, 1997.

83. Feldman EJ, Arnes D, Grossman MI: Epidermal growth factor stimulates ornithine decarboxylase activity in the digestive tract of the mouse. Proc Soc Exp Biol Med 159:400–402, 1978.

84. O'Loughlin E, Winter M, Shun A, et al: Structural and functional adaptation following jejunal resection in rabbits: Effects of epidermal growth factor. Gastroenterology 107:87–93, 1994.

85. Saxena SK, Thompson JS, Sharp JG: Role of epidermal growth factor in intestinal regeneration. Surgery 111:318–325, 1992.

86. Ko TC, Beauchamp RD, Townsend CM: Glutamine is essential for epidermal growth factor–stimulated intestinal cell proliferation. Surgery 114:147–154, 1993.

87. Shulman DI, Hu CS, Duckett G, Lavallee-Grey M: Effects of short-term growth hormone therapy in rats undergoing 75% small intestinal resection. J Pediatr Gastroenterol Nutr 14:3–11, 1992.

88. Inoue Y, Copeland EM, Souba WW: Growth hormone enhances amino acid uptake by the human small intestine. Ann Surg 219:715–724, 1994.

89. Christensen H, Jorgensen PH, Oxlund H: Growth hormone increases the mass, the collagenous proteins, and the strength of rat colon. Scand J Gastroenterol 25:1137–1143, 1990.

90. Iannoli P, Miller JH, Ryan CK, et al: Epidermal growth factor and human growth hormone accelerate adaptation after massive enterectomy in an additive, nutrient-dependent, and site-specific fashion. Surgery 122:721–728, 1997.

91. Steeb CB, Trahair JF, Thomas FM, Read LC: Prolonged administration of IGF peptides enhances growth of gastrointestinal tissues in normal rats. Am J Physiol 266:g1090–g1098, 1994.

92. Olanrewaju H, Patel L, Seidel ER: Trophic action of local intraileal infusion of insulin-like growth factor 1: Polyamine dependence. Am J Physiol 263:e282–e286, 1992.

93. Ziegler TR, Mantell MP, Rombeau JL, Smith RJ: Effects of glutamine and IGF-1 administration on intestinal growth and the IGF-1 pathway after partial small bowel resection. J Parenter Enteral Nutr 18(Suppl):20, 1994.

94. Drucker DJ, Erlich P, Asa SL, Brubaker PL: Induction of intestinal proliferation by glucagon-like peptide 2. Proc Natl Acad Sci U S A 93:7911–7916, 1996.

95. Fiore NF, Ledniczky G, Liu Q, et al: Comparison of interleukin-11 and epidermal growth factor on residual small intestine after massive small bowel resection. J Pediatr Surg 33:24–29, 1998.

96. Byrne TA, Morrissey TB, Nattakom TV, et al: Growth hormone, glutamine, and a modified diet enhance nutrient absorption in patients with severe short bowel syndrome. J Parenter Enteral Nutr 19:296–302, 1995.

97. Howard L, Heaphey LL, Timchalk M: A review of the current national status of home parenteral and enteral nutrition from the provider and consumer perspective. J Parenter Enteral Nutr 10:416–424, 1986.

98. Steiger E, Srp F: Morbidity and mortality related to home parenteral nutrition in patients with gut failure. Am J Surg 145:102–104, 1983.

99. Galea MH, Holliday H, Carachi R, et al: Short bowel syndrome: A collective review. J Pediatr Surg 27:592–596, 1992.

100. Grosfeld JL, Rescoria FJ, West KW: Short bowel syndrome in infancy and childhood. Analysis of survival in 60 patients. Am J Surg 151:41–46, 1986.

101. Wilmore DW: Factors correlating with a successful outcome following extensive intestinal resection in newborn infants. J Pediatr 80:88–95, 1972.

102. Ricotta J, Zuidema GD, Gadacz TR, et al: Construction of an ileocecal valve and its role in massive resection of the small intestine. Surg Gynecol Obstet 152:310–314, 1981.

103. Waddell WR, Kern F, Halgrimson CG, et al: A simple jejunocolic "valve" for relief of rapid transit and the short bowel syndrome. Arch Surg 100:438–444, 1970.

104. Panis Y, Messing B, Rivet P, et al: Segmental reversal of the small bowel as an alternative to intestinal transplantation in patients with short bowel syndrome. Ann Surg 225:401–407, 1997.

105. Thompson JS, Rikkers LF: Surgical alternatives for the short bowel syndrome. Am J Gastroenterol 82:97–106, 1987.

106. Tanner WA, O'Leary JF, Byrne PJ, et al: The effect of reversed jejunal segments on the myoelectrical activity of the small bowel. Br J Surg 65:567–571, 1978.

107. Glick PL, de Lorimier AA, Adzick NS, et al: Colon interposition: An adjuvant operation for short gut syndrome. J Pediatr Surg 19:719–723, 1984.

108. Lloyd DA: Colonic interposition between the jejunum and ileum after massive small bowel resection in rats. Prog Pediatr Surg 12:51–106, 1978.

109. Sidhu GS, Narasimharao V, Rani V, et al: Morphological and functional changes in the gut after massive small bowel resection and colon interposition in rhesus monkeys. Digestion 129:47–54, 1984.

110. Cullen JJ, Kelly KA: The future of intestinal pacing. Gastroenterol Clin North Am 23:391–402, 1994.

111. Gladen HE, Kelly KA: Electrical pacing for short bowel syndrome. Surg Gynecol Obstet 153:697–700, 1981.

112. Thompson JS: Surgical considerations in the short bowel syndrome. Surg Gynecol Obstet 176:89–101, 1993.

113. Thompson JS, Langnas AN, Pinch LW, et al: Surgical approach to short-bowel syndrome. Experience in a population of 160 patients. Ann Surg 222:600–607, 1995.

114. Weber TR, Vane DW, Grosfeld JL: Tapering enteroplasty in infants with bowel atresia and short gut. Arch Surg 117:684–688, 1982.

115. Bianchi A: Intestinal loop lengthening: A technique for increasing small intestinal length. J Pediatr Surg 15:145–151, 1980.

116. Bianchi A: Longitudinal intestinal lengthening and tailoring: Results in 20 children. J R Soc Med 90:429–432, 1997.

117. Figueroa-Colon R, Harris PR, Birdsong E, et al: Impact of intestinal lengthening on the nutritional outcome for children with short bowel syndrome. J Pediatr Surg 31:912–916, 1996.

118. Thompson JS, Pinch LW, Murray N, et al: Experience with intestinal lengthening for the short bowel syndrome. J Pediatr Surg 26:721–724, 1991.

119. Weber TR, Powell MA: Early improvement in intestinal function after isoperistaltic bowel lengthening. J Pediatr Surg 31:61–64, 1996.

120. Chen Y, Zhang J, Qu R, et al: An animal experiment on short gut lengthening. Chin Med J (Engl) 110:354–357, 1997.

121. Narayan D, Castro A, Jackson IT, Herschman B: Tissue expanders in the gut: A histologic and angiographic study. J R Coll Surg Edinb 37:402–404, 1992.

122. Printz H, Schlenska R, Requardt P, et al: Small bowel lengthening by mechanical distraction. Digestion 58:240–248, 1997.

123. Choi RS, Vacanti JP: Preliminary studies of tissue-engineered intestine using isolated epithelial organoid units on tubular synthetic biodegradable scaffolds. Transplant Proc 29:848–851, 1997.

124. Kimura K, Soper RT: A new bowel elongation technique for the short-bowel syndrome using the isolated bowel segment Iowa models. J Pediatr Surg 28:792–794, 1993.

125. Kawaguchi AL, Dunn JC, Fonkalsrud EW: In vivo growth of transplanted genetically altered intestinal stem cells. J Pediatr Surg 33:559–563, 1998.

126. Goulet O, Jan D, Brousse N, et al: Small-intestinal transplantation. Ballieres Clin Gastroenterol 11:573–592, 1997.

127. Grant D: Intestinal Transplantation: Report of the International Intestinal Transplant Registry. Transplantation 67:1061–1064, 1999.

128. Todo S, Reyes J, Furukawa H, et al: Outcome analysis of 71 clinical intestinal transplantations. Ann Surg 3:270–282, 1995.

129. Starzl TE, Demetris AJ, Murase N, et al: Cell migration, chimerism, and graft acceptance. Lancet 339:1579–1582, 1992.

130. Abu-Elmagd K, Reyes J, Todo, et al: Clinical intestinal transplantation: New perspectives and immunologic considerations. J Am Coll Surg 186:512–527, 1998.

131. Hadaway L: An overview of vascular access devices inserted via the antecubital area. J Intraven Nurs 13:297–306, 1990.

132. Collier PE, Goodman GB: Cardiac tamponade caused by central venous catheters perforation of the heart: A preventable complication. J Am Coll Surg 181:459–463, 1995.

133. Azizkhan RG, Taylor LA, MJaques PF, et al: Percutaneous translumbar and transhepatic inferior vena caval catheter for prolonged vascular access in children. J Pediatr Surg 12: 165–169, 1992.

134. DeCsepel J, Stanley P, Padua EM, et al: Maintaining long-term central venous access by repetitive hepatic vein cannulation. J Pediatr Surg 29:56–57, 1994.

135. Willard W, Coit D, Lucas A, et al: Long-term vascular access via the inferior vena cava. J Surg Oncol 46:162–166, 1991.

136. Gorman RC, Buzby GP: Difficult access problems. Surg Oncol Clin N Am 4:453–472, 1995.

137. Torosian MH, Meranze SA, Mullen JL, et al: Central venous access with occlusive superior venous thrombosis. Ann Surg 203:30–33, 1986.

138. Bennett JD, Papadouris D, Rankin RN, et al: Percutaneous inferior vena caval approach for long-term central venous access. J Vasc Inter Radiol 8:851–855, 1997.

139. Cunningham RS, Bonam-Crawford D: The role of fibrinolytic agents in the management of thrombotic complications associated with vascular access devices. Nurs Clin North Am 28:899–909, 1993.

140. Kraybill WG, Allen BT: Preoperative duplex venous imaging in the assessment of patients with venous access. J Surg Oncol 52:244–248, 1993.

141. Lowell JA, Bothe A: Central venous catheter related thrombosis. Surg Oncol Clin N Am 4:479–492, 1995.

142. Haire WD, Lieberman RP, Lund GB: Occluded central venous catheters: Restoring function with a 12 hour urokinase infusion of low dose urokinase. Cancer 66:2279–225, 1990.

143. Haire WD, Lieberman RP: Thrombosed central venous catheters: Restoring function with 6-hour urokinase infusion after failure of bolus urokinase. JPEN J Parenter Enteral Nutr 16:129–132, 1992.

144. Shulman RJ, Reed T, Pitre D, et al: Use of hydrochloric acid to clear obstructed central venous catheters. JPEN J Parenter Enteral Nutr 12:509–510, 1988.

145. Loughran SC, Borzatta M: Peripherally inserted catheters: A report of 2506 catheter days. JPEN J Parenter Enteral Nutr 19:133–136, 1995.

146. CDC HICPAC: Guidelines for the prevention of intravascular device-related infection. Infect Control Hosp Epidemiol 17:438–473, 1996.

147. Raad II, Darouiche RO: Catheter-related septicemia: Risk reduction. Infect Med 9:807–823, 1996.

148. Raad II, Coserton W, Sabharwal U, et al: Ultrastructural analysis of indwelling vascular catheters: A quantitative relationship between luminal colonization and duration of placement. J Infect Disease 168:400–407, 1993

149. Sitges-Serra, A, Linares J, Perez JL, et al: A randomized trial on the effect of tubing changes on hub contamination and catheter sepsis during parenteral nutrition. JPEN J Parenter Enteral Nutr 9:322–325, 1985.

150. Krzywda E, Andris DA, Edmiston CE, et al: Treatment of Hickman catheter sepsis using antibiotic lock technique. Infect Control Hosp Epidemiol 16:595–598, 1995.

151. Fishbein JD, Friedman HS, Bennett BB, et al: Catheter-related sepsis refractory to antibiotic treated successfully with adjunctive urokinase infusion. Pediatr Infect Dis J 9: 676–678, 1990

152. Jones GR, Konsler GK, Dunaway RP: Urokinase in the treatment of bacteremia and candidemia in patients with right atrial catheters. Am J Infect Control 24:160–166, 1996

153. Benet LZ, Kroetz DL, Sheiner LB: Pharmacokinetics: The dynamics of drug absorption, distribution, and elimination. *In* Hardman JG, Limbird LE (eds): Goodman and Gilman's The Pharmacological Basis of Therapeutics, 9th ed. New York, McGraw-Hill, 1996, pp 3–27.

154. Smyth DH: Alimentary absorption of drugs: Physiological considerations. *In* Binns TB (ed): Absorption and Distribution of Drugs. Baltimore, Williams & Wilkins, 1964, pp 1–15.

155. Ehrenpreis ED, Guerriero S, Nogueras JJ, et al: Malabsorption of digoxin tablets, gel caps, and elixir in a patient with an end jejunostomy. Ann Pharmacother 28:1239–1340, 1994

156. McFadden MA, DeLegge MH, Kirby DF: Medication delivery in the short-bowel syndrome. JPEN J Parenter Enteral Nutr 17:180–186, 1993.

15

◆ Trauma and Burns

Mette M. Berger, M.D., Ph.D.
René L. Chioléro, M.D.

◆ OVERVIEW

Trauma is a general term encompassing blunt or penetrating injury to any organ of the body, ranging from burns or isolated brain injury to complex extensive multiple injuries. Severely injured patients develop an extensive acute-phase response, very rapidly lose weight, and develop malnutrition. Although this has long been recognized, the metabolic support of the traumatized patient continues to attract considerable interest, as reflected by the 185 publications in 1998 found in MEDLINE using the key words *trauma* and *metabolism* or *nutrition*. The causes for this sustained interest are many. First, the number of trauma patients is large, and the social consequences are heavy. Injury is a major cause of disability and death throughout the world, the third most frequent cause of death in young adults, and accounts for 12.5% of male and 7.4% of female deaths worldwide.[1] Second, the patients who survive the initial insult are frequently critically ill for prolonged periods of time: they develop severe metabolic responses characterized by intensive catabolism that are not completely understood. Third, these patients frequently become dependent on nutritional support, as they require repeated surgical treatment and prolonged periods of rehabilitation. Fourth, research shows that changes in the timing and route of artificial nutritional provision and the proportion and type of nutrients may have a direct impact on the secondary insults and on the development of infections. Finally, as malnutrition is frequent after complicated trauma or surgery, optimization of nutritional management has been shown to decrease the complication rate[2] and to improve the outcome.[3]

Nowadays severely injured patients frequently survive the shock phase, and very soon metabolic support becomes a central preoccupation. This often means using artificial nutritional support because the patient rarely can eat enough food to meet the energy requirements. Moreover, the adaptation to fasting is altered by the critical illness.[4] In the late 1960s, before the introduction of total parenteral nutrition (TPN), significant weight losses, proportional to the extent of injury, were reported. Considering that clinically significant alterations in organ function occur rapidly during acute weight loss and that mortality from starvation added to injury may reach 40%,[5] the importance of nutritional support becomes obvious. Some major changes in the metabolic concepts underlying the nutritional support of trauma patients have occurred during the 1990s; they concern the choice of the route of delivery, the energy and micronutrient requirements, and substrate provision. All these topics continue to elicit extensive debate.

Does the Burn-Injured Patient Differ from Other Trauma Patients?

Burn-injured patients have frequently been separated from patients with other types of injuries. Indeed, some aspects of clinical course are specific: (1) the tissue surface to repair is extensive; (2) the infectious risk is elevated because of the loss of the skin barrier; (3) the patients suffer cutaneous exudative losses of fluids containing large quantities of proteins, minerals, and micronutrients, and this causes acute deficiency syndromes; (4) the venous access is more difficult because of the destruction of the skin at the punction sites, causing a higher infectious risk of catheter-related infection; and (5) compared with other trauma patients, burn patients stay for much longer periods in intensive care units (ICU), often many weeks, and require more prolonged nutritional support. But the similarities between burn and other trauma patients are more important than the differences. Additional morbidity from shock, acute respiratory distress syndrome, sepsis, and multiple organ dysfunction syndrome will occur in any severely injured patient, whatever the cause of the injury. Overall, the metabolic response is similar, the differences being limited to the intensity of the response. All are referred to as *trauma* patients hereafter, unless otherwise specified.

Why Do Severely Traumatized Patients Often Require Artificial Nutrition?

Victims of major trauma are usually unable to feed themselves for extended periods of time. This may be due to coma, impaired voluntary movements, or anorexia, which is invariably present in trauma patients. If the patient is able to eat by mouth, the magnitude of the lack of appetite is related to the severity of the injury[6] and to the use of opiates for analgesia. A prolonged reduction in spontaneous food intake predisposes to malnutrition, which is an important cause of low immunocompetence and reduced resistance to infection in animal and human studies.[7] Malnutrition results in altered organ function, abnormal blood chemistry results, reduced body mass, and outcomes below optimal expectations. Starvation studies have shown that alterations of immune function, muscle strength, and wound healing occur as soon as a subject has lost 5 to 10% of body weight[5] and that the risk of dying from the complications of malnutrition increases with added trauma. In severely injured hypermetabolic patients, catabolism is accelerated, resulting in earlier appearance of malnutrition. The presence of prior alterations of nutritional status extends the indications for artificial nutrition to categories of patients with less severe trauma. Some previously malnourished patients have a clinically evident reduction of the body mass index. These patients will experience high rates of complications, including muscle weakness, wound-healing delay, infections, and increased mortality. At the other extreme, obese patients appear healthy but frequently have an inadequate nutritional status. Indeed, obesity is associated with increased mortality after trauma,[8] although the place of artificial nutrition is still controversial in such patients.

Prevention of malnutrition motivates aggressive nutritional support, which frequently has to be delivered by the intravenous route. Like any medical technique, TPN has true indications but also limitations and complications. Some complications are directly related to the application of the TPN technique to patients without malnutrition or appropriate indications[9] or to improper formulation of the solution.[10] Others are due to the effects of TPN on the acute-phase response,[11] which is intense after trauma; TPN may worsen the outcome.[12] This can probably be ascribed to the deleterious effects of overfeeding. Strict adherence to actual recommendations and to nutritional protocols avoid most problems.

This chapter develops recent knowledge about the general responses to injury, the changes in energy expenditure, and the influence of starvation and stress on injured patients. The changes in substrate metabolism occurring after trauma and the impact of specific parenteral nutrition on these pathways are then discussed. Clinically relevant considerations regarding trauma patient categories, the impact of parenteral nutrition on the outcome, the specific indications for parenteral nutritional after trauma, and how to manage TPN are then detailed.

◆ METABOLIC CONSIDERATIONS

The metabolic response and the nutritional requirements of the injured patient have been under investigation since the 1930s, pioneered by Sir David Cuthbertson.[13] After the initial resuscitation, injured patients exhibit a biphasic response, characterized by a complex combination of humoral, endocrine, metabolic, and immune responses.[4] Muscle wasting, tissue catabolism, and increased energy expenditure are the characteristic features of this response. The association between weight loss, infection, and a poor outcome has long been recognized. It has become clear that full nutritional support is unable to completely reverse catabolism until convalescence. However, the place of specific nutrients remains debated.

Acute-Phase Response and Regulation Mechanisms

The acute-phase response is a highly orchestrated sequence of events involving local and systemic alterations. It constitutes a regulatory response that is essential for defense against injury and infection. This response is part of the systemic inflammatory response syndrome (SIRS) and is characterized by the production of numerous hormonal and nonhormonal mediators that modulate the metabolic,[14] immune, neural, and endocrine responses. The net result is a mobilization of endogenous body substrates, making them available for energy production, tissue repair, and immune defense.

Four types of mechanisms regulate the metabolic changes:

1. *Tissue factors* are particularly prominent in trauma. Local injury, whatever the mechanism, produces local inflammatory mediators: histamine, bradykinin, prostaglandins, and others produce local effects before the systemic changes, and this stimulates the neural afferences immediately.

2. *Cytokines* constitute a large group of peptides that elicit a wide range of systemic and local reactions. The synthesis of proinflammatory cytokines increases strongly after injury:[15, 16] Tumor necrosis factor and interleukin 6 (IL-6) levels are negatively correlated with the outcome, whereas IL-2 and IL-6 levels are correlated with the insult severity.[17] IL-6 initiates the reprioritization of hepatic protein synthesis toward the acute-phase proteins.[18] The cytokines are responsible for immunomodulatory effects and for cellular proliferation, growth, and differentiation. They have wide-ranging autocrine (cellular), paracrine (neighboring tissue), and endocrine (at a distance) effects and have direct impact on the different metabolic pathways: their effects on protein catabolism are particularly strong.[17–19] The first visible clinical chemistry manifestation of the acute-phase response is the serum or plasma protein changes, which start within 12 hours of injury: the C-reactive protein level increases sharply and remains elevated as long as SIRS persists. Thereafter, albumin, prealbumin, transferrin, and immunoglobulin levels decrease, whereas fibronectin, antitrypsin, ceruloplasmin, and α_1-acid glycoprotein levels increase. The changes last at least 3 weeks.[18, 20] Trace element distribution is also af-

fected in response to IL-6. Plasma concentrations of iron, selenium, and zinc decrease, whereas copper levels tend to increase.[21, 22] This response is further amplified by the losses through wound exudates, drains, and hemorrhage, which result in negative micronutrient balances.[23, 24]

3. *Endocrine changes* also occur. Catecholamine, cortisol, and glucagon levels increase strongly soon after injury. The catecholamines appear to be the first-line metabolism stimulators, particularly of energy metabolism and substrate release. Glucagon acts only on the liver by stimulating both glycogenolysis (transient) and gluconeogenesis (sustained effect). Cortisol exerts permissive effects on both liver and peripheral tissues. Nevertheless, studies in healthy subjects show that although administration of the triple hormone combination epinephrine, cortisol, and glucagon causes some of the classic hypermetabolic changes,[25] other mechanisms contribute to the full-blown picture.[26]

Insulin levels are normal to elevated in the flow phase (see next section). There is a peripheral resistance to insulin, with an elevated basal rate of endogenous glucose production despite normal or elevated insulin levels and high plasma glucose levels. Adrenergic blocking agents have no depressing effects on glucose production. Data show that there is an uncoupling of the growth hormone–insulin-like growth factor I (IGF-I) axis after burn injury, with an attenuation of the effects of insulin on IGF-binding protein-1.[27] Growth hormone secretion is increased but fails to support IGF-I secretion by the liver. IGF-I levels instead tend to decrease, through mechanisms that remain unexplained. The consequence is that high growth hormone concentrations mainly exert catabolic effects, such as the stimulation of lipolysis.

The thyroid axis is also affected, losing its predominant role in metabolic rate control, which is shifted toward the sympathoadrenal axis. Patients exhibit a euthyroid sick syndrome, also called *low T₃ syndrome*, with normal thyroid-stimulating hormone and free and total thyroxine (T_4) levels, low free and total triiodothyronine (T_3) levels, and increased reverse T_3 levels. The meaning of these changes is not understood, and the restoration of serum levels of T_4 or T_3 by supplementation fails to modify the level of hypermetabolism[28] and outcome.

4. Finally the *central nervous system* also contributes to the full development of the acute-phase response, because of its integrative functions at the hypothalamic and pituitary levels.[29]

Although the initial changes occurring after injury are perceived as beneficial, the persistence of this response pattern for prolonged periods causes a progressive loss of body cell mass, particularly of skeletal muscle; weakness; and increased susceptibility to infection. It favors organ dysfunction and eventually organ failure. Therefore, efforts have been made at modulating this response by nutritional means, and pharmaconutrition has been developed to address it. Nutritional intervention consists in the administration of two to seven times the usual amounts of selected normal dietary constituents;[30] this is discussed in the specific sections.

Energy Expenditure and Thermal Control

General

The metabolic response to trauma is essentially biphasic. Immediately after injury, there is a period of hemodynamic instability with reduced tissue perfusion and release of high levels of catecholamines. This initial sideration phase has classically been called the *ebb phase*.[13] It is characterized by lowered total oxygen consumption (Vo_2), decreased central core temperature, vasoconstriction, low cardiac output, and a low metabolic rate. Depending on the severity of injury and the success of the hemodynamic resuscitation, it lasts a few hours or persists for up to 72 hours.

This first phase is progressively replaced by the *flow phase*, characterized by high Vo_2, elevated resting energy expenditure, elevated substrate flows, and accelerated potassium and nitrogen losses. In burns, visceral blood flow and splanchnic oxygen consumption have been shown to increase with the total cardiac output and total Vo_2.[31] During this phase, the body's temperature is

generally increased and central thermoregulation is shifted upward, especially in severe burns. Metabolic studies carried out in burn patients at different ambient temperatures show that the core and skin temperatures as well as resting energy expenditure (REE) remain elevated despite a net reduction in heat loss by the increased ambient temperature. Coverage of burns with water-impermeable dressings in order to reduce water vapor release only moderately reduces the metabolic rate. These changes last until convalescence, often after the patient has been discharged from the hospital.

Assessing Energy Requirements

Accurately defining the patient's energy needs is the first step of nutritional support. Energy requirements of severely injured patients are specific and vary with the time elapsed since injury.[32] As both underfeeding and overfeeding have deleterious consequences, an accurate assessment of energy expenditure (EE) is desirable to adjust the individual caloric intake, particularly in patients with a prolonged and complicated course. Different approaches are possible. The EE may be measured or estimated clinically. The simplest way is to make a rough estimate, setting the requirements at 25 to 30 kcal/kg/day in nonburn injuries and 30 to 40 kcal/kg/day in burns depending on the extent of injury. Alternative methods are the use of (1) metabolic charts based on age, sex, and body surface, (2) the Harris-Benedict equation adjusted for activity and stress, or (3) any other standard equation.[31] Most of these equations overestimate the requirements (Table 15–1).

Indirect calorimetry is based on measurements of Vo_2, Vco_2, and nitrogen excretion, and the 24-hour EE is extrapolated from 30 to 60–minute measurements. It can be used in clinical settings in both pediatric and adult injured patients at different stages of their clinical course.[32, 33] To be reproducible, the technique requires a strict standard condition during the measurements.[34] Another method to determine Vo_2 in clinical settings is to use the pulmonary artery catheter, with the Fick equation in combination with the Weir equation to determine the nonprotein energy expenditure.[35] In critically ill patients, Vo_2 values determined by indirect calorimetry and those determined by the

Table 15-1. Methods to Estimate Energy Requirements with Some Specific Equations*

Method	Formula	Accuracy
Any patients		
Harris-Benedict equation	TEE = EBEE × activity factor × stress factor†	Overestimates
	where EBEE =	
	M: 66.5 + (13.8 × weight [kg]) + (5 × height [cm]) − (6.8 × age [years])	
	F: 655.1 + (9.6 × weight) + (1.8 × height) − (4.7 × age)	
Burn patients[31]	(20 kcal × kg body weight) + 40 kcal × % of BSA burned	Overestimates
Elderly burn patients[31]	Basal requirement + 65 kcal/ % of BSA burned	Overestimates
Trauma[169]	MEE = − 4343 + (10.5 × % of BSA burned) + (0.23 × CI) +	Reasonably
	(0.84 × EBEE) + (114 × T °C) − (4.5 × days after injury)	accurate
	TEE = MEE × activity factor	

*The majority overestimate requirements.
Major surgery, 1.0–1.2; skeletal trauma, 1.2–1.5; major burn, 1.4–1.8
†BSA, body surface area; EBEE, estimated basal energy expenditure from the Harris-Benedict equation; MEE, measured energy expenditure using indirect calorimetry; TEE, total energy expenditure; CI, caloric intake; T, temperature.

Fick equation, are well correlated, despite a large variability. Yet the use of this method for nutritional purposes remains controversial.[4]

The REE measured by indirect calorimetry corresponds to the rate of energy expenditure by patients under clinical conditions, that is, in a nonthermoneutral environment, under nonfasting conditions, or with drug or supportive treatment administration. Total energy expenditure (TEE) is the sum of REE and the thermic effect of food and physical activity. Nutrient metabolism consumes energy; in critically ill patients, the nutrient-induced thermogenesis accounts for approximately 10% of the calories given to the patients during nutritional support.[36] The relation of REE to TEE may vary under different physiologic conditions. If a critically ill trauma patient is studied under the previously mentioned standard conditions,[34] the metabolic rate is generally greater than the resting energy expenditure (REE) predicted from the Harris-Benedict equation: the increase in REE is proportional to the severity of injury[37] and is called *hypermetabolism*. Massive burn injuries are classically known to produce the most intense hypermetabolic responses, whereas elective surgery produces only minimal increases. The increase in REE plateaus by 55 to 70% of the body surface area burned.[31] In burned children, the TEE is 1.18 ± 0.17 times the measured REE and is significantly correlated with the REE (r^2 = .92).[38] If the determina-

tion of REE by indirect calorimetry is available, TEE can reasonably be estimated by multiplying the measured REE by a factor of 1.2. Present knowledge suggests that this is an optimal level of energy provision from both substrate maximization and clinical outcome standpoints in adults as well as in children.[38, 39]

Low REE determinations occur in critically ill patients. Technical error in the performance of indirect calorimetry is one of the more frequent causes of this type of result; volume leaks result in apparently decreased V_{O_2} and V_{CO_2}. But true hypometabolism may be present on occasions; the most common clinical causes include deep sedation and analgesia, muscle relaxant administration, hypothermia, and shock. Further, REE is particularly difficult to predict in some categories of trauma patients, for example, brain injury.

Finally, it is important to consider that the metabolic rate changes over time. In most types of injury, the maximal increase in the REE measured by indirect calorimetry occurs between the fifth and the 15th days.[40] During this period, many authors have measured values of REE varying between 1.2 and 1.5 times the predicted value. The alterations persist for at least 3 weeks and up to 2 to 3 months after severe burns. A weekly determination of REE is hence desirable in patients with persistent catabolism. The administration of fixed amounts of energy to critically ill trauma patients based on standardized equations is acceptable only when indirect calorimetry measurements are not available.[41]

Metabolic Response to Injury

Simple Versus Stress Starvation

Energy production is a constant phenomenon because of the very small adenosine triphosphate (ATP) reserve. In a resting condition, ATP stores are very limited, covering body energy requirements for 2 to 3 minutes only. Thus, a continuous flow of substrate to the tissue must be supplied for ATP synthesis. Healthy subjects can sustain prolonged periods of total starvation without irreversible harm, thanks to complex metabolic adaptations. During the first 12 to 24 hours, the provision of glucose is achieved by mobilization of hepatic glycogen stores. Thereafter, gluconeogenesis is stimulated. However, this initial response is inadequate in the long term, because the maintenance of a high gluconeogenesis rate would require the breakdown of large amounts of proteins, leading to wasting. This problem is solved by a metabolic adaptation consisting of preferential oxidation of endogenous fats associated with an intensive stimulation of hepatic ketone body synthesis, which massively increases their blood concentrations. Subsequently, as starvation progresses, body mass and energy expenditure gradually decrease, which further favors the economy of endogenous fuels.[6, 42] The most striking example of adaptation to total starvation in previously healthy young men was provided by the 30 Irish Republican Army hunger strikers in Northern Ireland (Fig. 15–1): in 60 to 70 days, they lost 38% of their body weight, and 10 died.[5]

Several features distinguish the metabolic response to starvation in severely injured patients. Glucose production is increased as a response to stress mediators (glucagon, cortisol, and epinephrine, as well as cytokines) and is essentially accounted for by gluconeogenesis. Glucose demand is concomitantly increased because of a continuous utilization by inflammatory cells and wounds. Net glucose production is fueled mainly by the conversion into glucose of amino acids derived from endogenous protein catabolism. Lipolysis is stimulated and releases large amounts of fatty acids, but hepatic ketogenesis is blunted and the provision of ketone bodies as an energy substrate for the brain fails to occur. As starvation progresses beyond 3 days, the protein catabolism persists (reflected by an elevated urinary nitrogen excretion) and is associated with a rapid loss of lean body mass. In addition, REE does not decrease as long as the acute-phase response persists. Consequently, starvation in the critically ill

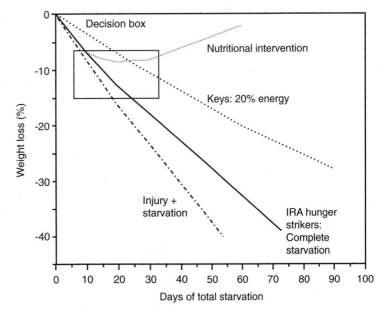

Figure 15–1. Effect of total or partial starvation on weight loss, and the effect of added injury. The figure shows the percentage weight loss in relation to the number of days of starvation. The decision box corresponds to a period during which nutritional management will reverse a deleterious outcome. IRA, Irish Republican Army. (Redrawn from Allison SP: Clin Nutr 11:319–330, 1992.)

trauma patient is associated with a high risk of protein-calorie malnutrition. Figure 15–1 shows how the addition of trauma worsens the outcome in the case of starvation.

The mechanisms responsible for the altered adaptation to starvation after injury are still incompletely understood. Many mediators are involved. Among them, the most important include the stress hormones, the cytokines, the tissue factors locally released from the injured areas, and several inflammatory mediators. In the healthy subject, starvation induces a finely tuned endocrine response. With prolonged starvation, the thyroid hormones regulate the total energy requirements and the T_3 concentration falls, leading to the low T_3 syndrome: proteolysis and lipolysis rates eventually fall, as do the rates of gluconeogenesis and ketogenesis. The hypothalamic-pituitary-adrenal axis is stimulated. The hypothalamic neuropeptide Y concentration increases in part because of low leptin levels, suppressing sympathetic activity and corticotropin-releasing hormone expression. In contrast, the response to injury involves a stimulation of hypothalamic corticotropin-releasing hormone release through the actions of cytokines and of the limbic nervous system. This leads to sympathetic activation, marked increases in epinephrine and cortisol levels, increased energy expenditure, and insulin resistance. As a consequence, blood glucose and insulin concentrations remain high, suppressing ketone body formation in the liver. The thyroid axis loses its predominant regulatory role. In addition, critically ill patients frequently receive small amounts of glucose as part of fluid resuscitation or drug delivery, and these amounts are possibly sufficient to inhibit ketogenesis.

Body Composition

The acute-phase response is associated with changes in body water content that are proportional to the severity of injury. These changes closely parallel body weight changes,[43] with early increases in total body weight of 15 to 20%, due mainly to the expansion of extracellular water compartment.

Trauma patients lose weight rapidly in the absence of nutrition, but a significant weight loss occurs even with full nutritional support because of persistent tissue catabolism. The response to artificial nutrition is altered after injury, particularly in the case of a complicated course. Patients with burns affecting less than 20% of the body surface area experience their maximal weight loss during the third week;[44] with burns exceeding 40% of the body surface area, the maximal weight loss (22%) is reached at 8 weeks after injury. The changes observed in other types of major injury are also important, leading to a progressive decrease in lean body mass. This is mainly related to a rapid decrease in the total body protein content, with a 10% loss of muscle mass after only 10 days, despite full artificial nutritional support. After 3 weeks, close to 20% of the total body protein is lost, 67% coming from skeletal muscle.[43] Proteolysis markedly reduces the body stores of proteins and free amino acids.[45] The loss worsens in cases of superimposed sepsis.

◆ SUBSTRATES

Proteins

Metabolism

Persistent muscle protein catabolism is a major problem in trauma patients. The net result is devastating. Over the first 21 days after injury, critically ill trauma patients lose 16% of their total body protein content despite full nutritional support.[46] During the first 10 days, close to two thirds of this protein loss come from skeletal muscle; thereafter it comes also from viscera. There are different theories to explain this increase in catabolism. The classic explanation is that it is initiated to provide amino acids for the synthesis of glucose via gluconeogenesis, for acute-phase protein synthesis and wound healing, and for direct oxidation to provide energy. An alternative explanation may be the imperative provision of glutamine for the immune cells (see later and Chapter 28).[47] Further, protein loss in major trauma is accompanied by progressive cellular dehydration[48] and altered muscle amino acid transport.[4] It has been hypothesized that the massive proteolysis is triggered and maintained by cell shrinkage secondary to cellular dehydration.[49] During the 1990s, it was recognized that whole-body protein turnover reflects only poorly the events occurring in the different organs: the kinetics of individual proteins may change in opposite directions.[50, 51] In the muscle compartment, protein turnover increases after injury, degradation predominating over synthesis, resulting in negative nitrogen balances. In the splanchnic area, protein turnover increases too, but synthesis is more important than catabolism, resulting in a positive balance in this area.

Protein Supply

The principal reason for artificial nutritional support after trauma is to reduce protein catabolism and to promote protein synthesis. Indeed, complete TPN increases whole-body protein synthesis and minimizes the rate of protein loss but does not suppress it.[52]

The amount of energy to be provided as amino acids to limit protein catabolism has been much debated and remains controversial. Protein losses are increased after injury because of additional losses from drains, collections, the gastrointestinal tract, and cutaneous exudative losses.[23, 46, 53] But increased losses do not necessarily mean increased requirements. During the 1970s and 1980s, the provision of 2 to 3 g of protein per kilogram per day was recommended after trauma and burns, based essentially on nitrogen balance data. In the 1980s, a poorly controlled study in burned children showed that the administration of large amounts of proteins was associated with an improved immune response, nutritional status, and clinical course;[54] 1.5 to 3.0 g of protein per kilogram of body weight per day were thereafter recommended, with a nonprotein energy-to-nitrogen ratio of about 100 kcal/g. The *calorie-to-nitrogen ratio* has long been a popular method to determine the protein intake on the basis of the caloric requirement, using the fact that 1 g of nitrogen is roughly equivalent to 6.25 g of protein. In the absence of organ failure, a range between 100 and 200 kcal/g of nitrogen has been recommended for the critically ill patient (liver and renal failure prompting reductions of the nitrogen load): a standard regimen is 150 kcal/g of nitrogen.

Animal data show that high levels of protein do not have positive effects on outcomes[55]: there is a ceiling effect. Human studies have also questioned aggressive protein feeding.[4] In burn patients, 1.3 to 1.4 g of protein per kilogram of body weight per day were effective to reduce endogenous protein breakdown, but the administration

of amino acids in excess of 1.5 g/kg/day failed to result in a further stimulation of protein synthesis. Excess amino acid intake may instead produce deleterious effects because of their large thermogenesis (20 to 25% of calories infused) and because of the generation of large amounts of nitrogenous waste products. Two well-controlled isotopic studies have shown, by comparing various levels of intake, that with the provision of more than 1.5 g of proteins per kilogram per day, further incorporation of nitrogen into protein does not occur in critically ill trauma patients.[40]

According to current knowledge, the clinician should obtain information on the pre-illness weight—that is, before the accumulation of water resulting from resuscitation and the acute-phase response—and prescribe 1.2 g/kg/day. If this information is not available, 1 g/kg/day measured on admission is a fair approximation.[41]

Albumin is a negative acute-phase marker. During periods of acute stress, its synthesis is depressed, and particularly in burns, increased vascular permeability leads to redistribution of albumin to extravascular spaces. This results in serum concentrations frequently below 20 g/L during the early phase after injury,[56] remaining between 25 and 30 g/L for many weeks (Fig. 15–2). This hypoalbuminemia is well tolerated, and TPN has no impact on it.[18, 57] There is no rationale for providing albumin to burn patients on a systematic basis. Outcome studies carried out in severely burned children have shown no benefit of supplementation.[56] Gastrointestinal complications, including the frequency of diarrhea, are unaffected. Moreover, in Europe supplementation with albumin is expensive.

Glutamine. The most abundant free amino acid in the body and muscles, glutamine constitutes 70 to 80% of the total body free amino acid pool. It is a nontoxic nitrogen shuttle to transport ammonia from peripheral tissues to visceral organs. Glutamine is a nitrogen donor for acute-phase proteins and, with alanine, is a major substrate for gluconeogenesis.[45] In severely injured patients, there is a rapid decrease in plasma and muscle glutamine levels. This is due to two independent phenomena: enhanced metabolic utilization and low exogenous glutamine supply. These changes participate in some of the immune system

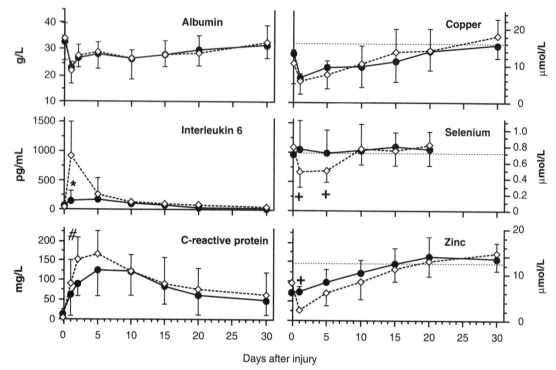

Figure 15–2. Changes observed in plasma proteins and trace elements during the acute-phase response in 20 severely burned patients (48% BSA burns), expressed as mean ± SD. The patients were randomized to receive a placebo solution (group C, --- ◇ ---) or large intravenous copper, selenium, and zinc supplements (group TE, —●—) from admission for 8 days (see doses in Table 15–2). The interleukin 6 production and C-reactive protein levels were significantly lower and the selenium and zinc concentrations significantly higher in the supplemented group. The dotted lines indicate the lower reference range values for trace elements BSA, body surface area; C, control; TE, trace element; *, $P < .001$; #, $P < .03$; +, $P < .05$. (From Berger MM, Spertini F, Shenkin A, et al: Trace element supplementation modulates pulmonary infection rates after major burns: a double-blind, placebo-controlled trial. Am J Clin Nutr 68:365–371, 1998.)

alterations characteristic of trauma. For reasons of solubility and stability in solution, glutamine cannot be included in standard amino acid mixtures. It can, however, be administered parenterally as a dipeptide (alanine-glutamine or glycine-alanine) that is hydrolyzed in the circulation.[58] Alternatively, the α-ketoglutamate analogues of glutamine can be administered. The provision of 10 to 30 g of this precursor per day increases muscle, hepatic, and plasma glutamine levels in surgical and cancer patients.[59, 60] In pediatric burn patients, glutamine supplementation has been reported to improve the bactericidal activity of the neutrophils.[61] In a randomized trial in critically ill patients including trauma patients, Griffiths and coworkers showed a marked reduction in the 6-month mortality and infectious complications after parenteral glutamine supplementation.[62] Further, a randomized trial using enteral glutamine in

patients with severe multiple trauma reported a significant reduction in infectious complications. Isocaloric and isonitrogenous jejunal nutrition was initiated within 48 hours of admission and continued until the patients tolerated oral feeding, but at least for 5 days. The frequency of pneumonia in the treatment versus the control group was 17% versus 45%, sepsis 3% versus 42%, and bacteremia 7% versus 42%.[63] In the control group, the infections occurred in the first 7 days. These very encouraging results prompt further research to define the place of glutamine supplements and their optimal route of delivery in trauma patients.

Arginine. Arginine is also conditionally essential. Like glutamine, it is used in large amounts by critically ill patients, and balance cannot be achieved by standard amino acid mixtures. It is the unique precursor of nitric oxide (NO). During sepsis, NO generation from arginine has been implicated in hemodynamic response and/or collapse, antibacterial defense, and systemic responses.

Plasma concentrations are severely reduced in burned children and adults. Arginine flux has also been shown to increase after injury,[64, 65] and balance cannot be achieved without an exogenous supply.[66] In animals with experimental burns, arginine supplementation during resuscitation has a favorable effect on cardiac function (less tachycardia, higher blood pressure, lower lactate levels) possibly through NO upregulation.[67] Animal data show that survival after burns is improved after supplementation.[47] Supplementation in nonseptic patients appears safe.[30] At this time, the impact of increased NO production on the immune defense has not been addressed, and the place of arginine supplementation has not yet been defined during the postinjury acute-phase response or in sepsis.

Glucose and Other Carbohydrates

Metabolism

After major injury, impaired glucose tolerance and peripheral insulin resistance with hyperglycemia and unsuppressed endogenous glucose production are constant findings. As early as the 1960s, the analogy between trauma and diabetes was made.[68] The similarities between type 2 diabetes and changes observed in critically ill patients

are many. The changes persist until convalescence and are aggravated in cases of infection. The endocrine changes underlying these alterations are complex: (1) insulin levels are low immediately after injury, then normal to elevated during the flow phase, the response to glucose challenge being unchanged or increased; (2) the levels of the counterregulatory hormones (glucagon, epinephrine, cortisol) are strongly increased.

Injury initiates a strong increase in endogenous glucose production (Fig. 15–3). The glucose turnover increases from 1.9 mg/kg/min in control subjects to 4.4 mg/kg/min in fed trauma patients.[37] This increased glucose flow is used by two main pathways: direct oxidation (brain and tissues) and glycolysis (inflammatory tissues). Glucose serves preferentially as cellular fuel for healing wounds and inflammatory tissues. Glucose oxidation rates increases to 130% above those of control subjects after trauma.[37] Administration of glucose, even in large amounts, fails to suppress endogenous glucose production (see Fig. 15–3), gluconeogenesis, and protein breakdown in trauma and burn patients. This has been attributed essentially to the insulin resistance induced by stress hormones and inflammatory mediators. Glucose itself is also a major regulator of glucose production.

Gluconeogenesis is the main mechanism behind increased glucose production and is under both hormonal and nonhormonal control. Nonhormonal control, which may

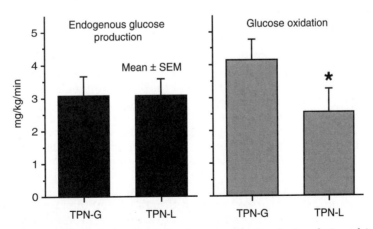

Figure 15–3. Absence of suppression of endogenous glucose production by isocaloric and isonitrogenous total parenteral nutrition (TPN) in 16 patients after major trauma. Glucose oxidation is decreased in the lipid-based TPN (TPN-L: 15% glucose, 15% protein, 70% lipid) compared with glucose TPN (TPN-G: 75% glucose, 15% protein, 10% lipid). *, $P < .05$ vs. TPN-G. (Adapted from Tappy L, Schwartz JM, Schneiter P, et al: Effects of isoenergetic glucose-based or lipid-based parenteral nutrition on glucose metabolism, de novo lipogenesis, and respiratory gas exchanges in critically ill patients. Crit Care Med 26:860–867, 1998.)

involve neural components, is documented in healthy subjects by the observation that hyperglycemia inhibits and severe hypoglycemia stimulates endogenous glucose production. This occurs even when changes in the major glucoregulatory hormones insulin, glucagon, and growth hormones are prevented and when the effects of sympathoadrenal hormones are pharmacologically inhibited.[69]

Carbohydrate Supply

Glucose. The administration of glucose as the sole or principal source of carbohydrate is of long standing in parenteral nutrition. Studies performed using indirect calorimetry have shown that graded glucose-insulin infusion results in a maximal glucose oxidation of about 4 mg/kg/min. Similar studies performed in critically ill patients using ^{13}C-labeled glucose led to a similar estimate of a maximal 4 to 5 mg/kg/min oxidation. The administration of exogenous glucose in excess of this maximal oxidative capacity may produce adverse effects by promoting exaggerated glycogen storage, de novo lipogenesis, and fatty infiltration of the liver. In addition, high glucose oxidation and de novo lipogenesis increase CO_2 production, which may have deleterious effects in patients with respiratory failure, particularly during weaning from mechanical ventilation. Stimulation of de novo lipogenesis has been long documented during the administration of hypercaloric, high-glucose TPN. More recently, it has been observed, using tracer methodology, that the stimulation of de novo lipogenesis also occurred during the administration of isocaloric TPN when glucose represented 75% of the calories.[70] Fatty infiltration of the liver is commonly observed in burn patients and other critically ill patients;[71–73] this is considered to be the consequence of de novo fatty acid synthesis from an excessive exogenous glucose supply, as reflected by respiratory quotients above 1. Based on these considerations, it is recommended to avoid a glucose supply exceeding 4 mg/kg/day and to consider glucose-lipid mixtures for patients without lipid intolerance, because of the previously mentioned maximal oxidizing capacity of glucose.[71, 74]

In past literature, there was a general perception that children can handle exogenous glucose better than adults. More recent data show that this is not correct. Consequently, the upper limit of glucose intake expressed in milligrams per kilogram is similar in children and in adults.[75]

Fructose. Already in 1968, it was proposed that trauma patients should be provided fructose as a carbohydrate source, considering the characteristic glucose intolerance.[68] Compared with glucose infusion, fructose infusion results in moderate glycemic increases. Although insulin is not required for its phosphorylation, it is necessary for the rest of its metabolism. It bypasses the rate-limiting hexokinase step, which may lead to the accumulation of fructose 1-phosphate. Lactic acidosis and hyperuricemia occur, depending on the rate of administration. The place of fructose in modern TPN is not defined in the absence of relevant literature.

Xylitol. This alcohol is a normal intermediate in the pentose phosphate cycle. It is mainly metabolized by insulin-dependent pathways in the liver to glucose via glucose-6-phosphate. After intravenous infusion, it results in modest increases in blood glucose levels in stressed patients.[76] There are no data in the literature to support the use of xylitol in TPN.

Lipids

Metabolism

The lipid profile is modified after injury.[77] High-density lipoprotein levels decrease drastically, low-density lipoprotein levels decrease slightly, and very low density lipoprotein levels increase. Total cholesterol levels decrease, whereas triglyceride levels increase.[78] The mechanisms responsible for these changes are complex, including cytokine and the stress hormones, mainly epinephrine via β_2-adrenergic stimulation.[79] After injury, lipolysis from the endogenous triglyceride stores is accelerated,[80] with a twofold increase in glycerol turnover and a doubling of the free fatty acid (FFA) oxidation rate.[52] But the FFA turnover is increased only 30% compared with controls, suggesting intracellular lipid oxidation. Ketogenesis is decreased or abolished.[81]

Unlike glucose release, FFA release may be completely dissociated from its rate of oxidation. Furthermore, the FFAs participate in the triacylglycerol–fatty acid cycle. Under normal conditions, about 50% of FFAs are re-esterified. In severely burned patients, this percentage is increased to about 65%, because of the intense stimulation of lipolysis.[4] Consequently, there are far more endogenous FFAs available as energy substrate than the organism can oxidize. Indeed, the exogenous fat supply does not affect the substrate metabolism significantly in burned children; the fats maintain peripheral lipid stores rather than being used as an energy source.[72] Lipid-containing TPN does not inhibit lipid mobilization in adult injured patients either.[37] In healthy individuals, it has been well documented that the protein and carbohydrate intake determine their own rate of oxidation, and that fat oxidation varies to make up the difference between the protein and carbohydrate supply and the total energy expenditure. Exogenous fat administration clearly does not promote fat oxidation by itself in healthy individuals. Similar data, however, are lacking in critically ill patients, and it remains possible that defective fat mobilization or utilization is present.

Lipid Supply

Fat emulsions have been largely used in critically ill patients, especially in those who are volume restricted. It was long proposed to combine fat and glucose,[73] especially in the case of respiratory failure, when high carbohydrate loads may increase CO_2 production.[82] Another rationale for providing some fat comes from the demonstration of essential fatty acid deficiency. In multiple-injury patients, pure carbohydrate and protein TPN results in signs of linoleic acid (n-6) deficiency after only 5 days (or increase in eicosatrienic acid and the triene-to-tetraene ratio) and a decreased α-linolenic acid level (n-3) after 7 days.[83] The minimal quantity of lipids required to avoid essential fatty acid deficiency is about 100 g weekly.

Although generally safe, the long-chain triglycerides (LCTs) have been associated with fatty infiltration of tissues, hypertriglyceridemia, impaired immune function, and interference with the reticulo-endothelial system.[30] The deleterious effects of lipids in artificial nutrition have been observed only after parenteral administration. Complications like sepsis, platelet dysfunction,[84] and alteration of pulmonary function[85] have been attributed to the lipids themselves. LCT emulsions are associated with reversible increases in mean pulmonary artery pressure and decreases of the PaO_2/FIO_2 in patients with acute respiratory failure;[86] this has been attributed to the release of vasoconstrictive prostaglandins. Some of the infectious complications of TPN have been attributed to the LCTs, although this aspect remains highly controversial. Considering the widely different methodologic approaches, it is difficult to determine which complications are truly related to lipids. Many of the problems can indeed be ascribed to central catheter infections, and others to overfeeding.

The amount of fat delivered may be critical in the generation of complications. The early studies, which showed an immune benefit from TPN, used smaller amounts of lipids (or none) than the studies published during the 1990s, in which fat constituted 25 to 45% of nonprotein energy. Controversial studies regarding neutrophil, lymphocyte, monocyte, and macrophage functions in vitro have led to the investigation of other types of fatty acid emulsions. Because trauma patients and many critically ill patients are at high septic risk, the immune consequences of intravenous lipid therapy are of utmost importance. A clinical trial using 25% energy from fat apparently showed an increase in infectious and respiratory complications in severely injured patients.[87] Unfortunately, TPN was not isocaloric, with a difference of 7 kcal/kg/day between the groups, resulting in a 25% difference in energy intake (target 30 kcal/kg/day in the lipid group, which may be excessive in many patients). The difference is thus possibly due to relative overfeeding. In bone marrow transplantation patients, a population at high septic risk, TPN providing 25 to 30% of the total energy because fat was not associated with any changes in bacterial or fungal infection rates when the energy target was set at 1.5 times the basal requirements.[88] Low-fat nutritional support (15% of the total energy) has been associated with reduced infectious morbidity and shorter hospital stays in burned patients compared with controls receiving 35% of the total energy as fat.[89]

Long- and Medium-Chain Fatty Acids

Different types of lipids are used, the composition of the emulsions reflecting the trends in lipid metabolism knowledge. The most widely used emulsions are soybean oil–based, hence rich in linoleic acid, an LCT containing n-6 polyunsaturated fatty acids. Medium-chain triglycerides (MCTs) with 6 to 10 carbons have been proposed as an alternative. They are water soluble (more soluble than LCTs), are hydrolized more rapidly, and contain no essential fatty acids. They are oxidized more rapidly and in larger quantities. Their hepatic oxidation leads to the synthesis of ketone bodies, but the rate of ketogenesis is reduced in the presence of carbohydrates.[90] MCTs have a low tendency to tissue incorporation and have a carnitine-independent fatty acid transport in contrast to LCTs.[91] In high doses, MCTs exert neurotoxic effects. LCT-MCT mixtures have only small effects on pulmonary hemodynamics and gas exchange, which can be an advantage in patients with acute respiratory distress syndrome requiring TPN.[92] In trauma patients, MCT-LCT solutions provoke greater fat oxidation and less fatty acid re-esterification, indicating a more rapid fuel utilization compared with LCTs.[91] Overall, MCTs appear to have energetic, metabolic, and immune advantages. Therefore, MCTs are proposed in combination with LCTs, solutions containing 50% of each. The place of such mixtures in clinical nutrition remains controversial.

n-3 Fatty Acids and Oleic Acid (n-9)

The interest in diets enriched with n-3 fatty acids, eicosapentaenoic acid (EPA, 20:5 n-3), and docosahexaenoic acid (DHA, 22:6 n-3) derive from the epidemiologic observation of lower atherosclerosis incidence and lower age-adjusted mortality in Eskimos compared with the general Danish population. Modifying the n-6/n-3 ratio has both rapid and persistent effects on inflammatory and immune responses.[93] In the unstressed state, EPA and DHA metabolites have lower proinflammatory effects than their n-6 counterparts.[94] Further, the leukotrienes derived from EPA (leukotriene B5 [LTB5] and LTC5) have less metabolic effects than their arachidonic acid–derived counterparts (LTB4, LTC4). But in the stressed state, the effects of n-3 fatty acids differ: delayed hypersensitivity is promoted when previously depressed by stress.[95] Supplements using fish oil as an n-3 source cause changes in the cytokine profile, with decreased IL-1 and tumor necrosis factor production. IL-6 production is unaffected.[96] In burned rats, TPN with n-6 fatty acids increases IL-6, IL-8, and IL-10 concentrations, whereas n-3–continuing TPN reduces the IL-8 and IL-10 levels (anti-inflammatory) and prevents the depression of delayed hypersensitivity.[97] In surgical patients, EPA–enriched solutions increased leukocytes' LTB5 and LTC5 production[98] without any increase in the bleeding tendency. In healthy subjects, increased n-3 intake from fish oil is associated with a reduction of platelet aggregation and increased bleeding times. Increasing the n-3 proportion produces significant platelet composition and functional changes within a few days of TPN.[99] Further studies are required to determine the place of n-3 supplements in trauma.

Oleic acid, an n-9 long-chain fatty acid, may offer a neutral alternative to some negative immune aspects of the n-6 fatty acids. It may attenuate some of the immune effects linked with the high intake of linoleic acid from soybean–derived emulsions. It is too early to consider systematic prescription in trauma patients, however, because large studies are yet not available.

Fat-to-Carbohydrate Ratio

In the normal Western diet, carbohydrates constitute about 50% of the total caloric load, fat making up 30 to 35%. Available data suggest that similar ratios should be used during TPN in most clinical conditions.[41] In burns, lower proportions of fat might be considered; enteral feeding providing only 15% of total calories as fat has resulted in lower infection complications rates,[89] using a fat-to-carbohydrate ratio of 1:4, which is significantly lower than the usual ratio of 0.8–1.1 to 1.

◆ NONENERGETIC NUTRIENTS

Water

Water metabolism is altered for prolonged periods after injury. Most of the initial body weight changes can be accounted for by changes in body water. At the end of the hemodynamic instability period, there is a net water accumulation, which varies between 4 and 13 L of total body water.[46, 48]

Intracellular water decreases relatively by 15 to 20%, whereas extracellular water increases. The correction of this expansion takes a variable time, lasting about 3 weeks in elderly patients and half this time in younger patients.

Burn patients exhibit the largest changes owing to the specific massive fluid resuscitation, which can reach 30 L in 24 hours. The water vapor barrier of skin is lost, and patients require nursing in a warm environment: unimpeded evaporative and exudative free water losses as well as insensible water losses increase, whereas the sodium losses are unchanged. Investigations in the early 1980s showed that water requirements were increased for medium-sized burns nursed in fluidized beds.[100] Further, burn patients have an elevated core temperature, and fever is frequent, increasing the evaporative losses.

Electrolytes

Trauma patients have some special requirements that distinguish them from other critically ill patients. Normal daily requirements are indicated in Table 15–2.

Sodium. Beyond the usual maintenance requirements, trauma patients have increased sodium requirements to achieve hemodynamic stability during the resuscitation phase. Fluid resuscitation results in a massive sodium intake during the first 24 to 48 hours, especially in burn patients. After stabilization, this extra sodium load is excreted, and hypernatremia may be observed. The severity of the alterations is roughly proportional to the severity of injury. Brain injury patients are another category of patients with important changes in salt and water metabolism: diabetes insipidus, syndrome of inadequate vasopressin secretion, and salt-wasting syndromes are frequent. In such cases, the sodium content of TPN solutions have to be adapted.

Potassium. Trauma patients frequently lose large amounts of potassium through the urine and tend to have higher requirements than normal. In cases of crash syndrome, rhabdomyolysis or acute renal failure, the reverse is true.

Calcium. Less than 1% of the total body calcium is found in the extracellular fluid. The biologically active form is free ionized calcium. Hypocalcemia is frequent in critically ill patients and in trauma patients, particularly because of alkalosis, renal failure, gastrointestinal bleeding, and blood transfusion. Whereas calcium supplements are usually not required during short-term TPN, they may be considered after 2 to 3 weeks.

Magnesium. Magnesium is the major intracellular divalent cation: 50% is found in bone, and 30% of the extracellular magnesium circulates bound to protein. Magnesium has a key role in cell energetics, because since it is essential for the activity of $Na^+, K^+,$-ATP-ase and neuromuscular function by regulating the release of acetylcholine by the presynaptic fibers. Hypomagne-

Table 15–2. Mineral Requirements in Adult Trauma Patients

Mineral	Normal Daily Requirements		Conditions That Modify Requirements	
Sodium	2–3 mmol/kg		↑ ↓	Early resuscitation phase: until 0–1 mmol/kg Mobilization of initial sodium load
Potassium	IV:	1–2 mmol/kg	↑ ↓	Diuretics, polyuria: until 2–4 mmol/kg Acute renal failure, rhabdomyolysis
Calcium	E: IV:	1200 mg 4 mmol	↑	Blood transfusion: until 15 mmol/day
Magnesium	E: IV:	400 mg 4 mmol	↑ ↑ ↑	Burns: until 20 mmol/day Nonburn trauma or with diuretics
Phosphate	E: IV:	1200 mg 3–4 mmol	↑ ↑ ↑	Burns, acute-phase response Glucose infusion, antacids: until 30 mmol/day

E, enteral route; IV, intravenous; ↑, increased; ↑ ↑, strongly increased; ↓, decreased.

semia is common in critically ill patients[101] and in trauma patients, who are characterized by increased losses from increased urinary excretion or cutaneous exudates.[102] Magnesium supplements should be considered early in the course of trauma, even before TPN. Spontaneous hypermagnesemia is rare in critically ill patients and results from renal failure.

Phosphate. Critically ill patients exhibit a high incidence of hypophosphatemia, which may affect 29% of patients admitted to the ICU.[103] The causes include a low-phosphate diet, malabsorption disorders, the use of phosphate-binding drugs (e.g., antacids), TPN without supplementation, exudative losses in burns,[102] and increased urinary losses.

Phosphate and glucose metabolism are intimately linked, and high glucose loads induce a decrease in plasma phosphate levels in up to 40% of patients.[104, 105] Considering the potentially severe effects of deficiency, such as impaired oxygen delivery to tissues owing to decreased 2,3-diphosphoglycerate levels, hemolytic anemia, glucose intolerance, muscle weakness, congestive myopathy, rhabdomyolysis, and consciousness impairment, the prevention and correction of hypophosphatemia are of utmost importance. In trauma patients, a systematic prescription of 20 to 25 mmol/1000 nonprotein calories has been shown to avoid hypophosphatemia during TPN.[106] A close follow-up of phosphate levels (two to three times weekly) is appropriate. Great attention should be given to the presence of hypocalcemia, which must be corrected first. Hyperphosphatemia is less usual and occurs mainly during renal failure involving loss of tubular function.

Micronutrients

In addition to their nutritional functions, which are detailed in Chapter 4, micronutrients, that is, trace elements and vitamins, have antioxidant functions, which have been largely investigated over the last two decades. These functions are of the utmost importance to trauma patients, who have strongly increased free radical production and lipid peroxidation.[107, 108] Further, it has been stressed in the later years that the micronutrients interact, especially as antioxi-

dants, and should therefore be provided in combination.

Trace Elements

Trace elements are involved in free radical scavenging as cofactors of the various antioxidant enzymes: copper-zinc and manganese superoxide dismutase, catalase, and the glutathione peroxidases.

Trauma and burn patients lose biologic fluids through wound exudates, drains, and hemorrhage, and this causes negative micronutrient balances, resulting in negative trace element balances during the first week after injury,[23, 24] the alterations being particularly marked for selenium. The alterations in trace element metabolism, are reflected by several things, including low plasma concentrations, which persist for many weeks after injury. The interpretation of the low plasma levels is complicated by the acute-phase response, which is present in any injured patient and characterized by decreased plasma levels of iron, selenium, and zinc. In a pure acute-phase response, copper levels are usually maintained or increased.[21, 22] It has been hypothesized that the redistribution of trace elements occurring during the acute-phase response may be deleterious if prolonged.

An acute trace element depletion decreases endogenous antioxidant defenses, thereby favoring secondary tissue injury; decreases cellular and humor immunity with increased infection rates; delays wound healing; and produces complex endocrine changes (including the low T_3 syndrome).[109]

Brain Injury. Providing patients with trace element supplements during the early phase may promote their delivery to "priority tissues," while preventing zinc depletion elsewhere in the body. This may particularly be the case in brain-injured patients, whose neurologic system is exposed to high levels of free radicals. A recent randomized trial showed that zinc supplementation during the immediate postinjury period was associated with improved neurologic recovery after severe closed head injury.[110] The patients were given 12 mg of elemental zinc per day for 15 days, followed by 22 mg for 3 months and were compared with patients given placebo. The benefits were first discernible after 2 weeks and were associated with increased serum concentrations of prealbumin and retinol-binding protein. Interestingly, the serum zinc levels were similar in the supplemented and control groups, confirming that the blood compartment is only a transition compartment, which does not reflect the tissue status.

Burns. Burn patients differ from other trauma patients in that they have lost the skin barrier on a variable proportion of their body, which causes characteristic exudative losses.[23] Burn patients have been shown to suffer significant trace element deficiencies involving predominantly copper, iron, selenium, and zinc.[111] The deficiencies are largely explained by extensive cutaneous exudative losses[23, 112] and to a lesser extent by urinary losses. Supplementation with quantities of trace elements, matched to compensate the exudative losses, restores serum concentrations, as well as related enzymatic activities,[113] to some extent (see Fig. 15–2). Some trace elements are involved in the immune response, which is severely depressed after major burns. Early supplementation with copper, selenium, and zinc achieves an earlier normalization of the plasma levels (see Fig. 15–2) and is associated with a significant reduction of pulmonary infectious complications.[114] The quantities used in this latter trial were above the actually recommended parenteral intakes (four times for copper, six times for selenium, and five times for zinc).

Burns are characterized by intense lipid peroxidation, which is explained partly by the direct effect of the burn on the lipids contained in skin, but also by increased free radical production. Therefore, antioxidant and anti-inflammatory treatments aimed at reducing the formation of lipid peroxidation products are part of the adjunctive therapies in major burns.[115] Further, large selenium supplements are associated with an earlier normalization of a lipid peroxidation end-product such as malonyldialdehyde,[116] confirming the importance of selenium provision for antioxidant defense.

Trace elements are also involved in wound healing;[117] manganese levels increase within scars, whereas copper, selenium, and zinc concentrations rise only marginally. The increase in levels of manganese, a trace element involved in mucopolysaccharide and glycoprotein synthesis, as well as in the mitochondrial antioxidant defense (manganese superoxide dismutase), is an indicator

of the importance of antioxidant function in wound healing. In burn injuries, secondary damage to tissues is partly attributed to lipid peroxide generation in the burn wound. Early wound excision has been advocated on this basis to reduce the quantities of lipid peroxide delivered to the distant tissues. The improved graft take observed in a human supplementation study using a combination of copper, selenium, and zinc[113] may be partly explained through an antioxidant mechanism. It remains unclear if the improvement is due to a direct effect on the wound or to an indirect effect associated with enhanced immunity.

Copper status alterations appear to be a particular problem in burns. Copper is involved in collagen synthesis and wound healing as a component of enzymes like lysyl oxidase, but also in antioxidant defense. Plasma copper levels remain low for many weeks after injury and are inversely correlated with the extent of burn injury.[118] The copper deficiency may be large enough to cause cardiac arrhythmia and even death.[119] After burns involving 30% of body surface or more, patients lose up to 40% of their body copper content within the first week of injury.[23] Intravenous copper supplementation using standard quantities for intravenous nutrition (20 μmol/day) is only marginally successful in restoring copper and ceruloplasmin levels toward normal.[120] Providing larger amounts intravenously, that is, four times the currently recommended quantities, is still insufficient to achieve complete correction.[114]

Vitamins

Since the 1940s, deficiencies in vitamin status have been known to occur in burn and trauma patients; the severity of the disturbances is proportional to the severity of the injury. Evidence is based mainly on low serum levels and reduced urinary excretion despite supplementation. As early as 1946, high-dose ascorbic acid supplementation (1–2 g/day) was advocated in association with thiamine, riboflavin, and nicotinic acid.[121] The group B vitamins will not be detailed here but are obviously essential in carbohydrate metabolism and wound healing, particularly thiamine (B_1), riboflavin (B_2), pantothenic acid (B_5), and pyridoxine (B_6). Proposed supplementation doses are summarized in Table 15–3.

Table 15–3. Trace Elements and Vitamins with Increased Requirements in Critically Ill Trauma Patients (Doses for Burn Patients in Parentheses): Proposed Daily Intravenous Supplements for Adults and Comparison with Actual Recommendations for Stable Surgical Patients*

	Trace Elements			Vitamins	
	Intravenous Dose	Comparison with Actual Recommendation		Intravenous Dose	Comparison with Actual Recommendation
Copper	2 mg	2×	Vitamin B₁	100 mg	30×
	(4 mg)	4×			
Selenium	150 μg	3×	Vitamin C	1000 mg	13×
	300 μg	6×			
Zinc	20 mg	3×	Vitamin A	10,000 IU	3×
	(30 mg)	4.5×			
			Vitamin E	100 mg	10×

*These supplements are to be administered in addition to the recommended multiple trace elements and vitamins. When provided in such large amounts, the supplements should be administered by separate infusion to avoid total parenteral nutrition instability. (Reprinted with permission from National Advisory Group on Standards and Practice Guidelines for Parenteral Nutrition: Safe practice for parenteral nutrition formulation. JPEN J Parenter Enteral Nutr 22:49–66, 1998.)

Vitamin C. This vitamin exerts antioxidant functions as a reducing agent.[122] There is convincing evidence from animal studies that the early provision of megadoses of ascorbic acid, corresponding to 10 to 15 g/day in humans, reduces fluid resuscitation requirements, probably through an antioxidant mechanism.[123, 124] Ascorbic acid is essential for the activity of proline and lysine hydroxylases. Wound healing is associated with increased requirements, the classic example of defective wound healing being scurvy, which is characterized by decreased accumulation of extracellular matrix, low collagen deposition, abnormal angiogenesis with hemorrhage, and marked delay in tensile strength gain. In healthy subjects, the effects of deficiency take many weeks to appear, whereas the vitamin C status deteriorates very early in critically ill patients: levels 50% of normal are observed after only 48 hours.[125] The optimal dose required for wound healing has long been discussed: 1 g/day was proposed in the 1940s.[121] The normal body pool is about 1500 mg, which can be expanded to 2800 mg by supplementation above daily recommended intakes.[126] There is a ceiling effect in healthy individuals above 200 mg/day,[127] at which level urinary excretion starts to increase. There are no known side effects after the ingestion of 1 g/day for a few weeks: considering the potential favorable impact on wound healing, such a dose can therefore be recommended in trauma patients.

Vitamin A. This vitamin is usually stored in the liver in large amounts. It affects cell morphology and ground substance production. The action on wound healing is only partially understood: it promotes overall immune responses and induces fibroblast differentiation and collagen secretion. Vitamin A counteracts the deleterious effects of corticosteroids on wound healing.[128] Supplementation increases the collagen content and breaking strength in experimental wounds.

Vitamin E. Plasma levels of vitamin E are low in burn patients[129] and in other categories of critically ill patients. Endogenous antioxidants are essential in inflammatory tissues to control the formation of granulation tissue: vitamin E and selenium together reduce collagen degradation.[130] After brain injury,[131] attempts at modulating the antioxidant defense with α-tocopherol supplements have been deceiving until now.[132]

◆ NONNUTRITIONAL MANIPULATIONS

The promotion of anabolism using endocrine factors has been intensively investigated during the 1980s and 1990s. Energy expenditure can also be influenced by many other non-nutritional factors, such as ambient temperature, analgesia and sedation, and supportive treatment.

Warm Ambient Temperature

The thermally injured patient, and to a lesser extent any injured patient, exhibits changes in thermoregulation. Severely burned patients have an elevated hypothalamic set-point, which makes them strive for a higher central temperature. They require an approximately 4° C higher ambient temperature to feel comfortable, compared with normal subjects. Increasing the temperature from 21 to 25° C reduces the metabolic rate by 10 to 20%.[31] The metabolic effects of these changes include decreased urinary nitrogen, catecholamine, and cortisol excretion.[100] The ambient temperatures of hospitals are adjusted to be a compromise between those required for energy restriction of the patients and those needed for the comfort of the hospital workers and visitors; this may impose cold stress on the patients. Hypothermia in critically ill burned patients is a worry, because a delay of recovery from hypothermia heralds a poor outcome.[133] The problem can be overcome by individual room temperature regulation or by overhead heaters.

Fluid Balance and Infection

Hypovolemia, dehydration, and sepsis are potent stimuli of catecholamine release. An adequate fluid therapy contributes to the reduction of this stress factor. Infection per se accentuates the resistance to nutrition and persistence of negative nitrogen balances. Treatment is essential for obvious reasons.

Wound Closure

In burns, early surgery decreases mortality and has also been shown to restore immunoglobulin M (IgM) synthesis.[134] The metabolic rate increases less with this type of management and helps facilitate nutritional management. Wound closure is followed by body weight stabilization within weeks regardless of the size of the burn wound.[44] However, the surgical sessions cause periods of fasting in enterally fed patients; combined TPN may be required to achieve nutritional targets.

Analgesia and Sedation

Pain and agitation increase energy expenditure, whereas adequate analgesia and sedation reduce both discomfort and metabolic requirements. Reducing pain, fear, and stress has been shown to reduce the urinary catecholamine excretion and metabolic rate.[100]

Physical Activity and Immobilization

Trauma patients generally spend a prolonged time totally immobilized, which lasts from a few days after skin grafting to many weeks in case of fractures involving the pelvis and the spine. Mechanical ventilation, monitoring devices, and sedation further confine critically ill patients. Muscle wasting is promoted by immobilization, even in healthy subjects normally eating. It is not possible to achieve positive nitrogen balances in the absence of physical activity. Activity favors muscle conservation or restoration. Burned patients in particular are frequently nursed in fluidized beds; the resulting immobility must be counteracted by intensive physical therapy.

Growth Factors

The section Practical Considerations has a comprehensive discussion of anabolic agents in artificial nutrition; the following sections focus on some specific aspects in trauma patients.

Growth Hormone and Insulin-like Growth Factor I

Recombinant human growth hormone (rhGH) therapy has been shown to improve nitrogen balance, to increase body cell mass in GH-deficient children, and bone formation.[135] Supplementation with rhGH corrects the hypoaminoacidemia observed after trauma.[136] But nitrogen metabolism resists rhGH treatment in the early phase after injury;[137] the supplements do not attenuate the reprioritization of acute liver protein synthesis in trauma patients or significantly affect immunoglobulin synthesis.[18] Studies in burned children have demonstrated that rhGH decreases the donor-site healing times.[138, 139] These results have not been repeated by others.

Using rhGH in critically ill patients deserves special attention considering the results from two European multicenter supplementation studies using a dose of 0.3 IU of rhGH per kilogram per day. Mortality was doubled in the supplemented patients; the deaths were mainly attributable to multiple organ dysfunction and to septic shock. The causes of these negative results are yet not clarified. They have been attributed to alterations of the immune function.[140] As long as the mechanism of the increased mortality in the European trials has not been elucidated, rhGH administration should probably be restricted to patients who either have proven GH deficiency or have passed the acute phase of their trauma.

Insulin

Insulin has well-known anabolic properties and promotes protein synthesis. In burn patients, high doses of intravenous glucose with insulin appear to be associated with shorter donor-site healing times.[141] In another trial in adult burn patients, the synthesis, breakdown, and inward transport of proteins were in balance during high-dose insulin administration in an isolated leg model compared with negative values under control conditions.[142] The doses of insulin (500–1000 U/day) and of glucose required to achieve this effect were far beyond normal requirements, resulting in a total energy intake of 60 kcal/kg/day. The generalized clinical application of this method is not straightforward considering the deleterious consequences of large glucose loads, which have been associated with fatty liver infiltration.[71]

Other Growth Factors

The most promising data come from the topical administration of growth factors. Various growth factors have been used to stimulate wound healing in experimental settings. Platelet-derived growth factor, a glycoprotein dimer regulating collagen synthesis, has been applied topically and shown to enhance chronic ulcer healing.[145] Topical fibroblast growth factor, transforming growth factor-β, and epidermal growth factor are all under investigation in relation to wound healing.[143] A human trial using recombinant bovine fibroblast growth factor in 600 patients has shown a significant reduction in healing time of second-degree burns.[144]

◆ PRACTICAL CONSIDERATIONS

Parenteral Versus Enteral Nutrition in Trauma

Trauma severity ranges from simple contusions to life-threatening injuries. Patients with the former type of injury recover very rapidly without any type of artificial nutrition, whereas the latter may require prolonged intensive care treatment and nutritional support. After the initial stabilization, that is, after 24 to 48 hours, enteral nutrition (EN) should be considered.[145] Although most nutrition specialists consider enteral feeding as the best route for nutritional support, many studies including one conducted in our multidisciplinary ICU[146] show that TPN remains the preponderant source of nutrients in 10 to 40% of the days during which patients require artificial nutrition (Fig. 15–4). The guidelines of the American Society for Parenteral and Enteral Nutrition (ASPEN) recommend using parenteral nutrition only after a failure of enteral feeding or in case of gut dysfunction.[147]

TPN differs from EN mainly in four aspects: TPN bypasses the gut and its protective "filtering" effects on diets containing an inappropriate proportion of nutrients; TPN must be prescribed in separate components; TPN has a higher risk of discrete nutrient deficiencies; and finally, TPN carries a high catheter-related septic risk. Therefore, the use of TPN requires strict rules.

Although using EN is desirable, the more severe the injury, the worse the patient's gut function and the more difficult the enteral feeding. Hemodynamic instability frequently aggravates the clinical course, particularly in older patients. This reduces splanchnic perfusion and may compromise the utilization of the gut for nutrition. Mechanical ventilation and septic problems further alter intestinal function. Many patients, especially burn patients, require repeated surgical sessions, with the nutritional consequences of repeated fasting, especially in cases of EN. The presence of gut injury may complicate the management. Some types of abdominal injuries such as pancreatic injuries are possibly best managed with bowel rest and TPN.[148] Most burned patients have an intact gut but exhibit some gastrointestinal problems that make EN difficult, such as paralytic ileus,

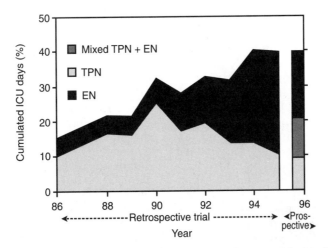

Figure 15–4. Place of total parenteral nutrition (TPN) in the nutritional support of critically ill patients including 12 to 15% trauma patients over a 10-year period. The vertical axis shows the proportion of all intensive care unit (ICU) treatment days with artificial nutrition. The retrospective study shows that pure TPN has stabilized at 25% of artificial nutritional support in the ICU. The last vertical bar shows the prospective results during a 6-month study in patients staying more than 3 days in the ICU: combined TPN and enteral nutrition (EN), which had not been analyzed in the retrospective study, was also studied and was shown to be present in 11% of ICU days. Altogether, this means that TPN was used in 21.3% of ICU days, that is, 54% of artificial-nutrition days. (Adapted from Berger MM, Chioléro RL, Pannatier A, Cayeux X, Tappy L: A 10-year survey of nutritional support in a surgical ICU: 1986–1995. Nutrition 13:870–877, 1997.)

gastrointestinal bleeding during the early and late courses of injury, acute pseudo-obstruction of the colon, and rarely, superior mesenteric artery syndrome.[149]

Brain injury patients are especially difficult to feed by the enteral route: in cases of elevated intracranial hypertension, gastric emptying is strongly decreased,[150] with significant regurgitation due to antiperistalsis.[151] Two studies of outcomes in brain-injured patients have shown beneficial effects of early TPN compared with EN.[152, 153] In both studies, EN resulted in marked underfeeding. In the first study, 38 head-injured patients were randomized to early TPN or to conventional enteral feeding.[152] The TPN group received 1800 kcal/day as mean intake, whereas the enteral nutrition group received only between 400 and 850 kcal/day for 2 weeks, resulting in elevated energy deficiency. Although the groups were similar initially, the outcomes differed significantly, with eight of the EN patients dying within 18 days of injury and no deaths in the TPN group. The study actually demonstrates how difficult it is to feed brain-injured patients by the enteral route and how rapidly malnutrition develops. In the second study by the same group,[153] the nasojejunal approach was used in the enteral

group to reduce the caloric deficit; but in this study too, which included 51 patients, the TPN group had a significantly higher cumulative mean protein and energy intake. The 3-month, 6-month, and 1-year neurologic outcomes differed significantly in favor of TPN. One further study after severe closed head injury, avoiding this underfeeding problem, showed similar outcomes and no increased infection rate with TPN in comparison with EN.[154]

Absorption of nutrients is not guaranteed; it has been shown that the gut absorptive capacity is severely depressed during the first week after trauma or sepsis, reverting to normal by 1 to 3 weeks after the event.[155] The risk of strongly negative energy balance is particularly elevated in EN,[151] as it frequently results in partial nutritional support, the mean delivery being 75% of the prescription.[146] A prolonged energy deficit invariably causes malnutrition.

The evidence in favor of EN may be less robust than apparent.[156] Even in the series of Kudsk and colleagues comparing both routes of nutrition, there were no significant differences in outcomes in patients with moderately severe injuries.[157] Studies performed in the 1980s showed no differences in outcomes between early EN and early

TPN in severely injured patients requiring laparotomy.[158] In addition, the benefits of EN shown in studies conducted by groups strongly motivated in favor of EN may not prove true in normal clinical settings.[145, 159, 160] There is indeed a major problem with EN: patients frequently suffer energy deficits for variable periods of time.

TPN remains an essential technique for nutritional support of severely traumatized patients, but its prescription requires a better knowledge of metabolism than necessary for EN. Errors in prescription and in translation of medical orders are frequent.[10, 161] The most commonly reported problems are incomplete TPN orders (missing components), a lack of laboratory control, and inappropriate orders. The technology of TPN and EN has changed considerably over the last 15 years. Some of the mediocre results of the TPN studies may be ascribed to the composition of the solutions. Huge efforts have been made to improve the composition of TPN, to facilitate its administration, and to take advantage of bypassing the intestinal barrier to manipulate the proportions of the different nutrients.

Effects of Total Parenteral Nutrition on Outcome

Many variables are involved in outcomes, making it difficult to control the studies for the direct effect of any form of nutritional support. In the general surgical population, two trials have clearly demonstrated that an elective preoperative nutritional TPN intervention is beneficial only in case of prior malnutrition, defined as a weight loss exceeding 10% of body weight.[9, 162] Both the Veterans Affairs' trial[9] and the Maastricht study[161] showed a significant reduction of noninfectious complications with TPN in the malnourished patients. In another large study involving 300 surgical patients, postoperative TPN did better than prolonged intravenous glucose (14 days), with a significantly lower mortality in the TPN group.[163] There are some older studies that showed benefit of TPN; these studies were unfortunately not well controlled for energy intake in the enteral group, leading to de facto malnutrition in that group. In brain injury, however, TPN appeared to have a favorable impact on outcomes, with a reduction in

mortality at 18 days and 1 year compared with delayed EN.[152]

The amount of energy provided and the specific nutrients may have an effect, hyperalimentation being deleterious whatever the feeding route. It stimulates de novo lipogenesis, with its negative consequences. In burn patients, Herndon and coworkers showed that providing a hypercaloric energy supply by means of TPN supplements worsened the outcome and failed to improve immunity.[72] The provision of early TPN using lipids (yielding relative hypercaloric nutrition) is associated with increased susceptibility to infection in severely injured patients when compared with no-fat isocaloric TPN groups.[87] All these data indicate that hypercaloric TPN should be avoided.

On the specific nutrient front, the news is better. Glutamine supplements are associated with better outcomes in an increasing number of controlled trials. In a well-designed prospective randomized trial in 84 critically ill patients with contraindications to EN, including severe trauma patients, TPN supplemented with glutamine reduced the 6-month mortality.[62] TPN was initiated either after 48 hours of intolerance to EN or in case of contraindication to EN. There were 18 deaths in the glutamine-supplemented group versus 28 in the control group ($P = .049$). Organ failure was the single most important cause of death and was less frequent in the glutamine group, with fewer cases of renal failure. The excess deaths occurred later in the control group; the total ICU and hospital costs per survivor were reduced by 50% in the glutamine group.

Micronutrient supplements are also efficient as shown by studies in burn patients and in brain-injured patients. Intravenous trace element supplements significantly reduced infectious complications and shortened ICU stays in severely burned patients receiving EN.[114] After brain injury, early zinc supplementation (12 mg/day) improved neurologic outcomes.[110]

Because the acute-phase response is very strong after trauma, its modulation by nutrients is worth considering. Every effort should be made to attenuate this response, which may precipitate organ failure. In healthy volunteers given artificial nutrition before an endotoxin challenge, cytokine production was facilitated by TPN compared with EN.[11] In patients with severe torso injuries, a significant blunting of the acute-phase response proteins has also been observed with EN compared with TPN,[164] and this has been confirmed in later studies.[145, 157] In this aspect, TPN may play a negative role, contributing to the amplification of the reaction; one explanation may be that the available studies were made with the "old" TPN solutions and did not include the glutamine-containing solutions, or the MCT-LCT mixtures. Considering the well-established severe effects of malnutrition in severely injured patients, all these studies show that parenteral nutritional intervention is required in patients intolerant to enteral feeding. At this stage, glutamine supplementation can be advocated, and early micronutrient administration appears advisable.

Indications for Total Parenteral Nutrition

The previously mentioned ASPEN guidelines[147] and a consensus statement of the American College of Chest Physicians[165] state that TPN in critically ill trauma patients should be used in three conditions: (1) when the enteral access cannot be obtained, (2) when enteral feeding fails to meet the nutritional requirements, and (3) when feeding into the gastrointestinal tract is contraindicated (major intra-abdominal sepsis, severe pancreatitis). Any severely injured patient with absent transit (defined as the passage of less than 500 mL of diet per 24 hours) present 4 to 5 days after injury should receive TPN.

Correcting a specific deficiency is an indication for selective parenteral supplementation; this is essentially the case with micronutrients. Supplements in addition to those provided by standard EN can be given intravenously.

Timing of Nutritional Intervention

It has been suggested that the need for parenteral repletion may be different for the various nutrients[41, 166]; micronutrients appear to be required earlier than energy, that is, proteins and fat (Fig. 15–5). Critically ill patients may express some functional defi-

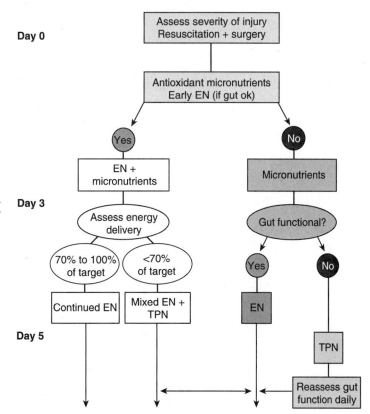

Figure 15–5. Nutritional algorithm for trauma patients. EN, enteral nutrition; TPN, total parenteral nutrition.

ciencies of selected electrolytes, minerals, vitamins, and trace elements within 24 to 48 hours, yet it will take many days before the body's stores are depleted. Some nutrients, like magnesium and phosphate, antioxidant vitamins, and trace elements, may be important early during the ebb phase, while full feeding is still not required in a previously well-nourished patient.[147]

We have found no data regarding the duration of starvation that can be tolerated without deleterious effects. Two weeks is too long, as shown by the results of a study in major surgery patients.[163] However, early TPN has no advantage over early EN in trauma patients.[160] Considering the enhancing effect of TPN on the acute-phase response, early TPN appears inadequate.[11, 164] Again, a 5-day delay before initiating full TPN seems to be appropriate.

Energy Supply

Defining nutritional requirements remains difficult. A food restriction to 90% of the usual predicted requirement results in a new balance, with a lower weight and a decreased substrate turnover. However, energy deficit results in malnutrition at a rate depending on the level of deficiency and the severity of injury. The fact that some degree of food restriction is beneficial in the absence of disease is supported by human observations during the World War II, during which large European populations were restricted to 70 to 90% of "normal intakes" and were in generally good health. In cases of infection, short-term food restriction is beneficial in animals, and anorexia appears as a defense mechanism.[167] The addition of trauma to an inadequate intake for days and weeks invariably results in malnutrition with its well-known consequences. There is a subtle edge that must not be crossed. Since the 1940s, the standard clinical management of severely burned patients has been based on high-calorie and high-protein feeding in order to maintain body weight and accelerated wound healing.[168] In the 1980s, the concept of hyperalimentation was extended to trauma patients in general. But for the last 15 years, the repeated calorimetric measurement of levels of REE below the values predicted by the various equations has prompted reassessment of the true requirements. The trend is now to provide either isocaloric or slightly hypocaloric nutrition during the ICU phase.

Indeed, exceeding the patient's caloric requirements with overfeeding promotes the release of catecholamines, with a subsequent potential metabolic and systemic overload. Overfeeding causes a series of deleterious side effects: hyperglycemia (hyperosmolar state, osmotic diuresis, dehydration), hypertriglyceridemia, respiratory failure, electrolyte imbalances, abnormal hepatic function (fatty liver),[72] acidosis, azotemia, and immune suppression.[41] The observation of these complications has prompted reflection about the real energy and protein requirements of the critically ill. Hyperalimentation in animals reduces resistance to infection and is associated with increased mortality.[7] The minimal level of energy and nutrient supply that will maintain the machinery during SIRS and sepsis without exposing the patients to the deleterious effects of malnutrition is unknown.

Other arguments in favor of underfeeding for limited periods are that achieving energy balance does not decrease protein catabolism and nitrogen loss.[169] Some authors therefore consider that 80% of the predicted energy requirement is a reasonable nutritional goal during the first 2 weeks.[41]

The prevailing attitudes in the severely injured patient are as follows. (1) Because the duration of tolerable fasting and the time of complete fasting required to cause biochemical alterations are not yet determined, one should limit fasting by empirical clinical considerations to 4 to 7 days. (2) One should consider the time elapsed since injury, because the requirements change along with the course of the illness.[43, 170] (3) One should avoid overfeeding. (4) One should consider an early micronutrient supply (antioxidants: vitamins, trace elements) and possibly glutamine provision. (5) One should assess nutrient delivery systematically and count the days with "permissive underfeeding"[171] to determine the cumulative deficit and avoid deleterious consequences. (6) One should assess the nutritional status in critically ill patients regularly, combining nutritional interventions to improve the status.

Venous Access

Trauma patients do not differ significantly from other critically ill patients regarding the ease of venous access (see Chapter 7). Peripheral nutrition is also possible, as peripheral veins are sometimes available. Burn patients differ in that central venous catheters are frequently the only available vascular access: catheters inserted through burned skin are at a higher infectious risk. Bloodstream infections related to vascular catheters are a constant threat to any trauma patient, and especially to the burned patient. When multiple perfusions and drug injections are required, there is an additional technical septic risk factor; to save one central venous catheter lumen for TPN in order to reduce the septic risk may be difficult. The risk of infection increases with the duration of the catheterization.

Effective preventive strategies include maximal sterile barriers during insertion: large sterile drapes, gloves, masks, gowns, and caps.[172] In burn patients, it is generally advocated to avoid the affected areas, but this is not always possible. Very early surgical débridement of the central venous line site (subclavian or femoral) with the insertion of the central venous line during surgery is possible in our experience. Antibiotic-coated and antiseptic-coated catheters reduce the rate of catheter colonization in high-risk patients, but the impact on the development of bacterial resistance might become a problem with the former. Moreover, these catheters are expensive. Nevertheless, high-risk critically ill trauma patients may benefit from antiseptic-coated catheters when they require prolonged ICU treatment.[173]

Our practice is to use standard central lines. We change them in case of a new unexplained episode of fever or in case of persistent fever without an obvious new infection site. Peripheral catheters are left in place no longer than 72 hours.

Prescription

In trauma patients without prior malnutrition, electrolytes and a small amount of calories are provided intravenously during the first days. But because such patients have early negative micronutrient balances, multiple–trace element and vitamin supplements should be given from admission (see Fig. 15–5). In Europe, this can be given in one vial of multiple trace element preparation, 100 mg of thiamine, and 500 mg of ascorbic acid in trauma patients. In burn patients, additional copper, selenium, and zinc supplements are infused (see Table 15–

3), with 1000 g of vitamin C and 100 mg of vitamin E given enterally. Brain-injured patients should be given extra zinc (additional 10 mg for a total of about 15 mg/day).

In the absence of gut function, parenteral nutrition should be initiated around the fifth day after injury. In the absence of indirect calorimetry measurement, energy requirement can be set at 30 kcal/kg/day (30–40 kcal/kg/day in severely burned patients); the delivery is escalated over 2 to 3 days.

The initial TPN solution should contain a mixture of carbohydrates and proteins. Optimal glucose provision is around 3 to 4 mg/kg/day. Such amounts of intravenous glucose are frequently associated with hyperglycemia. Since hyperglycemia is due to insulin resistance caused by the acute phase response, tight control of glycemia is not considered mandatory and is possibly even deleterious. In our ICU, insulin infusion is introduced at a rate of 1 to 4 U/h (more if required) to maintain a glycemia below 12 mmol/L. After brain injury, carbohydrate provision is subject to controversy, because of the potentially deleterious effects of hyperglycemia on compromised brain tissue; and tight control of glycemia is considered to be important.

Protein provision should not exceed 1.5 g/kg/day. Amino acid solutions containing glutamine supplements as dipeptides appear justified in any critically ill trauma patient; the optimal dose is still not determined but appears to be in the range of 20 to 25 g/day.[62]

In the absence of lung injury, lipids can be added as in any other critically ill patient. In the presence of acute lung injury, lipids are limited to the minimal amount that avoids essential fatty acid deficiency, that is, 100 g/wk in adults. Emulsions combining LCTs and MCTs appear preferable at this stage.

Electrolytes ought to be prescribed according to daily laboratory determinations. Vitamins and trace elements must be prescribed with TPN, using the standard recommendation for TPN, and adding the previously mentioned early supplements for about 2 weeks.

Combined Total Parenteral and Enteral Nutrition: Transition to Enteral

Enteral feeding is frequently difficult in critically ill patients. Insisting on pure EN frequently results in insufficient delivery of energy over prolonged periods. As EN appears to be associated with a reduction in infection rates, it would be interesting to determine the critical quantity of enteral nutrients required to get beneficial gut effects; this remains unknown. A study performed in the 1980s suggests that benefits are obtained when about one third (25 to 40%) of the nutrient requirement is delivered by this route.[174] Combined parenteral feeding is then required to provide adequate nutrient intake.

Combining the enteral and parenteral routes offers some advantages. If lower amounts of energy are to be delivered and in the absence of fluid restriction, peripheral nutrition can be used; this may be an advantage after the patient leaves the ICU. The enteral route, reducing the osmotic load given intravenously, can be used to deliver mineral and vitamin supplements. Further, there are intestinal absorption antagonisms. An example is the competition of zinc and copper for transmucosal transportation by metallothionin. In burn patients who require simultaneously high doses of copper and zinc, the provision by the enteral route fails to correct the trace element deficiency.[175] Using a separate intravenous infusion for the supplements while feeding the patient enterally avoids this problem.[115]

After TPN, EN is reintroduced when signs of gut intolerance decrease; a decrease in gastric residues and the appearance of bowel sounds or gases herald the return of intestinal function. Continuing TPN while initiating EN is safe and avoids the risk of energy deficit. The same is true with the reintroduction of oral feeding. As patients often have altered appetite for prolonged periods, maintenance on TPN while letting the patient eat progressively more is an acceptable way for both the patient and the nursing team and has the advantage of avoiding conflicts due to low food intake.

Monitoring

Clinical observation and subjective global assessment remain the best monitoring tools.[176]

Anthropometry

Looking for muscle wasting and obvious changes in body composition (edema, visible slimming) is part of the clinical assessment. Repeated determination of skin folds helps assess the degree of change. Further, although its place is not exactly determined, repeated bioelectric impedance analysis measurement is an additional tool that helps determine lean body mass and total body water.[177]

Body Weight

Fluid accumulation during critical illness complicates the estimation of the nutritional status, but assessing the body weight is difficult in this patient population.[40] In burned patients, daily body weight monitoring is particularly important during the acute phase because fluid changes occur rapidly; this can be done during the various transportation maneuvers required for hydrotherapy and surgery. The patient can be weighed twice weekly thereafter. In other trauma patients, nursing in air beds (e.g., Therapulse, Kinetic Concepts, Inc. [San Antonio, TX]) enables a fair estimation of body weight.

Clinical Chemistry

Blood determinations do not differ from those required in other critically ill patients on TPN, except for plasma phosphate and magnesium levels, which should be monitored closely (three times a week) in burn patients.[102]

Energy Expenditure

Energy expenditure should be measured whenever possible. Indirect calorimetry determination should be done once weekly in the critically ill patient with a prolonged ICU stay. Calculation of the oxygen consumption from a pulmonary artery catheter is an alternative.

Nitrogen Balance

Nitrogen balance has frequently been proposed as monitoring of nutritional adequacy; the usual goal is a balance of −5 to zero g/day during the first 2 weeks and then a positive balance. The determination requires a 24-hour urine collection (6 hours is acceptable). As nitrogen determination is not readily available in a hospital setting, it can be replaced by measurement of urinary urea, which constitutes about 80% of urinary nitrogen.[178] The following equation allows the conversion to nitrogen:

$$\text{N loss (g)} = \frac{\text{Urinary Urea (mmol/L)} \times \text{24-h Urine (L)} \times 0.06}{2.14} + 4\,\text{g}$$

Where

2.14 = Weight of nitrogen in the urea molecule

0.06 = Conversion of g/L to mmol/L

4 g = Other nitrogen losses (4 g/day in males and 3 g/day in females)

    2 g of fecal and cutaneous losses

    2 g for nonureic urinary N (mainly NH_4, uric acid, creatinine)

Many losses are not considered in this calculation: cutaneous exudates in burns, losses from drains, hemorrhage, upper gastrointestinal losses, and diarrhea may all considerably negate the nitrogen balance.

Nutrient Delivery

The knowledge of the quantity of nutrients actually delivered to the patient is crucial, because the mean difference between prescription and delivery is around 15% for TPN and 25 to 30% for EN.[146] This is also important during the transition toward enteral or oral feeding. Systematic protocols facilitate the prescription and administration of artificial nutritional support, whether enteral or parenteral. Errors in prescription are frequent[161] and can be reduced by continuous quality control programs.

◆ PERSPECTIVES

Many questions in the nutritional management of trauma patients are unresolved and deserve further research. The physiologic effects of starvation remain largely unknown in the critically ill trauma patient. How long is starvation tolerable? How long can hypocaloric nutrition be tolerated? Which is the optimal route for artificial feeding? Should nutritional support be dissociated with an early provision of micronutrients? What is the value of pharmaconutrition, and how early should specific nutrients such as glutamine or n-3 fatty acids be introduced? Which specific substrate should be given in trauma remains uncertain. Regarding clinical practice,

the use of combined parenteral and enteral nutrition, which is a rational way to avoid underfeeding, is not widespread; its advantages have not been investigated systematically. Regardless, whatever the answers to these questions, parenteral nutrition will remain a cornerstone in artificial nutrition in the severely injured patient during the first decade of the 21st century.

ACKNOWLEDGMENTS

We would like to thank Professor Luc Tappy, M.D. (Institute of Physiology, University of Lausanne), for careful revision of the manuscript.

REFERENCES

1. Murray CJL, Lopez AD: Mortality by cause for eight regions of the world: Global burden disease study. Lancet 349:1269–1276, 1997.
2. Bastow MD, Rawlings J, Allison SP: Benefits of supplementary tube feeding after fractured neck of femur: A randomized controlled trial. B M J (Clin Research Ed) 287:1589–1592, 1983.
3. Kudsk KA, Minard G, Crocce MA, et al: A randomized trial of isonitrogenous enteral diets after severe trauma. An immune-enhancing diet reduces septic complications. Ann Surg 224:531–543, 1996.
4. Wolfe RR: Relation of metabolic studies to clinical nutrition—The example of burn injury. Am J Clin Nutr 64:800–808, 1996.
5. Allison SP: The uses and limitations of nutritional support. Clin Nutr 11:319–330, 1992.
6. Bosagh Zadeh AR, Emery PW: Some aspects of metabolic response to surgical trauma. Proc Nutr Soc 57:225–229, 1998.
7. Petersen SR, Kudsk KA, Carpenter G, Sheldon GF: Malnutrition and immunocompetence: Increased mortality following an infectious challenge during hyperalimentation. J Trauma 21:528–533, 1981.
8. Choban PS, Weireter LJ Jr, Maynes C: Obesity and increased mortality in blunt trauma. J Trauma 31:1253–1257, 1991.
9. Veterans Affairs Total Parenteral Nutrition Cooperative Study: Perioperative total parenteral nutrition in surgical patients. N Engl J Med 325:525–532, 1991.
10. National Advisory Group on Standards and Practice Guidelines for Parenteral Nutrition: Safe practice for parenteral nutrition formulation. JPEN J Parenter Enteral Nutr 22:49–66, 1998.
11. Fong Y, Marano MA, Braber A, et al: Total parenteral nutrition and bowel rest modify the metabolic response to endotoxin in humans. Ann Surg 210:449–457, 1989.
12. Herndon DN, Barrow RE, Stein M, et al: Increased mortality with intravenous supplemental feeding in severely burned patients. J Burn Care Rehabil 10:309–313, 1989.
13. Cuthbertson DP: Post-shock metabolic response. Lancet 1:433–437, 1942.

14. American College of Chest Physicians / Society of Critical Care Medicine Consensus Conference: Definitions for sepsis and organ failure and guidelines for the use of innovative therapies in sepsis. Crit Care Med 20:864–874, 1992.

15. Drost AC, Burleson DG, Cioffi WG, et al: Plasma cytokines after thermal injury and their relationship to infection. Ann Surg 218:74–78, 1993.

16. Hoch RC, Rodriguez R, Manning T, et al: Effects of accidental trauma on cytokine and endotoxin production. Crit Care Med 21:839–845, 1993.

17. Kowal-Vern A, Walenga JM, Hoppensteadt D, et al: Interleukin-2 and interleukin-6 in relation to burn wound size in the acute phase of thermal injury. J Am Coll Surg 178:357–362, 1994.

18. Petersen SR, Jeevanandam M, Shahbazian LM, Holaday NJ: Reprioritization of liver protein synthesis resulting from recombinant human growth hormone supplementation in parenterally fed trauma patients: The effect of growth hormone on the acute-phase response. J Trauma 42:987–995, 1997.

19. DeBandt JP, Chollet-Martin S, Hernvann A, et al: Cytokine response to burn injury: Relationship with protein metabolism. J Trauma 36:624–628, 1994.

20. Young AB, Ott LG, Beard D, et al: The acute-phase response of the brain-injured patients. J Neurosurg 69:375–380, 1988.

21. Gaetke LM, McClain CJ, Talwalkar RT, Shedlofsky SI: Effects of endotoxin on zinc metabolism in human volunteers. Am J Physiol (Endocrinol Metab 35) 272:E952–E956, 1997.

22. Shenkin A: Trace elements and inflammatory response: Implications for nutritional support. Nutrition 11:100–105, 1995.

23. Berger MM, Cavadini C, Bart A, et al: Cutaneous zinc and copper losses in burns. Burns 18:373–380, 1992.

24. Berger MM, Cavadini C, Chioléro R, Dirren H: Copper, selenium, and zinc status and balances after major trauma. J Trauma 40:103–109, 1996.

25. Gore DC, Jahoor F, Wolfe RR, Herndon DN: Acute response of human muscle protein to catabolic hormones. Ann Surg 218:679–684, 1993.

26. Bessey PQ, Lowe KA: Early hormonal changes affect the catabolic response to trauma. Ann Surg 218:476–491, 1993.

27. Nygren J, Sammann M, Malm M, et al: Disturbed anabolic hormonal patterns in burned patients: The relation to glucagon. Clin Endocrinol 43:491–500, 1995.

28. Becker RA, Vaughan GM, Goodwin CW Jr, et al: Plasma norepinephrine, epinephrine, and thyroid hormone interactions in severely burned patients. Arch Surg 115:439–443, 1980.

29. Chioléro R, Berger MM: Endocrine response to brain injury. New Horiz 2:432–442, 1994.

30. De-Souza DA, Greene LJ: Pharmacological nutrition after burn injury. J Nutr 128:797–803, 1998.

31. Goodwin CW: Metabolism and nutrition in the thermally injured patient. Crit Care Clin 1:97–117, 1985.

32. Cunningham JJ, Hegarty MT, Meara PA, Burke JF: Measured and predicted calorie requirements of adults during recovery from severe burn trauma. Am J Clin Nutr 49:404–408, 1989.

33. Allard JP, Jeejeebhoy KN, Whitwell J, et al: Factors influencing energy expenditure in patients with burns. J Trauma 28:199–202, 1988.

34. Chioléro R, Bracco D, Revelly JP: Does indirect calorimetry reflect energy expenditure in the critically ill patient? In Willmore D, Carpentier Y (eds): Metabolic support of the critically ill subject, Vol 17. New York, Springer-Verlag, 1993, pp 95–118.

35. Cobean RA, Gentilello LM, Parker A, et al: Nutritional assessment using a pulmonary artery catheter. J Trauma 33:452–456, 1992.

36. Carlson GL: Nutrient induced thermogenesis. Baillières Clin Endocrinol Metab 11:603–615, 1997.

37. Long CL, Nelson KM: Nutritional requirements based on substrate fluxes in trauma. Nutr Res 13:1459–1478, 1993.

38. Goran MI, Peters EJ, Herndon DN, Wolfe RR: Total energy expenditure in burned children using the doubly labeled water technique. Am J Physiol 259:576–585, 1990.

39. Prelak K, Cunningham JJ, Sheridan RL, Tompkins RG: Energy and protein provision for thermally injured children revisited; an outcome-based approach for determining requirements. J Burn Care Rehabil 18:177–181, 1997.

40. Ishibashi N, Plank LD, Sando K, Hill GL: Optimal protein requirement during the first 2 weeks after the onset of critical illness. Crit Care Med 26:1529–1535, 1998.

41. DeBiasse MA, Wilmore DW: What is optimal nutritional support? New Horiz 2:121–130, 1994.

42. Cahill GF, Owen OE: Starvation and survival. Trans Am Clin Climatol Assoc 79:13–20, 1968.

43. Monk DN, Plank LD, Franch-Arcas G, et al: Sequential changes in the metabolic response in critically injured patients during the first 25 days after blunt trauma. Ann Surg 223:395–405, 1996.

44. Newsome TW, Mason AD, Pruitt BA: Weight loss following thermal injury. Ann Surg 178:215–217, 1973.

45. Gamrin L, Essén P, Fosberg AM, et al: A descriptive study of skeletal muscle metabolism in critically ill patients: Free amino acids, energy-rich phosphates, protein, nucleic acids, fat, water and electrolytes. Crit Care Med 24:575–583, 1996.

46. Hill GL: Implications of critical illness, injury, and sepsis on lean body mass and nutritional needs. Nutrition 14:557–558, 1998.

47. Newsholme E, Hardy G: Supplementation of diets with nutritional pharmaceuticals. Nutrition 13:837–839, 1997.

48. Finn PJ, Plank LD, Clark MA, et al: Progressive cellular dehydration and proteolysis in critically ill patients. Lancet 347:654–656, 1996.

49. Häussinger D, Lang F, Gerok W: Regulation of cell function by the cellular hydration state. Am J Physiol (Endocrinol Metab 30) 267:E343–E355, 1994.

50. Essén P, McNurlan MA, Gamrin L, et al: Tissue protein synthesis rates in critically ill patients. Crit Care Med 26:92–100, 1998.

51. Soeters PB, De Blaauw I, Van Acker BAC, et al: In vivo inter-organ protein metabolism of the splanchnic region and muscle during trauma, cancer and enteral nutrition. Baillieres Clin Endocrinol Metab 11:659–677, 1997.

52. Shaw JHF, Wolfe RR: An integrated analysis of glucose, fat, and protein metabolism in severely traumatized patients. Ann Surg 209:63–72, 1989.

53. Waxman K, Rebello T, Pinderski L, et al: Protein

loss across burn wounds. J Trauma 27:136–140, 1987.

54. Alexander JW, McMillan BG, Stinnett JD, et al: Beneficial effects of aggressive protein feeding in severely burned children. Ann Surg 192:505–517, 1980.

55. Markley K, Smallman E, Thornton SW: The effect of diet protein on late mortality. Proc Soc Exp Biol Med 135:94–99, 1970.

56. Sheridan RL, Prelak K, Cunningham JJ: Physiologic hypoalbuminemia is well tolerated by severely burned children. J Trauma 43:448–452, 1997.

57. Spiess A, Mikalunas V, Carlson S, et al: Albumin kinetics in hypoalbuminemic patients receiving total parenteral nutrition. JPEN J Parenter Enteral Nutr 20:424–428, 1996.

58. Fürst P: New parenteral substrates in clinical nutrition. Part II: New substrates in lipid nutrition. Eur J Clin Nutr 48:681–691, 1994.

59. DeBandt JP, Coudray-Lucas C, Lioret N, et al: A randomized controlled trial of the influence of the mode of enteral ornithine α-ketoglutarate administration in burn patients. J Nutr 128:563–569, 1997.

60. LeBricon T, Coudray-Lucas C, Lioret N, et al: Ornithine α-ketoglutarate metabolism after enteral administration in burn patients: Bolus compared with continuous infusion. Am J Clin Nutr 65:512–518, 1997.

61. Ogle CK, Ogle JD, Mao JX, et al: Effect of glutamine on phagocytosis and bacterial killing by normal and pediatric burn patient neutrophils. JPEN J Parenter Enteral Nutr 18:1128–1133, 1994.

62. Griffiths RD, Jones C, Palmer TEA: Six-month outcome of critically ill patients given glutamine-supplemented parenteral nutrition. Nutrition 13:295–302, 1997.

63. Houdijk APJ, Rijnsburger ER, Wesdorp RIC, et al: Randomised trial of glutamine-enriched enteral nutrition on infectious morbidity in patients with multiple trauma. Lancet 352:772–776, 1998.

64. Yu YM, Ryan CM, Burke JF, et al: Relations among arginine, citrulline, ornithine, and leucine kinetics in adult burn patients. Am J Clin Nutr 62:960–968, 1995.

65. Yu YM, Sheridan RL, Burke JF, et al: Kinetics of plasma arginine and leucine in pediatric burn patients. Am J Clin Nutr 64:60–66, 1996.

66. Yu YM, Young VR, Castillo L, et al: Plasma arginine and leucine kinetics and urea production rates in burn patients. Metabolism 44:659–666, 1995.

67. Horton JW, White J, Maass D, Sanders B: Arginine in burn injury improves cardiac performance and prevents bacterial translocation. J Appl Physiol 84:695–702, 1998.

68. Allison SP, Hinton P, Chamberlain MJ: Intravenous glucose-tolerance, insulin, and free-fatty acid levels in burned patients. Lancet 2:1113–1116, 1968.

69. Courtney Moore M, Connoly CC, Cherrington AD: Autoregulation of hepatic glucose production. Eur J Endocrinol 138:240–248, 1998.

70. Tappy L, Schwarz JM, Schneiter P, et al: Effects of isoenergetic glucose-based or lipid-based parenteral nutrition on glucose metabolism, de novo lipogenesis, and respiratory gas exchanges in critically ill patients. Crit Care Med 26:860–867, 1998.

71. Burke JF, Wolfe RR, Mullany CJ, et al: Glucose requirements following burn injury. Ann Surg 190:274–285, 1979.

72. Herndon DN, Stein M, Rutan R, et al: Failure of TPN supplementation to improve liver function, immunity, and mortality in thermally injured patients. J Trauma 27:195–203, 1987.

73. Meguid MM, Schimmel E, Johnson WC, et al: Reduced metabolic complications in total parenteral nutrition: Pilot study using fat to replace one-third of glucose calories. JPEN J Parenter Enteral Nutr 6:304–307, 1982.

74. Sheridan RL, Yu YM, Prelak K, et al: Maximal parenteral glucose oxidation in hypermetabolic young children. JPEN J Parenter Enteral Nutr 22:212–216, 1998.

75. Wolfe RR: Maximal parenteral glucose oxidation in hypermetabolic young children. JPEN J Parenter Enteral Nutr 22:190, 1998.

76. Georgieff M, Pscheidl E, Götz H, et al. Untersuchung zum Mechanismus der Reduktion der Proteinkatabolie nach Trauma und Sepsis durch Xylit. Anaesthesist 40:85–91, 1991.

77. Coombes EJ, Shakespeare PG, Batstone GF: Lipoprotein changes after burn injury in man. J Trauma 20:971–975, 1980.

78. Gordon BR, Parker TS, Levine DM, et al: Low lipid concentrations in critical illness: Implications for preventing and treating endotoxemia. Crit Care Med 24:584–589, 1996.

79. Aarsland A, Chinkes D, Wolfe RR, et al: Beta-blockade lowers peripheral lipolysis in burn patients receiving growth hormone. Ann Surg 223:777–789, 1996.

80. Cetinkale O, Yazici Z: Early postburn fatty acid profile in burn patients. Burns 23:392–399, 1997.

81. Birkhahn RH, Long CL, Fitkin DL, et al: A comparison of the effects of skeletal trauma and surgery on ketosis of starvation in man. J Trauma 21:513–519, 1981.

82. Askanazi J, Nordenström J, Rosenbaum SH, et al: Nutrition of the patient with respiratory failure. Anesthesiology 54:373–377, 1981.

83. Adolph M, Hailer S, Echart J: Serum phospholipid fatty acids in severely injured patients on total parenteral nutrition with medium chain/long chain triglyceride emulsions. Ann Nutr Metab 9:251–260, 1995.

84. Goulet O, Girot R, Maier-Redelsperger M, et al: Hematologic disorders following the prolonged use of intravenous fat emulsions in children. JPEN J Parenter Enteral Nutr 10:384–388, 1986.

85. Järnberg PO, Lindholm M, Eklund J: Lipid infusion in critically ill patients. Acute effects on hemodynamics and pulmonary gas exchange. Crit Care Med 9:27–31, 1981.

86. Hwang TL, Huang SL, Chen MF: Effects of fat intravenous emulsion on respiratory failure. Chest 97:934–938, 1990.

87. Battistella FD, Widergren JT, Anderson JT, et al: A prospective, randomized trial of intravenous fat emulsion administration in trauma victims requiring total parenteral nutrition. J Trauma 43:52–60, 1997.

88. Lenssen P, Bruemer BA, Bowden RA, et al: Intravenous lipid dose and incidence of bacteremia and fungemia in patients undergoing bone marrow transplantation. Am J Clin Nutr 67:927–933, 1998.

89. Garrel DR, Razi M, Larivière F, et al: Improved clinical status and length of care with low-fat nutrition support in burn patients. JPEN J Parenter Enteral Nutr 19:482–491, 1995.

90. Ball MJ: Parenteral nutrition in the critically ill: Use of medium chain triglyceride emulsion. Intensive Care Med 19:89–95, 1993.

91. Jeevanandam M, Holaday NJ, Voss T, et al: Efficacy of a mixture of medium-chain triglyceride (75%) and long-chain triglyceride (25%) fat emulsions in the nutritional management of multiple-trauma patients. Nutrition 11:275–284, 1995.

92. Smirniotis V, Kostopangiotou G, Vassiliou J, et al: Long chain versus medium chain lipids in patients with ARDS: Effects on pulmonary hemodynamics and gas exchange. Intensive Care Med 24:1029–1033, 1998.

93. Endres S, Ghorbani R, Kelley VE, et al: The effects of dietary supplementation with n-3 polyunsaturated fatty acids on the synthesis of interleukin-1 and tumor necrosis factor by mononuclear cells. N Engl J Med 320:265–271, 1989.

94. Kinsella JE, Lokesh B: Dietary lipids, eicosanoids, and the immune system. Crit Care Med 18:S94–S113, 1990.

95. Alexander JW, Saito H, Trocki O, Ogle CK: The importance of lipid type in the diet after burn injury. Ann Surg 204:1–8, 1986.

96. Bernier J, Jobin N, Emptoz-Bonneton A, et al: Decreased corticosteroid-binding globulin in burn patients: Relationship with interleukin-6 and fat in nutritional support. Crit Care Med 26:452–460, 1998.

97. Hayashi N, Tashiro T, Yamamori H, et al: Effects of intravenous ω-3 and ω-6 fat emulsion on cytokine production and delayed type hypersensitivity in burned rats receiving total parenteral nutrition. JPEN J Parenter Enteral Nutr 22:363–367, 1998.

98. Morlion BJ, Torwesten E, Lessire H, et al: The effect of parenteral fish oil on leukocyte membrane fatty acid composition and leukotriene-synthesizing capacity in patients with postoperative trauma. Metabolism 45:1208–1213, 1996.

99. Roulet M, Frascarolo P, Pilet M, Chapuis G: Effects of intravenously infused fish oil on platelet fatty acid phospholipid composition and on platelet function in postoperative trauma. JPEN J Parenter Enteral Nutr 21:296–301, 1997.

100. Ryan DW: The fluidised bed. Intensive Care Med 21:270–276, 1995.

101. Hamill-Ruth RJ, McGory R: Magnesium repletion and its effects on potassium homeostasis in critically ill adults: Results of a double-blind, randomized, controlled trial. Crit Care Med 24:38–45, 1996.

102. Berger MM, Rothen C, Cavadini C, Chioléro RL: Exudative mineral losses after serious burns: A clue to the alterations of magnesium and phosphate metabolism. Am J Clin Nutr 65:1473–1481, 1997.

103. Zazzo JF, Troch AEG, Ruel P, Maintenant J: High incidence of hypophosphatemia in surgical intensive care patients: Efficacy of phosphorus therapy on myocardial function. Intensive Care Med 21:826–831, 1995.

104. Clark CL, Sacks GS, Dickerson RN, et al: Treatment of hypophosphatemia in patients receiving specialized nutrition support using a graduated dosing scheme: Results from a prospective clinical trial. Crit Care Med 23:1504–1511, 1995.

105. McLeod DB, Montoya DR, Fick GH, Jessen KR: The effects of 25 grams IV glucose on serum inorganic phosphate. Ann Emerg Med 23:524–528, 1994.

106. Sheldon GF, Grzyb S: Phosphate depletion and repletion: Relation to parenteral nutrition and oxygen transport. Ann Surg 182:683–689, 1975.

107. Demling RH, Picard L, Campbell C, Lalonde C: Relationship of burn-induced lung lipid peroxidation on the degree of injury after smoke inhalation and body burn. Crit Care Med 21:1935–1943, 1993.

108. Ikeda Y, Long DM: The molecular basis of brain injury and brain edema: The role of oxygen free radicals. Neurosurgery 27:1–11, 1990.

109. Berger MM, Lemarchand-Béraud T, Cavadini C, Chioléro R: Relations between the selenium status and the low T_3 syndrome after major trauma. Intensive Care Med 22:575–581, 1996.

110. Young B, Ott L, Kasarskis E, et al: Zinc supplementation is associated with improved neurologic recovery rate and visceral protein levels of patients with severe closed head injury. J Neurotrauma 13:25–34, 1996.

111. Shakespeare PG: Studies on the serum levels of iron, copper and zinc and the urinary excretion of zinc after burn injury. Burns 8:358–364, 1982.

112. Berger MM, Cavadini C, Bart A, et al: Selenium losses in 10 burned patients. Clin Nutr 11:75–82, 1992.

113. Berger MM, Cavadini C, Chioléro R, et al: Influence of large intakes of trace elements on recovery after major burns. Nutrition 10:327–334, 1994.

114. Berger MM, Spertini F, Shenkin A, et al: Trace element supplementation modulates pulmonary infection rates after major burns: A double blind, placebo controlled trial. Am J Clin Nutr 68:365–371, 1998.

115. LaLonde C, Knox J, Daryani R, et al: Topical flurbiprofen decreases burn wound–induced hypermetabolism and systemic lipid peroxidation. Surgery 109:645–651, 1991.

116. Berger MM, Chioléro R: Relations between copper, zinc and selenium intakes and malondialdehyde excretion after major burns. Burns 21:507–512, 1995.

117. Bang RL, Dashti H: Keloid hypertrophic scars: Trace element alteration. Nutrition 11:527–531, 1995.

118. Gosling P, Rothe HM, Sheehan TMT, Hubbard LD: Serum copper and zinc concentrations in patients with burns in relation to burn surface area. J Burn Care Rehabil 16:481–486, 1995.

119. Sampson B, Constantinescu MA, Chandarana I, Cussons PD: Severe hypocupraemia in a patient with extensive burn injuries. Ann Clin Biochem 33:462–464, 1996.

120. Cunningham JJ, Lydon MK, Emerson R, Harmatz PR: Low ceruloplasmin levels during recovery from major burns injury–Influence of open wound size and copper supplementation. Nutrition 12:83–88, 1996.

121. Lund CC, Levenson SM, Green RW, et al: Ascorbic acid, thiamine, riboflavin and nicotinic acid in relation to acute burns in man. Arch Surg 55:557–583, 1946.

122. Herbaczynskacedro K, Wartanowicz M, Panczenkokresowska B, et al: Inhibitory effect of vitamins C and E on the oxygen free radical production in

human polymorphonuclear leucocytes. Eur J Clin Invest 24:316–319, 1994.

123. Matsuda T, Tanaka H, Reyes H, et al: Antioxidant therapy using high dose vitamin C: Reduction of postburn resuscitation fluid volume requirement. World J Surg 19:287–291, 1995.

124. Tanaka H, Matsuda H, Shimazaki S, et al: Reduced resuscitation fluid volume for second-degree burns with delay initiation of ascorbic acid therapy. Arch Surg 132:158–161, 1997.

125. Schorah CJ, Downing C, Piripitsi A, et al: Total vitamin C, ascorbic acid, and dehydroascorbic acid concentrations in plasma of critically ill patients. Am J Clin Nutr 63:760–765, 1996.

126. Levine M, Dhariwal KR, Welch RW, et al: Determination of optimal vitamin C requirements in humans. Am J Clin Nutr 62 (Suppl):1347S–1356S, 1995.

127. Blanchard J, Tozer TN, Rowland M: Pharmacokinetic perspectives of megadoses of ascorbic acid. Am J Clin Nutr 66:1165–1171, 1997.

128. Omori M, Chytil F: Mechanism of vitamin A action. J Biol Chem 23:14370–14374, 1982.

129. Mingjian Z, Qifang W, Lanxing G, et al: Comparative observation of the changes in serum lipid peroxides influenced by the supplementation of vitamin E in burn patients and healthy controls. Burns 18:19–21, 1992.

130. Åsman B, Wijkander P, Hjerpe A: Reduction of collagen degradation in experimental granulation tissue by vitamin E and selenium. J Clin Periodontol 21:45–47, 1994.

131. Chan PK: Antioxidant-dependent amelioration of brain injury: role of CuZn-superoxide dismutase. J Neurotrauma 9:S417–S423, 1992.

132. Stoffel M, Berger S, Staub F, et al: The effect of dietary α-tocopherol on the experimental vasogenic edema. J Neutrotrauma 14:339–348, 1997.

133. Shiozaki T, Kishikawa M, Hiraide A, et al: Recovery from postoperative hypothermia predicts survival in extensively burned patients. Am J Surg 165:326–330, 1993.

134. Yamamoto H, Siltharm S, deSerres S, et al: Immediate burn wound excision restores antibody synthesis to bacterial antigen. J Surg Res 63:157–162, 1996.

135. Klein GL, Wolf SE, Langman CB, et al: Effect of therapy with recombinant human growth hormone on insulin-like growth factor system components and serum levels of biochemical markers of bone formation in children after severe burn injury. J Clin Endocrinol Metab 83:21–24, 1998.

136. Jeevanandam M, Ali MR, Holaday NJ, Petersen SR: Adjuvant recombinant human growth hormone normalizes plasma amino acids in parenterally fed trauma patients. JPEN J Parenter Enteral Nutr 19:137–144, 1995.

137. Roth E, Valentini L, Semsroth M, et al: Resistance of nitrogen metabolism to growth hormone treatment in the early phase after injury of patients with multiple injuries. J Trauma 38:136–141, 1995.

138. Gilpin DA, Barrow RE, Rutan RL, et al: Recombinant human growth hormone accelerates wound healing in children with large cutaneous burns. Ann Surg 220:19–24, 1994.

139. Herndon DN, Barrow RE, Kunkel KR, et al: Effects of recombinant human growth hormone on donor-site healing in severely burned children. Ann Surg 212:424–429, 1990.

140. Takala J, Ruokonen E, Webster NR, et al: Increased mortality associated with growth hormone treatment in critically ill adults. N Engl J Med 341:785–792, 1999.

141. Pierre EJ, Barrow RE, Hawkins HK, et al: Effects of insulin on wound healing. J Trauma 44:342–345, 1998.

142. Sakurai Y, Aarsland A, Herndon DN, et al: Stimulation of muscle protein synthesis by long-term insulin infusion in severely burned patients. Ann Surg 222:283–297, 1995.

143. Muller MJ, Gilpin DA, Herndon DN: Modulation of wound healing and the postburn response. *In* Herndon D (ed). Total Burn Care. Philadelphia, WB Saunders, 1996, pp 223–236.

144. Fu X, Shen Z, Chen Y, et al: Randomised placebo-controlled trial of use of topical recombinant bovine basic fibroblast growth factor for second-degree burns. Lancet 252:1661–1664, 1998.

145. Kudsk KA: Gut mucosal support: Enteral nutrition as primary therapy after multiple system trauma. Gut 35:S52–S54, 1994.

146. Berger MM, Chioléro RL, Pannatier A, et al: A ten year survey of nutritional support in a surgical ICU: 1986–1995. Nutrition 13:870–877, 1997.

147. ASPEN Board of Directors: Guidelines for the use of parenteral and enteral nutrition in adult and pediatric patients. JPEN J Parenter Enteral Nutr 17:1SA–51SA, 1993.

148. Shilyansky J, Sena LM, Kreller M, et al: Nonoperative management of pancreatic injuries in children. J Pediatr Surg 33:343–349, 1998.

149. Lescher TJ, Sirinek KR, Pruitt BA Jr: Superior mesenteric artery syndrome in thermally injured patients. J Trauma 19:567–571, 1979.

150. Kao CH, ChangLai SP, Chieng PU, Yen TC: Gastric emptying in head-injured patients. Am J Gastroenterol 93:1108–1112, 1998.

151. Weekes E, Elia M: Observation on the patterns of 24-hour energy expenditure changes in body composition and gastric emptying in head-injured patients receiving nasogastric tube feeding. JPEN J Parenter Enteral Nutr 20:31–37, 1996.

152. Rapp RP, Young B, Twyman D, et al: The favourable effect of early parenteral feeding on survival in head-injured patients. J Neurosurg 58:906–911, 1983.

153. Young B, Ott LG, Twyman D, et al: The effect of nutritional support on outcome from severe head injury. J Neurosurg 67:668–676, 1987.

154. Borzotta AP, Pennings J, Papasadero B, et al: Enteral versus parenteral nutrition after severe closed head injury. J Trauma 37:459–468, 1994.

155. Singh G, Harkema JM, Mayberry AJ, Chaudry IH: Severe depression of gut absorptive capacity in patients following trauma or sepsis. J Trauma 36:803–809, 1994.

156. Lipman TO: Grains or veins: Is enteral nutrition really better than parenteral nutrition? A look at the evidence. JPEN J Parenter Enteral Nutr 22:167–182, 1998.

157. Kudsk KA, Croce MA, Fabian TC, et al: Enteral versus parenteral feeding. Ann Surg 215:503–513, 1992.

158. Adams S, Dellinger P, Wertz MJ, et al: Enteral versus parenteral nutritional support following laparotomy for trauma: A randomized prospective trial. J Trauma 26:882–890, 1986.

159. Moore FA, Moore EE, Jones TN, McCroskey BL:

TEN versus TPN following major abdominal trauma—Reduced septic morbidity. J Trauma 29:916–923, 1989.

160. Moore FA, Feliciano DV, Andrassy RJ, et al: Early enteral feeding, compared with parenteral, reduces postoperative septic complications. Results of a meta-analysis. Ann Surg 216:172–182, 1992.

161. Quercia RA, Keating KP: A CQI program for prescribing and dispensing total parenteral nutrition. Nutr Clin Pract 13:219–224, 1998.

162. Von Meyenfeldt MF, Meijerink WJHJ, Rouflart MMJ, Builmaasen MTHJ, Soeters PB. Perioperative nutritional support: a randomized clinical trial. Clin Nutr 11:180–186, 1992.

163. Sandström R, Drott C, Hyltander A, et al: The effect of postoperative intravenous feeding (TPN) on outcome following major surgery evaluated in a randomized study. Ann Surg 217:185–195, 1993.

164. Peterson VM, Moore EE, Jones TN, et al: Total enteral nutrition versus total parenteral nutrition after major torso injury: Attenuation of hepatic protein repriorization. Surgery 104:199–207, 1988.

165. Cerra FB, Benitez MR, Blackburn GL, et al: Applied nutrition in ICU patients. A consensus statement of the American College of Chest Physicians. Chest 111:769–778, 1997.

166. Berger MM: Role of trace elements and vitamins in perioperative nutrition. Ann Franc Anesth Reanim 14:82–94, 1995.

167. Murray MJ, Murray AB: Anorexia of infection as a mechanism of host defense. Am J Clin Nutr 32:593–596, 1979.

168. Cunningham JJ: Factors contributing to increased energy expenditure in thermal injury: A review of studies employing indirect calorimetry. JPEN J Parenter Enteral Nutr 14:649–656, 1990.

169. Frankenfield DC, Smith JS, Cooney RN: Accelerated nitrogen loss after traumatic injury is not attenuated by achievement of energy balance. JPEN J Parenter Enteral Nutr 21:324–329, 1997.

170. Allard JP, Pichard C, Hoshino E, et al: Validation of a new formula for calculating energy requirements of burn patients. JPEN J Parenter Enteral Nutr 14:115–118, 1990.

171. Zaloga GP, Roberts P: Permissive underfeeding. New Horiz 2:257–263, 1994.

172. Raad I: Intravascular-catheter-related infections. Lancet 351:893–898, 1998.

173. Veenstra DL, Saint S, Saha S, et al: Efficacy of antiseptic-impregnated central venous catheters in preventing catheter-related bloodstream infection. A meta-analysis. JAMA 281:261–267, 1999.

174. Border JR, Hassett J, LaDuca J, et al: The gut origin septic states in blunt multiple trauma (ISS = 40) in the ICU. Ann Surg 206:427–448, 1986.

175. Pochon JP, Klöti J: Zinc and copper replacement therapy in children with deep burns. Burns 5:123–126, 1979.

176. Manning EMC, Shenkin A: Nutritional assessment in the critically ill. Crit Care Clin 11:603–634, 1995.

177. Frankenfield DC, Cooney RN, Smith JS, Rowe WA: Bioelectrical impedance analysis of body composition in critically injured and health subjects. Am J Clin Nutr 69:426–431, 1999.

178. Milner EA, Cioffi WG, Mason AD, et al: Accuracy of urea nitrogen for predicting total urinary nitrogen in thermally injured patients. JPEN J Parenter Enteral Nutr 17:414–416, 1993.

16

◆ Parenteral Nutrition and Cardiopulmonary Disease

Michael S. Sherman, M.D.

Cardiopulmonary diseases are the most common causes of admission to medical intensive care units. Despite a long history of parenteral nutritional support dating back to at least 1656, when Sir Christopher Wren infused wine intravenously in a canine model, there is a paucity of well-designed studies to prove that parenteral nutrition improves outcomes in this group of patients. Parenteral nutrition is commonly used in patients admitted for cardiopulmonary disease who have a nonfunctional gastrointestinal tract. Prescriptions of parenteral nutrition must take into consideration the effects of the nutritional intervention on the underlying cardiac and pulmonary disease process.

◆ UNDERNUTRITION AND PULMONARY DISEASE

The interaction between undernutrition and pulmonary disease is most evident in chronic obstructive lung disease (COPD). Patients with COPD are commonly undernourished.[1, 2] Both the prevalence and the severity of undernutrition are increased in patients with COPD who present with respiratory failure and carbon dioxide retention.[3, 4] Patients with COPD and profound weight loss have been shown to have a significantly lower survival than controls without weight loss who were matched for the severity of pulmonary function.[5, 6]

The cause of weight loss in patients with lung disease is not totally known. Malnutrition correlates only weakly with the degree of pulmonary impairment. Patients with COPD have resting energy expenditures (REEs) that are higher than predicted.[7–9] Some of this increase may be related to the increased work of breathing in these patients, which incurs a lower efficiency and an increased caloric cost.[10] In particular, patients with emphysema have a significantly

higher cost of breathing than patients with chronic bronchitis, which may explain, in part, why emphysema patients are more prone to being malnourished.[11] Goldstein and coworkers demonstrated that patients with COPD had a higher diet-induced thermogenesis, suggesting another possible mechanism for the overall increase in energy expenditure.[8] However, a follow-up study by Dore and associates showed no significant difference in diet-induced thermogenesis between undernourished and eutrophic patients with COPD.[12] Gray-Donald and colleagues demonstrated that postprandial dyspnea was no greater in underweight patients with COPD than in normal-weight patients and that the postprandial increases in minute ventilation, oxygen consumption, and carbon dioxide production were the same in both groups.[13]

Regardless of the mechanism, protein-calorie malnutrition can have significant adverse effects on lung parenchyma, respiratory muscles, respiratory drive, and immunologic defense mechanisms.

◆ LUNG PARENCHYMA

Mild starvation or protein deficiency has not been observed to cause pathologic changes or lung abnormalities.[14] Severe starvation has been shown to affect the synthesis of matrix proteins. Animal models of severe starvation show structural changes in the lung, characterized by reductions in alveolar number, increases in alveolar size with dilation of terminal air spaces, and fragmentation of elastin fibers.[14] The lung weight is also reduced, and there is a reduction in elastic recoil.[15] These changes are morphologically and physiologically consistent with emphysema. In a human study, necropsy examinations of young, otherwise normal adults who died of starvation also showed an unusually high rate of emphysema. Specific nutrient deficiencies such as copper, zinc, ascorbic acid, and vitamin A may also adversely affect parenchymal lung tissue.[15]

Starvation is also associated with a loss of surfactant.[16] Surfactant is a surface-active chemical that stabilizes alveoli and prevents atelectasis; a lack of surfactant may lead to areas of lung collapse and decreased lung compliance.

◆ RESPIRATORY MUSCLES

Ventilation is accomplished through the work of the inspiratory muscles, predominantly the diaphragm, but also external intercostal muscles and strap muscles in the neck. In an autopsy study, Arora and Rochester demonstrated that patients with profound weight loss had a proportional loss of diaphragmatic muscle mass.[17] Similarly, nutritional depletion was associated with a reduction in diaphragmatic muscle mass that was proportional to reductions in limb muscle mass.[15] Undernourished patients were also shown to have an evenly distributed loss of muscle strength between inspiratory and expiratory muscles.[18] These studies suggest that there is no "sparing" of respiratory muscles during starvation. Indeed, patients with emphysema tended to have their diaphragmatic mass reduced out of proportion to their degree of weight loss.[19] Thus, the effect of malnutrition on respiratory muscles of patients with COPD may potentially be more profound than in the general population.

The loss of diaphragmatic muscle mass is accompanied by changes in function. The contractile strength of individual fibers has been shown to be reduced.[20] Fast-twitch fibers are affected more than slow-twitch oxidative fibers,[21] which may explain in part the paradoxical preservation of diaphragmatic endurance in the presence of a loss of diaphragmatic muscle mass.[22] Globally, malnutrition was associated with reductions in inspiratory muscle strength, measured vital capacity, and maximal voluntary ventilation (a measure of endurance).[18, 21] Vital capacity and pulmonary function increase when these malnourished patients gain weight.[21] Similarly, inspiratory muscle strength was shown to correlate with increased weight in surgical patients fed parenterally.[21] Conversely, Marks and colleagues reported no difference in respiratory

muscle function between malnourished patients with cystic fibrosis and well-nourished asthmatic patients.[23]

Data regarding the effects of refeeding of malnourished patients with COPD on respiratory muscle function are limited. Whittaker and associates fed six such patients 1000 kcal/day above their usual intake for 16 days and found significant improvements in mean inspiratory and maximal expiratory pressures compared with baseline and controls.[24] Wilson and coworkers gave supplemental feeding to six malnourished patients with emphysema and showed improvements in peak inspiratory pressure, transdiaphragmatic pressure, and handgrip strength but did not show improvements in spirometry, lung volume measurements, or diffusion capacity.[25] Efthimiou and colleagues demonstrated an improvement in respiratory muscle strength, inspiratory muscle fatigability, and the 6-minute walking distance in patients fed a supplemental diet associated with significant weight gain.[26] Again, no significant changes in pulmonary function tests were seen.

◆ RESPIRATORY DRIVE

Starvation is characterized by a decrease in the basal metabolic rate. The subsequent decrease in carbon dioxide production leads to a decrease in minute ventilation and tidal volume.[27] A decrease in sigh volume and frequency has also been noted. Decreased sighs may lead to atelectasis in the bases of the lungs, which may cause areas of ventilation-perfusion mismatch and shunt. Atelectasis may also reduce lung compliance.

Doekel and associates demonstrated that normal volunteers with semistarvation had a decreased respiratory drive as evidenced by a reduced response to hypoxia.[28] A blunted ventilatory response to carbon dioxide has also been demonstrated in healthy persons fed a protein-free diet for 7 days.[29] Refeeding has been shown to restore the depressed respiratory drive to normal.[28, 30]

◆ IMMUNOLOGY

Malnutrition is associated with an increase in the incidence and severity of pneumonia. Indeed, data from Holocaust victims showed that the majority of non-murder deaths were associated with pneumonia.[31, 32] The incidence of postoperative pneumonia is also higher in patients with preoperative malnutrition.[31] The prevalence of pneumonia is likely due to the effects of malnutrition on pulmonary defense mechanisms.

Protein-calorie malnutrition is associated with a reduction in the ratio of T helper to T suppressor cells, a decrease in ciliary movement, and a decreased secretory immunoglobulin A (IgA) antibody response.[15] Nutritionally depleted patients have higher bacterial adherence to tracheal cells than do controls,[33, 34] especially with *Pseudomonas* species. Cell-mediated immunity is impaired, in part because the conversion of monocytes to alveolar macrophages is inhibited[35] and macrophage function is impaired.[36] Macrophages phagocytize microorganisms and also are involved in presenting antigens to lymphocytes to initiate cellular immune responses. Reduced immunoglobulin concentrations including secretory IgA, decreased T lymphocytes and T cell subsets, decreased complement formation, and a decrease in interferon levels have also been described.[37] In an interesting corollary, an allergic response to antigen was found to be reduced in an animal model of protein-calorie malnutrition owing to the reduction in IgE levels.[38] Specific nutrient deficiencies may also impair the resistance to infection.

◆ UNDERNUTRITION AND CARDIAC DISEASE

Hippocrates first described the association of severe malnutrition with advanced congestive heart failure (CHF). This syndrome of cardiac cachexia is associated with a poor outcome, especially in surgical patients,[39] and is classically associated with patients with chronic rheumatoid valvular heart disease. The etiology of cardiac cachexia is multifactorial; suggested explanations include anorexia, malabsorption, hypermetabolic state, and impaired nutrient and oxygen delivery.

Anorexia may be due in part to the reactive depression associated with chronic illness. Chronic passive congestion of gastric and small intestinal mucosa can cause postprandial discomfort and early satiety.[40] Additionally, medications used for the treatment of CHF (such as digitalis and diuretics) may cause anorexia or nausea. Electrolyte imbalances due to diuretics may have an adverse effect on taste. Finally, the prescription of bland low-sodium diets may contribute to the problem.

Fat malabsorption has been described in patients with CHF.[40, 41] In a study comparing women with CHF and cardiac cachexia, women with normal weight and CHF, and healthy volunteers, fat absorption was reduced in the cachexia group only. Fat malabsorption was found to be related to the severity of heart failure as well as to the disease duration. There was no evidence for bacterial overgrowth as the cause, suggesting that bowel edema or other mechanisms were the cause.[41, 42]

There are several hypothesized causes for a hypermetabolic state in severe CHF. High levels of circulating catecholamines may play a role. Elevated levels of tumor necrosis factor-α (TNF-α) in CHF were first observed by Levine and colleagues.[43] Subsequently, investigators have demonstrated that concentrations of TNF-α were higher in cachectic patients with CHF compared with eutrophic controls and suggested that TNF-α may be a factor contributing to reduced body weight.[44, 45] An increase in concentrations of TNF-α along with its soluble receptors was found to correlate with the severity of heart failure and with body mass.[45, 46] This increase was also found to correlate with a rise in the plasma cortisol-to-dehydroepiandrosterone ratio (a measure of the endocrine balance between catabolism and anabolism), which suggests a possible causal relationship between the elevated TNF-α levels and weight and muscle loss in chronic CHF.[46]

◆ EFFECTS OF UNDERNUTRITION ON CARDIAC FUNCTION

Undernutrition is associated with a reduction in cardiac mass and function. Myocardial muscle loss has been shown to be proportional to the loss of skeletal muscle; like the diaphragm, cardiac muscle is not spared.[42] Myocardial atrophy has been documented in patients with anorexia nervosa, kwashiorkor, and low-calorie diets.[47] Morphologic changes have been described, including a significant decrease in myofibrillar diameter, myocardial atrophy, and interstitial edema.[48–50] In a canine model of protein-calorie malnutrition, a decrease in cardiac contractility was seen, along with a decrease in left ventricular compliance. A possibility of a vicious circle has been proposed, whereby the CHF causes malnutrition, which in turn exacerbates CHF.[48]

The loss in myocardial muscle mass is associated with a proportional decrease in cardiac output and stroke volume. Compensation to increased pressure and metabolic demands is also lessened.[51] To compensate, the blood pressure, heart rate, blood volume, and oxygen demand decrease.[42] The metabolic demand is also reduced in malnutrition because of diminished catecholamine levels and impairment in the conversion of thyroxine to triiodothyronine.[47]

Malnutrition has also been associated with arrhythmias. Sixty episodes of sudden death were reported in the "liquid protein" diets of the 1970s.[52] Isner and coworkers reported QT prolongation and ventricular tachycardia in a cohort of obese patients undergoing aggressive weight loss with this diet as well.[53]

Malnourished patients with heart disease have a higher mortality rate from surgery than their normally nourished controls.[54, 55] Abel and coworkers showed a 16% mortality in a group of malnourished patients versus no mortality in their well-nourished control group.[54] Morbidity is also more frequent, with a higher rate of pulmonary complications, renal failure, and sternal wound complications in malnourished patients. Hospital stays are also prolonged.[47] Paccagnella and colleagues gave patients with cardiac cachexia who were scheduled for cardiac surgery enteral and parenteral nutritional support 2 weeks before and 3 weeks after the surgical procedure. They observed improvement in hemodynamic and immunologic parameters, and all subjects survived.[56] Earlier observations also report survival in cachectic patients undergoing cardiac surgery after nutritional support.[57] These reports lack a control group for comparison; it is certainly possible that the improved mortality rates observed by Paccagnella and colleagues may be due to improvements in medical and surgical techniques. Based on limited data, Ulciny suggests that preoperative correction of malnutrition is prudent in these patients.[47] Further controlled studies are clearly needed.

◆ INDICATIONS FOR PARENTERAL NUTRITION

Nutrition should be given enterally if at all possible. When compared with parenteral feeding, enteral feeding is lower in cost, prevents intestinal villous atrophy, maintains mucosal integrity of the gastrointestinal tract, and has been demonstrated to have lower rates of bacterial translocation in animal models. Evidence supporting the presence of bacterial translocation in humans is more controversial. Studies have shown increased gut permeability in critical illness, trauma, and burns; endotoxin has also been found in organ specimens from nontraumatized organ donors who had received no feeding.[58] The development of systemic inflammatory response syndrome, multiple organ failure, or dysfunction is also less in critically ill patients fed enterally, rather than parenterally. Enteral feeding also reduces the risk of catheter-related sepsis and pneumothorax and the risk of gastrointestinal bleeding.[59–61] Several randomized trials in intensive care units showed that early enteral feeding within 3 days of illness is associated with an improved outcome.[62, 63] Parenteral nutrition has also been associated with atrophy of gut-associated lymphoid tissue, a phenomenon that does not occur with enteral feedings. Some of the adverse effects of parenteral feeding on the gastrointestinal tract have been ascribed to a lack of glutamine in this form of nutrition. Glutamine is thought to be an important fuel for the intestinal mucosa and a conditionally essential amino acid in stress situations. Supplemental glutamine has been demonstrated to reverse some of the adverse effects of parenteral feeding and has been shown to prevent villous atrophy, preserve the mucosal barrier, stimulate gut-associated lymphoid tissue, and increase IgA secretion.[64, 65] The beneficial effects of glutamine may be seen with either parenteral or enteral supplementation. Enteral glutamine enrichment has been demonstrated to reduce the incidence of pneumonia in trauma patients, possibly by decreasing bacterial translocation from the gastrointestinal tract.[66] Amino acid solutions containing supplemental glutamine are commercially available in Europe but not approved (as of this writing) in the United States. Further studies on the role of glutamine supplementation are clearly needed.

Parenteral nutrition may increase the infection rate. The Cooperative Veterans Affairs Total Parenteral Nutrition study showed a significant increase in infection rates in mild to moderately malnourished patients receiving parenteral nutrition preoperatively, compared with those fed enterally. A higher incidence of pneumonia was noted in the parenteral group.[67] Infectious complications were also noted to be higher in trauma patients randomized to parenteral nutrition.[63]

A number of studies have addressed the effects of parenteral nutrition on immune function. In an animal study, Shou and colleagues showed that parenterally fed rats developed impairments in pulmonary macrophage function with decreased superoxide production, decreased phagocytosis, decreased pulmonary clearance of bacteria, and decreased macrophage production of TNF-α.[68] Long-chain polyunsaturated n-6 fatty acids are the usual lipid source in parenteral nutrition. The n-6 fatty acids are precursors of prostaglandin E_2, which can suppress cell-mediated immunity, increase suppressor T cell activity, inhibit complement synthesis, and increase superoxide production. Preparations containing medium-chain triglycerides have been advocated as being less immunosuppressive; however, clinical data comparing these preparations to long-chain lipid sources are equivocal.[69] Human newborns fed parenterally had reduced bactericidal activity in an in vitro, whole-blood assay and the TNF-α release after bacterial challenge was also reduced. The addition of small amounts of enteral feeding improved both the bactericidal activity and the cytokine response.[70]

Parenteral nutrition may also have direct adverse effects on the lung. The U.S. Food and Drug Administration issued a safety alert in response to two deaths and two cases of respiratory distress believed to have been caused by pulmonary emboli secondary to calcium phosphate precipitates in three-in-one parenteral nutrition admixtures.[71,72] Similar admixtures were infused in an animal model, and an invisible precipitate consisting of calcium, phosphorus, and organic material was isolated from the solution. Infusion of this solution into healthy pigs resulted in sudden death; this was thought to be due to microvascular pulmonary emboli.[73] After these reports, the use of peripheral parenteral nutrition was reviewed in a retrospective study. Infusion of calcium phosphate precipitate was felt to be responsible for a variety of respiratory events that ranged from interstitial infiltrates to sudden death. Shay and colleagues reported that the amino acid source had an effect on the stability of these solutions.[74] Infusions of parenteral nutrition mixtures containing lipid emulsion have been shown to decrease arterial oxygen tension and diffusion capacity and increase dead space; this effect is abolished by filtration of the mixture. Possible causes of this phenomenon include direct disruption of the alveolar capillary membrane[75] and changes in pulmonary vascular tone mediated by the lipid-induced increases in eicosanoid production.[76] These changes may cause hypoxia by reversing hypoxic-induced vasoconstriction, which can worsen ventilation-perfusion mismatch. Long-term lipid infusions have been associated causally with pulmonary hypertension in an animal model.[77]

Right atrial thrombus and pulmonary thromboembolism are potentially fatal complications of long-term parenteral nutrition. This may be of more concern in the pediatric population. A retrospective study showed that 26% of deep venous thrombosis cases in children were associated with central venous lines, in contrast to an incidence of less than 2% in adults.[78] In an evaluation of 32 children undergoing long-term parenteral feeding, 12 had major thrombi or pulmonary emboli. Four of these patients died of pulmonary emboli.[79] Thrombus can form as a fibrin sheath around the tip of the central catheter or as a larger clot, which can adhere to the superior vena cava or atrium and subsequently embolize to the lung. Although these clots may form on central catheters in the absence of parenteral nutrition, there are studies suggesting that hypertonic parenteral nutrition solutions induce a procoagulant state and that lipid infusions may increase thrombin production, thus activating platelets.[80, 81]

Parenteral nutrition is thus a distant second-best choice, to be used for patients without a functional gastrointestinal tract. In general, this situation would most likely be seen in a critically ill intensive care unit patient with cardiopulmonary disease. The instinctive reaction of the clinician is that all such patients unable to receive enteral feedings be started on parenteral feeding. However, data to confirm that aggressive early nutritional support improves outcomes in critically ill patients with cardiopulmonary disease are lacking. The empirical behavior of starting nutrition is based on observations that many hospitalized patients are malnourished; that for equal severity of illness, malnourished patients have a worse clinical outcome; and that many abnormalities associated with malnutrition improve with refeeding.[82] However, a case can be made for delaying full nutritional support in nonmalnourished patients until the enteral route can be used in order to avoid the complications associated with parenteral feeding. Indeed, some have advocated "permissive underfeeding"—the concept that nutritional repletion may actually worsen the clinical outcome, and that underfeeding may be beneficial in certain disease states.[83]

In general, most studies involving nutrition in the intensive care unit setting have been performed on surgical patients, and thus our ability to apply these studies to medical patients with cardiopulmonary diagnoses is limited. A reasonable approach to patients unable to be fed enterally (based on limited data) is to feed parenterally within 3 to 5 days of an intensive care unit admission and to consider earlier intervention for malnourished individuals. Many of these patients will be able to tolerate limited enteral feedings, and supplementation with parenteral nutrition may be helpful.

◆ CALORIC REQUIREMENTS FOR CRITICALLY ILL PATIENTS WITH CARDIOPULMONARY DISEASE

Caloric requirements are usually estimated using weight-based estimates or predictive equations. A common approach is to use 25 kcal/kg/day for mechanically ventilated patients with respiratory or cardiac disease with no other medical problems, 25 to 30 kcal/kg/day for moderate levels of physiologic stress, 35 to 45 kcal/kg/day for severe stress situations (such as sepsis or trauma), and 45 to 50 kcal/kg/day for overwhelming infection, major burns, and major trauma. Of the predictive equations, the Harris-Benedict equation[84] is the best known:

Males: REE = 66.47 + 13.75 (Weight in kg) + 5 (Height in cm) − 6.76 (Age in yr)

Females: REE = 655.1 + 9.56 (Weight in kg) + 1.8 (Height in cm) − 4.68 (Age in yr)

Stress factors are then added to the REE based on the severity of the patient's illness. An average stress factor of 1.2 can be assumed for mechanically ventilated patients with respiratory or cardiac disease with no other medical problems. Hypermetabolic patients with overwhelming infection or a major burn affecting a body surface area over 40% may have a stress factor above 2.

Although these estimates of caloric requirements work well for patients who are not critically ill, predictive equations and stress factors become increasingly more inaccurate as the disease severity increases. Several studies have shown that both gross overfeeding and underfeeding may occur when predictive equations are used to estimate caloric need in the intensive care unit setting.[85–87] Several measurements have been used to more accurately determine caloric expenditure in this clinical setting.

Indirect Calorimetry

Indirect calorimetry is measured with a metabolic cart. Oxygen consumption and carbon dioxide production are measured and the metabolic rate is then calculated using the Weir equation:[88]

$$REE = [(3.9 \times V_{O_2}) + (1.1 \times V_{CO_2})] \times 1.44$$

where V_{O_2} and V_{CO_2} are in kilocalories per minute. An additional 20 to 30% may be added as an activity factor in patients who are not paralyzed or sedated.[89] Indirect calorimetry is usually performed for a 20- to 30-minute period with the patient at rest, and a 24-hour figure is extrapolated.

Although this technique has been recommended as the most accurate means to determine caloric requirements, it does have some limitations. Differences between expired and inspired volumes (due in part to the respiratory exchange ratio, R) are measured indirectly by the Haldane transformation. This method is generally inaccurate at inspired oxygen tensions greater than 50% F_{IO_2}. Inaccuracies can also occur if there are leaks in the circuitry, if care is not taken to remove water and water vapor from the circuitry, if there is metabolic activity within the lung parenchyma (e.g., pneumonia or acute respiratory distress syndrome [ARDS]), or if there is interconversion of fuels.[90, 91] Finally, extrapolation of REE from a 20-minute sample to a 24-hour determination may be an added source of inaccuracy.

Pulmonary Artery Catheter Technique

Oxygen consumption may be calculated using a pulmonary artery catheter. Measurements of cardiac output are obtained using thermodilution techniques. The arterial–mixed venous oxygen difference is measured by co-oximetry, and Vo_2 is calculated by a modification of the Fick equation:

$$Vo_2 = \text{Cardiac Output (Arterial Oxygen Content} - \text{Mixed Venous Oxygen Content)}$$

where content is $1.34 \times$ hemoglobin (g/Dl) $\times$ oxygen saturation.

REE is then calculated by assuming an average respiratory quotient (RQ) of 0.83. The caloric cost of oxygen at an RQ of 0.83 is 4.81 kcal/L of oxygen consumed. Substituting appropriately, REE can then be calculated by the Liggett–St. John–Lefrak equation:

$$\text{REE (kcal/day)} = \text{Cardiac Output (L/min)} \times \text{Hemoglobin (g/dl)} \times (\text{Arterial Saturation \%} - \text{Venous Saturation \%}) \times 95.18$$

Limitations to the technique include the inability to measure R, which can be useful in determining whether a patient is underfed or overfed, and the inaccuracies inherent in thermodilution measurements of cardiac output.[90] The use of an assumed value for R may also cause inaccuracies if a patient is at the extremes of physiologic respiratory quotients and is either ketotic (and has a low R) or overfed (with a high R). Nonetheless, Ligett and colleagues found good correlation between this method and indirect calorimetry.[92] (Note that R is the respiratory exchange ratio of expired carbon dioxide production over oxygen consumption; R can be measured using inspired and expired gas. RQ is the ratio of the metabolic production of carbon dioxide over the metabolic consumption of oxygen. RQ cannot be measured clinically; instead we try to ensure steady-state conditions and assume that RQ is equal to R.)

Expired Carbon Dioxide Technique

In a similar derivation to the thermodilution technique, carbon dioxide production can be measured and the energy expenditure calculated. When an average R of 0.83 is assumed, the caloric equivalent of carbon dioxide is 5.8 kcal/L of carbon dioxide produced. REE can then be calculated by the Sherman equation:[93]

$$\text{REE} = \text{Pe}_{\text{CO}_2} \times \text{Minute Ventilation} \times 9.27$$

Pe_{CO_2} can be measured by collecting expired gas from the expiratory port of the ventilator in a bag and running it through a blood gas analyzer. Minute ventilation should be measured by an external spirometer (such as a Wright spirometer, used by respiratory therapists to confirm the accuracy of a ventilator), as the ventilator's internal pneumotachometer may become inaccurate when contaminated by expired gases, especially over a prolonged period of time.[94]

The expired carbon dioxide technique can be performed without a metabolic cart and without a pulmonary artery catheter. As with the thermodilution technique, this method is less accurate at extremes of physiologic R. Inaccuracies may occur if there are air leaks in the system and if minute ventilation is not measured accurately. However, it has been shown to correlate well with the results of indirect calorimetry by metabolic cart.[93]

Although caloric expenditure can be measured with reasonable accuracy using these methods, optimal nutrient intake has not been established. While many clinicians prescribe full nutritional repletion based on estimated or measured caloric expenditure, restricted caloric intake in the early stages of critical illness has not been shown to be harmful and may indeed be beneficial.[83] Further studies are needed in this population.

◆ PRESCRIPTIONS FOR PARENTERAL NUTRITION: CONSIDERATIONS FOR SPECIFIC CARDIOPULMONARY DISEASES

Chronic Obstructive Pulmonary Disease

COPD is a comprehensive term describing a number of disease entities that are characized by air flow obstruction that does not improve to normal with bronchodilator therapy. A broad definition would include chronic bronchitis, emphysema, bronchiectasis, chronic persistent asthma, and cystic fibrosis. However, COPD usually refers to bronchitis and emphysema. Chronic bronchitis is defined clinically as a persistent cough for 3 months per year for 2 consecutive years. Obstructive chronic bronchitis is chronic bronchitis associated with airflow obstruction. Pathologically, airways of patients with chronic bronchitis are narrowed with inflammation, mucus, and hypertrophy of the mucous gland layer. Emphysema is defined pathologically as an abnormal permanent enlargement of the acini with destruction of alveolar walls without fibrosis. Obstruction is caused by collapse of the bronchi during expiration (premature airway closure) and by a decrease in the elastic recoil of the lungs.[95]

Patients with COPD, especially those who are malnourished, are often hypermetabolic.[9, 96–98] Schols and coworkers noted that the caloric intake in patients with COPD and weight loss was similar to the caloric intake in patients with COPD and stable weight, suggesting that the weight loss was due to the hypermetabolic condition in a segment of this population.[97, 98] Thus, increased caloric intake may be required in some patients with COPD. Wilson and associates found values approximately 15% above Harris-Benedict–predicted values in malnourished COPD patients.[9] In evaluating only emphysema patients, Fu and colleagues noted values approximately 15% above the predicted values in normally nourished patients and 20% above predicted in malnourished patients.[99]

Overfeeding, however, must also be avoided. A significant rise in carbon dioxide production has been demonstrated with increasing caloric intake in patients on mechanical ventilation.[100] This effect is felt to be due to lipogenesis, the process whereby carbohydrates given in excess of caloric needs are stored as fat. The RQ value of this reaction is approximately 8.0. This elevation in R is associated with an increase in carbon dioxide production and thus, secondarily, an increase in minute ventilation. Several studies have shown that patients with COPD who are receiving mechanical ventilation have increased minute ventilation and are difficult to wean when provided calories in excess of their requirements.[101, 102]

Ideally, indirect calorimetry would be helpful in these patients to determine their caloric needs. If indirect calorimetry is not available, a stress factor of 10 to 20% above the predicted value based on the Harris-Benedict equation would be prudent in patients with COPD who require parenteral nutrition, using the higher end of this range in patients with emphysema and/or in those who are malnourished.

In a normal individual, minimal protein requirements may be as little as 0.5 to 0.8 g/kg/day. The stress of illness can increase these requirements because of increased utilization and decreased utilization efficiency. As a rough rule of thumb, patients in the intensive care unit setting usually are given 1.5 to 2 g/kg/day. Patients with large body surface area burns and major trauma may need up to 3 g/kg/day. However, protein requirements for patients with COPD are generally not radically elevated and a protein intake of 1 to 1.5 g/kg/day is usually adequate. This translates to a calorie-to-nitrogen ratio of about 20 to 30 kcal/g of protein. Optimal protein intake in this population, as in others, can be determined through measurements of nitrogen balance. Nitrogen balance measurements may be erroneous due to extrarenal losses of nitrogen and to miscalculations of nitrogen intake.[103, 104] A sustained rise in plasma protein levels (e.g., albumin, prealbumin, and retinol-binding protein) can also be used to indicate a positive nitrogen balance. However, in the intensive care unit setting, these protein levels may be altered by non-nutritional factors such as capillary leak syndrome, liver disease, or nonspecific acute-phase reactions. Changes in these protein levels may reflect a change in the severity of illness, rather than anabolism.

The need to meet protein requirements must be balanced against the effects of protein ingestion and amino acid infusions on ventilation. Zwillich and coworkers showed that the ingestion of egg albumin was followed by an increase in minute ventilation and oxygen consumption, as well as an increased ventilatory response to both hypoxia and hypercapnia.[105] Weissman and coworkers infused amino acids into semistarved healthy subjects and demonstrated a rise in the resting minute ventilation, in inspiratory flow rates, and in the ventilatory response to inhaled carbon dioxide.[30] Askenazi and colleagues varied the amino acid intake in malnourished patients and found an increase in minute ventilation, a decrease in arterial carbon dioxide levels, and an increase in the ventilatory response to carbon dioxide at higher levels of infused nitrogen.[106] Further studies by this group showed that the effect of amino acids on respiratory drive was more pronounced in solutions rich in branched-chain amino acids.[107] Although this property has been used therapeutically,[108] the increase in minute ventilation may be an unwanted side effect in patients with COPD who may not be able to meet the increased respiratory demand. Care should be taken to avoid overfeeding protein in these individuals.

Approximately 100 g of carbohydrate intake per day is needed to provide caloric substrate for the brain and prevent endogenous protein breakdown. Absolute requirements for lipid intake are also small—enough to avoid essential fatty acid deficiency (about 10 to 20 g/day). These minimums are hardly enough to supply adequate nutrition, and a decision on the substrate mix of carbohydrates and lipids for specific disease processes is a complex one.

Adverse effects of lipids on pulmonary function have been reviewed earlier in this chapter. Carbohydrate feeding also may have pulmonary consequences. Carbohydrate metabolism has an RQ of 1, compared with about 0.83 for a mixed substrate diet and 0.7 for fat oxidation. In theory, the use of high-carbohydrate nutrition should increase carbon dioxide production compared with a calorically equivalent low-carbohydrate diet. A number of studies have addressed this effect.

Efthimiou and colleagues administered a high-caloric high-carbohydrate oral load to patients with COPD and found significant increases in carbon dioxide production, oxygen consumption, RQ, and minute ventilation; these increases were higher than changes seen with a calorically equivalent high-fat load.[109] Postoperative patients receiving gradually increasing amounts of intravenous dextrose demonstrated increases in carbon dioxide production; infusions at the highest level of 9 mg/kg/min was associated with a measured R of greater than 1.[110] Rodriguez and associates infused four normal subjects and four trauma patients with low- and high-glucose infusions. Increasing glucose intake was associated with a parallel increase in minute ventilation.[111] Similarly, Liposky and Nelson found a correlation between carbohydrate intake and carbon dioxide production, and between carbohydrate intake and alveolar ventilation in critically ill patients.[112] This study did not separate the effects of overfeeding total calories from increased carbohydrate load.

The observation that carbohydrate feeding increases minute ventilation led to the hypothesis that high-fat low-carbohydrate feedings could reduce RQ, decrease carbon dioxide production, and thus decrease minute ventilation. Angelillo and colleagues found that COPD patients fed high-fat low-carbohydrate enteral diets had significantly lower carbon dioxide production, R, and arterial PCO_2 levels than patients fed moderate- or high-carbohydrate diets.[113] High-fat low-carbohydrate enteral feedings were also given to patients with ventilatory failure receiving mechanical ventilation. These studies have shown a reduction in R and carbon dioxide production[114–116] and a decreased time of weaning off mechanical ventilation.[117] In a parenteral study, R and minute ventilation increases were again noted when patients were given 100% dextrose compared with a 50% dextrose, 50% lipid formula.[118]

Conversely, Talpers and colleagues showed that in patients given isocaloric regimens containing varied percentages of carbohydrate, carbon dioxide production did not differ. These findings suggest that although total calories had an affect on carbon dioxide production (and, by extension, on minute ventilation), the percentage of carbohydrate calories actually had a minimal effect when the caloric intake was constant.[100] And although studies quoted earlier suggest that an improvement in weaning can occur with a change to a lipid-based diet, others have not demonstrated a salient effect that is independent of a total calorie effect.[100] No large-scale controlled trials have been performed that can support recommendations for lipid-predominant or carbohydrate-predominant feedings in this population. Recommendations are thus somewhat empirical. A reasonable substrate mix, given the data reviewed earlier, is a 60% carbohydrate 40% lipid balance of nonprotein calories. Consideration should be given to increasing the lipid for patients with COPD who have severe respiratory failure and carbon dioxide retention, especially those who are difficult to wean off mechanical ventilation.

Acute Respiratory Distress Syndrome

ARDS is a clinical syndrome comprising severe hypoxia and diffuse pulmonary infiltrates with pulmonary edema, without clinical evidence of CHF.[119] Pathologically, ARDS is characterized by an initial phase of lung edema associated with swelling of endothelial cells and hyaline membranes and inflammation. A second proliferative phase is characterized by resolution of the neutrophilic inflammation and an increase in cellular proliferation. Most patients who survive have normal pulmonary architecture; some develop interstitial fibrosis. Mortality is usually due to the underlying disease.

ARDS is associated with a variety of clinical disorders. ARDS may follow a direct insult to the lung, such as aspiration pneumonia, near-drowning, or toxic gas inhalation. ARDS may also occur in association with a number of systemic illnesses. The most common of these include severe sepsis, trauma, acute pancreatitis, and drug overdose.[120] Patients with ARDS are almost invariably mechanically ventilated and often have multiple organ system failure, especially those who have sepsis syndrome as the underlying cause. As these conditions may also affect the gastrointestinal tract, parenteral nutrition may be necessary for some patients with ARDS.

The caloric requirements of patients with ARDS vary with the underlying cause. Many of the causes of ARDS are associated with hypermetabolic states. These patients frequently have tachycardia, an increased cardiac output, increased oxygen consumption, and fever, all of which are associated with increased metabolic expenditure and thus increased caloric requirements. Patients with ARDS often have malnutrition due to the metabolic response to injury, as opposed to starvation.[121] The response to injury, inflammation, and infection is manifested by hormone and cytokine release. The hormonal response includes release of glucocorticoids, catecholamines, glucagon, and growth hormone. These agents can increase the metabolic rate, cause stress diabetes, and worsen the nitrogen balance. Cytokines, including interleukins 1, 2, 6, and 8 and TNF-α have been shown to independently increase fever and the metabolic rate as well as produce anorexia. TNF-α and interleukin 1 have both been shown to down-regulate the albumin gene, thus decreasing albumin production in stressed individuals.[122] Protein catabolism occurs, in part stimulated by catecholamine effects on gluconeogenesis.

Because of these effects, stress factors for ARDS are traditionally high—20 to 40% of REE in the hypermetabolic phase.[123, 124] However, in nonsurgical patients with ARDS not caused by sepsis, Liggett and Renfro reported only a 13% increase in caloric requirements over those calculated with the Harris-Benedict equations, which was not statistically significant. Patients with sepsis had an increase of approximately 20% over predicted values.[92] Because estimates of caloric requirements in patients with critical illness may vary greatly from actual requirements,[85, 92, 123] a method of indirect calorimetry (metabolic cart, thermodilution technique, or expired gas technique) should be considered in these patients.

The net protein catabolic rate was significantly higher in septic patients than in controls; protein intake partially counteracted the catabolism by modest increases in protein synthesis.[125] However, studies have shown that providing excessive protein does not further prevent protein loss,[126] likely because increasing protein intake has little or no effect on decreasing protein catabolism. Reasonable protein intake for a stressed patient with ARDS is about 1.5 to 2.0 g/day.

Parenteral branched-chain amino acids may have a beneficial effect on protein balance. Branched-chain amino acids have been shown to decrease protein catabolism and increase hepatic and muscle synthesis of protein.[127] Cerra and colleagues demonstrated improved nitrogen balance when surgical intensive care unit patients were administered branched-chain amino acids. Additionally, they showed that the increase in nitrogen balance was proportional to the increase in branched-chain amino acid intake.[128] Garcia-de-Lorenzo and colleagues showed increases in prealbumin and retinol-binding protein synthesis in septic patients given branched-chain amino acid–enriched parenteral nutrition. They also demonstrated improved mortality in the supplemented group but did not show any difference in the length of stay.[129] Conversely, Vente and coworkers found no improvement in nitrogen balance in a mixed group of septic and trauma patients randomized to branched-chain–enriched amino acids versus standard amino acid regimens. Plasma total protein and prealbumin levels rose significantly in both groups, and there was no difference between groups.[130] Currently, the role of branched-chain amino acid supplementation is controversial. Most of the patients studied were critically ill trauma or surgery patients; the application of these findings to patients with nonsurgical causes of ARDS is not clear.

Cystic Fibrosis

Cystic fibrosis (CF) is an autosomal recessive disease affecting all exocrine glands. CF is caused by mutations in the cystic fibrosis transmembrane conductance regulator (CFTR) gene. The frequency of this gene mutation is approximately 1 in 25 persons of northern European ancestry; the incidence of disease in the United States white population is approximately 1 in 3000 live births. The gene is less common in other ethnic groups, with a disease frequency of about 1 in 15,000 live births in African Americans. More than 600 CF gene mutations have been reported, although the majority of disease occurs with only a few, more common mutations. CFTR functions as a chloride channel; dysfunction causes decreased chloride and water secretion, resulting in dehydrated mucus. CFTR also affects ATP transport and endosomal pH and may have an effect on intracellular membranes.

Chronic pulmonary disease is a hallmark of CF. Respiratory involvement is characterized by the production of thick, viscid mucus with chronic bacterial infection. Infection is typically *Staphylococcus aureus* early in the course of the disease. *Pseudomonas* species predominate later in life. Neutrophilic inflammation is found in the lower airways. Bronchiectasis and fibrosis occur as the result of recurrent infection and ongoing inflammation. Bronchodilation and bronchoconstriction may be present in CF, but to a much lesser degree than in patients with asthma. Chest radiographs show minimal peribronchial thickening early in the disease. Bronchiectasis, atelectasis, cystic lesions, and honeycombing are seen later in the disease.

CF may present as a meconium ileus in infancy. Pancreatic function may be normal at birth; however, the thick viscid exocrine secretions progressively obstruct the pancreatic ducts. Pancreatic enzymes, unable to pass through the ducts, digest the pancreas, leading to cystic destruction and secondary fibrosis of the pancreas. Infants may develop failure-to-thrive syndrome; older children and adults may present with bulky malodorous stools with steatorrhea and fat malabsorption. CF may also affect the mucous glands and goblet cells in the bowel, causing further problems with malabsorption.

CF is often diagnosed by the sweat test; the defects in chloride channels cause high concentrations of sodium and chloride in sweat. Genetic testing is also available; however, at this writing, only screening for the most common alleles is available. A negative genetic test therefore does not rule out the diagnosis.

Patients with CF are frequently malnourished.[131] Chronic malnutrition in CF is associated with a slower rate of growth in children with the disease, a worse prognosis, and a more rapid deterioration in lung function.[132, 133] Malnutrition in CF is felt to be multifactorial. Baseline energy expenditure is increased in CF, although the measured elevations in REE have varied from as little as 4% above predicted to as much as 26%.[134–138] The elevation in REE has been ascribed to the primary CF genetic defect,[131–133] chronic and acute inflammation and infection,[139] and a decrease in total body fat. Three studies showed that elevations in REE declined during hospitalization for acute flares of CF. These findings suggest that pulmonary exacerbations increase energy expenditure, possibly from an increased caloric cost of breathing.[140, 141] In contrast, Stallings and colleagues showed no significant changes in REE with an acute exacerbation, although an elevation in baseline REE was confirmed. However, the patients studied by Stallings and colleagues had milder pulmonary dysfunction than the earlier studies.[138] Malabsorption from gastrointestinal involvement also contributes to malnutrition in CF. Recommendations to increase caloric consumption by 20% to as much as 100% above predicted values have been promoted to improve the nutritional status of patients with CF;[142, 143] however, patients often fail to meet these aggressive goals.[144]

The role of parenteral nutrition in CF has not been well defined. Elliott and Robinson reported that parenteral lipids given to a child improved sweat tests and found improvement in sweat tests and pancreatic function.[145] Chase and associates supplemented CF patients with lipid and found greater height and weight gain in the lipid group compared with controls.[146] Several studies have shown improved weight gain with parenteral nutrition supplementation in CF patients.[147–149] Mansell and colleagues demonstrated improvement in respiratory muscle strength but no improvement in pulmonary function in parenterally supplemented CF patients.[148] Shepherd and coworkers noted significantly fewer pulmonary infections in their parenterally supplemented group and noted significant improvements in clinical scores and pulmonary function.[149] Conversely, Kussofsky and associates found no improvement in pulmonary function.[150] Kirvela and coworkers found that only a subgroup of patients had pulmonary function improvements with parenteral nutrition.[151] This subgroup was characterized by a detectable rise in serum dihomo-γ-linolenic acid concentrations during parenteral feeding. Parenteral nutrition has also been reported to improve oxygenation[152] and exercise tolerance[153] in case studies.

Oral nutritional supplementation, enteral feeding, and parenteral feeding interventions have all been shown to promote weight gain and improve nutritional status in patients with CF. A 1998 meta-analysis analyzed 18 studies of nutritional intervention on weight gain in CF.[154] Behavioral interventions, oral supplementation, enteral supplementation, and parenteral supplementation were all demonstrated to be effective at producing weight gain. Moreover, a univariate analysis showed no significant differences in the effect size for weight gain between these interventions. Analysis also indicated that behavioral intervention had a greater effect on caloric intake than oral supplementation. These findings suggest that the least invasive intervention, behavioral modification, had at least equal efficacy in improving nutritional status as oral supplements and the more invasive enteral and parenteral feedings.

Given these findings, the evidence does not support the routine use of parenteral nutrition in CF. Parenteral nutrition may be required when there is a nonfunctional gastrointestinal tract. High lipid-to-carbohydrate ratios are rational as they decrease R and also supplement essential fatty acids, which may be depleted in CF because of the pancreatic insufficiency. Care must be given to avoid overfeeding because of the effect on R and increasing minute ventilation. A caloric intake of 20 to 50% above that predicted is a reasonable estimate of the requirements; indirect calorimetry may be helpful in the more severely malnourished patients as their REE may exceed predicted values by over 100%.[155]

Congestive Heart Failure

CHF is a syndrome characterized by symptoms of shortness of breath, dyspnea on exertion, edema, and (when severe) end-organ dysfunction. It occurs when the left ventricular "pump" either cannot meet metabolic demands of the body or can only meet these demands at the expense of elevated filling pressures.

CHF affects approximately 1 to 2% of the general population. It is more common among men than women, and the incidence increases with age. Mortality is high and rivals that of many cancers, with a 5-year survival rate of 25% in males and 38% in females. Despite improvements in our understanding of the pathophysiology of CHF and new modalities of treatment, mortality rates have not significantly improved over the past four decades.[156]

The most common cause of CHF is ischemic heart disease, accounting for up to 70% of cases. Hypertension accounts for about 15% of cases. Other causes include valvular heart disease, dilated cardiomyopathy, restrictive cardiomyopathy, hypertrophic obstructive cardiomyopathy, and pericardial disease.[157] CHF is often divided by pathophysiology into systolic dysfunction and diastolic dysfunction. Patients with systolic dysfunction have a reduced contractility of the left ventricle and reduced left ventricular ejection fractions. Patients with diastolic dysfunction have impaired ventricular relaxation and stiff, poorly compliant ventricles in diastole.

Specific therapy for CHF may depend on the cause. In general, patients with diastolic dysfunction are treated with medications that improve the compliance of the ventricle, such as calcium channel blockers, β-blockers, or angiotensin-converting enzyme inhibitors. Diuretics are also used when fluid overload is present. Patients with systolic dysfunction are treated with diuretics to reduce pulmonary and peripheral congestion, angiotensin-converting enzyme inhibitors (or other vasodilators) to reduce afterload and improve cardiac output, and digitalis to improve cardiac contractility.[158] Carvedilol, a β-blocker with vasodilator properties, has been shown to decrease sympathetic tone and improve morbidity and mortality.[159] All patients with heart failure are sodium- and fluid-restricted to decrease intravascular volume.

Most patients with CHF can be fed enterally with gains in lean body mass and no adverse effects on cardiac performance.[160] When enteral feeding is not possible, the parenteral nutrition prescription should be tailored to minimize fluid intake. A reasonable goal is to restrict the total volume to 1.5 L/day and to restrict sodium intake to 1.5 to 2 g/day. Adequate caloric intake is required to prevent myocardial atrophy. Intravenous fat emulsions are often used in these patients as a high-caloric-density energy source to maintain adequate calories and decrease fluid intake. Fat emulsions were reported to decrease cardiac output in a canine model.[161] However, no hemodynamic effects were noted in human patients with CHF given 10% fat emulsion.[162] In patients who underwent coronary bypass surgery, a 20% fat emulsion had no effect on cardiac function at 1 mL/min, but cardiac output decreased at higher infusion rates of 2 mL/min,[163] a rate higher than that normally used clinically. A 20% fat emulsion is thus safe to use at clinically relevant infusion rates. Concentrated amino acid (10% or higher) and glucose (70% dextrose) solutions provide a higher caloric density than standard solutions and can be utilized to decrease fluid intake. The use of high concentrations of glucose may cause hyperglycemia, requiring the addition of insulin to the parenteral nutrition solutions.

Careful monitoring and replacement of electrolytes is necessary due to the effects of the loop diuretics used to treat this condition. Natriuresis, kaliuresis, and a loss of magnesium accompany the diuresis. Hypokalemia and hypomagnesemia are associated with ventricular arrhythmias, especially if patients are receiving digitalis. Diuretic use is also associated with a metabolic alkalosis, which can be corrected by repletion of potassium and chloride in the parenteral nutrition solution. Slow nutritional repletion and careful monitoring of phosphate and other electrolytes are particularly important in patients with cardiac cachexia, who may be prone to the refeeding syndrome.

Acute Coronary Syndromes

Acute coronary syndromes are a leading cause of hospitalization and death in industrialized nations. Acute coronary syndromes are classified into three entities: unstable angina, non–Q-wave myocardial infarction, and Q-wave myocardial infarction. These ischemic syndromes are caused by thrombus formation at the site of ruptured plaques in atherosclerotic coronary arteries. Unstable angina is thought to be due to intermittent arterial occlusion with or without vasoconstriction. Non–Q-wave infarctions are thought to be due to complete occlusion followed by early reperfusion, frequently with collateral circulation preserving tissue in the territory supplied by the affected vessel. Q-wave infarctions are thought to be due to persistent thrombotic occlusion causing a transmural myocardial infarct.[164]

Treatment strategies are aimed at restoring perfusion to the occluded coronary arteries. Heparin and aspirin decrease the chance of myocardial infarction and reduce mortality in patients with unstable angina. Medical management with β-blockers, nitrates, and calcium antagonists can improve the balance between vascular supply and the metabolic demands of the heart. Reperfusion for acute myocardial infarction should be done more acutely. Thrombolysis or immediate angioplasty have been shown to improve survival; early intervention improves the outcome. Heparin and aspirin are used to prevent rethrombosis. Nitrates and β-blockers may be used as adjunctive therapy. Complications include arrhythmias, hypotension, valvular heart disease, and CHF.[165]

The isolated heart can use any substrate for energy metabolism. Although the normal heart uses glucose predominantly, free fatty acids are used in the fasting state, ketones in diabetic ketoacidosis, and lactate plus all other available fuels during exercise. In the anoxic and ischemic heart, glucose is used in anaerobic glycolysis; fatty acids are poorly utilized and are thought to accumulate. Substrates used for myocardial metabolism can affect myocardial oxygen consumption. In ischemic animal hearts, circulating free fatty acids increase oxygen consumption, depress cardiac output, and increase myocardial injury. Because of these changes, the use of glucose-insulin-potassium (GIK) solutions was studied in the 1970s and early 1980s for patients with acute coronary syndromes.

Infusion of GIK solutions has been shown to increase myocardial glucose uptake by up to 200% and reciprocally decrease fatty acid uptake by up to 100%.[166] GIK was subsequently studied in patients with acute myocardial infarction. Infusion of GIK was associated with a significant reduction in ventricular arrhythmias,[167] a reduction in pulmonary capillary occlusion pressures, an increase in cardiac output,[168] and an elevation in the ejection fraction compared with controls given placebo infusions. GIK administration was shown to reduce wall motion abnormalities and preserve cardiac ejection fraction compared with controls; a retrospective study also noted that GIK recipients had a lower hospital mortality.[169] The solution has also been demonstrated to decrease chest pain frequency in patients with unstable angina.

Several mechanisms have been proposed to explain the beneficial effects of GIK. GIK solution depresses levels of circulating free fatty acids, which have a toxic effect on myocardial membranes. Glucose and insulin administration increases glucose metabolism and decreases fatty acid metabolism by ischemic myocardial cells. Insulin stabilizes myocardial cells and increases the fibrillation threshold in ischemic myocardial cells. GIK infusion also increases arachidonic acid levels, which may increase prostacyclin production.[169]

The use of GIK infusion has waned in the current age of thrombolytic therapy, and its use in conjunction with revascularization therapy has not been studied. When parenteral nutrition is needed in patients with acute cardiac syndrome, a substrate mix of 80% carbohydrate and 20% lipid would be reasonable. Whether GIK solutions should be used as an adjunct to current therapy is not known and may be worth further study.

Careful monitoring of fluid status and glucose and potassium levels is warranted, and limitation of fluid intake may be needed when CHF is present.

REFERENCES

1. Braun SR, Keim NL, Dixon RM, et al: The prevalence and determinants of nutritional changes in chronic obstructive pulmonary disease. Chest 4:558–563, 1984.
2. Hunter ALB, Carey MA, Larsh HW: The nutritional status of patients with chronic obstructive pulmonary disease. Am Rev Respir Dis 123:376–381, 1981.
3. Driver AG, McAlevy MT, Smith JL, et al: Nutritional assessment of patients with chronic obstructive pulmonary disease and acute respiratory failure. Chest 82:568–571, 1982.
4. Fiaccadori E, Del Canale S, Coffrini E, et al: Hypercapnic-hypoxemic chronic obstructive pulmonary disease (COPD): Influence of severity of COPD on nutrition status. Am J Clin Nutr 48:680–685, 1988.
5. Wilson DO, Rogers RM, Wright EC, et al: Body weight in chronic obstructive pulmonary disease: The National Institutes of Health intermittent positive-pressure breathing trial. Am Rev Respir Dis 139:1435–1438, 1989.
6. Vandenbergh E, Van de Woestijne K, Gyselen A: Weight changes in the terminal stages of chronic obstructive lung disease. Am Rev Resp Dis 95:556–566, 1967.
7. Openbrier DR, Irwin MM, Dauber JH, et al: Factors affecting nutritional status and the impact of nutritional support in patients with emphysema. Chest 85:67S, 1984.
8. Goldstein S, Askanazi J, Weissman C, et al: Energy expenditure in patients with chronic obstructive pulmonary disease. Chest 91:222–224, 1987.
9. Wilson DO, Donahoe M, Rogers RM, et al: Metabolic rate and weight loss in chronic obstructive lung disease. JPEN J Parenter Enterol Nutr 14:7–11, 1990.
10. Cherniack RM: The oxygen consumption and efficiency of the respiratory muscles in health and emphysema. J Clin Invest 38:494–499, 1959.
11. Jounieaux V, Mayeux I: Oxygen cost of breathing in patients with emphysema or chronic bronchitis in acute respiratory failure. Am J Respir Crit Care Med 152:2181–2184, 1995.
12. Dore MF, Laaban JP, Orvoen-Frija E, et al: Role of the thermic effect of malnutrition of patients with chronic obstructive pulmonary disease. Am J Respir Crit Care Med 155:1535–1540, 1997.
13. Gray-Donald K, Carrey Z, Martin JG: Postprandial dyspnea and malnutrition in patients with chronic obstructive pulmonary disease. Clin Invest Med 21:135–141, 1998.
14. Edelman NH, Rucker RB, Peavy HH: Nutrition and the respiratory system: Chronic obstructive pulmonary disease. Am Rev Respir Dis 134:347–352, 1986.
15. Sahebjami H, Vassallo CL: Effects of starvation and refeeding on lung mechanics and morphometry. Am Rev Respir Dis 119:443–451, 1979.
16. Faridy E: Effect of food and water deprivation on

surface activity of lungs of rats. J Appl Physiol 29:493–498, 1970.

17. Arora NS, Rochester DF: Effect of body weight and muscularity on human diaphragm muscle mass, thickness, and area. J Appl Physiol 52:64–70, 1982.

18. Arora NS, Rochester DF: Respiratory muscle strength and maximal voluntary ventilation in undernourished patients. Am Rev Respir Dis 126:5–8, 1982.

19. Thurlbeck WM: Diaphragm and body weight in emphysema. Thorax 33:483–487, 1978.

20. Kelsen SG, Ference M, Kapoor S: Effects of prolonged undernutrition on structure and function of the diaphragm. J Appl Physiol 58:1354–1359, 1985.

21. Kelly SM, Rosa A, Field S, et al: Inspiratory muscle strength and composition in patients receiving total parenteral nutrition therapy. Am Rev Respir Dis 130:33–37, 1984.

22. Rochester DF: Body weight and respiratory muscle function in chronic obstructive pulmonary disease. Am Rev Respir Dis 134:646–648, 1986.

23. Marks J, Pasterkamp H, Tal A, et al: Relationship between respiratory muscle strength, nutritional status, and lung volume in cystic fibrosis and asthma. Am Rev Respir Dis 133:4114–4117, 1986.

24. Whittaker JC, Ryan CF, Buckley PA, et al: The effects of refeeding on peripheral and respiratory muscle function in malnourished chronic obstructive pulmonary disease patients. Am Rev Respir Dis 142:283–288, 1990.

25. Wilson DO, Rogers RM, Sanders MH, et al: Nutritional intervention in malnourished patients with emphysema. Am Rev Respir Dis 134:672–677, 1986.

26. Efthimiou J, Fleming J, Gomes C, Spiro SG: The effect of supplementary oral nutrition in poorly nourished patients with chronic obstructive pulmonary disease. Am Rev Respir Dis 137:1075–1082, 1988.

27. Rosenbaum SH, Askanazi J, Hyman AI, et al: Respiratory patterns in profound nutritional depletion. Anesthesiology 51:S366, 1979.

28. Doekel RC, Zwillich CW, Scoggin CH, et al: Clinical semi-starvation: Depression of the hypoxic ventilatory response. N Engl J Med 295:358–361, 1976.

29. Askenazi J, Weissman C, La Sala PA, et al: Effect of protein intake on ventilatory drive. Anesthesiology 60:106–110, 1984.

30. Weissman C, Askanazi J, Rosenbaum S, et al: Amino acids and respiration. Ann Intern Med 98:41–44, 1983.

31. Mowatt-Larssen CA, Brown RO: Specialized nutritional support in respiratory disease. Clin Pharm 12:276–292, 1993.

32. Dmochowski JR, Moore FD: Choroba Godowa. N Engl J Med 293:356–357, 1975.

33. Niederman MS, Merrill WW, Ferranti RD, et al: Nutritional status and bacterial binding in the lower respiratory tract in patients with chronic tracheostomy. Ann Intern Med 100:795–800, 1984.

34. Niederman MS, Mantovani R, Schoch P, et al: Patterns and routes of tracheobronchial colonization in mechanically ventilated patients. The role of nutritional status in colonization of the lower airway by *Pseudomonas* species. Chest 95:155–161, 1989.

35. Jakab GJ, Warr GA, Astry CL: Alteration of pulmonary defense mechanisms by protein depletion diet. Infect Immun 34:610–622, 1981.

36. Browder W, Williams D, Pretus H, et al: Beneficial effect of enhanced macrophage function in the trauma patient. Ann Surg 211:605–612, 1990.

37. Scrimshaw NS, SanGiovanni JP: Synergism of nutrition, infection and immunity: An overview. Am J Clin Nutr 66:464S–477S, 1997.

38. Cunha MG, Naspitz CK, Macedo-Soares F, et al: Malnutrition and experimental lung allergy. Clin Exp Allergy 27:1212–1218, 1997.

39. Abel RM, Fischer JF, Buckley M, et al: Malnutrition in cardiac surgical patients. Arch Surg 111:45–50, 1976.

40. Jones RV: Fat malabsorption in congestive cardiac failure. BMJ 1:1276, 1961.

41. King D, Smith ML, Chapman TJ, et al: Fat malabsorption in elderly patients with cardiac cachexia. Age Ageing. 25:144–149, 1996.

42. Circulation and cardiac function. *In* Keys A, Brosek J, Henschel A, et al: The Biology of Human Starvation. Minneapolis, University of Minnesota Press, 1950, pp 607–634, 1950.

43. Levine B, Kalner J, Mayer L, et al: Elevated circulating levels of tumor necrosis factor in severe congestive heart failure. N Engl J Med 323:236–241, 1990.

44. McMurray J, Abdullah I, Dargie HJ, et al: Increased concentrations of tumour necrosis factor in "cachectic" patients with severe chronic heart failure. Br Heart J 66:356–358, 1991.

45. Zhao SP, Zeng LH: Elevated plasma levels of tumor necrosis factor in chronic heart failure with cachexia. Int J Cardiol 58:257–261, 1997.

46. Anker SD, Clark AL, Kemp M, et al: Tumor necrosis factor and steroid metabolism in chronic heart failure: Possible relation to muscle wasting. J Am Coll Cardiol 30:997–1001, 1997.

47. Ulicny KS, Hiratzka LF: Nutrition and the cardiac surgery patient. Chest 101:836–842, 1992.

48. Abel RM, Grimes JB, Alonso D, et al: Adverse hemodynamic and ultrastructural changes in dogs' hearts subjected to protein-calorie malnutrition. Am Heart J 97:733–744, 1979.

49. Rossi MA, Pissaia O, Cury Y, Oliveira JSM: Noradrenaline levels and morphologic alterations in myocardium in experimental protein-calorie malnutrition. J Pathol 131:83–93, 1980.

50. Rossi MA, Zucoloto S: Ultrastructural changes in nutritional cardiomyopathy of protein-calorie malnourished rats. Br J Exp Pathol 63:242–253, 1982.

51. Kyger ER, Block WJ, Roach G, Dudrick SJ: Adverse effects of protein malnutrition on myocardial function. Surgery 84:147–156, 1978.

52. Liquid Protein Diets. Publication No. EPI-78-11-2. Atlanta, Centers for Disease Control, 1979.

53. Isner JM, Sours HE, Paris AL, et al: Sudden unexpected death in avid dieters using the liquid protein modified fast diet: Observation in 17 patients and the role of the prolonged QT interval. Circulation 60:1401–1412, 1979.

54. Abel RM, Fischer JE, Buckley MJ, et al: Malnutrition in cardiac surgical patients: Results of a prospective, randomized evaluation of early postoperative parenteral nutrition. Ann Surg 111:45–50, 1976.

55. Gibbons GW, Blackburn GL, Harken DE, et al:

Pre and postoperative hyperalimentation in the treatment of cardiac cachexia. J Surg Res 19:439–444, 1976.

56. Paccagnella A, Calo MA, Caenaro G, et al: Cardiac cachexia: Preoperative and postoperative nutrition management. JPEN J Parenter Enteral Nutr 18:409–416, 1994.

57. Gibbons GW, Porter K: Cardiac cachexia. *In* Blackburn GL, Bell SJ, Mullen JL (eds): Nutritional Medicine: A Case Management Approach. Philadelphia, WB Saunders, 1989, pp 87–91.

58. O'Leary MJ, Coakley JH: Nutrition and immunonutrition. Br J Anaesth 77:118–127, 1996.

59. Mizock B, Troglia S: Nutritional support of the hospitalized patient. Dis Mon 43:357–425, 1997.

60. Hadfield RJ, Sinclair DG, Houldsworth PE, et al: Effects of enteral and parenteral nutrition on gut mucosal permeability in the critically ill. Am J Respir Crit Care Med 152:1545–1548, 1995.

61. Pingleton SK, Hadzima SK: Enteral alimentation and gastrointestinal bleeding in mechanically ventilated patients. Crit Care Med 11:13–17, 1983.

62. Adams S, Dellinger EP, Wertz MJ, et al: Enteral versus parenteral nutritional support following laparotomy for trauma: A randomized prospective trial. J Trauma 26:882–886, 1986.

63. Kudsk KA, Croce MA, Fabian TC, et al: Enteral vs parenteral feeding: Effects on septic morbidity after blunt and penetrating abdominal trauma. Ann Surg 215:503–510, 1992.

64. Ziegler TR, Smith RJ, Byrne TA, et al: Potential role of glutamine supplementation in nutritional support. Clin Nutr 12(Suppl 1):S82–S90, 1993.

65. Alverdy JC: Effects of glutamine-supplemented diets on immunology of the gut. JPEN J Parenter Enterol Nutr 14(Suppl):109S–113S, 1990.

66. Houdijk AP, Rijnsburger ER, Jansen J, et al: Randomised trial of glutamine-enriched enteral nutrition on infectious morbidity in patients with multiple trauma. Lancet 352:772–776, 1998.

67. The Veterans Affairs Total Parenteral Nutrition Cooperative Study Group. Perioperative total parenteral nutrition in surgical patients. N Engl J Med 325:525–532, 1991.

68. Shou J, Lappin J, Daly JM: Impairment of pulmonary macrophage function with total parenteral nutrition. Ann Surg 219:291–297, 1994.

69. Ulrich H, Pastores SM, Katz DP, Kvetan V: Parenteral use of medium chain triglycerides: A reappraisal. Nutrition 12:231–238, 1996.

70. Okada Y, Klein N, van Saene HK, Pierro A: Small volumes of enteral feedings normalize immune function in infants receiving parenteral nutrition. J Pediatr Surg 33:16–19, 1998.

71. Food and Drug Administration: Safety alert: Hazards of precipitation associated with parenteral nutrition. Am J Hosp Pharm 51:427–428, 1994.

72. McKinnon BT: FDA safety alert: hazards of precipitation associated with parenteral nutrition. Nut Clin Prac 11:59–65, 1996.

73. Hill SE, Heldman LS, Goo ED, et al: Fatal microvascular pulmonary emboli from precipitation of a total nutrient admixture solution. JPEN J Parenter Enteral Nutr 20:81–87, 1996.

74. Shay DK, Fann LM, Jarvis WR: Respiratory distress and sudden death associated with receipt of a peripheral parenteral nutrition admixture. Infect Control Hosp Epidemiol 18:814–817, 1997.

75. Greene HL, Hazlett D, Demaree R: Relationship between intralipid-induced hyperlipidemia and pulmonary function. Am J Clin Nutr 29:127–135, 1976.

76. Skeie B, Askanazi J, Rothkopf MM, et al: Intravenous fat emulsions and lung function: A review. Crit Care Med 16:183–194, 1988.

77. Aksenes J, Schmidt H, Hall C, Nordstrand K: Long term lipid-based parenteral nutrition causes pulmonary hypertension in pigs. Eur J Surg 162:649–656, 1996.

78. David M, Andrew M: Venous thromboembolic complications in children. J Pediatr 123:337–346, 1993.

79. Dollery CM, Sullivan ID, Bauraind O, et al: Pulmonary embolism and long term central venous access for parenteral nutrition. Lancet 344:1043–1045, 1994.

80. Wakefield A, Cohen Z, Craig M, et al: Thrombogenicity of total parenteral nutrition solutions. Gastroenterology 97:i210–i219, 1989.

81. Hebuterne X, Frere AM, Bayle J, Rampal P: Priapism in a patient treated with total parenteral nutrition. JPEN J Parenter Enteral Nutr 16:171–174, 1992.

82. Mizock, B, Troglia S: Nutritional support of the hospitalized patient. Dis Mon 43:349–426, 1997.

83. Zakloga GP, Roberts P: Permissive underfeeding. New Horiz 2:257–263, 1994.

84. Harris JA, Benedict FG: A Biometric Study of Basal Metabolism in Man. Pub No. 297. Washington, DC, Carnegie Institute of Washington, 1919.

85. Makk LL, McClave SA, Creech PW, et al: Clinical application of the metabolic cart to the delivery of total parenteral nutrition. Crit Care Med 18:1320–1327, 1990.

86. Weissman C, Kemper M, Askanazi J, et al: Resting metabolic rate of the critically ill patient: Measured versus predicted. J Anesth 64:673–679, 1986.

87. Foster GD, Knox LS, Dempsey DT, Mullen JL: Caloric requirements in total parenteral nutrition J Am Coll Nutr 6:231–253, 1987.

88. Weir JB de V: New methods for calculating metabolic rate with special reference to protein metabolism. J Physiol (London) 109:1–9, 1949.

89. Bursztein S: The theoretical framework of indirect calorimetry and energy balance. *In* Bursztein S, Elwyn DH, Askanazi J, Kinney JM (eds): Energy metabolism, indirect calorimetry and nutrition. Baltimore, Williams & Wilkins, 1989:27–83.

90. Sherman MS, Kosinski R, Paz, H, Campbell D: Measuring cardiac output in critically ill patients: Disagreement between thermodilution, calculated, expired gas and oxygen consumption based methods. Cardiology 88:19–25, 1997.

91. McClave SA, Snider HL: Use of indirect calorimetry in clinical nutrition. Nutr Clin Pract 7:207–221, 1992.

92. Liggett SB, Renfro AD: Energy expenditures of mechanically ventilated nonsurgical patients. Chest 98:682–686, 1990.

93. Sherman MS: A predictive equation for determination of resting energy expenditure in mechanically ventilated patients. Chest 105:544–549, 1994.

94. Sherman MS, Kaulback M, Brodman K: Ventilators are inaccurate at measuring tidal volumes and respiratory pressures. Chest 102:163S, 1992.

95. Fishman AP: Chronic obstructive lung disease: Overview. *In* Fishman AP, Elias JA, Fishman JA,

et al (eds): Fishman's Pulmonary Diseases and Disorders, 3rd ed. New York, McGraw-Hill, 1998, pp 645–658.

96. Goldstein S, Askanazi J, Weissman C, et al: Energy expenditure in patients with chronic obstructive pulmonary disease. Chest 91:222–224, 1987.

97. Schols AM, Soeters PB, Mostert R, et al: Energy balance in chronic obstructive pulmonary disease. Am Rev Respir Dis 413:1246–1252, 1991.

98. Schols AM, Fredrix EW, Soeters PB, et al: Resting energy expenditure in patients with chronic obstructive pulmonary disease. Am J Clin Nutr 54:983–987, 1991.

99. Fu A, Yoneda T, Yoshikawa M, et al: Energy expenditure in patients with pulmonary emphysema. Nihon Kokyuki Gakkai Zasshi 36:10–17, 1998.

100. Talpers SS, Romberger DJ, Bunce SB, et al: Nutritionally associated increased carbon dioxide production. Excess total calories vs high proportion of carbohydrate calories. Chest 102:551–555, 1992.

101. Askanazi J, Elwyn DH, Silverberg PA, et al: Respiratory distress secondary to a high carbohydrate load. Surgery 87:596–598, 1980.

102. Covelli HD, Black JW, Olson MS: Respiratory failured precipitated by high carbohydrate loads. Ann Intern Med 95:579–581, 1981.

103. Hegsted DM: Assessment of nitrogen requirements. Am J Clin Nutr 21:1669–1677, 1978.

104. Konstantinides FN, Konstantinides NN, Li JC, et al: Urinary urea nitrogen: too insensitive for calculating nitrogen balance studies in surgical clinical nutrition. JPEN J Parenter Enteral Nutr 15:189–193, 1991.

105. Zwillich CW, Sahn SA, Weil JV: Effects of hypermetabolism on ventilation and chemosensitivity. J Clin Invest 60:900–906, 1977.

106. Askanazi J, Weissman C, LaSala PA, et al: Effect of protein intake on ventilatory drive. Anesthesiology 60:106–110, 1984.

107. Takala J, Askanazi J, Weissman C, et al: Changes in respiratory control induced by amino acid infusions. Crit Care Med 16:465–469, 1988.

108. Blazer S, Reinersman GT, Askanazi J, et al: Branched-chain amino acids and respiratory pattern pattern and function in the neonate. J Perinatol 14:290–295, 1994.

109. Efthimiou J, Mounsey PJ, Benson DN, et al: Effect of a carbohydrate-rich versus fat-rich loads on gas exchange and walking performance in patients with chronic obstructive pulmonary disease. Thorax 47:451–456, 1992.

110. Wolfe RR, O'Donnell TF Jr, Stone MD, et al: Investigation of factors determining the optimal glucose infusion rate in total parenteral nutrition. Metabolism 29:892–900, 1980.

111. Rodriguez JL, Askanazi J, Weissman C, et al: Ventilatory and metabolic effects of glucose infusions. Chest 88:512–518, 1985.

112. Liposky JM, Nelson LD: Ventilatory response to high caloric loads in critically ill patients. Crit Care Med 22:796–802, 1994.

113. Angelillo VA, Bedi S, Durfee D, et al: Effects of low and high carbohydrate feedings in ambulatory patients with chronic obstructive lung disease and chronic hypercapnia. Ann Intern Med 103:883–885, 1985.

114. Garfinkel F, Robinson RD, Price C: Replacing carbohydrate calories with fat calories in enteral feeding for patients with impaired respiratory function. JPEN J Parenter Enteral Nutr 9:106, 1985.

115. Lathrop JC, Bommarito A, Letson JA, et al: The effects of a high fat enteral feeding formula on patients requiring mechanical ventilation. Pharm Pract News 32:1, 1986.

116. Van den Berg B, Bogaard JM, Hop WCJ: High fat, low carbohydrate enteral feeding in patients weaning from the ventilator. Intensive Care Med 20:470–475, 1994.

117. Al-Saady NM, Blackmore CM, Bennett ED: High fat, low carbohydrate, enteral feeding lowers $PaCO_2$ and reduces the period of ventilation in artificially ventilated patients. Intensive Care Med 15:290–295, 1989.

118. Askanazi J, Nordenstrom J, Rosenbaum SH, et al: Respiratory changes induced by the large glucose loads of total parenteral nutrition. JAMA 243:1444–1447, 1980.

119. Bernard GR, Artigas A, Brigham KL, et al and the Consensus Committee: The American-European Consensus Conference on ARDS: Definitions, mechanisms, relevant outcomes, and clinical trial coordination. Am J Respir Crit Care Med 149:818–824, 1994.

120. Hudson LD, Milberg JA, Anardi D, Maunder RJ: Clinical risks for development of the acute respiratory distress syndrome. Am J Respir Crit Care Med 151:293–301, 1995.

121. McMahon MM, Farnell MB, Murray MJ: Nutritional support of critically ill patients. Mayo Clin Proc 68:911–920, 1993.

122. Perlmutter DH, Dinarello CA, Punsal PI, Colten HR: Cachexin/tumor necrosis factor regulates hepatic acute-phase gene expression. J Clin Invest 78:1349–1354, 1986.

123. Carlsson M, Nordenstrom J, Hendstierna G: Clinical implications of continuous measurement of energy expenditure in mechanically ventilated patients. Clin Nutr 3:103–107, 1984.

124. Weissman C, Kemper M, Askanazi J, et al: Resting metabolic rate of the critically ill patient: Measured vs predicted. Anesthesiology 64:673–679, 1985.

125. Shaw JH, Wildbore M, Wolfe RR: Whole body protein kinetics in severely septic patients. The response to glucose infusion and total parenteral nutrition. Ann Surg 205:288–294, 1987.

126. Streat SJ, Beddoe AH, Hill GL: Aggressive nutritional support does not prevent protein loss despite fat gain in septic intensive care patients. J Trauma 27:262–266, 1987.

127. Freund HR, James JH, Fischer JE: Nitrogen sparing mechanism of singly administered branch-chain amino acids in the injured rat. Surgery 90:237–243, 1981.

128. Cerra FB, Mazuski J, Teasley K, et al: Nitrogen retention in critically ill patients is proportional to the branched chain amino acid load. Crit Care Med 11:775–778, 1983.

129. Garcia-de-Lorenzo A, Ortiz-Leyba C, Planas M, et al: Parenteral administration of different amounts of branch-chain amino acids in septic patients: Clinical and metabolic aspects. Crit Care Med 25:418–424, 1997.

130. Vente JP, Soeters PB, von Meyenfeldt MF, et al: Prospective randomized double-blind trial of

branched chain amino acid enriched versus standard parenteral nutrition solutions in traumatized and septic patients. World J Surg 15:128–132, 1991.

131. FitzSimmons SC: Cystic fibrosis patient registry annual data report, 1995. Bethesda, Md, Cystic Fibrosis Foundation, 1996.

132. Corey M, McLaughlin FJ, Williams M, Leninson H: A comparison of survival, growth and pulmonary function in patients with cystic fibrosis. J Clin Epidemiol 41:588–591, 1988.

133. Kraemer R, Rudeberg A, Hadorn B, Rossi E: Relative underweight in cystic fibrosis and its prognostic value. Acta Paediatr Scand 67:33–37, 1978.

134. Fried M, Durie P, Tsui L, et al: The cystic fibrosis gene and resting energy expenditure. J Pediatr 119:913–916, 1991.

135. O'Rawe A, McIntosh I, Dodge JA, et al: Increased energy expenditure in cystic fibrosis is associated with specific mutations. Clin Sci 82:71–76, 1992.

136. Shepherd R, Vasques-Velasquez L, Prentice A, et al: Increased energy expenditure in young children with cystic fibrosis. Lancet 1:1200–1203, 1988.

137. Girardet JP, Tounian P, Sardet A, et al: Resting energy expenditure in infants with cystic fibrosis. J Pediatr Gastroenterol Nutr 18:214–219, 1994.

138. Stallings VA, Fung EB, Hofley PM, Scanlin TF: Acute pulmonary exacerbaton is not associated with increased energy expenditure in children with cystic fibrosis. J Pediatr 132:483–489, 1998.

139. Buchdahl R, Cox M, Fulleylove C, et al: Increased energy expenditure in cystic fibrosis. J Appl Physiol 64:1810–1816, 1988.

140. Naon H, Hack S, Shelton MT, et al: Resting energy expenditure. Chest 103:1819–1825, 1993.

141. Steinkamp G, Drommer A, von der Hardt H: Resting energy expenditure before and after treatment for *Pseudomonas aeruginosa* infection in patients with cystic fibrosis. Am J Clin Nutr 57:685–689, 1993.

142. Michel SH, Mueller DH: Practical approaches to nutrition care of patients with cystic fibrosis. Top Clin Nutr 2:10–17, 1987.

143. MacDonald A, Holden C, Harris G: Nutritional strategies in cystic fibrosis: Current issues. J R Soc Med 84(Suppl 18):28–35, 1991.

144. Stark LJ, Jelalian E, Mulvihill MM, et al: Eating in preschool children with cystic fibrosis and healthy peers: A behavioral analysis. Pediatrics 95:210–215, 1995.

145. Elliot RB, Robinson PG: Unusual clinical course in a child with cystic fibrosis treated with fat emulsion. Arch Dis Child 50:76–78, 1975.

146. Chase HP, Cotton EK, Elliott RB: Intravenous linoleic acid supplementation in children with cystic fibrosis. Pediatrics 64:207–213, 1979.

147. Lester LA, Rothberg RM, Dawson G, et al: Supplemental parenteral nutrition in cystic fibrosis. JPEN J Parenter Enterol Nutr 10:289–295, 1986.

148. Mansell AL, Andersen JC, Muttart CR, et al: Short term pulmonary effects of total parenteral nutrition in children with cystic fibrosis. J Pediatr 104:700–705, 1984.

149. Shepherd R, Cooksley WG, Cooke WD: Improved growth and clinical, nutritional, and respiratory changes in response to nutritional therapy in cystic fibrosis. J Pediatr 97:351–357, 1980.

150. Kussofsky E, Strandvik B, Troell S: Prospective study of fatty acid supplementation over 3 years

151. Kirvela O, Stern RC, Askanazi J, et al: Long-term parenteral nutrition in cystic fibrosis. Nutrition 9:119–126, 1993.

152. Antonelli M, Capello G, Cortinovis AM, et al: Beneficial effect of prolonged total parenteral nutrition in a very malnourished cystic fibrosis patient. Acta Univ Carol Med (Praha) 36:174–176, 1990.

153. Skeie B, Askanazi J, Rothkopf MM, et al: Improved exercise tolerance with long-term parenteral nutrition in cystic fibrosis. Crit Care Med 15:960–962, 1987.

154. Jelalian E, Stark LJ, Reynolds L, Seifer R: Nutritional intervention for weight gain in cystic fibrosis: A meta analysis. J Pediatr 132:486–492, 1998.

155. Cropp GJA, Rosenberg PN: Energy costs of breathing in cystic fibrosis and their relation to severity of pulmonary disease. Monogr Paediatr 14:91–94, 1981.

156. Ho KKL, Pinsky JL, Kannel WB, Levy D: The epidemiology of heart failure: The Framingham Study. J Am Coll Cardiol 22(Suppl A):6A–13A, 1993.

157. McAlister FA, Teo KK: The management of congestive heart failure. Postgrad Med J 73:194–200, 1997.

158. Cohn JN: Overview of the treatment of heart failure. Am J Cardiol 80(11A):2L–6L, 1997.

159. Konstam MA, Remme WJ: Treatment guidelines in heart failure. Prog Cardiovasc Dis. 48(1Suppl 1):65–72, 1998.

160. Heymsfield SB, Casper K: Congestive heart failure: Clinical management by use of continuous nasoenteric feeding. Am J Clin Nutr 50:539–544, 1989.

161. Grimes JB, Abel RM: Hemodynamic effects of fat emulsion in dogs. JPEN J Parenter Enteral Nutr 3:40–44, 1979.

162. Fisch D, Abel RM: Hemodynamic effects of intravenous fat emulsions in patients with heart disease. JPEN J Parenter Enteral Nutr 5:402–405, 1981.

163. Abel RM, Fisch D, Grossman ML: Hemodynamic effects of intravenous 20% soy emulsion following coronary bypass surgery. JPEN J Parenter Enter Nutr 7:534–540, 1983.

164. Yun DD, Alpert JS: Acute coronary syndromes. Cardiology 88:223–237, 1997.

165. ACC and AHA Task Force: ACC/AHA guidelines for management of patients with acute myocardial infarction. J Am Coll Cardiol 28:1328–1428, 1996.

166. Rogers WJ, Russell RO Jr, McDaniel HG, Rackley CE: Acute effects of glucose-insulin-potassium infusion on myocardial substrates, coronary blood flow and oxygen consumption in man. Am J Cardiol 40:421–425, 1977.

167. Rogers WJ, Segal PH, McDaniel HG, et al: Prospective randomized trial of glucose-insulin-potassium in acute myocardial infarction. Am J Cardiol 43:801–806, 1979.

168. Mantle JA, Rogers WJ, Smith LR, et al: Clinical effects of glucose-insulin-potassium on left ventricular function in acute myocardial infarction: Results from a randomized clinical trial. Am Heart J 102:313–324, 1981.

169. Rackley CE, Russell RO Jr, Rogers WJ, et al: Clinical experience with glucose-insulin-potassium therapy in acute myocardial infarction. Am Heart J 102:1038–1049, 1981.

17

◆ Total Parenteral Nutrition: Effects on the Small Intestine

Howard T. Wang, M.D.
Harry C. Sax, M.D., F.A.C.S.

Total parenteral nutrition (TPN) dramatically affects the morbidity and mortality of patients with a wide range of diseases. With short-term use, TPN can enhance the nutritional state of patients until enteral nutrition can be resumed. In certain situations, prolonged or lifetime TPN becomes necessary, increasing the chances of significant complications. These include catheter-related sepsis, metabolic derangement, and organ dysfunction.[1, 2] The lack of enteral stimulation can also lead to significant changes in small bowel morphology and function with both short- and long-term implications.

Short bowel syndrome, a leading indication for long-term TPN, is a devastating clinical condition resulting from surgical removal of the small bowel owing to vascular disease, intestinal volvulus, ischemic bowel, inflammatory bowel disease, or abdominal sepsis. After massive enterectomy, important changes that enable the patient to improve nutrient absorption occur in the small bowel, such as an increase in villous height and intestinal length through hypertrophy and hyperplasia.[1–3] Alterations in nutrient transport can also improve the efficiency of uptake for individual nutrients.[4, 5] The process of adaptation may take up to 2 years before maximal tolerance of enteral nutrition is reached.[3] During this time, TPN plays a critical role in supporting the dietary requirements of patients with varied degrees of malabsorption. TPN alone, however, cannot stimulate optimal adaptation. Enteral nutrition is trophic toward the gut and enhances compensatory hypertrophy and hyperplasia. The combination of enteral and parenteral diets usually results in better adaptation than either route alone.[6]

A better understanding of how TPN affects the small bowel can lead to insight on improving enterocyte function. Such knowledge can be used to decrease patients' dependence on TPN and reduce gut-related complications such as immune dysfunction or bacterial translocation (BT). The gut is a large reservoir for bacteria, and their escape may be the source of sepsis in critically ill patients. This chapter examines gut-specific TPN effects and suggests strategies to minimize potential morbidity.

◆ ADAPTATION

The human small bowel possesses tremendous adaptive capacity. In normal adults, the small bowel length ranges from 300 to 800 cm depending on the state of contraction or relaxation. Resection of up to 50% can be tolerated within a short time, whereas 70% resection requires a period of adaptation before full volitional feedings are possible. The preservation of certain segments of bowel such as the terminal ileum, ileocecal valve, and pylorus increases the size of resection that a patient will tolerate by slowing the transit time and allowing additional digestion and absorption.[1–3] Short bowel syndrome, however, is not defined by an exact length of bowel resected. Rather, it is defined as the onset of clinical symptoms consistent with malabsorption such as intractable diarrhea, steatorrhea, weight loss, dehydration, electrolyte disturbances, and malnutrition. Paramount in the treatment of these patients is minimizing the metabolic consequences arising from these symptoms.

The effect of enterectomy depends on not only the size of the resection but also its location. The jejunum and ileum are distinct morphologic and physiologic entities. The small bowel lumen contains circular folds (valvulae conniventes), villi, and microvilli, which greatly increase the absorptive surface area. These structures are more prominent in the jejunum, where the majority of digestion and absorption of nutrients occurs. The ileum, in contrast, is the primary site of vitamin B_{12} and bile salt absorption and also contains more lymphoid tissue.[1, 2]

The adaptive process has been well documented in animals. In a rabbit model, 1 month after 70% enterectomy, brush-border membrane nutrient transport of amino acids and glucose is decreased with a concomitant increase in villous and mucosal heights. The organism attempts to increase the surface area to compensate for not only the loss of bowel but also a decrease in nutrient uptake efficiency. After 3 months, both the nutrient uptake and the morphology return to normal.[4] Furthermore, jejunal and ileal uptake of nutrients can vary in a site-specific manner in response to both surgical stress and the site of resection.[7]

In humans, the adaptive period is more prolonged. Up to 2 months after resection, patients may experience metabolic derangement such as electrolyte and fluid imbalance secondary to intractable diarrhea. After these symptoms subside, the goal is to define maximal oral nutritional tolerances. At 2 years, adaptation reaches steady state, and at this point, the patient who is still on TPN may be so for life.[3]

TPN can have a beneficial effect on outcomes by providing essential nutrients during periods of malabsorption. In an animal model, parenterally fed enterectomized puppies that were also offered enteral nutrition showed normal growth and development. Animals fed exclusively by enteral nutrition lost or failed to gain weight during the same time period. Furthermore, parenterally fed dogs exhibited normal stools after weaning to full enteral nutrition, whereas the enterally fed dogs continued to have watery diarrhea even at 6 to 8 months of age. Although all animals showed increases in morphologic adaptation, it was thought that the enterally fed animals adapted poorly because massive resection prevented adequate nutrient absorption from the gut lumen.[8] *No matter how trophic oral feedings may be, the organism must be nutritionally repleted in order to benefit from enteral nutrition.*

Although lifesaving for many patients, TPN alone cannot stimulate optimal adaptation in the small bowel. Short gut rats fed standard chow exhibited significantly greater increases in villous height, crypt depth, DNA and RNA content, and sucrase activity compared with animals fed exclusively by parenteral nutrition. These changes were reversible, however. After the resumption of enteral nutrition for 4 weeks, TPN-supported animals achieved similar body weights and greater intestinal length compared with animals fed enterally from the start.[9]

Not every form of enteral nutrition, however, can enhance adaptation. Elemental feedings are not as effective as complex diets in stimulating trophic changes in the residual bowel. Several studies showed decreased adaptation, mucosal weight, DNA, and protein content in rats fed an elemental diet.[10–12] Although human studies on this matter are sparse, a case report from Italy examined a patient who underwent a subtotal colectomy and was given 30 days of TPN postoperatively.[13] After being refed a regular diet for 14 days, the patient exhibited a reversion of hypoplasia (villous height and crypt depth) to hyperplasia in the small bowel.

The mechanisms by which enteral feedings effect changes in the intestine are unclear. Many current studies concentrate on endogenous growth factors. One such example is epidermal growth factor (EGF), a 53–amino acid, 6-kd polypeptide secreted by the salivary glands and Brunner's glands of the duodenum. EGF is known to enhance adaptation after massive enterectomy.[14–16] It has been demonstrated that the intragastric administration of alcohol can increase mucosal EGF and EGF receptor expression.[17] Whether alcohol increases EGF release through injuring the bowel or stimulating the bowel as a nutrient, a signaling process must occur to affect EGF release at the salivary and/or Brunner's glands. Increased EGF, in turn, could enhance adaptation. Neurotensin, found mainly in the central nervous system and mucosal endocrine cells, has also been shown to increase microvillous height after massive resection and reverse the deleterious effects seen with an elemental diet.[12, 15] Understanding how nutrients can stimulate the release of growth factors and hormones will provide a mechanistic knowledge of these processes. As we discuss later in the chapter, hormones alone can affect small bowel physiology in a manner similar to that of oral nutrition.

◆ IMMUNE RESPONSE AND BACTERIAL TRANSLOCATION

A major complication in critically ill patients is sepsis. The intestine is a reservoir for microorganisms and toxins and is a potential source of bacteremia. This could occur secondary to disease processes such as trauma, perforated viscus, and necrosis of the bowel. At one end of the spectrum, perforation secondary to disease or penetrating trauma may directly release bacteria into the peritoneal cavity. However, nonpenetrating trauma, burns, and intestinal obstruction have also been implicated as possible causes for BT.[18–21] Such injuries can lead to alterations in the normal gut flora, intestinal permeability, and host immune response.[21–24] Many of these patients may require short-term TPN until they are able to resume a normal diet. This further compounds the problem, because although protein malnutrition itself does not induce BT, TPN can.[25, 26] Malnutrition also leads to impaired immune responses and increases the susceptibility of the patient to infectious complications.[27] Thus, critically ill patients may have multiple factors that are additive in increasing the chance of sepsis.

The gut represents an enormous surface area by which the body is exposed to the external environment. Food includes bacteria and other potential pathogens, and its ingestion adds these bacteria to the already-numerous colonies of endogenous bacteria that normally reside within the healthy gastrointestinal tract. The ability of the gut to defend against such insults is complicated by the need to absorb nutrition while preventing the absorption of bacteria and toxins. Low gastric pH helps reduce the bacterial load in the proximal intestinal tract, whereas gut motility prevents bacterial overgrowth, which occurs secondary to stagnation. The gut also represents a rich environment for immune defenses of the body. The major intestinal antibody is immunoglobulin A (IgA). It is secreted by plasma cells contained in the lamina propria of the intestine. IgA then crosses the mucosa via protein carriers. These secretory antibodies inhibit bacteria proliferation, viral cell adhesion, and the absorption of endotoxins. The immune response in the intestine is further buttressed by a rich network of lymphoid tissue such as the mesenteric lymph nodes and Peyer's patches in the ileum.[28, 29]

Enteral stimulation is a necessary component in normal gastrointestinal immunity. IgA levels were reduced in rats infused with TPN formulations compared with rats fed

an isonitrogenous, isocaloric diet enterally.[30] The form of oral nutrition (elemental vs. complex) necessary to induce changes, however, is not entirely clear. In the previous study, IgA levels were influenced by the presence of enteral nutrition regardless of whether the diet was elemental.[30] This is in distinct contrast to other reports, which show an increase in BT and decreased immune function as a result of parenteral or enteral feeding of TPN formulations. In mice, a decrease in lamina propria, intraepithelial space, Peyer's patch lymphocytes, and B cells was seen in oral and intravenous TPN groups compared with chow-fed groups.[31] Only intestinal IgA, however, was significantly decreased with oral and intravenous TPN feeding. Serum and biliary IgA remained unaffected. In contrast, a complex enteral diet, Nutren, preserved lymphocyte populations. Other animal models confirm these findings. In rats, 7 days of oral feeding of TPN formulations reduced the blastogenic response of blood and splenic lymphocytes to mitogens and increased BT. The animals' resistance to a *Staphylococcus aureus* challenge was also reduced. Within 3 days of refeeding with a standard enteral diet, however, the immune response recovered (Fig. 17–1).[32] A similar effect was seen in mice with a rapid return of gut-associated lymphoid tissue cellularity (GALT) after enteral refeeding following a TPN-only diet.[33]

Although glutamine is important in maintaining the gut mucosa (discussed later), its role in preserving immune function is controversial. Results vary based on the species and experimental model. Burke and colleagues demonstrated a reduction in BT and an increase in IgA levels with glutamine-supplemented TPN.[34] Furthermore, TPN resulted in a decrease in B and T cells, whereas glutamine supplementation helped preserve cell populations.[35] Oral glutamine supplementation was also noted to reduce BT in rats after radiation injury.[36] However, the immune response in healthy rats fed an elemental enteral diet was not improved by oral glutamine supplementation. An elemental diet, with or without glutamine, decreased the blastogenic response in lymphocytes harvested from the blood, spleen, and mesenteric lymph nodes.[37]

BT is affected by nutrition in a manner similar to that of the immune system. Both elemental enteral diet and intravenous TPN have been shown in many animal studies to

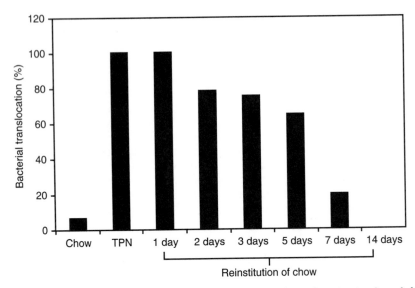

Figure 17–1. Bacterial translocation after reinstitution of diet. Bacterial translocation in chow-fed and oral–total parenteral nutrition (TPN)–fed animals for 7 days are compared with animals fed 7 days of oral-TPN and reinstitution of chow. There is a steady decrease of bacterial translocation with the number of days after the reinstitution of chow, reaching to zero percent at 2 weeks. (From Mainous M, Xu D, Lu Q, et al: Oral-TPN-induced bacterial translocation and impaired immune defenses are reversed by refeeding. Surgery 110:279, 1991.)

be associated with increased bacterial escape from the intestine.[26, 32, 37] Refeeding animals with a normal enteral diet reversed both the increase in BT and the decrease in immune function.[32] Unfortunately, results of animal studies have not been consistently duplicated in humans. In critically ill trauma patients, infectious complications and outcomes were not related to intraoperative mesenteric lymph node culture results. In fact, BT to mesenteric lymph nodes could not be demonstrated in any of the trauma patients (n = 25) undergoing laparotomy.[38] In another study, portal or systemic bacteremia within the first 5 days after injury could not be confirmed despite an eventual 30% incidence of multiple organ failure.[39]

Further studies have elucidated specific components of a complex diet that may be beneficial. Fiber supplementation decreased BT and improved immune function in animals supported with parenteral and elemental oral diets.[40] The addition of cellulose powder decreased the incidence of BT to 8% in groups fed TPN formulations orally and 0% in intravenous TPN–fed groups in rats compared with 60% in those fed TPN without fiber formulations orally or intravenously. This was not seen in conjunction with decreased TPN-induced bacterial overgrowth or decreased mucosal proteins (a reflection of mucosal mass).[41] More specifi-

cally, BT decreased only when bulk-forming fiber was administered and not when citrus pectin (non–bulk-forming) was given. Gram-negative enteric overgrowth was also less with bulk-forming fiber compared with citrus pectin.[42] Bacterial overgrowth, however, has not been consistently shown to be correlated with BT.[25, 26, 41, 42] The evidence suggests that fiber may exert its effect by preventing mucosal abnormalities induced by TPN.[41]

The mechanisms by which enteral nutrition affects BT may be through the induction of hormones. Bombesin and somatostatin are considered the "on" and "off" switches of the gut by regulating the release of other gut hormones and peptides.[29] In mice fed an elemental enteral diet, bombesin was as effective as dietary fiber in reducing BT. The somatostatin analogue sandostatin in contrast, blocked the beneficial effect of fiber. The mucosal mass and gut flora, however, did not consistently correlate with hormonal treatment.[43] A similar effect was seen in rats (Fig. 17–2). Bombesin appears to decrease mucosal injury in animals fed either an elemental enteral or a parenteral diet.[44] In terms of clinical applicability, bombesin was effective in decreasing BT in animals fed three different commercially available liquid enteral diets including the elemental enteral diet Vivonex.[45]

Although enteral nutrition can reverse the detrimental effects of TPN, it appears that the composition of the enteral diet is extremely important. Elemental enteral diets can induce the same alterations as TPN in terms of mucosal atrophy, BT, and immune dysfunction. Refeeding with polymeric enteral diets usually reversed any adverse changes caused by TPN. Fiber, bombesin, and glutamine can have trophic effects on intestinal physiology when the resumption of a normal diet is not possible.

◆ SMALL BOWEL MUCOSAL BARRIER AND BACTERIAL TRANSLOCATION

Although much has been established about BT, its clinical applicability and its relation to mucosal integrity remain unclear. Theoretically, bacteria might translocate more easily if atrophy or mucosal injury were to occur. Barrier function may affect BT independent of the overall immune response. This section examines the effects of specific factors on mucosal integrity and BT.

Although considered a nonessential amino acid, glutamine has been shown to be extremely important to small intestinal metabolism. It is the primary oxidative fuel for the dividing enterocyte.[46–48] The role of glutamine in small bowel injury has been well established, and under conditions of stress, it becomes an essential amino acid.[49] Oral glutamine has been shown to be beneficial in rats receiving whole-abdomen radiation, reducing the number of complications such as bloody diarrhea and bowel perforation while increasing mucosal villous height.[50] Furthermore, the gut switches from an organ of glutamine release to one of uptake after enterectomy, indicating an increased need for this nutrient.[51]

The absence of enteral nutrition inhibits adaptive hyperplasia after massive enterectomy.[9] Furthermore, commercially available amino acid solutions, which are used in the formulation of TPN solutions, do not contain glutamine. In intact rats, glutamine-supplemented TPN increased jejunal wet weight, DNA, protein, mucosal thickness, and villous height when compared with those of rats fed an isonitrogenous glycine preparation.[52] In addition, glutamine dipeptide–supplemented TPN was shown to be as effective as glutamine in maintaining mucosal thickness, villous height, and nitrogen balance in healthy as well as 50% enterectomized rats.[53] Similar benefits were seen

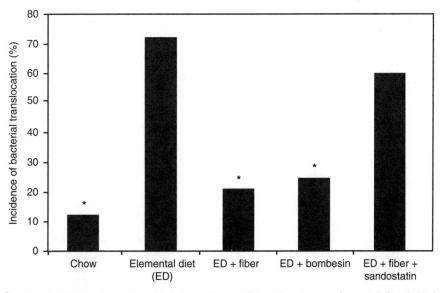

Figure 17–2. Effects of bombesin and sandostatin on bacterial translocation in elemental diet (ED)–fed rats. The incidence of bacterial translocation was significantly decreased with the addition of fiber or bombesin to the elemental diet. Sandostatin reversed the beneficial effects of fiber. *$P < .01$ vs. elemental diet and $P < .05$ vs. ED + fiber + sandostatin. (From Haskel Y, Xu D, Lu Q, Deitch EA: The modulatory role of gut hormones in elemental diet and intravenous total parenteral nutrition–induced bacterial translocation in rats. JPEN J Parenter Enteral Nutr 18:161, 1993.)

in rats with glutamine-enriched TPN after endotoxin infusion. Nitrogen balance was improved and mucosal atrophy was decreased when compared with animals receiving an isonitrogenous glycine preparation.[54] Human studies have shown an increase in D-xylose excretion after a modified D-xylose test (a measure of absorption efficacy of the duodenum) in groups receiving glutamine dipeptide–supplemented TPN compared with conventional TPN.[55] While glutamine's role in immune function is not entirely clear, it is an integral part of maintaining the gut mucosa. In addition, TPN formulations without additional glutamine may not meet the increased demands of rapidly dividing enterocytes after bowel injury.

Hormonal influences also play an important role. EGF enhances the adaptive response of the small intestine after massive enterectomy, whereas bombesin decreases BT.[14, 15, 43, 44] Other gut peptides have been examined such as glucagon-like peptide-2. Coinfusion of glucagon-like peptide-2 with TPN in rats was able to reverse the reduction in intestinal mass, protein, and DNA.[56] The question that remains is how these hormonal influences are related to enteral nutrition, fiber, and glutamine supplementation in adaptation. One possible mechanism is that enteral nutrition stimulates the endogenous release of hormones, facilitating the maintenance of the mucosal barrier.

Sugars have been demonstrated to be trophic when given as an enteral supplementation to TPN. Glucose, fructose, mannose, and mannitol, representing different forms of transport (active, nonactive, and carrier-mediated), all were able to stimulate mucosal growth. In addition, phlorhizin, an inhibitor of glucose transport, did not significantly affect fructose-induced mucosal growth.[57] These findings raise the question of whether the presence of substrates in the lumen of the intestine, regardless of the type of nutrient, can increase mucosal mass.

Before bacteria can translocate, they must penetrate the intestinal mucus and attach to the underlying mucosa. It would seem logical that a breakdown in the mucosal barrier may allow bacteria to escape and bypass the lymph nodes, where the immune system can clear the pathogens. In a study examining the role of bacterial adherence and the mucous barrier in BT, protein-malnourished rats were compared with endotoxin-treated rats. Protein malnutrition is associated with changes in morphology but not BT. In contrast, endotoxin challenge is associated with BT but not morphologic changes. The adherence of bacteria, the first step in BT, was decreased in malnourished rats, whereas it was increased in endotoxin-challenged rats. Furthermore, increased binding of *Escherichia coli* to insoluble mucus was noted in rats receiving endotoxin. Therefore, BT appears to be closely related to bacterial adherence to mucosa and its associated mucous layer but not to changes in morphology.[58]

The next step in bacterial translocation is for the pathogen to effectively cross the enterocyte and/or paracellular junctions, a measure of which is intestinal permeability. TPN and elemental enteral diet–fed rats showed significant increases in BT *in vitro* in a model measuring gut permeability. The magnitude of *E. coli* and phenol red transmucosal passage in Ussing chambers was significantly higher in TPN or elemental enteral diet–fed rats compared with chow-fed rats. The electric potential differences across the membrane remained unchanged although the resistance in TPN and elemental enteral diet–fed rats was significantly lower than in chow-fed rats. This suggests that permeability is affected by diet and is correlated with BT.[59]

Other studies contradict this finding and suggest that permeability and BT are independent variables. In vivo permeability to lactulose was increased significantly in TPN-fed rats and was related to gut atrophy. This was not associated with increased BT.[60] Partial enteral nutrition with a polymeric diet at 25% of the total calories decreased BT and improved nitrogen balance in TPN-supported rats (Fig. 17–3). There was no associated change in gut permeability.[61]

Although nutritional factors are important in maintaining the mucosal barrier, there is no clear and convincing evidence that this translates to decreased BT. Endotoxin increases BT without any significant change in gut morphology. Direct mucosal injury has been implicated as a possible mechanism, although how exactly this leads to increased BT is not clear. Rather, BT is probably a multifactorial event. Immune function, the mucosal barrier, permeability, mucus production, and bacterial adherence are apparently additive in their ability to promote or prevent BT (Fig. 17–4).

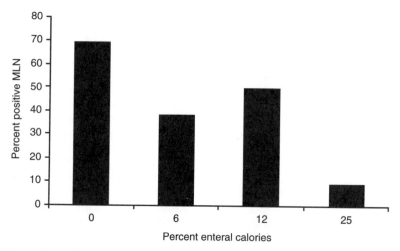

Figure 17–3. Effects of partial enteral nutrition on bacterial translocation. Partial enteral nutrition decreased bacterial translocation, with the most dramatic effect seen in animals fed 25% of calories with enteral nutrition ($P < .03$). (From Sax HC, Illig KA, Ryan CK, Hardy DJ: Low-dose enteral feeding is beneficial during total parenteral nutrition. Am J Surg 171:589, 1996.)

Many of the studies examined BT by measuring the presence of bacteria in the mesenteric lymph nodes. However, this does not necessarily lead to an increased incidence of sepsis, multiple organ failure, or death. One theory is that bacterial sampling in the mesenteric lymph nodes is a normal component of the immune response. This helps to better focus the plasma cell response to commonly encountered antigens. The lymph nodes prevent further egress of the bacteria into the body by trapping and eliminating the bacteria. Under pathologic conditions, bacteria may escape at a greater rate to the mesenteric lymph nodes without necessarily increasing the systemic exposure to such pathogens.

◆ ENDOTOXEMIA

Endotoxin is a lipopolysaccharide-protein complex normally found in the cell wall of gram-negative bacteria. Its release from the cell wall can result in adverse systemic effects through activation of biologic pathways (complement system, cytokines, coagulation) of the host organism.[62] Many

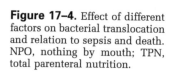

Figure 17–4. Effect of different factors on bacterial translocation and relation to sepsis and death. NPO, nothing by mouth; TPN, total parenteral nutrition.

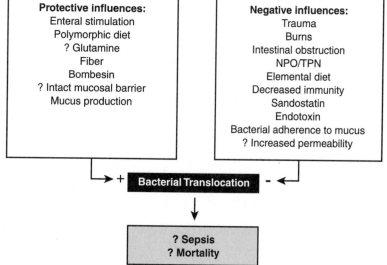

critically ill patients who require parenteral nutrition also suffer from gram-negative sepsis. As discussed earlier, TPN affects the immune system, and this may change the clinical outcome for septic patients. The source of infection (gut vs. nongut) is less important since the route of nutrition can alter the systemic immune function. This section explores how TPN affects organisms with endotoxemia.

The first concern is TPN's effects on the gut's barrier function. Increases in gut permeability may increase endotoxin escape, leading to activation of cytokine pathways and subsequent systemic effects. Studies show increases in permeability in TPN-fed animals as well as humans,[59, 60] although a correlation with increased BT or a worsened clinical outcome was not demonstrated.[63] Endotoxin exposure in humans has also been correlated with a transient increase in gut permeability, despite no differences being noted between the TPN and the enteral nutrition groups.[64] Human studies do not consistently show increased morbidity in endotoxemia with TPN usage.[63–66] TPN-supported humans exposed to endotoxin showed increased symptomatology, tumor necrosis factor (TNF), and acute-phase reactant proteins compared with controls fed a standard oral supplement.[65] Another study on TPN usage in humans, in contrast, demonstrated decreased plasma interleukin-6 and platelet responses with no change in TNF levels or symptoms.[63] Nevertheless, it does appear that TPN or the lack of enteral nutrition can alter mediators of systemic inflammatory responses.

Glutamine, through its ability to maintain the gut mucosa, is also thought to be of benefit in endotoxemia. Glutamine supplementation decreases mucosal atrophy as evidenced by increased jejunal mucosal wet weight, protein content, villous height, crypt depth, and wall thickness and assists in the maintenance of the mucosal barrier function in endotoxemia.[54] TPN decreases cytokine release and increases mucosal injury, which is improved by glutamine dipeptide in rats with hemorrhagic shock.[67] However, glutamine supplementation in elemental enteral diet–fed endotoxemic rats improved mucosal architecture with no effect on survival.[68]

Other components of TPN that may be influential in endotoxemia include the dietary fats. Fatty acids are precursors to eicosanoids, including leukotrienes, thromboxanes, and prostaglandins, which are known to mediate inflammation, coagulation, and the immune response. The essential fatty acid used in available preparations of TPN is linoleic acid (n-6). The primary concern is that linoleic acid is the precursor of arachadonic acid, which can be converted to thromboxanes and proinflammatory and immunosuppressive prostaglandins via cyclooxygenase. These eicosanoids have powerful systemic effects, producing clinically apparent changes. The n-3 fatty acids (linolenic acid), which are commonly found in fish oil, in contrast, produce less proinflammatory eicosanoids and can compete with the n-6 fatty acids in the arachadonic acid pathway. The significance is that the n-3 fatty acids may reduce the negative effects exhibited by the n-6 fatty acids. Since traditional TPN formulations include only n-6 fatty acids, such preparations may dangerously promote inflammatory and immunosuppresive mediators in critically ill patients.[69] Although this topic strays from the focus of this chapter (TPN's effect on the small bowel), immune system changes can have serious consequences on bacterial and endotoxin translocation.

In rats given 4 days of fish oil, olive oil, or corn oil concurrently with endotoxin, fish oil decreased the percentage of linoleic acid and arachadonic acid in hepatic Kupffer and endothelial cells in comparison with controls. Olive oil decreased only linoleic acid levels.[70] Rats that were subjected to both endotoxin and a 30% body surface area burn given TPN supplemented with linolenic acid showed increases in anti-inflammatory eicosanoid precursors compared with rats without supplementation.[71] In terms of morbidity, fish oil–supplemented TPN decreased lactic acidosis induced by endotoxin in guinea pigs compared with soybean oil supplementation.[72]

Long-chain triglycerides (LCTs) widely used in TPN preparations are less well oxidized and block reticuloendothelial system functions when compared with medium-chain triglycerides (MCTs). Thus, using MCTs may help blunt some of the negative effects of LCTs and confer metabolic advantages. Gollaher and colleagues examined fish oil–MCT structured triglyceride diets in rats stressed by burn and endotoxin.[73] Rats fed parenterally, supplemented with zero, 5, 15, or 30% of the non-nitrogen diet with structured triglycerides, showed maximal whole-body protein synthesis at 15% supplementation. Furthermore, structured triglyceride–supplemented TPN usage in endotoxemia appears to reduce bacterial sequestration in the lungs accompanied by increased sequestration of bacteria in the liver and spleen. There was also less fatty infiltration in the liver compared with a physical mixture of LCTs and MCTs.[74]

Other nutrients that are not commonly found in TPN but may have beneficial effects include arginine and nucleoside-nucleotide mixtures. Arginine-supplemented TPN, thought to be advantageous from an immunologic standpoint,[75] has been shown to improve histone and fibrinogen synthesis in septic rats compared with glycine-supplemented controls.[76] Oral arginine supplementation did not, however, influence lymphocyte proliferation in endotoxemic rats.[77]

Dietary nucleotides may be helpful in preserving immune function[69] as well as being trophic to the gut. In nucleoside-nucleotide supplemented endotoxemic mice fed a protein-free diet, there was decreased BT along with increased villous height, crypt depth, and wall thickness compared with the unsupplemented group.[78] Although nucleotides are not usually thought of as essential nutrients, this study suggests possible beneficial effects of such compounds in diet.

Host organisms' response to endotoxin appears to be mediated by cytokines or paracrine functions and can be altered by local signaling. Systemic signaling has also been implicated as a factor in endotoxemia. Specifically, the effect of insulin-like growth factor-I (IGF-I) has been studied. IGF-I improved nitrogen balance in endotoxemic TPN-fed rats compared with groups not given IGF-I.[79] Furthermore, enteral nutrition appears to ameliorate the decrease in IGF-I, IGF-I protein, and mRNA seen with TPN usage in endotoxemia. This increase in the enteral nutrition group was correlated with a decrease in TNF levels.[80] IGF-I also preserved mucosal integrity in septic rats receiving TPN.[81]

An issue previously explored with BT is the effect of bacterial overgrowth in TPN usage. An increased bacterial count in the colon may translate into an increase in endotoxin release and escape. Polymyxin B has been used in an attempt to decrease the bacterial count as well as block endotoxin activity and TNF production. Rats given

TPN, TPN with oral polymyxin B, or TPN with intravenous polymyxin B showed decreased levels of total fat and triglycerides as well as TNF production in the latter antibiotic groups. This was correlated with a decrease in the cecal bacterial count.[82]

In summary, although few studies demonstrate a significant improvement in morbidity and mortality in either animal studies or human trials, it appears that dietary manipulations do affect an organism's response to endotoxin. The concern, of course, is whether any nutritional supplementation in TPN or hormonal or antimicrobial manipulation actually leads to improvements of patients' health. The applicability of animal trials is further examined in the next section.

◆ CLINICAL STUDIES

The translation of results from animal studies to humans regarding TPN's effects has been inconsistent. In a study comparing villous changes, children aged 9 months to 5 years receiving TPN were compared with age-matched controls. Only in the case of long-term (>9 months) TPN usage was any villous atrophy noted. In addition, the atrophy was considered mild in three of four patients.[83] In adults who had at least 10 days of preoperative TPN without any enteral nutrients, no significant decrease in villous height or increase in BT were noted compared with those on a regular diet preoperatively.[84] Guedon and coworkers performed biopsies in the duodenum of seven adults (all with inflammatory bowel disease) before TPN, after about 3 weeks of TPN, and after discontinuing TPN and restarting oral feedings.[85] They noted no change in gross villous morphology with only a moderate decrease in microvillous height after 21 days of TPN. Major enzyme activities (sucrase, maltase, lactase, and so forth) were decreased after 21 days of TPN but returned to normal after oral feeding.[85] A study examining eight healthy volunteers did see decreases in villous height after 2 weeks of TPN usage. Although the changes were significant, the decrease was much smaller than changes noted in animal studies.[86]

In terms of physiologic changes, TPN decreases amino acid and glucose transport in the brush-border membrane of the enterocyte. In this study, six surgical patients were randomized to receive 1 week of preoperative TPN and seven patients were randomized to receive a regular diet. At celiotomy, ileal or jejunal samples were then obtained and transport studies performed on the brush-border membranes. TPN-treated patients showed decreases in methylamino isobutyric acid, L-alanine, L-arginine, L-leucine, and D-glucose transport. Paradoxically, glutamine transport was preserved, supporting its central role in the enterocyte.[87]

◆ TREATMENTS

The jump from the laboratory bench to the bedside can be a long one. Nevertheless, certain factors that can improve intestinal mucosal growth, such as glutamine and enteral stimulation, may in fact be beneficial regardless of their effect on BT as seen by numerous trauma studies with better outcomes in enterally supported patients.[88–90] A large number of TPN-dependent patients have short bowel syndrome. Enteral nutrition and glutamine can improve the overall immune function of the patient leading to decreased septic complications. Bombesin, EGF, fiber, and other trophic factors may improve gut function and adaptation, allowing patients to be weaned from TPN sooner and resulting in reduced TPN related morbidity.

Wilmore's group has applied these concepts in long-term TPN patients.[91] The combination of exogenous growth hormone, glutamine, and a high-carbohydrate, low-fat diet improved the absorption of protein by 39% with a 33% decrease in stool output. In the long-term study, 40% of the patients receiving this treatment remained off TPN; an additional 40% of the patients had decreased TPN requirements.[91]

◆ PERSPECTIVES

Appropriately applied, TPN can be of great benefit to patients. It allows the physician time to treat disease while providing adequate nourishment to patients who cannot tolerate full enteral nutrition. One must be cognizant, however, of the potential adverse changes TPN can induce in the intestine that may affect the outcome. This chapter has examined the role of enteral nutrition, glutamine, fiber, and bombesin on ameliorating some of the detrimental effects of TPN on intestinal mucosa and physiology. Although the most dramatic effects are seen in animal models, there is great excitement in the application of these techniques to improvements in patient outcomes.

REFERENCES

1. Wilmore DW, Byrne TA, Persinger RL: Short bowel syndrome: New therapeutic approaches. Curr Probl Surg 34:391–444, 1997.
2. Vanderhoof JA, Langnas AN: Short-bowel syndrome in children and adults. Gastroenterology 113:1767–1778, 1997.
3. Dudrick SJ, Latifi R, Fosnocht DE: Management of the short bowel syndrome. Surg Clin North Am 7:625–643, 1991.
4. Sarac TP, Seydel AS, Ryan CK, et al: Sequential alterations in gut mucosal amino acid and glucose transport after 70% small bowel resection. Surgery 120:503–508, 1996.
5. Klimberg VS, Souba WW, Salloum RM, et al: Intestinal glutamine metabolism after massive small bowel resection. Am J Surg 159:27–33, 1990.
6. Al-Jurf AS, Younoszai MK, Chapman-Furr F: Effect of nutritional method on adaptation of the intestinal remnant after massive bowel resection. J Pediatr Gastroenterol Nutr 4:245–252, 1985.
7. Wang HT, Miller JH, Avissar N, Sax HC: Amino acid transport after massive enterectomy is dependent on the site of resection. Surg Forum 49:166–168, 1998.
8. Wilmore DW, Dudrick SJ, Daly JM, Vars HM: The role of nutrition in the adaptation of the small intestine after massive resection. Surg Gynecol Obstet 132:673–680, 1971.
9. Ford WD, Boelhouwer RU, King WWK, et al: Total parenteral nutrition inhibits intestinal adaptive hyperplasia in young rats: Reversal by feeding. Surgery 96:527–534, 1984.
10. Young EA, Cioletti LA, Winborn WB, et al: Comparative study of nutritional adaptation to defined formula diets in rats. Am J Clin Nutr 33:2106–2118, 1980.
11. Morin CL, Ling V, Bourassa D: Small intestinal and colonic changes induced by a chemically defined diet. Dig Dis Sci 25:123–128, 1980.
12. Evers BM, Izukura M, Townsend CM Jr, et al: Neutotensin prevents intestinal mucosal hypoplasia in rats fed an elemental diet. Dig Dis Sci 37:426–431, 1992.
13. Biasco G, Callegari C, Lami F, et al: Intestinal morphological changes during oral refeeding in a patient previously treated with total parenteral nutrition for small bowel resection. Am J Gastroenterol 79:585–588, 1984.
14. Chaet MS, Arya G, Ziegler MM, Warner BW: Epidermal growth factor enhances intestinal adaptation after massive small bowel resection. J Pediatr Surg 29:1035–1039, 1994.
15. Ryan CK, Miller JH, Seydel AS, et al: Epidermal growth factor and neurotensin induce microvillus hypertrophy following massive enterectomy. J Gastrointest Surg 1:467–473, 1997.

16. Heitz PU, Kasper M, Van Noorden S, et al: Immunohistochemical localisation of urogastrone to human duodenal and submandibular glands. Gut 19:408–413, 1978.
17. Tarnawski A, Lu SY, Stachura J, Sarfeh IJ: Adaptation of gastric mucosa to chronic alcohol administration is associated with increased mucosal expression of growth factors and their receptor. Scand J Gastroenterol Suppl 193:59–63, 1992.
18. Deitch EA, McIntyre Bridges R: Effect of stress and trauma on bacterial translocation from the gut. J Surg Res 42:536–542, 1987.
19. Deitch EA: Intestinal permeability is increased in burn patients shortly after injury. Surgery 107:411–416, 1990.
20. Deitch EA: Simple intestinal obstruction causes bacterial translocation in man. Arch Surg 124:699–701, 1989.
21. Deitch EA, Bridges WM, Ma JW, et al: Obstructed intestine is a reservoir for systemic infection. Am J Surg 159:394–401, 1990.
22. Deitch EA, Maejima K, Berg R: Effect of oral antibiotics and bacterial overgrowth on the translocation of the gastrointestinal tract microflora in burned rats. J Trauma 25:385–392, 1985.
23. Berg RD: Inhibition of *Escherichia coli* translocation from the gastrointestinal tract by normal cecal flora in gnotobiotic or antibiotic-decontaminated mice. Infect Immun 29:1073–1081, 1980.
24. Deitch EA, Winterton J, Berg R: Thermal injury promotes bacterial translocation from the gastrointestinal tract in mice with impaired T-cell-mediated immunity. Arch Surg 121:97–101, 1986.
25. Deitch EA, Winterton J, Berg R: Effect of starvation, malnutrition, and trauma on the gastrointestinal tract flora and bacterial translocation. Arch Surg 122:1019–1024, 1987.
26. Alverdy JC, Aoys E, Moss GS: Total parenteral nutrition promotes bacterial translocation from the gut. Surgery 104:185–190, 1988.
27. Chandra RK: Nutrition, immunity, and infection: Present knowledge and future directions. Lancet 8326(1):688–691, 1983.
28. Ashley SW, Evoy D, Daly JM: Stomach. *In* Schwartz SI, Shires GT, Spencer FC, et al (eds): Principles of Surgery, 7th ed. New York, McGraw-Hill, 1999, pp 1181–1215.
29. Evers BM, Townsend CM, Thompson JC: Small intestine. *In* Schwartz SI, Shires GT, Spencer FC, et al (eds): Principles of Surgery, 7th ed. New York, McGraw-Hill, 1999, pp 1217–1263.
30. Alverdy J, Chi HS, Sheldon GF: The effect of parenteral nutrition on gastrointestinal immunity. The importance of enteral stimulation. Ann Surg 202:681–684, 1985.
31. Li J, Kudsk KA, Gocinski B, et al: Effects of parenteral and enteral nutrition on gut-associated lymphoid tissue. J Trauma 39:44–51, 1995.
32. Mainous M, Xu D, Lu Q, et al: Oral-TPN-induced bacterial translocation and impaired immune defenses are reversed by refeeding. Surgery 110:277–284, 1991.
33. Janu P, Li J, Renegar KB, Kudsk KA: Recovery of gut-associated lymphoid tissue and upper respiratory tract immunity after parenteral nutrition. Ann Surg 225:707–717, 1997.
34. Burke DJ, Alverdy JC, Aoys E, Moss GS: Glutamine-supplemented total parenteral nutrition improves gut immune function. Arch Surg 124:1396–1399, 1989.
35. Alverdy JA, Aoys E, Weiss-Carrington P, Burke DA: The effect of glutamine-enriched TPN on gut immune cellularity. J Surg Res 52:34–38, 1992.
36. Souba WW, Klimberg VS, Hautamaki RD, et al: Oral glutamine reduces bacterial translocation following abdominal radiation. J Surg Res 48:1–5, 1990.
37. Xu D, Qi L, Thirstrup C, et al: Elemental diet–induced bacterial translocation and immunosuppression is not reversed by glutamine. J Trauma 35:821–824, 1993.
38. Peitzman AB, Udekwu AO, Ochoa J, Smith S: Bacterial translocation in trauma patients. J Trauma 31:1083–1086, 1991.
39. Moore FA, Moore EE, Poggetti R, et al: Gut bacterial translocation via the portal vein: A clinical perspective with major torso trauma. J Trauma 31:629–636, 1991.
40. Xu D, Lu Q, Deitch EA: Elemental diet–induced bacterial translocation associated with systemic and intestinal immune suppression. JPEN J Parenter Enteral Nutr 22:37–41, 1998.
41. Spaeth G, Berg RD, Specian RD, Deitch EA: Food without fiber promotes bacterial translocation from the gut. Surgery 108:240–247, 1990.
42. Spaeth G, Specian RD, Berg RD, Deitch EA: Bulk prevents bacterial translocation induced by the oral administration of total parenteral nutrition solution. JPEN J Parenter Enteral Nutr 14:442–447, 1990.
43. Haskel Y, Xu D, Lu Q, Deitch E: Elemental diet–induced bacterial translocation can be hormonally modulated. Ann Surg 217:636–643, 1993.
44. Haskel Y, Xu D, Lu Q, Deitch E: The modulatory role of gut hormones in elemental diet and intravenous total parenteral nutrition–induced bacterial translocation in rats. JPEN J Parenter Enteral Nutr 18:159–166, 1994.
45. Haskel Y, Xu D, Lu Q, Deitch E: Bombesin protects against bacterial translocation induced by three commercially available liquid enteral diets: A prospective, randomized, multigroup trial. Crit Care Med 22:108–113, 1994.
46. Souba WW, Klimberg VS, Plumley DA, et al: The role of glutamine in maintaining a healthy gut and supporting the metabolic response to injury and infection. J Surg Res 48:383–391, 1990.
47. Windmueller HG: Glutamine utilization by the small intestine. Adv Enzymol 53:201–237, 1982.
48. Windmueller HG, Spaeth AE: Respiratory fuels and nitrogen metabolism in vivo in small intestine of fed rats. J Biol Chem 255:107–112, 1980.
49. Smith RJ, Wilmore DW: Glutamine nutrition and requirements. JPEN J Parenter Enteral Nutr 14:94S–99S, 1990.
50. Klimberg VS, Salloum RM, Kasper M, et al: Oral glutamine accelerates healing of the small intestine and improves outcome after whole abdominal radiation. Arch Surg 125:1040–1045, 1990.
51. Souba WW, Roughneen PT, Goldwater DL, et al: Postoperative alterations in interorgan glutamine exchange in enterectomized dogs. J Surg Res 42:117–125, 1987.
52. O'Dwyer ST, Smith RJ, Hwang TL, Wilmore DW: Maintenance of small bowel mucosa with glutamine-enriched parenteral nutrition. JPEN J Parenter Enteral Nutr 13:579–585, 1989.

53. Jiang Z, Wang L, Qi Y, et al: Comparison of parenteral nutrition supplemented with L-glutamine or glutamine dipeptides. JPEN J Parenter Enteral Nutr 17:134–141, 1993.

54. Chen K, Okuma T, Okamura, et al: Glutamine-supplemented parenteral nutrition improves gut mucosa integrity and function in endotoxemic rats. JPEN J Parenter Enteral Nutr 18:167–171, 1994.

55. Tremel H, Kienle B, Weilemann LS, et al: Glutamine dipeptide–supplemented parenteral nutrition maintains intestinal function in the critically ill. Gastroenterology 107:1595–1601, 1994.

56. Chance WT, Foley-Nelson T, Thomas I, Balasubramaniam A: Prevention of parenteral nutrition–induced gut hypoplasia by coinfusion of glucagon-like peptide-2. Am J Physiol 273:G559–G563, 1997.

57. Weser E, Vandeventer A, Tawil T: Stimulation of small bowel mucosal growth by midgut infusion of different sugars in rats maintained by total parenteral nutrition. J Pediatr Gastroenterol Nutr 1:411–416, 1982.

58. Katayama M, Xu D, Specian RD, Deitch EA: Role of bacterial adherence and the mucus barrier on bacterial translocation. Ann Surg 225:317–326, 1997.

59. Deitch EA, Xu D, Naruhn MB, Deitch DC, et al: Elemental diet and IV-TPN–induced bacterial translocation is associated with loss of intestinal mucosal barrier function against bacteria. Ann Surg 221:299–307, 1995.

60. Illig KA, Ryan CK, Hardy DJ, et al: Total parenteral nutrition–induced changes in gut mucosal function: Atrophy alone is not the issue. Surgery 112:631–637, 1992.

61. Sax HC, Illig KA, Ryan CK, Hardy DJ: Low-dose enteral feeding is beneficial during total parenteral nutrition. Am J Surg 171:587–590, 1996.

62. Howard RJ: Surgical infections. In Schwartz SI, Shires GT, Spencer FC, et al (eds): Principles of Surgery, 7th ed. New York, McGraw-Hill, 1999, pp 123–153.

63. Santos AA, Rodrick ML, Jacobs DO, et al: Does the route of feeding modify the inflammatory response? Ann Surg 220:155–163, 1994.

64. Reynolds JV, Kanwar S, Welsh FK, et al: 1997 Harry M Vars Research Award. Does the route of feeding modify gut barrier function and clinical outcome in patients after major upper gastrointestinal surgery? JPEN J Parenter Enteral Nutr 21:196–201, 1997.

65. Fong Y, Marano MA, Barber A, et al: Total parenteral nutrition and bowel rest modify the metabolic response to endotoxin in humans. Ann Surg 210:449–457, 1989.

66. Lowry SF: The route of feeding influences injury responses. J Trauma 30(12 Suppl.):S10–S15, 1990.

67. Schroder J, Kahlke V, Fandrich F, et al: Glutamine dipeptides–supplemented parenteral nutrition reverses gut mucosal structure and interleukin-6 release of rat intestinal mononuclear cells after hemorrhagic shock. Shock 10:26–31, 1998.

68. Barber AE, Jones WG II, Minei JP, et al: Harry M Vars Award. Glutamine or fiber supplementation of a defined formula diet: Impact on bacterial translocation, tissue composition, and response to endotoxin. JPEN J Parenter Enteral Nutr 14:335–343, 1990.

69. Alexander JW: Immunonutrition: An emerging strategy in the ICU. J Crit Care Nutr 1:21–32, 1993.

70. Palombo JD, Bistrian BR, Fechner KD, et al: Rapid incorporation of fish or olive oil fatty acids into rat hepatic sinusoidal cell phospholipids after continuous enteral feeding during endotoxemia. Am J Clin Nutr 57:643–649, 1993.

71. Karlstad MD, DeMichele SJ, Leathem WD, Peterson MB: Effect of intravenous lipid emulsions enriched with gamma-linolenic acid on plasma n-6 fatty acids and prostaglandin biosynthesis after burn and endotoxin injury in rats. Crit Care Med 21:1740–1749, 1993.

72. Pomposelli JJ, Flores E, Hirschberg Y, et al: Short-term TPN containing n-3 fatty acids ameliorate lactic acidosis induced by endotoxin in guinea pigs. Am J Clin Nutr 52:548–542, 1990.

73. Gollaher CJ, Fechner K, Karlstad M, et al: The effect of increasing levels of fish oil–containing structured triglycerides on protein metabolism in parenterally fed rats stressed by burn plus endotoxin. JPEN J Parenter Enteral Nutr 17:247–253, 1993.

74. Pscheidl E, Hedwig-Geissing M, Winzer C, et al: Effects of chemically defined structured lipid emulsions on reticuloendothelial system function and morphology of liver and lung in a continuous low-dose endotoxin rat model. JPEN J Parenter Enteral Nutr 19:33–40, 1995.

75. Barbul A, Wasserkrug HL, Yoshimura NN, et al: High arginine levels in intravenous hyperalimentation abrogate post-traumatic immune suppression. J Surg Res 36:620–624, 1984.

76. Leon P, Redmond P, Stein TP, et al: Harry M Vars Research Award. Arginine supplementation improves histone and acute-phase protein synthesis during gram-negative sepsis in the rat. JPEN J Parenter Enteral Nutr 15:503–508, 1991.

77. Torre PM, Ronnenberg AG, Hartman WJ, Prior RL: Oral arginine supplementation does not affect lymphocyte proliferation during endotoxin-induce inflammation in rats. J Nutr 123:481–488, 1993.

78. Adjei AA, Yamamoto S: A dietary nucleoside-nucleotide mixture inhibits endotoxin-induced bacterial translocation in mice fed protein-free diet. J Nutr 125:42–48, 1995.

79. Dickerson RN, Manzo CB, Charland SL, et al: The effect of insulin-like growth factor-1 on protein metabolism and hepatic response to endotoxemia in parenterally fed rats. J Surg Res 58:260–266, 1995.

80. Wojnar MM, Fan J, Li YH, Lang CH: Endotoxin-induced changes in IGF-1 differ in rats provided enteral vs parenteral nutrition. Am J Physiol 276:E455–E464, 1999.

81. Chen K, Okuma T, Okamura K, et al: Insulin-like growth factor-1 prevents gut atrophy and maintains intestinal integrity in septic rats. JPEN J Parenter Enteral Nutr 19:119–124, 1995.

82. Pappo I, Bercovier H, Berry EM, et al: Polymyxin B reduces total parenteral nutrition–associated hepatic steatosis by its antibacterial activity and by blocking deleterious effects of lipopolysaccharide. JPEN J Parenter Enteral Nutr 16:529–532, 1992.

83. Rossi TM, Lee PC, Young C, Tjota A: Small intestinal mucosa changes, including epithelial cell proliferative activity, of children receiving total parenteral nutrition (TPN). Dig Dis Sci 38:1608–1613, 1993.

84. Sedman PC, Macfie J, Palmer MD, et al: Preoperative total parenteral nutrition is not associated with mucosal atrophy or bacterial translocation in humans. Br J Surg 82:1663–1667, 1995.

85. Guedon C, Schmitz J, Lerebours E, et al: Decreased brush border hydrolase activities without gross morphologic changes in human intestinal mucosa after prolonged total parenteral nutrition of adults. Gastroenterology 90:373–378, 1986.
86. Buchman AL, Moukarzel AA, Bhuta S, et al: Parenteral nutrition is associated with intestinal morphologic and functional changes in humans. JPEN J Parenter Enteral Nutr 19:453–460, 1995.
87. Inoue Y, Espat NJ, Frohnapple DJ, et al: Effect of total parenteral nutrition on amino acid and glucose transport by the human small intestine. Ann Surg 217:604–612, 1993.
88. Grahm TW, Zadrozny DB, Harrington T: The benefits of early jejunal hyperalimentation in the head-injured patient. Neurosurgery 25:729–735, 1989.
89. Kudsk KA, Croce MA, Fabian TC, et al: Enteral *versus* parenteral feeding: Effects on septic morbidity after blunt and penetrating abdominal trauma. Ann Surg 215:503–511, 1992.
90. Moore FA, Moore EE, Jones TN, et al: TEN versus TPN following major abdominal trauma-reduced septic morbidity. J Trauma 29:916–923, 1989.
91. Byrne TA, Persinger RL, Young LS, et al: A new treatment for patients with short-bowel syndrome. Ann Surg 222:243–255, 1995.

18

◆ Renal Failure and Parenteral Nutrition

T. Alp Ikizler, M.D.
Raymond M. Hakim, M.D., Ph.D.

Despite substantial improvements in the science and technology of renal replacement therapy, the morbidity and mortality of patients with renal failure remain excessively high.[1–4] Among the many factors that adversely affect patient outcomes, protein-calorie malnutrition has been shown to be highly associated with increased morbidity and mortality in the population of patients with chronic renal failure (CRF) and end-stage renal disease (ESRD). (Patients with CRF are those with advanced renal disease but not yet on renal replacement therapy [dialysis, transplantation]. Patients with ESRD are those with advanced renal disease and on renal replacement therapy [hemodialysis, peritoneal dialysis, transplantation].).[5–8] Chronic or acute uremia per se as well as renal replacement therapy may predispose the renal failure patient to multiple nutritional complications and hence protein-calorie malnutrition. In this chapter, we attempt to define the importance of nutrition on the outcome of CRF and acute renal failure (ARF) patients and explore the possible mechanisms that cause and/or promote poor nutritional status in these patients. We discuss measures to prevent malnutrition in stable chronic dialysis patients, as well as several treatment options, in particular the use of parenteral nutrition in patients who are already malnourished. However, it is important to note that although ARF and CRF patients may be predisposed to protein-calorie malnutrition for many common reasons, the assessment, management, and outcome of these two patient populations may differ significantly with regard to nutrition. It is therefore more practical to discuss these conditions separately in certain sections throughout the text.

◆ ASSOCIATION OF NUTRITION AND OUTCOME IN RENAL FAILURE

A number of studies have documented the increased mortality and morbidity in renal failure patients with malnutrition.[8, 9] This direct relationship between poor nutrition and outcomes is also observed in patient populations other than renal failure patients, particularly in acutely ill and elderly patients.[10–12] It is interesting to note that in the CRF and ESRD patient, malnutrition is rarely documented as a cause of death. Nevertheless, there is a body of evidence to suggest that the nutritional status of CRF patients plays a major role in the outcome of these patients. In fact, the first apparent indication of suboptimal nutrition and related poor outcomes in chronic dialysis patients came from the analysis of the National Cooperative Dialysis Study results.[5] In this well-known comprehensive study of 262 chronic hemodialysis (CHD) patients divided into four groups, the patient group with the lowest protein catabolic rate (PCR), which presumably reflects the dietary protein intake in stable CHD patients, had the highest treatment failure and dropout rate. In addition, this group of patients had the highest death rate after the termination of the study. This observation was later confirmed in a study by Acchiardo and colleagues, who suggested that CHD patients with a PCR below 0.63 g/kg/day had a higher mortality and hospitalization rate compared with patients with a PCR above 0.93 g/kg/day.[13]

The most comprehensive study on the association of nutrition and outcome in CRF patients was reported by Lowrie and Lew.[7] In their cross-sectional analysis of more than 12,000 CHD patients, they identified serum albumin concentration as the most powerful indicator of mortality. The risk of death in patients with serum albumin concentration below 2.5 g/dL was close to 20-fold greater than patients with serum albumin levels of 4 to 4.5 g/dL, which is considered to be the reference range. When compared with this reference range, even serum albumin values of 3.5 to 4 g/dL resulted in a twofold increase in the relative risk of death. It is important to note that this latter value of albumin is in the range of "normal" for many laboratories. Therefore, a small difference in serum albumin concentrations, even when they are in the "normal" range, may adversely affect the relative mortality risk in CHD patients. In addition to serum albumin levels, Lowrie and Lew were able to define a close relationship between mortality and other biochemical markers of nutrition. Specifically, low blood urea nitrogen and serum cholesterol concentrations, indicators of low protein and energy intake, as well as low levels of serum creatinine, an indicator of decreased muscle mass, were also associated with an increased risk of death in this patient population. In a 1994 report, they also included the anion gap and the relative fraction (expressed in percent) of ideal body weights of these patients as significant predictors of death; based on their extensive analysis, four of the six most significant predictors of death in CHD patients, namely, serum creatinine levels, albumin levels, the anion gap, and the percentage of ideal body weight, were nutritional factors.[14]

These observations were later confirmed by many other studies in different patient populations that have also highlighted the association of nutritional markers with morbidity and mortality.[6, 15–17] Specifically, serum levels of transferrin, prealbumin, and insulin-like growth factor I (IGF-I), as well as total lymphocyte counts and abnormal plasma amino acid profiles, have been associated with an increased risk of death in ESRD patients.[7, 11, 18–20] However, most of these studies were performed on smaller study populations, and their validity, or relationship to serum albumin levels, remains to be determined.

Similar observations can be made in peritoneal dialysis (PD) patients. Several studies reported that the serum albumin level was the best predictor of death and a strong predictor of hospitalization days.[21–23] Most recently, Lowrie, Huang, and Lew reported their findings for death risk predictors among 1522 PD patients.[24] In this regard, it is important to note that the relative risk of death for patients with low serum albumin levels was the same for CHD and PD patients, suggesting that peritoneal losses of albumin do not militate against serum albumin levels as a prognostic factor of the patients' mortality. Avram and colleagues reported the independent association of serum albumin, prealbumin, and creatinine levels with an increased risk of death in their patient population, which was followed up to 7 years.[25] The importance of initial (i.e., at the time of initiation of dialysis) nutritional parameters including serum albumin levels with regard to subsequent survival in PD patients was also reported by the large multicenter (CANUSA) study.[26]

Even though malnutrition is highly prevalent in ARF patients, the question whether malnutrition per se is a predictor of outcome in ARF patients has been evaluated by only a limited number of studies. Indeed, the first indication for such a relation came from the early studies by Abel and coworkers[27] and Baek and associates,[28] who separately showed a reduction in mortality of ARF patients who received supplemental nutritional support in a combination of essential and/or nonessential amino acids and glucose compared with patients receiving glucose alone. After these early reports, multiple investigators have evaluated the impact of aggressive nutritional support in ARF patients. In a series of studies in which they measured the energy balance in surgical intensive care unit patients, Bartlett and colleagues have shown that cumulative energy deficit over the hospitalization period was significantly worse in ARF patients who died in comparison with patients who survived.[29, 30] Furthermore, they postulated that the extent of nutritional support may also affect their survival.

The importance of malnutrition in patients with ARF is further emphasized in a 1999 report by Fiaccadori and colleagues, who reported on a group of 187 consecutive patients admitted to an intermediate renal care unit with the diagnosis of ARF.[31] Patients with malnutrition at the time of admission (using the subjective global assessment) had a 48% mortality rate, versus a 29% mortality rate for those patients without malnutrition. The subjective global assessment also correlated with significantly lower levels of serum albumin and prealbumin, the total lymphocyte count, and anthropometric measurements. Logistic regression analysis revealed malnutrition as a statistically significant independent predictor of mortality. Nevertheless, although the extent of malnutrition and extent of catabolism are widely considered to be important factors in determining the outcome of patients with ARF, there are very few studies that systematically examine the cause and severity of malnutrition.

◆ INDICES OF NUTRITIONAL STATUS

Although practical methods to assess nutritional status are imperative, the appropriate interpretation of nutritional markers in renal failure patients remains a challenge. Various anthropometric and biochemical indices are routinely used to monitor the nutritional status of patients with varying disease states. Although a significant relationship has been established between the nutritional state of the patients and the various markers, the variance of the association is large, and renal failure patients are no exception. Further, several markers used for nutritional purposes are influenced by many non-nutritional factors, especially in renal failure patients. We shall briefly mention the important clinical aspects of several nutritional indices. A list of commonly used indices of malnutrition (along with their advantages and disadvantages) in renal failure patients is given in Table 18–1.

Biochemical Markers

In renal failure patients, relatively simple biochemical measures reflecting the visceral protein stores, such as levels of serum albumin, creatinine, and blood urea nitrogen, as well as more complex and not readily available parameters such as levels of transferrin, prealbumin, and IGF-I, have been proposed as nutritional indices.[32–35] The serum albumin level is probably the most extensively examined nutritional index in almost all patient populations, probably due to its easy availability and strong association with outcomes.[11, 32, 36–39] These observations have led to the general concept that an abnormal serum albumin concentration by itself is usually sufficient to diagnose protein-energy malnutrition in renal failure patients. However, it should be kept in mind that the serum albumin concentration may also be affected by other coexisting problems in addition to malnutrition. Specifically, serum albumin is a negative acute-phase reactant, and its serum concentration decreases sharply in response to inflammation and

thus may not necessarily reflect the changes in nutritional status in acutely and/or chronically ill patients. Therefore, when serum albumin levels are used, the inflammatory state should also be considered.[12, 40] The serum albumin concentration in chronic dialysis patients may also be affected by other non-nutritional factors, such as external losses (i.e., proteinuria, dialytic losses), intra- and extravascular fluid shifts, and other illnesses, that is, liver disease. In acutely ill ARF patients, the serum albumin concentration is determined by the level of synthesis, the degree of catabolism, and the level of nutritional support. However, because the half-life of serum albumin is relatively long (20 days), the changes in its concentration in response to malnutrition as well as refeeding are rather late in the acute disease processes. Indeed, in a 1996 study by Spiess and associates, it was shown that the half-life of serum albumin can be as short as 7 days in critically ill patients.[41] Although affected by several mechanisms, the serum albumin concentration is likely to be an important metabolic and nutritional marker in acutely ill ARF patients.

Serum transferrin and prealbumin levels are also used for the assessment of nutritional status in renal failure patients. Both have shorter half-lives compared with serum albumin, which makes them more advantageous as an early indicator of visceral serum protein concentrations. However, both these markers are also negative acute-phase reactants. In addition, serum transferrin concentrations are also affected by iron stores, and serum prealbumin concentrations may be falsely elevated in patients with reduced renal function because its main route of excretion is the kidneys.[42]

Body Composition Analysis

The simplest, but unfortunately the least reliable, technique for body composition analysis is an anthropometric study. This relatively easy but largely subjective test is a readily available method that may be tried as a confirmatory analysis in any patient with suspected protein-energy malnutrition. More reliable and accurate methods of body composition analysis, such as prompt neutron activation analysis, which measures total body nitrogen content, and dual-energy x-ray absorptiometry, require expensive

Table 18–1. Indices of Malnutrition in Chronic Dialysis Patients and Their Advantages and Disadvantages

Advantages	Disadvantages
Biochemical Parameters	
Serum Albumin (<4 g/dL)	
Easy to measure	Negative acute-phase reactant
Good predictor of outcome	Long (20-day) half-life
Serum Transferrin (<200 mg/dL)	
Readily available	Dependent on iron stores
Early response	Negative acute-phase reactant
Serum Prealbumin (<20 mg/dL)	
Good predictor of outcome	Falsely elevated in renal failure
Good and early response to nutritional support	Negative acute-phase reactant
Serum IGF-I (<200 ng/dL)	
Good association with other markers	Not readily available for clinical use
Short half-life	Not validated in large-scale studies
Body Composition Techniques	
Anthropometric Measures	
Useful if followed longitudinally in same patient	Crude marker and large variations
	Operator dependent
Bioelectric Impedance Analysis	
Easy to measure	Affected by fluid status
Good predictor of outcome	Not clinically validated in large studies
DEXA	
Good association with other methods	Affected by fluid status
	Expensive and not readily available
	Operator dependent
Dietary Assessment	
Protein cataboic rate (<1 g/kg/day)	Related to short-term dietary intake
	Not well-established association with other nutritional markers
Subjective Global Assessment	
Includes objective data (disease state, weight changes)	Heavy reliance on clinical judgment
Easy applicability	Inability to tailor a specific nutritional intervention.

DEXA, dual-energy x-ray absorptiometry; IGF-I, insulin-like growth factor I.

equipment and are available only in specialized centers, and their validity needs to be confirmed with further studies. A promising method of nutritional assessment is bioelectric impedance analysis, which has been proposed as an accurate and reproducible measure of body composition in various patient populations including renal failure patients.[43] Although this method provides a good correlation of total body water and lean body mass in healthy subjects, the variance in renal failure patients may be large. This is partly because bioelectric impedance analysis does not detect acute changes in body composition, particularly in relationship to dialysis when large fluid shifts occur. Therefore, for consistency and accuracy, it is suggested that the measurements be done before dialysis or 30 minutes after dialysis in hemodialysis patients. Other issues that have not been clarified include the validity of the results in moderately or severely malnourished renal failure patients and its usefulness in prospective studies.

Subjective global assessment is a proposed method to evaluate the nutritional status of chronic hemo- and peritoneal dialysis patients.[44] It was originally designed for general surgery patients but is being used for renal failure patients also. Its advantage is that it includes objective data (disease state, weight changes), several manifestations of poor nutritional status, and the clinical judgment of the involved physician. The limitations are a heavy reliance on clinical judgment and an inability to tailor a specific nutritional intervention. Its use as a standard nutritional tool in renal failure is yet to be determined.

Nutritional indices are also important for identifying the malnourished ARF patient and designing appropriate nutritional support as well as assessing the response to nutritional supplementation. It should be kept in mind that in ARF the major process contributing to poor nutritional status is the metabolic response to ongoing morbidity or catabolism, whereas in other states, malnutrition is largely a response to chronic starvation. The nutritional markers that correlate best with the efficacy of nutritional therapy and patient outcomes may be considerably different in these two separate disease states and have not been well delineated in the ARF patient population.

Among the several dynamic markers that can be used in ARF patients, urea nitrogen appearance is a specific indicator of catabolic stress. Nitrogen balance measurement derived from the difference of dietary protein intake and PCR calculated from urea nitrogen appearance is considered to be a marker of catabolic stress and determines the changes in intracellular protein content. Similarly, the measurement, or at least estimation, of energy expenditure to calculate calorie balance in acutely ill patients may be a useful method in both predicting outcomes and tailoring the nutritional supplementation regimen in these patients.

Traditional measures of body composition such as anthropometry have limited application in acutely ill patients. Although anthropometry is a simple and safe method, it fails to detect short-term changes in the functional capacity of lean body mass. In addition, due to major shifts in body water, its use in ARF patients is usually limited. Creatinine kinetics and total body potassium are other important markers of body composition, although their use is significantly hampered by concurrent renal failure and its effect on creatinine and potassium

metabolism. As mentioned earlier, bioelectric impedance analysis may be a useful tool for measuring the metabolically active component of the body in renal failure patients. Its major limitations in ARF patients include its dependency on weight and fluid status, which may be inaccurate in these patients, and a lack of ARF-specific regression equations from which body composition can be estimated. However, bioelectric impedance analysis remains a promising technique because it is a noninvasive, safe, and easy-to-perform bedside method of monitoring body composition.

◆ EXTENT OF MALNUTRITION IN RENAL FAILURE PATIENTS

Virtually every study that has evaluated the nutritional status of ESRD patients has reported some degree of malnutrition in this population. The prevalence of malnutrition has been estimated to range from approximately 20 to 50% in different renal failure patient populations using various nutritional parameters. Lowrie and Lew reported serum albumin concentrations less than 3.7 g/dL in 25% of their patient population, which included more than 12,000 CHD patients.[7] Similar findings with regard to serum albumin levels are found in a 1995 report by the Health Care Financing Administration.[45] In an analysis of all networks in the United States, 53% of the CHD patients were reported to have a serum albumin concentration between 3.5 and 3.9 g/dL, and 22% of the patients had a serum albumin concentration of 3.4 g/dL and below.

Analysis of body composition with different techniques has also shown evidence of malnutrition in chronic dialysis patients.[46, 47] Rayner and associates reported that body protein depletion was detected in up to 26% of their patients who were considered to be nutritionally normal by other indices of nutrition.[48] A 1995 report by Pollock and coworkers suggested that 76% of their chronic dialysis patient population had a nitrogen index lower than the predicted value (observed nitrogen/predicted normal nitrogen) when analyzed with prompt neutron activation analysis.[49] Malnutrition appears to be even more prevalent in PD patients. In 1991, a multicenter international study reported severe to moderate malnutrition in 40% of the PD patients as evaluated by subjective nutritional assessment.[44] Interestingly, in 1995, Cianciaruso and associates reported the extent of malnutrition in PD patients (42.3%) to be higher than in their CHD population (30.8%).[50]

◆ FACTORS AFFECTING THE NUTRITIONAL STATUS OF END-STAGE RENAL DISEASE PATIENTS

Considering the magnitude of the problem, it is likely that multiple factors play important roles in the evolution of malnutrition in renal failure patients. Many of these factors act simultaneously in the progression from suboptimal nutrition to apparent malnutrition. A list of these factors is given in Table 18–2.

Decreased Dietary Nutrient Intake

One of the most significant clinical indicators of advanced uremia is an apparent decrease in appetite. Although this has not been well studied, it has been generally thought that anorexia worsens as the renal failure progresses. Even though there has been a clear association between decreased dietary protein intake and outcomes in ESRD patients, the mechanism by which this apparent decline in dietary protein intake occurs has not been defined. Animal

Table 18–2. Factors Associated with Decreased Nutritional Status of Chronic Renal Failure Patients

Increased protein and energy requirements
  Losses of nutrients (amino acids and/or proteins)
    during dialysis
  Increased resting energy expenditure
Decreased protein and calorie intake
  Anorexia
  Frequent hospitalizations
  Inadequate dialysis dose
  Comorbidities (diabetes mellitus, gastrointestinal
    diseases, ongoing inflammatory response)
  Multiple medications
Increased catabolism and/or decreased anabolism
  Dialysis-induced catabolism
    Bioincompatible hemodialysis membranes
  Amino acid abnormalities
  Metabolic acidosis
  Hormonal derangements
    Hyperparathyroidism
    Insulin and growth hormone resistance

studies suggested that accumulation of a low-molecular-weight (<5 kd) substance isolated from uremic plasma ultrafiltrate and normal urine may be a potential marker of this decreased food intake in uremia, because it induces a dose-dependent suppression of appetite after injection into otherwise normal rats.[51]

Decreased dietary nutrient intake may also be related to factors other than the accumulation of toxins. Indeed, it was suggested that the actual daily protein and energy intake of CHD patients admitted to a regular ward is at very low levels (0.55 ± 0.33 g/kg/day); simultaneous calculations of PCR by urea kinetics revealed a negative nitrogen balance in 80% of these hospitalized patients.[52] Serum albumin concentrations showed a significant decrease with hospitalizations in the same patients. Therefore, frequent hospital admissions may also be an insidious and important cause of poor dietary intake in chronic dialysis patients.[53] Specific comorbid conditions can also facilitate the development of malnutrition in chronic dialysis patients. Patients with renal failure secondary to diabetes mellitus, which is the leading cause of ESRD in the United States, have a higher incidence of malnutrition compared with patients who are not diabetic. The cause of this observation is probably multifactorial. Diabetic patients are likely to be more prone to malnutrition because of dietary restrictions, gastrointestinal symptoms such as gastroparesis, nausea and vomiting, bacterial overgrowth in the gut, and pancreatic insufficiency, as well as the high occurrence of nephrotic syndrome and related complications.[9]

Depression, which is commonly seen in ESRD patients, is also associated with anorexia. In addition, renal failure patients are usually prescribed a large number of medications, particularly sedatives, phosphate binders, and iron supplements, which are also associated with gastrointestinal complications. Finally, the socioeconomic status of the patients, their lack of mobility, and their age are other factors in the development of malnutrition in renal failure patients.

Amino Acid Abnormalities in Chronic Renal Failure Patients

CRF patients have well-defined abnormalities in their plasma and to a lesser extent in their muscle amino acid profiles. Commonly, essential amino acid concentrations are low and nonessential amino acid concentrations are high. The etiology of this abnormal profile is multifactorial. The progressive loss of renal tissue, in which metabolism of several amino acids takes place, is an important factor that alters the plasma concentrations. Specifically, glycine and phenylalanine concentrations are elevated and serine and tyrosine concentrations are decreased. Because histidine concentrations are also decreased because of decreased synthesis, histidine is considered to be an essential amino acid in renal failure patients. Plasma and muscle concentrations of branched-chain amino acids (valine, leucine, and isoleucine) are reduced in chronic dialysis patients. Among branched-chain amino acids, valine displays the greatest reduction. In contrast, plasma levels of citrulline, cystine, aspartate, methionine, and both 1- and 3-methylhistidine are increased.

The overall decrease in essential amino acid concentrations suggests that protein malnutrition is an additional factor in abnormal amino acid profiles. However, certain abnormalities occur even in the presence of adequate dietary nutrient intake, indicating that the uremic milieu has an additional effect on amino acid profiles. Indeed, it has been suggested that metabolic acidosis, which is commonly seen in uremic patients, plays an important role in increased oxidation of branched-chain amino acids. Further, there is a direct relationship between predialysis plasma bicarbonate concentrations and intracellular valine concentrations. Although there are no specific interventions other than adequate dietary nutrient intake for the correction of abnormal amino acid profiles, treatment of metabolic acidosis may be a potential maneuver to improve at least branched-chain amino acid concentrations (see later).

Metabolic and Hormonal Derangements

Multiple metabolic and hormonal abnormalities related to the loss of renal tissue as well as to the loss of renal function become apparent in CRF patients. Metabolic acidosis, which commonly accompanies progressive renal failure, also promotes malnutrition by increased protein catabolism.

Detailed experimental in vitro and animal model studies suggest that muscle proteolysis is stimulated by an ATP-dependent pathway involving ubiquitin and proteasomes during metabolic acidosis.[54, 55] More recently, it has been reported that metabolic acidosis of 7 days' duration induced with high doses of NH_4Cl (4.2 mmol/kg) significantly reduced albumin synthesis and induced negative nitrogen balance in otherwise healthy subjects.[56] It has also been shown that correction of metabolic acidosis actually improves muscle protein turnover in a small number of CHD and/or PD patients.[57, 58] Two 1997 studies in CHD and PD patients also showed improvements in anthropometric measurements and body weight.[59, 60] However, there are several other cross-sectional as well as prospective studies that showed no difference in nutritional parameters, most importantly in serum albumin in CHD patients.[61, 62] Therefore, although the evidence suggests that correction of metabolic acidosis may be nutritionally beneficial in chronic dialysis patients, large-scale studies are still warranted.

Several hormonal derangements including insulin resistance, increased glucagon concentrations, and secondary hyperparathyroidism are also implicated as factors in the development of malnutrition in CRF.[55, 63] A postreceptor defect in insulin responsiveness of tissues is the most likely cause of insulin resistance and associated glucose intolerance in uremia.[64] However, it is not clear to what extent this insulin resistance affects protein metabolism in CRF. It has also been suggested that hyperparathyroidism usually seen in advanced renal failure is, at least in part, responsible for decreased insulin secretion by pancreatic β-cells.[63, 65] Increased concentrations of parathyroid hormone have also been implicated as a catabolic factor that promotes protein metabolism in uremia by enhancing amino acid release from muscle tissue.[66] Finally, there are several abnormalities in thyroid hormone profiles of uremic patients, characterized by low thyroxine and triiodothyronine concentrations.[67] These changes resemble those seen in prolonged malnutrition in other patient populations,[68] and it has been suggested that the thyroid hormone profile of malnutrition[69] and possibly of renal failure is a maladaptive response to decreased energy intake in an effort to preserve overall energy balance.

More recently, abnormalities in the growth hormone and IGF-I axis have been suggested as an important factor in the development of malnutrition in uremic patients.[70] Growth hormone is the major promoter of growth in children and exerts several anabolic actions in adults, such as enhanced protein synthesis, increased fat mobilization, and increased gluconeogenesis, with IGF-I as the major mediator of these actions.[71–73] Although plasma concentrations of growth hormone actually increase during the progression of renal failure, probably due to its reduced renal clearance, evidence suggests that uremia per se is associated with the development of resistance to growth hormone action at cellular levels.[74] In experimental settings, uremia is characterized by reduced hepatic growth hormone receptor messenger RNA (mRNA) as well as hepatic IGF-I mRNA expression.[75, 76] This blunted response would be expected to attenuate the anabolic actions of these hormones. Interestingly, these abnormalities can also be observed with decreased food intake, as well as in experimental metabolic acidosis.[77] Clinically, metabolic acidosis and decreased dietary protein and energy intake are also associated with decreased IGF-I levels, although it is not clear which is the primary effect and which is the secondary response.[56, 78, 79] Thus, the current evidence suggests an interesting, ill-defined interrelationship among these hormonal, metabolic, and nutritional factors that are involved in the evolution of malnutrition in renal failure patients. With this information, the use of anabolic growth factors such as recombinant growth hormone and recombinant human IGF-I at pharmacologic doses has been proposed as a potential intervention for the treatment of chronic dialysis patients who are already malnourished in spite of preventive strategies.

Nutrient Losses

Hemodialysis

Hemodialysis has long been considered a catabolic process, and inevitable loss of nutrients during hemodialysis is an important component of dialysis-related catabolism. Earlier studies by Kopple and associates and Wolfson and colleagues have documented a loss of 5 to 8 g of free amino acids during each hemodialysis session when low-flux dialyzers are used.[80, 81] With the use of high-flux membranes, these losses further increase by 30% because of the larger surface area of the membranes and higher blood flows used.[82] Simultaneous changes in plasma amino acid concentrations suggested that these patients catabolized approximately 25 to 30 g of body protein to compensate for these losses.

Similarly, there is a considerable amount of amino acid and protein loss when continuous renal replacement therapies are used.[83] These losses range between 7 and 50 g/day depending on the dialyzer used, the total amount of ultrafiltrate, the nature of the solute removal, and the serum protein amino acid concentrations.[84, 85] This continuous unavoidable loss of nutrients repetitively predisposes the ARF patient to negative nitrogen balance, especially in the presence of inadequate intake, which is a common finding in these patients.

Peritoneal Dialysis

Losses of proteins and amino acids into the dialysate fluid have long been identified as a catabolic factor in PD patients. Several studies have reported a loss of 5 to 12 g of proteins into the dialysate daily.[86] A large amount of these losses consists of albumin, along with immunoglobulins and amino acids. Free amino acid losses have been estimated to be in the range of 2 to 4 g/day according to different studies.[87] Most importantly, during episodes of peritonitis, these losses of proteins and amino acids increase substantially.[86] The generally lower serum albumin concentrations, as well as several abnormalities in plasma amino acid profiles seen in PD patients, are presumed to be a result of these inevitable losses. Nevertheless, the continuous unavoidable loss of nutrients repetitively predisposes the PD patients to negative nitrogen balance, especially in the presence of inadequate intake.

Conversely, the amount of energy intake, at least indirectly, is relatively higher in PD patients, due to the absorption of glucose from the dialysate fluid. This absorption usually provides energy in the range of 5 to 20 kcal/kg daily in many patients and is possibly the explanation for the relatively lower resting energy expenditure (REE) levels observed in this patient population.[88] Unfortunately, this absorption of glucose may also predispose these patients to further anorexia due to the development of satiety, in addition to the feeling of fullness related to the fluid in the peritoneal cavity. The extensive presence of protein malnutrition in these patients, in spite of this increased energy consumption, is probably related to their inadequate intake of dietary protein because protein intake affects nitrogen balance more profoundly than the overall energy intake.[89]

Dose of Dialysis

One of the most important factors that affect the nutritional status of dialysis patients is the dose of dialysis.[90] In a study of 55 hemodialysis patients, Lindsay and Spanner were able to show a significant linear relationship between the dose of dialysis and the PCR (a marker for dietary protein intake).[91] Moreover, the attempts to increase the dietary protein intake of these patients by dietary counseling were unsuccessful unless the dose of dialysis was first increased. Bergstrom and Lindhom have also reported a significant linear relationship between the dose of dialysis and PCR, all consistent with anorexia related to underdialysis.[92] In a further study of their patient population, Lindsay and coworkers prospectively analyzed the effects of increasing the dialysis dose in a group of patients with PCR values less than 1 g/kg/day.[93] Their results showed that PCR increased significantly in the group of patients whose doses of dialysis were increased, whereas there was no change in PCR values in the group of patients whose doses of dialysis remained the same. In studies by Acchiardo and colleagues and Burrowes and coworkers, significant increases in serum albumin concentrations were demonstrated in CHD patients when their doses of dialysis were increased to adequate levels.[94, 95] Hakim and associates have performed a prospective 4-year study in which the dose of dialysis was increased intentionally to 1.33 (by delivered Kt/V) in 130 CHD patients.[96] (Kt/V is the term used to quantify the dose of dialysis, where K is urea clearance of dialyzer, t is time of dialysis session, and V is volume of distribution of urea.) They observed that when the nutritional parameters of patients with yearly average Kt/V values below 0.86 and above 1.21 were identified, statistically significant differences were found between serum albumin, transferrin, and PCR measurements.

Similar conclusions with regard to the dose of dialysis are reported in PD patients in several studies.[21, 97] Lindsay and colleagues have hypothesized the same association between the dose of dialysis and dietary protein intake in PD patients.[93] Bergstrom and Lindholm have also reported similar findings with regard to their dialysis patients, with the additional observation that PD patients required a lower dialysis dose than hemodialysis patients did to achieve a given dietary protein intake.[92] They have postulated that better removal of uremic toxins at the middle molecule range (1 K–5 K daltons), which are thought to be the causal factor in the anorexia associated with uremia, is the explanation for this relationship.

An important report on this issue is the cross-sectional analysis of an international study on the nutritional status of PD patients. In this study, a higher incidence of malnutrition was observed in patients who were treated with PD for longer than 3 months compared with patients who were treated for less than 3 months, suggesting that as residual renal function decreases (a major contributor to total clearance in PD patients), indices of malnutrition become more evident.[44]

Most recently, the results of a large multicenter study have been published and have suggested a positive relationship between the adequacy of dialysis and nutritional status in PD patients.[26] It was reported that decreasing serum albumin concentrations and worsening nutrition according to subjective global assessment were predictive of worsening mortality and increasing hospitalizations. A further analysis of the data showed that the estimates of adequacy of dialysis and nutritional status are positively correlated in these patients.[98]

All the available evidence in chronic dialysis patients confirms the close association between the dialysis dose and nutrition. It is important to note, however, that the specific level of optimal dose of dialysis after which no further improvement in nutritional status is observed has not been established. Several prospective studies are under way to evaluate this question. Studies suggest a relationship between the dose of dialysis and outcomes in ARF patients also. Whether nutritional status plays a role in this relationship has not been studied in detail.

Biocompatibility

Another well-defined (at least experimentally) cause of inappropriate protein catabolism in dialysis patients is the adverse consequence (or enhanced inflammatory response) resulting from the contact between blood and foreign material during hemodialysis, that is, the effects of bioincompatibility.[99] It is now well established that the type of dialysis membrane used affects protein metabolism in CHD patients. Specifically, bioincompatible membranes that vigorously activate the complement system also induce net protein catabolism compared with dialysis membranes that do not activate this inflammatory response.[82, 100] Although both membranes induce net protein catabolism due to amino acid losses observed during hemodialysis, this catabolism is more intense with bioincompatible membranes[82] and can be observed at 6 hours after the initiation of dialysis in healthy subjects.[101]

In spite of the extensive experimental and cross-sectional studies highlighting the catabolic and anorectic effects of bioincompatible membranes,[100, 102] it is still not clearly established whether long-term use of biocompatible membranes per se can improve the nutritional markers in CHD patients. In fact, the first evidence that supports the argument that biocompatible hemodialysis membranes favorably affect the nutritional status of CHD patients was reported in 1996 by our laboratory.[103] In a prospective randomized study of 159 new hemodialysis patients randomized to either a low-flux biocompatible membrane or a low-flux bioincompatible membrane, we measured the effects of biocompatibility on several nutritional parameters, including estimated dry weight, serum albumin levels, and IGF-I over 18 months. Our results showed that the biocompatible group had a mean increase in their dry weight by 4.36 ± 8.57 kg at the end of the study, whereas no change in average weight was observed in the bioincompatible group. In addition, the biocompatible group had an earlier (6 vs. 12 months) and more marked increase in serum albumin concentrations compared with the bioincompatible group, as well as consistently higher IGF-I values.

The mechanism by which the bioincompatibility and activation of the complement pathway enhance protein catabolism is not clear. The production of cytokines, such as interleukin 1 and tumor necrosis factor-α, may induce muscle protein degradation and excess amino acid release.[104, 105] In studies by Gutierrez and associates, the release of amino acids during dialysis with bioincompatible membranes was most prominent at 6 hours after the initiation of hemodialysis,[100] a time period consistent with the activation of monocytes and subsequent release of cytokines, followed by their action on muscle cells.[106] Complement activation has been shown to result in increased transcription of the tumor necrosis factor-α, and in a 1994 study by Canivet and coworkers, increased serum concentrations of tumor necrosis factor-α were reported in CHD patients dialyzed with a complement-activating membrane.[107]

Reports from the U.S. Renal Data System have suggested that the use of bioincompatible membranes is associated with an increased risk of death in comparison with biocompatible membranes.[108] Whether altered nutritional status plays a role in this process is not clear. However, a 1996 analysis of the cause of death in these two groups of patients dialyzed with biocompatible versus bioincompatible membranes highlighted the significant increase in infection-related deaths in the bioincompatible group.[109] It is possible that poor nutritional status may increase the prevalence of infectious episodes in patients dialyzed with bioincompatible membranes and eventually increase the risk of death. Nevertheless, further studies are required to evaluate the cause-and-effect relationship between these factors.

◆ NUTRITIONAL REQUIREMENTS OF RENAL FAILURE PATIENTS

Protein Requirements

In general, the "minimal" daily protein requirement is one that maintains a neutral nitrogen balance and prevents malnutrition; this has been estimated to be a daily protein intake of approximately 0.6 g/kg in healthy individuals, with a "safe level" of protein intake equivalent to the minimal requirement plus 2 standard deviations, or approximately 0.75 g/kg/day.[110, 111] This suggested intake of protein for healthy individuals does not necessarily apply to CRF patients, who may require higher levels due to concurrent abnormalities. Indeed, it has been shown that for chronic dialysis patients, a protein intake of 1.4 g/kg/day is needed to maintain a positive or neutral nitrogen balance during nondialysis days, and even this intake may not be adequate for dialysis days.[112] Very few other studies have systematically evaluated the actual protein requirements of dialysis patients.[113] Nevertheless, a minimum of 1.2 g/kg/day is suggested as a safe level of dietary protein intake for both CHD and PD patients based on several metabolic balance studies.[114] These suggested levels of dietary protein intake are clearly much higher (almost twofold) than in the healthy population.

Energy Requirements

The minimal energy requirements of chronic dialysis patients are less well defined. This requirement is dependent on the REE, the activity level of the patient, and other ongoing illnesses. Several earlier studies on this issue reported that the REE in CRF and ESRD patients was similar to that in matched healthy controls.[115–117] However, more recent studies have reported that the REE is actually higher in CHD patients, especially after adjusting the REE for fat-free mass, where the majority of energy expenditure occurs, compared with age-, sex-, and body mass index–matched healthy controls.[118] This higher level of REE was evident on nondialysis days and further increased during the hemodialysis procedure, when the nutrient losses and catabolism are at a maximum. This increase in the REE during nondialysis periods as well as during hemodialysis may constitute an additional increase of 10 to 20% of the REE compared with healthy individuals. However, the cause of this increased REE in CHD patients is not well defined.

Although there are not many studies with regard to the REE in PD patients, a study conducted in our laboratories indicated that the increase in REE of PD patients is comparable to the increase in CHD patients.[119] The same study also showed that the REE of CRF patients who are not yet on dialysis was actually lower than predicted. With the available information, a minimum of 30 to 35 kcal of energy intake per kilogram per day is usually suggested for chronic dialysis

patients. This level of energy intake is for stable patients, and if there is concurrent illness, especially if hospitalization is required, this intake may be increased.

Protein and Calorie Requirements in Acute Renal Failure Patients

The nutritional hallmark of ARF is the excessive catabolism seen in these patients. Multiple studies have shown that the PCR in ARF patients requiring dialytic support is much higher than that seen in other patient populations and can be massive at times.[120] Indeed, daily PCRs ranging between 1.4 and 1.8 g/kg/day have been reported in several different studies.[121–124] Our own experience with regard to the extent of catabolism in ARF patients confirms a high PCR that averaged 1.74 g/kg/day.[125]

Several factors have been postulated as the underlying mechanism for this extensive protein catabolism observed in ARF patients. The concurrent illness commonly seen in these patients can initiate a sequence of catabolic events through multiple cascades that may lead to the previously mentioned observations. Specific cytokines including interleukins and tumor necrosis factor-α are stimulated during catabolic conditions such as sepsis. Careful in vitro studies have shown that interleukin 1 can increase skeletal muscle breakdown.[126] Tumor necrosis factor-α is also shown to increase whole-body protein breakdown.[127] Furthermore, Horl and colleagues have speculated that circulating proteases from granulocytes in patients with hypercatabolism can also further stimulate catabolism.[128] In addition to increased catabolism, ARF patients may also encounter a diminished utilization and incorporation of available nutrients.

Because protein and energy requirements are increased in patients with ARF, it seems logical to supply aggressive nutritional supplementation in these patients. However, there are several limitations to this approach that also predispose to poor nutrition in ARF patients. In clinical practice, the patients' actual nutritional needs are frequently not determined; the measurement of actual urea nitrogen appearance, which reflects protein catabolism, may be cumbersome in clinical settings, as is the measurement of energy expenditure. The utilization of predetermined formulas for energy expenditure may substantially underestimate the actual energy needs of the ARF patients because these formulas are usually derived from healthy individuals and rely on normal body fluid distribution.[129] The actual fluid distribution and the fat-free mass may be considerably altered in ARF patients, especially during the oliguric-anuric phase. Clark and colleagues have measured creatinine kinetics in patients with ARF and demonstrated a lower-than-expected lean body mass, compared with either healthy individuals or ESRD patients.[130]

Another limitation of nutritional supplementation is the potential side effects of this treatment. Specifically, in the presence of diminished utilization and clearance, excessive protein supplementation results in increased accumulation of end-products of protein and amino acid metabolism. In addition, larger quantities of nutrient provision require more fluid infusion and may predispose the patients to fluid overload. Aggressive nutrition may also cause hyperglycemia, hyperlipidemia, hypernatremia, or hyponatremia in ARF patients.[131] Finally, multiple abnormalities in amino acid profiles in ARF patients who have been aggressively supplemented, particularly with essential amino acids as the sole source of nitrogen, have been reported and resulted in significant neurologic complications as well as death.[83] Although most of these abnormalities can be managed by complementary dialytic support, the initiation, intensity, and dose of dialysis treatment is an area of controversy in itself,[123] and in some cases even dialysis cannot fully prevent the development of these abnormalities in patients treated with parenteral nutrition.[83] These observations along with conflicting results of several clinical studies on nutritional supplementation have led most clinicians to be conservative in the nutritional management of patients with complicated ARF that may further aggravate the poor nutrition in these patients.

Vitamin and Trace Element Requirements

Vitamins

The concentration of many vitamins is altered in chronic dialysis patients, and both decreased and increased concentrations can be found in these patients. A list of vitamins with their relevance to chronic dialysis patients is shown in Table 18–3. We will briefly discuss the clinically important vitamins.

Vitamin A concentrations are usually elevated in chronic dialysis patients, and even small amounts lead to excessive accumulation. There have been several reports of vitamin A toxicity in chronic dialysis patients, and therefore vitamin A should not be supplemented in these patients. Vitamin E levels in chronic dialysis patients have not been defined, and there have been reports of increased, decreased, or unchanged concentrations. Therefore, it is not clear whether vitamin E supplementation is required in chronic dialysis patients. However, there have not been any studies reporting adverse effects of vitamin E supplementation, with several short-term studies reporting decreased lipid peroxidation. Vitamin K supplementation is usually not recommended in chronic dialysis patients unless they are at high risk for developing deficiency, such as if they are undergoing prolonged hospitalizations with poor dietary intake.

A well-known complication of advanced renal failure is the development of renal osteodystrophy. The kidney plays an important role in mineral homeostasis by maintaining an external balance for calcium, phosphorus, magnesium, and pH. A combination of factors plays a role in the development of renal osteodystrophy. As renal function falls to levels less than 20% of normal, hypocalcemia develops because of hyperphosphatemia, decreasing renal synthesis of 1,25-dihydroxyvitamin D (calcitriol) and worsening hyperparathyroidism with resistance to peripheral actions of parathyroid hormone. The resulting conditions, which may range from osteitis fibrosa and osteomalacia to mixed and adynamic bone lesions, are important, long-term complications that subsequently affect ESRD patients while on dialysis.

In early renal failure, phosphorus control can be achieved by moderate dietary phosphorus restriction. This usually increases calcitriol to near-normal levels. Calcitriol also enhances the absorption of calcium from the gut to correct hypocalcemia. Once the glomerular filtration rate is less than 20 to 30 mL/min, phosphorus restriction is not enough to stimulate calcitriol production, and gastrointestinal phosphorus-binding agents are required. The use of aluminum-

Table 18–3. Vitamins and Trace Elements in Chronic Renal Failure Patients

Vitamin*	Function	Clinical Syndrome	Requirements
A† (=/↑)	Vision, immune response	CNS toxicity, ↑ Ca^{2+}	None
E† (=/↑/↓)	Antioxidant	None	Not clear
K† (=/↑/↓)	Coagulation	↑ Prothrombin time, bleeding	None
B$_1$ (=)	Coenzyme	Beriberi (rare)	1–5 mg/day‡
B$_2$ (=/↑)	Oxidation-reduction	None	1.2–1.7 mg/day‡
B$_6$ (=/↓)	Coenzyme	↑ Hyperoxalemia, hyperhomocysteinemia ↓ Decreased immune response	10 mg/day‡
B$_{12}$ (=)	Myelin synthesis Folic acid metabolism	Pernicious anemia	2 µg/day‡
C (=/↓)	Antioxidant Collagen synthesis	↑ Hyperoxalemia ↓ Scurvy	60 mg/day‡
Folic acid (=/↓)	DNA synthesis	Anemia (macrocytic)	1–5 mg/day
Niacin (=/↑)	Enzymatic reactions	Pellagra	13–19 mg/day‡
Biotin (=/↑)	CO$_2$ carrier, coenzyme	Depression, dermatitis, muscle pain	30–100 µg/day‡
Pantothenic acid (=/↓)	Synthesis of fatty acids, cholesterol, amino acids	Retarded growth (animals), fatigue	4–7 mg/day‡

Trace Element	Normal Serum Levels*	Possible Toxic Effects§
Aluminum	1.0–6.0 µg/L (↑)	↑ Encephalopathy, osteomalacia
Arsenic	0.09–5.49 µg/L (↑)	↑ Cancer, anemia
Cadmium	< 0.20 µg/L (↑)	↑ Cancer, osteomalacia
Cobalt	0.04–0.40 µg/L (↑)	↑ Heart failure
Copper	0.98–1.07 µg/L (=/↑)	↑ Fever, myocardial infarction
Iron	0.79–1.63 mg/L (↑)	↑ Pancytopenia, ischemic heart disease ↑ Hepatotoxicity, cardiac ischemia ↓ Anemia
Mercury	0.55–2.10 µg/L (↑)	↑ Hypertension
Selenium	0.081–0.185 mg/L (=/↓)	↑ Cardiomyopathy, cancer, anemia, immune dysfunction
Zinc	0.69–1.21 mg/L (↓)	↓ Sexual dysfunction, decreased taste and smell acuity

*Arrows in parentheses indicate the levels reported in chronic dialysis patients.
†Lipid soluble.
‡Recommended daily allowance.
§Arrows indicate levels associated with toxicity.

containing binders should be avoided as much as possible because it is known that in the long term the absorption of this metal can predispose dialysis patients to aluminum-related osteomalacia. Calcium acetate is the most commonly used phosphate binder. It is most effective when given with meals. Because there is patient-to-patient as well as within-patient variability of phosphorus intake from meal to meal, the dose frequency and timing should be adjusted for each individual meal. For CRF patients who have low calcium concentrations and/or parathyroid hormone levels that are high (>300 pg/mL), calcitriol administration should be considered. This approach may alleviate the symptoms and development of renal osteodystrophy. However, the patients must be monitored closely for hypercalcemia and hyperphosphatemia. A "calcium × phosphorus" product above 65 to 70 should be avoided because it may predispose patients to soft tissue calcifications. Newer phosphate binders (calcium-free cross-linked polyallylamine) and vitamin D_3 analogues tend not to cause hypercalcemia and may be used to treat hyperphosphatemia and vitamin D_3 deficiency.

The serum concentrations of any of the water-soluble vitamins are reported to be low in chronic dialysis patients mainly due to decreased dietary intakes and increased clearances by diffusion during hemodialysis. The use of daily multivitamin prescriptions that are specifically designed for ESRD patients usually alleviates these low concentrations. Nevertheless, it is important to recognize that the daily requirements of vitamin B_6, folic acid, and ascorbic acid are usually higher in chronic dialysis patients and that their levels may need to be followed for patients at risk, such as those who require prolonged hospitalizations. Furthermore, the effects of high-flux and high-efficiency dialyzers on water-soluble vitamins are not clearly defined.

Trace Elements

The concentrations of most of the trace elements are mainly dependent on the degree of renal failure. Although there is an extensive list of trace elements that may have altered concentrations in body fluids in chronic dialysis patients, only a few of these compounds are thought to be important in this patient population. A list of trace ele-

ments with their relevance to chronic dialysis patients is given in Table 18–3. We will briefly discuss the clinically important trace elements.

Serum aluminum is the most important trace element in chronic dialysis patients because elevated levels have been shown to be associated with *dialysis dementia* as well as aluminum-related bone disease. The first reports of aluminum intoxication were recognized in patients who were dialyzed with untreated water sources. These untreated water resources are usually in areas where the soil is rich in minerals and/or in industrial areas where environmental precautions are not employed vigorously. This scenario is mostly eliminated in developed countries, where the use of reverse osmosis for water purification eliminates aluminum; however, the risk still continues in many developing countries. Another source of aluminum is the use of phosphate binders that contain aluminum hydroxide. In ESRD patients with poor control of phosphate intake, prolonged use may be a risk for aluminum intoxication; therefore, these patients' aluminum concentrations should be monitored carefully and frequently. A serum aluminum concentration well below 30 µg/L is the desired level in ESRD patients. Finally, the concomitant use of aluminum-containing phosphate binders and citrate-containing preparations is contraindicated because citrate increases aluminum absorption and predisposes that patient to acute aluminum intoxication.

Selenium deficiency has been associated with cardiovascular disease through increased peroxidative damage to the cells. Decreased concentrations of selenium have been observed in ESRD patients, probably secondary to inadequate dietary intake. However, whether selenium supplementation to correct concentrations would be beneficial is not well defined. Similarly, low concentrations of zinc have been reported in ESRD patients. Zinc deficiency is associated with impotence and anorexia. However, the beneficial effects of supplemental zinc therapy have not been confirmed in dialysis patients.

Carnitine

Carnitine has a number of well-established roles in intermediary metabolism. It is an obligate cofactor for the oxidation of long-chain fatty acids by mitochondria and is also a buffer for the coenzyme A pool. Carnitine is derived from dietary sources and from endogenous biosynthesis. Carnitine homeostasis is altered in renal failure. Specifically, the serum pool is redistributed in favor of acylcarnitine, and the muscle total carnitine content is low. The important functions of carnitine and its altered homeostasis in renal failure have led to an interest in therapeutic studies of carnitine supplementation.

Carnitine supplementation is thought to improve several biochemical abnormalities and symptoms and signs that are commonly seen in ESRD patients. These include hypertriglyceridemia, intradialytic symptoms such as hypotension and cramping, skeletal muscle atrophy and poor exercise tolerance, left ventricular dysfunction, and anemia. Although several preliminary studies have suggested beneficial effects of carnitine, well-controlled studies with a larger number of patients are lacking. Currently there are no absolute indications for supplemental carnitine therapy in ESRD patients, and one should consider the clinical appropriateness (presence of signs and symptoms) as well as the financial implications of the therapy when prescribing carnitine supplementation.

Lipid Metabolism

Dyslipidemia is quite common in renal failure patients, and abnormalities in lipid profiles can be detected in patients once renal function begins to deteriorate, suggesting that uremia is associated with lipid disorders. The presence of nephrotic syndrome or other comorbidities such as diabetes mellitus and liver disease as well as the use of medications altering lipid metabolism further contributes to the dyslipidemia seen in renal failure.

Dyslipidemia in Hemodialysis Patients

In hemodialysis patients, the most common abnormalities are elevated levels of serum triglycerides and very low density lipoproteins and decreased levels of low- and high-density lipoproteins. The increased triglyceride component is thought to be related to increased levels of apolipoprotein C-III, an inhibitor of lipoprotein lipase. In addition, there is a defect in the lipolytic metabolic step (postprandial lipoprotein metabolism) resulting in the accumulation of chylomicron remnants. A substantial number of CHD patients also have elevated lipoprotein (a) levels.

Dyslipidemia in Peritoneal Dialysis Patients

Patients on PD exhibit higher concentrations of serum cholesterol, triglyceride, LDL cholesterol, and apolipoprotein B even though the mechanisms that alter the lipid metabolism are similar to those of CHD patients. This is thought to be related to an increased amount of protein losses through the peritoneum and glucose load from the dialysate. They also exhibit higher concentrations of lipoprotein (a). Whether these differences in dyslipidemia are clinically significant remains to be clarified.

Dyslipidemia and Cardiovascular Risk in Dialysis Patients

Cardiovascular events are the leading cause of death in chronic dialysis patients. Hypercholesterolemia and other abnormalities in the lipid profile have been associated with an increased risk of atherosclerosis and cardiovascular events in the general population. However, whether this relationship applies to chronic dialysis patients has not been well established. Indeed, large cross-sectional studies have identified low cholesterol concentrations, rather than high cholesterol concentrations, with an increased risk of death in chronic dialysis patients. In contrast, a large multicenter study showed that in a cohort of diabetic patients on CHD, the ones who died from a cardiovascular event had a higher median cholesterol level, LDL cholesterol level, LDL/HDL ratio, and apolipoprotein B concentration at the time of initiation of dialysis.[132]

Such findings can be explained with the data that indicate that the development of atherosclerosis begins early at the stage of mild to moderate CRF. In addition, the extensive prevalence of protein-calorie malnutrition in chronic dialysis patients also complicates the use of serum cholesterol levels as a risk factor for atherosclerosis.[133] Nevertheless, it is generally accepted that chronic dialysis patients with known risk factors for atherosclerosis and cardiovascular events should be treated with an appropriate regimen including lipid-lowering agents when indicated. A cholesterol concentration higher than 240 mg/dL and/or LDL concentration higher than 130 mg/dL in the presence of other risk factors should be treated in chronic dialysis patients. Whether this approach influences the overall outcome in these patients remains to be answered with further studies.

◆ STRATEGIES FOR TREATMENT OF MALNUTRITION IN RENAL FAILURE PATIENTS

A list of general measures to prevent and/or to treat malnutrition in different stages of ESRD is presented in Table 18–4. Figure 18–1 shows a proposed protocol for the assessment and treatment of malnourished CRF patients.

Conventional Nutritional Therapy

Considering the catabolic nature of chronic uremia, it is clear that attempts to encourage patients to maintain an adequate protein and calorie intake must be actively maintained in chronic dialysis patients. Most of these patients continue their predialysis diets while on chronic renal replacement therapy. It is important to ensure that the dietary protein and calorie intake of these patients fulfills the increased requirements after the initiation of dialysis. Repetitive

Table 18–4. Interventions to Prevent and/or Treat Malnutrition

---

Nutritional counseling to encourage increased intake
Appropriate amount of dietary protein (>1.2 g/kg/day) and calories (>30 kcal/kg/day)
Optimal dose of dialysis (Kt/V > 1.4 or URR > 70%)
Use of biocompatible dialysis membranes
Oral nutritional supplements
Intradialytic parenteral nutritional supplements for hemodialysis patients; amino acid dialysate for peritoneal dialysis patients
Enteral nutritional supplementation (PEG tube)
Growth factors (experimental)
　Recombinant human growth hormone
　Recombinant human insulin-like growth factor I

Kt/V, dose of dialysis (see text for description); PEG, percutaneous endoscopic gastrostomy; URR, urea reduction ratio.

comprehensive dietary counseling by an experienced dietitian is an important step to improve dietary intake, as well as the detection of early signs of malnutrition. Similar efforts should be spent not only in outpatient settings but also during hospitalizations of these patients. These hospitalized patients should be closely followed by experienced renal dietitians during their frequent and sometimes long hospital admissions, because these patients have even lower dietary protein and calorie intake.

Enteral and Intradialytic Parenteral Nutrition

Dietary counseling to improve the nutritional status unfortunately is usually unsuccessful in optimizing the dietary intake in most of the malnourished ESRD patients.[134] For these patients, other forms of supplementation such as enteral (including oral protein, amino acid tablet, and energy supplementation;[135–137] nasogastric tubes;[63] percutaneous endoscopic gastroscopy or jejunostomy tubes;[138]) and intradialytic parenteral nutrition (IDPN) need to be considered. Only a limited number of studies evaluating the effects of enteral supplementation in malnourished ESRD patients are available.[136, 137, 139, 140] Furthermore, most of these studies are not controlled and are small in scope, and the degree of success is variable. Therefore, for the nephrologist, it is usually a challenge to determine whether an enteral form of supplementation is effective and to know when to try further, relatively more expensive and invasive measures such as IDPN.

　Several reports have emphasized the effective use of IDPN as a therapeutic intervention in malnourished CHD patients.[141] This mode of treatment has been advocated after a trial of enteral nutritional supplementation. The early studies by Heidland and Kult, as well as several subsequent studies, reported positive effects of intradialytic infusions of nutrients on several nutritional parameters.[39, 142] In contrast, other studies were not able to show any benefit of IDPN.[143, 144] A list of studies using parenteral nutrition in CHD patients is given in Table 18–5. All these studies had drawbacks in their designs and patient populations, and therefore no definitive conclusions could be made. Of the few studies that suggested a

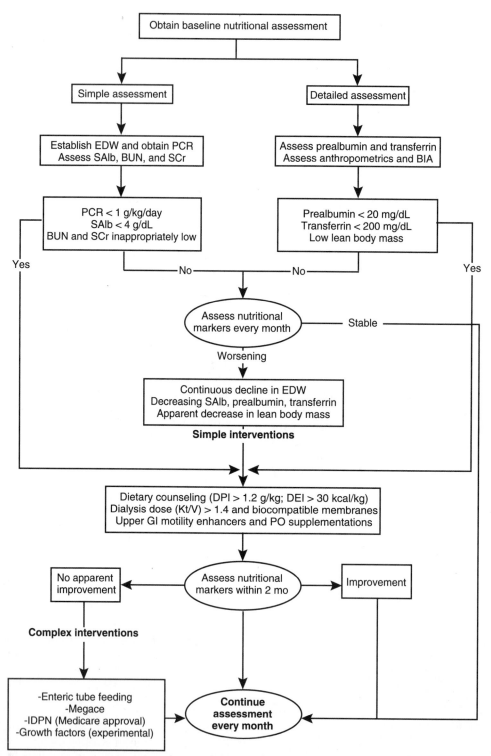

Figure 18–1. A proposed schematic diagram of nutritional assessment and management of chronic renal failure patients. BIA, bioelectric impedance analysis; BUN, blood urea nitrogen; DEI, dietery energy intake; DPI, dietary protein intake; EDW, estimated dry weight; GI, gastrointestinal; IDPN, intradialytic parenteral nutrition; Kt/V, dose of dialysis (see text definition); PCR, protein catabolic rate; PO, orally; SAlb, serum albumin; Scr, serum creatinine.

Table 18–5. Studies Using Supplemental Nutrition in Chronic Renal Failure Patients

Study	Supplement*	Design	No. of Patients	Duration	Outcome
Heidland and Kult[142]	EAAs	Not controlled	18	60 wk	Improved Salb, transferrin, C3
Guarnieri et al.[39]	EAAs vs. NEAAs	Controlled	18	2 mo	Minimal improvement in body weight
Piraino et al.[167]	EAAs ± NEAAs	Not controlled	21	20 wk	Improved body weight
Moore and Acchiardo[168]	EAAs + NEAAs	Not controlled	8	3 mo	Improved Salb
Toigo et al.[169]	EAAs ± NEAAs	Controlled and randomized	21	6 mo	No significant improvement in nutritional markers
Cano et al.[145]	GAAs + lipids	Controlled and randomized	26	3 mo	Increase in Salb, Prealb, AMC, creatinine appearance
Madigan et al.[170]	No glucose arm GAAs + lipids	Not controlled	9	2 mo	Improved Salb and body weight
Matthys et al.[171]	EAAs	Not controlled	10	3 mo	Increase in body weight, improved general condition
Snyder et al.[172]	GAAs + lipids	Not controlled	6	3 mo	No significant effect
Vehe et al.[173]	?	Not controlled	13	7–28 day	Increase in Prealb, IGF-I, fibronectin
Schulman et al.[162]	GAAs + lipids vs IDPN + rhGH	Not controlled	7	3 mo	Increase in transferrin, Salb with IDPN and rhGH
Capelli et al.[174]	+ control group	Controlled	81	9 mo	Improvement in survival and Salb in treated group
Chertow et al.[146]	No randomization ?	Controlled retrospective	1679 vs. 22,517	1 yr	Better survival in treated group (More significant in patients with Scr < 8 mg/dL and low Salb)
Smolle et al.[175]	GAAs	No control group	16	16 wk	Improvement in Salb, Prealb, TLC, cholinesterase
Mortelmans et al.[176]	GAAs + lipids	No control group	16	9 mo	Improvement in body weight and triceps skinfold
Cranford[177]	GAAs + lipids	Retrospective	43	6 mo	Improvement in Salb, BUN, and hospitalization cost

*Compared with glucose infusion unless otherwise stated.

EAAs, essential amino acids; NEAAs, nonessential amino acids; Salb, serum albumin; Prealb, serum prealbumin; AMC, arm muscle circumference; IGF-I, insulin-like growth factor I; IDPN, intradialytic parenteral nutrition; rhGH, recombinant human growth hormone; Scr, serum creatinine; TLC, total lymphocyte count; BUN, blood urea nitrogen.

positive impact of parenteral nutrition, Cano and colleagues, in a randomized controlled study, reported improvements in multiple nutritional parameters with IDPN in a group of 26 malnourished CHD patients.[145] In a retrospective analysis of more than 1500 CHD patients treated with IDPN, Chertow and associates have reported a decreasing risk of death with the use of IDPN, particularly in patients with serum albumin concentrations below 3.5 g/dL and serum creatinine concentrations below 8 mg/dL.[146] They were able to show substantial improvements in these parameters after the use of IDPN. These findings suggested that this mode of treatment is probably most useful in patients with moderate to severe malnutrition.

Studies using amino acid dialysate (AAD) in PD patients have also provided conflicting results. In studies that suggested a benefit from AAD, serum transferrin and total protein concentrations increased and plasma amino acid profiles tended toward normal with one or two exchanges of AAD.[147, 148] However, an increase in blood urea nitrogen concentrations associated with exacerbation of uremic symptoms as well as worsening metabolic acidosis remains as a complication of AAD.[147–149] Kopple and coworkers reported significant short-term improvements in nitrogen balance as well as serum total protein and transferrin concentrations in 19 malnourished continuous ambulatory peritoneal dialysis (CAPD) patients treated with AAD.[150] In a more recent study, Jones and colleagues reported significant improvements in serum albumin and prealbumin concentrations in malnourished CAPD patients, particularly in those who had serum albumin concentrations within the lowest tertile.[151] These results are consistent with the reports in CHD patients, suggesting that these interventions are probably most useful in patients with severe malnutrition.

In the aggregate, the available evidence suggests that IDPN and AAD may be useful in the treatment of malnourished ESRD patients and offer an alternative method of nutritional intervention in a group of dialysis patients in whom oral or enteral intake cannot be maintained. However, most of the studies evaluating IDPN are retrospective, uncontrolled, and short term. Furthermore, there are no clear data to prove that aggressive nutritional supplementation through the gastrointestinal tract is actually inferior to parenteral supplementation in dialysis patients. Until a controlled study comparing various forms of nutritional supplementation in similar patient groups is completed, one should be cautious in choosing highly costly nutritional interventions; thus, there is an urgent need to initiate prospective studies to evaluate the long-term effects of IDPN and compare it to different forms of enteral nutrition.

Given the clinical complexity of the patient with complicated ARF, one can expect conflicting results in studies evaluating the parenteral nutritional treatment in such patients. Indeed, the available literature on this issue has been full of studies with a wide range of treatment protocols and no clear-cut results to guide the practicing clinicians.[27, 28, 121, 152–155] A selected list of these studies is provided in Table 18–6. The results of these studies have been subject to detailed and comprehensive reviews by several authors.[120, 156–158] The consensus of these reviews is that because of their limitations and drawbacks, no definitive conclusions can be made with regard to the effects of nutritional supplementation on the recovery of renal function and mortality. It is also our belief that the results of the available studies on nutritional supplementation are inconclusive and that decisions on optimal timing, route, composition, and amount of nutritional replacement for patients with ARF must be individualized at present. However, this should not preclude clinicians' performing more comprehensive and larger-scale studies, because this approach seems to be the only potential way to provide reliable information on the effects of optimal nutritional supplementation in complicated ARF patients.

Experimental Nutritional Therapies

As previously mentioned, growth hormone and its major mediator IGF-I have several anabolic properties. With the availability of recombinant forms of these agents, recombinant human growth hormone (rhGH) has been used in multiple patient populations at pharmacologic doses to promote net anabolism.[73] Consequently, with the recognition of alterations in the growth hormone–IGF-I axis in ESRD patients, rhGH has been proposed as a potential anabolic agent in this patient population.[159] Several animal studies

Table 18–6. Studies Using Supplemental Nutrition in Acute Renal Failure Patients

Study	Supplement*	Design	No. of Patients	Duration (days)	Outcome	Complications
Abel et al.[27]	Glu + EAAs	Pr randomized	53	13.5 vs. 10.8	Improved recovery and survival	Infections (3)
Baek et al.[28]	Glu + EAAs + NEAAs	Pr observational	29	NR	Lower mortality and morbidity	None
McMurray et al.[152]	Glu + EAAs + NEAAs	Retrospective	49	NR	Improved survival in complicated patients	
Pelosi et al.[154]	Glu + EAAs + NEAAs	Pr observational	46	NR	No change in survival; improved NB	
Mirtallo et al.[153]	EAAs vs. GAAs	Pr randomized	45	11 vs. 17	No difference in survival and NB	Hyperglycemia and sepsis (3)
Feinstein et al.[121]	Glu + EAAs + NEAAs	Pr randomized	30	31/2–36	No change in survival and/or renal function	No major complications
Fiaccadori et al.[155]	Enteral supplementation only	Observational	14	14 ± 2	Improvement in nutritional markers; No survival data	Tube obstruction

*Compared with glucose infusion unless otherwise stated.
Glu, glucose; EAAs, essential amino acids; GAAs, generalized amino acids; NB, nitrogen balance; NEAAs, nonessential amino acids; Pr, prospective; NR, not reported.

have suggested that rhGH induces a net anabolic action in uremic rats and also improves food utilization.[160] Furthermore, a preliminary short-term study in CHD patients by Ziegler and associates demonstrated a decrease in the predialysis blood urea nitrogen concentrations by approximately 25% and a significant reduction in net urea generation and PCR with rhGH administration.[161] In a subsequent study by our laboratory in which rhGH was given to seven malnourished hemodialysis patients in association with IDPN, the combination of IDPN with rhGH resulted in significant improvements in serum albumin, transferrin, and IGF-I concentrations.[162]

Similar net anabolic actions of rhGH have also been observed in PD patients. In a controlled prospective study by Ikizler and associates, rhGH treatment was shown to induce a substantial (29%) decrease in net urea generation in 10 PD patients.[163] Interestingly, these changes were associated with concurrent statistically significant decreases in serum potassium and phosphorus concentrations, as well as an increase in serum creatinine concentrations, suggestive of a net anabolic process in muscle mass. In a subsequent analysis of amino acid (AA) profiles of the same patients, the net anabolic processes induced by rhGH reflected a shift in AA metabolism towards peripheral muscle tissues.[87] Other studies in abstract form also suggested consistent results with rhGH administration in PD patients.[164]

Because IGF-I is the major mediator of growth hormone action, recombinant human IGF-I has also been proposed as an anabolic agent. Preliminary nitrogen balance studies in PD patients are consistent with this hypothesis; however, the side-effect profile of this agent, at least as observed in CRF patients, may impede its widespread use at this time.[165] Interestingly, the combined utilization of these agents in healthy subjects seems to provide the most efficient anabolic action with the fewest side effects.[166] It is unknown whether the long-term use of these agents in malnourished CHD and PD patients would result in improved nutritional parameters and hence in better outcomes.

ACKNOWLEDGMENT

This work is supported in part by NIH Grant No. DK-45604-07, DK53413-01 and FDA Grant No. FD-R-000943-5.

REFERENCES

1. United States Renal Data System: Excerpts from United States Renal Data System 1995 annual data report. Am J Kidney Dis 26(Suppl 2):S69–S84, 1995.
2. Fenton S, Desmeules M, Copleston P, et al: Renal replacement therapy in Canada: A report from the Canadian Organ Replacement Register. Am J Kidney Dis 25:134–150, 1995.
3. Teraoka S, Toma H, Nihei H, et al: Current status of renal replacement therapy in Japan. Am J Kidney Dis 25:151–164, 1995.
4. Mallick NP, Jones E, Selwood N: The European (European Dialysis and Transplantation Association—European Renal Association) Registry. Am J Kidney Dis 25:176–187, 1995.
5. Parker TFI, Laird NM, Lowrie EG: Comparison of the study groups in the National Cooperative Dialysis Study and a description of morbidity, mortality, and patient withdrawal. Kidney Int 23(Suppl 13):S42–S49, 1983.
6. Owen WF Jr, Lew NL, Liu Y, et al: The urea reduction ratio and serum albumin concentrations as predictors of mortality in patients undergoing hemodialysis. N Engl J Med 329:1001–1006, 1993.
7. Lowrie EG, Lew NL: Death risk in hemodialysis patients: The predictive value of commonly measured variables and an evaluation of death rate differences between facilities. Am J Kidney Dis 15:458–482, 1990.
8. Kopple JD: Effect of nutrition on morbidity and mortality in maintenance dialysis patients. Am J Kidney Dis 24:1002–1009, 1994.
9. Hakim RM, Levin N: Malnutrition in hemodialysis patients. Am J Kidney Dis 21:125–137, 1993.
10. Horber FF, Hoppeler H, Herren D, et al: Altered skeletal muscle ultrastructure in renal transplant patients on prednisone. Kidney Int 30:411–416, 1986.
11. Verdery RB, Goldberg AP: Hypocholesterolemia as a predictor of death: A prospective study of 224 nursing home residents. J Gerontol 46:M84–M90, 1994.
12. Law MR, Morris JK, Wald NJ, Hale AK: Serum albumin and mortality in the BUPA study. British United Provident Association. Int J Epidemiol 23:38–41, 1994.
13. Acchiardo SR, Moore LW, Latour PA: Malnutrition as the main factor in morbidity and predictors of mortality on hemodialysis. Kidney Int 24 (Suppl 16):S199–S203, 1983.
14. Lowrie EG, Huang WH, Lew NL, Liu Y: The relative contribution of measured variables to death risk among hemodialysis patients, In Friedman EA (ed): Death on Hemodialysis. Amsterdam, Kluwer Academic, 1994, p 121.
15. Churchill DN, Taylor DW, Cook RJ, et al: Canadian hemodialysis morbidity study. Am J Kidney Dis 19:214–234, 1992.
16. Iseki K, Kawazoe N, Fukiyama K: Serum albumin is a strong predictor of death in chronic dialysis patients. Kidney Int 44:115–119, 1993.
17. Collins AJ, Ma JZ, Umen A, Keshavia HP: Urea index and other predictors of hemodialysis patient survival. Am J Kidney Dis 23:272–282, 1993.
18. Goldwasser P, Michel MA, Collier J, et al: Prealbumin and lipoprotein(a) in hemodialysis: Relation-

ships with patient and vascular access survival. Am J Kidney Dis 22:215–225, 1993.

19. Goldwasser P, Mittman M, Antignani A, et al: Predictors of mortality on hemodialysis. J Am Soc Nephrol 3:1613–1622, 1993.

20. Oksa H, Ahonen K, Pasternack A, Marnela KM: Malnutrition in hemodialysis patients. Scand J Urol Nephrol 25:157–161, 1991.

21. Teehan BP, Schleifer CR, Brown JM, et al: Urea kinetic analysis and clinical outcome on CAPD. A five year longitudinal study. Adv Perit Dial 6:181–185, 1990.

22. Blake PG, Flowerdew G, Blake RM, Oreopoulos DG: Serum albumin in patients on continuous ambulatory peritoneal dialysis—Predictors and correlations with outcomes. J Am Soc Nephrol 3:1501–1507, 1993.

23. Rocco MV, Jordan JR, Burkart JM: The efficacy number as a predictor of morbidity and mortality in peritoneal dialysis patients. J Am Soc Nephrol 4:1184–1191, 1993.

24. Lowrie EG, Huang WH, Lew NL: Death risk predictors among peritoneal dialysis and hemodialysis patients: A preliminary comparison. Am J Kidney Dis 26:220–228, 1995.

25. Avram MM, Mittman N, Bonomini L, et al: Markers for survival in dialysis: A seven-year prospective study. Am J Kidney Dis 26:209–219, 1995.

26. Canada-USA (CANUSA) Peritoneal Dialysis Study Group: Adequacy of dialysis and nutrition in continuous peritoneal dialysis: Association with clinical outcomes. J Am Soc Nephrol 7:198–207, 1996.

27. Abel RM, Beck CH, Abot WM: Improved survival from acute renal failure after treatment with intravenous essential L-amino acids and hypertonic glucose. N Engl J Med 288:695, 1973.

28. Baek SM, Makabali GG, Bryan-Brown CW, et al: The influence of parenteral nutrition on the course of acute renal failure. Surg Gynecol Obstet 141:405–408, 1975.

29. Bartlett RH, Mault JR, Dechert RE, et al: Continuous arteriovenous hemofiltration: Improved survival in surgical acute renal failure? Surgery 100:400–408, 1986.

30. Mault JR, Dechert RE, Lees P, et al: Continuous arteriovenous filtration: An effective treatment for surgical acute renal failure. Surgery 101:478–484, 1987.

31. Fiaccadori E, Lombardi M, Leonardi S, et al: Prevalence and clinical outcome associated with preexisting malnutrition in acute renal failure: a prospective cohort study. J Am Soc Nephrol 10:581–593, 1999.

32. Blumenkrantz MJ, Kopple JD, Gutman RA, et al: Methods for assessing nutritional status of patients with renal failure. Am J Clin Nutr 33:1567–1585, 1980.

33. Young GA, Swanepoel CR, Croft MR, et al: Anthropometry and plasma valine, amino acids, and proteins in the nutritional assessment of hemodialysis patients. Kidney Int 21:492–499, 1982.

34. Cano N, Feinandez JP, Lacombe P, et al: Statistical selection of nutritional parameters in hemodialysis patients. Kidney Int 32(Suppl 22):S178–S180, 1987.

35. Jacob V, Carpentier JEL, Salzano S, et al: IGF-1, a marker of undernutrition in hemodialysis patients. Am J Clin Nutr 52:39–44, 1990.

36. Anderson CF, Wochos DN: The utility of serum albumin values in the nutritional assessment of hospitalized patients. Mayo Clin Proc 57:181–184, 1982.

37. Herrmann FR, Safran C, Levkoff SE, Minaker KL: Serum albumin level on admission as a predictor of death, length of stay, and readmission. Arch Intern Med 152:125–130, 1992.

38. Sullivan DH, Carter WJ: Insulin-like growth factor I as an indicator of protein-energy undernutrition among metabolically stable hospitalized elderly. J Am Coll Nutr 13:184–191, 1995.

39. Guarnieri B, Faccini L, Lipartiti T, et al: Simple methods for nutritional assessment in hemodialyzed patients. Am J Clin Nutr 33:1598–1607, 1980.

40. O'Keefe SJ, Dicker J: Is plasma albumin concentration useful in the assessment of nutritional status of hospital patients? Eur J Clin Nutr 42:41–45, 1988.

41. Spiess A, Mikalunas V, Carlson S, et al: Albumin kinetics in hypoalbuminemic patients receiving total parenteral nutrition. JPEN J Parenter Enteral Nutr 20:424–428, 1996.

42. Avram MM, Goldwasser P, Erroa M, Fein PA: Predictors of survival in continuous ambulatory peritoneal dialysis patients: The importance of prealbumin and other nutritional and metabolic markers. Am J Kidney Dis 23:91–98, 1994.

43. Chertow GM, Lowrie EG, Wilmore DW, et al: Nutritional assessment with bioelectrical impedance analysis in maintenance hemodialysis patients. J Am Soc Nephrol 6:75–81, 1995.

44. Young GA, Kopple JD, Lindholm B, et al: Nutritional assessment of continuous ambulatory peritoneal dialysis patients: An international study. Am J Kidney Dis 17:462–471, 1991.

45. Health Care Financing Administration: Opportunities to improve care for adult in-center hemodialysis patients. Am J Kidney 26:2:S69–S84, 1995.

46. Biasioli S, Petrosino Z, Cavalli L, et al: Bioelectrical impedance for the assessment of body composition of dialyzed patients [Letter]. Clin Nephrol 31:274–275, 1989.

47. Stenver DI, Gotfredsen A, Hilsted J, Nielsen B: Body composition in hemodialysis patients measured by dual-energy x-ray absorptiometry. Am J Nephrol 15:105–110, 1995.

48. Rayner HC, Stroud DB, Salamon KM, et al: Anthropometry underestimates body protein depletion in haemodialysis patients. Nephron 59:33–40, 1991.

49. Pollock CA, Ibels LS, Ayass W, et al: Total body nitrogen as a prognostic marker in maintenance dialysis. J Am Soc Nephrol 6:82–88, 1995.

50. Cianciaruso B, Brunori G, Kopple JD, et al: Cross-sectional comparison of malnutrition in continuous ambulatory peritoneal dialysis and hemodialysis patients. Am J Kidney Dis 26:475–486, 1995.

51. Anderstam B, Mamoun AH, Sodersten P, Bergstrom J: Middle-sized molecule fractions isolated from uremic ultrafiltrate and normal urine inhibit ingestive behavior in the rat. J Am Soc Nephrol 7:2453–2460, 1996.

52. Ikizler TA, Yenicesu M, Greene JH, Wingard RL, Hakim RM: Nitrogen balance in hospitalized chronic hemodialysis patients. Kidney Int 50(Suppl 57):553–556, 1996.

53. Sanders HN, Narvarte J, Bittle PA, Ramirez G:

Hospitalized dialysis patients have lower nutrient intakes on renal diet than on regular diet. J Am Diet Assoc 91:1278–1280, 1991.

54. May RC, Kelly RA, Mitch WE: Mechanisms for defects in muscle protein metabolism in rats with chronic uremia: The influence of metabolic acidosis. J Clin Invest 79:1099–1103, 1987.

55. Mitch WE, Walser M: Nutritional therapy of the uremic patient. *In* Brenner BM, Rector FC (eds): The Kidney. Philadelphia, WB Saunders, 1991, p 2186.

56. Ballmer PE, McNurlan MA, Hulter HN, et al: Chronic metabolic acidosis decreases albumin synthesis and induces negative nitrogen balance in humans. J Clin Invest 95:39–45, 1995.

57. Graham KA, Reaich D, Channon SM, et al: Correction of acidosis in CAPD decreases whole body protein degradation. Kidney Int 49:1396–1400, 1996.

58. Graham KA, Reaich D, Channon SM, et al: Correction of acidosis in hemodialysis decreases whole body protein degradation. J Am Soc Nephrol 8:632–637, 1997.

59. Williams AJ, Dittmer ID, McArley A, Clarke J: High bicarbonate dialysate in haemodialysis patients: Effects on acidosis and nutritional status. Nephrol Dial Transplant 12:2633–2637, 1997.

60. Walls J: Effect of correction of acidosis on nutritional status in dialysis patients [Review]. Miner Electrolyte Metab 23:234–236, 1997.

61. Brady JP, Hasbargen JA: Correction of metabolic acidosis and its effect on albumin in chronic hemodialysis patients. Am J Kidney Dis 31:35–40, 1998.

62. Uribarri J: Moderate metabolic acidosis and its effects on nutritional parameters in hemodialysis patients. Clin Nephrol 48:238–240, 1997.

63. Bergstrom J: Nutritional requirements of hemodialysis patients. *In* Mitch WE, Klahr S (eds): Nutrition and the Kidney. Boston, Little Brown, 1993, p 263.

64. Defronzo RA, Alvestrand A, Smith D, et al: Insulin resistance in uremia. J Clin Invest 67:563–568, 1981.

65. Mak RHK, Bettinelli A, Turner C, et al: The influence of hyperparathyroidism on glucose metabolism in uremia. J Clin Endocrinol Metab 60:229–233, 1985.

66. Garber AJ: Effects of parathyroid hormone on skeletal muscle protein and amino acid metabolism in the rat. J Clin Invest 71:1806–1821, 1983.

67. Kaptein EM, Feinstein EI, Massry SG: Thyroid hormone metabolism in renal disease. Contrib Nephrol 33:122–135, 1982.

68. Waterlow JC: Endocrine changes in severe PEM. *In* Waterlow JC (ed): Protein-Energy Malnutrition. London, Edward Arnold, 1992, p 112.

69. Waterlow JC: Metabolic adaptation to low intakes of energy and protein. Ann Rev Nutr 6:495–526, 1986.

70. Krieg JRJ, Santos F, Chan JCM: Growth hormone, insulin-like growth factor and the kidney. Kidney Int 48:321–336, 1995.

71. Chwals WJ, Bistrian BR: Role of exogenous growth hormone and insulin-like growth factor 1 in malnutrition and acute metabolic stress: A hypothesis. Crit Care Med 19:1317–1322, 1991.

72. Wilmore DW: Catabolic illness: Strategies for enhancing recovery. N Engl J Med 325:695, 1991.

73. Kaplan SL: The newer uses of growth hormone in adults. Adv Intern Med 38:287–301, 1993.

74. Veldhuis JD, Johnson ML, Wilkowski MJ, et al: Neuroendocrine alterations in the somatotrophic axis in chronic renal failure. Acta Paediatr Scand 379:12–22, 1991.

75. Chan W, Valerie KC, Chan JCM: Expression of insulin-like growth factor-1 in uremic rats: Growth hormone resistance and nutritional intake. Kidney Int 43:790–795, 1993.

76. Tonshoff B, Eden S, Weiser E, et al: Reduced hepatic growth hormone (GH) receptor gene expression and increased plasma GH binding protein in experimental uremia. Kidney Int 45:1085–1092, 1994.

77. Challa A, Chan W, Krieg RJ Jr, et al: Effect of metabolic acidosis on the expression of insulin-like growth factor and growth hormone receptor. Kidney Int 44:1224–1227, 1993.

78. Underwood LE, Clemmons DR, Maes M, et al: Regulation of somatomedin-C/insulin-like growth factor I by nutrients. Hormone Research 24:166–176, 1986.

79. Thissen JP, Ketelslegers JM, Underwood LE: Nutritional regulation of the insulin-like growth factors. Endocr Rev 15:80–101, 1994.

80. Kopple JD, Swendseid ME, Shinaberger JH, Umezawa CY: The free and bound amino acids removed by hemodialysis. Trans Am Soc Artif Intern Organs 19:309–313, 1973.

81. Wolfson M, Jones MR, Kopple JD: Amino acid losses during hemodialysis with infusion of amino acids and glucose. Kidney Int 21:500–506, 1982.

82. Ikizler TA, Flakoll PJ, Parker RA, Hakim RM: Amino acid and albumin losses during hemodialysis. Kidney Int 46:830–837, 1994.

83. Kopple JD: The nutrition management of the patient with acute renal failure. JPEN J Parenter Enteral Nutr 20:3–12, 1996.

84. Davies SP, Reaveley DA, Brown EA, Kox WJ: Amino acid clearances and daily losses in patients with acute renal failure treated by continuous arteriovenous hemodialysis. Crit Care Med 19:1510–1515, 1991.

85. Mokrzycki MH, Kaplan AA: Protein losses in continuous renal replacement therapies. J Am Soc Nephrol 7:2259–2263, 1996.

86. Kopple JD, Hirschberg R: Nutrition and peritoneal dialysis. *In* Mitch WE, Klahr S (eds): Nutrition and the Kidney. Boston, Little, Brown, 1993, p 290.

87. Ikizler TA, Wingard RL, Flakoll PJ, et al: Effects of recombinant human growth hormone on plasma and dialysate amino acid profiles in CAPD patients. Kidney Int 50:229–234, 1996.

88. Lindholm B, Bergstrom J: Nutritional management of patients undergoing peritoneal dialysis. *In* Nolph KD (ed): Peritoneal Dialysis. Dordrecht, Kluwer Academic, 1989, p 230.

89. Bursztein S, Elwyn DH, Askanazi J, et al: Nitrogen balance. *In* Bursztein S, Elwyn DH, Askanazi J, Kinney JM (eds): Energy Metabolism, Indirect Calorimetry, and Nutrition. Baltimore, Williams & Wilkins, 1989, p 85.

90. Schoenfeld PY, Henry RR, Laird NM, Roxe DM: Assessment of nutritional status of the national cooperative dialysis study population. Kidney Int 23:80–88, 1983.

91. Lindsay RM, Spanner E: A hypothesis: The protein catabolic rate is dependent upon the type and amount of treatment in dialyzed uremic patients. Am J Kidney Dis 132:382–389, 1989.

92. Bergstrom J, Lindholm B: Nutrition and adequacy of dialysis. How do hemodialysis and CAPD compare? Kidney Int 43(Suppl 40):S39–S50, 1993.

93. Lindsay R, Spanner E, Heidenheim P, et al: Which comes first, Kt/V or PCR—Chicken or egg? Kidney Int 42(Suppl 38):S32–S37, 1992.

94. Acchiardo SR, Moore L, Smith SO, et al: Increased dialysis prescription improved nutrition [Abstract]. J Am Soc Nephrol 6:571, 1995.

95. Burrowes DD, Lyons TA, Kaufman AM, Levin NW: Improvement in serum albumin with adequate hemodialysis. J Renal Nutr 3:171–176, 1993.

96. Hakim RM, Breyer J, Ismail N, Schulman G: Effects of dose of dialysis on morbidity and mortality. Am J Kidney Dis 23:661–669, 1994.

97. Lameire NH, Vanholder R, Veyt D, et al: A longitudinal, five year survey of kinetic parameters in CAPD patients. Kidney Int 42:426–432, 1992.

98. Churchill DN: Adequacy of peritoneal dialysis: How much dialysis do we need? Kidney Int 48:S2–S6, 1997.

99. Hakim RM: Clinical implications of hemodialysis membrane biocompatibility. Kidney Int 44:484–494, 1993.

100. Gutierrez A, Alvestrand A, Wahren J, Bergstrom J: Effect of in vivo contact between blood and dialysis membranes on protein catabolism in humans. Kidney Int 38:487–494, 1990.

101. Gutierrez A, Bergstrom J, Alvestrand A: Protein catabolism in sham-hemodialysis: The effect of different membranes. Clin Nephrol 38:20–29, 1992.

102. Lindsay RM, Spanner E, Heidenheim P, et al: PCR, Kt/V, and membrane. Kidney Int 43(Suppl 41):S268–S273, 1993.

103. Parker TF III, Wingard RL, Husni L, et al : Effect of the membrane biocompatibility on nutritional parameters in chronic hemodialysis patients. Kidney Int 49:551–556, 1996.

104. Flores EA, Bistrian BA, Pomposelli JJ, et al: Infusion of tumor necrosis factor/cachectin promoted catabolism in the rat. J Clin Invest 83:1614–1622, 1989.

105. Himmelfarb J, Hakim RM: Biocompatibility and risk of infection in hemodialysis patients. Nephrol Dial Transplant 9:138–144, 1994.

106. Himmelfarb J, Lazarus JM, Hakim RM: Reactive oxygen species production by monocytes and polymorphonuclear leukocytes during dialysis. Am J Kidney Dis 17:271–276, 1991.

107. Canivet E, Lavaud S, Wong T, et al: Cuprophane but not synthetic membrane induces increases in serum tumor necrosis factor-alpha levels during hemodialysis. Am J Kidney Dis 23:41–46, 1994.

108. Hakim RM, Held PJ, Stannard DC, et al: Effects of the dialysis membrane on mortality of chronic hemodialysis patients. Kidney Int 50:566–570, 1994.

109. Bloembergen WE, Port FK, Hakim RM, et al: Relationship of dialysis membrane and cause-specific mortality. Am J Kidney Dis 33:1–10, 1994.

110. Maroni BJ: Nutritional requirements of normal subjects and patients with renal insufficiency. In Jacobson HR, Striker GE, Klahr S (eds): The Principles and Practice of Nephrology. Philadelphia, BC Decker, 1991, p 708.

111. Young VR: Nutritional requirements of normal adults. In Mitch WE, Klahr S (eds): Nutrition and the Kidney. Boston, Little, Brown, 1993, p 1.

112. Borah MF, Schoenfeld PY, Gotch FA, et al: Nitrogen balance during intermittent dialysis therapy of uremia. Kidney Int 14:491–500, 1978.

113. Bergstrom J, Furst P, Alvestrand A, Lindholm B: Protein and energy intake, nitrogen balance and nitrogen losses in patients treated with continuous ambulatory peritoneal dialysis. Kidney Int 44:1048–1057, 1993.

114. Blumenkrantz MJ, Kopple JD, Moran JK, Coburn JW: Metabolic balance studies and dietary protein requirements in patients undergoing continuous ambulatory peritoneal dialysis. Kidney Int 21:849–861, 1982.

115. Schneeweiss B, Graninger W, Stokenhuber F, et al: Energy metabolism in acute and chronic renal failure. Am J Clin Nutr 52:596–601, 1990.

116. Monteon FJ, Laidlaw SA, Shaib JK, Kopple JD: Energy expenditure in patients with chronic renal failure. Kidney Int 30:741–747, 1986.

117. Olevitch LR, Bowers BM, Deoreo PB: Measurement of resting energy expenditure via indirect calorimetry among adult hemodialysis patients. J Renal Nutr 4:192–197, 1994.

118. Ikizler TA, Wingard RL, Sun M, et al: Increased energy expenditure in hemodialysis patients. J Am Soc Nephrol 7:2646–2653, 1996.

119. Neyra RN, Chen K, Sun M, et al: Resting energy expenditure and energy balance in chronic renal failure, peritoneal dialysis and hemodialysis patients [Abstract]. J Am Soc Nephrol 8:223A, 1997.

120. Shuler CL, Wolfson M: Nutrition in acute renal failure. In Rombeau JL, Caldwell MD (eds): Clinical Nutrition: Parenteral Nutrition, 2nd ed. Philadelphia, WB Saunders, 1993, p 667.

121. Feinstein EI, Blumenkrantz MJ, Healy H: Clinical and metabolic responses to parenteral nutrition in acute renal failure. A controlled double-blind study. Medicine 60:124,1981.

122. Clark WR, Mueller BA, Alaka KJ, Macias WL: A comparison of metabolic control by continuous and intermittent therapies in acute renal failure. J Am Soc Nephrol 4:1413–1420, 1994.

123. Himmelfarb J: Dialytic therapy in acute renal failure: No reason for nihilism. Semin Dial 9:230–234, 1996.

124. Chima SC, Meyer L, Hummell C, et al: Protein catabolic rate in patients with acute renal failure on continuous arteriovenous hemofiltration and total parenteral nutrition. J Am Soc Nephrol 3:1516–1521, 1993.

125. Ikizler TA, Greene JH, Wingard RL, Hakim RM: Nitrogen balance in acute renal failure (ARF) patients [Abstract]. J Am Soc Nephrol 6:466, 1995.

126. Flores EA, Istfan N, Pomposelli JJ, et al: Effect of interleukin-1 and tumor necrosis factor/cachectin on glucose turnover in the rat. Metabolism 39:738–743, 1990.

127. Flores EA, Bistrian BR, Pomposelli JJ, et al: Infusion of tumor necrosis factor/cachectin promotes muscle catabolism in the rat. A synergistic effect with interleukin 1. J Clin Invest 83:1614–1622, 1989.

128. Horl WH, Heidland A: Enhanced proteolytic activity—Cause of protein catabolism in acute renal failure. Am J Clin Nutr 33:1423–1427, 1980.

129. Burnstein S, Elwyn DH, Askanazi J, et al: Theoreti-

cal framework of indirect calorimetry and energy balance. *In* Burstein S, Elwyn DH, Askanazi J, Kinney JM (eds): Energy Metabolism, Indirect Calorimetry, and Nutrition. Baltimore, Williams & Wilkins, 1989, p 27.

130. Clark WR, Mueller BA, Kraus MA, et al: Estimation of lean body mass by creatinine kinetics in critically ill patients with acute renal failure [Abstract]. J Am Soc Nephrol 7:1369, 1996.

131. Sax HC: Complications of total parenteral nutrition and their prevention. *In* Rombeau JL, Caldwell MD (eds): Clinical Nutrition: Parenteral Nutrition, 2nd ed. Philadelphia, WB Saunders, 1993, p 367.

132. Tschope W, Koch M, Thomas B, Ritz E: Serum lipids predict cardiac death in diabetic patients on maintenance hemodialysis. Results of a prospective study. The German Study Group Diabetes and Uremia. Nephron 64:354–358, 1993.

133. Ikizler TA, Hakim RM: Nutrition in end-stage renal disease. Kidney Int 50:343–357, 1996.

134. Compher C, Mullen JL, Barker CF: Nutritional support in renal failure. Surg Clin North Am 71:597–608, 1991.

135. Hecking E, Port FK, Brehm H, et al: A controlled study on the value of oral supplementation with essential amino acids and keto analogues in chronic hemodialysis. Proc Dial Transplant Forum 7:157–161, 1977.

136. Hecking E, Kohler H, Zobel R, et al: Treatment with essential amino acids in patients on chronic hemodialysis: A double blind cross-over study. Am J Clin Nutr 31:1821–1826, 1978.

137. Tietze IN, Pedersen EB: Effect of fish protein supplementation on amino acid profile and nutritional status in haemodialysis patients. Nephrol Dial Transplant 6:948–954, 1991.

138. Ponsky JL: Percutaneous endoscopic stomas. Surg Clin North Am 69:1227–1236, 1989.

139. Allman MA, Stewart PM, Tiller DJ, et al: Energy supplementation and the nutritional status of hemodialysis patients. Am J Clin Nutr 51:558–562, 1990.

140. Mastroiacovo P, Pace V, Sagliaschi G: Amino acids for dialysis patients. Clin Ther 15:698–704, 1993.

141. Ikizler TA, Wingard RL, Hakim RM: Interventions to treat malnutrition in dialysis patients: The role of the dose of dialysis, intradialytic parenteral nutrition, and growth hormone. Am J Kidney Dis 26:256–265, 1995.

142. Heidland A, Kult J: Long-term effects of essential amino acids supplementation in patients on regular dialysis treatment. Clin Nephrol 3:234–239, 1975.

143. Foulkes CJ, Goldstein DJ, Kelly MP, Hunt JM: Indications for the use of intradialytic parenteral nutrition in the malnourished hemodialysis patient. Renal Nutr 1:23–33, 1991.

144. Wolfson M: Use of intradialytic parenteral nutrition in hemodialysis patients [Editorial; Comment]. Am J Kidney Dis 23:856–858, 1994.

145. Cano N, Labastie-Coeyrehourq J, Lacombe P, et al: Perdialytic parenteral nutrition with lipids and amino acids in malnourished hemodialysis patients. Am J Clin Nutr 52:726–730, 1990.

146. Chertow GM, Ling J, Lew NL, et al: The association of intradialytic parenteral nutrition with survival in hemodialysis patients. Am J Kidney Dis 24:912–920, 1994.

147. Bruno M, Bagnis C, Marangella M, et al: CAPD with an amino acid dialysis solution: A long-term, cross-over study. Kidney Int 35:1189–1194, 1989.

148. Arfeen S, Goodship THJ, Kirkwood A, Ward MK: The nutritional/metabolic and hormonal effects of 8 weeks of continuous ambulatory peritoneal dialysis with a 1% amino acid solution. Clin Nephrol 33:192–199, 1990.

149. Young GA, Dibble JB, Hobson SM, et al: The use of an amino-acid-based CAPD fluid over 12 weeks. Nephrol Dial Transplant 4:285–292, 1989.

150. Kopple JD, Bernard D, Messana J, et al: Treatment of malnourished CAPD patients with an amino acid based dialysate. Kidney Int 47:1148–1157, 1995.

151. Jones M, Hagen T, Boyle CA, et al: Treatment of malnutrition with 1.1% amino acid peritoneal dialysis solution: Results of a multicenter outpatient study. Am J Kidney Dis 32:761–769, 1998.

152. McMurray SD, Luft FC, Maxwell DR, et al: Prevailing patterns and predictor variables in patients with acute tubular necrosis. Arch Intern Med 138:950–955, 1978.

153. Mirtallo JM, Schneider PJ, Mavko K, et al: A comparison of essential and general amino acid infusions in the nutritional support of patients with compromised renal function. JPEN J Parenter Enteral Nutr 6:109–113, 1982.

154. Pelosi G, Proietti R, Arcangeli A, et al: Total parenteral nutrition infusate. An approach to its optimal composition in post-trauma acute renal failure. Resuscitation 9:45–51, 1981.

155. Fiaccadori E, Leonardi S, Lombardi M, et al: Enteral nutrition in patients with acute renal failure: Nutritional effects and adequacy of nutrient intakes [Abstract]. J Am Soc Nephrol 7:1372, 1996.

156. Sponsel H, Conger JD: Is parenteral nutrition therapy of value in acute renal failure? Am J Kidney Dis 25:96–102, 1995.

157. Alkhuaizi AM, Schrier RW: Management of acute renal failure: New perspectives. Am J Kidney Dis 28:315–328, 1996.

158. Conger JD: Interventions in clinical acute renal failure: What are the data? Am J Kidney Dis 26:565–576, 1995.

159. Kopple JD: The rationale for the use of growth hormone or insulin-like growth factor-1 in adult patients with renal failure. Miner Electrolyte Metab 18:269–275, 1992.

160. Mehls O, Ritz E, Hunziker EB, Eggli P, et al: Improvement of growth and food utilization by human recombinant growth hormone in uremia. Kidney Int 33:45–52, 1988.

161. Ziegler TR, Lazarus JM, Young LS, et al: Effects of recombinant human growth hormone in adults receiving maintenance hemodialysis. J Am Soc Nephrol 2:1130–1135, 1991.

162. Schulman G, Wingard RL, Hutchinson RL, et al: The effects of recombinant human growth hormone and intradialytic parenteral nutrition in malnourished hemodialysis patients. Am J Kidney Dis 21:527–534, 1993.

163. Ikizler TA, Wingard RL, Breyer JA, et al: Short-term effects of recombinant human growth hormone in CAPD patients. Kidney Int 46:1178–1183, 1994.

164. Kang DH, Lee SW, Kim HS, et al: Recombinant human growth hormone (rhGH) improves nutritional status of undernourished adult CAPD patients [Abstract]. J Am Soc Nephrol 5:494, 1994.

165. Peng S, Fouque D, Kopple J: Insulin-like growth factor-1 causes anabolism in malnourished CAPD patients [Abstract]. J Am Soc Nephrol 4:414,1993.

166. Kupfer SR, Underwood LE, Baxter RC, Clemmons DR: Enhancement of the anabolic effects of growth hormone and insulin-like growth factor I by use of both agents simultaneously. J Clin Invest 91:391–396, 1993.

167. Piraino A, Tirpo J, Powers D: Prolonged hyperalimentation in catabolic chronic dialysis therapy patients. J Parenter Enteral Nutr 5:463–477, 1981.

168. Moore L, Acchiardo S: Aggressive nutritional supplementation in chronic hemodialysis patients. CRN Q 11:14, 1987

169. Toigo G, Situlin R, Tamaro G, et al: Effect of intravenous supplementation of a new essential amino acid formulation in hemodialysis patients. Kidney Int Suppl 27:S278–S281, 1989.

170. Madigan KM, Olshan A, Yingling DJ: Effectiveness of intradialytic parenteral nutrition in diabetic patients with end-stage renal disease. J Am Diet Assoc 90:861–863, 1990.

171. Matthys DA, Vanholder RC, Ringoir SM: Benefit of intravenous essential amino-acids in catabolic patients on chronic maintenance hemodialysis. Acta Clin Belg 46:150–158, 1991.

172. Snyder S, Bergen C, Sigler MH, Teehan BP: Intradialytic parenteral nutrition in chronic hemodialysis patients. ASAIO Trans 37:M373–M375, 1991.

173. Vehe KL, Brown RO, Moore LW, et al: The efficacy of nutrition support in infected patients with chronic renal failure. Pharmacotherapy 11:303–307, 1991.

174. Capelli JP, Kushner H, Camiscioli TC, et al: Effect of intradialytic parenteral nutrition on mortality rates in end-stage renal disease care. Am J Kidney Dis 23:808–816, 1994.

175. Smolle KH, Kaufmann P, Holzer H, Druml W: Intradialytic parenteral nutrition in malnourished patients on chronic haemodialysis therapy. Nephrol Dial Transplant 10:1411–1416, 1995.

176. Mortelmans AK, Duym P, Vanderbroucke J, et al: Intradialytic parenteral nutrition in malnourished hemodialysis patients: A prospective long-term study. JPEN J Parenter Enteral Nutr 23:90–95, 1999.

177. Cranford W: Effectiveness of IDPN therapy measured by hospitalizations and length of stay. Nephrol News Issues 12:33–39, 1998.

19

◆ Liver Disease and Parenteral Nutrition

Sheung-Tat Fan, M.S., M.D., F.R.C.S.(Ed & Glasg),
F.A.C.S.
Ronnie Tung-Ping Poon, M.S., F.R.C.S.(Ed)

◆ METABOLIC FUNCTIONS OF LIVER

The liver plays a central role in regulating the nutrition of the body by an array of biochemical pathways responsible for the metabolism of carbohydrate, lipid, and protein. Its main blood supply comes from the portal circulation, through which it receives nutrients absorbed from the gut. The nutrients are metabolized, stored, or redistributed to the peripheral tissues. The blood supply from the hepatic artery is the major source of oxygen for the liver. In the fasted state it also conveys nutrients from the storage tissues, mainly amino acids from the muscles and fatty acids from adipose tissues, to the liver for metabolism to provide fuels for peripheral tissues. A basic knowledge of the metabolic functions of the liver is essential to the understanding of metabolic disturbances and nutritional management in liver disease.

The most important function of the liver in carbohydrate metabolism is to provide a constant supply of glucose, which is the main fuel for the central nervous system. Glucose absorbed from the gut after a meal is converted into glycogen for storage in the liver (glycogenesis), and in the fasted state, glucose is produced by a combination of breakdown of glycogen (glycogenolysis) and conversion of amino acids or glycerol from storage tissues (gluconeogenesis). The enzyme glucose-6-phosphatase is unique to the liver and plays the key role of dephosphorylation of glucose and liberation of free glucose into the bloodstream. These metabolic processes are regulated by the interaction of insulin and glucagon in the fed state (hyperinsulinemia and hypoglucagonemia) or fasting state (hypoinsulinemia and hyperglucagonemia) to maintain a constant blood glucose level. These hormones themselves are catabolized by the liver. Carbohydrate metabolism in the liver is also influenced by other hormones including growth hormone, catecholamines, thyroxine, and glucocorticoids, which contribute to the regulation of blood glucose levels under different physiologic situations such as stress.

Dietary fat is digested into free fatty acids and glycerol in the gut and is re-esterified within the mucosal cell, then bound with apolipoproteins and phospholipids to form chylomicrons, which are absorbed through lymphatic channels rather than the portal circulation into the systemic bloodstream. Medium-chain fatty acids in the gut can be absorbed directly into the portal circulation. The liver allows the liberation of free fatty acids from chylomicrons in the peripheral tissues by adding apolipoproteins to form lipoproteins. The liver also metabolizes free fatty acids released from adipose tissues, which can be esterified into triglycerides or undergo β-oxidation to produce ATP and acetoacetate. The latter can be utilized by some body tissues, such as heart muscles, the kidney, or the brain, as an energy source, especially during starvation. The liver can also synthesize fatty acids de novo from pyruvate. In the fed state, de novo fatty acid synthesis and the esterification of fatty acids are the dominating processes. In the fasting state, fatty acid synthesis and esterification are inhibited, whereas β-oxidation is increased. In addition to triglyceride and fatty acid metabolism, the liver is also a site of synthesis of cholesterol, which in turn is a substrate for bile acid synthesis.

The liver has essential functions in amino acid metabolism through its interaction with muscles in fed and fasting states. Amino acids from the portal circulation after a meal undergo interconversion by transamination and other reactions in the liver. They can be recirculated to peripheral tissues, especially muscles, to replenish protein loss and can be incorporated into other molecules such as purines and pyrimidines or used for protein synthesis. During the fasting state, amino acids are derived from protein breakdown in muscles; most of the amino acids received by the liver are converted into glucose by gluconeogenesis, but some may be used for other purposes such as protein synthesis or oxidized to produce energy after conversion into ketoacids. The deamination of amino acids for gluconeogenesis results in the formation of ammonia, which is normally removed by urea formation. Branched-chain amino acids (BCAAs; valine, leucine, and isoleucine) are catabolized mainly in the muscles. The amino groups released are bound to glutamate to form glutamine, which is transported by the bloodstream to intestines and muscles for utilization. Aromatic amino acids (AAAs; phenylalanine, tyrosine, tryptophan) and sulfur amino acids, however, have to be transported to the liver for catabolism, because their oxidative enzymes are located solely in the liver.[1] This explains the increased concentration of AAAs in the bloodstream in liver failure, while deamination of BCAAs in the muscles continues, resulting in an increased serum AAA/BCAA ratio.

In addition to its central role in the metabolism of nutrients, the liver has other important functions. Many of the plasma proteins are synthesized in the liver, including albumin, α- and β-globulins, fibrinogen, and clotting factors II, VII, IX, and X. The synthesis of these clotting factors requires vitamin K. The liver is the storage organ for many vitamins, and it contributes to the digestion of fats and absorption of fat-soluble vitamins by secreting bile. The liver is also responsible for the detoxification and excretion of toxins from the gut. Hence the liver is the central metabolic organ of the body, and failure of its functions in acute or chronic liver disease can result in complex metabolic problems.

◆ PATHOPHYSIOLOGY OF LIVER FAILURE

Hepatic failure can be described as either acute or chronic, although some patients may have a combination of both. Fulminant hepatic failure is the result of acute diffuse hepatocellular injury usually caused by viral infection or drugs in a previously healthy person.[2] It is manifested by rapidly progressive jaundice, markedly elevated transaminase levels, and a loss of liver synthetic function with a prolonged prothrombin time and is always characterized by hepatic encephalopathy.[3] The latter is manifested by neuropsychiatric symptoms, which vary in severity from subtle behavioral changes to coma. Fulminant hepatic failure is seldom reversible and has a very poor prognosis with a mortality rate in excess of 60%.[4] Liver transplantation has become an established treatment of fulminant liver failure,[4, 5] and bioartificial liver support is under clinical trial as a temporizing measure to allow transplantation or natural recovery by liver regeneration.[6, 7] Artificial nutritional support could be important in optimizing the patient's condition before transplantation or in promoting liver regeneration.

Chronic liver failure is more common and occurs in chronic liver disease most frequently due to alcoholism or chronic viral infection. Cirrhosis is the usual underlying abnormality and is accompanied by the manifestations of portal hypertension such as esophageal variceal bleeding and ascites. Portosystemic shunting allows toxins from the gut to bypass the hepatic filter and results in the accumulation of toxic substances in the systemic circulation. Patients with chronic liver disease are prone to septic complications because of an impairment of immunocompetence that is in part the result of associated chronic malnutrition.[8, 9] Acute-on-chronic liver failure may develop in cirrhotic patients secondary to an acute insult such as gastrointestinal bleeding, infection, and starvation. Regenerating nodules in cirrhotic liver are deprived of portal blood supply and are hence particularly vulnerable to ischemia resulting from reduced hepatic arterial blood supply during states of dehydration, shock, or sepsis.[10, 11] The development of hepatic encephalopathy is a poor prognostic sign in patients with chronic liver disease. For patients with end-stage chronic liver failure, liver transplantation is the only effective treatment. Nutritional support to enhance the nutritional status may improve the results of liver transplantation.[12, 13]

◆ NUTRITIONAL AND METABOLIC DISTURBANCES IN LIVER DISEASE

Protein-calorie malnutrition is a common phenomenon of chronic liver disease. Studies of nutritional assessment in cirrhosis have found some signs of malnutrition in up to 65% of patients depending on the severity of the liver disease.[14-16] The cause of nutritional deficiency in chronic liver disease is multifactorial. Decreased dietary intake is certainly an important factor.[17] Reduced appetite is common, but the dietary restriction imposed by the physicians for the management of hepatic encephalopathy may also contribute. Impaired digestion and absorption of nutrients may be another factor. Exocrine pancreatic insufficiency and intestinal malabsorption have been documented in patients with chronic liver disease.[18, 19] Malabsorption can be aggravated in patients with cholestasis, such as those with primary biliary cirrhosis, as bile salts are necessary for the absorption of fat and fat-soluble vitamins.[20] Drugs prescribed for patients with liver disease may also aggravate malnutrition. For example, the use of lactulose and cholestyramine may exacerbate fat malabsorption. Reduced synthesis of plasma transport protein can affect the transport of nutrients such as trace elements, and the storage of vitamins in the liver is decreased in chronic liver disease.[21] Nutritional deficiencies may perpetuate liver damage, resulting in further impairment of liver function.[22, 23] Malnutrition has been shown to induce increased liver fibrosis in rats in combination with alcohol and is likely to be an important factor in the development of fibrosis in alcoholic liver disease.[24]

Chronic liver disease is frequently associated with hypermetabolism. Studies have confirmed increased energy expenditure and substrate oxidation in cirrhotic patients that may contribute to malnutrition in these patients.[25, 26] Specific disturbances in nutrient metabolism in chronic liver disease are well established. Table 19–1 summarizes the main abnormalities in carbohydrate, fat, and amino acid metabolism.

The key abnormality in carbohydrate metabolism in chronic liver failure is glucose intolerance, which is usually associated with normal or raised insulin levels, indicating that insulin resistance rather than deficiency is responsible.[27] The levels of both insulin and glucagon may increase owing to decreased hepatic degradation, but there is a decrease in the effective insulin-to-glucagon ratio as a result of glucagon predominance, insulin resistance, or both.[28] There is a re-

Table 19–1. Metabolic Disturbances in Chronic Liver Failure

Carbohydrate Metabolism

Glucose intolerance
Accelerated gluconeogenesis
Decreased glycogen store
Hypoglycemia (end-stage)

Lipid Metabolism

Decreased apoprotein synthesis
Reduced clearance of long-chain triglycerides
Increased serum free fatty acids

Amino Acid and Protein Metabolism

Increased plasma AAAs
Decreased plasma BCAAs
Decreased ureagenesis
Increased plasma NH_3 level
Decreased protein synthesis
Increased muscle proteolysis

AAAs, aromatic amino acids; BCAAs, branched-chain amino acids.

duced insulin sensitivity predominantly of muscle tissues. The exact pathogenesis of insulin resistance in liver cirrhosis is unknown, but a receptor or postreceptor dysfunction probably exists.[29] Protein-calorie malnutrition could be responsible in part for insulin resistance in chronic liver disease, and a 1992 study demonstrated improved insulin sensitivity after nutritional support in patients with alcoholic liver disease.[30] Increased gluconeogenesis occurs in cirrhotic liver, and it has been postulated that hyperglucagonemia together with increased catecholamine and corticosteroid levels as a result of impaired degradation produce a state of sustained gluconeogenesis.[31]

Hypoglycemia is more common in cases of massive hepatocellular injury as in fulminant hepatic failure, but it can occur in end-stage chronic liver failure. Reduced glycogenesis and accelerated glycogenolysis cause a chronic depletion of glycogen storage, resulting in hypoglycemia after only a short period of fasting. In fulminant hepatic failure, gluconeogenesis may fail and contribute to profound hypoglycemia. The occurrence of glucose intolerance in chronic liver disease and of hypoglycemia in acute liver failure has practical implications in the nutritional management of these patients. Cirrhotic patients may not be able to tolerate a large amount of glucose as the primary energy source in nutritional supplements, and additional alternative energy substrates such as lipid are useful. In patients with fulminant liver failure, an adequate supply of glucose must be provided.

Alterations in lipid metabolism also occur in liver disease and can have implications for the nutritional management of these patients. The liver plays a major role in the metabolism of long-chain triglycerides (LCTs), and investigations have found a reduced clearance of LCTs in cirrhosis.[32] This is probably the result of reduced synthesis of apolipoprotein C-II, albumin, hepatic triglyceridase, and carnitine, which are required in the liver metabolism of LCTs.[33–35] Some authors have advised against the use of LCTs in cirrhotic patients because of reduced metabolic clearance.[36, 37] However, others believe that fat emulsions should not be withheld in cirrhotic patients.[38] Medium-chain triglycerides (MCTs) have been developed as an energy substrate for parenteral nutritional therapy.[39, 40] They are readily oxidized by all body tissues, little is deposited in the liver, and they are less dependent on albumin, apolipoprotein C-II, and carnitine for metabolic clearance.[41, 42] MCTs thus appear to be an ideal energy substrate for cirrhotic patients. However, MCTs do not contain significant amounts of essential fatty acids, so a mixture of MCTs and LCTs is commonly given. We performed a study to determine the metabolic clearance of a fat emulsion containing a mixture of MCTs and LCTs in 28 cirrhotic patients.[43] By using an intravenous fat tolerance test, we found that the clearance of serum triglycerides in cirrhotic patients is as rapid as that in healthy control subjects, indicating that the clearance of MCT-LCT blend emulsion is not impaired in cirrhotic patients.[43] The use of lipid emulsion is particularly helpful for advanced cirrhotic patients, as they are more in need of nutritional therapy and are frequently intolerant of large amounts of glucose.

Decreased esterification of fatty acids results in increased serum free nonesterified fatty acids in cirrhotic patients. This may be important with respect to hepatic encephalopathy. Nonesterified fatty acids circulate in the blood at least partially bound to albumin, and increased serum fatty acids may result in displacement of bound tryptophan from albumin, resulting in an increased amount of tryptophan available to cross the blood-brain barrier.[44] Serum cholesterol levels may be increased in chronic liver disease because of reduced excretion. However, in patients with severe malnutrition, serum levels of both fatty acids and cholesterol may be reduced.[45]

Derangement of amino acid metabolism is of particular importance. In chronic and acute-on-chronic liver failure, a characteristic imbalance of amino acids with decreased plasma levels of BCAAs and increased levels of AAAs is observed.[46, 47] Decreased serum BCAAs in cirrhosis can be due to an augmented uptake of BCAAs in muscles as a result of hyperinsulinemia.[48] Acute-on-chronic liver failure is frequently associated with sepsis, which can increase the peripheral consumption of BCAAs for energy and further decrease plasma level of BCAAs.[49, 50] Elevation in the AAA levels is due to reduced hepatic metabolism in liver failure. In addition, increased muscle protein breakdown occurs in chronic or acute liver failure and results in the increased release of AAAs into the plasma.[51] The alteration in the amino acid pattern is thought to play a central role in the pathogenesis of hepatic encephalopathy.

An increased serum ammonia level is another characteristic feature of severe liver failure. Hyperammonemia results in part from a diminished capacity of liver for urea production. Another important cause in chronic liver disease is portosystemic shunting of ammonia produced by intraluminal deamination of amino acids in the gut. Ammonia has been implicated as one of the toxic metabolites that acts as a direct cerebral toxin in the pathogenesis of hepatic encephalopathy.[52] However, there is a lack of evidence of a direct effect of ammonia in hepatic encephalopathy, and it may be merely an indicator of disturbed nitrogen metabolism.[53]

◆ AMINO ACID IMBALANCE AND HEPATIC ENCEPHALOPATHY

The characteristic pattern of amino acid imbalance has formed the basis for the formulation of amino acid solutions used in parenteral nutritional therapy in liver disease. An understanding of the relation of amino acid imbalance and hepatic encephalopathy is crucial to the rational use of amino acid solutions.

The exact mechanism of hepatic encephalopathy is unknown, but currently it is viewed as a disorder in the balance of central neurotransmitters, particularly those of the aminergic system.[53-55] AAAs are precursors of aminergic neurotransmitters, and excessive brain concentrations of these AAAs can result in an imbalance of these aminergic neurotransmitters. Excessive accumulation of AAAs in the brain results directly from the increased plasma levels. A reduced serum level of BCAAs also contributes indirectly to the increased brain concentrations of AAAs as BCAAs compete with AAAs for the same carrier system to cross the blood-brain barrier.[56] Both animal and human studies have shown that a change in brain concentrations of aminergic neurotransmitters such as noradrenaline, dopamine, and serotonin correlates closely with the presence of hepatic encephalopathy.[57-60] The administration of BCAAs to rats with portacaval shunts has been shown to reduce the concentration of tryptophan, serotonin, and 5-hydroxyindoleacetic acid in the brain tissue, suggesting that amino acid imbalance contributes to derangement in aminergic neurotransmitters in the brain.[61]

Ammonia may play a role in the pathogenesis of hepatic encephalopathy by increasing the rate of transport of AAAs across the blood-brain barrier rather than by direct central nervous system toxicity. In the brain, ammonia combines with glutamate to form glutamine, which is exchanged for BCAAs and AAAs by the same carrier system across the blood-brain barrier.[53] An increase in brain ammonia would hence increase the rate of exchange of glutamine for other neutral amino acids.

The disturbances of the levels of neurotransmitters in chronic liver disease may not reach the threshold for symptomatic manifestations, but the brain is sensitized so that encephalopathy may ensue if the amino acid imbalance is exacerbated. Acute stress conditions, such as starvation, sepsis, and gastrointestinal bleeding, cause an increase in muscle protein catabolism and hence an increase in plasma AAA levels and a decrease in plasma BCAA levels. The exacerbation of amino acid imbalance in such conditions may then precipitate hepatic encephalopathy. Figure 19-1 summarizes the current concept of the role of amino acid imbalance in the pathogenesis of hepatic encephalopathy; this is the most widely accepted hypothesis.

Another theory of the pathogenesis of hepatic encephalopathy is an imbalance between excitatory amino acid neurotransmission mediated by glutamate and inhibitory amino acid neurotransmission mediated by γ-aminobutyric acid (GABAergic theory); another is increased cerebral concentrations of an endogenous benzodiazepine-like substance (benzodiazepine theory).[62] Although there is some evidence in support of these theories, the exact role of these mechanisms in hepatic encephalopathy remains to be elucidated.

◆ PARENTERAL NUTRITION IN LIVER DISEASE—GENERAL CONSIDERATIONS

The role of nutritional therapy in chronic liver disease is well established. There is growing evidence that the prognosis of patients with severe liver disease correlates with the severity of the malnutrition, and nutritional supplementation can improve the nutritional status, immunologic status, and liver function in these patients.[63] Enteral feeding is a more physiologic route for nutritional supplementation with known beneficial trophic effects on the gut and the liver resulting from the first-pass effects of nutrients. However, in patients with severe liver disease, there is often insufficient oral intake due to anorexia and chronic encephalopathy. Adequate provision of protein is important in correcting protein malnutrition and supporting protein synthesis and liver regeneration, but an enteral protein load is poorly tolerated, with a risk of exacerbation of encephalopathy. Hence, parenteral nutrition may be necessary in patients with severe liver disease, especially in those with acute liver failure or severe malnutrition or in perioperative situations.

The use of amino acid–enriched solutions is one of the cornerstones in the modern parenteral nutritional therapy of liver disease. Protein restriction was previously the mainstay of treatment to prevent encephalopathy. The emphasis is now on sufficient protein to promote a positive nitrogen balance. It has been estimated that amino acid requirements are double the normal level in patients with hepatic failure, which represents a hypercatabolic state.[64, 65] In general,

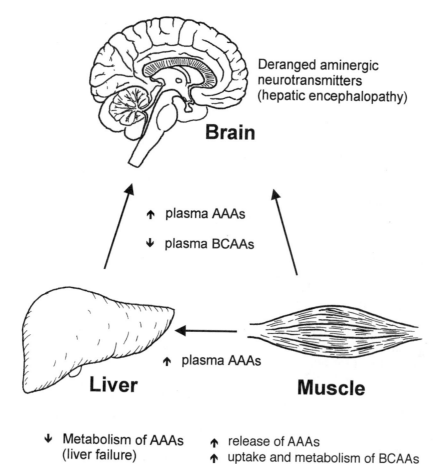

Deranged aminergic
neurotransmitters
(hepatic encephalopathy)

Brain

↑ plasma AAAs

↓ plasma BCAAs

Liver　　　　**Muscle**

↑ plasma AAAs

↓ Metabolism of AAAs　　↑ release of AAAs
(liver failure)　　　　　↑ uptake and metabolism of BCAAs
　　　　　　　　　　　　　　(stress, starvation, sepsis)

Figure 19–1. Relationship between amino acid imbalance and hepatic encephalopathy. AAA, aromatic amino acid; BCAA, branched-chain amino acid.

patients should receive at least 1 g of amino acids per kilogram per day; in protein-depleted patients, 1.5 g/kg/day may be given. Formulas enriched in BCAAs are accepted by many as the preferable amino acid supplements in patients with liver failure, despite the controversy on its advantage over the standard amino acid formula.[63] The administration of BCAAs corrects the amino acid imbalance and could be helpful in preventing encephalopathy. In addition, BCAAs have been found to decrease muscle catabolism, increase hepatic protein synthesis, and increase the synthesis of immune defense proteins in critically ill and septic patients.[66–68] BCAAs also have an anticatabolic effect in cirrhotic patients.[69] A 1995 animal study showed that a BCAA-enriched solution rather than the standard amino acid formula was effective in increasing protein synthesis in rats with liver failure.[70]

The main rationales for the use of BCAAs in patients with liver disease are summarized in Table 19–2. As BCAA-enriched formulas are more expensive than conventional

Table 19–2. Rationales for the Use of Branched-Chain Amino Acids in Liver Disease

BCAAs compete with AAAs for transport across blood-brain barrier
BCAAs decrease plasma level of AAAs by suppressing efflux from muscle
BCAAs increase hepatic protein synthesis
BCAAs decrease muscle proteolysis
BCAAs provide amino group for glutamine synthesis
BCAAs could be utilized directly by muscle, heart, brain, and liver to provide up to 30% of energy supply when glucose utilization and ketogenesis are depressed

AAAs, aromatic amino acids; BCAAs, branched-chain amino acids.

amino acid formulas, some authors have recommended the use of conventional amino acid formulas as nutritional supplements in liver disease patients who are not in hepatic encephalopathy.[63] However, we prefer BCAA-enriched solutions in patients with severe chronic liver disease who require short-term parenteral nutritional supplementation even when they are not in hepatic encephalopathy because of the anticatabolic effect of BCAAs. A prospective randomized study has demonstrated a significant benefit of BCAA-enriched solution when compared with standard amino acid infusions in promoting a positive nitrogen balance in the short-term nutritional support of patients with uncomplicated chronic liver disease.[71]

It has been shown that up to 125 g of BCAA-enriched solution is well tolerated in patients with hepatic encephalopathy.[64] Supplementation with BCAAs alone would not improve the nitrogen balance, as all essential amino acids are needed. Several amino acids including cystine, taurine, and tyrosine can normally be synthesized from precursors and hence are not essential in healthy subjects. In the cirrhotic state, however, the production of these amino acids may be insufficient because of metabolic defects, and they become "conditionally essential" amino acids.[63] The value of supplementation with these amino acids in liver disease remains to be studied.

Glutamine is another amino acid of intense interest in parenteral nutrition. Glutamine is the most abundant free amino acid in healthy humans. It is a precursor for protein synthesis and is an intermediate in many metabolic pathways. Of clinical importance is its preferential use by cells of gut mucosa, repair, and immune systems as an energy source. In the liver, it is essential for the synthesis of the antioxidant glutathione.[72] Hypercatabolic states such as sepsis and trauma are characterized by a profound depletion of glutamine when its requirement is increased because of the increased activity of immune and repair cells. Depletion of glutamine in the hypercatabolic state could contribute to severe clinical consequences such as poor wound healing, infection, increased intestinal permeability, endotoxemia, and multiple organ failure.[73, 74] Standard commercial parenteral amino acid solutions do not contain glutamine because of its instability. Glutamine supplementation in parenteral nutrition has been shown to have trophic effect on the gut and immune system in hypercatabolic patients.[75–77] Hence, glutamine is considered a conditionally essential amino acid in the hypercatabolic state. In cirrhosis, there is reduced intestinal uptake of glutamine, and in advanced cases, intracellular muscle glutamine concentrations are reduced.[78, 79] It has been postulated that glutamine may also be a conditionally essential amino acid in cirrhotic patients.[80] Glutamine supplementation in cirrhotic patients may promote muscle protein synthesis, help preserve the gut barrier, and help reduce endotoxemia, which is common in cirrhosis.[81, 82] Glutamine supplementation could potentially increase the production of ammonia, but this may represent a small proportion of the maximal capacity of ammonia detoxification in cirrhotic patients.[80] Because of the blood-brain barrier, it is also unlikely that increased plasma glutamine concentrations will increase levels of brain glutamine, which has been hypothesized to precipitate encephalopathy by enhancing the synthesis of γ-aminobutyric acid.[80] BCAAs increase glutamine synthesis in the muscles. This may be one of its beneficial effects in liver failure and stress conditions. The role of glutamine in the nutritional management of cirrhotic patients remains to be investigated by clinical trials.

The administration of adequate calories is essential in advanced liver disease patients in a hypercatabolic state. For most patients, the daily caloric requirement should be 1.2 to 1.4 times the resting energy expenditure as calculated by the Harris-Benedict equation (equivalent to about 30 kcal/kg of body weight).[63, 83] Sufficient caloric intake is critical for the efficient use of amino acids to achieve a positive nitrogen balance.

The caloric requirement can be provided by a combination of hypertonic glucose solution and fat emulsion. The use of lipid-based parenteral nutrition has been previously implicated in increased postoperative complications in surgical patients.[84, 85] Increased complications from lipid-based parenteral nutrition are likely to be the result of excessively rapid infusion rates.[86] There has been a particular concern about the use of lipid emulsions in cirrhosis because of decreased metabolic clearance of LCTs. Our previous study has shown that the metabolic clearance of an MCT-LCT blend solution is not impaired in cirrhotic patients.[43] Another study showed that the use of a parenteral nutrition regimen with the inclusion of an MCT-LCT lipid emulsion reduces postoperative complications in patients undergoing hepatectomy.[87] MCTs are readily oxidized by all body tissues for energy, and little is deposited in the liver.[43] The use of an MCT-LCT lipid emulsion reduces the requirement for glucose in cirrhotic patients, who are usually intolerant to a high glucose load. In general, 30 to 35% of the caloric requirement can be given as fat emulsion with good tolerance in patients with liver disease.[63, 88]

In cirrhotic patients, special attention should be paid to the volume of fluid and the amount of electrolytes prescribed in parenteral nutrition. These patients often have ascites and edema associated with secondary hyperaldosteronism, and sodium restriction may be necessary. Electrolyte disturbances should be avoided as they can precipitate hepatic encephalopathy. In patients with hepatorenal syndrome, extra care should be taken in the administration of fluid volume and nitrogen, although renal dialysis usually allows parenteral nutrition to be continued.

Other important considerations in cirrhotic patients include the provision of adequate vitamins and trace elements, as these patients are frequently malnourished. In patients with severe cholestasis, vitamin K_1 may need to be administered parenterally to correct coagulopathy. Adequate trace elements such as zinc are essential for effective protein synthesis in the liver.[89] The importance of zinc supplementation in cirrhotic patients deserves particular emphasis. Zinc deficiency is common in cirrhosis and is caused mainly by an increased loss in the urine.[90] There is evidence that zinc deficiency may contribute to the development of hepatic encephalopathy as some enzymes involved in the metabolism of amino acids and ammonia are zinc dependent, and zinc supplementation may have beneficial effects on liver function and encephalopathy in cirrhotic patients.[91, 92]

Hypertonic solutions of amino acids, glucose, and fat emulsion should be administrated by a central vein, although less concentrated solutions can be given by a peripheral vein as short-term supplements in patients who have a reasonable dietary intake. Cirrhotic patients are particularly prone to septic complications. Even short-term administration of parenteral nutrition by a conventional central venous line could result in central line sepsis, which could be fatal for these immunocompromised patients. Hence it is advisable to insert a subcutaneously tunneled single-lumen catheter for parenteral nutrition should it be required for more than 4 days, and extra care should be taken to prevent line sepsis.

◆ USE OF PARENTERAL NUTRITION IN SPECIFIC LIVER CONDITIONS

Hepatic Encephalopathy

A conventional treatment regimen for hepatic encephalopathy in cirrhotic patients includes dietary protein restriction and purgatives such as lactulose and neomycin. Recent emphasis on the management of hepatic encephalopathy has shifted to the need to correct amino acid imbalances and to provide sufficient protein for repair and regeneration. The use of BCAAs in liver disease originated from their effect on patients with hepatic encephalopathy.[93] The first randomized controlled trial of parenteral BCAA therapy for hepatic encephalopathy was reported in 1982, with 40 patients randomized to receive either 60 g of BCAAs in hypertonic glucose solution or oral lactulose with equivalent hypertonic glucose for at least 4 days.[94] Awakening of patients occurred in 70% of the BCAA group compared with 47% in the lactulose group, but the difference was not statistically significant. Several subsequent randomized trials have demonstrated that awakening from encephalopathy is more likely and occurs more rapidly in patients given BCAA-enriched solutions compared with those receiving lactulose and neomycin.[95–98] In two of these trials, an improvement in the survival of patients receiving BCAA-enriched solution was observed.[95, 96] However, in two other trials, no significant difference was found in the treatment results of BCAA-enriched solution compared with standard amino acid solution or glucose solution alone as control.[99, 100] In contrast to other studies that used glucose as the main energy source, the latter two studies used fat as the major energy source (50 and 60%, respectively). The exact cause of such a difference in response to BCAAs in relation to the use of different energy sources is uncertain.

A meta-analysis of five randomized controlled studies published in 1989 showed a significant improvement in mental recovery and a reduction in mortality with BCAA-enriched solutions.[101] Although there is still some controversy, it appears from these trials that BCAA-enriched solution is useful in hepatic encephalopathy at least in terms of mental recovery, but further randomized trials are needed to clarify its overall benefit.

Fulminant Hepatic Failure

Fulminant hepatic failure is a rare condition. Although hepatic encephalopathy is a common feature of fulminant hepatic failure, its management should be considered separately from hepatic encephalopathy in patients with chronic liver disease. In fulminant hepatic failure, hepatic encephalopathy is a very poor prognostic sign and usually indicates the need for liver transplantation.[102] Timely liver transplantation is the only hope for these patients, but nutritional therapy can be important in supporting the patients awaiting liver transplantation, and in less severe cases, it can promote liver regeneration.

The role of parenteral nutrition in the management of fulminant hepatic failure is not well studied, and there is a lack of randomized trials. In the past, emphasis has been placed on protein restriction to reduce ammonia production. However, a study showed that even in the presence of massive hepatic necrosis, significant amino acid oxidative loss continues, especially in fasted patients, suggesting a continuing need for amino acid supplementation.[103] Although amino acid oxidation rates are reduced, patients with fulminant hepatic failure may tolerate up to 60 g of standard amino acid solutions per day.[103] The role of BCAA-enriched solutions in fulminant hepatic failure is more controversial. Unlike in chronic or acute-on-chronic liver failure, in fulminant hepatic failure, serum BCAA levels are kept relatively normal by the opposing effects of increased release from the liver and increased uptake by peripheral tissues, whereas there is a gross elevation of all other amino acids including AAAs as a result of increased release from massive hepatocyte necrosis.[46, 104] BCAA-enriched solution may not be adequate to normalize the amino acid pattern, and no clear benefit of its use in fulminant hepatic failure has been demonstrated. However, there may be a potential advantage of BCAA-enriched formulas over standard amino acid formulas in the presence of excessive AAAs, and there is anecdotal evidence of a beneficial effect of BCAA-enriched solution in fulminant hepatitis.[105]

There is a need to provide a constant infusion of glucose solution to prevent hypoglycemia in patients with fulminant hepatic failure because of reduced glycogen storage and impaired glycogenolysis and gluconeogenesis. Up to 1000 kcal/day should be provided as 10 to 20% glucose solution. However, excessive glucose should be avoided to prevent fatty liver changes that could further aggravate the liver function impairment. Excessive lipid should also be avoided because of the impaired clearance of lipid, especially LCTs. It seems logical to use an MCT-LCT blend, as MCT can be metabolized easily by other body tissues. There has been little documentation of the use of lipid in fulminant hepatic failure, but a study has shown that most patients can tolerate 500 ml of 10% fat emulsions daily and many patients can tolerate 20% emulsions.[106] It would probably be reasonable to provide 25 to 30% of calories with an MCT-LCT blend solution in patients with fulminant hepatic failure.

Alcoholic Hepatitis

Alcoholic hepatitis is almost invariably associated with significant malnutrition, and parenteral nutrition may have a role in the management of severe alcoholic hepatitis patients who are in a hypercatabolic state.[107] Seven trials have been published on the use of supplementary parenteral nutrition in alcoholic hepatitis.[108–115] All these trials use standard amino acid solutions for intravenous supplementation. A review of these trials has shown that parenteral nutritional supplementation improved the nitrogen balance and the serum levels of visceral proteins such as serum albumin, prealbumin, and transferrin.[63] However, none of the studies have demonstrated a survival benefit in these patients with severe alcoholic hepatitis, although the earliest study by Nasrallah and Galambos did show a favorable trend in mortality.[108] The role of BCAA-enriched solution in alcoholic hepatitis has not been studied. Further studies are needed to clarify the benefits of parenteral nutrition in patients with alcoholic hepatitis.

Hepatectomy for Hepatocellular Carcinoma

Hepatectomy for hepatocellular carcinoma is a procedure with significant risk because the majority of patients have underlying cirrhosis and are often malnourished and immunocompromised. Animal studies have shown that the administration of BCAA-enriched solutions promotes liver regeneration and improves liver function after hepatectomy.[116, 117] It has also been shown in hepatectomized rats that a fat emulsion containing 50% MCT and 50% LCT significantly enhances visceral protein synthesis after hepatectomy.[118] Based on the results of these animal studies, we have performed a clinical randomized trial to evaluate the effect of parenteral nutritional support in patients undergoing hepatectomy for hepatocellular carcinoma.[87]

In our study, we randomized 124 patients undergoing hepatectomy for hepatocellular carcinoma to receive either perioperative nutritional support in addition to their oral diet or just an oral diet. The parenteral nutritional therapy consisted of a solution enriched with 35% BCAAs at a dosage of 1.5 g of amino acids per kilogram per day, and dextrose solution plus a lipid emulsion containing 50% MCT and 10% LCT to provide 30 kcal/kg/day. There was no significant difference in mortality, but a significant reduction in postoperative morbidity was found in the nutritional support group compared with the control group (34% vs. 55%, $P < .05$), mainly because of a lower incidence of septic complications (17% vs. 37%, $P < .05$). In the nutritional support group, there was also a lower rate of ascites requiring diuretics, less weight loss after hepatectomy, and less deterioration of liver function, especially in the patients who underwent major hepatectomy with underlying cirrhosis.

Our study has shown a definite benefit of perioperative nutritional support in patients undergoing hepatectomy, but there are still issues that remain to be studied. Animal studies have demonstrated that glutamine-supplemented parenteral nutrition can also promote protein synthesis and liver regeneration after hepatectomy and can attenuate

enterocyte malnutrition thereby reducing enteral bacterial translocation.[119, 120] As discussed previously, the role of glutamine supplementation in cirrhotic patients remains unclear. The relative benefit of glutamine and BCAA supplementation cannot be known without a randomized trial. Whether parenteral nutrition represents the best route for nutritional support in hepatectomized patients is also uncertain. Some animal studies have indicated that enteral nutritional supplementation may be better than total parenteral nutrition in promoting liver regeneration, preserving intact intestinal mucosa, and reducing bacterial translocation.[121, 122] A randomized trial involving 26 patients showed no significant difference in the nutritional parameters between patients receiving early enteral nutrition and those receiving parenteral nutrition, but the former group had a higher immunocompetence.[123] Further larger randomized trials should be carried out to clarify the relative benefit of parenteral and enteral nutrition. Until further evidence is available, we will use total parenteral nutrition with BCAA-enriched solutions routinely for nutritional supplementation in patients with severe cirrhosis after a major hepatectomy, but also encourage early dietary intake to allow the trophic effects of enteral nutrients on gut mucosa and the regenerating liver.

Liver Transplantation

Patients requiring liver transplantation usually have severe malnutrition, which is a significant risk factor for post-transplant outcomes.[13] Correction of the malnutritional status with enteral nutritional therapy in these patients with end-stage liver failure while waiting for a liver graft is conceivably difficult to achieve. Hence, postoperative parenteral nutritional support may be more practical to reduce the effect of malnutrition on the postoperative outcome, especially with a functioning transplanted liver, which should be more effective in replenishing the nutritional deficiency.

A prospective randomized trial has compared total parenteral nutrition using standard amino acids and total parenteral nutrition using BCAA-enriched solutions with no nutritional support for 7 days after the transplantation.[124] Both groups with nutritional supplementation could be weaned away from the ventilator earlier, had a shorter stay in the intensive care unit, and had a significantly better improvement in nitrogen balance compared with the control group. The total hospital charges were the highest in the control group. In both groups with nutritional supplementation, 1.5 g of amino acids per kilogram per day was given; this amount was well tolerated without an increase in ammonia levels or clinical measurements of encephalopathy. This study did not demonstrate any significant benefit by using a BCAA-enriched solution.

In a prospective study evaluating the caloric and protein requirements of adult patients after liver transplantation, it was found that the resting energy expenditure did not increase compared with preoperative values, but there was a significant increase in nitrogen catabolism from the muscles, which persisted for 28 days postoperatively.[83] Based on the findings of this study, it was recommended that the caloric intake should be the amount calculated by the Harris-Benedict equation at ideal body weight plus 20%, and parenterally or enterally administered protein of more than 1.2 g/kg/day should be provided.

The controversy of enteral versus parenteral nutrition also exists regarding nutritional supplementation after liver transplantation. A randomized trial in 24 patients comparing enteral feeding by a nasojejunal tube and total parenteral nutrition after liver transplantation did not show any significant difference in the number of days on a ventilator, the postoperative hospital stay, nutritional parameters, and the intestinal permeability.[124] Further larger randomized trials are needed for a more definite conclusion.

Post–liver transplantation patients require special care in the management of parenteral nutrition because of frequent coexisting problems such as sepsis, acute renal failure, and possible interactions of immunosuppressive drugs. Particular attention is needed to prevent central line sepsis, which could be highly fatal in these immunocompromised patients. The use of steroids may lead to difficulty in controlling blood glucose levels when hypertonic glucose solution is administered. The use of cyclosporine may lead to a disproportionate increase in serum urea levels. Dialysis may be necessary in patients with renal failure to allow the use of parenteral nutrition. Deterioration of liver function is usually the

result of sepsis or rejection, although one has to bear in mind the possibility of liver function impairment induced by total parenteral nutrition.

SUMMARY

The need for nutritional support in patients with liver disease is now well recognized as a result of numerous studies in the last two decades. In acute or acute-on-chronic liver conditions such as hepatic encephalopathy and fulminant liver failure, and in perioperative periods of hepatectomy or liver transplantation, parenteral nutrition has been shown to reduce morbidity and may potentially improve the survival of the patients. The understanding of amino acid imbalance and the proven value of BCAA-enriched solutions have resulted in dramatic improvements in parenteral nutritional therapy in liver disease. The use of mixed MCT-LCT lipid emulsions for more efficient energy utilization in liver disease represents another major advance.

There are still many controversies in this area. Some authorities are not yet fully convinced of the benefit of BCAAs over standard amino acids, because there is a lack of support from large and well-conducted trials. A significant survival benefit with the use of parenteral nutrition in patients with severe liver disease remains to be demonstrated. The relative roles of enteral and parenteral nutrition need to be established. The value of glutamine supplementation in liver disease is a new area to be studied. Although further clinical trials will help to clarify these issues, continuing research to unveil the basic mechanisms of the nutritional and metabolic disturbances down to the molecular level in various kinds of liver disease is important to establish the best nutritional therapy for the patients.

REFERENCES

1. Felig P: Amino acid metabolism in man. Ann Rev Biochem 44:933–955, 1975.
2. Hoofnagle JH, Carithers RL Jr, Shapiro C, Ascher N: Fulminant hepatic failure: Summary of a workshop. Hepatology 21:240–252, 1995.
3. Bernstein D, Tripodi J: Fulminant hepatic failure. Crit Care Clin 14:181–197, 1998.
4. Kramer DJ, Aggarwal S, Martin M, et al: Management options in fulminant hepatic failure. Transplant Proc 23:1895–1898, 1991.

5. Goss JA, Shackleton CR, Maggard M, et al: Liver transplantation for fulminant hepatic failure in the pediatric patient. Arch Surg 133:839–846, 1998.

6. Yoshiba M, Inoue K, Sekiyama K, Koh I: Favorable effect of new artificial liver support on survival of patients with fulminant hepatic failure. Artif Organs 20:1169–1172, 1996.

7. Watanabe FD, Mullon CJ, Hewitt WR, et al: Clinical experience with a bioartificial liver in the treatment of severe liver failure. A phase I clinical trial. Ann Surg 225:484–491, 1997.

8. O'Keefe SJD, El Zayadi A, Carraher TE, et al: Malnutrition and immunocompetence in patients with liver disease. Lancet 2:615–617, 1980.

9. Ledesma Castano F, Echevarria Vierna S, Lozano Polo JL, et al: Interleukin-1 in alcoholic cirrhosis of the liver: The influence of nutrition. Eur J Clin Nutr 46:527–533, 1992.

10. Alison MR: Regulation of hepatic growth. Physiol Rev 66:499–541, 1986.

11. Saadia R, Schein M, MacFarlane C, et al: Gut barrier function and the surgeon. Br J Surg 77:487–492, 1990.

12. DiCecco SR, Wieners EJ, Wiesner RH, et al: Assessment of nutritional status of patients with end-stage liver disease undergoing liver transplantation. Mayo Clin Proc 64:95–102, 1989.

13. Lowell JA: Nutritional assessment and therapy in patients requiring liver transplantation. Liver Transpl Surg 2(5 Suppl 1):79–88, 1996.

14. Lautz HU, Selberg O, Korber J, et al: Protein-calorie malnutrition in liver cirrhosis. Clin Investig 70:478–486, 1992.

15. Lolli R, Marchesini G, Bianchi G, et al: Anthropometric assessment of the nutritional status of patients with liver cirrhosis in an Italian population. Ital J Gastroenterol 24:429–435, 1992.

16. Caregaro L, Alberino F, Amodio P, et al: Malnutrition in alcoholic and virus-related cirrhosis. Am J Clin Nutr 63:602–609, 1996.

17. Porayko MK, DiCecco S, O'Keefe SJD: Impact of malnutrition and its therapy on liver transplantation. Semin Liver Dis 11:305–314, 1991.

18. Van Goidsenhoven GE, Henke WJ, Vacca JB, Knight WA: Pancreatic function in cirrhosis of the liver. Am J Dig Dis 8:160–173, 1963.

19. Mezey E: Intestinal function in chronic alcoholism. Ann N Y Acad Sci 252:215–227, 1975.

20. Munoz SJ, Heubi JE, Balistreri WF, et al: Vitamin E deficiency in primary biliary cirrhosis: Gastrointestinal malabsorption, frequency and relationship to other lipid-soluble vitamins. Hepatology 9:525–531, 1989.

21. Herman RH: Metabolism of the vitamins by the liver in normal and pathological conditions. In Zakim D, Boyer PD (eds): Hepatology, 2nd ed. Philadelphia, WB Saunders, 1990, pp 96–114.

22. Mendenhall CL: Protein-calorie malnutrition associated with alcoholic hepatitis. Veterans Administration Cooperative Study Group on Alcoholic Hepatitis. Am J Med 76:211–222, 1984.

23. Mendenhall CL, Tosch T, Weesner RE, et al: VA cooperative study on alcoholic hepatitis. II: Prognostic significance of protein-calorie malnutrition. Am J Clin Nutr 43:213–218, 1986.

24. Bosma A, Seifert WF, van Thiel de Ruiter GC, et al: Alcohol in combination with malnutrition causes increased liver fibrosis in rats. J Hepatol 21:394–402, 1994.

25. Muller MJ, Lautz HU, Plogmann B, et al: Energy expenditure and substrate oxidation in patients with cirrhosis: The impact of cause, clinical staging and nutritional state. Hepatology 15:782–794, 1992.

26. Greco AV, Mingrone G, Benedetti G, et al: Daily energy and substrate metabolism in patients with cirrhosis. Hepatology 27:346–350, 1998.

27. Marchesini G, Zoli M, Angiolini A, et al: Muscle protein breakdown in liver cirrhosis and the role of altered carbohydrate metabolism. Hepatology 1:294–299, 1981.

28. Soeters PB, Fischer JE: Insulin, glucagon, amino acid imbalance, and hepatic encephalopathy. Lancet 2:880–882, 1976.

29. Nolte W, Hartmann H, Ramadori G: Glucose metabolism and liver cirrhosis. Exp Clin Endocrinol Diabetes 103:63–74, 1995.

30. Wahl DG, Dollet JM, Kreher M, et al: Relationship of insulin resistance to protein-energy malnutrition in patients with alcoholic liver cirrhosis: Effect of short-term nutritional support. Alcohol Clin Exp Res 16:971–978, 1992.

31. Sherwin R, Joshi P, Hendler R, et al: Hyperglucagonemia in Laennec's cirrhosis. The role of portalsystemic shunting. N Engl J Med 290:239–242, 1974.

32. Muscaritoli M, Cangiano C, Cascino A, et al: Exogenous lipid clearance in compensated liver cirrhosis. JPEN J Parenter Enteral Nutr 10:599–603, 1986.

33. Lutz O, Lave T, Frey A, et al: Activities of lipoprotein lipase and hepatic lipase on long- and medium-chain triglyceride emulsions used in parenteral nutrition. Metabolism 38:507–513, 1989.

34. Bolzano K, Krempler F, Sandhofer F: "Hepatic" and "extrahepatic" triglyceride lipase activity in post-heparin plasma of normals and patients with cirrhosis of the liver. Horm Metab Res 7:238–241, 1975.

35. Wolfram G: Die Bedeutung von Karmitin im Fettstoffwechsel. In Exkart J, Wolfram G (eds): Fett in der parenteralen Ernahrung. Vol 2. Munich, W Zuckschwerdt, 1982, pp 28–43.

36. Dudrick SJ: Parenteral nutrition. In Committee on Preoperative and Postoperative Care, American College of Surgeons (eds): Manual of Preoperative and Postoperative Care. Philadelphia, WB Saunders, 1983, pp 86–105.

37. Watters JM, Freeman JB: Parenteral nutrition by peripheral vein. Surg Clin North Am 61:593–604, 1981.

38. Nagayama M, Takai T, Okuno M, Umeyama K: Fat emulsion in surgical patients with liver disorders. J Surg Res 47:59–64, 1989.

39. Eckart J, Adolph M, van der Muhlen U, Naab V: Fat emulsions containing medium chain triglycerides in parenteral nutrition of intensive care patients. JPEN J Parenter Enteral Nutr 4:360–366, 1980.

40. Sailer D, Muller M: Medium chain triglycerides in parenteral nutrition. JPEN J Parenter Enteral Nutr 5:115–119, 1981.

41. Deckelbaum RJ, Carpentier Y, Oliverona T, Moser A: Hydrolysis of medium vs long chain triglycerides in pure and mixed intravenous lipid emulsions by purified lipoprotein lipase in vitro. Clin Nutr 5(Suppl):54, 1986.

42. Bach AC, Babayan VK: Medium-chain triglycer-

ides: An update. Am J Clin Nutr 36:950–962, 1982.

43. Fan ST, Wong J: Metabolic clearance of a fat emulsion containing medium-chain triglycerides in cirrhotic patients. JPEN J Parenter Enteral Nutr 16:279–283, 1992.

44. Cummings MG, James JH, Soeters PB, et al: Regional brain study of indoleamine metabolism in the rat in acute hepatic failure. J Neurochem 27:741–746, 1976.

45. Gonzalez J, Periago JL, Gil A, et al: Malnutrition-related polyunsaturated fatty acid changes in plasma lipid fractions of cirrhotic patients. Metabolism 41:954–960, 1992.

46. Fischer JE, Yoshimura N, James JH, et al: Plasma amino acids in patients with hepatic encephalopathy. Effects on amino acid infusions. Am J Surg 127:40–47, 1974.

47. Morgan MY, Milsom JP, Sherlock S: Plasma ratio of valine, leucine and isoleucine to phenylalanine and tyrosine in liver disease. Gut 19:1068–1037, 1978.

48. Munro HN, Ferstrom JD, Wurtmann RJ: The plasma amino acid imbalance, and hepatic coma. Lancet 1:722–724, 1975.

49. Freund HR, Ryan JA Jr, Fischer JE: Amino acid derangements in patients with sepsis: Treatment with branched chain amino acid rich infusions. Ann Surg 188:423–430, 1978.

50. Vary TC, Siegel JH, Aechnich A, et al: Pharmacological reversal of abnormal glucose regulation, BCAA utilization, and muscle catabolism in sepsis by dichloroacetate. J Trauma 28:1301–1311, 1988.

51. O'Keefe SJD, Abraham R, El Zayadi A, et al: Increased plasma tyrosine concentrations in patients with cirrhosis and fulminant hepatic failure associated with increased plasma tyrosine flux and reduced hepatic oxidation capacity. Gastroenterology 81:1017–1024, 1981.

52. Zieve FJ, Zieve L, Doizaki WM, Gilsdorf RB: Synergism between ammonia and fatty acids in the production of coma: Implications for hepatic coma. J Pharmacol Exp Ther 191:10–16, 1974.

53. James JH, Ziparo V, Jeppsson B, Fischer JE: Hyperammonemia, plasma amino acid imbalance, and blood-brain amino acid transport: A unified theory of portal-systemic encephalopathy. Lancet 2:772–775, 1979.

54. Fraser CL, Arieff AI: Hepatic encephalopathy. N Engl J Med 313:865–873, 1985.

55. Echizen H, Ishizaki T, Oda T: Amino acid metabolism in liver failure: Its etiologic role in hepatic encephalopathy. In Yoshida A, Naito H, Niiyama Y, Suzuki T (eds): Nutrition: Proteins and Amino Acids. Tokyo, Japan Science Society Press and Berlin, Springer-Verlag, 1990, pp 233–243.

56. Oldendorf WH: Brain uptake of radiolabeled amino acids, amines and hexoses after arterial injection. Am J Physiol 221:1629–1639, 1971.

57. Dodsworth JM, James JH, Cummings MG, Fischer JE: Depletion of brain norepinephrine in acute hepatic coma. Surgery 75:811–820, 1974.

58. Knell AJ, Davidson AR, Williams R, et al: Dopamine and serotonin metabolism in hepatic encephalopathy. BMJ 1:549–551, 1974.

59. Faraj BA, Camp VM, Ansley JD: Evidence for central hypertyraminemia in hepatic encephalopathy. J Clin Invest 67:395–402, 1981.

60. Borg J, Warter JM, Schlienger JL, et al: Neurotransmitter modifications in human cerebrospinal fluid and serum during hepatic encephalopathy. J Neurol Sci 57:343–356, 1982.

61. Cummings MG, Soeters PB, James JH, et al: Regional brain indoleamine metabolism following chronic portacaval anastomosis in the rat. J Neurochem 27:501–509, 1976.

62. Maddison JE: Hepatic encephalopathy. Current concepts of the pathogenesis. J Vet Intern Med 6:341–353, 1992.

63. Nompleggi DJ, Bonkovsky HL: Nutritional supplementation in chronic liver disease: An analytical review. Hepatology 19:518–533, 1994.

64. Freund H, Dienstag J, Lehrich J, et al: Infusion of branched-chain amino acid–enriched solution in patients with hepatic encephalopathy. Ann Surg 196:209–220, 1982.

65. Marchesini G, Zoli M, Dondi C, et al: Anticatabolic effect of branched-chain amino acid–enriched solutions in patients with liver cirrhosis. Hepatology 2:420–425, 1982.

66. Sakamoto A, Moldawer LL, Usui S, et al: In vivo evidence for the unique nitrogen-sparing mechanism of branched-chain amino acid administration. Surg Forum 30:67–69, 1979.

67. Bower RH, Muggia Sullam M, Vallgren S, et al: Branched chain amino acid–enriched solutions in the septic patients. A randomized, prospective trial. Ann Surg 203:13–20, 1986.

68. Sax HC, Talamini MA, Fischer JE: Clinical use of branched-chain amino acids in liver disease, sepsis, trauma, and burns. Arch Surg 121:358–366, 1986.

69. Maddrey WC: Branched chain amino acid therapy in liver disease. J Am Coll Nutr 4:639–650, 1985.

70. Miwa Y, Kato M, Moriwaki H, et al: Effects of branched-chain amino acid infusion on protein metabolism in rats with acute hepatic failure. Hepatology 22:291–296, 1995.

71. Rocchi E, Cassanelli M, Gibertini P, et al: Standard or branched-chain amino acid infusions as short-term nutritional support in liver cirrhosis? JPEN J Parenter Enteral Nutr 9:447–451, 1985.

72. Hong RW, Rounds JD, Helton WS, et al: Glutamine preserves liver glutathione after lethal hepatic injury. Ann Surg 215:114–119, 1992.

73. Wilmore DW: Catabolic illness. Strategies for enhancing recovery. N Engl J Med 325:695–702, 1991.

74. Souba WW: Glutamine: A key substrate for the splanchnic bed. Annu Rev Nutr 11:285–308, 1991.

75. Van der Hulst RR, van Kreel BK, von Meyenfeldt MF, et al: Glutamine and the preservation of gut integrity. Lancet 341:1363–1365, 1993.

76. Calder PC: Glutamine and the immune system. Clin Nutr 13:2–8, 1994.

77. Morlion BJ, Stehle P, Wachtler P, et al: Total parenteral nutrition with glutamine dipeptide after major abdominal surgery: A randomized, double-blind, controlled study. Ann Surg 227:302–308, 1998.

78. Dejong CH, Deutz NEP, Soeters PB: Intestinal glutamine and ammonia metabolism during chronic hyperammonemia induced by liver insufficiency. Gut 92:2834–2840, 1993.

79. Plauth M, Egberts EH, Abele R, et al: Characteristic pattern of free amino acids in plasma and skeletal muscle in stable hepatic cirrhosis. Hepatogastroenterology 37:135–139, 1990.

80. Teran JC, Mullen KD, McCullough AJ: Glutamine—A conditionally essential amino acid in cirrhosis? Am J Nutr 62:897–900, 1995.

81. Fukui H, Brauner B, Bode JC, et al: Plasma endotoxin concentrations in patients with alcoholic and non-alcoholic liver disease: Re-evaluation with an improved chromogen assay. J Hepatol 12:162–169, 1971.

82. Bode C, Fukui H, Bode JC: "Hidden" endotoxin in plasma in patients with alcoholic liver disease. Eur J Gastroenterol Hepatol 5:257–262, 1993.

83. Plevak DJ, DiCecco SR, Wiesner RH, et al: Nutritional support for liver transplantation: Identifying caloric and protein requirements. Mayo Clin Proc 69:225–230, 1994.

84. Elwyn DH, Kinney JM, Askanazi J: Energy expenditure in surgical patients. Surg Clin North Am 61:545–556, 1981.

85. Muller JM, Keller HW, Brenner U, et al: Indications and effects of preoperative parenteral nutrition. World J Surg 10:53–63, 1986.

86. Niles JM: Intravenous fat emulsions in nutritional support. Curr Opin Gastroenterol 7:306–311, 1991.

87. Fan ST, Lo CM, Lai ECS, et al: Perioperative nutritional support in patients undergoing hepatectomy for hepatocellular carcinoma. N Engl J Med 331:1547–1552, 1994.

88. Nagayama M, Takai T, Okuno M, Umeyama K: Fat emulsion in surgical patients with liver disorders. J Surg Res 47:59–64, 1989.

89. Bates J, McClain CJ: The effect of severe zinc deficiency on serum levels of albumin, transferrin, and prealbumin in man. Am J Clin Nutr 34:1655–1660, 1981.

90. Keeling PWN, Jones RB, Hilton PJ, Thompson RPH: Reduced leucocyte zinc in liver disease. Gut 21:561–564, 1980.

91. Van der Rijt CC, Schalm SW, Schat H, et al: Overt hepatic encephalopathy precipitated by zinc deficiency. Gastroenterology 100:1114–1118, 1991.

92. Marchesini G, Fabbri A, Bianchi G, et al: Zinc supplementation and amino acid-nitrogen metabolism in patients with advanced cirrhosis. Hepatology 23:1084–1092, 1996.

93. Fischer JE, Rosen HM, Ebeid AM, et al: The effect of normalization of plasma amino acids on hepatic encephalopathy in man. Surgery 80:77–91, 1976.

94. Rossi Fanelli F, Riggio O, Cangiano C, et al: Branched-chain amino acids vs lactulose in the treatment of hepatic coma: A controlled study. Dig Dis Sci 27:929–935, 1982.

95. Gluud C, Dejgaard A, Hardt F, et al: Preliminary treatment results with balanced amino acid infusion to patients with hepatic encephalopathy [Abstract]. Scand J Gastroenterol 18(Suppl 86):19, 1983.

96. Fiaccadori F, Ghinelli F, Pedretti G, et al: Branched chain amino acid enriched solutions in the treatment of hepatic encephalopathy: A controlled trial. In Capocaccia L, Fischer JE, Rossi Fanelli F (eds): Hepatic encephalopathy in chronic liver failure. New York, Plenum Press, 1984, pp 323–333.

97. Cerra FB, Cheung NK, Fischer JE, et al: Disease specific amino acid infusion (F080) in hepatic encephalopathy: A prospective, randomized, double-blind, controlled trail. JPEN J Parenter Enteral Nutr 9:288–295, 1985.

98. Strauss E, Santos WR, Cartapatti E, et al: A randomized controlled clinical trial for the evaluation of the efficacy of an enriched branched chain amino acid solution compared to neomycin in hepatic encephalopathy [Abstract]. Hepatology 3:862, 1983.

99. Wahren J, Denis J, Desurmont P, et al: Is intravenous administration of branched chain amino acids effective in the treatment of hepatic encephalopathy? A multicenter study. Hepatology 3:475–480, 1983.

100. Michel H, Pomier Layrargues G, Aubin JP, et al: Treatment of hepatic encephalopathy by infusion of a modified amino acid solution: Results of a controlled study of 47 cirrhotic patients. In Capocaccia L, Fischer JE, Rossi Fanelli F (eds): Hepatic Encephalopathy in Chronic Liver Failure. New York, Plenum Press, 1984, pp 323–333.

101. Naylor CD, O'Rourke K, Detsky AS, Baker JP: Parenteral nutrition with branched-chain amino acids in hepatic encephalopathy. A meta-analysis. Gastroenterology 97:1033–1042, 1989.

102. O'Grady JG, Alexander GJ, Hayllar KM, Williams R: Early indicators of prognosis in fulminant hepatic failure. Gastroenterology 97:439–445, 1989.

103. O'Keefe SJD, Abraham R, El Zayadi A, et al: Increased plasma tyrosine concentrations in patients with cirrhosis and fulminant hepatic failure associated with increased plasma tyrosine flux and reduced hepatic oxidative capacity. Gastroenterology 81:1017–1024, 1981.

104. Rosen HM, Yoshimura N, Hodgeman JM, Fischer JE: Plasma amino acid patterns in hepatic encephalopathy of differing etiology. Gastroenterology 72:483–487, 1977.

105. Fryden A, Weiland O, Martensson J: Successful treatment of hepatic coma with balanced solution of amino acids. Scand J Infect Dis 14:177–180, 1982.

106. Forbes A, Wicks C, Marshall W, et al: Nutritional support in fulminant hepatic failure: The safety of lipid solutions. Gut 38:1347–1349, 1998.

107. Marsano L, McClain CJ: Nutrition and alcoholic liver disease. JPEN J Parenter Enteral Nutr 15:337–344, 1991.

108. Nasrallah SM, Galambos JT: Amino acid therapy of alcoholic hepatitis. Lancet 2:1276–1277, 1980.

109. Diehl AM, Boitnott JK, Herlong HF, et al: Effect of parenteral amino acid supplementation in alcoholic hepatitis. Hepatology 5:57–63, 1985.

110. Naveau S, Pelletier G, Poynard T, et al: A randomized clinical trial of supplementary parenteral nutrition in jaundiced alcoholic cirrhotic patients. Hepatology 6:270–274, 1986.

111. Achord JL: A prospective randomized clinical trial of peripheral amino acid–glucose supplementation in acute alcoholic hepatitis. Am J Gastroenterol 82:871–875, 1987.

112. Simon D, Galambos JT: A randomized controlled study of peripheral parenteral nutrition in moderate and severe alcoholic hepatitis. J Hepatol 7:200–207, 1988.

113. Bonkovsky HL, Fiellin DA, Smith GS, et al: A randomized, controlled trial of treatment of alcoholic hepatitis with parenteral nutrition and oxandrolone. I: Short-term effects on liver function. Am J Gastroenterol 86:1200–1208, 1991.

114. Bonkovsky HL, Singh RH, Jafri IH, et al: A randomized, controlled trial of treatment of alcoholic

hepatitis with parenteral nutrition and oxandrolone. II: Short-term effects on nitrogen metabolism, metabolic balance, and nutrition. Am J Gastroenterol 86:1209–1218, 1991.

115. Mezey E, Caballeria J, Mitchell MC, et al: Effect of parenteral amino acid supplementation on short-term and long-term outcomes in severe alcoholic hepatitis: A randomized controlled trial. Hepatology 14:1090–1096, 1991.

116. De Caterina M, Piccolboni D, Alfieri R, et al: Effects of total parenteral nutrition enriched with branched chain amino acid infusion on liver function and serum amino acid pattern in dogs undergoing hepatectomy. Ric Clin Lab 15:79–88, 1985.

117. Rigotti P, Peters JC, Tranberg KG, Fischer JE: Effects of amino acid infusions on liver regeneration after partial hepatectomy in the rat. JPEN J Parenter Enteral Nutr 10:17–20, 1986.

118. Farriol M, Balsells J, Schwartz S, et al: Influence of fat emulsions in parenteral nutrition on visceral protein synthesis: Study in hepatectomized rats. Rev Esp Fisiol 46:297–302, 1990.

119. Yoshida S, Yunoki T, Aoyagi K, et al: Effect of glutamine supplement and hepatectomy on DNA and protein synthesis in the remnant liver. J Surg Res 59:475–481, 1995.

120. Yamaguchi T, Minor T, Isselhard W: Effect of glutamine or glucagon-insulin enriched total parenteral nutrition on liver and gut in 70% hepatectomized rats with colon stenosis. J Am Coll Surg 185:156–162, 1997.

121. Aoi T: Influence of enteral nutrition on hepatic regeneration and small intestinal epithelium after hepatectomy in rat—Comparative assessment with TPN. Nippon Geka Gakkai Zasshi 96:295–300, 1995.

122. Qiu JG, Delany HM, Teh EL, et al: Contrasting effects of identical nutrients given parenterally or enterally after 70% hepatectomy: Bacterial translocation. Nutrition 13:431–437, 1997.

123. Shirabe K, Matsumata T, Shimada M, et al: A comparison of parenteral hyperalimentation and early enteral feeding regarding systemic immunity after major hepatic resection—The results of a randomized prospective study. Hepatogastroenterology 44:205–209, 1997.

124. Reilly J, Mehta R, Teperman L, et al: Nutritional support after liver transplantation: A randomized prospective study. JPEN J Parenter Enteral Nutr 14:386–391, 1990.

20

◆ Nutritional Support of the Obese Patient

Steven B. Heymsfield, M.D.
Patricia S. Choban, M.D.
David B. Allison, Ph.D.
Louis Flancbaum, M.D.

Over one third of adult Americans are obese and are thus at increased risk of developing comorbid conditions such as diabetes, high blood pressure, gout, and some malignancies.[1] Because obesity is so prevalent and obese individuals are at increased risk for many diseases, it is not unexpected that obesity is also very common in hospitalized patients. In a review of elective surgical patients at a tertiary care hospital, 37% of patients were found to have a body mass index (BMI) over 27 kg/m², with a BMI less than 25 kg/m² considered normal weight.[2] In a review of patients evaluated over a 1-year period by the nutritional support service at the same institution, 64 of 243 patients (26.3%) had a body weight 30% in excess of ideal.[2]

Nutritional management of the obese patient differs from that of patients who are at or near their desirable body weight. Although there are relatively few objective data concerning nutritional support of the obese patient, there is a growing consensus on the major issues related to evaluation and clinical management. The aim of this chapter is to provide the specialist in nutritional support with an overview of the important concepts in obesity practice with an emphasis on clinical assessment and nonvolitional feeding.

◆ DIAGNOSIS

Obesity can have its onset at any point in life ranging from infancy to old age. Usually no single mechanism causes excess weight gain. Genetic, nutritional, sociologic, psychological, and other factors are known to contribute to the long-term development of positive energy balance and fat deposition.[1]

Although a diagnosis of obesity would optimally include an estimate of total body fat, for clinical purposes, weight adjusted for stature is usually satisfactory to confirm the presence of excess adiposity. Two weight-stature indices are practical to use clinically. The first is desirable weight, a concept that has evolved over the last 80 years and represents the patient's risk of morbidity over that of an established reference group.[1] Usually, two reference tables, the 1959 and 1983[3] Metropolitan Life Insurance Company tables of desirable weights, are used. According to both tables, mortality is significantly increased in patients who are at or above about 120% of desirable weight (i.e., [patient's weight/desirable weight for height] × 100), and the tables give similar results for patients in this heavier range. A National Institutes of Health consensus panel recommended using the 1959 desirable weight table in preference to the 1983 table, particularly when patients present with a family history of obesity or a current medical problem related to excess adiposity.[4, 5] The ideal body weight concept is useful in the context of obesity as it is also widely used to diagnose malnutrition.

The second method of diagnosing obesity from weight-stature indices is BMI, which is weight in kilograms divided by height in meters squared (Fig. 20–1). The morbidity function for BMI is similar to that for desirable weight in that it is curvilinear and increases rapidly above about 30 kg/m² (Fig. 20–2).[6] A normal BMI is considered between 18.5 and 24.9 kg/m², overweight 25 kg/m² or greater, obesity 30 kg/m² or greater, and morbid obesity 40 kg/m² or greater.[1]

Total body weight or adiposity alone does not account for all the excess morbidity of obesity. Fat distribution also influences the

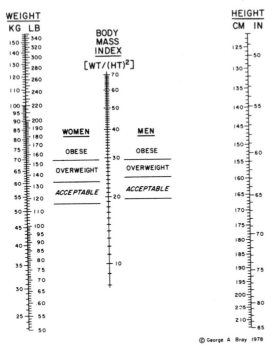

Figure 20–1. A nomogram for determining body mass index. To use this nomogram, place a ruler or other straight edge between the body weight in kilograms or pounds (without clothes) located on the left-hand line and the body weight in centimeters or in inches (without shoes) located on the right-hand line. The body mass index is read from the middle of the scale and is in metric units. (Copyright 1978 by George A. Bray, M.D.)

risk of excess weight, with upper body and central fat carrying a higher morbidity than lower body and peripheral fat. The more specific anatomic locations of upper and lower body fat are the intra-abdominal cavity and subcutaneous compartment of the buttocks and thighs, respectively.[7–9]

In addition to morphologic differences among obese individuals, there are also metabolic and hormonal characteristics of upper and lower body obesity. Although the specific mechanism resulting in variations in fat distribution remains unknown, patients with upper body obesity have higher levels of circulating insulin,[10] a lower hepatic insulin extraction,[11] greater insulin resistance,[7, 10] elevated levels of serum triglyceride,[12] and reduced serum levels of high-density lipoprotein.[13] Taken collectively, these abnormalities predispose the patient with upper body obesity to glucose intolerance,[7] diabetes,[9, 13] high blood pressure,[14] and coronary artery disease.[15]

The clinical evaluation of fat distribution

is usually made by measuring the waist circumference.[16] A high waist circumference (males >102 cm and females >88 cm) suggests upper body adiposity and increased cardiovascular risk of obesity.[17] The metabolic and hormonal derangements of upper body obesity are similar to some of the abnormalities characteristic of acute stress or injury. It is unknown at present if fat distribution influences the metabolic response to injury or outcome after an acute stress.

◆ COMPLICATIONS

As described in the previous section, excess body weight and adipose tissue are associated with an increased risk of several acute and chronic illnesses. A brief description of metabolic differences between patients with upper and lower body obesity was also provided. The following discussion summarizes the major pathophysiologic abnormalities associated with obesity. Social and psychological consequences of obesity are also discussed.

Hyperinsulinemia and Insulin Resistance

Glucose intolerance and type 2 diabetes are more common in obese than in nonobese patients.[18] These clinical findings correspond to two well-documented abnormalities in patients with excess body weight: elevated circulating insulin levels and insu-

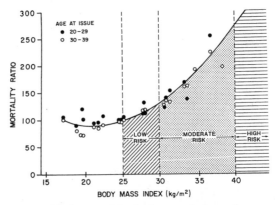

Figure 20–2. Use of the body mass index and excess mortality to provide an estimate of risk from obesity. Solid circles show persons aged 20 to 29 years, and open circles show persons aged 30 to 39 years. (Copyright 1976 by George A. Bray, M.D.)

lin resistance. Pancreatic secretion of insulin is increased in obese persons,[19] and because insulin clearance does not rise proportionately, serum levels in the basal state and after a glucose challenge also increase.[20] The specific mechanism leading to increased pancreatic secretion of insulin is unknown, although abnormalities in glucagon metabolism, in the release of insulinotropic hormone and gastric inhibitory peptide, and in feedback inhibition of insulin synthesis are suggested possibilities.[21]

Insulin resistance is a characteristic feature of obesity.[20] Resistance to the action of insulin may be present in obese patients even in the absence of glucose intolerance and is more marked in peripheral tissue compared with hepatic tissue.[22] Insulin's action is related to both cellular receptors and postreceptor processes, and both are implicated in the insulin resistance of obesity.[22] Although the mechanism of insulin resistance is unknown, suggested causes include a down-regulation of insulin receptors secondary to hyperinsulinemia, a reduced capacity of the increased skeletal muscle mass of obese patients to utilize glucose, and inhibition of insulin action secondary to elevated circulating free fatty acids.[23–25]

Critical illness, especially with infectious or traumatic causes, exacerbates insulin resistance. The obese critically ill patient is especially apt to develop hyperglycemia during nutritional support. Parenteral insulin can be provided to control serum glucose levels during nutritional support, although usually the amount of energy supplied as glucose is restricted by reducing the obese patient's total caloric intake to below the maintenance requirement. A later section on nutritional support of the obese patient suggests an approach to prescribing energy as glucose.

Abnormal Serum Lipids

Hypertriglyceridemia and low circulating high-density lipoprotein levels frequently accompany obesity, particularly when excess adipose tissue is deposited in the intra-abdominal compartment.[26, 27] Serum triglyceride levels are increased because of a high hepatic production rate of very low density lipoprotein. The augmented release of very low density lipoprotein may be secondary to the increased hepatic delivery of insulin, glucose, and free fatty acids.

Elevated levels of serum triglycerides before or during parenteral lipid infusion may limit the use of exogenous lipids as a source of calories in the obese patient, although no published studies have examined this possibility.

High Blood Pressure

High blood pressure is more common in the obese person,[28] and weight gain in young adults is an important risk factor for developing hypertension.[28] Weight reduction lowers blood pressure, and weight loss is a major component of antihypertensive therapy in obese patients who have high blood pressure.[28] The mechanisms of high blood pressure in obese patients are multifactorial and include increased circulating fluid volume, elevated cardiac output, increased peripheral vascular resistance, and endocrine abnormalities, including insulin resistance and increased activity of the sympathetic nervous system.[28]

Chronic poorly controlled hypertension can lead to cardiac hypertrophy and congestive heart failure, particularly in the obese patient.[29, 30] This is because obesity alone causes eccentric enlargement of the left ventricle, and when combined with high blood pressure, the additional mechanical work produces concentric hypertrophy.[30] These abnormalities in cardiac anatomy and function may predispose the obese patient to congestive heart failure during nutritional support.

Severe or chronic high blood pressure also causes collagenous fibrosis and luminal narrowing of renal arterioles, reduced renal blood flow, and impaired tubular function.[31]

Abnormal Hepatic Function

Steatosis occurs in 60 to 90% of obese patients, and fatty infiltration of the hepatic parenchyma is a linear function of relative body weight.[32, 33] Morbidly obese persons frequently have elevated serum transaminase levels and marked hepatic steatosis.[34] A possible relation exists between fatty infiltration of the liver in obesity, elevated circulating insulin levels, and increased very low density lipoprotein synthesis.[35]

Fatty liver is also a problem observed during nutritional support, particularly with high total caloric infusions and large amounts of glucose. Excess hepatic glucose stimulates the synthesis of hepatic acetyl-CoA decarboxylase and fatty acid synthetase, which together with elevated insulin levels promotes triglyceride deposition in the liver.[36] The risk of worsening or producing new fatty changes within the liver of obese patients during nutritional support again suggests a prudent use of glucose as a source of nonprotein energy.

Increased Risk of Cholelithiasis

Cholesterol output in bile is increased in the obese patient secondary to an elevated rate of hepatic cholesterol production.[37] The increase in the whole-body cholesterol synthetic rate is a function of body weight and adiposity.[37] Bile acid secretion does not increase in proportion to the release of excess cholesterol, and the result is a supersaturated solution that favors precipitation of cholesterol crystals.[38] Other factors, such as increased gallbladder volume and impaired contractility,[39] may also contribute to the increased risk of cholesterol gallstone formation in the obese population. One third of obese women over the age of 60 years have cholesterol gallstones.[6]

Long-term nutritional support is associated with an increased risk of cholesterol gallstones,[40] probably due to an interruption of the normal enterohepatic circulation with fasting and a corresponding rise in bile lithogenicity.[40] Other factors, such as the underlying disease process, may also contribute.

Weight loss during treatment with very low calorie diets is known to be associated with an increase in bile lithogenicity and an increase in the rate of cholesterol gallstone formation.[41] The risk of gallstones also increases with the weight loss that follows obesity surgery.[42]

No information is available on changes in biliary lipids during nutritional support of obese patients, particularly those who are maintained on hypocaloric infusions and are losing weight. This increased risk can be nearly eliminated by the use of ursodeoxycholic acid (600 mg/day) for the first 6 months after gastric bypass.[43]

Abnormal Pulmonary Function

Vital capacity, expiratory reserve volume, and maximal voluntary ventilation are all impaired in severely obese persons.[44] Abnormal respiratory muscle function, the increased mechanical work of moving the extra chest weight, and other factors may contribute to the abnormalities in pulmonary function that accompany obesity.[44, 45]

Obesity hypoventilation syndrome, sleep apnea, or a combination of the two were found in 10% of patients referred for surgical management of morbid obesity.[46] Obesity hypoventilation syndrome is associated with markedly abnormal ventilatory responses to hypercapnia and hypoxia, and chronic hypoxemia can lead to pulmonary artery vasoconstriction, pulmonary hypertension, polycythemia, and changes in cardiac morphology and function.[45, 46] These physiologic derangements may further increase the risk of congestive heart failure in the severely obese patient receiving nutritional support.

Weight loss, particularly in morbidly obese patients, improves arterial blood oxygenation; reduces carbon dioxide retention; increases forced vital capacity, expiratory reserve volume, and total lung capacity; and reduces apnea frequency.[46]

Obese patients with respiratory insufficiency are at significantly increased anesthetic risk and may require prolonged intubation after surgery.[46]

Thromboembolic Disease

Obese patients have elevated fasting plasma fatty acid levels that accelerate coagulation by several mechanisms including activation of Hageman's factor, which in turn causes endothelial damage and the initiation of the clotting cascade.[47] In addition, obesity predisposes patients to decreased levels of circulating fibrinolytic activity. Because of these physiologic changes, obesity is assumed to be a predisposing factor for postoperative thrombophlebitis, deep venous thrombosis (DVT), and pulmonary embolism (PE). However, the actual clinical incidence of DVT in obese patients is difficult to quantify. An increased incidence of obesity was observed in patients with DVT and PE in several retrospective and autopsy series.[48] Several studies have used I^{131}-labeled fibrinogen scans to confirm the increased presence of DVT in obese patients,[49] although these findings are not confirmed in all studies.[50] The incidence of clinical thrombosis was 0.7% in a review of several series of morbidly obese patients who underwent gastric bypass surgery for weight loss.[51] In other populations at high risk for DVT and PE, such as those undergoing total hip or knee arthroplasty, obesity has not been shown to increase the risk of DVT[52] or PE.[53]

The incidence of PE in obese patients after elective surgery is low. In several combined series of patients undergoing gastric bypass or gastroplasty for weight loss, PE was observed in 0.6% of patients.[51] Obese patients have an increased incidence of pulmonary hypertension, especially those with obesity hypoventilation syndrome and obstructive sleep apnea, which appears to increase the risk of fatal pulmonary embolism.[54]

Neoplasia

The risk of some malignancies is increased in obese patients; endometrial, breast, and gallbladder cancers are more prevalent in obese women, and colon and prostate cancers are more prevalent in obese men.[55] Benign neoplastic conditions such as myoma and fibroma of the uterus and ovarian cysts are also more frequent in overweight women.[56] One hypothesized mechanism for the development of these tumors is the conversion of estriol to androstenedione in the enlarged adipose tissue mass,[57] and androstenedione purportedly then acts as a metabolic stimulus for benign and malignant neoplasia.[57]

Musculoskeletal Abnormalities

The increased mechanical load produced by excess weight increases the obese patient's risk of osteoarthritis in weight-bearing joints and the spine.[55] Physical activity may be limited due to osteoarthritis, which makes weight control measures such as increased physical activity difficult to implement. Special exercise or rehabilitation programs may be needed in patients with limited mobility due to joint disease.

Obesity and Surgical Procedures

Obesity is often cited as a risk factor for a poor outcome from a variety of surgical procedures. The actual extent of the risk is difficult to determine. There appears to be an increased risk associated with anesthesia, and there are more wound and wound-healing problems. With elective procedures, there are few data to support the suggestion that the obese patient is at an increased risk beyond these two areas.[58]

Anesthetic Risks

Obese patients often have short, thick necks and heavy chest walls that can make oro- or nasotracheal intubation and ventilation difficult. Therefore, issues related to airway control are a major concern to anesthesiologists when confronted with the need to provide general anesthesia to obese patients. Additionally, arterial and venous access may be difficult due to indistinct landmarks resulting from the increase in subcutaneous adiposity. The loss of anatomic landmarks also contributes to difficulty in the positioning of catheters for regional anesthetics.[59]

Obese patients have elevated gastric residual volumes with lower intragastric pH than do their nonobese counterparts, placing them at greater risk for pulmonary aspiration and pneumonitis. A multicenter study of patient outcomes after general anesthesia found obesity to be a predictor of severe adverse respiratory outcomes.[60]

In addition to anatomic factors are pharmacologic considerations related to the predictability of distribution and the effect of many of the agents used during anesthesia in the obese patient. There is a theoretical difficulty in properly maintaining, and appropriately withdrawing, anesthesia because of the lipid solubility of volatile anesthetics and the increased distribution of lipophilic agents in obese patients. However, when inhalation agents were compared with narcotic–nitrous oxide (i.e., balanced) anesthetic techniques for general anesthesia in morbidly obese patients, Cork and associates found no significant differences in clinical postoperative anesthetic outcomes.[61] Finally, the increased intra-abdominal pressure observed in obese patients shifts blood from the inferior vena cava to the epidural venous system, thereby decreasing the volume of epidural and subarachnoid spaces.[62]

This makes the dosing of regional anesthetics more difficult because the spread of local anesthetics injected into the epidural or subarachnoid space is increased.

Wound Problems

After gastric bypass or gastroplasty, wound infection is the most common cause of morbidity in obese patients.[51] The incidence of wound complications is also significantly greater in obese patients undergoing duodenal ulcer surgery,[63] cholecystectomy,[64] hysterectomy,[65] cesarean section,[66] coronary artery bypass grafting,[67, 68] and renal transplantation.[69–71]

Minor wound problems, such as superficial wound disruption, seromas, hematomas, and fat necrosis, also occur with increased frequency in obese patients.[72] These wound problems are multifactorial in origin. Local changes in the surrounding tissues, such as the presence of a relatively avascular adipose tissue mass with poor infection resistance, an increase in local trauma related to retraction of the large abdominal wall, and an increase in operative time due to the patient's size, contribute to these problems. Additionally, systemic factors, including insulin resistance and hyperglycemia, are associated with impaired wound healing. Obesity has also been associated with changes in cell-mediated and humoral immunity.[73] Although many of these changes resolve with weight reduction,[74] it is not clear if improvements are related to the reduction in adipose tissue mass or to the improved profile of ingested dietary lipids.[75]

Although obesity is a recognized risk factor for wound dehiscence,[76] this has not been a major clinical problem. In five series of patients undergoing surgical treatment for morbid obesity, the incidence of fascial dehiscence ranged between 0.3 and 1.2%, with an average of 0.4%,[51] and was similar to the 1% rate noted in a large 5-year review of major intra-abdominal operations.[76] The reported incidence of incisional hernias in a series of patients undergoing gastric bypass for clinically severe obesity has been compared with the incidence in a group of patients undergoing total proctocolectomy for inflammatory bowel disease.[77] The incidence in the obese patients was 20% (198/968) compared with 4% (7/171) in the inflammatory bowel disease patients even

though 60% of these intestinal disease patients were taking corticosteroids. This observation supports studies that suggest that obese patients may have a higher incidence of incisional hernia, although most of these retrospective studies examined the incidence of obesity in patients with incisional hernias and not the incidence of incisional hernias in obese patients. The incidence of obesity ranges between 25 and 48% in patients with incisional hernia.

Increased Trauma Risk

Although the data on trauma risk are limited, the available information suggests that obese patients are at increased risk of traumatic injury.[78, 79] Moreover, the mortality rate appears higher in the obese population after blunt trauma, possibly related to pulmonary complications.[80]

Thermal Injury Outcome

Compared with normal-weight subjects, obese patients appear at increased risk of postoperative sepsis, bacteremia, and clinical sepsis after thermal injury.[81] After thermal injury, ventilator times are longer in the obese patient than in the nonobese patient.[82]

Altered Drug Metabolism

The enlarged adipose tissue mass of obesity increases the volume of distribution for some lipid-soluble drugs and anesthetic gases.[59–61] The increased free fatty acid level often found in obese patients can displace drugs such as morphine and phenytoin from their binding proteins. The hepatic clearance of prednisolone, ibuprofen, and some other medications is increased in obese patients.[59–61]

Negative Societal Attitudes

Finally, obesity is associated with significant problems of a social nature.[83] Obese patients are less likely to be rented apartments,[84] less sought after as mates,[85, 86] less likely to be offered employment[87] or admission to college despite equal qualifications,[88] and less likely to be offered favors.[89] Negative atti-

Table 20–1. Complications of Obesity

Hyperinsulinemia and insulin resistance
   Glucose intolerance
   Diabetes mellitus
Abnormal serum lipid levels
   Hypertriglyceridemia
   Low HDL-cholesterol
High blood pressure
Cardiac abnormalities
   Right and/or left ventricular hypertrophy
   Propensity toward coronary artery disease
   Congestive heart failure
   Premature ventricular contractions
Abnormal hepatic function
   Hepatic steatosis
Increased risk of cholelithiasis
Abnormal pulmonary function
   Sleep apnea
   Alveolar hypoventilation
Increased risk of thromboembolism
Increased neoplasia risk
   Endometrial and possibly breast cancer
Musculoskeletal abnormalities
   Osteoarthritis of the knees
   Aggravation of other postural faults
Increased surgical risk
Possible increased trauma risk
Altered drug metabolism
Impaired reproductive and sexual function
   Increased obstetric risks
   Menstrual irregularities
   Reduced fertility
Negative societal attitudes
   Impairment of self-image with feeling of inferiority
   Social isolation
   Subject to discrimination
   Loss of mobility

HDL, high-density lipoprotein.
Adapted from Clinical Guidelines on the Identification, Evaluation, and Treatment of Overweight and Obesity in Adults: The Evidence Report. No. 98-4083. Washington, DC, U.S. Department of Health and Human Services, 1998.

tudes toward obese people are held not only by laypeople but by health professionals as well.[90, 91] Lastly, obese persons themselves have negative attitudes toward obese individuals, which may be a partial cause of the low self-esteem frequently noted among obese people.[91–93]

The complications of obesity are summarized in Table 20–1.

◆ BODY COMPOSITION

The increased body weight of obese subjects consists of two main components, adipose tissue and adipose tissue–free mass. The adipose tissue–free mass consists of visceral organs, skin, skeletal muscle, and skeleton,

all of which are increased in obese subjects.[94]

Another approach to subdividing body weight is the chemical model in which four compartments are recognized: fat, protein, water, and mineral.[95, 96] The weight of all four chemical components is increased in obese subjects, and some generalities on the proportional changes in each compartment are accepted by most investigators. Excess weight is considered to be all the extra body mass above that of a hypothetical subject who has only fat-free body mass (i.e., sum of water + protein + mineral) and no fat.[97] The composition of excess weight is approximately one fourth the fat-free body mass and three fourths fat.[97] This is generally the recommended composition of weight change during hypocaloric diet therapy.

◆ ENERGY EXPENDITURE

As obese patients have an increase in nonadipose tissue and fat-free body mass, they also have a higher energy expenditure.[98] Three components of total energy expenditure are recognized: (1) the fasting and resting energy expenditure, usually referred to as the resting metabolic rate (RMR); (2) the thermic effect of food (TEF); and (3) the energy expended in physical activities.[99] In the following discussion, the term *RMR* is used in reference to *fasting resting metabolic rate.* Other terms are used to describe the energy expenditure measured in patients who are resting but not fasting.

The RMR is increased in obese patients in direct relation to the enlarged fat-free body mass.[98] Studies vary, but usually the correlation r between the RMR and the fat-free body mass is .7 and .9 for mixed groups of subjects who differ in age, gender, and BMI.[99] Thus, 50 to 80% of between-individual differences in RMR can be explained by variations in body composition.

Many studies have examined the TEF in obese patients, and most investigators agree that this small component of total daily thermogenesis is either normal or low in weight-stable obese patients.[100] Under usual dietary conditions, the TEF accounts for about 5 to 10% of the total daily energy expenditure.[100]

Of more relevance to specialized nutritional support is thermogenesis during the continuously fed state, which differs from the cyclic heat production observed with fasting and feeding.[101] With continuous formula infusion, a steady state heat production exists that has a magnitude related to the caloric infusion rate.[101]

The thermic response to continuous feeding is similar in normal-weight and obese subjects. Vernet and associates studied isocaloric continuous intragastric and intravenous infusions in lean and obese subjects.[102] The infusion rate in both groups of subjects was twice the measured RMR. Although the time to reach steady state was longer with intragastric feeding, both infusions produced an equivalent increase in thermogenesis (Fig. 20–3). Obese subjects had a higher initial RMR, although the relative steady state thermic response was equivalent to that of lean subjects.

Thus, absolute RMR is increased in obese subjects in relation to their larger metabolically active cell mass, and their relative thermic response to continuous infusion is similar to that of subjects who are at a normal body weight.

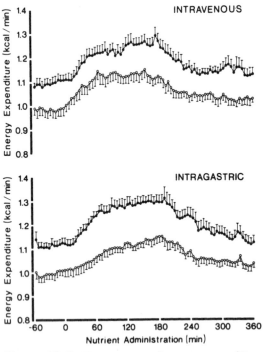

Figure 20–3. Time course of energy expenditure (*closed circles*, obese group; *open circles*, lean group). At all times, the energy expenditure of the obese group was significantly greater (*P* < .05 to .001) than that of the lean group. (From Vernet O, Christin L, Schutz Y, et al: Enteral versus parenteral nutrition: Comparison of energy metabolism in lean and moderately obese women. Am J Clin Nutr 43:194–209, 1986. © Am J Clin Nutr American Society for Clinical Nutrition.)

The energy cost of various physical activities per kilogram of body weight is the same in obese subjects as in lean individuals.[98] The total energy expended in physical activity is thus higher in otherwise healthy obese subjects compared with their lean counterparts.

Obese subjects as a group have a significantly increased total 24-hour energy expenditure.[98, 99] Although each component of total thermogenesis was known to be either unchanged or increased in obese subjects, improved calorimetry techniques were required to confirm the existence of an elevation in daily heat production. Both the respiratory chamber–indirect calorimeter and doubly-labeled water methods demonstrate a high correlation between 24-hour energy expenditure and fat-free body mass (r = .7–.8) and body weight (r = .4–.6).[103] A useful index is the ratio of the total energy expenditure to the RMR, which allows an estimation of the daily energy production from a resting measurement. For healthy ambulatory obese subjects living in industrialized nations, the ratio is about 1.6 to 1.8.[99]

In summary, obese subjects appear to require a higher energy intake to maintain their body weight and tissue composition compared with normal-weight individuals.

A more complex question is how to estimate the energy requirement of hospitalized patients, particularly those who are obese. The most direct approach is to measure the RMR using bedside indirect calorimetry. Several measurements spread over the day and under different conditions would give a reasonable estimate of the subject's energy requirement for weight maintenance.

The more practical, but less accurate, approach is to approximate the patient's energy requirement from the individual components of energy expenditure. The factorial method, in which the total energy expenditure is the sum of RMR + TEF + energy expended in physical activity + injury factor, is usually used.[104] Limited data suggest that the relative increase in energy expenditure with injury is similar in obese and nonobese subjects. In one study, obese subjects and nonobese subjects with a similar burn size had nonsignificantly different elevations in measured energy expenditure.[105]

Several prediction equations for RMR are in use, and all involve factors such as age, stature, and gender (Table 20–2).[106, 107] The first equation in Table 20–2 uses the

Table 20–2. Equations Used for Estimating the Energy Requirements of Obese Patients

Author	Equation
1. Harris-Benedict[106]	Males RMR = 66 + (13.7 × BW) + (5 × Ht) − (6.8 × Age)
	Females RMR = 65 + (9.6 × BW) + (1.7 × Ht) − (4.7 × age)
2. ADA Manual[109]	Adjusted BW = [(ABW − IBW) × 0.25] + IBW
3. Owen et al.[113]	Males RMR = 879 + 10.2 × BW
	Females RMR = 795 + 7.2 × BW
4. Ireton-Jones and Francis[81]	(v): 1,784 − 11A + 5W + 244G + 239T + 804B
	(s): 629 − 11 9A + 25W − 6,090
5. Glynn et al.[112]	RMR = HB × 1.3

ABW, actual body weight; A, age (years); BW, body weight (kg); B, burn; T, trauma; W, weight; Ht, height (m); HB, Harris-Benedict equation (use average of actual and ideal BW); IBW, ideal body weight; RMR, resting metabolic rate (kcal/day); G, gender (male, 1; female, 0); (v), ventilator dependent; (s), spontaneously breathing.

classic Harris-Benedict equations, one of which is for males and the other for females.[106] Age, stature (i.e., height), and body weight are used in these two equations to estimate RMR. Harris and Benedict developed their equations using normal-weight subjects, giving rise to the problem of inaccuracy when applied to obese patients. We and others have found systematic deviations between the RMR measured by indirect calorimetry and the RMR predicted by the Harris-Benedict and other similar equations.[107, 108] In addition, the standard error of the estimate of the RMR based on such factors as weight, stature, and age is relatively large. For example, the correlation coefficient r for the RMR calculated using the Harris-Benedict and other similar equations is .6 to .7, meaning that weight, stature, and age account for less than half of the variance in the observed RMR. Similarly, observations of a systematic bias and wide confidence interval between measured and predicted RMRs was made by Pavlou and coworkers[108] in moderately obese males. The predicted RMR was 7 to 8% above the measured RMR if the actual body weight was used in the equation, and 10 to 15% below the measured RMR if the ideal body weight was used.

In order to overcome this discrepancy between observed and predicted energy expenditures when using the actual body weight versus the ideal body weight, one group recommends calculating an adjusted body weight by assuming that one fourth of the weight above the ideal or desirable weight is metabolically active.[109] The second equation in Table 20–2 is then used to calculate an adjusted weight for use in the Harris-Benedict equations. This is an interesting suggestion, but there is little evidence that when used in the available equations an adjusted weight improves the prediction of RMR.[110–112]

Glynn and associates have found that the best correlate of the measured energy expenditure in a population of acutely ill hospitalized patients is the energy expenditure predicted by the Harris-Benedict equation in which the body weight is empirically set at the average of the actual and the ideal body weight.[112] The ideal body weight was calculated using the Hamwi formulas: males (pounds) = 106 + 6 × height (inches); females (pounds) = 100 + 5 × height (inches). The calculated result is then multiplied by an injury factor of 1.3 (see Table 20–2).

Another pair of equations in Table 20–2 were developed by Owen and his colleagues in groups of men and women who ranged widely in BMI.[113, 114] These investigators found that age contributed little to the prediction of RMR and that the body weight was highly correlated with more complex body composition estimates. No significant correlation was observed between RMR and adipose tissue distribution. Owen's equations require only the measured body weight and had in the original study an r of about .7 for the body weight versus the RMR. This is similar to the correlation observed by Harris and Benedict between age, height, and weight in their gender-specific equations and RMR. We also found significant systematic differences between the RMR measured in our patients and Owen's equations.[115]

The first comprehensive examination of energy expenditure in obese hospitalized patients was carried out by Ireton-Jones and colleagues.[105, 116] Two equations were developed (see Table 20–2), one for ventilator-dependent obese patients and the other for spontaneously breathing patients.. The hospitalized patients had diagnoses including burns, trauma, and other catabolic states of varied severity. The term *energy expenditure* is used here to distinguish the measured quantity from the RMR, as some of Ireton-Jones' patients were resting, but not fasting, at the time of study. Significant predictors in the equation for ventilator-dependent patients include age, sex (male = 1, female = 0), actual weight (body weight), and type of injury. The r for both equations is similar to those previously mentioned, about .6 to .8. Ireton-Jones and Francis subsequently tested the equations in a prospective study and found good agreement between the observed and the predicted energy expenditures.[81] Amato and coworkers came to a similar conclusion but found large differences between predicted and observed energy expenditures in some subjects.[111]

In summary, estimating the energy requirements of hospitalized obese patients can be accomplished either by measurement using indirect calorimetry or by calculation using one of the several alternatives outlined in Table 20–2. When RMR equations (Equations 1, 3, or 5) are used, there may be a need to adjust for additional factors, such as the severity of injury. Glynn and associates apply an injury factor of 1.3 for acutely ill hospitalized patients,[112] and they also use the average of actual and ideal body weights in their prediction model (see Table 20–2). The factorial approach to estimating energy requirements is inexact and has received very little formal study in obese hospitalized patients. This is an important area for future research. Exact values for energy expenditure may not be needed when managing obese patients, and a pragmatic approach to providing energy during nutritional support is suggested in a later section.

◆ PROTEIN METABOLISM

Healthy obese patients have an increase in total body protein mass, which is maintained at a constant level by a higher protein intake, equivalent protein turnover, and increased excretion of the catabolic end-product of amino acid metabolism, urea.[117] With fasting, healthy obese patients are more ef-

ficient in conserving body nitrogen than are subjects of normal body weight, and their relative rate of weight loss is also slower.[118, 119] Forbes and Drenick[119] and others have shown that the ratio of nitrogen loss to weight loss during an extended fast is inversely related to the body fat content. For example, the $\Delta N/\Delta BW$ (where N is nitrogen and BW is body weight) in nonobese people during a prolonged fast is 20 g/kg and for obese people with a total body fat mass of greater than 50 kg is 10 g/kg.[119] This suggests that healthy obese patients can endure a fast longer without complications than subjects who are at a normal body weight.

Marked individual variability exists, however, in individual nitrogen losses during a total or partial fast. Yang and VanItallie found that obese subjects who had the greatest lowering of serum T_3 levels during weight reduction, an adaptive response to negative energy balance, also had the lowest nitrogen loss.[120]

Other factors are also known to influence nitrogen losses during weight reduction treatment, including the amount of total energy and nitrogen provided, the source of nonprotein energy, the quality of protein in the diet, and the subject's level of physical activity.[121]

◆ METABOLIC RESPONSE TO INJURY

Nonobese Patients

With a severe injury, food intake is curtailed, and therefore endogenous substrates serve as a source of fuel and as the precursors for new protein synthesis. This process is mediated by the counter-regulatory hormones—epinephrine, glucagon, cortisol, and growth hormone—which, combined with monokines, regulate the flow of endogenous substrates between organs and tissues.[122]

Fuel needed to support energy requirements is derived from the oxidation of carbohydrate, fat, and, to a lesser extent, protein. Carbohydrate stores, mainly in the form of glycogen, are limited, and depletion occurs within hours of the acute injury. Organs that require glucose as a fuel are supplied by de novo glucose synthesis from glucogenic amino acids and glycerol, an end-product of triglyceride catabolism. Lipolysis of stored triglyceride provides a source of free fatty acids, which are readily oxidized by most tissues. Over 80% of energy requirements during acute stress are supplied by free fatty acids released during lipolysis of adipocyte triglyceride stores.[123] Amino acids, derived mainly from skeletal muscles, can be used directly as a source of fuel, and some amino acids can also be converted to glucose. Amino acid oxidation results in the release of the metabolic end-product urea. The result is that fat and protein oxidation rates are increased in the early phase of injury, glycerol and free fatty acid levels rise in plasma, urinary urea excretion is increased, and nitrogen balance is negative in the absence of nutritional support. The use of endogenous substrates is minimized and nitrogen balance is improved with the addition of nutritional support during the acute phase of an injury, although overall net protein catabolism is usually not eliminated.[124]

Adequate wound healing requires an increase in the synthesis of proteins involved in tissue repair, immune function, and other vital processes. Amino acids, released mainly from skeletal muscle, serve as precursors for the synthesis of these proteins. Severe injury is usually characterized by an increase in whole-body protein turnover, a small increase in protein synthesis, and a significant elevation in protein breakdown.[125]

The increase in levels of counter-regulatory hormones after injury produces hyperglycemia, skeletal muscle catabolism (providing precursors for protein and glucose synthesis), negative nitrogen balance, and lipolysis. A detailed description of the metabolic response to injury is presented in Chapter 2.

Obese Patients

Limited evidence suggests that the metabolic response to injury in the obese patient differs from that in the normal-weight individual. Jeevanandam and his colleagues investigated the metabolic response to severe multiple trauma in seven obese (BMI > 30 kg/m²) and 10 nonobese patients who had an equivalent level of injury, immediately after admission to the intensive care unit

after stabilization of fluid balance.[126] All the patients were on assisted ventilation at the time of evaluation. Kinetic studies and gas exchange measurements were used to evaluate energy expenditure and substrate flux.

Jeevanandam and colleagues found that the RMR in the obese patients (2550 ± 172 kcal/day) was equivalent to that in the normal-weight control subjects (2538 ± 162 kcal/day). The source of endogenous metabolic fuels differed significantly in Jeevanandam's obese and nonobese patients. The nonobese patients had the expected increase in net fat oxidation (Fig. 20–4), whereas the obese patients had a significantly lower percentage of their energy requirements derived from fat oxidation. Additionally, plasma glycerol levels were significantly reduced in the obese patients, plasma free fatty acids were significantly increased, and their whole-body lipolytic rate was reduced, al-

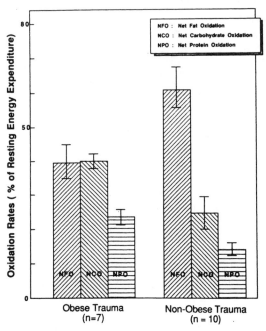

Figure 20–4. Whole-body net oxidation rates (as a percentage of resting energy expenditure) of net fat oxidation (NFO), net carbohydrate oxidation (NCO), and net protein oxidation (NPO) in obese (n = 7) and nonobese (n = 10) trauma patients. $P = .01$ for NFO; $P = .05$ for NCO; and $P = .025$ for NPO (obese versus nonobese trauma patients). From Jeevanandam M, Young DH, and Schiller WR: Obesity and the metabolic response to severe multiple trauma in man. Reproduced from the Journal of Clinical Investigation 87:262–269, 1991 by copyright permission of the American Society for Clinical Investigation.)

though not significantly. Jeevanandam and his colleagues hypothesized that obese patients have both a reduced ability to mobilize fat stores after an acute injury and a limited capacity to oxidize fat.[126]

As fat oxidation was reduced in the injured obese patients, energy was produced instead from oxidation of carbohydrate and protein (both increased vs. nonobese, $P <$ .05; see Fig. 20–4). The rates of whole-body protein turnover and synthesis were higher in the obese patients, but the differences were not statistically significant. Urinary nitrogen losses were significantly increased in the obese patients (22.2 $\pm$ 3.2 g/day) compared with the nonobese control patients (14.3 $\pm$ 1.7 g/day). One of the main concerns in this study is how to express results relative to body composition. For example, was lipolysis reduced in the obese injured patients relative to total body fat?

The investigators had no measures of body composition and made some approximations that allowed them to examine these questions, but a definitive answer could not be provided. Thus, although some questions exist regarding the interpretation of these results, one finding is clear: obese patients do not "spare" protein after a severe injury. Absolute nitrogen losses are increased and nitrogen balance is more negative after severe trauma in fasting obese patients compared with their lean counterparts.

Hormone levels in the obese trauma patients, including levels of insulin, glucagon, cortisol, epinephrine, and norepinephrine, were not significantly different from levels observed in the nonobese trauma patients.[126] Plasma levels of C-peptide, a marker of insulin secretion, were significantly elevated in the obese patients, although the significance of this finding remains uncertain.

A comparison between the metabolic response to trauma in the fasting state, the metabolic profile of a representative fasting obese patient, and the two conditions combined, as reported by Jeevanandam and others, is presented in Table 20–3. Although some trends are evident in obese versus nonobese traumatized patients, additional studies on larger groups of subjects are needed to validate these initial results.

The study by Jeevanandam and his colleagues is important because this is the first examination of how obese and nonobese patients differ in their metabolic response to

Table 20–3. Comparative Physiologic and Metabolic Effects of Trauma, Obesity, and Combined Obesity-Trauma

Physiologic-Metabolic Indices	Condition		
	Trauma	Obesity	Trauma + Obesity
Resting energy expenditure	+[93]	+[125]	+ (NS)[126]
Fasting glucose	+[1]	±[125]	+ (NS)[126]
Insulin secretion	+[19]	+[125]	+[126]
Plasma free fatty acids	+[126]	+[125]	+[126]
Urinary nitrogen excretion	+[117]	+[125]	+[126]

+, significant increase; ±, increase or no change; NS, nonsignificant difference for trauma versus nontrauma, obese versus lean, and traumatized obese versus traumatized lean.

an equally severe injury. Questions remain regarding interpretation of these results, and no mechanism has yet been established that explains why the presence of excess adipose tissue alters the metabolic response to injury. Nevertheless, this study emphasizes that the protection offered by a large adipose tissue mass during weight reduction therapy may not extend directly to the concept that obese people are equally resistant to depletion of lean tissues after severe multiple trauma. An important and unanswered question is how the traumatized obese patient's lipid, carbohydrate, and protein metabolism responds to nutritional support.

◆ NUTRITIONAL SUPPORT

Attitudes Toward the Obese

Professional staff who make decisions regarding medical and surgical therapies of obese patients should be aware of some important attitudinal biases and ethical issues. Unfortunately pejorative attitudes toward obese persons are not limited to laypeople. For example, over 24% of a sample of registered nurses agreed or strongly agreed with the statement "Caring for an obese patient usually repulses me."[127] Maiman and co-workers found that over 50% of a group of health professionals, comprising primarily nutritionists, held disparaging attitudes toward obese persons.[128] Derogatory attitudes toward obese persons have also been found among rehabilitation counseling students[129] and mental health professionals.[130]

In a 1969 survey of 100 physicians, more than half the respondents described obese patients as "weak willed," "ugly," and "awkward."[90] Moreover, these physicians indicated that they generally preferred not to manage obese patients. Similar negative attitudes have been found among physicians and medical students in three more surveys that, combined, included a total of 856 subjects.[131–133] Sadly, attitudes do not seem to have improved. In fact, Young and Powell report that younger professionals hold more negative attitudes than do their older counterparts.[130]

It would be nice to believe that professional clinical decisions are made on wholly objective grounds and are not influenced by the personal attitudes of the professional. Unfortunately, both common sense and research suggest the contrary. Breytspraak and associates, [134] Young and Powell,[130] and Kaplan[129] have all clearly demonstrated that the perception of a patient as obese influences treatment decisions and recommendations independent of clinically relevant data.

Does the belief that obese patients should lose weight encourage physicians to provide reduced caloric intake during periods of nutritional support? Does this belief influence decisions about nutritional support independent of empirical data (or the lack thereof) on the relative cost and benefits of various caloric intakes during nutritional support? Do some physicians, with the best of intentions, provide reduced nutritional support for the injured obese patient as a form of reducing diet, disregarding the fact that the patient did not seek hospitalization as a treatment for obesity and may not even wish to lose weight? The answers to these questions are unknown. However, given the available data on attitudes toward obese persons, affirmative answers to each are plausible. It is hoped that awareness of, and attention to, these attitudinal biases will alert physicians to potential distortions in their clinical decision making regarding obese patients. Such attention and awareness may help to derail prejudicial reactions and facilitate treatment protocols based on clinically relevant information and empirical findings.

Vascular Access

Subclavian and internal jugular catheters may be difficult to place in obese patients. When this is the case, the internal jugular site is associated with fewer and less serious complications than subclavian catheterization.[65]

Nutritional Support Protocol

The purpose of nutritional support of obese patients who cannot maintain their voluntary maintenance food intake is to provide adequate protein, energy, and other essential nutrients in order to facilitate wound healing, aid in the preservation and recovery of vital physiologic functions, and optimize outcomes.

Under ideal conditions, nutritional support of the obese patient would be similar to that of hospitalized patients who are not obese. It is important to recognize that providing obese patients with a maintenance energy requirement will preserve the integrity of their lean tissues and should not lead to positive fat balance and accumulation of new adipose tissue.

Although maintenance support is desirable, two problems are encountered that suggest that a reduced caloric intake is desirable in obese patients receiving nonvolitional feeding. First, the exact level of energy required for maintenance support is difficult to estimate accurately for the reasons described earlier. Second, it is often difficult to meet the obese patient's full energy requirement because of (1) glucose intolerance secondary to insulin resistance, (2) a sensitivity to fluid administration due to cardiac dysfunction caused by comorbid conditions such as coronary artery disease, high blood pressure, obesity hypoventilation syndrome, and diabetes, and (3) sensitivity of the respiratory system and liver to excess carbohydrate related to the presence of underlying pulmonary disease and fatty infiltration of the liver, respectively.

Greenberg and Jeejeebhoy[135] and later Dickerson and his colleagues[136] attempted to overcome these barriers to maintenance nutritional support by hypocaloric feeding that optimized protein intake and continued to supply adequate amounts of other essential nutrients. According to this approach, lean tissue preservation is facilitated while endogenous fat serves as an additional source of energy. Hypocaloric diets can be classified into two types: those that are ketogenic and consist primarily of protein and those that are designed to provide submaintenance energy with a balanced fuel profile consisting mainly of fat, protein, and carbohydrate sources.

Ketogenic Hypocaloric Diet

A hypocaloric diet is a reasonable choice at the outset of treatment if the main goal is weight loss, fluid mobilization, and relief of respiratory and cardiac dysfunction. A ketogenic parenteral feeding protocol (65 g of protein per day plus other noncalorie essential nutrients) was used by Collier and Walker in a patient with morbid obesity and acute respiratory failure secondary to Prader-Willi syndrome.[137] This or similar very low energy feeding programs should be used for only minimally stressed obese patients who are extremely sensitive to higher levels of calorie and fluid intake and in whom the primary goal of nutritional support is weight loss.

Although there were early suggestions that parenteral amino acids had direct central stimulatory effects on ventilation, a study by Abbott and his colleagues found in postoperative morbidly obese patients no advantage of a hypocaloric amino acid (3.5%) infusion over dextrose (5%) in a wide range of pulmonary and metabolic indices.[138] The beneficial effects of amino acids on the respiratory system should therefore not be used as a rationale for infusing only amino acids, not other energy sources.

Balanced Hypocaloric Diet

For obese patients who are moderately or severely stressed and in whom weight reduction is not the primary therapy, most investigators suggest attempting to reach a maintenance or submaintenance energy intake by prioritizing protein intake, then carbohydrate, and finally lipid.

Semistarvation or hypocaloric feeding has been successfully used as a treatment for obesity in otherwise healthy individuals for some time. Adaptive changes during starvation reduce energy requirements and allow fat depots to be used for energy while sparing muscle protein from excessive catabolism. In this setting, the administration of adequate amounts of exogenous protein (i.e., 1 g/kg of ideal body weight) results in nitrogen equilibrium or positive nitrogen balance.[135, 136]

In one early study, Greenberg and Jeejeebhoy evaluated the response to two different levels of protein intake in 12 obese patients.[135] The patients had diagnoses including peptic ulcer disease, intestinal fistulas, pancreatitis, carcinoma of the bowel, and other illnesses believed to be associated with mild or moderate stress. The subjects were relatively young (mean age 45 years), although the degree of obesity could not be ascertained as no body weight information was provided. Amino acids fed through a central venous line for 7 days served as the sole source of calories and nitrogen. Patients were randomized either to an average of 0.83 g of amino acids per kilogram of ideal body weight or to 1.83 g of amino acids per kilogram of ideal body weight. Sufficient amounts of electrolytes, vitamins, and trace elements were provided. Ketosis was not present in either group of obese patients receiving the amino acid infusions.

Each patient's nitrogen balance was followed over the next week. Both groups excreted about 100 g of nitrogen in urine. Because the nitrogen intake differed between the two groups, retention of nitrogen was greater in the high amino acid group (16.3 ± 6.7 g vs. −26.1 ± 11.5 g, $P < .025$). The findings were qualitatively similar if the nitrogen balance results were adjusted for cutaneous and other unmeasured losses. The investigators suggested providing obese patients with 2 g of amino acids per kilogram of ideal body weight to achieve positive nitrogen balance during hypocaloric feeding.

Data concerning the safety of hypocaloric nutritional regimens in acutely ill obese patients are accumulating, and three prospective studies have been performed to date. The first report, by Dickerson and colleagues,[136] demonstrated that nitrogen balance can be achieved in mild to moderately stressed obese patients receiving total parenteral nutrition containing approximately 51% of measured resting energy expenditure as nonprotein calories. The source of the nonprotein calories was predominantly dextrose, and intravenous lipid was provided intermittently.[136] The study of Dickerson and colleagues included morbidly obese surgical patients who were 208 ± 114% (range 117 to 577%) of ideal body weight as calculated according to the formula of Devine.[138] The nonprotein caloric intake averaged 881 ± 393 kcal/day, and the protein intake was 2.13 ± 0.59 g/kg of ideal body weight. The patients were maintained on this regimen for an average of 48 days. Serum levels of albumin and total iron-binding capacity improved significantly, and all subjects had complete tissue healing. A treatment goal was negative energy balance, and the subjects lost weight, from 120 ± 60 kg at baseline to 110 ± 33 kg at follow-up.

Based on the study of Dickerson and colleagues,[136] Flancbaum and associates carried out two prospective randomized double-blind trials of hypocaloric nutritional support in obese hospitalized patients.[139, 140] Eligible patients were greater than 130% of ideal body weight and were expected to require parenteral nutritional support for greater than 10 days. As the protocol required the administration of a large amount of protein (1.5 to 2.0 g/kg of ideal body weight per day), patients with renal and/or hepatic dysfunction were excluded. In the first study, patients in the intensive care unit and with pre-existing diabetes mellitus were excluded, although they were not excluded in the second study. Two parenteral formulas, shown in Table 20–4, were used in both studies.

Energy expenditure in the first study was measured using indirect calorimetry, and the total parenteral nutrition formulas were administered at a rate to provide 100% of measured energy expenditure as nonprotein calories to the control subjects or 50% of measured energy expenditure as nonprotein calories to the hypocaloric group. The second study was performed in an attempt to eliminate the need for indirect calorimetry, making this approach more widely applica-

ble. The same two "three-in-one" formulas were used (see Table 20–4), although the infusion rate was based on the protein component to initiate treatment at 2 g of protein per kilogram of ideal body weight per day. Urinary urea nitrogen was then periodically monitored over 24 hours and the infusion rate increased if patients were in negative nitrogen balance. In both studies, the length of time on the study formula was kept at or less than 14 days, after which the patient was transitioned to a standard formula. The main assessment of efficacy was nitrogen balance. Three-in-one solutions were chosen because providing all the nonprotein calories as dextrose may increase the risk of metabolic and respiratory complications. The outcome, in terms of overall average nitrogen balance and the number of patients who remained in negative nitrogen balance in the hypocaloric and control groups, is shown in Table 20–5. Both studies showed that most patients (>90%) achieved positive nitrogen balance without adverse effects. In addition, there was no difference in the probability of a patient's reaching positive nitrogen balance regardless of the formula received.

Although weight loss was a primary treatment goal for the population of Dickerson and colleagues,[136] it was not an objective of the studies by Burge and associates[139] and Choban and coworkers.[140] Their aim was to show comparable nitrogen balance and safety and avoid the risks inherent in overfeeding. These two studies were of much shorter duration than that of Dickerson and colleagues (average, 9.6 vs. 48 days). Although the methods used to determine the rate of formula administration differed in the first and second studies, the final daily amounts of protein and energy provided were similar (see Table 20–5). Study 1 used indirect calorimetry to guide treatment, and in study 2, treatment was based on the pa-

Table 20–4. Hypocaloric and Control TPN Formulas Used in the Study of Burge et al.[139]

Formula	Amino Acids (g/L)	Dextrose (g/L)	Lipid (g/L)	NP Energy/N (kcal/g)	Total energy/N (kcal/g)
Hypocaloric TPN	60	75	20	46:1	75:1
Control TPN	60	150	40	93:1	150:1

NP, nonprotein; TPN, total parenteral nutrition.

Table 20–5. Main Demographic and Outcome Characteristics of Two Hypocaloric Randomized Controlled Feeding Trials

Feeding	Hypocaloric		Control	
	1	*2*	*1*	*2*
Reference	Burge et al.[139]	Choban et al.[140]	Burge et al.[139]	Choban et al.[140]
Subject number	9	16	7	14
kcal/day (per kg IBW)	1285 ± 374	1290 ± 299	2492 ± 298	1940 ± 198
	(22 ± 6.9)	(22 ± 2.8)	(42 ± 7.2)	(36 ± 4.3)
NP kcal/day (per kg IBW)	585 ± 170	814 ± 153	1972 ± 235	1508 ± 164
	(10 ± 3.1)	(14 ± 2.8)	(33 ± 6)	(28 ± 3.9)
Protein (g/day) (g/kg IBW)	111 ± 32	108 ± 14	130 ± 15.5	120 ± 26.8
	(2.0 ± 0.6)	(2.0 ± 0.11)	(2.2 ± 0.4)	(1.97 ± 0.13)
Initial UUN (g/day)	10.7 ± 10.2	8.2 ± 5.9	8.1 ± 5.5	8.2 ± 5.9
ΔN (g/day)	+1.3 ± 3.6	+4.0 ± 4.2	+2.8 ± 6.9	+3.6 ± 4.1
Negative ΔN	1	2	1	1
(%)	(11)	(12.5)	(14.3)	(7)

NP, nonprotein; IBW, ideal body weight; UUN, urinary urea nitrogen.

tient's ideal body weight and adjusted based on the nitrogen balance. The daily protein and energy delivered in these two studies as well as those from the study by Dickerson and colleagues are summarized in Table 20–6.

Formula Infusion Rate and Composition

The main techniques for estimating maintenance energy requirements and their limitations were described earlier. An additional hypocaloric approach was suggested by Pasulka and Kohl, who recommend feeding obese patients a "maximal" caloric intake as actual body weight (kg) × 25.[141] Baxter and Bistrian suggested that patients should be fed about 300 to 500 kcal/day less than their maintenance requirement, which the inves-

tigators estimated as actual body weight (kg) × 18 to 22 for females and × 22 to 25 for males.[142]

To meet caloric requirements, the protein intake should be maintained at 1.5 to 2 g/kg of ideal body weight, as originally described by Greenberg and Jeejeebhoy.[135] Baxter and Bistrian recommend adding a minimum of 150 g of dextrose per day in order to prevent ketosis and to provide additional calories, with a maximal carbohydrate intake of 300 g/day.[142] The upper limit is suggested because of the aforementioned problems with glucose tolerance. Choban and associates begin their formula (see Table 20–4) infusion at a rate of 2 g/kg of ideal body weight per day and alter the intake according to monitored nitrogen balance (g), that is, $\Delta N = N$ intake $- (UUN\ [g] + 0.2[UUN] + 2)$, where N is nitrogen and UUN is urinary urea nitrogen.[140]

Table 20–6. Summary of Nutritional Support Studies of Obese Patients

Study	Study Type	N (H/C)	Protein (g/kg/day) (H/C)	Total kcal/kg/day (H/C)	Nonprotein kcal/kg/day (H/C)	End-Point +NB (H/C)
Dickerson et al.[136]	Prospective	13/0	2.1 IBW 1.2 ABW		15 IBW 6.9 ABW	8
Burge et al.[139]	Prospective DB Randomized	9/7	2.0/2.2 IBW 1.2/1.3 ABW	22/42 IBW 14/25 ABW	10/33 IBW 7/20 ABW	8/6
Choban et al.[140]	Prospective DB Randomized	16/14	2.0/2.0 IBW 1.2/1.2 ABW	22/36 IBW 13.5/22.4 ABW	14/28 IBW 17.5/8.6 ABW	13/13

ABW, actual body weight; C, control; DB, double-blind; H, hypocaloric; IBW, ideal body weight; kcal, kilocalories; +NB, positive nitrogen balance.

There is no evidence that additional calories supplied by lipid are needed in order to prevent essential fatty acid deficiency. About 10% of fat stores consist of linoleic acid, and therefore the 2- to 3.5-g requirement for linoleic acid per day can be obtained from mobilization of 20 to 35 g/day (<350 kcal/day) of endogenous fat. Stegink and his colleagues demonstrated maintenance of plasma linoleic acid levels after 10 to 14 days of an amino acid infusion (1.5 g of protein per kilogram per day) in nonobese postsurgical patients.[143] Longer periods of nutritional support may require the provision of lipid, as Dickerson and his colleagues detected clinical signs that suggested essential fatty acid deficiency (dry scaly skin) in one of their obese patients who received no exogenous essential fatty acids for 20 days.[136] Moreover, the studies of Jeevanandam and associates suggested an inhibition of lipolysis in the severely injured obese patient.[126] The question of exogenous essential fatty acid requirements in the hypocalorically fed acutely ill obese patient remains an important topic for future research.

Parenteral lipid is useful in providing calories to obese patients who are severely catabolic and therefore require higher energy intakes. The advantages of parenteral lipids over glucose as a source of nonprotein calories in the stressed obese patient include a reduced need for pancreatic insulin secretion in the presence of insulin resistance and hyperglycemia, a lower risk of producing fatty infiltration of the liver with associated abnormalities in liver function tests, a diminished rate of carbon dioxide production and therefore reduced ventilatory demands, and a smaller fluid volume per calorie infused.

Important clinical considerations and a suggested approach for managing the acutely injured or stressed obese patient that summarizes the information in this section is presented in Figure 20–5. If the goal is weight maintenance, caloric levels approaching requirements are fed by combining lipid, carbohydrate, and protein calories as guided by the presence of the conditions outlined in the figure. A nutritional support program designed specifically for weight loss has a severely reduced energy content that is derived mainly from protein and, to a lesser extent, glucose.

Although parenteral nutritional support is the main focus of this chapter, several useful concepts regarding enteral feeding of the obese patient emerge from the previous discussion. These include a rationale for and appropriate amounts of prescribed total energy, protein, carbohydrate, and fluid.

Two choices are usually available when deciding on the specific enteral formula to administer. The first choice is to select a commercially prepared enteral solution that approximates the patient's nutrient require-

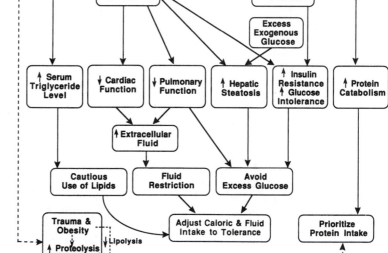

Figure 20–5. Considerations when providing nutritional support to the critically ill obese patient.

ments. If protein is prioritized for the stressed obese patient as suggested earlier, a high-nitrogen formula with a calorie-to-nitrogen ratio of about 100 to 125 would be optimal for the delivery of 80 to 120 g of protein per day, and 1500 to 2000 kcal of total energy per day with 1.5 to 2 L of fluid. An example is a 100-kg severely injured obese male patient who has an ideal body weight of 70 kg and an estimated energy requirement of 2300 kcal/day (i.e., 23 kcal/kg of actual body weight). An intake of 1800 kcal/day is prescribed, which results in a negative energy balance of 500 kcal/day. Protein intake is set at 1.5 g/kg of ideal body weight, or a total of 105 g/day. A formula that has a calorie-to-nitrogen ratio of 107:1 would satisfy this requirement.

The second choice with respect to enteral formula prescription is to create a modular solution following similar nutrient guidelines to those suggested above for parenteral formulas.

Technical details regarding enteral support of the obese patient are similar to those described for hospitalized patients in general.

Monitoring

A critical issue is determining whether the level of nutritional support is optimal for maximizing the patient's outcome. This is always a difficult question to answer but is particularly so in the obese patient who is intentionally being underfed for all the reasons mentioned earlier. A practical approach is to regularly monitor the systems or functions known to be at risk from prolonged negative nutrient balance: cardiac, respiratory, immune, and wound healing. Decisions to change the level of nutritional support must be balanced against results obtained from monitoring diet-sensitive metabolic factors, such as serum ketone and glucose levels, respiratory indices such as arterial PcO_2 and pH, and functional or indirect markers of hepatic and renal function. Respiratory gas analysis (e.g., the respiratory quotient), serum protein levels, and nitrogen balance are additional studies that should be considered in selected patients.

There are several other important surgical concerns in the critically ill obese patient. Obese patients are at increased risk of aspiration pneumonia[65] and have a significantly higher residual gastric volume and a lower pH of gastric fluid compared with nonobese controls.[144] These findings may be explained by a delayed gastric emptying and elevated acid secretory capacity in obese people.[145] As acidity and volume are the two major factors that influence pulmonary injury with aspiration,[146] additional care should be taken in the obese patient to reduce the risk of or to prevent aspiration.

Obesity is a major risk factor for the development of pneumonia. Pain medication, particularly sedatives, can cause severe respiratory depression in the obese person.[65] Early ambulation, chest physical therapy, and the cautious use of narcotics and sedatives are suggested preventive measures.[65]

Pulmonary embolism, as mentioned earlier, is an important cause of morbidity and mortality in obese patients. Pulmonary embolism was the most frequent pulmonary complication in postsurgical morbidly obese patients undergoing a variety of operative procedures.[147] Deep vein thrombosis after gynecologic surgery is most common in patients with excess body weight.[147, 148] Glucose infusion should be beneficial in preventing thromboembolism by reducing the hemoconcentration and by inhibiting lipolysis, which lowers serum acid levels.[65] External pneumatic compression is a safe antithrombotic measure in the obese patient and may reduce peripheral venous pooling and stimulate the release of fibrinolytic factors.[65] Leg compression combined with the semirecumbent position has the additional beneficial effect of improving respiratory function. The use of intermittent compression stockings is probably as effective as low-dose heparin in preventing pulmonary emboli and is not associated with the increased risk of hematoma.[65]

SUMMARY

Medical, surgical, and nutritional management of the obese patient requires knowledge and an approach distinct from that applied to the nonobese patient. Considering the very large and increasing population of obese patients in the United States, remarkably little information is available on the specifics of nutritional support in this group. Our review is designed to provide an overview of obesity and to present the limited information on nutritional management of the obese hospitalized patient. More importantly, we attempted to reveal the large gaps in our present understanding of this area. Finally, we attempted to enlighten the reader about the potential biases that might interfere with medical and nutritional management of the obese patient.

REFERENCES

1. Clinical Guidelines on the Identification, Evaluation, and Treatment of Overweight and Obesity in Adults: The Evidence Report. No. 98-4083. Washington, DC, U.S. Department of Health and Human Services, 1998.
2. Choban PS, Heckler R, Burge J, Flancbaum L: Nosocomial infections in obese surgical patients. Am Surg 61:1001–1005, 1995.
3. Metropolitan Life Foundation: Height and weight tables. New York, Metropolitan Life Insurance Company, 1983.
4. Kral JG, Heymsfield S: Morbid obesity: Definitions, epidemiology, and methodological problems. Gastroenterol Clin North Am 16:197–205, 1987.
5. Olmstead SL: Obese, overweight, desirable, ideal: Where to draw the line in 1986? J Am Diet Assoc 86:1702–1704, 1986.
6. Bray GA, Angeles L: Complications of obesity. Ann Intern Med 103:1052–1062, 1985.
7. Kissebah AH, Vydelingum N, Murray R, et al: Relation of body fat distribution to metabolic complications of obesity. J Clin Endocrinol Metab 54:254–260, 1982.
8. Fried SK, Kral JG: Adipose tissue of morbidly obese patients: Clinical implications of distribution, morphology, and metabolism. Gastroenterol Clin North Am 16:207–213, 1987.
9. Fujioka S, Matsuzawa Y, Tokunaga K, Tarui S: Contribution of intra-abdominal fat accumulation to the impairment of glucose and lipid metabolism in human obesity. Metabolism 36:54–59, 1987.
10. Despres J-P, Nadeau A, Tremblay A, at al: Role of deep abdominal fat in the association between regional adipose tissue distribution and glucose tolerance in obese women. Diabetes 38:304–309, 1989.
11. Peires AN, Mueller RA, Struve MF, et al: Relationship of androgenic activity to splanchnic insulin metabolism and peripheral glucose utilization in premenopausal women. J Clin Endocrinol Metab 64:162–169, 1987.
12. Ferland M, Despres J-P, Nadeau A, et al: Contribution of glucose tolerance and plasma insulin levels to the relationships between body fat distribution and plasma lipoprotein levels in women. Int J Obes Relat Metab Disord 15:677–688, 1991.
13. Haffner S, Stern MP, Hazuda HP, et al: Do upper-body and centralized adiposity measure different aspects of regional body-fat distribution? Relationship to non-insulin dependent diabetes mellitus, lipids, and lipoproteins. Diabetes 36:43–51, 1987.
14. Schmieder RE, Messerli FH: Obesity hypertension. Med Clin North Am 71:991–1001, 1987.
15. Harty A, Grubb B, Wild R, et al: The association of waist hip ratio and angiographically determined coronary artery disease. Int J Obes Relat Metab Disord 14:657–665, 1990.
16. Houmard JA, Wheeler WS, McCammon MR, et al: An evaluation of waist to hip ratio measurement methods in relation to lipid and carbohydrate metabolism in men. Int J Obes Relat Metab Disord 15:181–188, 1991.
17. Bjorntorp P: Regional patterns of fat distribution. Ann Intern Med 103:994–995, 1985.
18. Pi-Sunyer FX: Health implications of obesity. Am J Clin Nutr 53:1595S–1603S, 1991.
19. Karam JH, Grodsky GM, Forsham PH: Excessive insulin response to glucose in obese subjects as measured by immunochemical assay. Diabetes 12:197–204, 1963.
20. Peiris A, Kissebah A: Endocrine abnormalities in morbid obesity. Gastroenterol Clin North Am 16:389–398, 1987.
21. Sirinek KR, O'Dorisio TM, Howe B, McFee AS: Pancreatic islet hormone response to oral glucose in morbidly obese patients. Ann Surg 201:690–694, 1985.
22. Kolterman OG, Insel J, Saekow M, Olefsky JM: Mechanisms of insulin resistance in human obesity. J Clin Invest 65:1272–1284, 1980.
23. Bar RS, Harrison LC, Muggeo M, et al: Regulation of insulin receptors in normal and abnormal physiology in humans. Adv Intern Med 24:23–52, 1979.
24. Grundy SM, Barnett JP: Metabolic and health complications of obesity. Dis Mon 36:641–696, 1990.
25. Meylan M, Henny C, Temler E, et al: Metabolic factors in the insulin resistance in human obesity. Metabolism 36:256–261, 1987.
26. Kesaniemi YA, Grundy SM: Increased low density lipoprotein production associated with obesity. Arteriosclerosis 3:170–177, 1983.
27. Egusa G, Belz WF, Grundy SM, Howard BV: Influence of obesity on the metabolism of apolipoprotein B in humans. J Clin Invest 76:596–603, 1985.
28. Dustan HP: Obesity and hypertension. Ann Intern Med 103:1047–1049, 1985.
29. Messerli FH, Sundgaard-Riise K, Reisin ED, et al: Dimorphic cardiac adaptation to obesity and arterial hypertension. Ann Intern Med 99:757–761, 1983.
30. Messerli FH, Sundgaard-Riise K, Reisin ED, et al: Disparate cardiovascular effects of obesity and arterial hypertension. Am J Med 74:808–812, 1983.
31. Shafrir E, Bergman M, Felig P: The endocrine process: Diabetes mellitus. In Felig P, Bacter JD, Broadus AE, Frohman LA (eds): Endocrinology and Metabolism, 2nd ed. New York, McGraw-Hill, pp 1043–1178.
32. Braillon A, Capron JP: Foie et l'obesite. Gastroenterol Clin Biol 7:627–634, 1983.
33. Buchwald H, Lober PH, Varco RL: Liver biopsy findings in seventy-seven consecutive patients undergoing jejunoileal bypass for morbid obesity. Am J Surg 127:48–52, 1974.
34. Kral JG: Morbid obesity and related health risks. Ann Intern Med 103:1043–1047, 1985.
35. Kral JG, Lundholm K, Bjorntorp P, et al: Hepatic lipid metabolism in severe human obesity. Metabolism 26:1025–1031, 1977.

36. Baker AL, Rosenberg IH: Hepatic complications of total parenteral nutrition. Am J Med 82:489–497, 1987.

37. Nestel PJ, Schreibman PH, Ahrens EH Jr: Cholesterol metabolism in human obesity. J Clin Invest 52:2389–2397, 1973.

38. Mabee TM, Meyer P, DenBester L, Mason E: The mechanism of increased gallstone formation in obese human subjects. Surgery 79:460–468, 1976.

39. Maryio L, Capore F, Neri, M, et al: Gallbladder kinetics in obese patients. Dig Dis Sci 33:4–9, 1988.

40. Pitt HA, King W III, Mann LL, et al: Increased risk of cholelithiasis with prolonged total parenteral nutrition. Am J Surg 145:106–112, 1983.

41. Liddle RA, Goldstein RB, Saxton J: Gallstone formation during weight-reduction dieting. Arch Intern Med 149:1750–1753, 1989.

42. Shiffman ML, Sugerman HJ, Kellum JM, et al: Gallstone formation after rapid weight loss: A prospective study in patients undergoing gastric bypass surgery for treatment of morbid obesity. Am J Gastroenterol 86:1000–1005, 1991.

43. Sugerman HJ, Brewer WH, Shiffman ML et al.: A multicenter, placebo-controlled, randomized, double-blind, prospective trial of prophylactic ursodiol for the prevention of gallstone formation following gastric-bypass–induced rapid weight loss. Am J Surg 169:91–97, 1995.

44. Ray CS, Sue DY, Bray G, et al: Effects of obesity on respiratory function. Am Rev Respir Dis 128:501–506, 1983.

45. Sharp JT, Barrocas M, Chokroverty S: The cardiorespiratory effects of obesity. Clin Chest Med 1:103–118, 1980.

46. Sugerman HJ: Pulmonary function in morbid obesity. Gastroenterol Clin North Am 16:225–237, 1987.

47. Connor WZ: The acceleration of thrombus formation by certain fatty acids. J Clin Invest 41:1199–1206, 1962.

48. Coon WW: Risk factors in pulmonary embolism. Surg Gynecol Obstet 143:385–390, 1976.

49. Borrow M, Goldson H: Postoperative venous thrombosis evaluation of five methods of treatment. Am J Surg 141:245–251, 1981.

50. Printen KJ, Miller EV, Mason EE, Barnes RW: Venous thromboembolism in the morbidly obese. Surg Gynecol Obstet 147:63–64, 1978.

51. Pasulka PS, Bistrian BR, Benotti PN, Blackburn GL: The risks of surgery in obese patients. Ann Intern Med 104:540–546, 1986.

52. Stern SH, Insall JN: Total knee arthroplasty in obese patients. J Bone J Surg 72A:1400–1404, 1990.

53. Lemos MJ, Sutton D, Hozack WJ, et al: Pulmonary embolism in total hip and knee arthroplasty. Risk factors in patients on warfarin prophylaxis: An analysis of the prothrombin time as an indicator of warfarin's prophylactic effect. Clin Orthop 282:158–163, 1992.

54. Sugerman HJ: Gastric surgery for morbid obesity. In Cameron J (ed): Current Surgical Therapy, 4th ed. St Louis, Mosby–Year Book, 1992, pp 67–72.

55. Kral JG: Surgical risks in obese patients. In Schettler G, Gotto AM, Middelhoff G, et al (eds): Atherosclerosis VI. Berlin, Springer- Verlag, 1983, pp 955–959.

56. Pitkin RM: Abdominal hysterectomy in obese women. Surg Gynecol Obstet 143:532–536, 1976.

57. Nimrod A, Ryan KJ: Aromatization of androgens by human abdominal and breast fat tissue. J Clin Endocrinol Metab 40:367–372, 1975.

58. Choban PS, Flancbaum L: The impact of obesity on surgical outcomes: A review. J Am Coll Surg 185:593–603, 1977.

59. Fox G, Whalley DG, Bevan DR: Anaesthesia for the morbidly obese: Experience with 110 patients. Br J Anaesth 53:811–816, 1981.

60. Forrest JB, Rehder K, Cahalan MK, Goldsmith CH: Multicenter study of general anesthesia III. Predictors of severe perioperative adverse outcomes. Anesthesiology 76:3–15, 1992.

61. Cork RC, Vaughn RW, Bentley JB: General anesthesia for morbidly obese patients—An examination of postoperative outcomes. Anesthesiology 54:310–313, 1981.

62. Taivainen T, Tuominen M, Rosenberg PH: Influence of obesity on the spread of spinal analgesia after injection of plain 0.5% bupivacaine at the L3–4 or L4–5 interspace. Br J Anesthesia 64:542–546, 1990.

63. Postlethwait RW, Johnson WD: Complications following surgery for duodenal ulcer in obese patients. Arch Surg 105:438–440, 1972.

64. Pemberton LB, Manax WG: Relationship of obesity to postoperative complications after cholecystectomy. Am J Surg 121:87–90, 1971.

65. Kral JG, Strauss RJ, Wise L: Perioperative risk management in obese patients. In Deitel M (ed): Surgery of the Morbidly Obese Patient. Philadelphia, Lea & Febiger, 1988, pp 55–65.

66. Edwards LE, Dickes WF, Alton IR, et al: Pregnancy in the massively obese: Course, outcome and obesity prognosis of the infant. Am J Obstet Gynecol 131:479–483, 1978.

67. Prasad US, Walker WS, Sang CTM, et al: Influence of obesity on the early and long term results of surgery for coronary artery disease. Eur J Cardiothorac Surg 5:67–73, 1991.

68. Fasol R, Schindler M, Schumacher B, et al: The influence of obesity of perioperative morbidity: Retrospective study of 502 aortocoronary bypass operations. Thorac Cardiovasc Surg 40:126–129, 1992.

69. Holley JL, Shapiro R, Lopatin WB, et al: Obesity as a risk factor following cadaveric renal transplantation. Transplantation 49:387–389, 1990.

70. Merion RM, Twork AM, Rosenberg L, et al: Obesity and renal transplantation. Surg Gynecol Obstet 172:367–376, 1991.

71. Gill IS, Hodge EE, Novick AC, et al: Impact of obesity on renal transplantation. Transplant Proc 25:1047–1048, 1993.

72. Sugerman HJ: Surgical infections in the morbidly obese patient. Infect Med Nov:37–52, 1991.

73. Stallone DD: The influence of obesity and its treatment on the immune system. Nutr Rev 52:37–50, 1994.

74. Tanaka S, Inoue S, Isoda F et al: Impaired immunity in obesity: Suppressed but reversible lymphocyte responsiveness. Int J Obes Relat Metab Disord 17:631–636, 1993.

75. Maki PA, Newberne PM: Dietary lipids and immune function. J Nutr 122:610–614, 1992.

76. Riou JA, Cohen JR, Johnson H: Factors influencing wound dehiscence. Am J Surg 163:324–330, 1992.

77. Sugerman HJ, Kellum JM Jr, Reines HD, et al: Greater risk of incisional hernia with morbidly

obese than steroid-dependent patients and low recurrence with prefascial polypropylene mesh. Am J Surg 171:80–84, 1996.

78. Drenick EJ, Bale GS, Seltzer F, Johnson DG: Excessive mortality and causes of death in morbidly obese men. JAMA 243:443–445, 1980.

79. Pirson J: A study of the influence of body weight and height on military parachute landing injuries. Mil Med 155:383–385, 1990.

80. Choban PS, Weireter LJ, Maynes C: Obesity and increased mortality in blunt trauma. J Trauma 31:1253–1257, 1991.

81. Ireton-Jones CS, Francis C: Obesity: Nutrition support practice and application to critical care. Nutr Clin Pract 10:144–149, 1995.

82. Gottschlich MM, Mayes T, Khoury JC, et al: Significance of obesity on nutritional, immunologic, humoral, and clinical outcome parameters in burns. J Am Diet Assoc 93:1261–1268, 1993.

83. Allon N: The stigma of overweight in everyday life. In Wolman BB (ed): Psychological Aspects of Obesity: A Handbook. New York, Van Nostrand Reinhold, 1982, pp 130–174.

84. Karris L: Prejudice against obese renters. J Soc Psychol 101:159–160, 1977.

85. Davis JM, Wheeler RW, Willy E: Cognitive correlates of obesity in a nonclinical population. Psychol Rep 67:879–884, 1987.

86. Harris MB: Is love seen as different for the obese? J Appl Soc Psychol 20:1209–1224, 1990.

87. Larkin JE, Pines HA: No fat persons need apply. Sociol Work Occup 6:312–327, 1979.

88. Canning H, Mayer J: Obesity—Its possible effects on college admissions. N Engl J Med 275:1172–1174, 1966.

89. Rodin J, Slochower J: Fat chance for a favor: Obese-normal differences in compliance and incidental learning. J Pers Soc Psychol 29:557–565, 1974.

90. Maddox GL, Liederman V: Overweight as a social disability with medical implications. J Med Educ 44:214–220, 1969.

91. Allison DB, Basile VC, Yuker HE: The measurement of attitudes toward and beliefs about obese persons. Intern J Eat Disord 10:599–607, 1991.

92. Davis S: Men as success objects and women as sex objects: A study of personal advertisements. Sex Roles 23:43–50, 1990.

93. Stein RF: Comparison of self-concept of nonobese and obese university junior female nursing students. Adolescence 22:77–90, 1987.

94. Nacye RL, Roode P: The sizes and numbers of cells in visceral organs in human obesity. Am J Clin Pathol 54:251, 1970.

95. Heymsfield SB, Lichtman S, Baumgartner RN, et al: Body composition of humans: Comparison of two improved four-compartment models that differ in expense, technical complexity, and radiation exposure. Am J Clin Nutr 52:52–58, 1990.

96. Heymsfield SB, Lichtman S, Baumgartner RN, et al: Assessment of body composition: An overview. In Bjorntorp P, Brodoff BN(eds): Obesity. Philadelphia, JB Lippincott, 1992, pp 37–54.

97. Webster JD, Hesp R, Garrow JS: The composition of excess weight in obese women estimated by body density, total body water, and total body potassium. Human Nutr Clin Nutr 38:299–306, 1984.

98. Ravussin E, Bogardus C: Relationship of genetics, age, physical fitness to daily energy expenditure and fuel utilization. Am J Clin Nutr 41:753–759, 1985.

99. Ravussin E, Lillioja S, Anderson TE, et al: Determinants of 24-hour energy expenditure in man: Methods and results using a respiratory chamber. J Clin Invest 78:1568–1578, 1986.

100. Segal KR, Edano A, Blando L, Pi-Sunyer FX: Thermic effect of a meal over 3 and 6 hours in lean and obese men. Metabolism 39:985–992, 1990.

101. Heymsfield SB, Erbland M, Carper K, et al: Enteral nutrition support: Metabolic, cardiovascular pulmonary interrelations. Clin Chest Med 7:41–67, 1986.

102. Vernet O, Christin L, Schutz Y, et al: Enteral versus parenteral nutrition: Comparison of energy metabolism in lean and moderately obese women. Am J Clin Nutr 43:194–209, 1986.

103. Schoeller DA, Fjeld CR: Human energy metabolism: What we have learned from the doubly-labeled water method. Ann Rev Nutr 11:355–373, 1991.

104. Long CL: The energy and protein requirements of the critically ill patient. In Wright RA, Heymsfield S, McManus CB (eds): Nutritional Assessment. Boston, Blackwell Scientific, 1984, pp 157–181.

105. Ireton-Jones CS, Turner WW, Liepa GU, Baxter CR: Equations for estimating energy expenditures in burned patients with special reference to ventilatory status. J Burn Care Rehabil 13:330–333, 1992.

106. Harris JA, Benedict FG: Biometric studies of basal metabolism in man. Carnegie Institute of Washington, publication No. 270. Washington, DC, Carnegie Institute, 1919.

107. Heshka S, Yang M, Wang J, et al: Weight loss and change in resting metabolic rate. Am J Clin Nutr 52:981–986, 1990.

108. Pavlou KN, Hoefer MA, Blackburn GL: Resting energy expenditure in moderate obesity—predicting velocity of weight loss. Ann Surg 203:136–141, 1986.

109. The American Dietetic Association: Manual of Clinical Dietetics. Chicago, ADA, 1988.

110. Ireton-Jones CS, Turner WW: Actual or ideal body weight: Which should be used to predict energy expenditure? J Am Diet Assoc 91:193–195, 1991.

111. Amato P, Keating KP, Quercia RA, Karbonic J: Formulaic methods of estimating calorie requirements in mechanically ventilated obese patients: A reappraisal. Nutr Clin Pract 10:229–232, 1995.

112. Glynn CC, Greene GW, Winkler MF, Albina JE: Predictive versus measured energy expenditure using limits-of-agreement analysis in hospitalized, obese patients. JPEN J Parenter Enteral Nutr 23:147–154, 1999.

113. Owen OE, Holup JL, D'Alessio DA, et al: A reappraisal of the caloric requirements of men. Am J Clin Nutr 46:875–885, 1987.

114. Owen OE, Kavle E, Owen RS, et al: A reappraisal of caloric requirements in healthy women. Am J Clin Nutr 44:1–19, 1986.

115. Heshka S, Feld K, Yang M,et al: Resting energy expenditure in the obese: A cross-validation and comparison of prediction equations. J Am Diet Assoc 93:1031–1036, 1993.

116. Ireton-Jones CS: Evaluation of energy expenditures in obese patients. Nutr Clin Pract 4:127–129, 1989.
117. Munro HN, Crim MC: The proteins and amino acids. *In* Shils ME, Young VR (eds): Modern nutrition in health and disease. Philadelphia, Lea & Febiger, 1988, pp 1–37.
118. Forbes GB: Weight loss during fasting: Implications for the obese. Am J Clin Nutr 23:1212–1219, 1970.
119. Forbes GB, Drenick EJ: Loss of body nitrogen on fasting. Am J Clin Nutr 32:1570–1574, 1979.
120. Yang MU, VanItallie TB: Variability in body protein loss during protracted, severe caloric restriction: Role of triiodothyronine and other determinants. Am J Clin Nutr 40:611–622, 1984.
121. Wadden TA, Stunkard AJ, Brownell KD: Very low calorie diets: Their efficacy, safety, future. Ann Intern Med 99:675–684, 1983.
122. McMahon MM, Bistrian BR: The physiology of nutritional assessment and therapy in protein-calorie malnutrition. Dis Mon 36:373–417, 1990.
123. Editorial: Nutrition and the metabolic response to injury. Lancet 1:995–997, 1989.
124. Shaw JHF, Wolfe RR: An integrated analysis of glucose, fat, and protein metabolism in severely traumatized patients. Ann Surg 209:63–72, 1989.
125. Jeevanandam M, Young DH, Schiller WR: Endogenous protein-synthesis efficiency in trauma victims. Metabolism 38:967–973, 1989.
126. Jeevanandam M, Young DH, Schiller WR: Obesity and the metabolic response to severe multiple trauma in man. J Clin Invest 87:262–269, 1991.
127. Bagley CR, Conklin DN, Isherwood RT, et al: Attitudes of nurses toward obesity and obese patients. Percept Mot Skills 68:954, 1989.
128. Maiman LA, Wang LW, Becker MH, et al: Attitudes toward obesity and the obese among professionals. Research 74:331–336, 1979.
129. Kaplan SP: Rehabilitation counseling students' perceptions of obese male and female clients. Rehabil Counseling Bull 27:172–181, 1984.
130. Young LM, Powell B: The effects of obesity on the clinical judgements of mental health professionals. J Health Soc Behav 26:233–246, 1985.
131. Blumberg P, Mellis LP: Medical students' attitudes toward the obese and the morbidly obese. Int J Eat Disord 4:169–175, 1980.
132. Najman JM, Munro C: Patient characteristics negatively stereotyped by doctors. Soc Sci Med 16:1781–1789, 1982.
133. Price JH, Desmond SM, Krol RA, et al: Family practice physicians' beliefs, attitudes, and practices regarding obesity. Am J Prev Med 3:339–345, 1987.
134. Breytspraak LM, McGee J, Conger JC, et al: Sensitizing medical students to impression formation processes in the patient interview. J Med Educ 52:47–54, 1977.
135. Greenberg GR, Jeejeebhoy KN: Intravenous protein-sparing therapy in patients with gastrointestinal disease. JPEN J Parenter Enteral Nutr 3:427–432, 1979.
136. Dickerson RN, Rosato EF, Mullen JL: Net protein anabolism with hypocaloric parenteral nutrition in obese stressed patients. Am J Clin Nutr 44:747–755, 1986.
137. Collier SB, Walker WA: Parenteral protein-sparing modified fast in an obese adolescent with Prader-Willi syndrome. Nutr Rev 49:235–238, 1991.
138. Abbott WC, Bistrian BR, Blackburn GL: The effect of dextrose and amino acids on respiratory function and energy expenditure in morbidly obese patients following gastric bypass surgery. J Surg Res 41:225–235, 1986.
139. Burge JC, Goon A, Choban PS, Flancbaum L: Efficacy of hypocaloric total parenteral nutrition in hospitalized obese patients: A prospective, double-blind randomized trial. JPEN J Parenter Enteral Nutr 18:203–207, 1994.
140. Choban PS, Burge JC, Scales D, Flancbaum L: Hypoenergetic nutrition support in hospitalized obese patients: A simplified method for clinical application. Am J Clin Nutr 66:546–550, 1997.
141. Pasulka PS, Kohl D: Nutrition support of the stressed obese patient. Nutr Clin Pract 4:130–132, 1989.
142. Baxter JK, Bistrian BR: Moderate hypocaloric parenteral nutrition in the critically ill, obese patient. Nutr Clin Pract 4:133–135, 1989.
143. Stegink LD, Freeman JB, Wispe J, Connor WE: Absence of the biochemical symptoms of essential fatty acid deficiency in surgical patients undergoing protein sparing therapy. Am J Clin Nutr 30:388–393, 1977.
144. Vaughan RW, Bauer S, Wise L: Volume and pH of gastric juice in obese patients. Anesthesiology 43:686–689, 1975.
145. Horowitz M, Collin PJ, Cook DJ, et al: Abnormalities of gastric emptying in obese patients. Int J Obes Relat Metab Disord 7:415–421, 1983.
146. Teabeaut JR II: Aspiration of gastric contents: An experimental study. Am J Pathol 28:51–67, 1952.
147. Clayton JK, Anderson JR, McNicol GP: Preoperative prediction of postoperative deep vein thrombosis. Br J Med 2:910–912, 1976.
148. Racokzi I, Chamone D, Collen D, et al: Prediction of post operative leg-vein thrombosis in gynaecological patients [Letter]. Lancet 1:509–510, 1978.

21

◆ Parenteral Nutrition in the Elderly Patient

James M. Watters, M.D., F.R.C.S.C.

The purpose of this chapter is to describe the ways in which parenteral nutrition in elderly patients differs from that in younger ones. Elderly persons represent a sizable and increasing proportion of the U.S. population in general and of hospitalized patients in particular. Separate consideration is important because elderly patients differ biologically from younger patients in ways that are relevant to their nutritional care. The basic principles of nutritional assessment and support do not depend on the age of the patient, but there are predictable, age-related changes in body composition, pre-existing nutritional status, and tolerance of glucose and protein loads that have important implications for nutritional care. These changes suggest the need to begin nutritional support early, to give particular attention to the choice and rates of substrate administration, and to monitor closely the clinical course and biochemistry of elderly patients.

◆ THE ELDERLY POPULATION

The elderly population is commonly considered to include all persons aged 65 years or more, although our expectations about the health and activities of those in their 60s and early 70s have evolved significantly. This segment of the population has increased both proportionally and in absolute numbers during recent decades, in significant part because of increases in life expectancy. For example, life expectancy at birth for women in the United States was 65 years in 1940 and had increased to 79 years by 1994; life expectancy for men increased from 61 years to 72 years in the same period.[1] Individuals reaching older ages have a significant number of years of life remaining, on average. Current expectations for 70-year-old men and women are an additional 12.5 and 15.3 years of life, and for 85-

year-old men and women, 5.3 and 6.3 years, respectively.[2] Of course, clinical application of these average values for the population must be tempered by a consideration of the individual's health and other factors, which may influence longevity. Many elderly people maintain high levels of physical, social, and intellectual function and live independently, whereas others have multiple medical problems and impaired function, and some may require institutional care. Individuals aged 65 or older represent a heterogeneous group with a tremendous range from the most fit to the most frail. This variability needs to be taken into account in clinical decision making and treatment planning.

There are more or less predictable changes in virtually every physiologic function and organ system that accompany normal aging. These changes are typically gradual and occur throughout adult life, although the extent to which they occur may vary considerably among individuals as a result of genetic, dietary, lifestyle, and other factors. Maximal levels of physiologic function tend to decline (e.g., maximal cardiac output), and the difference between resting and maximal levels (*physiologic reserve*) decreases (e.g., minute ventilation). Greater deviations from homeostatic norms are necessary to trigger physiologic sensors (e.g., baroreceptors), and the mechanisms to restore homeostasis are less efficient (e.g., renal conservation of sodium and water). The result is that deviations from those norms are more marked than in younger individuals. These physiologic limitations in older patients predispose them to clinical complications and demand our close attention to avoid or identify and correct abnormalities related to nutritional support.

◆ STUDIES OF THE ELDERLY POPULATION

Studies of aging may be longitudinal, that is, individuals are assessed at intervals, typically over a period of years. Such studies have made major contributions to our knowledge but are challenging to conduct and are not suited to addressing some questions. Many more research studies are cross-sectional in design, for example, comparing young and older subjects or patients at a single point in time. This and other elements of study design are relevant to determining whether the findings described in a given research report are pertinent to one's own clinical practice. Perhaps most important is a clear description of the individuals studied. The elderly population is heterogeneous in terms of functional status, comorbidity, and even the differences in physiology between healthy young-old persons (65 to 74 years) and the oldest-old (≥85 years of age). Potential study subjects may have been screened to exclude the effects of overt or occult disease, and the extent of screening can influence the findings considerably.

Several biases may occur in cross-sectional studies of aging. For example, elderly subjects are an unavoidably select group by virtue of their having survived to an advanced age, whereas others of their original young cohort have died. Referral bias is common, may take several forms, and needs to be considered in reports of institutional experience. For example, elderly patients referred for major surgical procedures are, in general, likely to be particularly fit; such therapy is not likely to be considered in the frail elderly patient. By contrast, for some clinical problems, patients referred to tertiary care institutions may be less fit than those whose care is undertaken at secondary institutions.

Since individuals obviously cannot be randomly assigned to being young or old, cross-sectional comparisons of age groups are observational. The importance of this is that variables other than age that can influence the outcomes of interest may be both unbalanced between groups and unmeasured.[3] The limitations imposed by study design need to be recognized, but important age-related information can nonetheless be derived and applied to the clinical care of elderly patients.

◆ NUTRITIONAL ASSESSMENT

In conceptual terms, nutritional status may be considered to represent the structural and functional consequences of the balance between nutrient intake and requirements. There is therefore a continuum of nutritional status from normally nourished to profoundly malnourished.[4] The translation of this concept to the clinical assessment of nutritional status is complicated by the range of macro- and micronutrients that may be in inadequate supply, the balance of any one or more of which may be demonstrably inadequate, difficult to determine, or inappropriate to label broadly as malnutrition. The problem of identifying a suitable instrument to measure nutritional status is further complicated by the multiplicity of structural and functional effects of inadequate nutrient intake. It is thus perhaps not surprising that there is no one "gold standard" measure of nutritional status and that a variety of anatomic, biochemical, and functional measures have been employed for different purposes and, in some instances, combined using multivariate statistical techniques.[5] Additionally, nutrient requirements may change with age in individuals in good health, and they change further during acute illness. The desirable attributes of a nutritional assessment tool depend in part on the uses to which the information will be put and in part on the population being assessed. The focus of this chapter is on the elderly patient in whom decisions about parenteral nutritional therapy must be made, most often during a period of hospitalization.

There is ample evidence that malnutrition, variously defined, is accompanied by worse clinical outcomes in elderly patients than occur in a normal nutritional state (see later). We therefore have a practical need to identify those who are malnourished or at risk of becoming so, in order to provide them the nutritional therapy that we believe will improve their clinical outcomes. The attributes of a nutritional assessment instrument that are desirable for use in hospitalized patients are that it be (1) practical in the clinical setting (rapid, cheap, safe, easy to administer, not uncomfortable); (2) predictive of clinical outcomes; (3) reproducible; and (4) responsive, that is, reflecting changes in nutritional status.

Body weight is a simple, aggregate measure of the mass of all tissue compartments. Significant weight loss is a widely used marker of impaired nutritional status and is generally superior to a single weight measurement compared with normal values. Unintentional weight loss of 10% or more is associated with impairments in muscle strength (especially respiratory muscle strength), immune function, wound healing, and thermoregulation.[6] It has been suggested that, in contrast to that in young and middle-aged adults, a weight loss of 5% is clinically significant in elderly individuals.[7] Unfortunately, the accuracy of assessing previous weight by recall, and thus weight change, is limited. In addition, the interpretation in nutritional terms of body weight and weight change measured in the hospital can be confounded by the marked changes in the sizes of body water compartments that can occur during acute illness and treatment. Moreover, although body weight does not change to any great extent with aging, the proportion that is fat tends to increase, whereas lean body mass, body cell mass, and muscle mass tend to decline.

The body mass index normalizes body weight by height (calculated as weight in kilograms divided by height in meters squared). Very low values (14 to 15 kg/m²) are associated with increased mortality.[4] Tables of weight for height for individuals up to the age of 94 years are also available.[8] However, aging is often accompanied by a gradual loss of height, and height may be difficult to measure accurately in patients with limited mobility or kyphosis.

A structured clinical assessment can be completed rapidly, is reliable, and is among the most useful tools for nutritional assessment. Subjective Global Assessment is one such approach that incorporates relevant features of the history and physical examination.[9] Subjective Global Assessment has been demonstrated to have predictive value for nutrition-associated complications and mortality in elderly residents of a long-term care facility that is superior to that of hypoalbuminemia.[10] The features of the history that are elicited are weight change, dietary intake, gastrointestinal symptoms, functional capacity, and the primary disease process in terms of its metabolic demands. Physical examination assesses losses of subcutaneous fat, muscle wasting, dependent edema, and ascites. On this basis, patients are considered to be well nourished (rating A), moderately or suspected of being malnourished (B), or severely malnourished (C). In practice, ratings are most affected by a history of weight loss and losses of subcuta-

neous fat and of muscle. Decubitus ulcers may also be an indicator of malnutrition in institutionalized elderly persons.[11]

The most important component of lost weight in the malnourished patient is protein.[12] It is argued that it is the effect of this loss on various physiologic functions that adversely affects outcomes, and that measures of such functions serve as useful indicators of nutritional status.[13] These include skeletal muscle function (both voluntary and involuntary muscle), respiratory function, and wound healing. In surgical patients with both a recent weight loss of 10% or more and physiologic impairments, the incidence of postoperative pneumonia and septic complications was greater and hospital stays longer than in those patients without weight loss. The same patients were also significantly older on average, and many were elderly, consistent with the loss of muscle mass that accompanies usual aging and underscoring the greater risk of nutrition-related complications in elderly patients.

Muscle mass is typically much reduced in elderly compared with young individuals. It can be assessed in several ways. Endogenous creatinine is derived from the hydrolysis of creatine that is found primarily in skeletal muscle in the form of creatine phosphate.[14] With a number of assumptions, creatinine excretion can be used as an index of muscle mass, 1 g of creatinine being derived from approximately 18 to 20 kg of skeletal muscle. Timed (usually 24-hour) urine collections must be complete, renal function stable, and dietary creatinine ideally avoided. These requirements may be challenging to fulfill in elderly persons, or indeed in patients of any age. Anthropometric measures such as midarm muscle circumference and triceps skin fold thickness are relatively easy to perform. Age-specific norms are available, but the reliability of these measures in individual patients and their ability to detect mild to moderate malnutrition is limited. They are probably most suited to population studies.[4]

Decreased muscle mass in older persons is accompanied by decreased strength. Maximal voluntary handgrip strength has been reported to be a useful predictor of postoperative complications and the length of hospital stay after elective surgical procedures and hip fracture.[15-19] Some reports relate measurements in patients to age- and sex-standardized norms. In some instances, grip strength has been a superior predictor of outcomes when compared with various other indices of nutritional status including weight loss, hypoalbuminemia, and the Prognostic Nutritional Index. Involuntary muscle function, that is, independent of patient cooperation, can be assessed by measuring the characteristics of contraction and relaxation of the adductor pollicis in response to electric stimulation of the ulnar nerve.[4] Muscle function measured in this way appears more sensitive to nutrient restriction and to refeeding than available techniques for the assessment of body composition.

Serum protein concentrations, commonly albumin, are often obtained as markers of visceral protein status. Serum albumin reflects the net result of its rates of synthesis and catabolism, its distribution between intravascular and extravascular compartments, the intravascular volume in which it is distributed, and other factors. Although hypoalbuminemia is a predictor of poor outcomes in hospitalized patients, the relationship is an association rather than a cause-and-effect one. Hypoalbuminemia appears to be a better marker of the severity of acute illness or metabolic stress than it is of nutritional status.

The focus of nutritional assessment is most often on the identification of inadequate protein-calorie intake and malnutrition, but elderly persons are also at risk for micronutrient deficiencies. The clinical signs and symptoms and laboratory assessment of trace element and vitamin status do not differ in elderly persons and are discussed in Chapter 4.

◆ MALNUTRITION IS COMMON

Elderly persons are at risk for malnutrition for several reasons, even before an acute illness. Cross-sectional studies have demonstrated striking decreases in the intake of all nutrients with increasing age.[20] A reduction in caloric intake may be appropriate in relation to decreased physical activity and resting energy expenditure, but the intake of all nutrients tends to decline in parallel. Thus, older individuals are at risk for an inadequate intake of calcium, iron, and other minerals and vitamins. The dietary range of the elderly person may be limited by a lack of awareness of the importance of a balanced diet, poverty, physical and cognitive disabilities, poor dentition, social isolation, and the effects of medication on appetite, taste, nutrient absorption, and metabolism. Low nutrient intake in elderly persons has been associated with a greater likelihood of having disability and comorbidity, but whether the former is a result of the latter remains to be demonstrated.[20] Thus, chronic illness, disability, and the other risk factors noted should raise suspicion and lead to a careful nutritional assessment when identified in an elderly patient. Pre-existing deficiencies in nutrient intake may contribute to the development or progression of acute problems necessitating hospitalization in community-dwelling elderly persons.[21]

Many studies have been conducted to evaluate dietary intake and nutritional status in the elderly population.[22] The prevalence of overt protein-calorie malnutrition among community-dwelling elderly persons is modest,[23] but intakes of specific minerals and vitamins may be less than recommended levels. The efficiency of absorption of some minerals and vitamins may decline with advancing age, and since lean body mass declines as well, their stores may also be smaller.[24, 25] Although requirements for micronutrients in elderly persons are not fully defined, many elderly individuals may have marginal stores or deficiencies that become clinically significant in the face of the increased demands that accompany acute illness. This concept is supported by clinical trials of vitamin and trace element supplementation in elderly persons: daily supplementation in healthy, community-dwelling, elderly subjects resulted in improved immune function and a lower incidence of clinical infections compared with placebo in one study.[26] Comparable findings have been reported in institutionalized elderly subjects.[27]

Malnutrition is more common in elderly residents of nursing homes and other long-term care facilities than in community-dwelling individuals. Reported rates vary considerably, presumably as a result of variation in the specific measures used and in the prevalence of disability, chronic illness, and other factors among the resident populations. Rates from 37 to 85% have been reported.[28–30] Thus, residence in a long-term care facility is a risk factor for malnutrition: an elderly resident who develops a medical or surgical problem necessitating transfer to an acute care hospital should undergo a careful nutritional assessment.

Protein-calorie malnutrition is common among elderly patients in acute care hospitals but is often not recognized or treated.[31] In one study of elderly medical and surgical patients, 39% were considered to be at high risk of having clinically significant malnutrition, but no patient had a diagnosis of malnutrition recorded and very few received any form of nutritional therapy.[32] Low serum albumin levels, the total lymphocyte count, the weight for height, or the body mass index defined the risk of malnutrition. Among patients screened for the Veterans Affairs Total Parenteral Nutrition Cooperative Study of perioperative parenteral nutrition, which included many elderly patients, the prevalence of malnutrition (the Subjective Global Assessment and the Nutritional Risk Index) was 40% or more.[33, 34] Volitional intake in the hospital is frequently inadequate, and weight loss and other markers of nutritional status tend to decline progressively throughout the hospital stay in the absence of nutritional therapy.[31, 35] The most marked ongoing weight loss occurs in those who are most malnourished at admission.[31] A number of factors undoubtedly contribute to inadequate dietary intake, among them decreased appetite. Marked impairment of appetite persists for several weeks in elderly patients after hip fracture, for example.[36]

It is apparent that malnutrition is common among elderly patients with acute medical or surgical problems, that it is frequently not recognized, and that the provision of nutritional therapy is uncommon.[37] Malnutrition is consistently associated with adverse outcomes in elderly, hospitalized patients, and intervention studies in a variety of patient populations provide evidence that nutritional therapy of malnourished patients improves their clinical outcomes.[35, 38–41] All these observations indicate that assessment of nutritional status should be routine in elderly patients admitted to an acute care hospital.

◆ NUTRITIONAL THERAPY SHOULD BE INSTITUTED EARLY IN THE HOSPITALIZED ELDERLY PATIENT

The elderly patient is at significant risk of being malnourished at the time of admission to the hospital and of a worsening nutritional state subsequently unless specific attention is given to the situation. Nutritional assessment should be an integral part of initial and subsequent assessments, not only because the need for nutritional therapy arises frequently but also because it should be begun early, that is, when malnutrition is identified on the initial assessment or when an inadequate nutrient intake is identified or anticipated. Early recognition and therapy are important for two reasons. Elderly patients, even if well-nourished initially, will develop clinically important malnutrition more rapidly during acute illness than will younger patients, and restoration of a normal nutritional state is more difficult to achieve in older patients once malnourished.

Body cell mass declines progressively with age, both in absolute terms and as a proportion of lean body mass. The decrease can be accounted for in large part by a decrease in muscle mass that is as much as 40 to 45% comparing a person 70 years of age with a young adult (Fig. 21–1). Comparable declines in the strength of many muscle groups occur and have functional consequences. For example, by the age of 80 years, the average woman is at the threshold of quadriceps strength for rising from a low armless chair, having lost the considerable reserve strength of earlier years.[42] Thus, the strength of elderly patients is very likely to fall rapidly below important clinical thresh-

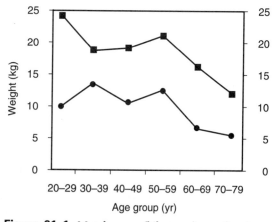

Figure 21–1. Muscle mass (kilograms) as a function of age in males (squares) and females (circles). (Data from Cohn SH, Vartsky D, Yasumura S, et al: Compartmental body composition based on total-body nitrogen, potassium, and calcium. Am J Physiol 1980; 239:E524–E530, 1980.)

olds during even brief periods of inadequate nutrition, physical inactivity, or acute illness. Mobility and respiratory muscle strength will be impaired, and the likelihood of clinically recognized complications increased proportionately. The problem is compounded for the elderly patient by moderate to severe acute illness, the metabolic responses to which are characterized by skeletal muscle catabolism, rapid erosion of lean tissue, and negative nitrogen balance.[43]

Early implementation of nutritional therapy is also important because the establishment of effective nutritional support is typically more challenging in the elderly patient and malnutrition more difficult to correct. Older patients may be less tolerant of fluid loads, especially if coronary artery disease is present and ventricular function is impaired. Glucose intolerance is common among older individuals, and the glucose intolerance that arises during acute illness is exaggerated in elderly patients (see later). Insulin responses to glucose loading are impaired in acutely ill elderly patients, contributing both to glucose intolerance and to ongoing catabolism. In addition, the restoration of body cell mass in malnourished patients receiving parenteral nutrition occurs more slowly in elderly patients than in younger patients receiving similar calorie and protein loads.[44]

◆ DECIDING TO INITIATE PARENTERAL NUTRITION

When malnutrition or inadequate nutrient intake is identified in the elderly patient, first consideration is given to optimizing volitional intake. Volitional intake is commonly inadequate in hospitalized patients, but only a small proportion of malnourished elderly patients are able increase their intake sufficiently to correct their nutritional deficit.[45] The use of oral protein-calorie supplements may allow the target intake to be reached in some patients. For others, especially when voluntary intake is less than one half of requirements, the establishment of enteral access and feeding should be considered.[34] A number of options are available to accomplish this.

The decision to initiate parenteral nutrition in an elderly patient is based on the same principles as in younger patients, with the distinction that the *threshold* for insti-

tuting nutrition support (whether enteral or parenteral) should be lower in the elderly patient for the reasons discussed earlier. The enteral route is superior in concept and practice in a number of ways, but obtaining reliable access may present problems or undue risks. Enteral feeding may also not be well tolerated or may take some time to establish at desired rates. Parenteral nutrition offers an immediate, reliable nutrient supply and should be initiated when nutritional support is required and the enteral route is expected to be unreliable or undesirable. Especially in the elderly patient, it should be considered as an interim measure when there is significant question about the likelihood of promptly establishing effective enteral feeding. The use of peripheral vein catheters and solutions or peripherally inserted central catheters may be useful for this purpose. Continued use of the gastrointestinal tract is advantageous even when nutrient requirements cannot be met: parenteral nutrition may be useful as an adjunct in this setting in order to allow nutrient targets to be reached.

Ideally, the primary medical problem of the patient for whom parenteral nutrition is under consideration is being actively treated and there is an identifiable end-point for parenteral support. If it is apparent from the outset that a patient is likely to require long-term, possibly home, parenteral nutrition, then the initial assessment should include consideration of placement options and the availability of assistance at home.[34] Enteral nutrition is much simpler than parenteral nutrition at home or in a long-term care institution. Decisions about home parenteral nutrition (see later) should normally be based more on the underlying diagnosis, the wishes of the patient, and the ability to manage the therapy than on the age of the patient.

◆ PROVIDING PARENTERAL NUTRITION

Venous Access and Solutions

Deciding on the use of peripheral or central venous solutions and peripheral, peripherally inserted central, or single- or multilumen central vein catheters is similar in elderly and younger patients. Since parenteral support should be started as an adjunctive or interim measure more frequently in elderly patients, the use of peripheral parenteral nutrition may be more common. In situations in which fluid restriction is a high priority, the more concentrated nutrient solutions tolerated only by central veins or the use of lipid as the primary calorie source may be advantageous. When multilumen catheters are used, it is important to ensure that the end of the lumen used for hypertonic nutrient solutions is within the superior vena cava. The second and third lumens may end several centimeters from the tip of the catheter and may not provide the blood flow, mixing, and dilution that are necessary if they are situated too proximally. In very frail or cachectic patients, regardless of age, the pleura may lie very close to the clavicle, increasing the risk of puncture and pneumothorax.[34] The incidence of line sepsis is not notably greater in the elderly patient.

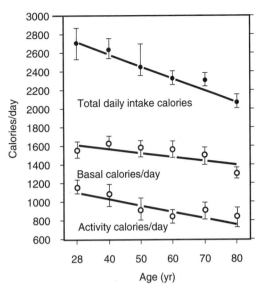

Figure 21–2. Total daily calorie intake and daily expenditure attributable to resting metabolism and activity in normal males. (From Shock NW: Energy metabolism, caloric intake and physical activity of the aging. *In* Carlson LA (ed): Nutrition in Old Age. 10th Symposium of the Swedish Nutrition Foundation. Uppsala, Almqvist and Wiksell, 1972, pp 12–23. Data of McGandy RB, Barrows CH Jr, Spanias A, et al: Nutrient intakes and energy expenditure in men of different ages. J Gerontol 21:587, 1966.)

Caloric Requirements

Energy expenditure is predictably lower in healthy elderly subjects than in younger subjects, since both resting energy expenditure and energy expenditure in physical activities decline (Fig. 21–2). The decrease in resting energy expenditure is approximately 1 to 2% per decade in adults aged 20 to 75 years and can be estimated as metabolic rate (kcal/m^2/hr) = 37 − ([age (yr) − 20]/10).[46 (p 27)] This decline is related principally to age-related changes in body composition, and the widely cited Harris-Benedict equations incorporate weight, height, sex, and age:[47]

Heat Production in Men (kcal/day) =
66.473 + 13.7516 × Weight (kg) +
5.003 × Height (cm) − 6.775 × Age (yr)

Heat Production in Women (kcal/day) =
655.0955 + 9.5634 × weight (kg) +
1.8496 × Height (cm) − 4.6756 × Age
(yr)

Fat mass tends to increase and lean body mass to decrease with advancing age, whereas body weight changes relatively little. Lean body mass comprises extracellular mass and body cell mass. The body cell mass is the component "containing the oxygen-consuming, potassium-rich, glucose-oxidizing, work-performing tissue."[48] The body cell mass decreases with age, even in

relation to a reduced lean body mass.[48] The resting energy expenditure is closely related to the lean body mass and to the body cell mass: when expressed in terms of body weight, the resting energy expenditure decreases in parallel with the changes in body composition that accompany normal aging.[49, 50] Utilizing the regression equations of Moore and colleagues,[48 (p 158)] the decrease in lean body mass in healthy individuals is approximately 12% between ages 30 and 80 years for both males and females. This difference is similar to the difference in basal energy expenditure observed over the same age range.[51] These values represent group means for healthy individuals, however, and estimates of body composition and resting energy expenditure made in the clinical setting must take into account the considerable interindividual variability among elderly patients. For example, a frail elderly woman with limited mobility and multiple medical problems will have a lean body mass, body cell mass, and skeletal muscle mass that are very small even relative to other women of the same age. The body composition of a healthy elderly man who has maintained a high level of physical activity on a lifelong basis is likely to be "youthful" relative to that of his more sedentary peers.[52]

Expenditure in physical activities is also a major contributor to the total daily energy expenditure. An average difference approaching 45% in energy expenditure has been described in older research comparing men aged 20 to 34 years with those 75 to 99 years.[51] With the combined effects of body composition and physical activity, the difference in total daily energy expenditure between healthy young and older men was approximately 22%, estimated as a decrease of 12.4 kcal/day/yr using dietary records.[51] More recent work suggests that age-related changes in levels of activity still persist, although patterns of activity and gender roles have altered significantly.[53]

The observation that energy expenditure for routine activities in healthy individuals declines with age may not be wholly relevant to the hospitalized elderly patient, whose level of physical activity is often quite limited. However, energy expenditure does increase significantly in relation to the accelerated metabolic activity and increased cardiopulmonary work of acute illness. Age-related variation in the increases in energy expenditure following the moderate stress of major elective abdominal surgery can be accounted for by differences in body composition.[54] Age-related changes in the maximal energy expenditure during exercise may provide some insight into the maximal responses to severe, acute illness. Maximal oxygen consumption declines consistently with age and does so as a function of the habitual level of activity.[55, 56] For example, the rate of decline is approximately 12% per decade among sedentary males and 5.5% among master athletes.[55] Whether there are clinical consequences of lower maximal energy expenditure in elderly patients is not known.

In summary, the influence of the patient's age on energy expenditure results principally from its association with changes in body composition. A knowledge of these changes and the use of predictive equations are useful, but there is considerable heterogeneity among elderly patients, and individual nutrient prescriptions must be tempered by careful clinical assessment of the patient for whom parenteral nutrition is being considered. Appropriate targets for providing calories to the elderly patient are often in the range of 20 to 25 kcal/kg/day. Derivation of energy expenditure from the measurement of respiratory gas exchange using a metabolic cart may be helpful on occasion. As discussed later, elderly patients often tolerate fluid and nutrient loads less well than younger patients do. For this reason, parenteral nutrient administration should be begun at a modest rate, providing perhaps one half of the caloric target initially. Rates can then be increased with careful biochemical monitoring, ongoing evaluation of the patient's clinical course, adjustment of both nutrient mixture and target values as appropriate, and the use of adjunctive measures such as exogenous insulin. Regardless of the initial estimate of their nutrient requirements, elderly patients are at particular risk for serious and even life-threatening adverse effects when parenteral nutrients are administered in excessive quantities.

Glucose

Glucose commonly serves as the major parenteral calorie source in the elderly patient as it does in younger ones, but elderly patients are more likely to become hyperglycemic for several reasons. Predictable changes in carbohydrate metabolism that accompany normal aging include increased blood glucose levels, decreased glucose tolerance, and decreased insulin sensitivity. These changes interact in clinically important ways with the alterations in glucose homeostasis that accompany acute illness, usually to the detriment of the elderly patient.

Ten percent of the U.S. population aged 65 or older have diagnosed diabetes mellitus, and the prevalence of undiagnosed diabetes is similar.[57] Altogether, 40% of those aged 65 or older have either diabetes mellitus or impaired glucose tolerance (Fig. 21–3). Even in normal individuals, there is a progressive age-related increase in the hyperglycemia that follows oral or intravenous glucose loads.[58] Several factors contribute to this decline in glucose tolerance. Non–insulin-mediated glucose disposal is reduced in older subjects.[59] The ultradian oscillations of insulin secretion in older subjects are similar to those of diabetic patients and suggest a decreased pancreatic β-cell responsiveness to glucose changes.[60] In addition to these factors, many studies have suggested that impaired sensitivity of tis-

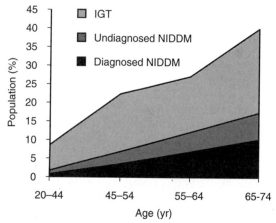

Figure 21–3. Prevalence of undiagnosed and diagnosed diabetes mellitus and impaired glucose tolerance. IGT, impaired glucose tolerance. (From Kenny SJ, Aubert RE, Geiss LS: Prevalence and incidence of non-insulin-dependent diabetes. *In* National Diabetes Data Group (eds): Diabetes in America, 2nd ed. Washington, DC, National Institutes of Health, National Institute of Diabetes and Digestive and Kidney Diseases, 1995, pp 47–68.)

sues to the effects of insulin is an important factor.[58, 59, 61–64] Renal clearance of glucose is normally an important defense against hyperglycemia. The renal glucose threshold increases with age, however, making elderly patients even more prone to hyperglycemia and a hyperosmolar state.[65]

Older age influences the changes in carbohydrate metabolism that typically follow injury or accompany acute illness. Blood glucose values following injury increase as a function of both age and the severity of injury.[66] Plasma insulin responses to glucose loading have been compared in young and older trauma patients and similarly aged healthy subjects using the hyperglycemic glucose clamp technique (Table 21–1).[67] Both age and injury effects on glucose tolerance were observed, such that the disposal of exogenous glucose was least in older patients, approximately one third that in young controls.[67] Plasma insulin values were markedly lower in the older trauma patients in comparison with those of the young patients. Lower plasma and urine C-peptide values suggest that the diminished plasma insulin responses of older patients result from diminished insulin secretion.[67] A similar age-related increase in plasma glucose levels and reduction in the plasma insulin response to the glucose loading of parenteral nutrition has been observed in a variety of patient groups.[68, 69] Increases in endogenous glucose production during acute illness are well recognized and increase as a function of both the patient's age and the severity of injury.[70] Presumably age-related exaggeration of the increases in endogenous glucose production contributes to more frequent and marked hyperglycemia in older patients receiving glucose loads and results from their higher serum cortisol concentrations and lesser pancreatic insulin secretion.[66, 68, 70–72]

Thus, increases in blood glucose levels during parenteral nutrition are more marked in older patients, and their risk of significant hyperglycemia and hyperosmolar states is greater.[68] Hyperglycemia adversely affects phagocytosis by polymorphonuclear leukocytes, and chemotaxis, phagocytosis, and intracellular killing are impaired in diabetic subjects.[73, 74] Such immunologic defects may contribute to higher incidences of surgical wound infections in diabetic patients.[75] Effective control of blood glucose levels in diabetic surgical patients is associated with a severalfold reduction in nosocomial infections.[76] Hyperglycemia can result in glycosylation of proteins and impairment of their functions. Glycosylation of immunoglobulins may contribute to the development of infections, and glycosylation of collagen can impair wound healing. Wound healing is adversely affected both by wound infection and by interference of hyperglycemia in ascorbate transfer into fibroblasts and leukocytes.[77] Acute hyperglycemia increases vascular tone and reduces blood flow in regional tissue beds, in association with

Table 21–1. Exogenous Glucose Disposal and Serum Insulin Levels During 20% Glucose Infusion After Injury*

	Glucose Disposal† (mg/kg/min)	Plasma Insulin† (pmol/L)
Young subjects	10.5 ± 3.8	432 ± 172
Older subjects	5.0 ± 1.4	393 ± 249
Young patients	5.4 ± 1.8	880 ± 375
Older patients	3.6 ± 1.0	233 ± 134

*Whole-body disposal of exogenous hypertonic (20%) glucose during fixed hyperglycemia, i.e., glucose tolerance, is impaired by both injury and older age. Serum insulin levels in young patients increase rapidly and are markedly higher than those of older patients.
†Mean ± SD.
Data from Watters JM, Moulton SB, Clancey SM, et al: Aging exaggerates glucose intolerance following injury. J Trauma 37:786–791, 1994.

increases in catecholamine release and oxidative stress.[78–80] Uncontrolled hyperglycemia resulting from either an enteral or a parenteral glucose load may give rise to hyperosmolar nonketotic coma, in which serum osmolarity and glucose levels are markedly elevated in association with a solute diuresis, dehydration, coma, and inappropriately low insulin and ketone levels.

Because of the predisposition to hyperglycemia, the administration of parenteral solutions with hypertonic glucose should be initiated at a modest rate in the elderly patient and increased gradually as tolerance is confirmed. A maximal rate of glucose administration of 4 mg/kg of body weight per minute has been advocated, regardless of the patient's age.[81] The use of alternative calorie sources such as 10 or 20% lipid is often helpful in reaching target values for calorie administration. Blood glucose levels should be monitored using reagent strips or other means for at least 24 to 48 hours after initiating parenteral nutrition, particularly if previous levels have been elevated. Mild hyperglycemia may possibly be beneficial in promoting glucose uptake by inflammatory cells and other tissues of healing wounds, but glucose concentrations above 10 mmol/L are increasingly likely to be accompanied by the adverse effects described earlier. When significant hyperglycemia occurs despite appropriate glucose infusion rates, then it should be corrected with insulin. This can be accomplished by intermittent subcutaneous injections of regular insulin using a scale based on glucose values from reagent strips. Once an estimate of insulin requirements is made, then more effective control can often be achieved by adding insulin to the parenteral solution. Separate intravenous insulin infusion may be useful in critical care or other areas with close nursing supervision when fluctuating insulin requirements are anticipated. Insulin has anabolic effects and can diminish the negative nitrogen balance associated with injury and other major stresses.[82–84] Fatty liver may occur with excessive glucose and insulin administration.

Lipid

Lipid emulsions are a useful parenteral calorie source in elderly patients and provide essential fatty acids. They are calorie dense and thus are useful in minimizing the fluid volumes necessary to reach caloric goals and when hyperglycemia limits glucose administration. They can be infused by a peripheral vein and serve as the principal calorie source for peripheral parenteral nutrition. Plasma triglyceride levels should be monitored regularly when lipid is infused since they tend to increase with normal aging and because lipid clearance may be altered.[85] Lipid turnover increases during acute illness, and clearance mechanisms may become overloaded, resulting in hypertriglyceridemia.

Protein

Protein prescriptions in elderly patients are generally similar to those in younger patients although attention must be given to alterations in renal function. Age-related declines in the glomerular filtration rate and creatinine clearance are significant and predictable even though serum creatinine values are relatively unchanged. Since muscle mass, that is, the principal source of creatinine, decreases with increasing age, serum creatinine values tend to remain within the laboratory normal range despite a considerable reduction in creatinine clearance. Age-related decreases in renal function may lead, on occasion, to azotemia in elderly patients receiving protein in amounts that would be well tolerated in younger patients.[86] For this reason, blood urea nitrogen values should be monitored on a regular basis. Whereas healthy adults can maintain normal protein economy ingesting protein at levels of 0.8 g/kg/day, requirements are greater during acute illness, and an initial target of 1 to 1.5 g/kg/day is appropriate for most elderly hospitalized patients. The protein prescription should be adjusted in patients with renal or hepatic insufficiency and reassessed in all patients as their biochemical tolerance and clinical course are followed. Skeletal muscle wasting and negative nitrogen balance are exacerbated by inactivity. Recovering and maintaining optimal muscle function in the elderly patient often requires an active promotion of and assistance with physical activity.[87]

Fluid Administration

Alterations in renal, cardiovascular, and endocrine function make close attention to fluid and electrolyte management mandatory in the elderly patient receiving parenteral nutrition, especially so in patients with coexisting cardiac or renal disease. Homeostatic mechanisms in younger patients are quite effective in maintaining the constancy of the internal milieu despite a wide range of physiologic insults. By contrast, elderly patients are less sensitive to disturbances of electrolyte, fluid, and acid-base status, and they have less effective compensatory mechanisms for restoring and maintaining homeostatic norms. Insensible fluid losses through the thinned skin of elderly individuals are greater than in younger subjects, resulting in an increased minimal requirement for water. Older subjects are less able to decrease urine flow and to increase urine osmolarity in response to water deprivation, and the time required to achieve sodium equilibrium in the presence of sodium restriction is prolonged. Elderly persons also have a decreased ability to excrete acute loads of water or salt and thus are likely to experience relatively prolonged extracellular fluid volume expansion with such loads. They are prone to excessive secretion of antidiuretic hormone, especially during the stress of acute illness, and to hyponatremia. Hyponatremia and water intoxication can be manifest as lethargy, confusion, weakness, and, if severe, seizures or coma. Restoration of normal body water compartments during recovery from acute illness is less rapid in older than in younger patients.[88]

Vitamins and Trace Elements

Vitamin and trace element administration in elderly patients is similar to that in younger patients. Our knowledge of requirements for inorganic elements in the elderly patient is incomplete, but their intake tends to be reduced in parallel with decreased energy intake.[24] Absorption from the gastrointestinal tract may also be reduced and stores diminished since lean body mass is decreased.[89] Deficiencies may therefore arise in elderly patients because of increased requirements during acute illness, even though their usual diet provides adequate vitamins and trace elements in the absence of stress. Increased requirements for a number of vitamins and trace elements have been identified during acute illness.[90] These have potential effects on immune function (vitamins A, C, D, E,

and B_6, pantothenic acid, folic acid, and zinc), wound healing (vitamins A, C, and B_2, pantothenic acid, and selenium), and defenses against free radical injury (vitamins A, C, and E). Even in healthy elderly subjects, daily supplementation with physiologic quantities of micronutrients has been shown to enhance immune function and reduce clinical infections.[26] Thus, with increased requirements during acute illness and the possibility that stores are diminished because of prior low dietary intake and alterations in body composition, micronutrient administration is of special importance in the elderly patient.

Growth Factors

Growth hormone is a potent anabolic agent with properties that suggest it as an attractive adjunct to nutritional therapy in the elderly patient, at least in concept.[12, 69] Growth hormone promotes muscle protein synthesis, the preservation of muscle strength, accelerated wound healing, and increased fat lipolysis.[91] However, its use can be accompanied by impaired glucose tolerance and the retention of sodium and water. Growth hormone has been associated with increased mortality in a large study of critically ill adults but not in another of pediatric burn patients.[92, 93] Many of the anabolic effects of growth are mediated by insulin-like growth factor I (IGF-I). The capacity for the liver to synthesize IGF-I seems to be necessary for the anabolic effects of growth hormone and may be insufficient in severely ill patients. Additionally, in young trauma patients, nutritional support is accompanied by increased circulating IGF-I levels; this response is impaired in elderly patients.[94] IGF-I administration is not accompanied by the hyperglycemia observed with growth hormone, and its potential clinical use is the subject of ongoing investigation.

◆ INFLUENCE OF PARENTERAL NUTRITION ON OUTCOMES

The early initiation of nutritional therapy in hospitalized elderly patients who are malnourished or at risk is reasonable since it seems very likely that nutrition-related morbidity and mortality are clinically important and can be reduced. However, evidence documenting the postulated improvements in clinical outcomes resulting from parenteral nutrition is limited. Few studies have included significant numbers of elderly patients, and fewer still have focused on them. Perhaps the most compelling data are from the Veterans Affairs Total Parenteral Nutrition Cooperative Study, a randomized clinical trial of perioperative parenteral nutrition in middle-aged and elderly patients (63 ± 10 years, mean ± SD) undergoing major elective noncardiac surgery.[33] A net clinical benefit was identified but only in the most severely malnourished patients, who had fewer noninfectious complications than control patients did. Recent progress in our understanding of energy, protein, and micronutrient requirements and of the potential roles of specific nutrients such as glutamine and arginine suggest that current nutritional therapy should achieve outcomes in appropriately selected patients that are comparable or superior.[5]

Hospitalized elderly patients are predisposed to respiratory complications, impaired oxygen transport, and respiratory failure for many reasons.[95] Parenteral nutrition was associated with a restoration of body cell mass and an improvement in respiratory muscle strength in a study of malnourished patients as old as 86 years.[96]

◆ HOME PARENTERAL NUTRITION

Home parenteral nutrition can be an effective therapy in the elderly patient and is much more cost-effective than providing the same support in the hospital. Among home parenteral nutrition patients, both the pediatric and geriatric groups have increased more rapidly than the overall number of patients.[97] The principles of care are similar to those in younger patients, although elderly patients are usually more dependent on another adult in the household or a professional caregiver. Home parenteral nutrition is most appropriate in patients with benign diagnoses. Most deaths in patients receiving home parenteral nutrition are attributable to the primary disease, whereas relatively few are related to nutritional therapy.[97] Therapy-related complications are no more frequent than in younger adults and are less common than in pediatric patients. In a recent study of patients with short bowel syndrome

maintained on long-term parenteral nutrition, successful bowel rehabilitation was independent of the patients' age.[98] Age appears to adversely affect outcomes in patients receiving home parenteral nutrition, specifically survival during therapy, but not to the extent that age per se should be a major determinant of the use of home parenteral nutrition.[97]

SUMMARY

Hospitalized elderly patients are a heterogeneous population, but they are at significant risk for presenting to the hospital with or developing both protein-calorie and micronutrient deficiencies. Nutritional assessment should be routine at admission and at intervals thereafter. In elderly patients requiring nutritional support, parenteral nutrition is indicated when the early establishment of effective enteral nutrition cannot be relied on and should be initiated early in the hospital course. Peripheral parenteral nutrition can be a valuable interim measure when the clinical course and volitional or enteral intake are uncertain. The physiologic and metabolic changes of aging compound those that accompany acute illness and predispose the elderly patient to complications from parenteral nutrition. Energy requirements, but not requirements for protein or micronutrients, are reduced in elderly persons. Parenteral nutrition should be initiated at a modest rate in the elderly patient and increased gradually, with careful clinical and biochemical monitoring.

REFERENCES

1. Singh GK, Kochanek KD, MacDorman MF: Advance report of final mortality statistics, 1994. [Abstract]. Monthly Vital Statistics Report 45(3)Suppl: Sept 30, 1996, p 19. Hyattsville, Md, National Center for Health Statistics.
2. Ventura SJ, Peters KD, Martin JA, Maurer JD: Births and Deaths: United States 1996, Vol 46, No 1, Suppl 2. Hyattsville, Md, National Center for Health Statistics, 1997.
3. Brennan P, Croft P: Interpreting the results of observational research: Chance is not such a fine thing. BMJ 309:727–730, 1994.
4. Jeejeebhoy KN: Nutritional Assessment. Gastroenterol Clin North Am 27:347–369, 1998.
5. Klein S, Kinney J, Jeejeebhoy K, et al: Nutrition support in clinical practice: Review of published data and recommendations for future research di-

rections. JPEN J Parenter Enteral Nutr 21:133–156, 1997.

6. Allison SP: Cost-effectiveness of nutritional support in the elderly. Proc Nutr Soc 54:693–699, 1995.

7. Beck AM, Ovesen L: At which body mass index and degree of weight loss should hospitalized elderly patients be considered at nutritional risk? Clin Nutr 17:195–198, 1998.

8. Master AM, Lasser RP, Beckman G: Tables of average weight and height of Americans aged 65 to 94 years. JAMA 172:658–662, 1960.

9. Detsky AS, McLaughlin JR, Baker JP, et al: What is Subjective Global Assessment of nutritional status? JPEN J Parenter Enteral Nutr 11:8–13, 1987.

10. Sacks G, Dearman K, Replogle B, Canada T: Evaluation of malnutrition with Subjective Global Assessment in geriatric longterm care facility patients. JPEN 22:S11, 1998.

11. Allman RM, Laprade CA, Noel LB, et al: Pressure sores among hospitalized patients. Ann Intern Med 105:337–342, 1986.

12. Wilmore DW: Does loss of body protein determine outcome in patients who are critically ill? Ann Surg 228:143–145, 1998.

13. Windsor JA, Hill GL: Weight loss with physiologic impairment. A basic indicator of surgical risk. Ann Surg 207:290–296, 1988.

14. Lukaski H: Sarcopenia: Assessment of muscle mass. J Nutr 127:994S–997S, 1997.

15. Klidjian AM, Foster KJ, Kammerling RM, et al: Relation of anthropometric and dynamometric variables to serious postoperative complications. BMJ 281:899–901, 1980.

16. Webb AR, Newman LA, Taylor M, Keough JB: Hand grip dynamometry as a predictor of postoperative complications. Reappraisal using age standardized grip strengths. JPEN J Parenter Enteral Nutr 13:30–33, 1989.

17. Kalfarentzos F, Spiliotis J, Velimezis G, et al: Comparison of forearm muscle dynamometry with nutritional prognostic index, as a preoperative indicator in cancer patients. JPEN J Parenter Enteral Nutr 13:34–36, 1989.

18. Twiston Davies CW, Moody Jones D, Shearer JR: Hand grip—A simple test for morbidity after fracture of the neck of femur. J R Soc Med 77:833–836, 1984.

19. Hunt DR, Rowlands BJ, Johnston D: Hand grip strength—A simple prognostic indicator in surgical patients. JPEN J Parenter Enteral Nutr 9:701–704, 1985.

20. Exton-Smith AN: Nutritional status: Diagnosis and prevention of malnutrition. *In* Exton-Smith AN, Caird FI (eds): Metabolic and Nutritional Disorders of the Elderly. Bristol, John Wright & Sons, 1980, pp 66–76.

21. Mowe M, Bohmer T, Kindt E: Reduced nutritional status in an elderly population (> 70 years) is probable before disease and possibly contributes to the development of disease. Am J Clin Nutr 59:317–324, 1994.

22. Ausman LM, Russell RM: Nutrition and aging. *In* Schneider EL, Rowe JL (eds): Handbook of the Biology of Aging, 3rd ed. San Diego, Academic Press, 1990, p 384–406.

23. Department of Health and Social Security: A Nutrition Survey of the Elderly. Reports on Health and Social Subjects. Report No. 16. London, HMSO, 1979.

24. Mertz W: Trace elements in the elderly. Nutrition 12:549–550, 1996.

25. Russell RM: Micronutrient requirements of the elderly. Nutr Rev 50:463–466, 1992.

26. Chandra RK: Effect of vitamin and trace-element supplementation on immune responses and infection in elderly subjects. Lancet 340:1124–1127, 1992.

27. Girodon F, Lombard M, Galan P, et al: Effect of micronutrient supplementation on infection in institutionalized elderly subjects: A controlled trial. Ann Nutr Metab 41(2):98–107, 1997.

28. Pinchcofsky-Devin GD, Kaminski MV: Incidence of protein-calorie malnutrition in the nursing home patient. J Am Coll Nutr 6:109–112, 1987.

29. Rudman D, Feller AG, Nagruj HS, et al: Relation of serum albumin concentration to death rate in nursing home men. JPEN J Parenter Enteral Nutr 11:360–363, 1987.

30. Shaver HJ, Loper JA, Lutes RA: Nutritional status of nursing home patients. JPEN J Parenter Enteral Nutr 4:367–370, 1980.

31. McWhirter JP, Pennington CR: Incidence and recognition of malnutrition in hospital. BMJ 308:945–947, 1994.

32. Sullivan DH, Moriarty MS, Chernoff R, Lipschitz DA: Patterns of care: An analysis of the quality of nutritional care routinely provided to elderly hospitalized veterans. JPEN J Parenter Enteral Nutr 13:249–254, 1989.

33. Veterans Affairs Total Parenteral Nutrition Cooperative Study Group: Perioperative total parenteral nutrition in surgical patients. N Engl J Med 325:525–532, 1991.

34. Rolandelli RH, Ullrich JR: Nutritional support in the frail elderly surgical patient. Surg Clin North Am 74:79–92, 1994.

35. Larsson J, Unosson M, Ek AC, et al: Effect of dietary supplement on nutritional status and clinical outcome in 501 geriatric patients—A randomised study. Clin Nutr 9:179–184, 1990.

36. Older MWJ, Edwards D, Dickerson JWT: A nutrient survey in elderly women with femoral neck fractures. Br J Surg 67:884–886, 1980.

37. Allison SP: Outcomes from nutritional support in the elderly. Nutrition 14:479–480, 1998.

38. Del Savio G, Zelicof SB, Wexler LM, et al: Preoperative nutritional status and outcome of elective total hip replacement. Clin Orthop 326:153–161, 1996.

39. Volkert D, Hübsch S, Oster P, Schlierf G: Nutritional support and functional status in undernourished geriatric patients during hospitalization and 6-month follow-up. Aging Clin Exp Res 8:386–395, 1996.

40. Bastow MD, Rawlings J, Allison SP: Benefits of supplementary tube feeding after fractured neck of femur: A randomised controlled trial. BMJ 287:1589–1592, 1983.

41. Potter J, Langhorne P, Roberts M: Routine protein energy supplementation in adults: Systematic review. BMJ 317: 495–501, 1998.

42. Young A: Exercise physiology in geriatric practice. Acta Med Scand Suppl 711:227–232, 1986.

43. Plank LD, Connolly AB, Hill GL: Sequential changes in the metabolic response in severely septic patients during the first 23 days after the onset of peritonitis. Ann Surg 228:146–158, 1998.

44. Shizgal HM, Martin MF, Gimmon Z: The effect of age on the caloric requirement of malnourished individuals. Am J Clin Nutr 55:783–789, 1992.

45. Lipschitz DA: Nutrition and health in the elderly. Curr Opin Gastroenterol 7:277–283, 1991.

46. Wilmore DW: The Metabolic Management of the Critically Ill. New York, Plenum Press, 1977.

47. Harris JA, Benedict FG: A Biometric Study of Basal Metabolism in Man. Philadelphia, JB Lippincott, 1919, pp 40–44.

48. Moore FD, Olesen KH, McMurrey JD, et al: The Body Cell Mass and Its Supporting Environment. Philadelphia, WB Saunders, 1963.

49. Kinney JM, Lister J, Moore FD: Relationship of energy expenditure to total exchangeable potassium. Ann N Y Acad Sci 110:711–722, 1963.

50. Tzankoff SP, Norris AH: Effect of muscle mass decrease on age-related BMR changes. J Appl Physiol 43:1001–1006, 1977.

51. McGandy RB, Barrows CH Jr, Spanias A, et al: Nutrient intakes and energy expenditure in men of different ages. J Gerontol 21:587, 1966.

52. Skrobak-Kaczynski J, Andersen KL: The effect of a high level of habitual physical activity in the regulation of fatness during aging. Int Arch Occup Environ Health 36:41–46, 1975.

53. Verbrugge LM, Gruber-Baldini AL, Fozard JL: Age differences and age changes in activities: Baltimore Longitudinal Study of Aging. J Gerontol B Psychol Sci Soc Sci 51B: (S30–S41), 1996.

54. Watters JM, Redmond ML, Desai D, March RJ: Effects of age and body composition on the metabolic responses to elective colon resection. Ann Surg 212:89–96, 1990.

55. Rogers MA, Hagberg JM, Martin WH III, et al: Decline in VO_2 max with aging in master athletes and sedentary men. J Appl Physiol 68:2195–2199, 1990.

56. Dehn MM, Bruce RA: Longitudinal variations in maximal oxygen intake with age and activity. J Appl Physiol 33:805–807, 1972.

57. Kenny SJ, Aubert RE, Geiss LS: Prevalence and incidence of non-insulin-dependent diabetes. In National Diabetes Data Group (ed): Diabetes in America, 2nd ed. Washington DC, National Institutes of Health, National Institute of Diabetes and Digestive and Kidney Diseases, pp 47–68, 1995.

58. Davidson MB: The effect of aging on carbohydrate metabolism. Metabolism 28:688–705, 1979.

59. Meneilly GS, Elahi D, Minaker KL, et al: Impairment of noninsulin-mediated glucose disposal in the elderly. J Clin Endocrinol Metab 63:566–571, 1989.

60. Scheen AJ, Sturis J, Polonsky KS, Van Cauter E: Alterations in the ultradian oscillations of insulin secretion and plasma glucose in aging. Diabetologia 39:564–572, 1996.

61. Andres R, Tobin JD: Aging and the disposition of glucose. Adv Exp Med Biol 61:239–249, 1975.

62. Rowe JW, Minaker KL, Pallotta JA, Flier JS: Characterization of the insulin resistance of aging. J Clin Invest 71:1581–1587, 1983.

63. DeFronzo RA: Glucose intolerance and aging: Evidence for tissue insensitivity to insulin. Diabetes 28:1095–1101, 1979.

64. Chen M, Bergman RN, Pacini G, Porte D Jr: Pathogenesis of age-related glucose intolerance in man: Insulin resistance and decreased beta-cell function. J Clin Endocrinol Metab 60:13–20, 1985.

65. Butterfield WJH, Keen H, Whichelow MJ: Renal glucose threshold variations with age. BMJ 4:505–507, 1967.

66. Desai D, March RJ, Watters JM: Hyperglycemia following trauma increases with age. J Trauma 29:719–723, 1989.

67. Watters JM, Moulton SB, Clancey SM, Blakslee JM, Monaghan R: Aging exaggerates glucose intolerance following injury. J Trauma 37:786–791, 1994.

68. Watters JM, Kirkpatrick SM, Hopbach D, Norris SB: Aging exaggerates the blood glucose response to total parenteral nutrition. Can J Surg 39:481–485, 1996.

69. Jeevanandam M, Ramias L, Shamos RF, Schiller WR: Decreased growth hormone levels in the catabolic phase of severe injury. Surgery 111:495–502, 1992.

70. Watters JM, Norris SB, Kirkpatrick SM: Endogenous glucose production following injury increases with age. J Clin Endocrinol Metab 82:3005–3010, 1997.

71. Bessey PQ, Watters JM, Aoki TT, Wilmore DW: Combined hormonal infusion simulates the metabolic response to injury. Ann Surg 200:264–281, 1984.

72. Barton RN, Weijers JWM, Horan MA: Increased rates of cortisol production and urinary free cortisol excretion in elderly women 2 weeks after proximal femur fracture. Eur J Clin Invest 23:171–176, 1993.

73. Valerius NH, Eff C, Hansen NE, et al: Neutrophil and lymphocyte function in patients with diabetes mellitus. Acta Med Scand 211:463–467, 1982.

74. Drachman RH, Root RK Jr, Wood WB: Studies on the effect of experimental non-ketotic diabetes on antibacterial defense. I: Demonstration of a defect in phagocytosis. J Exp Med 124:227–240, 1966.

75. Boyko EJ, Lipsky BA: Infection and diabetes. In National Diabetes Data Group (eds): Diabetes in America, 2nd ed. Washington, DC, National Institutes of Health, National Institute of Diabetes and Digestive and Kidney Diseases, 1995, pp 485–500.

76. Pomposelli JJ, Baxter JK III, Babineau TJ, et al: Early postoperative glucose control predicts nosocomial infection rate in diabetic patients. JPEN J Parenter Enteral Nutr 22:77–81, 1998.

77. Cohen IK, Diegelmann RF: Wound healing. In Greenfield LJ, Mulholland MW, Oldham KT, Zelenock GB (eds): Surgery: Scientific Principles and Practice. Philadelphia, JB Lippincott, 1993, pp 86–102.

78. Guigliano D, Marfella R, Coppola L, et al: Vascular effects of acute hyperglycemia in humans are reversed by L-arginine. Evidence for reduced availability of nitric oxide during hyperglycemia. Circulation 95:1783–1790, 1997.

79. Henry S, Schnieter P, Jequier E, Tappy L: Effects of hyperinsulinemia and hyperglycemia on lactate release and local blood flow in subcutaneous adipose tissue of healthy humans. J Clin Endocrinol Metab 81:2891–2895, 1996.

80. Ceriella A, dello Russo P, Amstad P, Cerutti P: High glucose induces antioxidant enzymes in human endothelial cells in culture. Evidence linking hyperglycemia and oxidative stress. Diabetes 45:471–477, 1996.

81. Schloerb PR, Henning JF: Patterns and problems of adult total parenteral nutrition use in US academic medical centers. Arch Surg 133:7–12, 1998.

82. Fellows IW, Woolfson AMJ: Effects of therapeutic intervention on the metabolic responses to injury. Br Med Bull 41:287–294, 1985.

83. Inculet RI, Finley RJ, Duff JH, et al: Insulin de-

creases muscle protein loss after operative trauma in man. Surgery 99:752–758, 1986.

84. Woolfson AMJ, Heatley RV, Allison SP: Insulin to inhibit protein catabolism after injury. N Engl J Med 300:14–17, 1979.

85. Buskirk ER, Hodgson JL: Age and aerobic power: The rate of change in men and women. Fed Proc 46:1824–1829, 1987.

86. Clevenger FW, Rodriguez DJ, Demarest GB, et al: Protein and energy tolerance by stressed elderly patients. J Surg Res 52:135–139, 1992.

87. Fiatarone MA, Oneill EF, Ryan ND, et al: Exercise training and nutritional supplementation for physical frailty in very elderly people. N Engl J Med 330:1769–1775, 1994.

88. Hill GL: Implications of critical illness, injury, and sepsis on lean body mass and nutritional needs. Nutrition 14:557–558, 1998.

89. Prasad AS, Fitzgerald JT, Hess JW, et al: Zinc deficiency in elderly patients. Nutrition 9:218–224, 1993.

90. DeBiasse MA, Wilmore DW: What is optimal nutritional support? New Horiz 2:122–130, 1994.

91. Jiang Z-M, He G-Z, Zhang S-I, et al: Low-dose growth hormone and hypocaloric nutrition attenuate the protein-catabolic response after major operation. Ann Surg 210:513–525, 1989.

92. Ramirez RJ, Wolf SE, Barrow RE, Herndon DN: Growth hormone treatment in pediatric burns. A safe therapeutic approach. Ann Surg 228:439–448, 1998.

93. Takala J, Ruokonen E, Webster NR, et al: Increased mortality associated with growth hormone treatment in critically ill adults. N Engl J Med 341:785–792, 1999.

94. Jeevanandam M, Holaday NJ, Shamos RF, Petersen SR: Acute IGF-1 deficiency in multiple trauma victims. Clin Nutr 11:352–357, 1992.

95. Watters JM, McClaran JC: The elderly surgical patient. *In* Wilmore DW, Cheung LY, Harken AH, et al (eds): Scientific American Surgery. New York, Scientific American, 1996.

96. Kelly SM, Rosa A, Field S, et al: Inspiratory muscle strength and body composition in patients receiving total parenteral nutrition. Am Rev Respir Dis 130:33–37, 1984.

97. Howard L, Hassan N: Home parenteral nutrition. 25 years later. Gastroenterol Clin North Am 27:481–512, 1998.

98. Wilmore DW, Lacey JM, Soultanakis RP, et al: Factors predicting a successful outcome after pharmacologic bowel compensation. Ann Surg 226:288–293, 1997.

22

◆ Acquired Immunodeficiency Syndrome and Parenteral Nutrition

Nancy Lau, M.D.
Donald P. Kotler, M.D.

Malnutrition and wasting are frequent signs in patients with human immunodeficiency virus (HIV) infection or acquired immunodeficiency syndrome (AIDS). Wasting is an AIDS-defining illness and in 1995 was the identifying sign in nearly 20% of newly diagnosed cases in the United States, as reported to the Centers for Disease Control and Prevention.[1-3] The definition of wasting, published by the Centers in 1987, is involuntary weight loss of 10% or greater of baseline body weight in the presence of chronic diarrhea (at least two loose stools per day for >30 days), or chronic weakness and fever (for ≥30 days, intermittent or constant) that is not attributable to other disease processes (Table 22–1).[4] Although weight loss in HIV infection may be involuntary, it may also accompany an identifiable secondary infection. In the past, the lifetime prevalence of malnutrition in AIDS was near universal.

The definition of AIDS wasting syndrome was based on early observations of weight loss in Africa, where HIV infection was known as *slim disease*. This definition may need revision because the criterion of 10% is not based on current scientific observations, the time frame is arbitrary, and symptoms of chronic diarrhea, weakness, and/or fever may not be present, in spite of weight loss. A study published in 1998 showed that weight loss of more than 5% predicts a worse outcome.[5] Newer criteria for AIDS wasting have been suggested in which involuntary loss of 3% from baseline in 1 month, 5% in 6 months, or 10% in 12 months may be sufficient for diagnosis.

The aims of this chapter are to describe the nutritional alterations associated with HIV infection, including patterns of weight loss, changes in body composition (macronutrients) and micronutrients, pathogenic mechanisms underlying malnutrition, nutri-

tional support, and adjunctive nutritional therapies.

◆ PATTERNS OF WEIGHT LOSS IN HIV INFECTION

Early observations indicated that once progression to advanced HIV disease occurred, weight loss was rapidly progressive and unremitting.[6] Macallan and associates analyzed patterns of weight change in a cohort of men with advanced HIV disease and described two distinct patterns of weight loss. Episodic, acute severe weight loss occurred in the presence of an opportunistic infection, with weight gain following recovery.[7] Weight loss accompanied cytomegalovirus infection, and a gain of weight and body cell mass (BCM) was demonstrated after specific treatment of cytomegalovirus infection, without additional nutritional therapy.[8] A second pattern was slow, progressive weight loss, a pattern that was associated with gastrointestinal disease and malabsorption.

◆ ADVERSE CONSEQUENCES OF WEIGHT LOSS

Malnutrition is common in HIV infection and has substantial effects on morbidity and

Table 22–1. Human Immunodeficiency Virus Wasting Syndrome

Involuntary weight loss >10% of baseline weight
plus
Chronic diarrhea (at least 2 stools/day for >30 days)
or
Chronic weakness and documented fever (for >30 days, intermittent or constant)
In the absence of concurrent illness or condition other than HIV infection that could explain the findings

HIV, human immunodeficiency virus.

mortality. Levels of weight loss ranging from 5 to 20% have been associated with an increased risk of mortality in several studies,[5, 9–12] with an effect independent of CD4+ lymphocyte counts.[9, 10, 12] Weight loss has been associated with an increased risk of hospitalization and an increased risk of developing an active opportunistic infection, effects also independent of CD4+ lymphocyte counts.[10, 12, 13]

Two studies correlated BCM depletion with decreased survival.[14, 15] In a prospective study,[15] BCM depletion was associated with shortened survival, an effect that was independent of the CD4+ count. In the other study, a decline in BCM mass and body weight, but not body fat, was progressive until death.[14] The results of that study suggested that the timing of death from wasting in AIDS was related to the degree of BCM depletion rather than the specific cause of the wasting process. In clinically stable HIV-infected patients, the BCM correlated with the quality of life, independently of the CD4+ count.[16] The aspect of quality of life that best correlated with nutritional depletion was decreased functional performance. In a longitudinal study, weight loss itself was associated with a decline in physical function.[17]

Malnutrition and its sequelae affect not only HIV-infected individuals but also the health care system and society. Malnutrition may increase fatigue, decrease physical activity, and decrease the level of contribution to society by the affected person. In addition, the increased use of health care resources in the need for custodial services, specialized nutritional support, hospitalizations, and medical care leads to higher health care costs.

◆ EFFECTS OF HIV INFECTION AND AIDS ON NUTRITIONAL STATUS

Macronutrients (Body Composition)

The choice of measure for assessing macronutrient status clinically remains controversial. Body weight is the simplest to measure, but it fails to distinguish between changes in lean or fat tissues. Such changes require at least a two-compartment model, which separates the body into fat and fat-free mass (FFM). However, the major clinical limitation of a two-compartment model is that changes to the FFM fail to differentiate between intra- and extracellular compartments. Thus, a three-compartment model, comprising fat, extracellular cell mass, and BCM, is favored. The BCM is the metabolically active tissue compartment and is responsible for oxygen consumption and carbon dioxide production. BCM is composed of the nonadipose tissue in skeletal muscle, organs, and the bloodstream. BCM depletion is associated with adverse outcomes in AIDS patients, as noted earlier, as well as in other clinical diseases, such as cancer.[14, 15, 18]

Body composition studies have extended our understanding of the patterns of weight loss and the extent and composition of tissue wasting. Ott and colleagues demonstrated BCM depletion without weight loss in asymptomatic HIV-infected patients relatively early in the disease course (before evidence of significant immunosuppression or opportunistic infections).[19] The results implied that alterations in body composition may occur as a direct effect of the underlying HIV infection itself.

Early body composition studies were performed in clinically ill AIDS patients. A disproportionate decrease in BCM, as assessed by total body potassium, relative to weight loss was documented. However, weight loss was masked by an expansion of the extracellular fluid compartment.[20] In the AIDS men studied, the magnitude of depletion of BCM was striking, because the body fat content was not severely depressed in many patients. Using a computed tomographic method, Wang and coworkers showed that approximately 50% of the weight difference between HIV-infected and control men could be attributed to skeletal muscle.[21] Other studies have confirmed these initial findings and have shown that the depletion of BCM is accompanied by depletion of total body nitrogen and skeletal muscle mass.[22] In contrast to men, HIV-infected women may exhibit progressive and disproportionate decreases in body fat relative to lean body mass (LBM) at all stages of wasting, although in the late stages of wasting, women also lose significant LBM and muscle mass.[23, 24] The reasons underlying gender-related differences are uncertain and may relate to hormonal differences.[24]

Body composition studies also have documented changes in hydration status in HIV infection. The alterations of body water volumes were contrasted in AIDS patients with either malabsorption or systemic infection.[25] Body water volumes were determined by probe dilution, and FFM by dual-energy x-ray absorptiometry. Wasting was associated with a decrease in intracellular water volume. Patients with malabsorption had greater depletion of total body water (TBW), compared with HIV-infected subjects without malabsorption and compared with controls. Subjects with systemic infections were overhydrated, with increased TBW/FFM ratios. The relative expansion of extracellular water during systemic infection increases body weight and thus masks clinical evidence of wasting. In contrast, patients with diarrhea and malabsorption are clinically dehydrated, with a low average TBW/FFM ratio.

In 1997, Mulligan and associates noted that although both fat and LBM were significantly lower in men with HIV-associated weight loss than in controls, fat was preferentially lost in patients who had more baseline fat.[26] In a longitudinal analysis, patients with baseline fat of more than 15% lost less LBM than did men with baseline fat of less than 15%. The difference between the results of Mulligan and associates and those of Kotler and coworkers[20] may be due in part to the fact that the data of Mulligan and associates were collected on ambulatory patients during periods of relative clinical stability, with no overt symptoms of opportunistic infection, whereas in the study of Kotler and coworkers, patients were studied during episodes of secondary infection. In addition, 10 years elapsed between the two studies, and the general health of HIV-infected patients has changed significantly during this period.

The disproportionate decrease in LBM in men with AIDS-associated wasting may be due to a decrease in a potent endogenous anabolic factor, testosterone. Testosterone and dehydroepiandrosterone sulfate deficiency may contribute to the decreased muscle mass found in women[27] and hypogonadal men with AIDS wasting.[28] The effects of testosterone replacement on body composition in HIV infection are discussed later in this chapter.

Several studies imply a direct association between HIV infection and weight loss, including BCM depletion in asymptomatic subjects;[19] between HIV infection and elevated resting energy expenditure in asymptomatic subjects;[29, 30] between recent weight loss and an elevated plasma HIV viral burden;[31] and between an elevated resting energy expenditure and both the plasma HIV viral burden[32] and clinical observations of weight gain during antiretroviral therapy.[33]

Current Trends in Macronutrient Status

With recent advances in antiretroviral therapies and in the prophylaxis and treatment of disease complications, the long-term outlook of patients with HIV has markedly improved, and serious malnutrition is less prevalent than in the past. Although the prevalence of severe malnutrition has fallen, the nutritional status does not return to normal in many people. A syndrome of truncal obesity and metabolic abnormalities has been described and is of concern. Characteristic alterations in body composition, notably the development of truncal (visceral) obesity and subcutaneous fat loss (lipodystrophy), as well as hyperlipidemia and insulin resistance, have been reported from many centers around the world, in both men and women.[34–37] The cause of these changes is unknown. The presence of central obesity, hyperlipidemia, and insulin resistance is a familiar triad in clinical medicine and occurs in several well-characterized medical syndromes, as well as in the absence of any other disease (syndrome X).[38] Its development during the course of an infectious disease (HIV infection) is distinctly unusual. The presence of these changes usually is a predictor of accelerated atherogenesis. Indeed, an increasing number of reports are describing the development of atherosclerotic cardiac disease with myocardial infarction in young HIV-infected subjects with these changes.[39]

There are two general hypotheses to explain the changes. The first states that the changes are a direct side effect of therapy with protease inhibitors, one class of antiretroviral agent, and a molecular mechanism to explain such changes has been published.[40] The alternative hypothesis states that the changes are indirectly related to therapy and somehow are unmasked by some effect of protease inhibitors, such as abolishing viral replication or promoting partial immune reconstitution. The second hypothesis is especially relevant in people who have developed some of the changes in the absence of protease inhibitor therapy.[41, 42] It is possible that the changes represent an altered stress response with mild chronic hypercortisolism in some people.[43, 44] This topic is under active investigation.

Micronutrients

Micronutrient deficiencies may occur relatively early in the disease course in HIV-infected individuals. Low to marginal serum levels of micronutrients have been reported in 57% of asymptomatic patients and in 87% of symptomatic patients. Overtly and marginally low blood levels of vitamin A, vitamin E, riboflavin, vitamin B_6, and vitamin B_{12}, together with copper and zinc, were documented in asymptomatic HIV-infected patients.[45]

Vitamin B_{12} is the most commonly recognized micronutrient to be deficient. Subnormal vitamin B_{12} levels have been shown in up to one third of patients.[46] In addition, some patients had absent intrinsic factor secretion as indicated by an abnormal part 1 Schilling test. In others, an abnormal part 2 of the Schilling test (vitamin B_{12} complexed to intrinsic factor) was found, implying ileal dysfunction. One study identified neuropsychological changes associated with low serum vitamin B_{12} concentrations, with normalization as a result of specific supplementation.[47] Another common B vitamin to be deficient is pyridoxine (vitamin B_6). Pyridoxine deficiency adversely affects lymphocyte responsiveness to mitogens and natural killer cell activity, independent of the $CD4^+$ cell count.[48] Vitamin B_6 deficiency in the general population has been associated with anorexia and decreased food intake. The clinical manifestations of vitamin B_6 deficiency include mouth soreness, glossitis, peripheral neuropathy, weakness, and mental status changes.

Low levels of vitamin A, zinc, and selenium are common and have been demonstrated to be associated with excess HIV-related mortality, independent of a $CD4^+$ cell count less than $200/mm^3$ at baseline, although in a multivariate analysis, only selenium deficiency was significantly associated with decreased survival.[49] Selenium deficiency is significantly associated with low body weight and body mass index, independent of the $CD4^+$ cell count, age, gender,

and race, suggesting that the selenium status may be a sensitive predictor of wasting in HIV-infected individuals.[50] Selenium deficiency may be associated with HIV cardiomyopathy. In one study, decreased selenium contents were found in cardiac tissue from autopsied AIDS patients.[51] Zinc deficiency has been associated with impairment in taste and olfaction. One study showed that serum zinc levels correlate with progression to AIDS in HIV-infected subjects, though a direct causal effect has not been demonstrated. Zinc may be sequestered in tissue as part of an acute-phase response; therefore, low levels may not represent an absolute deficiency.

Deficiencies of fat-soluble vitamins also occur and are likely related to fat malabsorption. Vitamin A deficiency was associated with increased mortality in a cohort of HIV-infected intravenous drug users.[52] In a study from Africa, Semba and colleagues showed that decreased serum concentrations of vitamin A in pregnant HIV-infected women was associated with an increased risk of maternal-fetal transmission of HIV.[53] Cunningham-Rundles and associates found that 70% of children congenitally exposed to HIV are vitamin A deficient in the first months of life compared with age-matched controls, whether these children are HIV infected or not.[54] Serum vitamin D concentrations are decreased in many symptomatic HIV-infected patients. In addition to its role in calcium and bone mineral metabolism, vitamin D also is recognized as having an immunoregulatory function. In in vitro studies, 1,25-vitamin D_3 has been shown to modulate the function of monocytes and lymphocytes.[55]

Decreased levels of glutathione have been observed in HIV-infected patients, suggesting that oxidative stress might play a role in HIV disease. Glutathione is a major intracellular defense against the production of reactive oxygen intermediates. Production of these oxidants depletes glutathione. Oxidative stress has been shown repeatedly to promote HIV replication in vitro, whereas N-acetylcysteine, a cysteine analogue that replenishes intracellular glutathione, inhibits HIV transcription and replication in vitro.[56] Decreased levels of plasma antioxidant micronutrients as well as increased lipid peroxidation indices have been observed in HIV-infected individuals, suggesting an increased oxidative stress.[57] Elevated serum levels of lipid peroxidation by-products such as hydroperoxides and malondialdehyde have been observed in HIV-infected patients and indicate the occurrence of membrane damage.[58] However, there is little evidence to link oxidative stress with a more rapid progression of immune deficiency. The clinical significance of oxidative stress to HIV disease progression needs further investigation.

The clinical implications of micronutrient deficiencies in HIV-infected individuals remain unclear. Micronutrient deficiencies are difficult to identify and quantify. Measured plasma concentrations may be inaccurate in the presence of an acute-phase response to infection and inflammation because of sequestration in tissue compartments. Racial, ethnic, and geographic differences may also confound micronutrient measurements. Further studies are needed to evaluate the clinical significance of these micronutrient deficiencies, especially in the current era, and to determine whether supplemental therapy is of clinical benefit.

◆ PATHOGENESIS OF WEIGHT LOSS

Weight loss is the consequence of negative energy balance. To maintain body weight, the total energy expenditure (TEE), which encompasses the resting energy expenditure (REE), the voluntary energy expenditure, and the energy expended in the digestive process, must match the caloric intake. The alterations in metabolism, oral intake, and nutrient absorption observed in HIV infection contribute to a negative caloric balance, leading to weight loss and wasting.

Alterations in Energy Expenditure

Studies of the various components of energy expenditure have yielded somewhat conflicting results. REE is the most studied component of energy expenditure. It might be expected that hypermetabolism and an increase in REE would significantly contribute to weight loss. An elevated REE has been demonstrated at all stages of HIV infection,[29, 30, 59, 60] although not all studies show this effect.[61] The REE was also found to be elevated in HIV-infected women in one study,[62] although another study found no

significant differences in either REE or body composition between HIV-positive women and controls.[63] However, despite significant increases in REE, patients did not show short-term weight loss in most studies.[30, 59–64]

Two studies specifically challenged the notion that hypermetabolism leads to weight loss and demonstrated that decreased food intake is quantitatively the most important factor in producing short-term weight loss. Grunfeld and colleagues studied groups of clinically stable and unstable HIV-infected subjects and controls.[60] Short-term weight loss occurred in AIDS patients with secondary infections who had a low caloric intake and an increased REE. However, in clinically stable HIV-infected and AIDS patients, short-term weight loss did not occur despite an equivalent increase in REE because of an adequate caloric intake.

Macallan and colleagues also studied energy balance in AIDS patients and examined the effects of secondary infections on energy expenditure.[64] Subjects whose weight remained stable had an adequate food intake, whereas patients who exhibited weight loss had a decreased intake. On the reasoning that weight loss ultimately is a consequence of negative caloric balance, the authors examined the TEE and energy intake in relation to weight changes. The TEE was reduced in patients undergoing weight loss, whereas the TEE was normal in patients who had either stable weights or weight gains. Thus, weight loss during acute disease occurred primarily as a result of decreased food intake and not because of hypermetabolism. Because the REE was either normal or elevated in the weight-losing subjects, the reduction in TEE during weight loss was attributed primarily to the reduction of energy expended for voluntary activity and may correlate with symptoms of fatigue and lethargy, which are common in HIV infection. Through an indirect argument, the authors convincingly showed that hypermetabolism (REE) is not the primary cause of weight loss in HIV-infected subjects; rather, weight loss occurs because the reduction in energy intake exceeds the reduction in TEE.

The observation that weight loss is more often associated with decreased caloric intake than with hypermetabolism raises the possibility that nutritional intervention might blunt the loss of weight. However, simply feeding the patient to reverse the wasting process is insufficient to replete the BCM, as discussed later in this chapter.

Altered Nutrient Metabolism

The metabolic alterations that occur in HIV infection include lipid, carbohydrate, and protein metabolism. Derangements in lipid metabolism are marked in HIV infection. High-density lipoprotein (HDL) and low-density lipoprotein (LDL) levels are decreased early in the course of HIV infection. Later in the course of HIV infection, triglyceride levels may be increased. Alterations in lipid metabolism include an increase in hepatic de novo fatty acid synthesis and esterification, increased very low density lipoprotein production, and decreased clearance of triglycerides from the blood. The relative increase in the synthesis of triglycerides from free fatty acids could lead to increased utilization of amino acids for energy, resulting in accelerated loss of lean body mass.[65]

There is evidence to suggest that protein metabolism may be disturbed in HIV infection. The tissue lost in HIV-related wasting consists disproportionately of lean tissue, including body protein. Increases in whole-body protein turnover, measured as [^{13}C] leucine turnover, were seen in advanced HIV infection, consistent with a catabolic process.[66, 67] However, another study, using [^{15}N]glycine as a tracer, found reduced rates of whole-body protein turnover,[68] consistent with starvation. Despite an observed increased whole-body protein turnover, an acute anabolic response to the provision of short-term intravenous parenteral nutrition was quantitatively normal in both stage II and stage IV HIV disease.[66, 69] That an acute anabolic response is observed with the provision of nutrition in HIV infection is in contrast to the response observed in acute sepsis. Septic animals failed to increase skeletal muscle protein synthesis in response to total parenteral nutrition (TPN),[70] and septic patients in the intensive care unit fed high-protein diets still lost body protein.[71]

Disturbances in metabolism and wasting may be attributed to the host response to infection, which is mediated by cytokines. Proinflammatory and other cytokines may produce symptoms such as fever, myalgia, anorexia, fatigue, and lethargy. The metabolic alterations observed in the host response to infection or inflammation may be mediated by cytokine activity. Tumor necrosis factor (TNF), interleukin 1 (IL-1), and the interferons have been shown to increase hepatic lipid synthesis in vivo and to decrease levels of lipoprotein lipase in certain adipose tissues in vitro and in vivo, which could result in a decrease in the rate of clearance of triglyceride-rich lipoproteins.[72, 73] One study showed a correlation between elevated levels of interferon-α and the presence of hypertriglyceridemia in AIDS.[74] Elevated levels of TNF were reported in one study of clinically ill AIDS patients.[75]

The role of cytokines is difficult to study, because they act predominantly via a paracrine mechanism. In addition, plasma levels may not reflect tissue activity. Cytokine activity may be modulated by natural antagonists as shown by Thea and associates in a study of Zairian women.[76] Asymptomatic subjects were clinically stable despite high circulating levels of the proinflammatory cytokines IL-1β and TNF-α. However, compared with late-stage subjects, the asymptomatic women had elevated levels of their natural inhibitors, IL-1 receptor antagonist and TNF-sRp55 (soluble form of the p55 [type 1] TNF-α receptor). The results suggested that chronic HIV induces immune activation, mediated by cytokines, and that cytokine activities are modulated by circulating inhibitors. In another cross-sectional study, African HIV-infected men with persistent diarrhea and severe malnutrition were examined to determine whether wasting might be related to intestinal opportunistic infection, untreated esophageal candidiasis, or increased cytokine activity.[77] Wasting in this group was not related to the presence of intestinal infection, esophageal candidiasis, or the duration of diarrhea but was strongly correlated with the TNF-sRp55 concentration in serum. The results implied that immune activation is associated with AIDS wasting in men. In a prospective study from France, elevated circulating levels of IL-1 receptor antagonist were associated with wasting in HIV-infected patients.[78] The authors suggested that IL-1 receptor antagonist accumulation was associated with intense systemic inflammation and may reflect a concerted activation of the immune system, although elevation of a single cytokine or a single cell system was not found.

Endocrine alterations have been documented in HIV-infected individuals. Serum testosterone and dihydroepiandosterone concentrations are low in many HIV-infected patients. In prior studies, hypogonadism was documented in 30 to 50% of men with AIDS.[79] Elevations in basal cortisol levels and loss of the normal diurnal periodicity,[80, 81] as well as a suboptimal cortisol response to the administration of synthetic corticotropin,[82] have been reported. Thyroid dysfunction, with low levels of reverse triiodothyronine (rT_3) and a normal T_3 level, has been observed,[83] as well as thyroid function tests suggestive of euthyroid sick syndrome (with high rT_3, low T_3).[84]

Alterations in Oral Intake

Decreased oral intake is common in HIV-infected patients and contributes significantly to weight loss and HIV-associated wasting, as discussed earlier.[85–87] Possible reasons for altered food intake are many and include oropharyngeal and esophageal abnormality, psychosocial and economic factors, fatigue, changes in mental status, and anorexia due to medications. Candidiasis is the most common infectious complication of HIV infection and may decrease taste sensations and affect swallowing, in addition to causing oral or substernal discomfort. Severe gingivitis or periodontitis as well as ulcerations due to aphthous ulcers, herpes simplex, or cytomegalovirus infection may cause pain and interfere with eating. The esophagus is affected by the same lesions as the oral cavity. A particularly striking lesion is the idiopathic esophageal ulcer, which may be large and produce debilitating symptoms.[88] No etiologic agent is found on biopsy of the ulcer, although cells containing HIV RNA may be present.[89] Other problems may affect food intake in the absence of oral or esophageal abnormality. Food intake may be reduced in response to intestinal malabsorption or systemic infection. Anorexia is a feature of systemic infections and may be mediated by cytokines. Patients with malabsorption do not overeat to compensate for the calories lost in the stool. About one half of the calculated energy deficit in patients with malabsorption can be ascribed to undereating (unpublished data of DP Kotler, J Nash). Many HIV patients fear embarrassment from stool incontinence or diarrhea and may consciously decrease their food intake in order to reduce stool frequency. Neurologic diseases due to mass lesions of the brain, such as toxoplasmosis or lymphoma, or dementia may decrease the perception of hunger and alter the ability to chew and swallow, thus decreasing voluntary food intake. Certain medications may cause anorexia.

The role of cytokines as mediators of anorexia has received considerable attention. In animal studies, TNF-α has been shown to decrease gastric motility, causing food retention in the stomach.[90] Many cytokines and chemokines exhibit anorectic effects on the central nervous system, including TNF, IL-1, IL-6, IL-8, interferon-α, and interferon-γ.[91] The specific site of cytokinic action is the hypothalamus. The anorectic effects induced by IL-1 are continuous in experimental animals, with a failure to maintain normal weight, while tachyphylaxis to the anorectic effect of TNF may occur. Cytokines enter the central nervous system from blood or lymphoid cells by way of the choroid plexus, near the third ventricle, where the blood-brain barrier is incomplete.

Malabsorption

Malabsorption may be defined as a decrease in the uptake of nutrients from the intestinal lumen with excessive losses in the stool. Malabsorption, often characterized by symptoms of chronic or recurrent diarrhea, is an important cause of weight loss and the HIV wasting syndrome. The most common type of malabsorption found in patients with AIDS is related to primary enterocyte injury, usually as a result of infection with protozoans such as cryptosporidia and microsporidia. Nutrient malabsorption may accompany severe small intestinal diseases and may be due to a diminution in intestinal surface area, cell defects from direct pathogen damage, and functional immaturity of villous epithelial cells related to rapid cell turnover.[92] Histologic studies show partial villous atrophy despite crypt hyperplasia. AIDS patients with cyptosporidiosis and microsporidiosis had decreased jejunal disaccharidase activities and xylose malabsorption compared with HIV-infected individuals and healthy controls.[93] Quantitative estimates of fecal losses due to intestinal cryptosporidiosis were about 20% for protein and fat (DP Kotler, personal observations, 1996).

Protein-losing enteropathy, or exudative enteropathy, is another mechanism for malabsorption seen in mycobacterial infections in AIDS patients, predominantly *Mycobacterium avium* complex.[93] Ileal dysfunction leading to bile salt wasting is another form of malabsorption seen in HIV infection. Cryptosporidia and microsporidia infect the ileum, as well as the upper small intestine. Infection with enteroadherent *Escherichia coli* is another cause of ileal dysfunction.[94] Infection with enteroaggregative *E. coli* organisms has been found in stool in HIV-infected patients with diarrhea more frequently than in HIV-infected adults without diarrhea.[95] In many patients, malabsorption and diarrhea occur without an identified pathogen. In these patients, it has been suggested that the malabsorption may be an effect of HIV itself.

◆ NUTRITIONAL SUPPORT AND OTHER THERAPIES

General Recommendations

Initial evaluation in the work-up of malnutrition should include a thorough history and physical examination that focuses on changes in body weight and shape; appetite; eating habits; and functional status. Determination of the etiologic disorders responsible for malnutrition and malabsorption may

be facilitated by using diagnostic algorithms.[96]

Dietary counseling and patient education may benefit HIV-infected patients who can voluntarily adjust their oral intake. It is prudent for any dietary regimen to provide at least the recommended dietary allowance for all nutrients, and three to four times the recommended daily allowance for vitamins and minerals. Otherwise, the recommended diet for HIV-infected individuals is not different from that of healthy individuals. Protein requirements, in the absence of secondary infection, are 1 to 1.2 g/kg of body weight, and as much as 2 g/kg may be helpful in patients with excess nutritional stresses.

In the following section, oral and parenteral nutritional support are discussed. Also, adjuvant therapies with anabolic agents and other therapies are reviewed. A comparison of various nutritional therapies is provided in Table 22–2.

Appetite Stimulants

Appetite stimulants have been used to treat AIDS-related anorexia and weight loss. Appetite stimulation is most beneficial in the absence of local pathologic lesions affecting chewing and swallowing, malabsorption syndromes, and active systemic infections. In two studies, megestrol acetate (Megace; Bristol-Myers Oncology Division, Princeton, N.J.) was shown to stimulate food intake and

Table 22–2. Body Composition Changes with Various Nutritional Therapies*

	Body Weight Change (mean, kg)	Body Fat Change (%)†	Lean Body Mass Change (%)†
Increased caloric intake			
Megestrol acetate‡[99]	+4.7	+76.6	+8.5
TPN§ [113]	+3.0	+130	+7
PEG‖ [108]	+3.0	+33	+14
Anabolic agents			
rhGH§ [127]	+1.6	−106	+187
Testosterone§ [132]	+0.9	−22	+133
Testosterone¶ [133]	+1.6	+56	+125
Nandrolone** [136]	+4	+10	+60

*Fat and lean body mass by dual energy absorptiometry or anthropometry, change in weight by scale.
†Kilograms gained or lost after treatment as a percentage of mean change.
‡Eight- to 12-week therapy.
§Twelve-week therapy.
‖Eight-week therapy.
¶Six-month therapy.
**Sixteen-week therapy.
PEG, percutaneous endoscopic gastrostomy; rhGH, recombinant human growth hormone; TPN, total parenteral nutrition.

promote weight gain.[97, 98] Although there were improvements in the quality of life, survival was not affected. Engelson and associates evaluated the effects of megestrol acetate on body composition and serum testosterone levels in a group of AIDS patients and in untreated HIV-infected controls.[99] Over 12 weeks, patients who received megestrol gained 4.7 kg, but the majority of the weight gained was fat; the BCM did not change. Serum testosterone concentrations decreased significantly during megestrol treatment but remained stable in HIV-infected controls. The preferential accumulation of fat may have been the result of a megestrol-induced decrease in testosterone secretion. A multicenter study to examine the separate and combined effects of megestrol and testosterone on weight gain is ongoing.

Dronabinol (Marinol) is a synthetic derivative of *Cannabis sativa* (marijuana) and is used to stimulate appetite in AIDS-related anorexia.[100, 101] Additional benefits include the drug's antiemetic effect and its purported ability to improve mood. Dronabinol's effect on the composition of weight gained has yet to be studied. The most common side effects of dronabinol involve the central nervous system and include drowsiness, anxiety, poor concentration, impairment of coordination, and confusion. In addition, tachycardia, palpitations, and vasodilation have been reported.

Oral Nutritional Supplementation

Commercial nutritional formulas differ widely in composition and palatability. Some formulas are low in residue, others are lactose-free or contain high contents of medium-chain triglycerides (MCTs) rather than long-chain triglycerides (LCTs), whereas others are semielemental or elemental or contain enhanced quantities of specific compounds.

Few studies have examined the effects of supplemental nutrition on weight and body composition, as well as the role of various nutritional compounds on immunologic status. In a small controlled double-blind crossover phase trial, stable HIV-infected men who consumed a formula fortified with n-3 polyunsaturated fatty acids (α-linolenic acid), L-arginine, and yeast-derived RNA showed a significant weight gain relative to the weight gained in those consuming a standard formula during a 4-month follow-up period, despite a similar total caloric intake.[102] No significant changes in anthropometric measures, parameters of body composition (fat mass, FFM, BCM), and serum total iron-binding capacity concentrations were observed. No changes in CD4[+] lymphocyte counts were observed. Ingestion of the study formula resulted in a significant increase in the serum concentrations of the soluble TNF receptor proteins. It was postulated that the increase in soluble TNF receptors modulates the negative effects of TNF.

A randomized double-blind controlled study that included a group of 64 HIV-positive ambulatory patients taking a balanced oral nutritional supplement with or without arginine and n-3 fatty acids for 6 months showed an increase in body weight and fat mass in both groups.[103] The addition of arginine and n-3 fatty acids did not improve CD4[+], CD8[+] lymphocyte counts, viremia, or the level of soluble TNF receptors.

Chlebowski and colleagues reported a weight gain and a decrease in hospitalizations in HIV-infected individuals who consumed a specialized formula compared with those who consumed a standard polymeric diet.[104] Their study formula was peptide based, containing an uncharacterized polypeptide, a mixture of carbohydrates and lipids, including MCTs, plus β-carotene, n-3 fatty acids, selected vitamins (B$_6$, B$_{12}$, C, E), minerals (iron, zinc, selenium), and soluble fiber.

A community-based study showed that patients who were infected with HIV, or in an early stage of AIDS without a secondary infection, were able to gain or maintain weight with dietary counseling and oral liquid nutritional supplements, which were high in energy and protein.[105] However, weight loss was observed in the majority of patients who developed a secondary infection, despite a greater consumption of oral supplements than those without a secondary infection.

In a small number of HIV-infected subjects with mild diarrhea, replacing a normal diet with full enteral feeding using an elemental diet containing MCTs and enzymatically hydrolyzed protein (Peptamen, Nestle Clinical Nutrition, Deerfield, Ill.) resulted in decreased stool frequency, stool volume, and fecal fat excretion.[106]

Intestinal dysfunction and fat malabsorption commonly affect the HIV-infected patient. Two studies examined the effect of fat composition on nutritional status. In a randomized double-blind trial, patients with AIDS and documented fat malabsorption for 12 days received full enteral feeding of either an oral formula containing 85% MCT/15% LCTs or the control formula containing 100% LCTs.[107] Subjects fed the MCT/LCT formula showed significantly decreased stool fat and stool nitrogen content and increased fat absorption, whereas those fed the LCT formula showed no significant changes.

Body weight and composition were analyzed in a 6-month prospective randomized double-blind multicenter study of clinically stable patients with advanced HIV disease (<100 CD4+ lymphocytes/mm³),[108] comparing MCT- and LCT-enriched oral formulas almost identical in composition to those of the previous study.[107] Both the MCT and LCT groups, on average, gained weight. However, the LCT group gained significantly more weight than the MCT group, possibly because of a greater intake of formula. Gains in BCM were small but similar in the two groups. Dropout rates were high in both groups, and subjects who dropped out were more likely to be losing BCM than those who continued on the study.

Larger studies with longer follow-up periods will be needed to further evaluate the effects of different nutritional formulations, the use of MCTs versus LCTs, and the additions of various micronutrients on HIV-associated weight loss.

◆ NONVOLITIONAL FEEDING

A reliable assessment of the clinical efficacy of TPN or enteral nutritional support in AIDS patients is difficult because relatively few studies have evaluated this issue. Most of the reported studies contain small numbers of subjects, and few were designed as prospective randomized controlled trials.

Gastrostomy Feeding

Indications for percutaneous endoscopic gastrostomy (PEG) in AIDS patients are the same as those in non–HIV-infected patients: the presence of a primary eating disorder and no objective evidence of severe malabsorption, systemic infection, or anatomic or motility barriers to enteral nutrition. PEG has been studied in AIDS patients by several groups of investigators. In a prospective case series, a commercially available enteral formula that was peptide based, consisting of 40% MCTs, was administered through an endoscopically placed gastrostomy tube for 2 months.[109] In this study of eight AIDS patients with severe eating disorders associated with systemic diseases and no malabsorption, the body weight rose, and increases in BCM, body fat content, serum albumin concentration, and serum iron-binding capacity were noted. Total lymphocyte counts increased significantly during the period of nutritional support in this study and were associated with an increase in the number of T suppressor (CD8+) lymphocytes but no changes in the number of T helper (CD4+) lymphocytes. In addition, functional improvements, including subjective improvements in cognitive function, were appreciated in patients receiving nutritional support.

Dowling and coworkers presented the results of a case series of AIDS patients fed via PEG for up to 15 months and reported weight gain and satisfaction with therapy in most patients.[110] Brantsma and associates reported that PEG feeding was cost-effective and improved nutritional status.[111] In a multicenter case control series compiled by Cappell and Godil,[112] the AIDS group gained weight and remained nutritionally stable while being fed via PEG feeding tubes. However, the number of serious complications was significantly higher in the AIDS patients than in the case controls and included infections at the PEG stomal site. Ockenga and colleagues reported that PEG feedings were as safe in AIDS patients as in non-AIDS patients.[113] PEG tube feedings led to increases in body weight, serum albumin levels, and iron-binding capacity. Survival was longer in patients who accepted PEG feedings compared with those who declined PEG feeding tubes.

Total Parenteral Nutrition

Parenteral nutrition should be considered when the gastrointestinal tract is nonfunctional and feedings cannot be taken through the oral or enteral route. The effect of TPN on body composition was analyzed in 12 AIDS patients.[114] In this study, although all patients gained body weight and body fat in response to prolonged TPN, significant repletion of the BCM was observed only in the five patients who were malnourished because of alterations in food intake or malabsorption, not in the seven patients who had serious systemic infections. The results showed a clear distinction between the effects of TPN in intestinal disease with malabsorption and the effects in untreated systemic infection. The poor response to nutritional repletion during active systemic infection may relate to the metabolic alterations, discussed earlier, associated with infection. The authors concluded that the response to TPN is related more to the clinical status of the patient receiving therapy than to the therapy itself.

In a recent prospective randomized controlled multicenter trial, the efficacy of 2-month treatment with home TPN was evaluated in malnourished severely immunodepressed AIDS patients without active secondary infection.[115] The group receiving TPN showed an increase in body weight, LBM, and BCM, whereas all parameters decreased in the control group who only received dietary counseling (DC). This is in agreement with the finding from whole-body protein kinetics studies that the acute anabolic response to intravenous nutrition is not quantitatively impaired by HIV infection. Patients in the TPN group had a higher Nutritional Subjective Global Assessment status and higher Karnofsky index and subjectively reported feeling better as a result of therapy. There was no difference in the survival rate between the TPN and the control groups during the short-term study.

However, improved survival by home TPN was found after prolonged follow-up.[116] After the initial 2-month trial, four patients in the DC group whose body weight continued to decline received TPN, and one patient initially receiving TPN declined further treatment. During the follow-up period, 18 of the 19 TPN-treated patients and all 12 patients who received DC died. However, a statistically significant increase in the median survival was noted in the TPN-treated group compared with the DC group (212 vs. 57 days, respectively, $P = .006$). When analysis was performed without the difference in the number of subjects in each group when therapy was altered, a statistically significant difference in median survival was still noted (199 days with TPN vs. 57 days with DC, $P = .01$).

Although TPN can improve nutritional status, the likely benefit is through increased caloric intake, rather than an intrinsic benefit from parenteral nutrition. In a randomized, controlled clinical trial that compared TPN with an oral semielemental diet (SED) in AIDS patients with documented malabsorption, the caloric intake, body weight, body composition, quality of life, survival, and medical costs were analyzed over a 3-month period.[117] The semielemental diet used was AlitraQ (Ross Laboratories, Columbus, Ohio), and patients in this group were encouraged to eat as little normal food as possible to adhere to the caloric target and not to interfere with the consumption of the SED. However, the TPN group consumed more total calories and gained more weight than the SED group. By multivariate analysis, changes in weight and body composition correlated with the caloric intake and not to whether the feeding was through the parenteral or the enteral route. Bioelectric impedance studies showed that the TPN group gained significantly more fat than the SED group, whereas the changes in BCM were similar and minimal in the two groups (Fig. 22–1). The SED group scored significantly better than the TPN group on a physical functioning subscale of quality of life (Medical Outcomes Survey, short form[118]). The peripheral blood CD4+ lymphocyte count and intestinal function were unaf-

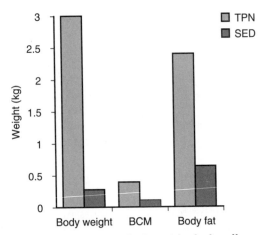

Figure 22–1. Change in body weight, body cell mass (BCM), and body fat in acquired immunodeficiency syndrome patients with malabsorption at the end of 3 months of treatment. TPN, total parenteral nutrition; SED, semi-elemental diet.

fected by either therapy. The median survival for the TPN group was 346 days (mean, 362 days), versus 481 days for the SED group (mean, 437 days). Survival did not differ between groups; however, survival was better in both groups than the average survival in patients with AIDS wasting in other published studies, before the use of protease inhibitors. The standardized costs of nutritional therapy were about four times higher for TPN than for the SED. Voluntary compliance with the SED was limited in some patients, although intestinal symptoms were associated more with the intake of food than with the formula (Kotler DP, personal observations).

Although these studies have evaluated TPN as a source of calories, a few studies have examined the effect of the lipid composition of TPN on immunologic function. The available data do not show striking effects. The effect on the immune response may be associated with the incorporation of different fatty acids into cell membranes and on the production of eicosanoids. Thus, modification of membrane lipids may be associated with altered lymphocytic function. In patients with clinical AIDS, Singer and associates studied the immunologic effects of lipid-based home parenteral nutrition in which 50% of nonprotein calories were given as fat.[119] After 2 months, an improved in vitro lymphocytic mitogenic response to phytohemagglutinin and to concanavalin A was noted, although the number of lymphocytes did not seem to be modified by the administration of intravenous lipids. In a prospective randomized double-blind multicenter trial, the immunologic effects of two lipid emulsions, LCTs or a balanced 50%-50% emulsion of LCTs and MCTs (LCT-MCT), were compared.[120] Patients were given a ternary mixture providing 1.5 g of protein per kilogram per day, a calorie intake of 30 kcal/kg, divided into 60% lipids and 40% carbohydrates. After 6 days of parenteral therapy, no changes in the lymphocyte count or different lymphocyte subpopulations were found in either group. However, an LCT intake of 2 g/kg/day seemed to induce decreased lymphocyte proliferation with different stimuli, although such abnormalities were not observed with LCT-MCT emulsion. No significant changes in T cell subset counts have been observed. Singer and associates did not observe any changes in viral cultures or in serum levels of p24 antigen.[119] Gelas and colleagues noted nonsignificant variations in the mean levels of p24: a decrease in the LCT-MCT group, and an increase in the LCT group.[120] Further studies with longer observation periods are needed to determine the effects of prolonged therapy with various lipid emulsions on the immune system and HIV disease.

Whether TPN predisposes HIV-infected patients to more catheter infections is a valid concern, with the literature showing mixed results (Table 22–3). A totally implantable central venous access device (port-A-Cath) appears to be safe for home infusion therapy in AIDS patients, without an additional risk of infection.[121] Early use

Table 22–3. Catheter-Related Complications and Infections in Patients with AIDS

Study	Complications/100 days	Infections/100 days
AIDS		
Altilio et al.,[123] 1988	—	1.19
Raviglione et al.,[122] 1989	—	0.47
Henry et al.,[147] 1989		0.31
Rosenthal et al.,[148] 1989		0.40
Saltzman et al.,[149] 1989		0.20
Skoutelis et al.,[150] 1989		0.19
Thurn et al.,[151] 1989		0.28
Singer et al.,[124] 1991	0.25	0.12
Van der Pijl and Frissen[121] 1992	0.40	0.13
Melchior et al.,[115] 1996	—	0.26
Non-AIDS		
Cancer[152]	0.30	
Crohn's disease[152]	0.25	
Ischemic bowel[152]	0.38	

AIDS, acquired immunodeficiency syndrome.

of Hickman catheters in AIDS patients receiving home parenteral therapy demonstrated an increased risk of catheter-related infections.[122, 123] Some studies of home parenteral nutrition in AIDS patients did not find higher risks of catheter-related sepsis or complications compared with other patient populations in which home parenteral nutrition is commonly applied,[115, 124] whereas in another study, increased rate of catheter-related infections were found.[125]

Adjuvant Therapies

Wasting is associated with a decreased quality of life and increased mortality. Decreased energy intake is a major contributing factor in the weight loss seen in AIDS patients. Increasing the total calories by appetite stimulants or enteral or parenteral hyperalimentation may result in weight gain but does not consistently result in an increase in LBM. In addition, improved physical performance may not occur with weight gain. For this reason, adjuvant therapy with anabolic agents is receiving increased attention due to its potential in increasing BCM. In the following section, the use of recombinant human growth hormone (rhGH), testosterone replacement, and other therapies is discussed.

Anabolic Agents

Pharmacologic doses of rhGH have previously been demonstrated to induce nitrogen retention both in acute catabolic conditions such as those seen after surgery and burns[126] and in otherwise healthy patients fed hypocaloric diets. On the basis of these results in other catabolic states, studies were undertaken to determine whether treatment with rhGH could produce an anabolic response in persons with HIV-associated weight loss.

In a small prospective randomized double-blind clinical trial, metabolic and anthropometric changes induced by "pharmacologic" versus "physiologic" doses of rhGH were examined.[127] The pharmacologic dose resulted in weight gain, increased LBM and total body water, and decreased fat mass and urinary nitrogen excretion. There was also an improvement in muscle power and endurance. However, these patients lost the weight gained 6 weeks after completion of

the study and termination of rhGH treatment. Minor positive changes in body composition were observed in the physiologic-dose rhGH group.

Administration of rhGH induced body weight increases and decreased urinary nitrogen and potassium excretion in a small group of patients who were hospitalized and fed a constant diet in a metabolic ward.[128] Subsequently, a randomized double-blind multicenter trial was performed to determine whether the protein-anabolic effect of a pharmacologic dose of rhGH could be sustained over a longer period in a larger group of patients.[129] Treatment with rhGH for 12 weeks resulted in a sustained and significant increase in weight and LBM, accompanied by a decrease in body fat. Although there was no significant difference in the overall quality of life and general health perception between the placebo and rhGH groups, a greater increase in treadmill work output was noted in the group receiving rhGH. There were no significant differences between the groups in clinical events, AIDS progression, or viral load. When components of energy metabolism were evaluated in patients treated with chronic rhGH, the REE and lipid oxidation increased, whereas protein oxidation decreased.[130] In a subset of patients who kept written food records, there were no significant effects of rhGH on the energy intake. A modest and nonsignificant trend for an increase in energy intake was obviated when adjusted for increases in weight, LBM, or REE. The study suggested that increases in weight and LBM occurred during rhGH treatment in the absence of significant sustained increases in energy intake.

Preliminary data suggested that rhGH can also be effective in limiting the acute weight loss associated with a systemic infection. In a placebo-controlled study in 20 patients beginning treatment for an opportunistic infection, patients randomized to rhGH experienced significant increases in LBM and reductions in protein oxidation during a 2-week course of treatment.[131]

The beneficial effects of rhGH on body composition and metabolism likely are mediated by insulin-like growth factor I (IGF-I). Limited studies of rhGH or recombinant human IGF-I (rhIGF-I) treatment alone in patients with AIDS have also resulted in an increase in circulating IGF-I levels, but with little effect on LBM and muscle function. In a randomized double-blind placebo-controlled trial, treatment with 12 weeks of rhGH, rhIGF-I, or both, was examined in patients with AIDS-associated wasting.[132] At 6 weeks, growth factors (rhGH and rhIGF-I) alone and in combination only modestly increased LBM and decreased total fat mass. No further improvements in body mass were seen after 12 weeks. Improvements in LBM persisted for 12 weeks only in the group that received both rhGH and rhIGF-I. Immunologic function did not improve in any group.

In normal men, supraphysiologic doses of testosterone (600 mg of testosterone enanthate intramuscularly weekly for 10 weeks), administered alone or in conjunction with strength training, increased FFM, muscle size, and strength.[133] Testosterone replacement has also been studied in HIV infection. Data suggest a significant benefit of physiologic testosterone replacement in the large subpopulation of androgen-deficient men and women with the AIDS wasting syndrome. Body composition was analyzed at baseline and after 12 weeks of open-label treatment with testosterone cypionate (Upjohn, Kalamazoo, Mich.) 400 mg biweekly intramuscularly, in HIV-infected men with sexual dysfunction.[134] Body composition by bioimpedance analysis (RJL Systems, Clinton Township, Mich.) showed that the increase in weight observed consisted of a significant increase in FFM, and a trend toward a decrease in body fat. The BCM increased by an average of 1.2 kg, which was statistically significant.

In the first randomized placebo-controlled study of physiologic testosterone administration in androgen-deficient men with the AIDS wasting syndrome, a net benefit of approximately 2.5 kg in LBM was demonstrated after 6 months of intramuscular testosterone enanthate administration at 300 mg intramuscularly every 3 weeks.[135] Patients receiving testosterone experienced significant improvement in the quality of life and overall well-being. Further study of this cohort for an additional 6 months during open-label administration demonstrated a sustained increase in LBM over the 12 months, with a net increase in LBM of 7.6% from baseline. The administration of physiologic doses of testosterone to women with the AIDS wasting syndrome has also been investigated. In a pilot study using an investigational skin patch system to deliver small quantities of testosterone appropriate for

women, a significant increase in weight was demonstrated.[136] Positive trends toward an improved quality of life were also demonstrated. Further studies involving androgen administration in women are needed, as well as in eugonadal men with the AIDS wasting syndrome.

Other anabolic steroids, such as nandrolone decanoate and oxandrolone, are also being evaluated for their efficacy in the treatment of wasting. Two studies using nandrolone decanoate for mild to moderate HIV wasting have shown increases in weight and LBM with short-term use.[137, 138] In a pilot study, oxymetholone (Anapolon, Syntex, Palo Alto, Calif.), a derivative of testosterone, was associated with weight gain and an improved quality of life.[139] In a multicenter double-blind study, oxandrolone (BTG Pharmaceuticals, Iselin, N.J.) resulted in weight gain and increased appetite and physical activity levels.[140] A study measuring body composition using bioeletric impedance in patients treated with oxandrolone had shown an increase in body weight and an increase in BCM, fat, and intracellular water.[141] In a large multicenter trial of oxandrolone in HIV-associated wasting, no significant effect on body composition at usual recommended doses was found, but evidence of liver toxicity was found at high doses (Carl Grunfeld, personal communication).

Other Therapies

Several agents have been proposed as cytokine inhibitors, including antioxidants, n-3 fatty acids, pentoxifylline (Trental, Hoechst-Roussel, Somerville, N.J.), and thalidomide (Celgene Corp., Warren, N.J.). Thalidomide (α-N-phthalimidoglutarimide) was developed in the late 1950s as a sedative in pregnancy but was soon shown to have teratogenic effects. Its current approved use is in the treatment of erythema nodosum leprosum. Thalidomide decreases TNF activity through enhancement of mRNA degradation. Short-term administration of thalidomide has been reported to induce weight gain in patients with HIV-associated wasting[142] and may be effective as therapy for aphthous ulceration of the mouth and oropharynx[143] and for diarrhea associated with cryptosporidiosis or microsporidiosis. The principal toxicities are drowsiness, rash, and peripheral neuropathy. There is concern about possible adverse effects of thalidomide on the HIV viral burden, and cotreatment with a highly active anti-HIV drug regimen should be considered. Effective contraceptive is mandatory for use in women.

Dietary supplementation with n-3 fatty acids has been proposed to modulate the inflammatory and immune process in HIV infection, as well as in other clinical states such as in cancer and burn patients; however, no apparent clinical benefit was observed in treatment studies.[144, 145]

In addition to the provision of adequate nutrition, exercise may become an important component of therapy to improve LBM. Scattered reports suggest that exercise training is feasible in HIV-infected individuals, including chronically ill subjects but not acutely ill subjects, and may lead to increased muscle strength. Progressive resistance exercise has been shown to improve skeletal muscle function and anthropometry in stable AIDS patients.[146]

SUMMARY

Proper nutritional management can have a positive impact on the clinical course of HIV-infected patients. With better treatment options and in the era of protease inhibitors, the nutritional status in HIV-infected individuals remains to be clarified. The role of HIV infection itself in the pathogenesis of malnutrition needs further evaluation. Further work is required to optimize therapy. Optimal therapy with combination treatments or other means of optimizing nutritional support require further investigation. Further studies directed at providing nutritional therapy during acute illnesses to minimize tissue depletion and debilitation associated with disease complications are needed.

REFERENCES

1. Nahlen BL, Chu SY, Nwanyanwu OC, et al: HIV wasting syndrome in the United States. AIDS 7:183–188, 1993.
2. Fleming PL, Cieleski CA, Byers RH, et al: Gender differences in reported AIDS indicative diagnoses. J Infect Dis 168:61–67, 1993.
3. Field-Gardner CA: Review of mechanisms of wasting in HIV disease. Nutr Clin Pract 10:167–176, 1995.
4. Centers for Disease Control: Revision of the CDC surveillance case definition for acquired immunodeficiency syndrome. MMWR 36:3S–15S, 1987.
5. Wheeler DA, Gibert CL, Launer CA, et al: Weight loss as a predictor of survival and disease progression in HIV infection. J Acquir Immune Defic Syndr Hum Retrovirol 18:80–85, 1998.
6. Chlebowski RT, Grosvenor MB, Bernhard NH, et al: Nutritional status, gastrointestinal dysfunction, and survival in patients with AIDS. Am J Gastroenterol 84:1288–1293, 1989.
7. Macallan DC, Noble C, Baldwin C, et al: Prospective analysis of patterns of weight change in stage IV HIV infection. Am J Clin Nutr 58:417–424, 1993.
8. Kotler DP, Tierney AR, Altilio D, et al: Body mass repletion during ganciclovir treatment of cytomegalovirus infections in patients with acquired immunodeficiency syndrome. Arch Intern Med 149:901–905, 1989.
9. Palenicek JP, Graham NMH, He YD, et al: Weight loss prior to clinical AIDS as a predictor of survival. J Acquir Immune Defic Syndr Hum Retrovirol 10:366–373, 1995.
10. Guenter PG, Muurahainen NE, Simons G, et al: Relationships among nutritional status, disease progression, and survival in HIV infection. J Acquir Immune Defic Syndr Hum Retrovirol 6:1130–1138, 1996.
11. Chlebowski RT, Grosvenor MB, Bernhard NH, et al: Nutritional status, gastrointestinal dysfunction, and survival in patients with AIDS. Am J Gastroentrol 84:1288, 1989.
12. Gibert C, Launer C, Bartsch G, et al: Body weight and percent weight change as predictors of mortality in AIDS [Abstract 215A]. Proceedings 35th ICAAC, 1995;I56.
13. Cohan GR, Muurahainen N, Guenter P, et al: HIV-related hospitalization, CD4 percent and nutritional markers [Abstract 3:67A]. Proceedings Eighth International Conference on AIDS, Amsterdam, The Netherlands, 1992.
14. Kotler DP, Tierney AR, Wang J, et al: Magnitude of body-cell-mass depletion and timing of death from wasting in AIDS. Am J Clin Nutr 50:444–447, 1989.
15. Suttmann U, Ockenga O, Selberg O, et al: Incidence and prognostic value of malnutrition and wasting in HIV-infected outpatients. J Acquir Immune Defic Syndr Hum Retrovirol 8:239–246, 1995.
16. Turner J, Muurahainen N, Terrell C, et al: Nutritional status and quality of life [Abstract]. Proc Tenth Int Conf AIDS, 1994; 2:35.
17. Wilson IB, Cleary PD: Clinical predictors of declines in physical functioning in persons with AIDS: Results of a longitudinal study. J Acquir Immune Defic Syndr Hum Retrovirol 16:343–349, 1997.
18. Heymsfeld SB, McManus C, Stevens V, et al: Muscle mass: Reliable indicator of protein-energy malnutrition severity and outcome. Am J Clin Nutr 35:1192–1199, 1982.
19. Ott M, Lembeke B, Fischer H, et al: Early changes of body composition in human immunodeficiency virus-infected patients: Tetrapolar body impedance analysis indicates significant malnutrition. Am J Clin Nutr 57:15–19, 1993.
20. Kotler DP, Wang J, Pierson RN: Studies of body

composition in patients with the acquired immunodeficiency syndrome. Am J Clin Nutr 42:1255, 1985.

21. Wang ZM, Visser M, Ma R, et al: Skeletal muscle mass: Validation of neutron activation and dual energy x-ray absorptiometry methods by computerized tomography. J Appl Physiol 80:824, 1996.

22. Kotler DP, Tierney AR, Dilmanian FA, et al: Correlation between total body potassium and total body nitrogen in patients with acquired immunodeficiency syndrome. Clin Res 39:549A, 1991.

23. Grinspoon S, Corcoran C, Miller K, et al: Body composition and endocrine function in women with acquired immunodeficiency syndrome wasting. J Clin Endocrinol Metab 82:1332–1337, 1997.

24. Kotler DP, Engelson E, Thea DM, et al: Relative influences of race, sex, environment, and HIV infection upon body composition in adults. Am J Clin Nutr, in press.

25. Babameto G, Kotler DP, Burastero S, et al: Alterations in hydration in HIV-infected individuals [Abstract]. Clin Res 42:279, 1994.

26. Mulligan K, Tai VW, Schambelan M: Cross-sectional and longitudinal evaluation of body composition in men with HIV infection. J Acquir Immune Defic Syndr Hum Retrovirol 15:43–48, 1997.

27. Grinspoon S, Corcoran C, Miller K, et al: Body composition and endocrine function in women with acquired immunodeficiency syndrome wasting. J Clin Endocrinol Metab 82:1332–1337, 1997.

28. Grinspoon S, Corcoran C, Lee K, et al: Loss of lean body and muscle mass correlates with androgen levels in hypogonadal men with acquired immunodeficiency syndrome and wasting. J Clin Endocrinol Metab 81:4051–4058, 1996.

29. Hommes MJ, Romijn JA, Godfried MH, et al: Increased resting energy expenditure in human immunodeficiency virus infected men. Metabolism 39:1186–1190, 1990.

30. Hommes MJT, Romijn JA, Endert E: Resting energy expenditure and substrate oxidation in human immunodeficiency (HIV)-infected asymptomatic men: HIV affects host metabolism in the early asymptomatic stage. Am J Clin Nutr 54:311–315, 1991.

31. Rivera S, Briggs W, Qian D, et al: Levels of HIV RNA are quantitatively related to prior weight loss in HIV associated wasting. J Acquir Immune Defic Syndr Hum Retrovirol 17:411–418, 1998.

32. Mulligan K, Tai VW, Schambelan M: Energy expenditure in HIV infection. N Engl J Med 336:70–71, 1997.

33. Fischl MA, Richman DD, Grieco MH, et al: The efficacy of azidothymidine (AZT) in the treatment of patients with AIDS and AIDS-related complex. N Engl J Med 317:185–191, 1987.

34. Carr A, Samaras K, Burton S, et al: A syndrome of peripheral lipodystrophy, hyperlipidemia, and insulin resistance in patients receiving HIV protease inhibitors. AIDS 12:F51–58, 1998.

35. Miller KD, Jones E, Yanovski JA, et al: Visceral abdominal-fat accumulation associated with use of indinavir. Lancet 351:871–875, 1998.

36. Dong KL, Bausserman LL, Flynn MM, et al: Changes in body habitus and serum lipid abnormalities in HIV-positive women on highly active antiretroviral therapy (HAART). J Acquir Immune Defic Syndr 21:107–113, 1999.

37. Walli RK, Herfort O, Michl GM, et al: Treatment with protease inhibitors associated with peripheral insulin resistance and impaired oral glucose tolerance in HIV-1 infected patients. AIDS 12:F167–173, 1998.

38. Bjorntorp P: Abdominal obesity and the development of noninsulin dependent diabetes mellitus. Diabetes Metab Rev 4:615–622, 1998.

39. Henry K, Melroe H, Huebsch J, et al: Severe premature coronary artery disease with protease inhibitors. Lancet 351:1328, 1998.

40. Carr A, Semaras K, Chisholm DJ, et al: Pathogenesis of HIV-1 protease inhibitor-associated peripheral lipodystrophy, hyperlipidemia, and insulin resistance. Lancet 131:1881–1883, 1998.

41. Lo JC, Mulligan K, Tai VW, et al: Buffalo hump in men with HIV-1 infection. Lancet 351:867–870, 1998.

42. Engelson EE, Kotler DP, Tan YX, et al: Fat distribution in HIV-infected patients reporting truncal enlargement quantified by whole-body magnetic resonance imaging. Am J Clin Nutr 69:1162–1169, 1999.

43. Miller KK, Daly PA, Sentochnik D, et al: Pseudo-Cushing's syndrome in human immunodeficiency virus–infected patients. Clin Infect Dis 27:68–72, 1998.

44. Kotler DP, Rosenbaum K, Wang J, et al: Studies of body composition and fat distribution in HIV-infected and control subjects. J Acquir Immune Defic Syndr 20:228–237, 1999.

45. Beach RS, Mantero-Atienza E, Shor-Posner G, et al: Specific nutrient abnormalities in asymptomatic HIV-1 infection. AIDS 6:701–708, 1992.

46. Harriman GR, Smith PD, McDonald KH, et al: Vitamin B$_{12}$ malabsorption in patients with the acquired immunodeficiency syndrome. Arch Intern Med 149:2039, 1989.

47. Beach RS, Morgan R, Wilkie F, et al: Plasma cobalamin levels as a potential cofactor in studies of HIV-1 related cognitive changes. Arch Neurol 49:501–506, 1992.

48. Baum MK, Mantero-Atienza E, Shor-Posner G, et al: Association of vitamin B$_6$ status with parameters of immune function in early HIV-1 infection. J Acquir Immune Defic Syndr Hum Retrovirol 4:1122, 1991.

49. Baum MK, Shor-Posner G, Lai S, et al: High risk of HIV-related mortality is associated with selenium deficiency. J Acquir Immune Defic Syndr Hum Retrovirol 15:370–374, 1997.

50. Baum MK, Shor-Posner G, Lu Y, et al: Micronutrients and HIV-1 disease progression. AIDS 9:1051–1056, 1995.

51. Dworkin BM, Antonecchia PP, Smith F: Reduced cardiac selenium content in the acquired immunodeficiency syndrome. JPEN J Parenter Enteral Nutr 13:644–647, 1989.

52. Semba RD, Graham NMH, Caiaffa WT, et al: Increased mortality associated with vitamin A deficiency during HIV-1 infection. Arch Intern Med 153:2149–2154, 1993.

53. Semba RD, Miotti PG, Chiphangwi JD, et al: Maternal vitamin A deficiency and mother-to-child transmission of HIV-1. Lancet 343:1593–1597, 1994.

54. Cunningham-Rundles S, Kim SH, Dnistrian A, et al: Micronutrient and cytokine interaction in congenital pediatric HIV infection. J Nutr 126:2674S–2679S, 1996.

55. Manolagas SC, Hustmyer FG, Yu XP: Immunomodulatory properties of 1,25 dihydroxy vitamin D₃. Kidney Int 38:S9, 1990.

56. Roederer M, Staal FJT, Raju PA, et al: Cytokine-stimulated HIV replication is inhibited by N-acetylcysteine. Proc Natl Acad Sci U S A 87:4884, 1990.

57. Allard JP, Aghdassi E, Chau J, et al: Oxidative stress and plasma antioxidant micronutrients in humans with HIV infection. Am J Clin Nutr 67:143–147, 1998.

58. Pace GW, Leaf CD: The role of oxidative stress in HIV disease. Free Radic Biol Med 19:523–528, 1995.

59. Melchior JC, Salmon D, Rigaud D, et al: Resting energy expenditure is increased in stable, malnourished HIV-infected patients. Am J Clin Nutr 53:437–441, 1991.

60. Grunfeld C, Pang M, Shimizu L, et al: Resting energy expenditure, caloric intake, and short-term weight change in human immunodeficiency virus infection and the acquired immunodeficiency syndrome. Am J Clin Nutr 55:455–460, 1992.

61. Kotler DP, Tierney AR, Brenner SK, et al: Preservation of short-term energy balance in clinically stable patients with AIDS. Am J Clin Nutr 57:7, 1990.

62. Grinspoon S, Corcoran C, Miller K, et al: Determinants of increased energy expenditure in HIV-infected women. Am J Clin Nutr 68:720–725, 1998.

63. Sharpstone D, Ross H, Hancock M, et al: Indirect calorimetry, body composition, and small bowel function in asymptomatic HIV-seropositive women. Int J STD AIDS 8:700–703, 1997.

64. Macallan DC, Noble C, Baldwin C, et al: Energy expenditure and wasting in human immunodeficiency virus infection. N Engl J Med 333:83–88, 1995.

65. Grunfeld C, Kotler DP: The wasting syndrome and nutritional support in AIDS. Semin Gastrointest Dis 2:25–36, 1991.

66. Macallan DC, McNurlan MA, Milne E, et al: Whole body protein turnover from leucine kinetics and the response to nutrition in HIV infection. Am J Clin Nutr 61:818–826, 1995.

67. Lieberman SA, Butterfield GE, Harrison D, et al: Anabolic effects of recombinant insulin-like growth factor-I in cachectic patients with the acquired immunodeficiency syndrome. J Clin Endocrinol Metab 78:404–410, 1994.

68. Stein TP, Nutinsky C, Condoluci D, et al: Protein and energy substrate metabolism in AIDS patients. Metabolism 39:876–881, 1990.

69. Selberg O, Suttman U, Melzer A, et al: Effect of increased protein intake and nutritional status on whole-body protein metabolism of AIDS patients with weight loss. Metabolism 44:1159–1165, 1995.

70. Ash SA, Griffin GE: Effect of parenteral nutrition on protein turnover in endotoxaemic rats. Clin Sci 76:659–666, 1989.

71. Streat SJ, Beddoe AH, Hill GL: Aggressive nutritional support does not prevent protein loss despite fat gain in septic intensive care patients. J Trauma 27:262–266, 1987.

72. Feingold KR, Grunfeld C: Tumor necrosis factor alpha stimulates hepatic lipogenesis in the rat in vivo. J Clin Invest 80:184–190, 1987.

73. Feingold KR, Soued M, Adi S, et al: The effect of interleukin-1 on lipid metabolism in the rat: Similarities to and differences from tumor necrosis factor. Arterioscler Thromb Vasc Biol 11:495–500, 1991.

74. Grunfeld C, Kotler DP, Shigenaga JK, et al: Circulating interferon-α levels and hypertriglyceridemia in the acquired immunodeficiency syndrome. Am J Med 90:154–162, 1991.

75. Lahdevirta J, Maury CPJ, Teppo AM, et al: Elevated levels of circulating cachetin/tumor necrosis factor in patients with acquired immunodeficiency syndrome. Am J Med 85:289–291, 1988.

76. Thea DM, Porat R, Nagimbi K, et al: Plasma cytokines, cytokine antagonists, and disease progression in African women infected with HIV-1. Ann Intern Med 124:757–762, 1996.

77. Kelly P, Summerbell C, Ngwenya B, et al: Systemic immune activation as a potential determinant of wasting in Zambians with HIV-related diarrhoea. Q J Med 89:831–837, 1996.

78. Rimaniol AC, Zylberberg H, Zavala F, et al: Inflammatory cytokines and inhibitors in HIV infection: Correlation between interleukin-1 receptor antagonist and weight loss. AIDS 10:1349–1356, 1996.

79. Dobs AS, Dempsey MA, Ladenson PW, et al: Endocrine disorders in men infected with HIV. Am J Med 84:611–616, 1988.

80. Coodley GO, Loveless MO, Nelson HD, et al: Endocrine function in the HIV wasting syndrome. J Acquir Immune Defic Syndr Hum Retrovirol 7:46, 1994.

81. Dobs AS, Dempsey MA, Landenson PW, et al: Endocrine disorders in men infected with human immunodeficiency virus. Am J Med 84:611, 1988.

82. Abbott M, Khoo SH, Hammer MR, et al: Prevalence of cortisol deficiency in late HIV disease. J Infect 31:1–4, 1995.

83. LoPresti JS, Fried JC, Spencer CA, et al: Unique alterations of thyroid hormone indices in the acquired immunodeficiency syndrome (AIDS). Ann Intern Med 110:970–975, 1989.

84. Grunfeld C, Pang M, Doerrier W, et al: Indices of thyroid function and weight loss in human immunodeficiency virus infection and the acquired immunodeficiency syndrome. Metabolism 42:1270–1276, 1993.

85. Sharkey SJ, Sharkey KA, Sutherland LR, Church DL. Nutritional status and food intake in HIV infection. J Acquir Immune Defic Syndr Hum Retrovirol 5:1091–1098, 1992.

86. Mercado I, Sharp V: Factors associated with malnutrition among HIV positive individuals [Abstract PO-B36–2377]. Presented at Ninth Int Conf AIDS; Berlin, 1993.

87. Chlebowski RT, Grosvenor M, Lillington L, et al: Dietary intake and counseling, weight maintenance, and the course of HIV infection. J Am Diet Assoc 95:428–432, 1995.

88. Kotler DP, Reka S, Orenstein JM, Fox CH: Chronic idiopathic esophageal ulceration in the acquired immunodeficiency syndrome: Characterization and treatment with corticosteroids. J Clin Gastroenterol 15:284–290, 1992.

89. Kotler DP, Wilson CS, Haroutounian G, Fox CH: Detection of HIV-1 RNA in solitary esophageal ulcers in two patients with the acquired immunodeficiency syndrome. Am J Gastroenterol 84:313–317, 1989.

90. Patton JS, Peters PM, McCabe J, et al: Development of partial tolerance to the gastrointestinal effects of high doses of recombinant tumor necrosis factor alpha in rodents. J Clin Invest 80:1587–1596, 1987.

91. Fantino M, Wieteska L: Evidence for a direct central anorectic effect of tumor necrosis factor alpha in the rat. Physiol Behav 53:477, 1993.

92. Roth RI, Owen RL, Keren DF, et al: Intestinal infection with Mycobacterium avium in acquired immunodeficiency syndrome (AIDS): Histological and clinical comparison with Whipple's disease. Dig Dis Sci 30:497, 1985.

93. Kotler DP, Reka S, Chow K, et al: Effects of enteric parasitoses and HIV infection upon small intestinal structure and function in patients with AIDS. J Clin Gastroenterol 16:10–15, 1993.

94. Kotler DP, Giang TT, Thiim M, et al: Chronic bacterial enteropathy in patients with AIDS. J Infect Dis 171:552–558, 1995.

95. Wanke CA, Mayer H, Weber R, et al: Enteroaggregative Escherichia coli as a potential cause of diarrheal disease in adults infected with human immunodeficiency virus. J Infect Dis 178:185–190, 1998.

96. Babameto G, Kotler DP: Malnutrition in HIV infection. Gastroenterol Clin North Am 26:393–415, 1997.

97. Von Roenn JH, Armstrong D, Kotler DP, et al: Megestrol acetate in patients with AIDS-related cachexia. Ann Intern Med 121:393–399, 1994.

98. Oster MH, Enders SP, Samuels SJ, et al: Megestrol acetate in patients with AIDS and cachexia. Ann Intern Med 121:400–408, 1994.

99. Engelson ES, Pi-Sunyer FX, Kotler DP: Effects of megestrol acetate on body composition and circulating testosterone in patients with AIDS. AIDS 9:1107–1108, 1995.

100. Gorter R, Seefried M, Volberding P: Dronabinol effects on weight in patients with HIV infection. AIDS 6:127, 1992.

101. Struwe M, Kaempfer SH, Geiger CJ, et al: Effect of dronabinol on nutritional status in HIV infection. Ann Pharmacol 27:827, 1993.

102. Suttmann U, Ockenga J, Schneider H: Weight gain and increased concentrations of receptor proteins for tumor necrosis factor after patients with symptomatic HIV infection received fortified nutrition support. J Am Diet Assoc 96:565–569, 1996.

103. Pichard C, Sudre P, Karsegard V: A randomized double-blind controlled study of 6 months of oral nutritional supplementation with arginine and n-3 fatty acids in HIV-infected patients. AIDS 12:53–63, 1998.

104. Chlebowski RT, Beall G, Grosvenor M, et al: Long-term effects of early nutritional support with new enterotropic peptide-based formula vs. standard enteral formula in HIV-infected patients: Randomized propective trial. Nutrition 9:507–512, 1993.

105. Stack JA, Bell SJ, Burke PA, et al: High-energy, high-protein, oral, liquid, nutrition supplementation in patients with HIV infection: Effect on weight status in relation to incidence of secondary infection. J Am Diet Assoc 96:337–341, 1996.

106. Salomon SB, Jung J, Voss T, et al: An elemental diet containing medium-chain triglycerides and enzymatically hydrolyzed protein can improve gastrointestinal tolerance in people infected with HIV. J Am Diet Assoc 98:460–462, 1998.

107. Craig CB, Darnell BE, Weinsier RL: Decreased fat and nitrogen losses in patients with AIDS receiving medium-chain triglyceride–enriched formula vs those receiving long-chain triglyceride-containing formula. J Am Diet Assoc 97:605–611, 1997.

108. Kotler DP, Tierney AR, Muurahainen N, et al: Nutritional supplements containing long- or medium-chain triglycerides: Effects upon body weight and composition in HIV-infected subjects with <100 CD4 + lymphocytes/mm³ [Abstract 42347]. Presented at 12th World AIDS Conference, Geneva, 1998.

109. Kotler DP, Tierney AR, Ferraro R, et al: Enteral alimentation and repletion of body cell mass in malnourished patients with acquired immunodeficiency syndrome. Am J Clin Nutr 53:149–154, 1991.

110. Dowling S, Kane D, Chua A, et al: An evaluation of percutaneous endoscopic gastrostomy feeding in AIDS. Int J STD AIDS 7:106, 1996.

111. Brantsma A, Kelson K, Malcom J: Percutaneous endoscopic gastrostomy feeding in HIV disease. Aust J Adv Nur 8:36, 1991.

112. Cappell MS, Godil A: A multicenter case controlled study of percutaneous endoscopic gastrostomy in HIV seropositive patients. Am J Gastroenterol 88:2059, 1993.

113. Ockenga J, Suttmann U, Selberg O, et al: Percutaneous endoscopic gastrostomy in AIDS and control patients: Risks and outcome. Am J Gastroenterol 91:1817, 1996.

114. Kotler DP, Tierney AR, Wang J, et al: Effect of home total parenteral nutrition upon body composition in AIDS. JPEN J Parenter Enteral Nutr 14:454–458, 1990.

115. Melchior JC, Chastang C, Gelas P: Efficacy of 2-month total parenteral nutrition in AIDS patients: A controlled randomized prospective trial. The French Multicenter Total Parenteral Nutrition Cooperative Group Study. AIDS 10:379–384, 1996.

116. Melchior JC, Gelas P, Carbonnel F, et al: Improved survival by home total parenteral nutrition in AIDS patients: Follow-up of a controlled randomized prospective trial. AIDS 12:336–337, 1998.

117. Kotler DP, Fogleman L, Tierney AR: Comparison of total parenteral nutrition and an oral, semielemental diet on body composition, physical function, and nutrition-related costs in patients with malabsorption due to acquired immunodeficiency sydrome. JPEN J Parenter Enteral Nutr 22:120–126, 1998.

118. Wachtel T, Piette J, Mor V, et al: Quality of life in persons with human immunodeficiency virus infection: Measurement by the medical outcomes survey instrument. Ann Intern Med 115:129–137, 1992.

119. Singer P, Rubinstein A, Askanazi J, et al: Clinical and immunologic effects of lipid-based parenteral nutrition in AIDS. JPEN J Parenter Enteral Nutr 16:165–167, 1992.

120. Gelas P, Cotte L, Poitevin-Later F, et al: Effect of parenteral medium- and long-chain triglycerides on lymphocytes subpopulations and functions in patients with acquired immunodeficiency syndrome: A prospective study. JPEN J Parenter Enteral Nutr 22:67–71, 1998.

121. Van der Pijl H, Frissen J: Experience with a totally implantable venous access device (Port-A-Cath) in patients with AIDS. AIDS 6:709–713, 1992.

122. Raviglione MC, Battan R, Pablos-Mendez A, et al: Infections associated with Hickman catheters in patients with acquired immunodeficiency syndrome. Am J Med 86:780–786, 1989.

123. Altilio D, Tierney AR, Kotler DP [Letter]. Nutr Clin Pract 3:171–172, 1988.

124. Singer P, Rothkopf MM, Kvetan V, et al: Risks and benefits of home parenteral nutrition in the acquired immunodeficiency syndrome. JPEN J Parenter Enteral Nutr 15:75–79, 1991.

125. Mukau L, Talamini MA, Sitzmann JV, et al: Long-term central venous access vs other home therapies: Complications in patients with acquired immunodeficiency syndrome. JPEN J Parenter Enteral Nutr 15:455–459, 1992.

126. Ponting GA, Halliday D, Teale JD, et al: Postoperative positive nitrogen balance with intravenous hyponutrition and growth hormone. Lancet 1:438–441, 1988.

127. Krentz AJ, Koster FT, Crist DM, et al: Anthropometric, metabolic, and immunological effects of recombinant human growth hormone in AIDS and AIDS-related complex. J Acquir Immune Defic Syndr Hum Retrovirol 6:245–251, 1993.

128. Mulligan K, Grunfeld C, Hellerstein MK, et al: Anabolic effects of recombinant human growth hormone in patients with wasting associated with human immunodeficiency virus infection. J Clin Endocrinol Metab 77:956–962, 1993.

129. Schambelan M, Mulligan K, Grunfeld C, et al: Recombinant human growth hormone in patients with HIV-associated wasting: A randomized, placebo controlled trial. Ann Intern Med 125:873–882, 1996.

130. Mulligan K, Tai VW, Schambelan M: Effects of chronic growth hormone treatment on energy intake and resting energy metabolism in patients with human immunodeficiency virus–associated wasting—A clinical research center study. J Clin Endocrinol Metab 83:1542–1547, 1998.

131. Paton NI, Newton PJ, Sharpstone DR, et al: Short-term growth hormone administration at the time of opportunistic infections in HIV-positive patients. AIDS 13:1195–1202, 1999.

132. Waters D, Danska J, Hardy K, et al: Recombinant human growth hormone, insulin-like growth factor 1, and combination therapy in AIDS-associated wasting: A randomized, double-blind, placebo controlled trial. Ann Intern Med 125:865–872, 1996.

133. Bhasin S, Storer TW, Berman N, et al: The effects of supraphysiologic doses of testosterone on muscle size and strength in normal men. N Engl J Med 335:1–7, 1996.

134. Engelson ES, Rabkin JG, Rabkin R, et al: Effects of testosterone upon body composition. J Acquir Immune Defic Syndr Hum Retrovirol 11:510–514, 1996.

135. Grinspoon S, Corcoran C, Askari H, et al: Effects of androgen administration in men with the AIDS wasting syndrome: A randomized, double-blind, placebo-controlled trial. Ann Intern Med 129:18–26, 1998.

136. Miller K, Corcoran C, Armstrong C, et al: Transdermal testosterone administration in women with acquired immunodeficiency syndrome wasting: A pilot study. J Clin Endocrinol Metab 83:2717–2725, 1998.

137. Bucher G, Berger DS, Fields-Gardner C, et al: A prospective study on the safety and effect of nandrolone decanoate in HIV-positive patients. Presented at Eleventh International Conference on AIDS, July 7–12, 1996, Vancouver, Canada.

138. Gold J, High HA, Li Y, et al: Safety and efficacy of nandrolone decanoate for treatment of wasting in patients with HIV infection. AIDS 10:745–752, 1996.

139. Hengge UR, Baumann M, Maleba R, et al: Oxymetholone promotes weight gain in patients with advanced HIV-1 infection. Br J Nutr 75:129–138, 1996.

140. Berger JR, Pall L, Hall CD, et al: Oxandrolone in AIDS-wasting myopathy. AIDS 10:1657–1662, 1996.

141. Poles MA, Meller JA, Lin A, et al: Oxandrolone as a treatment for AIDS-related weight loss and wasting. Presented at Infectious Disease Society of America Conference, 1996.

142. Haslett P, Hempstead M, Seidman C, et al: The metabolic and immunologic effects of short-term thalidomide treatment of patients infected with the human immunodeficiency virus. AIDS Res Hum Retroviruses 13:1047–1054, 1997.

143. Jacobson JM, Greenspan JS, Spritzler J, et al: Thalidomide for the treatment of oral aphthous ulcers in patients with human immunodeficiency virus infection. N Engl J Med 336:1487–1493, 1997.

144. Bell SJ, Chavali S, Bistrian BR, et al: Dietary fish oil and cytokine and eicosanoid production during human immunodeficiency virus infection. JPEN J Parenter Enteral Nutr 20:43–49, 1996.

145. Hellerstein MK, Wu K, McGrath M, et al: Effects of dietary n-3 fatty acid supplementation in men with weight loss associated with the acquired immune deficiency syndrome: Relation to indices of cytokine production. J Acquir Immune Defic Syndr Hum Retrovirol 11:258, 1996.

146. Spence DW, Galantino ML, Mossberg KA, et al: Progressive resistance exercise: Effective on muscle function and anthropometry of a select AIDS population. Arch Phys Med Rehabil 71:644–648, 1990.

147. Henry K, Thurn J, Johnson S: Experience with central venous catheters in patients with AIDS. N Engl J Med 320:1496, 1989.

148. Rosenthal J, Langley C, Lederman M: Sepsis from implanted catheters in patients with AIDS. Presented at Fifth International Conference on AIDS, June 4–9, 1989, Montreal, Quebec, Canada.

149. Saltzman B, Perlman D, Levey D, et al: Infections and complications of indwelling central venous catheters: Comparisons between patients with AIDS vs other illnesses. Presented at Fifth International Conference on AIDS, June 4–9, 1989, Montreal, Quebec, Canada.

150. Skoutelis A, Murphy R, MacDonell K, et al: Indwelling central venous catheter infections in patients with acquired immune deficiency syndrome. J Acquir Immune Defic Syndr Hum Retrovirol 3:335–342, 1990.

151. Thurn HK Jr, Johnson S: Experience with central venous catheters in patients with AIDS. N Engl J Med 320:1496, 1989.

152. Howard L, Ament M, Fleming CR, et al: Current use and clinical outcome of home parenteral and enteral nutrition therapies in the United States. Gastroenterology 109:355–365, 1995.

23

◆ Parenteral Nutrition in Neonates

Winston W. K. Koo, M.B.B.S., F.R.A.C.P.
Eugene E. Cepeda, M.D.

Parenteral nutrition (PN) is one of the major advances in neonatal medicine, and it can be used successfully for prolonged periods in infants who cannot be fed enterally. Early use of PN can minimize the adverse impact of multiple metabolic complications (Table 23–1) in part because it provides multiple nutrients that may target a common metabolic function through different metabolic pathways.[1, 2] For example, PN can optimize energy metabolism with the provision of three different substrates—dextrose, amino acids, and fatty acids—for energy, and vitamins such as thiamine and trace elements such as chromium in PN may optimize energy metabolism by improving the tolerance to dextrose. The early use of PN also helps to maintain an optimal nutritional state and allows the infant to better tolerate enteral feeding, which in turn is critical to the successful weaning of the infant from PN. In contrast, inadequate nutritional support may contribute to a delay in growth over the short term (until hospital discharge)[3] and over the long term by the persistence of growth delay into childhood,[4] particularly in small preterm infants. Nutrient intake during the first few weeks may also be crucial to subsequent neurodevelopment,[5, 6] and improvement in nutritional support after a period of inadequate nutritional support unfortunately does not guarantee normal catch-up growth and development. Thus, the early introduction of PN is essential in neonates for whom enteral nutrition support is inadequate.

The technique of PN is deceptively simple, but many gaps still exist in our knowledge, and it is not entirely free from side effects. Nonetheless, many aspects of PN are reasonably well understood but frequently are not applied in clinical practice or are applied inappropriately, that is, "too little too late" or "too much too quickly." The former often occurs when the infant is considered to be "too sick" or "too immature" to tolerate PN. The latter often occurs when there is unreasonable expectation of dramatic reversal of prior prolonged periods of inadequate nutritional support.

Successful PN is achieved only by rigorous attention to the infant's needs, under-

Table 23–1. Multiple Problems That May be Minimized with the Early Use of Parenteral Nutrition*

Problem	Direct Role of PN	Indirect Role of PN
Obligatory tissue catabolism of ~ 1 g protein/kg/day	Amino acids	Nonprotein energy sources
Essential fatty acid deficiency	Lipid	Adequate energy intake
Hypoglycemia, hypocalcemia, ± hypophosphatemia, hyperkalemia	Specific nutrients	Minimization of tissue catabolism, e.g., lowering of release of tissue potassium
Glucose intolerance	Nondextrose (gluconeogenic) nutrients	Gluconeogenic substrates and cofactors for glucose metabolism, e.g., thiamine and chromium
Delayed tolerance to full enteral feeding	? specific substrate for gut mucosa	Maintenance of general nutritional status

*For neonates unable to receive adequate enteral feeding, the use of parenteral dextrose water should be limited to the brief period pending the routine availability of PN.

PN, parenteral nutrition.

Adapted from Koo WWK, McLaughlin K, Saba M: Nutrition support for the preterm infant. *In* Merritt RJ (ed): The A.S.P.E.N. Nutrition Support Practice Manual, Chapter 26. Washington, DC, American Society for Parenteral and Enteral Nutrition, 1998, pp 1–16; and Koo WWK, Raju NV, Tan-Laxa MA: Infant nutrition. Hong Kong J Paediatr 3:103–121, 1998.

standing the potential interference to nutrient metabolism and utilization from underlying disease and its treatment, and constant monitoring with the prevention or correction of potential side effects associated with PN therapy.

◆ INDICATIONS

PN is indicated for infants who cannot or should not be fed, for example, infants with major gastrointestinal tract anomalies before corrective procedures. Even in patients who can be fed, the presence of any condition that interferes with the successful delivery, digestion, or absorption of enteral nutrients may necessitate a period of PN. For example, most preterm infants have immature gastrointestinal, respiratory, hepatic, renal, and neurobehavioral functions at birth that may interfere with successful enteral feeding. In general, the sicker and smaller the infant, the greater the stress on the minimal nutritional reserve and the greater the need for nutritional support. Thus, PN should commence simultaneously with enteral nutrition for any infant who is not expected to tolerate adequate amounts of feeds within 2 to 3 days of initiating enteral nutrition. In preterm neonates, particularly those with birth weights under 1000 g, PN should be initiated during the first 24 hours after birth because it normally takes some days before adequate enteral intake is ensured even in those with an uncomplicated postnatal course.

◆ REQUIREMENTS

The earlier concept to individualize the PN solution for the needs of each child is a gross simplification of the extent of information needed for this purpose. Nutrient requirements for PN are based on the data from enteral nutrient intake; mass balance studies; quantitative tissue measurements, for example, bone mineral content; and the functional and metabolic status of the infant. However, detailed information is lacking in all these aspects for each nutrient. Therefore, the most practical approach is the use of a few stock solutions with minimal manipulation of the nutrient content once the desired nutrients and fluid goal are achieved. This makes ordering the PN easier

with less likelihood of making errors during the ordering and preparation of PN.

Clinical circumstances may affect nutritional needs and tolerance of parenteral nutrients. Thus, sick preterm infants have greater physiologic demand for nutrients but often do not tolerate the delivery of large amounts of nutrients because of metabolic intolerance or lower excretory capacity, or both. There are numerous other examples of this paradox with the use of PN in neonates. The increased energy need is often accompanied by glucose intolerance, especially if the clinical course is complicated by sepsis. An increased fluid requirement is often accompanied by intolerance to high fluid intake because of poor renal excretory capacity and the risk of opening the ductus arteriosus.

Another situation is that found in infants with gastrointestinal malformation or dysmotility, in whom often large volumes of gastrointestinal aspirate or fistula drainage cannot be managed by simple replacement with the existing PN solution but require the use of specifically constituted fluid. Similarly, selective supplements, for example, protein, energy, electrolytes, and minerals, are also inappropriate for infants requiring PN. Protein supplementation without adequate total energy intake and vice versa results in suboptimal growth. Increased caloric intake alone can result in weight gain, but unless there is a balanced intake of all nutrients, the resultant weight gain constitutes only glycogen and fat. Furthermore, carbon dioxide production associated with fat synthesis can increase the work of respiration[7] with deleterious consequences. Overfeeding, particularly excessive energy intake, can occur even in critically ill patients.[8]

Therefore, nutritional support should take into account the pathophysiology of the underlying disease and its therapy, with an understanding of how each factor might interfere with nutrient metabolism and utilization. All preterm infants have greater need for multiple nutrients to compensate for the missed period of rapid in utero growth and for the illnesses that frequently coexist with prematurity.[1, 2, 9–11] This is further complicated by the need to use certain drugs such as steroids and diuretics, which have direct impact on the nutritional status of the infant. Steroid therapy is associated with glucose intolerance, negative nitrogen balance, and growth delay,[12–14] and chronic diuretic use may cause electrolyte and acid-base disturbances, growth delays, and disturbed bone mineralization.[15]

There are also aspects of PN support unique to the neonate, particularly the small preterm newborn. In order to achieve the maximal nutritional support for the neonate, there is no reason to use dextrose electrolyte infusion except for the few hours needed to prepare the PN infusate. At an infusion rate of 1 mL/h, the volume infused is equivalent to 48 mL/kg/day for a small preterm infant weighing 500 g. This is equivalent to one third of the daily fluid requirement; thus, the opportunity to deliver one third of all nutrient needs would be lost with the use of dextrose electrolyte solution alone. Therefore, it is critical to maintain PN solution in infants with a birth weight of less than 1000 g even at the minimal infusion rate.

The practice of interrupting PN for drug administration differs from institution to institution and may have significant impact on the optimal delivery of PN. Acyclovir, amphotericin B, metronidazole, and trimethoprim-sulfamethoxazole are incompatible with PN solution and are normally infused in dextrose water with the PN turned off. Any interruption of PN for the administration of "incompatible" medications should be minimized. This may be achieved by careful review with the pharmacy staff and the institution's PN committee to allow the delivery of these medications in the smallest volume of non-PN solution over the shortest time possible. For similar reasons, the practice of infusing dextrose electrolyte solution to maintain a second catheter for the administration of medications should be discouraged because it wastes precious fluid volume that can be given as PN. In this circumstance, the use of a heparin lock is generally preferable.

The parenteral requirement for some nutrients may be 10 to 20% less than that of enteral nutrient because it eliminates the digestive and absorptive losses associated with enteral intake. The major differences between the needs of the term versus preterm neonate, and between the stable versus stressed neonate, are in the quantities of energy and some nutrients, although the ability to tolerate the increased delivery of nutrients also may be compromised under these circumstances, as discussed earlier.

Table 23–2. Parenteral Fluid, Macronutrients, and Mineral Needs for Stable Neonates*

	Nutrients/kg/day
Water (mL)	100–160
Energy (kcal)	80–120
Protein (g)	1.5–4
Carbohydrate	
(g)	10–15
(%)	5–20
Fat (g)	0.5–3
Sodium (mEq)	2–4
Potassium (mEq)	2–4
Chloride (mEq)	2–4
Calcium (mg)	60–90†
Phosphorus (mg)	47–70†
Magnesium (mg)	4.3–7.2†

*Once the desired fluid goal is determined, the nutrient content can begin at 60 to 70% and increase progressively to goal over 2 to 3 days to allow for better metabolic adaptation. In general, the lower range of nutrients is used for term infants, and the reverse is true for preterm infants.
†Assuming a fluid intake of 120 to 150 mL/kg/day.
Adapted from references 1, 2, and 9 through 11.

Fluid Volume

The daily macronutrient and parenteral fluid requirements of clinically stable neonates are listed in Table 23–2. The ability to tolerate large amounts of fluid is limited in neonates, particularly in very small and sick infants. However, adequate amounts of nutrients can be delivered in the usual amounts of fluid that most neonates tolerate. The major constraint to the delivery of adequate amounts of parenteral nutrients is in situations in which severe fluid restriction is needed. Smaller volumes require a greater concentration of nutrient infusate, thus resulting in extremely high osmolarity and possibly exceeding the limits of solubility of calcium and phosphorus salts. In contrast, in situations of high fluid requirement (>200 mL/kg/day) in preterm infants with low renal thresholds for many nutrients, a diluted infusate must be provided to prevent the delivery of excessive nutrients, particularly dextrose. In this situation, the limiting factor is the ability to provide a dilute solution without being significantly hypotonic. A PN solution with dextrose concentration as low as 3% may be isotonic as long as there is also at least 1% amino acid with other standard additives. Some flexibility in manipulating the tolerance to the volume infused can be achieved by manipulating environmental factors. For example, caring for the neonate under a radiant warmer results in greater insensible fluid loss and allows the delivery of a larger volume of PN.[1]

Amino Acids

Synthetic crystalline amino acids are normally used in PN in neonates. Current amino acid solutions for parenteral use are effectively utilized in neonates.[16–24] They are based on the amino acid profile of human milk and on the postprandial plasma levels of breast-fed infants.[25] These pediatric amino acid formulations contain tyrosine, aspartic acid, and glutamic acid. They also contain conditionally essential amino acids including cysteine, taurine, histidine, and arginine. Cysteine is added during compounding to minimize its precipitation in the dimeric form. The addition of cysteine (40 mg/g of amino acid) also enhances the solubility of calcium and phosphorus. The pediatric amino acid formulations contain lower concentrations of methionine, glycine, and phenylalanine than those found in amino acid solutions intended for older patients. Preparations with other sources of nitrogen including dipeptides are being used experimentally.[26]

Neonates receiving only glucose during the immediate newborn period show an obligatory loss of about 1 g of endogenous protein per kilogram per day.[16–18, 20–24] The current amino acid preparations are well utilized as indicated by standard nitrogen balance studies[16, 18] and by stable isotope studies.[17–24] They show that tissue catabolism can be minimized with the provision of PN.[16–24] In clinically stable infants, the protein gain is linearly related to the protein intake extending over a range of net protein administration from 2 to 4 g/kg/day.[16] Generally, a lower intake of 2 to 3 g/kg/day results in nitrogen retention comparable to that observed in enterally fed infants, although higher protein intakes of about 4 g/kg/day may be needed for the smallest preterm infants with a gestational age less than 28 weeks.[11, 16]

Supplementation of a specific amino acid for a particular reason—for example, adding glutamine up to 25% of the total protein in PN to facilitate its role as the primary fuel for rapidly dividing cells[27] and to improve the immune function[28] of the infant—is being studied. However, not all studies reported beneficial effects from a glutamine-enriched diet.[29, 30] Catabolism of glutamine, which is by way of glutamate, requires disposal of twice as much ammonia compared with glutamate oxidation and thus requires more arginine for hepatic urea formation and more renal ammonia disposal. Furthermore, glutamine supplementation in animals even at 10% or less of total protein intake is associated with increased extracellular fluid rather than gains in lean tissue mass[31] and has potential neurotoxicity.[32, 33] The use of a single nutrient in large quantities could theoretically lead to metabolic imbalances and other unforeseen side effects. Thus, the use of high doses of glutamine should be avoided until definitive data are available to define its benefits and risks. The role of salvaged urea nitrogen for further metabolic interaction and its influence on protein requirement remains to be defined.[34] The use of growth factors and hormones during nutritional support remains experimental.[35]

Energy

The energy requirement during PN is 10 to 20% lower than during enteral nutrition. Consistent nitrogen accretion and weight gain can occur at an energy intake of about 70 kcal/kg/day and a protein intake of about 2 g/kg/day, although small preterm infants often require greater energy and protein intake to achieve an in utero rate of tissue accretion.[11, 16, 36] With suboptimal energy intake, the endogenous protein is used as an energy source, resulting in negative nitrogen balance, whereas higher energy intake results in sparing of the endogenous protein from tissue catabolism and in the optimal utilization of the exogenous protein for lean tissue gain.[16, 18] However, excess energy intake (>120 to 130 kcal/kg/day) is probably associated with increased fat deposition and possibly worsening of any underlying respiratory illness because of increased carbon dioxide release from fat synthesis.[7, 8, 36–38]

Carbohydrate

Many nonlipid energy sources have been used for PN in infants. These include glucose (dextrose), fructose, galactose, sorbitol, glycerol, and ethanol, but none have any advantage over dextrose as the carbohydrate source for use in PN. The glycerol present in lipid emulsions contributes only a small amount of carbohydrate calories. The major drawback in the use of dextrose is its hyperosmolarity and the need for central venous access when it is used at a concentration of greater than 12.5%. During periods of acute stress, for example, sepsis or steroid therapy, the infusion of dextrose at a much lower concentration of 3 to 5% may be needed to avoid hyperglycemia. Hyperglycemia is associated with glucosuria with osmotic diuresis and possibly intracranial hemorrhage leading to increased morbidity and mortality. Glucose restriction for infants is the usual treatment until the tolerance improves. Insulin has been used to treat persistent hyperglycemia,[38] but caution is required to avoid hypoglycemia. Insulin administration does not improve the overall nitrogen accretion and is associated with lactate accumulation and metabolic acidosis;[39] thus, the routine use of insulin to enhance growth is not recommended. High glucose intake from PN results in increased carbon dioxide production as early as the first few days after birth. When the glucose intake was greater than 18 g/kg/day, that is, from an infusion of 15% dextrose at 120 ml/kg/day, the nonprotein respiratory quotient was consistently greater than 1, indicating fat synthesis and carbon dioxide release.[37]

Lipids

Lipid emulsions available in the United States are from soy or a mixture of soy and safflower oil. They contain primarily triglycerides with linoleic and linolenic acids. In addition to the lipids' being the source of essential fatty acids, the use of lipid optimizes nitrogen utilization without further increase in carbon dioxide production[37] and allows the use of a lower dextrose load in PN.

Current commercial lipid emulsions are available in 10% and 20% concentrations. The 20% emulsion is more calorically dense (2 vs. 1.1 kcal/ml) without an additional phospholipid content. The risk of hypercholesterolemia and hyperphospholipidemia is lower at the same infusion rate with the use of the 20% rather than the 10% lipid emulsion because phospholipid inhibits lipoprotein lipase, the main enzyme for the clearance of intravenous lipid.[40, 41] Structured lipids in the form of long- and medium-chain triglyceride emulsions are available in Europe and have some theoretical advantages for metabolic utility. However, soy emulsions have been in use for more than 30 years, and there are no definitive studies to support the use of one preparation of lipid over another. In addition, none of the lipid preparations appear to maintain the normal intrauterine accumulation of very long chain polyunsaturated fatty acids of the n-3 and n-6 families in developing infant tissues.

Lipid emulsion can be given on the first day of PN at 0.5 to 1 g/kg/day and increased at 0.5 to 1 g/kg/day up to a maximum of 3 to 4 g/kg/day as long as serum triglyceride levels remain lower than 200 mg/dl. Smaller increments and a lower total dose may be prudent for acutely ill or very small preterm infants.[1, 2, 9–11] In the presence of an adequate energy intake, a minimal intake of 0.5 to 1 g of lipid per kilogram per day is necessary to avoid essential fatty acid deficiency. Continuous infusion of lipids over 18 to 24 hours allows better tolerance and minimizes the complications associated with an excess rate and volume of lipid administration.

Jaundice and sepsis are not absolute contraindications to the use of fat emulsions. Lipid emulsions can be continued if the serum bilirubin level is controlled with phototherapy. The dose probably should be in the range of 1 to 2 g/kg/day if the serum bilirubin level is more than half the exchange level and at the normal dose if the serum bilirubin level is less than 50% of the exchange level.

Carnitine plays an essential role in the metabolism of long-chain fatty acids, although there seems to be no convincing evidence of a clinical benefit from the addition of carnitine to the parenteral lipid infusions of infants. However, supplementation of about 2.4 to 4.8 mg (15 to 30 μmol) of L-carnitine per kilogram per day, that is, comparable to the amount provided by human milk and enough to support in utero rates of tissue accretion, may be appropriate for preterm infants receiving parenteral lipid.[42] High intakes of 48 mg (300 μmol) of L-carnitine per kilogram per day may be associated with an increased metabolic rate and decreased fat and protein accretion and may prolong the time to regain birth weight in preterm infants.[43]

Electrolytes and Minerals

Electrolytes and minerals are usually added to PN solutions as sodium and potassium salts of chloride, phosphate, or acetate. Acetate may be used as a source of base.[44] Salts of amino acids are other sources of anions. Magnesium (Mg) is provided as hydrated magnesium sulfate. Calcium (Ca) is usually provided as 10% Ca gluconate. The simultaneous addition of Ca and phosphorus (P) results in the precipitation of minerals, and the salts should be added sequentially. The specific procedures for predicting and maximizing the maintenance of Ca and P in PN solution are well known to pharmacists. The recommendation of higher amino acid intake and the addition of cysteine further enhance the ability of current PN solutions to maintain high Ca and P contents.[15]

Micronutrients and Vitamins

Current recommendations for parenteral intake of micronutrients and vitamins are shown in Tables 23–3 and 23–4, respectively. An incomplete knowledge of micronutrient and vitamin requirements in infants and the limited commercial potential are reflected in the relatively few commercial preparations.

Trace elements are commercially available individually or in combination. It has been stated that only zinc (Zn) is needed for "short"-term PN;[45] however, many institutions routinely add most of the currently

Table 23–4. Recommended Parenteral Intakes of Vitamins*

Vitamin	Term Infants (dose/day)	Preterm Infants† (dose/kg/day)
Lipid-soluble		
Vitamin A (μg)**	700	700–1500
Vitamin E (mg)	7	2.8–3.5
Vitamin K (μg)	200	8–10
Vitamin D (μg)	10	1–4
(IU)	400	40–160
Water-soluble		
Thiamine, B_1 (mg)	1.2	0.2–0.35
Riboflavin, B_2 (mg)	1.4	0.15–0.2
Pyridoxine, B_6 (mg)	1	0.15–0.2
Niacin (mg)	17	4–6.8
Pantothenate (mg)	5	1–2
Biotin (μg)	20	5–8
Folate (μg)	140	56
Cyanocobalamine, B_{12} (μg)	1	0.3
Ascorbic acid, C (mg)	80	15–25

*Maximum should not exceed one 5-mL vial of M.V.I. Pediatric, Astra Pharmaceutical Products, Inc., Westborough, Mass.
†Best estimate.
Adapted from references 9 through 11 and 45.

Table 23–3. Recommended Parenteral Intakes of Trace Minerals

Trace Mineral	Term Infant (μg/kg/day)	Preterm Infant (μg/kg/day)
Iron*	100	200
Zinc	250 <3 mo	400
	100 >3 mo	
Copper	20	20
Selenium	2	2
Iodide†	1	1
Manganese	1	1
Molybdenum	0.25	0.25
Chromium	0.2	0.2

*Normally not needed before second month. Adjust according to iron status.
†Normally consider for long-term total parenteral nutrition subjects. Topical disinfectants and detergents are sources of iodide.
Adapted from references 9 through 11, 45.

recommended trace minerals regardless of the expected duration of PN. Parenteral iron (0.1 to 0.2 mg/kg/day) as iron dextran should be considered if PN is provided exclusively for 2 months or more during infancy or if iron deficiency develops.[45–47]

There is no commercial parenteral multivitamin preparation that provides the amount of recommended daily intake for infants (see Table 23–4). The currently recommended daily intake of a multivitamin preparation (M.V.I. Pediatric, Astra Pharmaceutical Products, Westborough, Mass.), 2 ml/kg up to a complete 5-ml vial for infants weighing more than 3 kg[45] may provide an excess of some water-soluble vitamins[48] and inadequate amounts of some fat-soluble vitamins (e.g., vitamin A), especially for preterm infants.[49] However, none of the other commercial parenteral multivitamin preparations are designed for use in infancy, and the vitamin content is at an even greater discrepancy from the current recommendations.

◆ DELIVERY

The dextrose–amino acid solution and lipid emulsion can be provided separately and delivered together through a Y connector via a peripheral or central venous catheter (CVC), or through umbilical venous or arterial catheters. The effective usable duration for different catheters is variable but generally is on the order of hours to several days for peripheral venous catheters, 7 to 10 days for umbilical arterial or venous catheters, days to several weeks for small-bore percutaneously inserted Silastic catheters, and weeks to months for surgically placed larger-diameter Silastic catheters.

In neonates, the choice of the catheter depends on the expected duration of PN support and other needs for parenteral access. In general, most acutely ill neonates require an umbilical venous or arterial access for blood sampling and other purposes. Either umbilical catheter can be used safely in the delivery of standard PN solution. To minimize the risks of sclerosis and inflammation of the wall of the vein from peripheral intravenous infusion and to avoid the need for multiple attempts at peripheral venous catheter insertion, many institutions routinely employ a percutaneously inserted Silastic catheter for PN on discontinuation of the umbilical catheter, generally at 7 to 10 days after birth. For infants who require extensive surgical procedures, a larger-bore Silastic catheter for subsequent PN needs is often inserted during the primary surgery. Strict asepsis is mandatory during catheter placement, and the correct position of all central catheters including umbilical catheters must be confirmed before the infusion of PN solution.

PN solutions including lipid emulsion probably should be protected from direct exposure to phototherapy and other light sources to minimize the photodegradation[50] of certain nutrients and possibly the formation of toxic products[51] from light exposure. The use of an in-line 0.22-μm filter may be helpful to minimize infusion-related phlebitis,[52] and it should be changed with the daily change of PN solution. This filter cannot be used with the catheter delivering lipid emulsion because of the larger size of the lipid particles.

Heparin at a concentration of 1 to 2 U/ml of PN solution is frequently employed when a CVC, particularly a percutaneously inserted CVC, is being used to deliver the PN. Its use may prolong the catheter patency and has the potential advantage of stimulating lipoprotein lipase activity, thereby increasing intravenous lipid clearance.[40]

PN may begin with a volume of intake between 80 and 120 ml/kg/day, a protein intake of 1 g/kg/day, carbohydrate concentrations of 5 to 10% dextrose (providing about 7 mg of glucose load per kilogram per minute at an intake of 100 ml of 10% dextrose/kg/day), and a lipid intake of 0.5 to 1 g/kg/day. Continuous infusion of PN solution and prolonging the infusion of lipid emulsion over 18 hours or more each day allow better tolerance. The lipid emulsion should be delivered through a Y connection as close as possible to the catheter entry into the skin, and the hourly rate of infusion probably should not be less than 0.3 ml to minimize the risk of skimming (layering) of the lipid emulsion over the amino acid–dextrose solution and not being delivered to the circulation. The latter is an important practical issue in the delivery of lipid emulsion in the small neonate. Thus, the duration of lipid infusion may need to be shortened to maintain an infusion rate of greater than 0.3 mL/h because the total volume of lipid to be infused is very low, particularly during the initial phase when lipid intake is low.

Normally, adequate amounts of nutrients can be easily delivered in a total daily volume of 120 to 160 ml/kg/day, and a stepwise increase in the content of macronutrients over the first 2 to 3 days of PN therapy allows better metabolic adaptations to the parenteral nutrient load. However, there is no benefit in prolonging the duration of transition to full PN therapy in clinically stable neonates. The fluid goal and nutrient concentration should not be increased simultaneously to avoid excess nutrient load to the neonate. If PN is to be resumed after a period of adequate enteral intake, all the components of the PN can be infused at the desired goal without the use of a low nutrient concentration and then a stepwise increase in nutrient content unless there is clinical instability. A trace amount of glucosuria is not uncommon in small preterm infants less than 1000 g and is not an indication to reduce the dextrose intake if the blood glucose level is normal.

Some institutions deliver PN as a total nutrient admixture, that is, mixing all nutrient components in the same container. The disadvantages of a total nutrient admixture are that the stability of each component of the admixture is not completely defined, it is impossible to determine whether there is a precipitation of nutrients in the admixture,[53] and a standard 0.22-μm bacterial filter cannot be used with total nutrient admixture solutions.

◆ COMPLICATIONS AND MONITORING

Many potential complications directly related to the use of PN (Table 23–5) may be minimized by continual assessment of the infant's clinical status; awareness of the effect of underlying disease and its therapy on nutrient tolerance and utilization; the performance of intermittent systematic laboratory studies; and the use of enteral feeding at the earliest time and at whatever amount can be tolerated by the infant.[1, 2]

It is theoretically possible that problems may occur during the preparation of the PN solution from component nutrients. However, this is unlikely to occur if the preparation of the PN solution is done by a hospital pharmacist or commercial companies adhering strictly to the standard practice guidelines.[54]

Catheter-related complications, in particular, extravasation associated with peripheral infusion, are the most frequent complications in PN. Meticulous attention to catheter insertion; subcutaneous tunneling of surgically placed CVCs; confirmation of proper positioning and good catheter care; the use of an in-line filter; and even electively changing peripheral intravenous catheters after 48 hours of infusion can minimize the risk of catheter-related complications.[52]

CVC occlusion with thrombus, chemicals (e.g., calcium phosphate), and lipid-related materials may be cleared with urokinase, 0.1 N hydrochloric acid, and 70% ethanol, respectively.[1] Urokinase product safety issues raised by the Food and Drug Administration in 1999[55] have prompted reassessment of the use of alternative thombolytic therapy. Tissue plasminogen activator may be considered for the lysis of recently formed thrombus, but it is associated with significantly higher costs. However, unless the occlusions are detected early, removal of the catheter may be the only option to minimize further complications such as occlusion of the superior vena cava or sepsis.

Table 23–5. Complications of Parenteral Nutrition

A. Mechanical
  1. Kinking, compression, tearing, dislodgment of catheter
  2. Catheter occlusion from thrombosis, chemical precipitate, lipid
  3. Extravasation
     Local: peripheral catheter
     Pleural, pericardial, or peritoneal space: central venous catheter
B. Sepsis
  1. Catheter related: insertion site, subcutaneous tunnel, or line sepsis
  2. Non–catheter related: associated with underlying disease
C. Metabolic
  1. Decreased nutrient availability from
     a) Adsorption, e.g., adherence of vitamin A and insulin to bag and tubing
     b) Photodegradation especially from phototherapy, e.g., tryptophan, methionine, histidine, riboflavin, vitamin A
     c) Nutrient loss, e.g., electrolytes, minerals and trace metal loss from loop diuretic and also from thiazide diuretics, potassium loss with amphotericin B
     d) Toxic products formation, e.g., photoperoxidation of lipid emulsions, hydrogen peroxide production from presence of multivitamins, in particular riboflavin, in amino acid–dextrose solution
     e) Drug-nutrient interaction, e.g., amphotericin B precipitates with sodium chloride (NaCl) or parenteral nutrition (PN) solution; significant Na and Cl intake from NaCl flushes
     f) Nutrient-nutrient interaction, e.g., excessive inorganic calcium and phosphorus
  2. Disturbances of circulating concentrations of glucose, sodium, potassium, calcium, magnesium, phosphorus, and acid-base status
  3. Gallbladder sludging, gallstones, and cholestasis
  4. Metabolic bone disease
  5. Contamination with trace minerals, e.g., boron, aluminum
  6. Anemia: iatrogenic from excessive blood tests
  7. Refusal to feed with prolonged PN and lack of oral stimulation

Adapted from Koo WWK, McLaughlin K, Saba M: Nutrition support for the preterm infant. *In* Merritt RJ (ed): The A.S.P.E.N. Nutrition Support Practice Manual, Chapter 26. Washington, DC, American Society for Parenteral and Enteral Nutrition, 1998, pp 1–16; and Koo WWK, Raju NV, Tan-Laxa MA: Infant nutrition. Hong Kong J Paediatr 3:103–121, 1998.

Septic episodes may or may not be catheter related. In neonates, the clinical manifestation of sepsis is frequently nonspecific and presents as lethargy, hyperbilirubinemia, temperature instability, or metabolic alterations. Metabolic alterations may present as a progressive or sudden intolerance to a previously tolerated glucose or lipid load and are frequently an early, if not the only, manifestation of sepsis. The organisms involved are frequently endogenous in origin from mucocutaneous and gastrointestinal sources. Empirical antibiotic therapy should be started if sepsis is suspected, after a culture of blood drawn from the catheter, from a noncatheterized blood vessel, and from obvious sites of septic foci. Initial therapy should be based on the clinical status of the neonate and the antibiotic sensitivities of microbial organisms prevalent in the nursery. Fever alone is not an indication to remove the PN catheter. However, persistent positive cultures in spite of antibiotic therapy suggest bacterial colonization of the catheter and necessitate the removal of the catheter. Prolonged antibiotic therapy predisposes the infant to fungal infection, and some clinicians recommend catheter removal if there is evidence of a fungal infection.

Metabolic complications with PN may be a result of nutrient loss from adsorption to the delivery system[49] or photodegradation of selected amino acids and vitamins[50] before the nutrients are delivered into the circulation. The latter situation is probably unique to neonates because intense phototherapy is the mainstay of therapy for the treatment of neonatal hyperbilirubinemia. Additional nutrient loss can occur after the delivery of PN, for example, a loss of multiple minerals and trace metals from prolonged diuretic therapy.[15] The formation of toxic products in PN solution has been documented,[51] and its potential clinical effects warrant continued vigilance.

The most common metabolic complications, however, are generally related to excessive, imbalanced, or inadequate intake. Abnormally high or low circulating levels of almost every electrolyte, mineral, and trace mineral have been described. Excessive intake is usually relative to the infant's ability to tolerate the amount of nutrient delivered. Typical complications related to parenteral protein intake include hyperammonemia, acidosis, and azotemia. The latter two complications are infrequent with current amino acid preparations, compared with older protein hydrolysate preparations, but may still occur with excessive intake, particularly in the sick infant with hepatic and/or renal dysfunction. During periods of stress and certain treatments, for example, steroid therapy for the weaning of the infant from the ventilator, there may be decreased tolerance

even to the "normal" amount of a nutrient such as dextrose. Even in clinically stable neonates, sudden interruption of the delivery of PN with high glucose concentrations (usually >15%) can result in hypoglycemia. This complication can be minimized by starting nutritional support immediately after birth, thus avoiding the need to increase the glucose load to "catch up" after a period of inadequate nutritional support. In addition, the use of parenteral lipid allows the use of a relatively low glucose concentration in the PN solution. If there is associated impairment of metabolic and excretory capacities as in liver dysfunction, the currently recommended intake of certain trace minerals, for example, copper and manganese, may be in excess of the infant's needs, and toxicity may occur.[45, 56]

The classic scenario of metabolic complication from imbalanced intake is the administration of PN solution containing low or no phosphorus.[15] This results in hypophosphatemia, phosphate deficiency, and secondary hypercalcemia. Another possible scenario is the attempt to replace gastrointestinal fluid loss with an increased amount of PN solution. This results in the delivery of excessive amounts of many nutrients including protein and carbohydrate. Appropriate replacement fluids should be administered via a separate line piggybacked onto the PN infusion line.

Deficiencies of micronutrients and vitamins are rarely reported except in situations in which one or more components are inadvertently omitted from the PN solution or provided in a relatively inadequate amount.[45, 49, 57, 58] A shortage of multivitamin preparations has resulted in more than 30 cases of vitamin deficiency.[58] Inadequate replacement of nutrients, such as zinc[59] and magnesium,[60] lost from gastrointestinal fistulas, frequently results in their deficiency.

Contamination with trace minerals is still prevalent in current PN solutions.[61] This may have positive and negative results. There are increasing reports of the physiologic role of certain trace minerals such as boron, although their exact requirements remain ill defined. Thus, contamination with some trace minerals theoretically may have undefined benefits. With the increasing availability of highly purified nutrient components for PN and the limited number of trace minerals being added to the final solution, the potential exists for relative and absolute deficiencies of undefined micro-

Table 23–6. Guideline for Metabolic Monitoring During Parenteral Nutrition

Variable	Initial Period*	Later Period†
Growth‡		
Weight	Daily	Daily
Head circumference	Baseline	Weekly
Length	Baseline	Weekly
Intake and output	Every shift	Daily
Serum electrolytes	2–3 times/wk	q 1–2 wk
BUN/creatinine	2–3 times/wk	q 1–2 wk
Calcium, magnesium, phosphorus	2–3 times/wk	q 1–2 wk
Serum triglyceride§	Daily during dose increase	q 1–2 wk
Finger stick for blood and urine glucose	1–3 times/day	As indicated
Serum glucose	As indicated	As indicated
Total and direct bilirubin	Baseline	q 1–2 wk
Total protein and albumin	Baseline	q 2–3 wk
Alanine aminotransferase, aspartate aminotransferase, and alkaline phosphatase	Baseline	q 2–3 wk
Complete blood count	Baseline	q 2–3 wk
Vitamin and trace mineral status and other specific tests	As indicated	As indicated

*Period to reach maximal doses of glucose, amino acids, and lipid emulsion, or during any period of metabolic instability. This period normally lasts <1 week.

†Period of metabolic steady state. For clinically stable infants receiving the desired intake of nutrients, the interval between laboratory measurements may be increased beyond the above recommendations pending clinical progress.

‡All measurements should be plotted on a standard growth chart for term infants after adjustment for gestational age. Growth charts showing postnatal growth of preterm infants are biased for nutritional management regimens and probably should not be used.

§Target level is <200 mg/dL.

BUN, blood urea nitrogen.

Adapted from Koo WWK, McLaughlin K, Saba M: Nutrition support for the preterm infant. In Merritt RJ (ed): The A.S.P.E.N. Nutrition Support Practice Manual, Chapter 26. Washington, DC, American Society for Parenteral and Enteral Nutrition, 1998, pp 1–16; and Koo WWK, Raju NV, Tan-Laxa MA: Infant nutrition. Hong Kong J Paediatr 3:103–121, 1998.

nutrients in subjects on prolonged PN.[45] Aluminum (Al) toxicity is a potential complication of long-term PN, although the benefits of current PN solutions outweigh the potential risks of Al toxicity.[62]

The prevalence of hepatic[63, 64] and skeletal[65–67] complications is inversely proportional to birth weight and gestational age and directly proportional to the duration of PN. The best means to minimize these complications is the introduction of enteral feeding at the earliest opportunity. Once the complications have occurred, continued maintenance of the optimal nutritional status and the use of enteral feedings whenever possible are the cornerstones to the continued management of these complications. Specific management of PN-related cholestasis also includes restricting nutrients that require hepatic excretion, for example, copper and manganese. Cholecystokinin, ursodeoxycholic acid, and conjugated bile acid analogues such as cholesarcosine are being used on an experimental basis.[63, 64]

Another potential problem for infants who receive prolonged PN from birth is their refusal to feed. This problem may be minimized with non-nutritive sucking and early introduction of oral feedings.[68, 69]

Intestinal mucosal atrophy[70] and bacterial translocation[71] have been reported in association with total PN. The extent of changes appears to be greater in animals than in humans, although it seems a prudent measure to maintain optimal nutritional status with PN and/or enteral nutrition, in addition to the initiation of enteral feeding at the earliest opportunity to minimize these potential complications.

Certain laboratory tests are necessary for the successful use of PN (Table 23–6). However, the frequency and type of tests may need to be adjusted depending on the duration of PN and the amount of enteral nutrition tolerated.[1, 2, 11] In general, regardless of the duration of PN, laboratory tests can be significantly fewer if PN is used as a supplement to enteral nutrition.

SUMMARY

Meticulous attention to details; an understanding of the pathophysiology of the underlying illness and its therapy, and how the illness and its treatment affect nutrient metabolism and utilization; and early provision of an adequate and balanced nutrient intake, whether enterally and/or parenterally, are cornerstones to safe and successful nutritional support for all infants. Thus, to achieve the goal of maintaining the best possible physical and developmental outcome for the infant, it is not a matter of the infant's being too sick or too small to receive nutritional support but is a matter of how best to deliver it.

REFERENCES

1. Koo WWK, McLaughlin K, Saba M: Nutrition support for the preterm infant. *In* Merritt RJ (ed): The A.S.P.E.N. Nutrition Support Practice Manual, Chapter 26. Washington, DC, American Society for Parenteral and Enteral Nutrition, 1998, pp 1–16.
2. Koo WWK, Raju NV, Tan-Laxa MA: Infant nutrition. Hong Kong J Paediatr 3:103–121, 1998.
3. Hack M, Wright L, Shankaran S, et al: Very low birth weight outcomes of the National Institute of Child Health and Human Development Neonatal Network, November 1989 to October 1990. Am J Obstet Gynecol 172:457–464, 1995.
4. Hack M, Taylor HG, Klein N, et al: School age outcomes in children with birth weights under 750 g. N Engl J Med 331:753–759, 1994.
5. Lucas A, Morley R, Cole TJ, et al: Early diet in preterm babies and development status at 18 months. Lancet 335:1477–1481, 1990.
6. Lucas A, Morley R, Cole TJ, Gore SM: A randomised multicentre study of human milk versus formula and later development in preterm infants. Arch Dis Child 70:f141–f146, 1994.
7. Jones MO, Pierro A, Hammond P, et al: Glucose utilization in the surgical newborn infant receiving total parenteral nutrition. J Pediatr Surg 28:1121–1125, 1993.
8. Chwals WJ: Overfeeding the critically ill child: Fact or fantasy? New Horiz 2:147–155, 1994.
9. Tsang RC, Lucas A, Uauy R, Zlotkin S (eds): Nutritional Needs of the Preterm Infant: Scientific Basis and Practical Guidelines. Baltimore, Williams & Wilkins, 1993.
10. Tsang RC, Zlotkin SH, Nichols BL, Hansen JW (eds): Nutrition During Infancy: Principles and Practice, 2nd ed. Cincinnati, Digital Educational Publishing, 1997, pp 467–485.
11. Committee on Nutrition, American Academy of Pediatrics: Pediatrics Nutrition Handbook, 4th ed. Elk Grove Village, Ill, American Academy of Pediatrics, 1998.
12. Van Goudoever JB, Wattimena JDL, Carnielli VP, et al: Effect of dexamethasone on protein metabolism in infants with bronchopulmonary dysplasia. J Pediatr 124:112–118, 1994.
13. Weiler HA, Wang Z, Atkinson SA: Dexamethasone treatment impairs calcium regulation and reduces bone mineralization in infant pigs. Am J Clin Nutr 61:805–811, 1995.
14. Papile LA, Tyson JE, Stoll BJ, et al: A multicenter trial of two dexamethasone regimens in ventilator dependent premature infants. N Engl J Med 16:1112–1118, 1998.
15. Koo WWK, Tsang RC: Calcium, magnesium, phosphorus, and vitamin D. *In* Tsang RC, Lucas A, Uauy R, Zlotkin S (eds): Nutritional needs of the preterm infant: Scientific basis and practical guidelines. Baltimore, Williams & Wilkins, 1993, pp 135–155.
16. Micheli JL, Schutz Y: Protein. *In* Tsang RC, Lucas A, Uauy R, Zlotkin S (eds): Nutritional Needs of the Preterm Infant: Scientific Basis and Practical Guidelines. Baltimore, Williams & Wilkins, 1993, pp 29–46.
17. Rivera A Jr, Bell EF, Bier DM: Effect of intravenous amino acids on protein metabolism of preterm infants during the first three days of life. Pediatr Res 33:106–111, 1993.
18. Mitton SG: Amino acids and lipid in total parenteral nutrition for the newborn. J Pediatr Gastroenterol Nutr 18:25–31, 1994.
19. Denne SC, Karn CA, Liu YM, et al: Effect of enteral versus parenteral feeding on leucine kinetics and fuel utilization in premature newborns. Pediatr Res 36:429–435, 1994.
20. Van Goudoever JB, Colen T, Wattimena JL, et al: Immediate commencement of amino acid supplementation in preterm infants: Effect on serum amino acid concentrations and protein kinetics on the first day of life. J Pediatr 127:458–465, 1995.
21. Denne SC, Karn CA, Ahlrichs JA, et al: Proteolysis and phenylalanine hydroxylation in response to parenteral nutrition in extremely premature and normal newborns. J Clin Invest 97:746–754, 1996.
22. Battista MA, Price PT, Kalhan SC: Effect of parenteral amino acids on leucine and urea kinetics in preterm infants. J Pediatr 128:130–134, 1996.
23. Poindexter BB, Karn CA, Ahlrichs JA, et al: Amino acids suppress proteolysis independent of insulin throughout the neonatal period. Am J Physiol 272:e592–e599, 1997.
24. Clark SE, Karn CA, Ahlrichs JA, et al: Acute changes in leucine and phenylalanine kinetics produced by parenteral nutrition in premature infants. Pediatr Res 41:568–574, 1997.
25. Wu PY, Edwards N, Storm MC: Plasma amino acid patterns in normal term breast-fed infants. J Pediatr 109:347–349, 1986.
26. Furst P, Stehle P: Are intravenous amino acid solutions unbalanced? New Horiz 2:215–223, 1994.
27. Lacey JM, Crouch JB, Benfell K, et al: The effects of glutamine-supplemented parenteral nutrition in premature infants. JPEN J Parenter Enteral Nutr 20:74–80, 1996.
28. LeLeiko NS, Walsh MJ: The role of glutamine, short chain fatty acids, and nucleotides in intestinal adaptation to gastrointestinal disease. Pediatr Clin North Am 43:451–469, 1996.
29. Bark T, Svenberg T, Theodorsson E, et al: Glutamine supplementation does not prevent small bowel mucosal atrophy after TPN in the rat. Clin Nutr 13:78–84, 1994.
30. Bartolo RFP, Pencharz PB, Ball RO: A comparison of parenteral and enteral feeding in neonatal piglets, including an assessment of the utilization of a glutamine-rich, pediatric elemental diet. JPEN J Parenter Enteral Nutr 23:47–55, 1999.
31. House JD, Pencharz PB, Ball RO: Glutamine supplementation to total parenteral nutrition promotes extracellular fluid expansion in piglets. J Nutr 124:395–405, 1994.

32. Kizer JS, Nemeroff CB, Youngblood WW: Neurotoxic amino acids and structurally related analogs. Pharmacol Rev 29:301–318, 1978.

33. Murphy TH, Schnaar RL, Coyle JT: Immature cortical neurons are uniquely sensitive to glutamate toxicity by inhibition of cystine uptake. FASEB J 4:1624–1633, 1990.

34. Wheeler RA, Griffiths DM, Jackson AA: Urea kinetics in neonates receiving total parenteral nutrition. Arch Dis Child 69:24–27, 1993.

35. Meyer NA, Miller MJ, Herndon DN: Nutrient support of the healing wound. New Horiz 2:202–214, 1994.

36. Heird WC: Amino acid and energy needs of pediatric patients receiving parenteral nutrition. Pediatr Clin North Am 42:765–789, 1995.

37. Van Aerde JE, Sauer PJ, Pencharz PB, et al: Metabolic consequences of increasing energy intake by adding lipid to parenteral nutrition in full-term infants. Am J Clin Nutr 59:659–662, 1994.

38. Wilson DC, McClure G: Energy requirements in sick preterm babies. Acta Paediatr 405(Suppl):60–64, 1994.

39. Poindexter BB, Karn CA, Denne SC: Exogenous insulin reduces proteolysis and protein synthesis in extremely low birth weight infants. J Pediatr 132:948–953, 1998.

40. Innis SM: Fat. *In* Tsang RC, Lucas A, Uauy R, Zlotkin S (eds). Nutritional Needs of the Preterm Infant: Scientific Basis and Practical Guidelines. Baltimore, Williams & Wilkins, 1993, pp 65–86.

41. Goel R, Hamosh M, Stahl GE, et al: Plasma lecithin: Cholesterol acyltransferase and plasma lipolytic activity in preterm infants given total parenteral nutrition with 10% or 20% Intralipid. Acta Paediatr 84:1060–1064, 1995.

42. Larrson LE, Olegad R, Ljung A, et al: Parenteral nutrition in preterm neonates with and without carnitine supplementation. Acta Anaesthesiol Scand 34:501–505, 1990.

43. Sulkers EJ, Lafeber HN, Degenhart HJ, et al: Effects of high carnitine supplementation on substrate utilization in low-birth-weight infants receiving total parenteral nutrition. Am J Clin Nutr 52:889–894, 1990.

44. Peters O, Ryan S, Matthew L, et al: Randomized controlled trial of acetate in neonates receiving parenteral nutrition. Arch Dis Child 77:f12–f15, 1997.

45. Greene HL, Hambridge KM, Schanler R, Tsang RC: Guidelines for the use of vitamins, trace elements, calcium, magnesium and phosphorus in infants and children receiving total parenteral nutrition. Am J Clin Nutr 48:1324–1342, 1988. (Revised reprint December 1990.)

46. Leung FY: Trace elements in parenteral micronutrition. Clin Biochem 28:561–566, 1995.

47. Friel JK, Andrews WL, Hall MS, et al: Intravenous iron administration to very-low-birth-weight newborns receiving total and partial parenteral nutrition. JPEN J Parenter Enteral Nutr 19:114–118, 1995.

48. Moore MC, Greene HL, Phillips B, et al: Evaluation of a pediatric multiple vitamin preparation for total parenteral nutrition in infants and children. I: Blood levels of water-soluble vitamins. Pediatrics 77:530–538, 1986.

49. Greene HL, Phillips BL, Granck L, et al: Persistently low blood retinol levels during and after parenteral feeding of very low birth weight infants: Examina-

tion of losses into intravenous administration sets and a method of prevention by addition to a lipid emulsion. Pediatrics 79:894–900, 1987.

50. Neuzil J, Darlow BA, Inder TE, et al: Oxidation of parenteral lipid emulsion by ambient and phototherapy lights: Potential toxicity of routine parenteral feeding. J Pediatr 126:785–790, 1995.

51. Lavoie JC, Belanger S, Spalinger M, Chessex P: Admixture of a multivitamin preparation to parenteral nutrition: The major contributor to in vitro generation of peroxides. Pediatrics 99, 1997. http://www.pediatrics.org/cgi/content/full/3/eb.

52. Department of Health and Human Services, Centers for Disease Control and Prevention: Draft guideline for prevention of intravascular device-related infections. 60 (187) Federal Register 49978–50006 (1995).

53. Murphy S, Craig DQ, Murphy A: An investigation into the physical stability of a neonatal parenteral nutrition formulation. Acta Pediatr 85:1483–1486, 1996.

54. Deffenbaugh JH (ed): Quality assurance for pharmacy—Prepared sterile product. ASHP technical assistance bulletin on practice standards of ASHP 1997–1998. Bethesda, Md, American Society of Health System Pharmacists, 1997, pp 171–181.

55. Public Health Service, Food and Drug Administration: Important drug warning Jan 25, 1999.

56. Reynolds AP, Kiely E, Meadows N, et al: Manganese in long term pediatric parenteral nutrition. Arch Dis Child 71:527–528, 1994.

57. La Selve P, Demolin P, Holzapfel L, et al: Shoshin beriberi: An unusual complication of prolonged parenteral nutrition. JPEN J Parenter Enteral Nutr 10:102–103, 1986.

58. Nelson RE, Biberdorf RI: Nationwide drug shortage: It's time to take the lead. Nutr Clin Pract 13:295–297, 1998.

59. Wolman SL, Anderson GH, Marliss EB, Jeejeebhoy KN: Zinc in total parenteral nutrition. Requirement and metabolic effects. Gastroenterology 76:458–467, 1980.

60. Thoren L: Magnesium deficiency in gastrointestinal fluid loss. Acta Chir Scand 306(Suppl):1–65, 1963.

61. Pluhator-Murton MM, Fedorak RN, Audette RJ, et al: Extent of trace-element contamination from simulated compounding of total parenteral nutrient solutions. Am J Health Syst Pharm 53:2299–2303, 1996.

62. Koo WWK, Kaplan LA: Aluminum and bone disorders: With specific reference to aluminum contamination of infant nutrients. J Am Coll Nutr 7:199–214, 1988.

63. Briones ER, Iber FL: Liver and biliary tract changes and injury associated with total parenteral nutrition: Pathogenesis and prevention. J Am Coll Nutr 14:219–228, 1995.

64. Teitelbaum DH: Parenteral nutrition–associated cholestasis. Curr Opin Pediatr 9:270–275, 1997.

65. Koo WWK: Parenteral nutrition–related bone disease. JPEN J Parenter Enteral Nutr 16:386–394, 1992.

66. Prestridge LL, Schanler RJ, Shulman RJ, et al: Effect of parenteral calcium and phosphorus therapy on mineral retention and bone mineral. J Pediatr 122:761–768, 1993.

67. Lipkin EW: A longitudinal study of calcium regulation in a nonhuman primate model of parenteral nutrition. Am J Clin Nutr 67:246–254, 1998.

68. Bernbaum JC, Pereira GR, Watkins JB, Peckham GJ: Nonnutritive sucking during gavage feeding enhances growth and maturation in premature infants. Pediatrics 71:41–45, 1983.

69. Schauster H, Dwyer J: Transition from tube feedings to feedings by mouth in children: Preventing eating dysfunction. J Am Diet Assoc 96:277–281, 1996.

70. Buchman AL, Moukarzel AA, Bhuta S, et al: Parenteral nutrition is associated with intestinal morphologic and functional changes in humans. JPEN J Parenter Enteral Nutr 19:453–460, 1995.

71. Lipman TO: Bacterial translocation and enteral nutrition in humans: An outsider looks in. JPEN J Parenter Enteral Nutr 19:156–165, 1995.

24

◆ Pediatric Parenteral Nutrition

Richard A. Falcone, Jr., M.D.
Brad W. Warner, M.D.

Nutritional management of the pediatric patient is unique and cannot be based on the assumption that "children are just small adults." In pediatric patients, not only must baseline metabolic functions be maintained, but the extra anabolic needs of growth and the stress of illness must be addressed. Growing children have specialized needs requiring relatively more nutrients than adults, but they have a limited ability to deal with excesses.

Differences in body composition among premature, term, and older infants and children require an understanding of essential substrate, vitamin, mineral, and energy requirements. The impact of growth and how this influences the utilization of energy, protein, and fat is important because caloric and substrate deprivation during periods of rapid brain growth and development can be associated with irreversible neurologic injury or developmental delay.

In 1969, Dudrick and associates demonstrated the successful use of parenteral nutrition (PN) in a child with the short gut syndrome.[1] Later that year in a review of advances in pediatric surgery, Hendren and Henderson proclaimed that the advent of PN "will doubtless save countless number of babies."[2] Since that time, no one group of patients has benefited more from the advent of PN than the pediatric population.[3]

◆ INDICATIONS

The indications for PN support in pediatric patients are similar to those for the adult population with a few notable exceptions (Table 24–1). The decision to implement PN should be based on a thorough clinical evaluation. The gastrointestinal tract should be used whenever possible, and it is therefore necessary to first establish whether sufficient nutrients to meet the child's requirements can be provided by the enteral route.

Although enteral nutrition is preferred, there are several circumstances in infants and children in which this is not feasible.

PN is considered primary therapy for patients with multiple gastrointestinal fistulas, short bowel syndrome, and severe Crohn's disease. PN is used supportively for patients with protracted diarrhea and malnutrition and for patients with adynamic ileus after surgical correction of congenital gastrointestinal anomalies.

The second consideration when determining the need for PN is the anticipated length of time before full enteral nutrition can be achieved. Estimated endogenous calorie reserves are relatively lower and the survival time is shorter in children when compared with adults (Table 24–2). In-

Table 24–1. Common Indications for Parenteral Nutrition

Congenital
Esophageal atresia
Intestinal atresia
Gastroschisis and omphalocele
Surgical conditions
Short bowel syndrome
Prolonged postoperative ileus
Enterocutaneous fistula
Inflammatory
Crohn's disease
Ulcerative colitis
Pancreatitis
Postradiation enteritis
Neuromuscular disorders
Intestinal psuedo-obstruction
Total aganglionic Hirschsprung's disease
Respiratory disorders
Respiratory distress syndrome
Cystic fibrosis
Chylothorax
Hypercatabolic states
Severe burns
Major trauma
Sepsis

Modified from Hill ID, Madrazo-de la Garza JA, Lebenthal E: Parenteral nutrition pediatric patients. *In* Rombeau J, Caldwell MD (eds): Clinical Nutrition: Parenteral Nutrition, 2nd ed. Philadelphia, WB Saunders, 1993, pp 770–790.

Table 24–2. Estimated Survival Time After Complete Starvation

	Survival Time
Healthy adult	3 mo
Healthy 1-year-old	44 days
Healthy 1-month-old	30 days
Healthy preterm 2-kg infant	12 days

Modified from Heird WC, Driscoll JMJ, Schullinger JN, et al: Intravenous alimentation in pediatric patients. J Pediatr 80:351, 1972.

creased metabolic requirements due to the catabolism associated with sepsis, burns, trauma, and surgery also have to be taken into consideration.[4–7] When disease and starvation coexist, even for relatively short periods, an individual's poor baseline nutritional status can have profound adverse effects on mortality and morbidity. If after thorough consideration, it appears likely that an infant or child will need PN, it should be started without delay in order to prevent or delay deterioration in the patient's nutritional status.[8]

Pediatric surgical disorders in which PN is routinely used include gastroschisis, intestinal atresia, or meconium ileus in the newborn. The role of PN in these disorders is to support growth until the anomaly can be corrected or the ileus following correction resolves. In the case of gastroschisis or atresias, the intestinal length may be considerably shortened and PN may be required for prolonged periods of time and even indefinitely.

The short bowel syndrome results from the inability of the gastrointestinal tract to absorb sufficient nutrients to sustain life. This syndrome generally results from a deficiency of intestinal absorptive surface after massive resection. In the pediatric population, such massive resection results most commonly from neonatal necrotizing enterocolitis, followed in frequency by intestinal atresias, midgut volvulus, gastroschisis, and aganglionosis (Fig. 24–1).[9] Although all such children would have died in the past, the advent of PN has led to improved survival even with as little as 11 to 20 cm of small bowel.[10] Many of these children will require PN for extended periods, and the length of PN will depend on the remnant bowel length, degree of intestinal adaptation, and presence or absence of the ileocecal valve.[11]

PN has been used with success in the treatment of pediatric patients with inflammatory bowel disease, particularly those with Crohn's disease.[12–14] Indications for PN in the treatment of Crohn's disease include correction of malnutrition before surgery, promotion of healing of enterocutaneous fistulas, treatment of postoperative complications, and failure of aggressive medical management. With total parenteral nutrition (TPN), symptoms such as abdominal pain, anorexia, and diarrhea diminish, and positive nitrogen balance, accelerated linear growth, and an increase in the caloric intake, body weight, and lean body mass have been documented.[15–18]

The role of PN in patients with cystic fibrosis is controversial. Malnutrition in cystic fibrosis results from decreased nutrient ingestion due to anorexia; malabsorption due to pancreatic exocrine insufficiency; a diminished availability of bile salts; and increased caloric requirements due to chronic lung disease. A loss of lean body mass impairs the mechanics of lung function[19] and adversely alters immune function, bronchial mucosal integrity, and the composition of lung secretions.[20, 21] PN can improve a patient's nutritional status, but the effect of such an improvement on pulmonary function, morbidity, and mortality has yet to be defined.[22–24]

Another group of pediatric patients who may benefit from PN are those with cancer. Pediatric oncology patients are often cata-

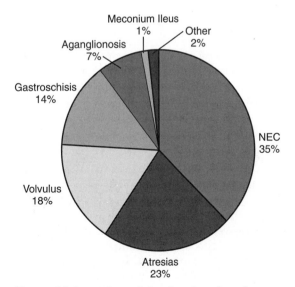

Figure 24–1. Etiology of the short bowel syndrome. NEC, necrotizing enterocolitis.

bolic, may have anorexia, and may have increased nutrient losses due to vomiting, malabsorption, diarrhea, or blood loss. Enteral nutrition in this patient population may often be difficult because of chemotherapy-induced mucositis. The risks of PN in oncology patients include the potential to enhance tumor growth, increased infection rates, and the propensity to cause metabolic derangements. PN is currently recommended for children receiving intensive chemotherapy, after bone marrow transplantation, or after major surgery in patients who are nutritionally depleted and unable to tolerate adequate enteral nutrition.[25, 26] The use of PN as an adjuvant therapy to control adverse effects of chemotherapy has increased markedly since the mid-1990s.[27]

◆ NUTRITIONAL REQUIREMENTS

In order to determine the nutritional needs of the pediatric patient, it is important not only to take into consideration basal metabolic needs but also to consider the unique requirements of growth and development. In addition, infants have specialized needs for both macro- and micronutrients and are less able to deal with excesses than older children. Finally, as with adult patients, the effect of disease and stress must be taken into consideration when nutritional requirements are calculated.

Fluids

The child receiving PN is dependent on the physician to fulfill fluid needs and must be monitored carefully to ensure adequate hydration. In contrast with adults, in whom the rate of the same concentration of PN is increased daily, in children, the rate stays the same, determined by fluid requirements, and the concentration of the solution is increased. Fluid requirements depend on the hydration status, the child's size, environmental factors (radiant warmers, ultraviolet light therapy), and the disease. Maintaining the desired fluid balance is essential because dehydration, hypernatremia, and hyperosmolarity may occur with inadequate fluid administration, and peripheral edema, pulmonary edema, and congestive heart failure can result from fluid overload. The margin

for error in children between these extremes is very slight.

For parenteral fluids, the standard formula of 100 mL/kg for the first 10 kg of body weight, 50 mL/kg for the second 10 kg, and 20 mL/kg for the third 10 kg of body weight is a reasonable starting point. Beyond 30 kg of body weight, it is more prudent to use body surface area (2000 mL/m²) as a means of calculating daily fluid requirements. As a rule of thumb, a 30-kg patient can be considered to be roughly 1 m².

Patients with underlying cardiac defects, head trauma, or renal compromise may require fluid restrictions to facilitate recovery or prevent exacerbation of the underlying disease. However, patients with a high urinary output, an increased ostomy output, diarrhea, and vomiting should be given appropriate replacement fluids. Replacement fluids are guided by the electrolyte content of the lost fluid. In fluids containing large amounts of protein (i.e., chylothorax), colloid must be replaced as Plasmanate or albumin. Careful monitoring of the urinary output and daily weights should be used to help assess the fluid status.

Energy

Energy requirements from birth through childhood include calories needed to maintain existing body tissues, to provide for growth, and to sustain energy expended during activity. Energy requirements decline from birth to the middle of the first year of life, likely as a reflection of reduced rates of growth (Table 24–3).[28] The energy require-

Table 24–3. Average Energy Requirements

Age (mo)	Average Energy Requirement (kcal/kg/day)
0–1	124
1–2	116
2–3	109
3–4	103
4–5	99
5–6	96.5
6–9	95
9–10	99
10–11	100
11–12	104.5

Adapted from Beaton GH: Nutritional needs during the first year of life. Some concepts and perspectives. Pediatr Clin North Am 32:275, 1985.

Table 24–4. Caloric Requirements on Parenteral Nutrition

Age (yr)	Caloric Requirement (kcal/kg/day)
0–1	90–120
1–7	75–90
7–12	60–75
12–18	30–60

Adapted from Wesley JR, Khalidi N, Faubion WC, et al: The University of Michigan Medical Center: Parenteral and Enteral Nutrition Manual (ed 6). North Chicago, IL, Abbott Laboratories Hospital Products Division, 1990.

ment is reduced when nutrition is administered intravenously compared to enterally, and adequate growth in neonates has been demonstrated with parenteral intakes in the range of 88 to 90 kcal/kg/day.[29–31]

Caloric requirements for older pediatric patients show a notable decline with increasing age (Table 24–4).[32] For all pediatric patients, the energy required for maintenance takes priority over growth. If the energy intake falls below maintenance levels, growth is halted. Additional energy is required to take into account the catabolic effects of stress and disease as discussed later. Sufficient nonprotein calories must be provided as carbohydrate or fat to meet basal metabolic energy demands, to ensure growth and development, and to prevent the use of protein from the PN, muscle, or visceral organs merely as an energy source.[33]

Carbohydrates

Dextrose (D-glucose), the major carbohydrate used in PN, provides most of the nonprotein calories. Minimal glucose infusion rates are critical, as hypoglycemia (blood glucose level <40 mg/dL) is associated with seizures and subsequent permanent neurologic injury.[32] Two major problems are associated with dextrose infusion in the pediatric age group. First, dextrose contributes most of the osmolality to the infusate, and when provided in concentrations exceeding 10%, it is associated with a high incidence of phlebitis of peripheral veins. In order to provide sufficient calories without giving an excess volume of water to children, it may be necessary to supply dextrose in concentrations of 20 to 25%. High-concentration dextrose can be infused only into central veins, where the blood flow is great enough to rap-

idly dilute the concentrated glucose. Second, young infants may be intolerant of high glucose infusions and develop hyperglycemia, which can lead to glucosuria with osmotic diuresis, dehydration, and intracranial hemorrhage.[34–36]

In order to combat both hypo- and hyperglycemia, it is crucial to know the glucose infusion rate for all young children receiving PN and to slowly advance the glucose infusion as tolerated. The minimal infusion rate for the prevention of hypoglycemia is 4 mg/kg/min. From a practical standpoint, infusion rates are begun at 6 mg/kg/min and advanced by 2 mg/kg/min each day until levels of 11 to 12 mg/kg/min are tolerated. This may take several days to achieve. Frequent monitoring of blood and urine glucose levels is required to prevent both hypo- and hyperglycemia in children as PN is administered. Higher rates of infusion may be required for adequate caloric supply but should be slowly increased as endogenous insulin production allows the maintenance of normoglycemia. If hyperglycemia prevents the administration of sufficient calories, insulin may be added to the parenteral solution. The addition of exogenous insulin must be performed cautiously as the infant's response may be extremely variable.[37]

Fats

Lipid infusions provide a low-volume, concentrated form of energy and are a source of essential fatty acids required for brain and somatic growth, skin integrity, immune function, and wound healing.[32, 38] Additionally, lipids are isotonic and can be administered by a peripheral vein. Intralipid (derived from soybean oil and stabilized with egg phospholipid) and Liposyn (derived from safflower oil) are the two primary lipid sources available.

In order to prevent essential fatty acid deficiency (EFAD), the Committee on Nutrition of the American Academy of Pediatrics has recommended intakes of 3.3 g of fat per 100 kcal, of which 300 mg should be n-6 fatty acids.[39] Although clinical evidence for essential fatty acid deficiency may take several weeks to months to develop in adults, signs may be evident as early as 1 week in infants[38] and include scaly dermatitis, sparse hair growth, increased susceptibility to infection, failure to thrive, and thrombocytopenia.[40, 41]

Another benefit of lipid administration in infants is more optimal nitrogen retention. Nose and associates noted lower basal metabolic rates, lower respiratory quotients, and higher nitrogen retention rates in infants and children receiving nonprotein calories as glucose plus lipid when compared with glucose alone.[42] Other investigators confirmed higher metabolic rates and higher respiratory quotients in infants receiving glucose alone as the source of nonprotein calories.[43, 44] Clearance of infused lipid is directly related to the gestational age of the infant, and tolerance improves with maturation. This is especially true with preterm and small-for-gestational-age infants as discussed in Chapter 23.

Infants have a poorly developed capacity to synthesize and store carnitine, which facilitates the transfer of free fatty acids across the mitochondrial membrane for β-oxidation.[33] In addition, children younger than 12 years may have an obligatory renal excretion of carnitine esters, which can lead to carnitine depletion in the absence of supplementation.[45] Supplementation with intravenous L-carnitine (10 mg/kg/day) in preterm infants or oral supplementation in infants on long-term PN have been advocated.[33] Despite these recommendations, the lack of carnitine in PN formulations has not been associated with the development of any particular clinical syndrome.

The use of intravenous lipids should be restricted in the presence of hyperlipidemia, because hyperlipidemia following lipid infusion may interfere with the pulmonary diffusing capacity[46] or induce pulmonary fat embolism.[47] The American Academy of Pediatrics recommended that serum triglyceride levels be maintained below 150 mg/dL.[48] It is therefore important that infants and children be monitored carefully during the administration of fat.

To prevent the development of ketonemia, no more than 60% of nonprotein calories should be administered as lipid,[49] and it has been recommended to limit the rate of lipid infusion to 3 g/kg/day.[48] Lipid should be infused over prolonged periods (18–24 hours), as intermittent administration results in wide fluctuations of plasma lipid fractions.[50] It is preferable to use a 20% rather than a 10% emulsion. Not only does this decrease the volume of fluid to be infused, but the lower phospholipid intake delivered with 20% lipid emulsion is associated with lower plasma triglyceride, cholesterol, and phospholipid concentrations.[51] In general, lipid infusions are started at 0.5 g/kg/day in premature infants or 1 g/kg/day in term infants and increased in daily increments of 0.25 to 0.5 g/kg/day until a maximum of 3 g/kg/day is reached.

Protein

Like energy requirements in children, protein requirements are relatively much greater in preterm and newborn infants and decline progressively with age. Proteins are needed for new tissue formation and the synthesis of enzymes, neurotransmitters, hormones, and bile salts.[8] Much of the information pertaining to protein requirements in pediatric patients has been obtained from studies with preterm infants, but the same principles are believed to apply to older children.

Proteins may be administered by the parenteral route as either protein hydolysates of fibrin or casein or as various mixtures of crystalline amino acids. Because of more optimal nitrogen utilization, a greater ability to vary individual amino acid concentrations, and a lower preformed ammonia load, crystalline amino acids are currently used.[52] Additional modifications in the composition of amino acid solutions, such as the use of basic salts of histidine and the substitution of acetate for chloride in the lysine salts, have eliminated the problem of hyperchloremic metabolic acidosis commonly encountered before these changes.

Not only do infants and children need relatively more protein than adults, but certain amino acids considered nonessential in adults are regarded as semiessential for young infants and children. Such semiessential amino acids in infants and children include cysteine, histidine, tyrosine, lysine, and arginine. Several amino acid solutions have been developed taking these differences into consideration.[53, 54] At present, it is not totally clear that these solutions justify their significantly greater cost. Increased weight gain and improved nitrogen balance were demonstrated in a group of postsurgical preterm infants using one of these special formulations (TrophAmine, Kendall McGaw Laboratories Inc., Irvine, Calif.) when compared with a standard formulation (FreAmine III, Kendall McGaw Laboratories Inc.).[55] Alternatively, no differences in nitrogen retention, weight gain, or biochemical parameters were found in other studies of specialized formulations (Neopham, Cutter Laboratories, Berkeley, Calif.)[56] It has been argued, however, that inadequate intake of the semiessential amino acids may not be recognized in terms of poor growth or nitrogen balance but rather as long-term deficits in neurologic function.[8]

The optimal quantity of each amino acid needed to meet the nutritional requirements of the growing child has yet to be determined. Although deficiencies of amino acids may result in growth failure and functional deficits, excesses can also cause adverse effects. For example, too much tryptophan may be hepatotoxic and contribute to PN-associated cholestasis,[57] and excess tyrosine in preterm infants may diminish intellectual performance.[58] Hyperammonemia during the PN of infants has been reported to occur up to 75% of the time.[59] Elevated levels of ammonia are usually associated with the overinfusion of protein and occur more commonly in the premature baby but may also be noted in full-term infants. Clinical signs of hyperammonemia include lethargy, which proceeds to muscle twitching and ultimately grand mal seizures. Treatment is to discontinue the parenteral protein, and resolution of symptoms generally follows.[60] Azotemia usually precedes hyperammonemia, and thus blood urea nitrogen levels should be serially followed. A rising blood urea nitrogen level in the absence of obvious renal failure or hypovolemia would be consistent with a low (<150:1) nonprotein-to-nitrogen calorie ratio.

From a practical standpoint, amino acid solutions are begun at a dose of 0.5 g of protein per kilogram per day and increased in increments of 0.5 g/kg/day to the maximal dose. In premature infants, an acceptable maximal dose is 2.5 to 3 g/kg/day. In older infants and children, a protein intake of 2 to 3 g/kg/day is appropriate.[61] If sufficient nonprotein calories are supplied to meet an individual's caloric requirements, then positive nitrogen retention in children occurs.[8]

Minerals, Trace Elements, and Vitamins
Minerals

The minerals known to play an essential role in nutrition support can be divided into

Table 24–5. Daily Electrolyte and Mineral Requirements

Electrolyte or Mineral	Daily Requirements
Sodium	2–4 mEq/kg
Potassium	2–3 mEq/kg
Chloride	2–3 mEq/kg
Acetate	1–4 mEq/kg
Magnesium	0.25–0.5 mEq/kg
Calcium	
Infant and child	100–200 mg/kg
Adolescent	50–100 mg/kg
Phosphate	
Infant and child	1 mM/kg
Adolescent	0.5–1 mM/kg

Adapted from Hill ID, Madrazo-de la Garza JA, Lebenthal E: Parenteral nutrition in pediatric patients. *In* Rombeau J, Caldwell MD (eds): Clinical Nutrition: Parenteral Nutrition, 2nd ed. Philadelphia, WB Saunders, 1993, pp 770–790.

two categories: minerals present in large quantities (e.g., calcium, magnesium, and phosphorus) and those present in only trace amounts (e.g., iron, zinc, and selenium).[3] The current recommendations for minerals, trace elements, and vitamins are derived from recommended dietary allowances for healthy people being fed enterally.[62] The needs of parenterally fed patients are therefore estimated from the enteral allowances, taking into consideration the efficiency of absorption. To allow for individual variations, the mineral requirements for children are usually given as a range (Table 24–5). Actual requirements for each child must be considered and are dependent on such factors as diuretic administration, increased electrolyte losses in gastrointestinal fluids (nasogastric tubes, diarrhea, various fistulas), renal function, and the degree of hydration. Serum electrolytes should be assessed daily for the first 2 to 3 days of PN and then every other day for about 4 days. After a week or more of therapy when the infant or child is stable and the electrolyte content of the PN is not being changed, electrolytes can be assessed weekly or every 2 weeks. If the electrolyte content of the PN solution is changing or if the patient is not stable, serum electrolytes should be monitored more frequently.[33]

It is especially important in pediatric patients to remember that electrolytes may be provided from other sources that are often overlooked. For example, some amino acid solutions supplemented with L-cysteine hydrochloride may provide an additional 0.5 to 1 mEq/kg/day of chloride.[63] Additionally, medications with a high electrolyte content (e.g., cabenicillin) may be used. Conversely, discontinuation of infusions or medications with an increased electrolyte content may result in a need to alter the electrolyte content of the PN solution.

Calcium is the most abundant mineral in the body. In very young infants, calcium and phosphorus are rapidly incorporated into bone matrix, and requirements during this period are relatively much greater than in older infants and children. Whereas phosphorus requirements are generally based on the amount required to maintain normal serum levels, serum calcium levels remain normal even in the presence of significant bone demineralization.[64] Calcium should therefore not be removed from the PN solution in the presence of normal serum levels. Clinically, bone demineralization is inferred by noting an increase in serum levels of alkaline phosphatase. The cause for this elevation may be difficult to determine because high levels are seen with PN-associated cholestasis as well as rapid growth. Fractionation of the alkaline phosphatase into heat-stable (liver) and heat-labile (bone) components may be useful.

The administration of calcium and phosphorus in high concentrations can lead to precipitation. It is for this reason that calcium gluconate is traditionally used instead of calcium chloride in parenteral fluids. The latter dissociates and precipitates with phosphorus more readily. During periods of fluid restriction, it is important not to inadvertently increase the concentration of calcium and phosphorus in the parenteral solution, because this may result in precipitation. Factors that reduce the solubility of calcium and phosphorus in parenteral solutions include a low amino acid or glucose content, a high pH, and prolonged exposure of intravenous tubing to the high temperatures of infant incubators.[65] Attempts to improve calcium and phosphate retention further by administering them in bolus fashion or sequentially have not proved to have advantages over continuous simultaneous infusion and may even be deleterious.[66, 67]

Trace Elements

Trace elements considered essential for normal metabolism in humans include chromium, molybdenum, manganese, iron, cobalt, copper, selenium, and zinc, and clinical

Table 24–6. Recommended Intravenous Intakes of Trace Elements

Element	Infants (g/kg/day)	Children (g/kg/day)
Zinc	250 <3 mo	50
	100 >3 mo	
Copper	20	20
Selenium	2.0	2.0
Chromium	0.2	0.2
Manganese	1.0	1.0
Molybdenum	0.25	0.25
Iodide	1.0	1.0

Adapted from Greene HL, Hambidge KM, Schanler R, Tsang RC: Guidelines for the use of vitamins, trace elements, calcium, magnesium, and phosphorus in infants and children receiving total parenteral nutrition: Report of the Subcommittee on Pediatric Parenteral Nutrient Requirements from the Committee on Clinical Practice Issues of the American Society for Clinical Nutrition. Am J Clin Nutr 48:1324, 1988. (Published errata appear in Am J Clin Nutr 49:1332; 50:560, 1989.)

deficiency syndromes in patients receiving PN have been described for most of these.[8] The problem of trace element deficiency in infants and children is especially important because normal growth and development depend on sufficient amounts in the diet. Recommended intakes of the various trace elements for the pediatric population are shown in Table 24–6.

Green and coworkers have suggested that zinc is the only trace element needed when PN is administered for only 1 to 2 weeks.[68] The other trace elements are considered essential if PN continues for longer than 4 weeks.[68]

Zinc is an essential component of multiple enzyme reactions. Increased losses may occur with persistent diarrhea or excessive gastrointestinal losses from fistulas or stomas. In infants, the earliest sign of deficiency is a decline in growth velocity. With more severe depletion, the infant becomes irritable, lethargic, or both, and a characteristic acro-orofacial rash develops with diarrhea and alopecia.

The addition of iron to PN infusates remains controversial. A concern is that excess iron will decrease the levels of antioxidants such as vitamin E and enhance the risk of gram-negative septicemia, particularly in the malnourished child, who may have low levels of transferrin.[69] The parenteral administration of iron is not usually recommended. Because the risk of iron overload does exist, when it is used, the dose administered should be monitored by regularly measuring serum iron and ferritin levels. Children receiving a dose greater than 100 μg/kg/day appear to be at risk for iron overload.[70]

Deficiency states of the other trace elements are extremely rare with long-term PN, even if these elements are not specifically added to the infusate. A certain amount of contamination of the amino acid mixture with trace elements occurs naturally, and blood or plasma infusions provide other sources of these metals.[71] Routine addition of commercially available trace element mixtures is advised, especially in children requiring TPN for greater than 2 to 3 weeks.

Vitamins

It is now generally accepted that all patients receiving PN should have vitamins added to the infusate. The need for separate adult and pediatric formulations for multivitamin supplements to PN solutions was first suggested in 1979 by the Nutrition Advisory Group of the American Medical Association.[72] More recently, a subcommittee of the American Society of Clinical Nutrition reviewed the existing data on the use of multivitamin preparations in pediatric patients and proposed new guidelines (Table 24–7).[68]

It is first important to recognize that the fat-soluble vitamins (A, D, E, and K) differ in several ways from the water-soluble vitamins in the pediatric population. Requirements for fat-soluble vitamins are more dependent on age and the degree of maturation, and because these vitamins are stored in body tissues, the potential for overdosage and toxicity exists. In contrast, body tissue stores of water-soluble vitamins are very limited, primarily due to efficient renal excretion, and toxicity occurs very rarely.[61]

A growing child has a limited hepatic reserve of vitamin A and therefore has a higher risk for the development of deficiency. Similarly, a relative state of vitamin E deficiency may exist in infants. Further, although vitamin D deficiency in adults may result in osteomalacia, vitamin D deficiency in infants and children is characterized by rickets, which includes the rachitic rib rosary, craniotabes, bowed legs, and muscle weakness.[73] It is important to appreciate the fact that infants and children with specific diseases may have higher or lower vitamin requirements. For example, in patients with cystic fibrosis, more fat-soluble vitamins may be required because of impaired fat absorption. Alternatively, children with renal impairment may require lower amounts of water-soluble vitamins because the ability to excrete vitamins in the urine may be compromised.[33] It is important that those caring for children on PN be aware of these differences and potential deficiency states.

Table 24–7. Suggested Intakes of Parenteral Vitamins in Infants and Children

Vitamin	Infants and Children (dose/day)
Lipid-soluble	
A (μg)	700
E (mg)	7
K (μg)	200
D (μg)	10
Water-soluble	
Ascorbic Acid (mg)	80
Thiamin (mg)	1.2
Riboflavin (mg)	1.4
Pyridoxine (mg)	1.0
Niacin (mg)	17
Pantothenate (mg)	5
Biotin (μg)	20
Folate (μg)	140
Vitamin B$_{12}$ (μg)	1.0

Adapted from Greene HL, Hambidge KM, Schanler R, Tsang RC: Guidelines for the use of vitamins, trace elements, calcium, magnesium, and phosphorus in infants and children receiving total parenteral nutrition: Report of the Subcommittee on Pediatric Parenteral Nutrient Requirements from the Committee on Clinical Practice Issues of the American Society for Clinical Nutrition. Am J Clin Nutr 48:1324, 1988. (Published errata appear in Am J Clin Nutr 49:1332, 50:560, 1989.)

◆ METABOLIC CHANGES IN CRITICALLY ILL PATIENTS

Acute protein-calorie malnutrition and deficient fat and protein stores have been identified in as many as 20% of childhood medical admissions to an intensive care unit.[74] Little is known, however, about children's metabolic response to critical illness. A study of adults has revealed increased metabolic requirements by as much as 100% during sepsis and after major trauma and burns.[75] In adults, critical illness is associated with changes in the metabolism of glucose, lipids, and proteins.[5] Hyperglycemia and glucose intolerance frequently occur during sepsis and injury, despite demonstrable increased insulin secretion. The insensitivity to insulin induced during trauma and sepsis may be further aggravated by high levels of the counter-regulatory hormones cortisol, norepinephrine, and glucagon.[76]

In stressed individuals, there is a progressive depletion of fat stores as the result of continued lipolysis despite high circulating levels of insulin.[77] Additionally, the protein contribution to the total caloric expenditure in critically ill patients is approximately doubled. Considerable amounts of data have established the source of most of the mobilized protein to be body musculature.[5] After minor injury or uncomplicated elective surgery, the catabolic phase is usually brief and of no serious consequences to a healthy, well-nourished patient. However, if this catabolic state occurs in individuals previously weakened by malnutrition or disease, or if the period of rapid catabolism is prolonged by a complicated injury, by infection, or by subsequent injury, then the large loss of body protein becomes a threat to the individual's survival.[5] Prolonged protein catabolism results in muscle weakness (contributing to inadequate pulmonary ventilation), reduced immune defenses, and eventually a loss of wound strength and poor healing.

In the absence of carbohydrates and fats, the provision of amino acids does not improve nitrogen balance in the critically ill patient. Together with adequate lipid and glucose infusions, however, amino acid infusions can limit the loss of lean body mass.[8] It is possible that nitrogen balance can be further improved by providing amino acid infusions that are enriched with branched-chain amino acids.[78, 79]

Pediatric patients are placed at a further disadvantage during critical illness because of their relatively smaller caloric reserve when compared with adults. It is essential in the management of children to limit the depletion of energy and protein reserves until a positive balance can be restored. In order to do this, calorie needs should ideally be measured; however, this is often not practically possible. An alternative is to estimate energy needs using the method developed by Souba and Wilmore in 1983.[80] This method uses known basal metabolic requirements (BMRs) together with various stress factors:

$$\text{Energy Needs (kcal/day)} = \text{BMR} \times \text{Stress Factor} \times 1.25$$

The factor 1.25 is included to allow for additional energy requirements resulting from

Table 24–8. Stress Factors for Calculating Energy Needs

Clinical Condition	Factor
Uncomplicated postoperative course	1.00–1.05
Malignancy	1.10–1.45
Sepsis	1.05–1.25
Major trauma, burns, and severe sepsis	1.30–1.55

From Shayevitz J, Weissman C: Nutrition and metabolism in the critically ill child. *In* Rogers M (ed): Textbook of Pediatric Intensive Care. Baltimore, Williams & Wilkins, 1987, pp 943–962.

stress related to treatment and hospital activity. In infants, the BMR is 70 kcal/kg, decreasing to 30 to 35 kcal/kg in growing children beyond infancy, and to 20 to 25 kcal/kg after the cessation of growth. Factors for the various forms of stress in children have yet to be determined, and until this information is known, figures for calculating the energy needs in adults should be used (Table 24–8). An additional 20 kcal/kg/day for infants and 5 to 10 kcal/kg/day for children should be added to allow for growth.[80]

The response to injury is quite variable in infants and depends on age, the degree of organ maturity, and the underlying nutritional status, as well as the severity of the insult.[81] For infants requiring surgery, the predominant stimulus of the energy response is the degree of insult from the underlying disease process. During the early postoperative phase in infants, there may actually be a decrease in energy requirements. Postoperatively, there is generally a reduction in activity and insensible losses in the sedated infant within a thermoneutral intensive care environment. Caloric requirements are therefore reduced to the amount necessary to meet basal metabolic needs alone. If caloric supplementation of these infants is based on their predicted energy requirements, many of these children will be overfed.[82] It is for these reasons that when caring for an infant, measured energy expenditure and the magnitude of stress resulting from surgery should be used to help direct nutritional support.[83]

◆ CATHETER PLACEMENT AND CARE

Primarily because of the body size and degree of physical activity of infants and children, the ability to safely secure and maintain reliable venous access in such patients poses many unique challenges. The first decision that needs to be made is whether the PN should be administered by the central or the peripheral route. Risks of anesthesia, technical and infectious complications, and limited venous access have all been cited as deterrents to the use of the central veins. On the other hand, the inability to reliably cannulate and maintain access for prolonged periods argues against peripheral access. Additionally, peripheral veins tend to thrombose as a result of the hypertonicity of the glucose solutions needed to provide sufficient calories without imposing an excessive water load. The maximal glucose concentration that can be infused by peripheral veins is 10 to 12.5%.

In addressing this issue, Ziegler and associates reviewed the records of 585 children receiving PN by either the central or the peripheral venous route.[84] In that study, central administration of PN resulted in a greater daily caloric intake (128 vs. 63 kcal/kg) for longer periods (33.7 vs. 11.4 days) and more weight gain (83% vs. 63%). Although infectious and metabolic complications were encountered more frequently in the group receiving central administration, technical complications were documented more often in the peripheral group. When the data were compared per day of therapy, no significant differences in complication rates were appreciated. Based on these results, it was recommended that the primary factor in deciding the method of therapy should be the caloric needs of the individual patient. Peripheral alimentation is suggested for nonstressed infants for brief courses of maintenance therapy when full growth and development are not the primary goal.

Several methods for achieving central venous access for PN are available. These methods are generally categorized into temporary (percutaneous) or permanent (tunneled) catheters, and the selection of an individual catheter depends on the needs and condition of the patient.

One of the more common techniques for long-term access involves the use of a Broviac catheter[85] inserted through a relatively large vein, with the catheter tip residing in the superior vena cava. Some of the available sites for central venous access in children are illustrated in Figure 24–2 and include the subclavian, internal jugular,

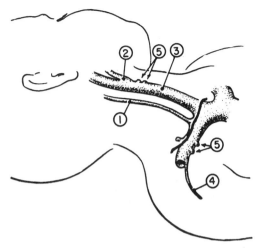

Figure 24–2. Sites for central venous access in infants, in order of preference. 1, external jugular vein; 2, facial vein; 3, internal jugular vein; 4, cephalic vein; 5, tributaries of subclavian and internal jugular veins. (Adapted from Kosloske AM, Klein MD: Techniques of central venous access for long term parenteral nutrition in infants. Surg gynecol obstet 154: 394, 1982.)

external jugular, facial, brachial, cephalic, and azygos veins. For percutaneously inserted catheters, the position of the guidewire (if used) should be confirmed before the larger peel-away sheath and introducer are inserted over the wire. For small catheters (<5 Fr), 1 to 2 mL of contrast material may be injected through the catheter to allow visualization during fluoroscopy. The catheter is then tunneled subcutaneously to exit at an area separate from the original incision and is usually on the anterior part of the chest. The inferior vena cava may also be used via a saphenous or femoral vein entrance site (Fig. 24–3). The exit site of the tunneled catheter may be either the lower thigh or the abdomen (above the diaper area).

Available sizes for Broviac catheters in children include 2.7, 3, 4.2, 5, 6.5, and 7 Fr. Broviac catheters in the pediatric population are associated with an incidence of catheter-related sepsis in the range of 6 to 9.8% and mechanical complications requiring removal of the catheter in 5 to 11.5%.[86, 87] Warner and associates reported the multiple-purpose use of these catheters for PN, replacement fluids, and medication administration in a group of 20 premature infants weighing less than 1000 g. The rates of catheter-associated sepsis and mechanical com-

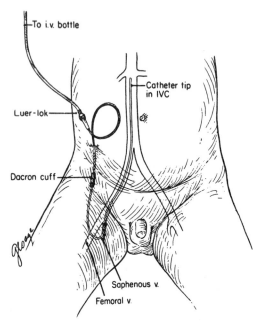

To i.v. bottle

Catheter tip
in IVC

Luer-lok

Dacron cuff

Saphenous v.

Femoral v.

Figure 24–3. A catheter is inserted into the inferior vena cava (IVC), with the tip placed at the level of the renal veins by saphenous venorrhaphy. The Dacron cuff on the catheter is placed in the subcutaneous tunnel at least 1 cm inferior to the catheter exit site on the abdominal wall. i.v., intravenous; v, vein. (Adapted from Fonkalsrud EW, Berquist W, Burke M, Amest ME: Long-term hyperalimentation in children through saphenous central venous catheterization. Am J Surg 143:209, 1982.)

plications in this high-risk group were 9 and 18%, respectively.

Other catheters used for PN include the Hickman and the Groshong (Bard Access Systems) catheters. The Groshong catheter has a specially designed valve at the tip to prevent reflux of blood into the catheter. The purpose of this particular valve is to reduce the incidence of catheter thrombosis. Although theoretically attractive, this catheter was associated with a greater risk of mechanical complications in a population of pediatric oncology patients.[89]

Percutaneous subclavian vein catherization is a frequent method of central venous access, even in small neonates, and offers the advantages of repeated catherization of the same vessel with the avoidance of surgical exposure and vessel ligation. The incidence of catheter-related sepsis with this technique is in the range of 2.5 to 15.9%, and mechanical complications are in the range of 12 to 31.8%.[90, 91] This method may be technically easier in older children; however, in infants and smaller children, it may

be associated with significant morbidity and mortality.[91, 92] Temporary PN catheters are not recommended for chronic use (> 3 wk) because of increased complication rates.[93] Regardless of the type of catheter (temporary or permanent), the placement of catheters in children is usually performed in the operating room. Exceptions to this rule include intubated neonates. The infections and mechanical complications are similar in this population regardless of the location of placement.[94]

Mechanical complications requiring catheter removal are fairly common and include catheter breaks, occlusion, and dislodgment. Catheter repair kits afford the opportunity to maintain larger-bore catheters; however, smaller catheters (2.7 or 3 Fr) are more easily injured and do not withstand repair as well as larger catheters. Catheter dislodgment may occur with greater frequency in younger children and appears to be directly related to the distance between the cuff of the catheter and the catheter exit site. A burst of saline that is injected through the catheter has been successful in repositioning these catheters in a fair percentage of patients.[95]

Peripherally inserted central catheters[96] have become more popular. The attractiveness of this method lies in the fact that no transportation to the operating room is required, no anesthesia is needed, and central venous access can be obtained by a nonsurgical physician or nurse. The overall incidence of sepsis and mechanical complications appear similar to those of other described methods.[93] This method has become an increasingly popular method of long-term venous access in pediatric patients requiring a relatively (< 3 wk) brief course of PN.

Once inserted, a central line provides a portal of entry for potentially fatal bacterial and fungal infection. To prevent such infection, it is necessary to develop protocols for catheter care and for changing the lines and infusates (Table 24–9). Strict adherence to the protocol is essential, and changes should be supervised by members of a support service with special interest and training in administering PN. Meticulous attention to aseptic technique is essential when changing the infusing solutions or opening the line for any reason. By adhering to an acceptable protocol, it is possible to keep the

Table 24–9. Catheter Care Protocol

Limit central line access to four times per 24 hours
Perform 15-second 70% alcohol preparation before
  access of injection ports
Perform 3-minute sterile scrub any time the central
  line is opened at the hub
Change dressing on tunneled central lines once a
  week (nonimmunosuppressed patient)
Change intravenous tubing for parenteral nutrition
  lipids every 24 hours

Adapted from the Children's Hospital Medical Center
Nursing Policy/Procedures Manual, 1998.

incidence of serious catheter infection to
less than 5%.[97]

◆ COMPLICATIONS OF PARENTERAL NUTRITION

Most complications related to parenteral nutrition in the pediatric patient are similar to
those that occur in adult patients, as discussed elsewhere in this book. The complications that do occur generally fall into one
of three categories: septic, technical (as related to placement and maintenance of the
catheter), and metabolic.

Septic Complications

Sepsis remains the most common complication of both short- and long-term PN, accounting for approximately 75% of all complications encountered in the pediatric age
group.[8] Current incidence rates range from
6 to 20%.[98] Not only does the PN delivery
system serve as source for introducing infections, but patients requiring this form of nutritional support are often critically ill or
have pre-existing nutritional depletion ren-
dering them more susceptible to infection.
As in adults, *Staphylococcus aureus* and
Staphylococcus epidermidis are most commonly isolated.[99] Children, like their adult
counterparts receiving PN, often receive
multiple courses of broad-spectrum antibiotics, predisposing them to fungal infections.

The prevention of sepsis in the pediatric
patient should be of utmost priority. This
requires education of all personnel involved
in the patient's management and strict adherence to standardized policies for catheter
care as discussed earlier. Formation of a formal nutritional support team to coordinate

every aspect of a patient's care has been
beneficial in reducing the rate of complications.[100] Accessing of central lines used for
PN should be kept to a minimum.

Because early diagnosis and treatment of
line sepsis is of utmost importance, fever
in a patient with a central line should be
attributed to catheter-related sepsis until
proved otherwise. In pediatric patients, the
onset of line sepsis may be insidious and
may manifest initially only as a change in
glucose tolerance, unexplained metabolic
acidosis, a failure to gain weight, or a worsening of their cholestasis. As with any patient with presumed sepsis, a thorough
physical examination is required to rule out
other sites of infection. Special attention
must be directed toward the catheter site,
looking for cellulitis or fluctuance. Blood
cultures from the central line as well as from
a peripheral site should be obtained in all
cases.

The decision to remove the central venous catheter must be based on sound clinical judgment and experience and supported
if possible by bacteriologic evidence. Historically, fever in a patient with a central line
would have mandated removal of the central
line. Automatic catheter removal is no
longer necessary because only a minority of
catheters removed for suspected sepsis are
actually infected;[97] further, many patients
respond to parenteral antibiotic treatment
without removal of the catheter.[101] Management of such patients should be based on
the patient's overall clinical condition and
the organism cultured. The initial therapy
for line sepsis in the absence of an associated tunnel infection begins with empirical
intravenous antibiotic therapy as soon as the
appropriate cultures have been obtained. A
trial of broad-spectrum antibiotics for 48
hours is acceptable for the patient who does
not appear septic. Persistence of fever after
this period constitutes a reason for removing
the central line.

Mechanical Complications

As discussed earlier with catheter care and
placement, mechanical complications are
associated both with the insertion of the
central line and with the catheter itself. Hematoma and pneumothorax are most likely
to complicate percutaneous attempts to cannulate a major vessel. Infants are more sus-

ceptible to pneumothorax than children or adults because the apex of the lung is higher in the thoracic inlet in infants.

Other potential mechanical complications include air embolism, venous thrombosis, and catheter malposition. Air embolus may occur during catheter insertion, intravenous set changes, and catheter removal. Air embolus through central lines may be a cause of stroke in children with congenital or acquired artero-venous communication. Thrombosis of major veins occurs secondary to the presence of a foreign body (the catheter) in the vessel. The use of newer silicone elastomer catheters has helped to reduce the incidence of this complication. Malposition of the central line can lead to extravasation of PN solutions; the catheter position should be confirmed by radiography at the time of placement and at any time there is a change in the external catheter position.

Various guidelines have been proposed to reduce the risk of technical complications, and Filston and Grant established safe criteria for subclavian catherization in infants and children.[90] A thorough preoperative evaluation should include a detailed history and physical examination as well as laboratory studies to identify thrombocytopenia (usually <50,000 platelets/ml) or other coagulopathies. In addition, in those patients having had multiple previous central lines, preoperative venous duplex ultrasonography may be used to more accurately assess the degree of thrombosis and/or central vein patency and to safely map sites for potential central line placement.

Metabolic Complications

Many metabolic complications related to PN in pediatric patients relate to glucose, fat, protein, vitamin, and mineral abnormalities as described earlier. One common, but poorly understood, complication in the pediatric population is cholestasis. In infants and young children, TPN-related cholestasis may lead to cirrhosis with end-stage liver failure and death. The liver dysfunction related to PN in older children and adults, however, seldom progresses beyond fatty infiltration.

The hepatobiliary complications of PN may be divided into three distinct clinical syndromes. The first syndrome is seen primarily in adults and is characterized by hepatic steatosis, steatohepatitis, and the infrequent occurrence of cholestasis. The second pattern is seen primarily in infants and is characterized predominantly by cholestasis. The third is common to both age groups and consists of the gallbladder-related problems of sludge formation and stones.[102]

PN-related cholestasis is most common in infants receiving PN for greater than 2 weeks, rising to 80% if parenteral therapy is continued for more than 60 days.[103] It is also noted to be more common in premature and low-birth-weight babies, with an incidence reported to be 50, 18, and 7% in infants with birth weights less than 1000, 1000 to 1500, and 1500 to 2000 g, respectively.[103] The onset is often insidious and initially detected only by changes in the biochemical profile. The earliest measurable changes appear to be an elevation in the concentration of the serum bile acids. Later, there is a rise in the transaminase, alkaline phosphatase, and bilirubin levels, progressing to clinical jaundice and hepatomegaly. In advanced cases, chronic liver damage with cirrhosis may occur.

Factors thought to play a role in TPN-related cholestasis include prematurity, low birth weight, sepsis, a lack of enteral nutrition, and gastrointestinal conditions that require operative intervention.[104] Immaturity of hepatocyte function with altered bile acid transport predisposes infants to cholestasis.[105] An excess or a deficiency of various amino acids has been implicated in the pathogenesis of PN-related cholestasis. Jaundice was demonstrated to occur more rapidly and to a greater extent in infants receiving PN solutions containing a higher protein content (3.6 vs. 2.3 g/kg/day).[106] A deficiency of certain amino acids, particularly taurine, may play a role, because standard amino acid solutions do not contain taurine. This amino acid may be considered essential in the neonate because of a reduced synthetic ability. In a controlled trial, however, taurine supplementation did not alter biochemical tests of hepatic toxicity.[107] Additionally, no reduction in the rate of PN-induced cholestasis was seen when two pediatric amino acid formulations were compared.[108]

Interference with the enterohepatic circulation of bile salts may also contribute to liver injury. Colonization of the gut with colonic-type bacteria because of intestinal stasis results in increased production of lithocholic acid, which has been shown to impair bile flow and induce cholestasis.[109] Further, pretreatment of patients with either oral metronidazole or gentamicin resulted in a reduced incidence of PN-related dysfunction.[110, 111] The beneficial effect of antibiotic administration may also be related to reducing the number of bacteria or bacterial by-products translocating across the gut mucosa and into the portal circulation.

It is important to emphasize that the diagnosis of TPN-induced cholestasis should be one of exclusion. The differential diagnosis of hyperbilirubinemia in the neonate is extensive. Sepsis from any cause should be ruled out. Noninvasive imaging of the biliary system should be done using ultrasonography, radionuclide scanning, or liver biopsy. In a study of 47 patients referred for evaluation of presumed PN-associated cholestasis, Farrell and Balistreri were able to make a definitive diagnosis of other disorders in 10% of the patients.[112]

After the diagnosis of PN-related cholestasis is confirmed, the best therapy is to begin or increase enteral feeding and wean the patient from PN as much as possible. Other maneuvers include reducing the amount of protein and decreasing the calorie-to-nitrogen ratio to roughly 150. In selected cases of severe chronic liver disease, transplantation of the liver with or without small bowel transplantation has been successful.[113, 114]

Another poorly understood metabolic complication of PN therapy in children is metabolic bone disease. This PN-related bone disease commonly presents as osteopenia in preterm infants and is likely a multifactorial condition.[115] Potential pathophysiologic mechanisms include inadequate calcium and phosphate supplementation, aluminum loading and toxicity, and possibly the provision of vitamin D.

◆ HOME PARENTERAL NUTRITION

Home parenteral nutrition (HPN) seeks to achieve positive nitrogen balance and weight gain and to improve the clinical outcome in nonhospitalized patients who lack adequate gastrointestinal tract function. A thorough discussion of the clinical outcome, technique, and finances of HPN are discussed in Chapter 25; we therefore attempt to summarize some of the unique features relevant to the pediatric patient.

Over the past two decades, the use of HPN has come to be accepted as a useful supportive and therapeutic technique for various gastrointestinal diseases and conditions. In the United States, it is estimated that approximately 40,000 patients are receiving HPN,[116] and of this group, between 5 and 20% are infants and children younger than 18 years.[117] At our institution over the past 1-year period, 153 children have required HPN for durations ranging from 3 days to a year. We are currently supporting one child who has required PN for 9 years because of short bowel syndrome.

Indications

HPN is indicated for any patient whose sole reason for remaining in the hospital is to receive parenteral support and who does not require nursing support beyond the capability of family members. The most common indications and conditions for instituting home HPN in children are shown in Table 24–10. In some patients, the purpose of HPN is to provide nutrition while the infant grows and the short small intestine adapts. In others, support will be indefinite, because the bowel is too short, the damage to the mucosal lining is irreversible, or, in the rarest instances, the villi fail to develop because of a congenital defect. Some of the patients require complete support, whereas others need only partial support.

Contraindications to HPN include a functional gastrointestinal tract such that enteral feeding is possible. Home therapy should also be avoided when no parent or family member is capable of or willing to learn and

Table 24–10. Common Indications for Home Parenteral Nutrition

---

Short gut syndrome
Gastroschisis
Total aganglionic Hirschsprung's disease
Intestinal pseudo-obstruction
Inflammatory bowel disease
Acute pancreatitis
Prolonged postoperative ileus
Cystic fibrosis
Preparation for transplant
Cancer patients

---

perform the daily techniques required for successful and safe administration of HPN.

Patient Preparation

Before the institution of HPN in a pediatric patient, discussions with the parents, and the child when possible, are essential. Both the benefits and risks for the patient should be discussed. The risk of complications, including catheter infection and sepsis, thrombosis of the catheter, hypoglycemia from stopping the infusion too rapidly, bleeding from separation of the tubing, and unknown and unforeseen metabolic complications, should be carefully addressed. Additionally, when possible, the likely duration of therapy should be discussed. The potential for intestinal adaptation and future surgical interventions should also be explained carefully.

Catheter Access

Details of catheter placement have been discussed earlier, and this section therefore emphasizes specific needs related to HPN. Access for long-term HPN should routinely be performed by a surgically placed tunneled catheter such as a Hickman or a Broviac catheter. Dual- and triple-lumen catheters may be used in pediatric patients, specifically in those with cancer requiring chemotherapy, and those undergoing transplantation. These catheters have a higher incidence of infection when compared with single-lumen catheters, and strict care is essential.[118] Totally implantable venous access systems such as Infuse-A-Port (Intermedics Infusaid Corporation, Norwood, Mass.) and port-A-Cath (Pharmacia Laboratories, Piscataway, N.J.) are devices that have a catheter attached to a subcutaneously placed injection port. These systems have been used for the administration of drugs (e.g., chemotherapy), blood products, and occasionally PN. There are several complications with this system that make it less suitable for HPN in the pediatric patient. The most unique complications include those related to the placement of the specially designed Huber needle. Potential problems include needle dislodgment, improper placement of the needle leading to extravasation, and catheter infection.

Infusion Schedules

In the hospital, the patient is initially established on a 24-hour infusion schedule. Once the maximal concentration of dextrose and fat has been reached, the number of hours of support may be decreased by 1 to 2 h/day. The rate of administration may then be increased, but the volume administered should remain constant. Gradually, over a period of 7 days, the number of hours of infusion can be decreased to 10 to 14 h/day.[119] The younger the infant is, the more hours the infusion is allowed to run. In school-aged children, it is beneficial to give the infusions over a 10-hour period. This schedule allows the child to have the maximal amount of time to be free of attachment to an infusion system. The rate of infusion must be slowly increased and decreased with the initiation and completion of daily infusions; this helps limit the risks of hyper- and hypoglycemia, respectively.

Home Catheter Care

Before discharge, an assessment should be done to identify who in the family will act as the primary caretaker for the child's home care, as well as to establish the adequacy of the home environment. Parents should first receive written instructions on HPN procedures and techniques and may benefit from viewing videotaped demonstrations of care. Parents may then begin working with mannequins or practice catheters and progress to working with their child in the hospital as they become more adept at the procedures for care. Parental education should include all aspects of care, including the care of solutions, infusion pump operation, catheter dressing care, and the identification of potential problems. The amount of time necessary to teach parents procedures for HPN care may vary from 5 days to 1 month. The average parent requires approximately 10 days of lessons to become independent in all aspects of care.[119]

Before the child's discharge from the hospital, the family should be linked to a reliable home care provider for the provision of solutions and supplies, and home care nursing after discharge. A home visit should be made before the child's discharge from the hospital if any problems are anticipated in terms of the family's ability to provide an adequate home environment for the storage of solutions and supplies and for safely carrying out HPN care procedures.

Complications of Home Parenteral Nutrition

Complications occurring with HPN include all the septic, mechanical, and metabolic complications described earlier for PN therapy. Some of these complications may become more evident with long-term home care and warrant further discussion. It is important that a team of physicians, nurses, and nutritionists experienced with HPN carefully monitor all children receiving HPN.

Long-term catheter use may result in catheters' becoming damaged at their external segments from repeated clamping and unclamping. Broken or disconnected catheters should be repaired emergently with catheter-specific repair kits. The repair should be done by a trained member of the nutritional support team under sterile conditions.

Although protocols for heparin flushing of catheters exist, catheter occlusion still occurs. If a long-term central venous catheter does become occluded or gives an indication that the infusion is slowing, 2500 U of urokinase per milliliter (appropriate volume to fill the catheter) should be slowly infused into the occluded catheter, and the catheter should be capped off. The urokinase should be allowed to remain in place for 3 hours and should then be aspirated back. A flushing solution of 100 U of heparin per milliliter can then be used to clear the catheter. Seventy-seven percent of acutely occluded catheters may be restored to patency by injection of a fibrinolytic agent.[120] Signs of impending catheter thrombosis that warrant urokinase administration include increased catheter resistance to infusion or flushing, slowing of a gravity drip infusion, and withdrawal occlusion.

Infectious complications remain the most frequent serious complication related to both in-hospital PN and HPN. It has been reported that there is an incidence of 1.66 catheter-related infections for 1000 days of inpatient catheter use, compared with 1.13 central venous catheter–related infections per 1000 days of PN in children who received long-term HPN.[121] This lower incidence of outpatient infectious complications is likely multifactorial, including factors such as sicker children with potentially depressed resistance likely compromising the inpatient group, and the level of experience of the patient's family with home care influencing the HPN group. It has been demonstrated that experience plays an important role, as catheter-related complications are higher in the first 2 years of HPN than in later years. It is important that each time a child receiving HPN develops a fever, parents be asked to bring the child in for an examination. Overall, 60% of children with a central venous catheter who present to the emergency room or walk-in clinic with fever are demonstrated to have a catheter-related infection.[119]

Catheter infections in patients receiving HPN are usually treated without removal of the catheter by administering parenteral antibiotics. Catheter removal is required in the presence of fungal infections, septic shock, endocarditis, persistent fever, or disseminated intravascular coagulation. In addition, infections of the tunnel tract usually require catheter removal. A new catheter may be replaced when the patient has been afebrile for 72 hours and blood cultures no longer contain the infectious organism.

As mentioned earlier in this chapter, trace element and vitamin deficiencies are potential problems with PN, and these problems are particularly relevant with long-term HPN. It is important to avoid deficiency states by following the recommended intravenous intakes shown in Table 24–5. With the use of multiple vitamin preparations that are added to the parenteral solution just before administration, vitamin deficiency should be exceedingly uncommon.[68]

For pediatric patients on HPN, it is necessary to be aware of potential gallbladder- and liver-related disease. Long-term studies of patients receiving PN have revealed cholelithiasis in as many as 10 to 40%.[122] Additionally, the chance of developing gallbladder sludge as a result of PN is almost 100% after patients have been receiving PN for 6 weeks. It is therefore important that any child who receives PN for greater than 30 days and develops abdominal pain be suspected of having cholecystitis. Early institution of some enteral feeding if possible may reduce the occurrence of PN-induced liver disease.

Long-Term Growth and Nutritional Status

A unique aspect of pediatric HPN compared with that of adults is the fact that pediatric patients are actively growing. Children receiving long-term PN can attain and maintain normal height, weight, and other anthropometric measurements of nutritional status. Growth retardation in children receiving PN may have various causes, including malnutrition resulting from suboptimal caloric support, essential fatty acid deficiency, and trace element deficiency.[119]

Besides physical growth, pediatric patients are growing developmentally and socially. Most children who have received HPN since infancy develop more slowly because of a prolonged hospitalization before discharge.[123] Prompt discharge from the hospital and successful treatment at home without rehospitalization provide the patient with the best chance for developing normally. The major developmental and social stumbling blocks for these children are likely related to their chronic illness and need for hospitalization and are not directly related to their HPN.

Home Parenteral Nutrition Team

Children receiving HPN need a multidisciplinary care team that is cognizant of the medical and metabolic complications of PN. Standards of practice for home nutritional support have been developed by the American Society of Parenteral and Enteral Nutrition.[124] The team should include a physician, a registered nurse, a registered dietician, a registered pharmacist, and a social worker, each of whom has appropriate education, specialized training, and experience in nutritional support.

The pharmacist is responsible for monitoring all patients receiving PN to promote appropriate use, optimal efficacy, and minimal complications. The HPN nurse is responsible for patient education, discharge planning, and assistance with the coordination of follow-up care. The nurse may also handle triage of outpatient care problems by telephone and may be available for catheter repair and "problem" catheter consultation on an outpatient basis. The dietician is responsible for calculating and recommending the appropriate amounts of parenteral glu-

cose, amino acid, lipid, minerals, and trace elements needed. Finally, the social worker provides counseling and support in dealing with the many emotional, economic, and social issues that confront patients receiving HPN and their families.

Expense

HPN is indeed expensive, with gross costs of greater than $20,000 per month. This cost, however, is substantially less both financially and developmentally than keeping a child hospitalized. In most states, government financial support is provided if insurance does not cover the cost.

SUMMARY

Pediatric PN has undoubtedly contributed to improved survival of patients with previously fatal conditions. The use of PN is, however, not without risk, including the potentially fatal complication of bacterial and fungal sepsis. PN, especially long-term PN, should be used only when it is impossible to provide adequate nutrition by an enteral route, and if used, PN should be discontinued as soon as the child can tolerate adequate enteral nutrition.

REFERENCES

1. Dudrick SJ, Wilmore DW, Vars HM, Rhoads JE: Can intravenous feeding as the sole means of nutrition support growth in the child and restore weight loss in an adult? An affirmative answer. Ann Surg 169:974, 1969.
2. Hendren WH, Henderson BM: Recent advances in pediatric surgery. Am J Surg 118:338, 1969.
3. Ford EG: Nutrition support of pediatric patients. Nutr Clin Pract 11:183, 1996.
4. Kurachi H, Oka T: Regulation of the level of epidermal growth factor by oestrogen in the submandibular gland of female mice. J Endocrinol 109:221, 1986.
5. Ryan NT: Metabolic adaptations for energy production during trauma and sepsis. Surg Clin North Am 56:1073, 1976.
6. Moront ML, Williams JA, Eichelberger MR, Wilkinson JD: The injured child. An approach to care. Pediatr Clin North Am 41:1201, 1994.
7. Rodriguez DJ: Nutrition in patients with severe burns: state of the art. J Burn Care Rehabil 17:62, 1996.
8. Hill ID, Madrazo-de la Garza JA, Lebenthal E: Parenteral nutrition in pediatric patients. *In* Rombeau J, Caldwell MD (eds): Clinical Nutrition: Par-

enteral Nutrition, 2nd ed. Philadelphia, WB Saunders, 1993, pp 770–790.

9. Warner BW, Ziegler MM: Management of the short bowel syndrome in the pediatric population. Pediatric Clin North Am 40:1335, 1993.

10. Iacono G, Carroccio A, Montalto G, et al: Extreme short bowel syndrome: A case for reviewing the guidelines for predicting survival. J Pediatr Gastroenterol Nutr 16:216, 1993.

11. Chaet MS, Farrell MK, Ziegler MM, Warner BW: Intensive nutritional support and remedial surgical intervention for extreme short bowel syndrome. J Pediatr Gastroenterol Nutr 19:295, 1994.

12. Kelly DG, Fleming, CR: Nutritional considerations in inflammatory bowel diseases. Gastroenterol Clin North Am 24:597, 1995.

13. Kleinman RE, Balistreri WF, Heyman MB, et al: Nutritional support for pediatric patients with inflammatory bowel disease. J Pediatr Gastroenterol Nutr 8:8, 1989.

14. Seidman EG, Roy CC, Weber AM, Morin CL: Nutritional therapy of Crohn's disease in childhood. Dig Dis Sci 32:82S, 1987.

15. Lin CH, Lerner A, Rossi TM, et al: Effects of parenteral nutrition on whole body and extremity composition in children and adolescents with active inflammatory bowel disease. JPEN J Parenter Enteral Nutr 13:366, 1989.

16. Strobel CT: Home parenteral nutrition in children with Crohn's disease [Letter]. Gastroenterology 77:1364, 1979.

17. Lake AM, Kim S, Mathis RK, Walker WA: Influence of preoperative parenteral alimentation on postoperative growth in adolescent Crohn's disease. J Pediatr Gastroenterol Nutr 4:182, 1985.

18. Layden T, Rosenberg J, Nemchansky B: Reveral of growth arrest in adolescents with Crohn's disease after parenteral alimentation. Gastroenterology 70:1017, 1976.

19. Arora NS, Rochester DF: Respiratory muscle strength and maximal voluntary ventilation in undernourished patients. Am Rev Respir Dis 126:5, 1982.

20. Harper TB, Chase HP, Henson J, Henson PM: Essential fatty acid deficiency in the rabbit as a model of nutritional impairment in cystic fibrosis. In vitro and in vivo effects on lung defense mechanisms. Am Rev Respir Dis 126:540, 1982.

21. Hopkins D, Witters R, Nesheim M: A respiratory disease syndrome in chickens fed essential fatty acid deficient diets. Proc Soc Exp Biol Med 114:82, 1963.

22. Farrell PM, Mischler EH, Engle MJ, et al: Fatty acid abnormalities in cystic fibrosis. Pediatr Res 19:104, 1985.

23. Mansell AL, Andersen JC, Muttart CR, et al: Short-term pulmonary effects of total parenteral nutrition in children with cystic fibrosis. J Pediatr 104:700, 1984.

24. Shepherd R, Cooksley WG, Cooke WD: Improved growth and clinical, nutritional, and respiratory changes in response to nutritional therapy in cystic fibrosis. J Pediatr 97:351, 1980.

25. Andrassy RJ, Chwals WJ: Nutritional support of the pediatric oncology patient. Nutrition 14:124, 1998.

26. Copeman MC: Use of total parenteral nutrition in children with cancer: A review and some recommendations. Pediatr Hematol Oncol 11:463, 1994.

27. Okada A: Clinical indications of parenteral and enteral nutrition support in pediatric patients. Nutrition 14:116, 1998.

28. Beaton GH: Nutritional needs during the first year of life. Some concepts and perspectives. Pediatr Clin North Am 32:275, 1985.

29. Cashore WJ, Sedaghatian MR, Usher RH: Nutritional supplements with intravenously administered lipid, protein hydrolysate, and glucose in small premature infants. Pediatrics 56:8, 1975.

30. Coran AG: The long-term total intravenous feeding of infants using peripheral veins. J Pediatr Surg 8:801, 1973.

31. Zlotkin SH, Bryan MH, Anderson GH: Intravenous nitrogen and energy intakes required to duplicate in utero nitrogen accretion in prematurely born human infants. J Pediatr 99:115, 1981.

32. Wesley JR, Khalidi N, Faubion WC, et al: The University of Michigan Medical Center: Parenteral and Enteral Nutrition Manual (ed 6). North Chicago, IL, Abbott Laboratories Hospital Products Division, 1990.

33. Cochran EB, Phelps SJ, Helms RA: Parenteral nutrition in pediatric patients. Clin Pharm 7:351, 1988. (Published erratum appears in Clin Pharm 11:750, 1992.)

34. Dweck HS, Cassady G: Glucose intolerance in infants of very low birth weight. I: Incidence of hyperglycemia in infants of birth weights 1,100 grams or less. Pediatrics 53:189, 1974.

35. Le DM: Intravenous glucose tolerance and plasma insulin studies in small-for-dates infants. Arch Dis Child 47:111, 1972.

36. Arant B, Gooch W: Effect of acute hyperglycemia on brains of neonatal puppies. Pediatr Res 13:448, 1979.

37. Goldman SL, Hirata T: Attenuated response to insulin in very low birthweight infants. Pediatr Res 14:50, 1980.

38. Friedman Z, Danon A, Stahlman MT, Oates JA: Rapid onset of essential fatty acid deficiency in the newborn. Pediatrics 58:640, 1976.

39. American Academy of Pediatrics Committee on Nutrition: Nutritional needs of low-birth-weight infants. Pediatrics 75:976, 1985.

40. Penn D, Ludwigs B, Schmidt-Sommerfeld E, Pascu F: Effect of nutrition on tissue carnitine concentrations in infants of different gestational ages. Biol Neonate 47:130, 1985.

41. Helms RA, Whitington PF, Mauer EC, et al: Enhanced lipid utilization in infants receiving oral l-carnitine during long-term parenteral nutrition. J Pediatr 109:984, 1986.

42. Nose O, Tipton JR, Ament ME, Yabuuchi H: Effect of the energy source on changes in energy expenditure, respiratory quotient, and nitrogen balance during total parenteral nutrition in children. Pediatr Res 21:538, 1987.

43. Sauer P, Van Aerde J, Smith J, et al: Substrate utilization of newborn infants fed intravenously with or without a fat emulsion [Abstract]. Pediatr Res 18:804, 1984.

44. Van Aerde J, Sauer P, Smith J, et al: Contribution of glucose and fat to the energy expenditure of parenterally fed neonates [Abstract]. Pediatr Res 19:322A, 1985.

45. Schmidt-Sommerfeld E, Penn D, Bieber LL, et al: Carnitine ester excretion in pediatric patients receiving parenteral nutrition. Pediatr Res 28:158, 1990.

46. Greene HL, Hazlett D, Demaree R: Relationship between intralipid-induced hyperlipemia and pulmonary function. Am J Clin Nutr 29:127, 1976.

47. Barson AJ, Chistwick ML, Doig CM: Fat embolism in infancy after intravenous fat infusions. Arch Dis Child 53:218, 1978.

48. American Academy of Pediatrics Committee on Nutrition: Use of intravenous fat emulsions in pediatric patients. Pediatrics 68:738, 1981.

49. Johnson JD, Albritton WL, Sunshine P: Hyperammonemia accompanying parenteral nutrition in newborn infants. J Pediatr 81:154, 1972.

50. Brans YW, Andrew DS, Carrillo DW et al: Tolerance of fat emulsions in very-low-birth-weight neonates. Am J Dis Child 142:145, 1988.

51. Haumont D, Deckelbaum RJ, Richelle M, et al: Plasma lipid and plasma lipoprotein concentrations in low birth weight infants given parenteral nutrition with twenty or ten percent lipid emulsion. J Pediatr 115:787, 1989.

52. Long CL, Zikria BA, Kinney JM, Geiger JW: Comparison of fibrin hydrolysates and crystalline amino acid solutions in parenteral nutrition. Am J Clin Nutr 27:163, 1974.

53. Imura K, Okada A, Fukui Y, et al: Clinical studies on a newly devised amino acid solution for neonates. JPEN J Parenter Enteral Nutr 12:496, 1988.

54. Kanaya S, Nose O, Harada T, et al: Total parenteral nutrition with a new amino acid solution for infants. J Pediatr Gastroenterol Nutr 3:440, 1984.

55. Helms RA, Christensen ML, Mauer EC, Storm MC: Comparison of a pediatric versus standard amino acid formulation in preterm neonates requiring parenteral nutrition. J Pediatr 110:466, 1987.

56. Chase HP, Nixt TL: A double-blind study comparing Neopham with FreAmine III in infants receiving parenteral nutrition. Acta Chir Scand Suppl 517:49, 1983.

57. Merritt RJ, Sinatra FR, Henton D, Neustein H: Cholestatic effect of intraperitoneal administration of tryptophan to suckling rat pups. Pediatr Res 18:904, 1984.

58. Menkes JH, Welcher DW, Levi HS, et al: Relationship of elevated blood tyrosine to the ultimate intellectual performance of premature infants. Pediatrics 49:218, 1972.

59. Seashore JH: Metabolic complications of parenteral nutrition in infants and children. Surg Clin North Am 60:1239, 1980.

60. Heird WC, Nicholson JF, Driscoll JMJ, et al: Hyperammonemia resulting from intravenous alimentation using a mixture of synthetic l-amino acids: A preliminary report. J Pediatr 81:162, 1972.

61. Warner B: Parenteral nutrition in the pediatric patient. In Fischer J (ed): Total Parenteral Nutrition. Boston, Little, Brown, 1991, pp 299–322.

62. National Research Council, F A N B: Recommended Dieterary Allowances, 9th ed. Washington, DC, National Academy of Sciences, 1980.

63. l-cysteine Hydrochloride Product Information. Irvine, Calif, Abbot Hospital Products, 1987.

64. Rose J, Gibbons K, Carlson SE, Koo WW: Nutrient needs of the preterm infant [see Comments]. Nutr Clin Pract 8:226, 1993.

65. Venkataraman PS, Brissie EOJ, Tsang RC: Stability of calcium and phosphorus in neonatal parenteral nutrition solutions. J Pediatr Gastroenterol Nutr 2:640, 1983.

66. Hoehn GJ, Carey DE, Rowe JC, et al: Alternate day infusion of calcium and phosphate in very low birth weight infants: Wasting of the infused mineral. J Pediatr Gastroenterol Nutr 6:752, 1987.

67. Kimura S, Nose O, Seino Y, et al: Effects of alternate and simultaneous administrations of calcium and phosphorus on calcium metabolism in children receiving total parenteral nutrition. JPEN J Parenter Enteral Nutr 10:513, 1986.

68. Greene HL, Hambidge KM, Schanler R, Tsang RC: Guidelines for the use of vitamins, trace elements, calcium, magnesium, and phosphorus in infants and children receiving total parenteral nutrition: Report of the Subcommittee on Pediatric Parenteral Nutrient Requirements from the Committee on Clinical Practice Issues of the American Society for Clinical Nutrition. Am J Clin Nutr 48:1324, 1988. (Published errata appear in Am J Clin Nutr 49:1332, 50:560, 1989.)

69. Porter KA, Bistrian BR, Blackburn GL: Guidewire catheter exchange with triple culture technique in the management of catheter sepsis. JPEN J Parenter Enteral Nutr 12:628, 1988.

70. Ben HM, Goulet O, De PS, et al: Iron overload in children receiving prolonged parenteral nutrition. J Pediatr 123:238, 1993.

71. Vanderhoof JA, Antonson DL: Trace elements in parenteral nutrition. In Lebenthal E (ed): Total Parenteral Nutrition. New York, Raven Press, 1986, pp 109.

72. Multivitamin preparations for parenteral use. A statement by the Nutrition Advisory Group. American Medical Association Department of Foods and Nutrition, 1975. JPEN J Parenter Enteral Nutr 3:258, 1979.

73. Specker B, Greer F, Tsang R: Nutrition in Infancy, 1st ed. Philadelphia, Hanley & Belfus, 1988.

74. Pollack MM, Wiley JS, Holbrook PR: Early nutritional depletion in critically ill children. Crit Care Med 9:580, 1981.

75. Elwyn DH, Kinney JM, Askanazi J: Energy expenditure in surgical patients. Surg Clin North Am 61:545, 1981.

76. Wilmore DW, Aulick LH, Mason AD, Pruitt BAJ: Influence of the burn wound on local and systemic responses to injury. Ann Surg 186:444, 1977.

77. Nordenstrom J, Carpentier YA, Askanazi J, et al: Metabolic utilization of intravenous fat emulsion during total parenteral nutrition. Ann Surg 196:221, 1982.

78. Weissman C, Askanazi J, Rosenbaum S, et al: Amino acids and respiration. Ann Intern Med 98:41, 1983.

79. Eriksson S, Hagenfeldt L, Wahren J: A comparison of the effects of intravenous infusion of individual branched-chain amino acids on blood amino acid levels in man. Clin Sci 60:95, 1981.

80. Souba W, Wilmore DW: Planning total parenteral nutrition. Clin Anesthesiol 1:663, 1983.

81. Chwals WJ: The metabolic response to surgery in neonates. Curr Opin Pediatr 6:334, 1994.

82. Letton RW, Chwals WJ, Jamie A, Charles B: Early postoperative alterations in infant energy use increase the risk of overfeeding. J Pediatr Surg 30:988, 1995.

83. Chwals WJ, Letton RW, Jamie A, Charles B: Stratification of injury severity using energy expenditure response in surgical infants. J Pediatr Surg 30:1161, 1995.

84. Ziegler M, Jakobowski D, Hoelzer D, et al: Route of pediatric parenteral nutrition: Proposed criteria revision. J Pediatr Surg 15:472, 1980.

85. Broviac JW, Cole JJ, Scribner BH: A silicone rubber atrial catheter for prolonged parenteral alimentation. Surg Gynecol Obstet 136:602, 1973.

86. Colombani PM, Dudgeon DL, Buck JR, et al: Multipurpose central venous access in the immunocompromised pediatric patient. JPEN J Parenter Enteral Nutr. 9:38, 1985.

87. Weber TR, West KW, Grosfeld JL: Broviac central venous catheterization in infants and children. Am J Surg 145:202, 1983.

88. Warner BW, Gorgone P, Schilling S, et al: Multiple purpose central venous access in infants less than 1,000 grams. J Pediatr Surg 22:820, 1987.

89. Warner BW, Haygood MM, Davies SL, Hennies GA: A randomized, prospective trial of standard Hickman compared with Groshong central venous catheters in pediatric oncology patients. J Am Coll Surg 183:140, 1996.

90. Filston HC, Grant JP: A safer system for percutaneous subclavian venous catheterization in newborn infants. J Pediatr Surg 14:564, 1979.

91. Groff DB, Ahmed N: Subclavian vein catheterization in the infant. J Pediatr Surg 9:171, 1974.

92. Eichelberger MR, Rous PG, Hoelzer DJ, et al: Percutaneous subclavian venous catheters in neonates and children. J Pediatr Surg 16:547, 1981.

93. Chung DH, Ziegler MM: Central venous catheter access. Nutrition 14:119, 1998.

94. Lally KP, Hardin WDJ, Boettcher M, et al: Broviac catheter insertion: Operating room or neonatal intensive care unit. J Pediatr Surg 22:823, 1987.

95. Warner BW, Ryckman FC: A simple technique to redirect malpositioned Silastic central venous catheters [see Comments]. JPEN J Parenter Enteral Nutr 16:473, 1992.

96. Dolcourt JL, Bose CL: Percutaneous insertion of silastic central venous catheters in newborn infants. Pediatrics 70:484, 1982.

97. Sanders RA, Sheldon GF: Septic complications of total parenteral nutrition. A five year experience. Am J Surg 132:214, 1976.

98. Taylor L, O'Neil J: Total parenteral nutrition in the pediatric patient. Curr Strat Surg Nutr 71:477, 1991.

99. Bozzetti F, Terno G, Bonfanti G, Gallus G: Blood culture as a guide for the diagnosis of central venous catheter sepsis. JPEN J Parenter Enteral Nutr 8:396, 1984.

100. Wesley JR: Efficacy and safety of total parenteral nutrition in pediatric patients. Mayo Clin Proc 67:671, 1992.

101. Schmidt-Sommerfeld E, Snyder G, Rossi TM, Lebenthal E: Catheter-related complications in 35 children and adolescents with gastrointestinal disease on home parenteral nutrition. JPEN J Parenter Enteral Nutr 14:148, 1990.

102. Briones ER, Iber FL: Liver and biliary tract changes and injury associated with total parenteral nutrition: Pathogenesis and prevention. J Am Coll Nutr 14:219, 1995.

103. Beale EF, Nelson RM, Bucciarelli RL, et al: Intrahepatic cholestasis associated with parenteral nutrition in premature infants. Pediatrics 64:342, 1979.

104. Quigley EM, Marsh MN, Shaffer JL, Markin RS: Hepatobiliary complications of total parenteral nutrition [see Comments]. Gastroenterology 104:286, 1993.

105. Novak DA, Balistreri WF: Management of the child with chronic cholestasis. Pediatr Ann 14:488, 1985.

106. Vileisis RA, Inwood RJ, Hunt CE: Prospective controlled study of parenteral nutrition–associated cholestatic jaundice: Effect of protein intake. J Pediatr 96:893, 1980.

107. Cooke RJ, Whitington PF, Kelts D: Effect of taurine supplementation on hepatic function during short-term parenteral nutrition in the premature infant. J Pediatr Gastroenterol Nutr 3:234, 1984.

108. Forchielli ML, Gura KM, Sandler R, Lo C: Aminosyn PF or TrophAmine: Which provides more protection from cholestasis associated with total parenteral nutrition? J Pediatr Gastroenterol Nutr 21:374, 1995.

109. Palmer RH, Ruban Z: Production of bile duct hyperplasia and gallstones by lithocholic acid. J Clin Invest. 45:1255, 1966.

110. Kubota A, Okada A, Imura K, et al: The effect of metronidazole on TPN-associated liver dysfunction in neonates. J Pediatr Surg 25:618, 1990.

111. Spurr SG, Grylack LJ, Mehta NR: Hyperalimentation-associated neonatal cholestasis: Effect of oral gentamicin. JPEN J Parenter Enteral Nutr 13:633, 1989.

112. Farrell MK, Balistreri WF: Parenteral nutrition and hepatobiliary dysfunction. Clin Perinatol 13:197, 1986.

113. Grant D, Wall W, Zhong R, et al: Experimental clinical intestinal transplantation: Initial experience of a Canadian centre. Transplant Proc 22:2497, 1990.

114. Williams JW, Sankary HN, Foster PF, et al: Splanchnic transplantation. An approach to the infant dependent on parenteral nutrition who develops irreversible liver disease JAMA 261:1458, 1989. (Published erratum appears in JAMA 262:210, 1989.)

115. Klein GL: Metabolic bone disease of total parenteral nutrition. Nutrition 14:149, 1998.

116. Collier S, Lo C: Advances in parenteral nutrition. Curr Opin Pediatr 8:476, 1996.

117. Howard L, Heaphey L, Fleming CR, et al: Four years of North American registry home parenteral nutrition outcome data and their implications for patient management. JPEN J Parenter Enteral Nutr 15:384, 1991.

118. McCarthy MC, Shives JK, Robison RJ, Broadie TA: Prospective evaluation of single and triple lumen catheters in total parenteral nutrition. JPEN J Parenter Enteral Nutr 11:259, 1987.

119. Moukarzel AA, Ament ME: Home parenteral nutrition in infants and children. In Rombeau J, Rolandelli R, (eds): Clinical Nutrition: Parenteral Nutrition. Philadelphia, WB Saunders, 1993, pp 791–813.

120. Winthrop AL, Wesson DE: Urokinase in the treatment of occluded central venous catheters in children. J Pediatr Surg 19:536, 1984.

121. Moukarzel AA, Haddad I, Ament ME, et al: 230 patient years of experience with home long-term

parenteral nutrition in childhood: Natural history and life of central venous catheters. J Pediatr Surg 29:1323, 1994.

122. Pitt HA, King W, Mann LL, et al: Increased risk of cholelithiasis with prolonged total parenteral nutrition. Am J Surg 145:106, 1983.

123. Ralston CW, O'Connor MJ, Ament M, et al: So-matic growth and developmental functioning in children receiving prolonged home total paren-teral nutrition. J Pediatr 105:842, 1984.

124. Guidelines for use of home total parenteral nutri-tion. A.S.P.E.N. Board of Directors. American So-ciety for Parenteral and Enteral Nutrition. JPEN J Parenter Enteral Nutr 11:342, 1987.

25

◆ Home Parenteral Nutrition: Clinical Outcome

Lyn Howard, M.B. (Oxon), F.R.C.P.
Margaret Malone, Ph.D., B.C.N.S.P., F.C.C.P.
Barbara Ehrenpreis
Allison Hilf

Home parenteral nutrition (HPN) was first attempted by Shils and colleagues in 1967,[1] and although this first patient survived only a few months, an important conceptual leap had been made. Now there are a growing number of patients who have survived over 20 years on this therapy.[2] It is an available life-support mechanism in most medically advanced countries. Initially, the use of HPN was confined to adults with severe short bowel syndrome due to relatively stable conditions such as Crohn's disease or mesenteric infarction.[3] In these individuals, HPN proved to be safe and associated with significant rehabilitation.[4–9] As experience with the therapy grew, so did the willingness to consider this option for patients with less stable, shorter-term conditions.[10] Currently in the United States and other medically advanced countries, HPN is recognized as a way to shift medical care to a less expensive setting. This implies a 180-degree turn from the early years when initiating HPN required special negotiation with a patient's third-party payer; in the present context, hospitals and insurance companies alike want to get *all* parenteral nutrition–dependent patients home whenever possible. Thus, it becomes the task of nutritional support professionals to help patients and families decide what they can manage at home and what they cannot. This requires familiarity with anticipated clinical outcomes and HPN-related psychosocial pressures.[11, 12] This chapter reviews the prevalence, cost, and clinical outcome on HPN therapy when used for different underlying diagnoses in both the United States and other medically advanced countries. It includes some discussion about the quality of life as assessed by professionals and from the viewpoint of a group of seasoned HPN patient-consumers. Finally, important unresolved issues are briefly presented.

◆ PREVALENCE OF HOME PARENTERAL NUTRITION

In the United States

Because there is no mandatory reporting of patients starting on HPN in the United States, there is no central source for measuring HPN prevalence in the general population. However, Medicare is the largest single payer for HPN therapy, and the Medicare yearly prevalence rate is known between 1989 and 1992.[11] During that 4-year period, HPN Medicare beneficiaries doubled from 4500 to 10,000, and the yearly prevalence rate increased from 136 to 288 per million Medicare population.

A second large database is the North American Home Parenteral and Enteral Nutrition (HPEN) Registry, which collected outcome information on over 12,000 HPN and home enteral nutrition patients from 217 nutrition support programs between 1985 and 1992. The HPN clinical outcome was assessed from the 5357 HPN patients who were reported to the registry during their first year on therapy.[13] Because the percentage of Medicare beneficiaries in the registry sample was consistently just over 25%, it is reasonable to assume that for every Medicare patient on HPN there were three non-Medicare patients in the general population. This translates to 18,000 HPN patients in 1989 increasing to 40,000 in 1992 in the general U.S. population and corresponds to a yearly prevalence rate of 70 per million general population in 1989, increasing to 150 per million in 1992.

In Other Medically Advanced Countries

In some European countries, for example Denmark and France, only nationally approved centers can initiate HPN and hence the total number of HPN patients is known. But in most European countries, the information is less complete. In seven European countries where it was estimated that 80% or more of the HPN activity was known, the prevalence on January 1, 1998, was 12.7 per million in Denmark, 3 to 4 per million in the United Kingdom, Netherlands, France, and Belgium, and less than 2 per million in Poland and Spain.[14] These European prevalence rates are much lower than the estimated prevalence in the United States. However, part of this is due to the difference between a yearly (United States) and 1-day (Europe) prevalence measurement. On both sides of the Atlantic, cancer patients are becoming high-volume users of HPN, and their average survival is 4 months. This means a 1-day point prevalence may capture only one out of three or four cancer patients per year. However, even if European prevalence rates are increased threefold or fourfold, their HPN utilization is still 5 to 10 times lower than utilization in the United States.[15] The reason for this discrepancy is not entirely clear, but it may reflect market forces in the U.S. health system, not present in countries with nationalized medical care (see the following discussion of cost).

◆ COST OF HOME PARENTERAL NUTRITION

In the United States

Again, in the area of cost, Medicare HPN payments are known, and they provide us with an estimate of the total dollars paid for this therapy in the United States.[11] In 1992, Medicare paid $156 million to support 10,000 Medicare beneficiaries on HPN. These dollars were 80% of the Medicare-allowable charge, the full amount being $195 million. Assuming HPN users in the general population consumed a similar amount of HPN, for a similar duration as Medicare patients, and assuming other third-party payers paid, on average, Medicare's allowable charge, then in 1992 the total national HPN dollars spent were $780 million.

It should be noted that this figure includes only the direct costs of providing the nutrient solution and infusion equipment. The costs of laboratory monitoring, outpatient follow-up visits to the physician, or the rehospitalization costs for a therapy-related complication are all reimbursed by other mechanisms and not factored into the direct cost of HPN.

In 1992, the Medicare mean allowable charge was $280/day[11] or approximately $100,000/yr. However, not all HPN patients received full nutritional support for 365 days a year. After a period of bowel adaptation, some patients can be sustained on just 3 to 4 days/wk of HPN; on other days they may infuse a simple hydration solution or be completely off therapy. In a retrospective chart review of one large program in 1996, the average cost for the intravenous solutions provided was $55,193/yr (range $9680 to $100,312). These costs were derived by adding each patient's monthly supplies, computing their cost from the Medicare-allowable charge, and then annualizing the data.[16]

Overall, it has been estimated that delivering parenteral nutritional support at home is less than half the cost of providing the same treatment in the hospital. But because the cost of the nutrient solution and infusion equipment is similar in the two settings, savings from home management chiefly reflect the fact that patients and families absorb most of the nursing costs. They also absorb transportation and lodging costs and lost income due to clinic visits. This patient and family contribution has never been financially evaluated.

From the viewpoint of the physician, the nutritional support team professionals, and their institutions, moving a complex patient from the hospital to the home also triggers many hidden costs. A study at the Cleveland Clinic analyzed these hidden costs and found they amounted to $2070 per HPN patient per year.[17] This included providing 24 hours of medical backup for these vulnerable patients, the time spent following up on laboratory values from tests obtained in the home setting, and the telephone calls to the patients, their home care suppliers, and home nursing services. These unreimbursed professional costs were initially one of a number of disincentives to transferring patients home. In the 1980s, infusion companies tried to remove this barrier by paying physicians management fees. These fees were later interpreted as financial "kickbacks" and deemed illegal.[18, 19] Certainly, these fees had a potential for encouraging an inexperienced physician to get involved in supervising an HPN patient and thereby blocking safer patient referrals. In 1996, Medicare moved to deal with the legitimate area of uncompensated professional time by introducing two reporting codes [99375 and 99376] allowing physicians to charge for documented care plan oversight services.*

Because the direct costs of HPN were generously reimbursed for many years, a large number of medical institutions opted to set up their own home infusion service. This led to an enormous proliferation of these services and concern about whether patients who were not contractually bound to a specific provider were being given freedom of choice. Since about 1994, managed care organizations have significantly ratcheted down the payment for HPN and other complex services and are increasingly requiring their selected contractor to provide all home services, from parenteral nutrition to respirators and other durable medical equipment, the so-called one-stop shop. This coalescing of services, often combined with shared financial risk, has eliminated many home care providers, both local and national.

What effect these organizational changes will have on the utilization of HPN in the United States remains to be seen.

In Other Medically Advanced Countries

In the United Kingdom, a cost analysis in 1995 found a direct cost for the first year on

---

*Care Plan Oversight Services: The work involved in providing very low intensity or infrequent supervision services is included in the pre and post encounter work for home, office/outpatient and nursing facility or domiciliary visit codes. Care plan oversight services provided which are less than 30 minutes during a 30-day period are considered part of patient evaluation and management and should not be reported separately.

99375 Physician supervision of patients under care of home health agencies, hospice or nursing facility patients (patient not present) requiring complex or multidisciplinary care modalities involving regular physician development and/or revision of care plans, review of subsequent reports of patient status, review of related laboratory and other studies, communication (including telephone calls) with other health care professionals involved in patient's care, integration of new information into the medical treatment plan and/or adjustments of medical therapy, within a 30 day period; 30–60 minutes.

99376 Over 60 minutes

Table 25–1. Underlying Diagnoses in Home Parenteral Nutrition Patients in the United States and Europe

	United States 1985–1992 (%)	Europe* 1993 (%)	Europe* 1997 (%)
Cancer	42	44	39
Crohn's disease	11	14	19
Ischemic bowel	6	13	15
Motility disorder	6	ND	ND
AIDS	5	4	2
Congenital bowel	4	ND	ND
Radiation enteritis	3	7	7
Other	23	18	18

*Children (>16 yr) not included in survey.
AIDS, acquired immunodeficiency syndrome; ND, no data provided.

HPN of $75,000 [44,288 pounds sterling].[20] This cost covered 3 weeks of in-hospital training, four outpatient-monitoring visits, infusion equipment, and nutrient solutions for six nights per week. This cost is comparable to that of 1 year on Medicare HPN for six nights per week [$87,000]. There is not much information available about the HPN cost in other European countries.

◆ DISEASE SPECTRUM OF PATIENTS RECEIVING HOME PARENTERAL NUTRITION

In the United States

In its early years, HPN was used almost exclusively for relatively stable patients with short bowel syndrome. In 1978, Shils reported the collective experience of 29 U.S. centers treating 168 HPN patients: 63% had Crohn's or ischemic bowel disease and only 17% had a resected malignancy.[3] As shown in Table 25–1, between 1985 and 1992, cancer had become by far the most common underlying diagnosis in HPN patients, followed by Crohn's disease, ischemic bowel, and motility disorders. Between 1985 and 1989, the growth in cancer patients accounted for over 90% of the HPN growth in U.S. programs (the percentage of reported patients with cancer in 37 large U.S. HPN programs in 1985 was 35%; in 1987, 43%; and in 1989, 46%).[10]

In Other Medically Advanced Countries

As shown in Table 25–1, two 1-year European surveys (1993 and 1997) of nine coun-

Table 25-2. Summary of Outcome of Home Parenteral and Enteral Nutrition

Diagnosis	No. of Patients	Age [yr (SD)]	Survival on Therapy [% (Observed Deaths/Expected Deaths)]*	Therapy Status at 1 Yr [% (SEM)]†			Rehabilitation Status in First Year [% (SEM)]‡			Complications§ (Per Patient Yr)	
				Full Oral Nutrition	Continued on HPEN Therapy	Died	Complete	Partial	Minimal	HPEN	Non-HPEN
Crohn's disease	562	36 (17)	96 (31/2.9)	70 (2)	25 (2)	2 (1)	60 (5)	38 (5)	2 (NA)	0.9	1.1
Ischemic bowel disease	331	49 (24)	87 (81/7.5)	27 (3)	48 (4)	19 (3)	53 (4)	41 (4)	6 (2)	1.4	1.1
Motility disorder	299	45 (22)	87 (81/3.1)	31 (3)	44 (4)	21 (3)	49 (4)	39 (4)	12 (3)	1.3	1.1
Congenital bowel defect	172	5 (14)	94 (20/1.6)	42 (6)	47 (6)	9 (3)	63 (6)	27 (5)	11 (4)	2.1	1.0
Hyperemesis gravidarum	112	28 (5)	100 (0/0.1)	100 (NA)	0 (NA)	0 (NA)	83 (4)	16 (4)	1 (NA)	1.5	3.5
Chronic pancreatitis	156	42 (17)	90 (9/0.6)	82 (3)	10 (3)	5 (2)	60 (5)	38 (5)	2 (NA)	1.2	2.5
Radiation enteritis	145	58 (15)	87 (47/3.2)	28 (5)	49 (5)	22 (4)	42 (6)	49 (6)	9 (3)	0.8	1.1
Chronic adhesive obstructions	120	53 (17)	83 (30/1.1)	47 (6)	34 (5)	13 (4)	23 (7)	68 (7)	10 (NA)	1.7	1.4
Cystic fibrosis	51	17 (10)	50 (254/0.05)	38 (7)	13 (5)	36 (7)	24 (6)	66 (7)	16 (5)	0.8	3.7
Cancer	2122	44 (24)	20 (1336/8.7)	26 (1)	8 (1)	63 (1)	29 (3)	57 (3)	14 (2)	1.1	3.3
AIDS	280	33 (12)	10 (182/0.8)	13 (3)	6 (2)	73 (4)	8 (NA)	63 (7)	29 (6)	1.6	3.3

*Survival rates on therapy are values at 1 year calculated by the life table method. This differs from the percentage listed as *died* under Therapy Status because all patients with known end-points are considered in this latter measure. The ratio of observed versus expected deaths is equivalent to a standard mortality ratio.
†Not shown are those patients who were readmitted to the hospital or who had changed the type of therapy by 12 months.
‡Rehabilitation is designated complete, partial, or minimal relative to the patient's ability to sustain normal age-related activity.
§Complications refer only to those complications that resulted in rehospitalization.
AIDS, acquired immunodeficiency syndrome; NA, not applicable because the group was too small; HPEN, home parenteral and enteral nutrition.
Data from the North American HPEN Patient Registry.[11]

tries show a diagnosis breakdown for HPN patients that is very similar to that in the United States.[14, 21] However, in Europe there are large intercountry differences in the use of HPN for cancer patients, from 60% of all patients in the Netherlands down to 5% in the United Kingdom. The more recent European survey shows a decrease in HPN use in acquired immunodeficiency syndrome (AIDS) patients, and this is thought to reflect the improved outcome for AIDS patients on newly released protease inhibitor drugs.

◆ CLINICAL OUTCOME ON HOME PARENTERAL NUTRITION

In the United States

The four outcome parameters measured by the North American HPEN Registry are described in detail elsewhere.[11] They include (1) the survival rate on HPN, (2) the therapy status after 1 year on treatment, (3) rehabilitation as assessed by the supervising professional, and (4) complications, HPN- and non-HPN–related, that required rehospitalization.

Table 25–2 summarizes the clinical outcomes for 11 diagnostic groups treated with HPN.[11] The number of patients within each group and their average age at HPN onset are given. Overall, there were approximately equal numbers of males and females; however, within particular groups this ratio was skewed, reflecting the gender distribution prevalent within certain disease categories. For example, there was a predominance of women (85%) with radiation enteritis, because of the use of radiotherapy for gynecologic malignancy. The majority of patients (90%) in the AIDS population were male.

Patients with relatively benign underlying diagnoses such as Crohn's disease, ischemic bowel disease, motility disorders, congenital bowel defects, hyperemesis gravidarum, and chronic pancreatitis all had good outcomes, with 87% or better one-year survival rates. In contrast, patients with cystic fibrosis or cancer had the poorest outcome in terms of survival. After 1 year, only 50% of cystic fibrosis and 20% of cancer patients were still alive on HPN. However, the outcome may not be as bleak as it appears to be, because 32% of cystic fibrosis and 25% of cancer patients came off HPN in the first

year and resumed oral nutrition. Although the registry patients with AIDS had a generally poor outcome, these data are from 1992 and predate the improved outlook for AIDS patients with new pharmacotherapeutic interventions, such as protease inhibitors.

The clinical outcome profiles presented in Table 25–2 and the survival curves shown in Figure 25–1 emphasize that the underlying diagnosis is the chief factor influencing the HPN outcome. However, even in disorders in which the overall prognosis is poor, there is a small percentage of patients who have a reasonable outcome. This means that the diagnosis alone cannot determine the appropriateness of initiating HPN, and a clinically predicted good quality of life at home for several months would seem to be the soundest justification.

The clinical outcome data show that HPN is relatively safe. Of those patients who died while receiving treatment, the HPN therapy

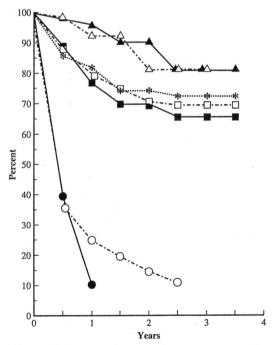

Figure 25–1. Survival curves of patients in seven disease categories who received home parenteral nutrition. Congenital bowel disorder (*open triangles*), n = 86; Crohn's disease (*solid triangles*), n = 388; ischemic bowel disease (*asterisks*), n = 179; motility disorders (*open squares*), n = 186; radiation enteritis (*solid squares*), n = 122; cancer (*open circles*), n = 1073; acquired immunodeficiency syndrome (*solid circles*), n = 91. (*Data from* North American Home Parenteral and Enteral Nutrition Patient Registry 1984–1988. Albany, NY, Oley Foundation.)

Table 25-3. Summary of Outcome of Home Parenteral and Enteral Nutrition by Age

Age Group	No. of Patients	Age [Yr (SD)]	Survival on Therapy [% (Observed Deaths/Expected Deaths)]*	Therapy Status at 1 Year [% (SEM)]†			Rehabilitation Status in First Year [% (SEM)]‡			Complications§ (Per Patient Yr)	
				Full Oral Nutrition	Continued on HPEN	Died	Complete	Partial	Minimal	HPEN	Non-HPEN
Pediatric	171	9 (7)	92 (7/0.5)	62 (4)	27 (4)	6 (2)	63 (6)	31 (6)	6 (NA)	1.8	1.1
Middle aged	370	45 (6)	90 (24/1.2)	48 (3)	42 (3)	8 (2)	62 (4)	34 (4)	3 (1)	0.9	0.9
Geriatric	204	72 (6)	67 (49/8)	34 (4)	31 (4)	29 (4)	38 (5)	47 (5)	15 (4)	0.9	0.7

Note: χ^2 analysis showed a statistically significant effect ($P < .01$) of age on the four measures of clinical outcome. The following were formed to identify differences more specifically: survival, pediatric = middle aged > geriatric; therapy status (resumption of full oral nutrition vs. continued on HPN or died), pediatric > middle age > geriatric; rehabilitation (complete vs. partial or minimal), pediatric = middle aged > geriatric; and complications due to HPN, pediatric > middle aged = geriatric.

*Survival rates on therapy are values at 1 year calculated by the life table method. This differs from the percentage listed as *died* under Therapy Status because all patients with known end-points are considered in this latter measure. The ratio of observed versus expected deaths is equivalent to a standard mortality ratio.

†Not shown are those patients who were readmitted to the hospital or who had changed the type of therapy by 12 months.

‡Rehabilitation is designated complete, partial, or minimal relative to the patient's ability to sustain normal age-related activity.

§Complications refer only to those complications that resulted in rehospitalization.

HPEN, home parenteral and enteral nutrition; HPN, home parenteral nutrition; NA, not applicable because the group was too small.

Data from the North American HPEN Patient Registry.[11]

was documented as the cause of death only 5% of the time. In fact, the likelihood of dying from an HPN complication depended on the primary diagnosis. In patients whose survival was measured in months, such as those with cancer, an HPN death was extremely rare (<2%); conversely, in those with long-term survival measured in years, such as Crohn's disease patients, 10% of deaths were related to HPN therapy.[10] In adults, an HPN complication leads to rehospitalization once a year; about half of these admissions were for confirmed or suspected sepsis.[11] To all physicians managing HPN patients, their low frequency of line sepsis is striking compared with the rates in traditional hospital-based patients. This lower sepsis rate could reflect the fact that home patients are out of the nosocomial environment; however, because the infecting organism in both settings is most often *Staphylococcus epidermidis*, a common skin commensal, the much lower infection rate in the home patient probably reflects better aseptic line care by the patient or close relative. Although a restored body composition and improved immunocompetence could also explain the lower frequency of infection, home-based cancer and AIDS patients, who are frequently immunosuppressed, also have a low incidence of line sepsis.

The impact of age on HPN outcome is an important issue because over the years there has been a widening of the age spectrum of persons starting this therapy. In 1978, 7.4% of patients were 10 years or younger and 5.9% were 65 years or older.[3] A decade later, 13.7% of patients were 10 years or younger and 19.4% were 65 years or older.[13] Because pediatric and geriatric patients are usually dependent on some adult relative or professional caregiver to administer their HPN infusion, this demographic change has far-reaching implications for family involvement and for community nursing. Table 25–3 describes the outcome in pediatric (age range zero to 18 years), middle-aged (age range 35 to 55 years), and geriatric (age range 65 years and older) patients receiving HPN for Crohn's disease, ischemic bowel, and motility disorders. These three diseases were chosen because they occur in all age groups and generally have long survival, making it possible to study the impact of age. The outcomes from these three diagnostic groups were pooled. As summarized in

Table 25–3, after 1 year on therapy, the survival, likelihood of resuming full oral nutrition, and rehabilitation all are better in children than these same parameters in adults. A therapy complication, however, was twice as frequent in children. The higher geriatric mortality is not explained by the higher expected mortality rate in an older subject. Expected mortality accounts for only a small fraction of the observed mortality even in the geriatric patients, which means that the need for HPN signals a significant degree of medical fragility.[22]

In Other Medically Advanced Countries

In the most recent European multicenter study,[14] mortality after 1 year on HPN was 4% in Crohn's disease, 13% in ischemic bowel, 21% in radiation enteritis, and 74% in cancer. These survival rates are very similar to those reported in the United States, as was the therapy status after 6 to 12 months on HPN.

In 1995 Elia reviewed HPN outcomes in the United Kingdom and Europe and noted reported HPN sepsis rates that varied from once every 11 months to once every 113 months.[15] In the North American Registry report, sepsis occurred once every 12 to 30 months depending on the diagnosis.[11] Messing reported 77 deaths in European HPN patients with nonmalignant chronic intestinal failure.[23] Ten percent of these deaths were due to an HPN complication, a frequency similar to that reported in Crohn's disease patients in the United States.[11]

Limited data on 231 Japanese HPN patients[24] and 14 Australian patients[25] showed outcomes similar to those of the United States and Europe.

◆ QUALITY OF LIFE ON HOME PARENTERAL NUTRITION

As Assessed by Health Care Professionals

In the majority of studies, the rehabilitation status has been assessed by the health professionals involved in the patients' care. There are just a few studies in which the patients' assessment or perspective on their quality of life has been formally evaluated.

In one such study, HPN patients and their caregivers were surveyed by a structured telephone interview and by mailed questionnaires.[26] These included the Quality of Life Index, a 70-item index that measures the person's perception of the importance of and satisfaction with health and function; socioeconomic status; and psychologic, spiritual, and family life. Also included were assessments of self-esteem, mental health, and life satisfaction; a measure that evaluated the caregiver's type of motivation to help the HPN patient; and a measure that assessed how the caregivers had adapted to caregiving, both positively and negatively. Last, a set of measures that assessed family relationships, coping, and adaptability were included. There were 116 respondents who had received HPN for a mean of 4.6 years. The majority of patients had Crohn's disease (n = 56), ischemic bowel, or radiation enteritis (n = 38). None of the patients had cancer or AIDS. Most caregivers spent around 4 hours a day (range 15 minutes to 24 hours) assisting the patient. Two thirds of patients reported a loss of friends, loss of employment, and depression. Both caregivers and patients reported problems with physical fatigue and depression. However, in spite of many difficulties, HPN was highly valued as life sustaining and of therapeutic benefit.

In a small study of 22 patients, the influence of HPN on lifestyle and general health status was assessed using the Medical Short Form-36, a general health status instrument.[16] All these patients had benign underlying diagnoses. In five of the eight domains of the short form, the health status of the HPN patients was significantly lower than that of age- and sex-matched persons in the general U.S. population. These perceived deficits were in the area of physical health, social functioning, vitality, and general health. Emotional status did not appear to be a significant area of impairment. The majority of patients did not perceive a worsening of their health when compared with the previous year, and in fact the majority felt their health had improved.

There are preliminary data from a study that compared two groups of short bowel HPN patients; 21 were affiliated with the Oley Foundation, a patient education and support network, and 22 were not associated with any support or educational group. The affiliated patients reported a better quality of life (P = .04), a lower mean depression score (P = .03), and fewer line infections. This emphasizes the importance of linking HPN patients with each other and to an educational support group.[27]

In a U.K. study, the quality of life was assessed in 51 HPN patients using two validated instruments, a general health status measure (Medical Short Form-36) and the EuroQol.[28] The health status profile was better in younger patients (<45 years) than in older patients. Patients who were addicted to narcotics had a poorer outcome based on these measures. These same authors conducted a cost-utility analysis of HPN using the EuroQol health status questionnaire to obtain a utility score and to calculate a "quality-adjusted life year (QALY)." The quality-adjusted life years gained were based on the assumption that life without HPN was not an option for patients with intestinal failure. The cost per quality-adjusted life year for an average patient was approximately $110,000. The provision of parenteral nutrition at home was estimated to be 65% more cost-effective than providing hospital-based care.

In 1997, the British Artificial Nutrition survey, sponsored by the British Association of Parenteral and Enteral Nutrition (BAPEN), described many aspects related to the quality of life in 95 HPN patients (16 to 75 years) with nonmalignant chronic intestinal failure. Although only 11% of these patients were employed, most were independent, self-caring, and able to undertake activities of daily living. Their quality of life improved significantly after HPN was initiated.[29]

The Patient-Consumer Perspective

The following points were made by a panel of seasoned HPN patients at a meeting in November 1998 organized by the Oley Foundation.* These points were intended to encourage a dialogue between clinicians and their HPN patients. It was felt that by describing some of the more common HPN experiences, the panel could help clinicians to better appreciate some of the psychoso-

---

*The Oley Foundation for Parenteral and Enteral Nutrition, a not-for-profit organization supporting patients and families who live on HPEN. Oley Foundation, Albany Medical Center, Albany, NY, 800-766-OLEY.

cial issues associated with HPN. In turn, the ability to recognize and manage these issues seems critical to ensuring patient compliance and maximizing rehabilitation.

The panel felt that the majority of long-term HPN users fall into two broad categories: those who were previously well and then experienced a catastrophic event that significantly affected their body's ability to absorb nutrients (e.g., mesenteric thrombosis or midgut volvulus) and those with chronic gastrointestinal medical conditions (e.g., Crohn's disease, intestinal pseudo-obstruction) who, because they have not adequately responded to less invasive therapies, are put on HPN as a "last-resort," lifesaving treatment. The differences between these two groups contribute in a major way toward a patient's *initial* acceptance of HPN. In the long run, however, acceptance and compliance appear unique not to the underlying disease or condition but to the individual.

Acceptance-Compliance

Many patients find it difficult to accept their dependence on HPN and all the restrictions that go along with it. This includes everything from scheduling work and activities around infusion times to the extra planning and precautions the patient needs to take before being able to enjoy activities such as swimming and traveling. As one patient describes it, "I find it difficult just to accept that something is wrong with me, let alone that I have to deal with the consequences of my illness. . . . maintaining my compliance is a daily battle. I infuse every day, but I'm very aware that I have to be compliant to do this." Viewed in this manner, acceptance is often an issue of control that needs to be addressed for the patient to successfully adjust to long-term use of HPN. This issue is compounded by the level of uncertainty most HPN patients face because of their medical condition; patients can't predict exacerbations of their disease, complications from their therapy, hospitalizations, absences from school or work, and so forth. Although the patients cannot "control" these events, they can control certain factors influencing them and hence minimize their occurrence and unpleasantness. It is not surprising, then, that compliance becomes less of an issue for patients if they are encouraged to exercise what control they realistically can have over their therapy. To do this, they need to become partners in the decision making. For example, whenever possible, patients should be given a choice of catheter device and infusion times. For this to work, the patients need to educate themselves about HPN and to develop a good working relationship with their physician. Being in touch with another HPN consumer to empathize and share experiences with can also make compliance easier.*

Sleeping Issues

One of the more difficult physical adjustments for HPN patients is how to regulate their sleep-wake cycle. Sleep deprivation, primarily from frequent nighttime bathroom visits, is an all-too-real occurrence that often exhausts not only the patient but also family members and caregivers. Some patients attempt to limit the disruption from frequent bathroom visits by keeping a portable commode next to the bed for easier night voiding.

Sleep can also be affected by the infusion process and equipment; some patients have trouble finding a comfortable sleeping position that minimizes the likelihood of tubing leaks and disconnections, or line occlusions and pump alarms. Although most of the newer, user-friendly infusion devices are relatively quiet, some noise is inevitable.

Additional sleep-related issues include morning fluid retention and nausea, particularly after nighttime lipid infusions. A few patients have coped with sleep-related disturbances by infusing some or all of their HPN during the day. One HPN patient who until recently infused only during the night describes her experience with daytime infusions: "The difference in how I feel is tremendous. I now sleep through the night, getting up only once or twice. . . . I have more energy and I no longer have those dark circles under my eyes." Besides being better rested, patients who infuse during the day feel they have more energy because HPN calories are immediately available to meet their energy requirements. They are also less likely to suffer from daytime dehydration and muscle cramps related to electrolyte shifts. Infusing during the day is a personal,

---

*1-800-776-OLEY; www:wizrat.net/oleyjdn; e-mail: bishopj@mail.amc.edu.

quality-of-life choice. Portable HPN pumps are readily available, yet many patients do not know that such an option exists. Barring any medical contraindications to daytime infusions, offering the patient the option of infusing at night or during the day has the additional benefit of permitting the patients to exercise some control over their condition.

Body Image

The central line catheter itself can be an issue for HPN patients, as it can be perceived as one more insult to a positive body image. This is especially true if the line was unexpected. The type and location of the catheter can make a difference in how the consumer accepts the catheter. An external catheter is a constant visual reminder of the patient's dependence on HPN and the underlying medical condition. It may restrict a patient's choice of clothing and complicate certain activities, such as showering, swimming, and participating in sports. An implanted port, on the other hand, is placed under the skin and is generally much less restrictive. (An implanted port is safer for showering and swimming only when the needle is out. A needle in the port is probably associated with the same risk of contamination as an externalized catheter.) With proper support, most patients' level of comfort with their body before HPN can carry forward into the HPN period.

Oral Nutritional Issues

Although a small percentage of HPN patients are unable to consume food orally, most HPN patients can eat, and this is usually encouraged by physicians, even when some dietary restrictions are necessary. Because our culture focuses many of its social gatherings around food, meals can be of great concern to patients who cannot eat or whose intake is limited. Not surprisingly, such patients find it difficult (at least initially) to enjoy a meal or a social occasion. Despite these barriers, many long-term patients find it is important for them and their families to maintain their participation in the "normal" family eating routine. Thus, many patients have a place set for themselves at the table and join the rest of the family for the social, if not nutritional, aspects of the meal. The patient's personal

level of comfort with modified eating often helps others to feel more comfortable about the patient's altered eating habits.

Parents and caregivers of children on HPN routinely express concern about their child's not wanting to eat. This often stems from the early period of life when a poorly working gastrointestinal tract frequently lead to vomiting. Several parents who have successfully cleared this hurdle preach patience, patience, and more patience. One intuitive parent states, "Training a child to eat falls under the category of art, not science. Some creativity must be in order to help the child to progress." Professional help is often needed for children who fail to develop eating skills.

Employment

Although some HPN patients can and do work, many others cannot. Paradoxically, HPN therapy often restores patients' health to a level at which they are physically able to work, at least part time, but they cannot return to work because they need "disability" insurance coverage to afford their HPN. Part-time work seldom offers insurance benefits. Additionally, the need for a generous insurance package to cover HPN may prohibit a patient from taking a full-time job or from being hired. For some patients, volunteer work is acceptable. For many, however, the question "What do you do?" is unsettling. Regardless of education, income, and social status, work itself has an intrinsic value that is difficult to relinquish. In the words of one patient, "I know I'm still the same professional, and volunteer work challenges my brain; yet, there is a part of me that feels inadequate in that I cannot continue to work on my terms. The innocent 'What do you do?' makes me teary-eyed." On a more positive note, several regulatory initiatives—such as the Health Insurance Portability and Accountability Act, the Work Initiative Incentive Act, and the broader interpretations of COBRA rights—are making health insurance more accessible and thus paid work a more viable option for HPN patients.

Friends and Family—When to Tell

Patients may find it difficult to discuss their condition with others because HPN is a relatively uncommon therapy, and because it includes bodily functions that most people consider private. For the single adult patient, discussing HPN may be particularly difficult with someone they may wish to date. Although how much they want to explain and when they feel comfortable discussing such matters depends primarily on the patient's personality, it also depends on the other person's curiosity and willingness to know. A common approach used by many patients is to give some form of a vague explanation, such as "My stomach cannot digest food" or "My intestines don't work." Such statements often spark the other person's curiosity, prompting questions, which then permit the patient to respond in a manner appropriate to the situation at hand. Some patients use this opportunity, through humor, to teach others about their unique way of eating. As one consumer likes to joke, "How many people do you know who can eat and have a root canal done at the same time?"

Sexual Relations

HPN therapy should not preclude a medically stable patient from having sexual relations, but it can be inhibiting both physically and psychologically. Because of the serious medical issues that are being addressed, this important topic is often innocently overlooked by the treating physician or it is left for discussion at "another time." Patients may be concerned about dislodging their catheter, conceiving while dependent on HPN, or engaging in intimate activities while they are "hooked up." Additionally, they may be uncomfortable with their body image or with discussing sexual issues with their partners. Support from a physician or other health care professionals (nurse, psychologist) can help patients become more comfortable with these issues. Because sexual relations can be a significant issue for the partner as well, couples should be encouraged to come together to an appointment to discuss their concerns.

Dependence on Home Parenteral Nutrition

HPN is not a disease; it is an "enabling" therapy that is the result of a traumatic accident or a symptom of chronic illness. For those patients who will never be able to sustain themselves without HPN, there are a multitude of never-ending stressful issues related to their dependency, from securing adequate insurance coverage for the therapy to retaining access sites to avoiding long-term complications such as bone and liver disease. As one patient vividly describes it: "HPN has been a double-edged sword. On the one hand, it has been nothing short of miraculous; I went from practically living in the hospital to really living. On the other hand, I can't help but worry about what will happen if I run out of access sites, or if my liver malfunctions, or if my insurance runs out." The fear of stopping HPN, whether out of necessity or by choice, is very real. Patients whose dependence on TPN is more borderline often have the same worries and additionally may need to overcome a "psychologic addiction" to HPN. Typically, patients with such addictions have experienced significant improvements in their quality of life since beginning HPN and think that without HPN their underlying condition will worsen and they will again become malnourished. Obviously, each case is unique, and getting over this addiction depends not only on the patient's past and present state of health but also on the quality of the doctor-patient relationship. Several patients also stress the importance of timing, stating that physicians often suggest stopping HPN when patients feel they need it most, for example, when they've been in the hospital for treatment of sepsis.

Finding Help

Although HPN patients who have chronic medical conditions are apt to adjust to life with HPN more easily than those who were previously well and experience a catastrophic event, most people on HPN experience what one patient describes as "an emotional roller coaster." For many, the "ups" and "downs" are most pronounced after hospitalization. In the words of one person, "Each time I return home from the hospital, no matter how happy and relieved I am to be free again, to be declared well, I re-experience my great vulnerability and I become depressed. I then get angry at myself for being depressed. While I understand my feelings, I can't escape them." Anger, fear, depression, and the whole gambit of emotions are common, but they need not be overwhelming. To deal with these emotions and the host of psychosocial issues causing them, many HPN patients seek professional help or reach out to others on HPN. Dealing with these issues and finding workable strategies not only improve patients' quality of life but can also improve their health by ensuring better compliance with the therapy. Physicians managing HPN patients should be able to recommend counseling resources in their community. In addition, the Oley Foundation for Home Parenteral and Enteral Nutrition can provide information and psychosocial support for HPN patients through a host of networking and information services.

◆ UNANSWERED QUESTIONS

Short-Term Use of Home Parenteral Nutrition

Short-term use of HPN relates to the terminal bowel-obstructed patient (expected survival <3 months), on the one hand, and the patient requiring preoperative buildup, on the other.

The appropriateness of HPN in a terminal patient is not clear. This clinical issue most often arises in cancer patients, and these patients are the largest diagnostic group of HPN users on both sides of the Atlantic. Two points can be made in this context: first, cancer cachexia is not readily redressed by parenteral nutrition,[30] and second, terminal patients rarely experience hunger. A study shows that providing artificial nutrition, or tray food for that matter, beyond that specifically requested by the patient does not contribute to a terminal patient's comfort.[31] Studies are needed to determine if simple hydration, rather than HPN, best meets the needs of the terminal bowel-obstructed patient. Although most physicians are comfortable providing just hydration to the terminal patient, the clinical quandary is always how to recognize when the terminal phase has been reached.

The appropriateness of HPN buildup for depleted patients going through major elective surgery is also not clear. Most of the time, the enteral approach can be used. There is one prospective randomized study of malnourished preoperative head and neck cancer patients showing a reduction in postoperative complications and the length of hospital stay after several weeks of preoperative home enteral nutrition.[32] Patients

with chronic pancreatitis and pseudocysts are often sent home on HPN while their cyst matures, in preparation for a drainage procedure; however, there are no randomized studies showing that this approach is safe and cost-effective.

Use of Home Parenteral Nutrition in Patients Without Primary Gastrointestinal Disease

The appropriateness of HPN in patients who have no major gastrointestinal disease but who suffer from severe nutritional depletion because of an inadequate oral intake is another unresolved issue. This can occur because of psychological or cognitive disorders such as anorexia nervosa or dementia. It can occur with metabolic disorders such as chronic renal and hepatic failure, which induce profound anorexia. It can occur if patients have to choose between eating and breathing as in severe pulmonary or cardiac dyspnea. In all these clinical situations, randomized prospective controlled trials are needed to determine if nutritional support in the nonhospital setting achieves nutritional repletion, and if it does, whether the nutritional repletion improves the quality of life and the overall cost efficiency of care. In disorders in which gastrointestinal dysfunction is not the primary disorder, home enteral nutrition, rather than HPN, is likely to be more appropriate.[11] The North American HPEN Registry information suggests that these types of patients account for about 20% of HPN currently being prescribed.[13]

Role of Small Bowel Transplantation

Small bowel transplantation was first attempted in dogs by Alexis Carrel in 1902. In the 1960s, the success of human kidney and liver transplantations led to a small bowel transplant in seven patients. All these early patients died within a few months, and it became clear that transplanting bowel presented a special challenge because of its large component of immunocytes and the consequent need for high-dose chronic immunosuppression. The immunosuppression led to serious post-transplant infections, particularly with cytomegalovirus and Epstein-Barr virus, the latter often leading to a B cell lymphoma.

In the late 1990s, several changes have improved bowel transplantation outcomes. These changes include the use of cytomegalovirus-negative donors for cytomegalovirus-negative recipients; constant monitoring for Epstein-Barr virus using the polymerase chain reaction and antiviral treatment if the test becomes positive; and exclusion of the colon from the intestinal allograft. These changes have led to an overall cumulative patient survival of 72% at 1 year and 48% at 5 years.[33] The outcome is better in children (aged 2 to 17 years) compared with adults. Although both isolated intestinal and multivisceral grafts have similar patient survival rates, graft survival is lower with the isolated intestine.

Although these improvements in intestinal transplantation are encouraging, they still do not compare well with the survival of patients with benign causes of short bowel syndrome managed on HPN. For this reason, the prevailing opinion is that transplantation should be reserved for HPN patients who run out of venous access or who develop severe parenteral nutrition–related liver disease.

Role of Certain Parenteral Nutrients

There is considerable uncertainty about the requirements in long-term HPN patients for certain nutrients that in healthy persons the body can synthesize. These nutrients, which may be essential for patients fed artificially, have been called *conditionally* essential nutrients and include many products of hepatic trans-sulfuration, such as lecithin, glutathione, choline, carnitine, and taurine.[34–38] Hepatic trans-sulfuration, is impaired in parenteral nutrition patients in part because precursor nutrients such as methionine are infused into the systemic circulation and not by the physiologic route, the portal vein. This systemic delivery leads to significant transamination of methionine to mercaptans in peripheral tissues. As a consequence, there is depletion of trans-sulfuration products, and this in turn may lead to the development of hepatic cholestasis, steatosis, and eventually cirrhosis and portal hypertension. Studies have described reversal of HPN cholestasis with ursodeoxycholate administration.[39] It is also widely recognized that both HPN cholestasis and gallbladder sludge are reduced by encouraging enteral feeding.

Concern has also been raised about contamination of certain additives with potentially toxic substances, for example aluminum, which may contribute to HPN bone disease,[40] and manganese, which may be another factor in hepatic dysfunction, especially in children.[41]

There have been deaths in parenteral nutrition patients caused by calcium and phosphate intravascular precipitation.[42–44] Studies have shown this is a risk if the pH of the base amino acid solution is high, if calcium and phosphate are added before the admixture is fully diluted, and if agitation during compounding is not constant. Unfortunately, intermittent agitation is a feature of most automated compounding equipment.[43]

Implications of Needleless Intravenous Access Devices

Needleless intravenous access devices have reduced needle-stick injuries in professional and family caregivers. They also limit the circulation of needles to people with the potential for drug abuse. However, a needleless system depends on valves, and it has been shown in vitro[45] that these are sites for bacterial adherence. Several programs have reported a significant increase in catheter-related bloodstream infections in HPN patients using needleless devices.[46–48]

Management of Thrombotic Events

It is not yet clear whether anticoagulation using low-dose warfarin or heparin reduces the incidence of catheter-related thrombotic events.[49–51]

There is evidence in oncology patients with an indwelling catheter that a urokinase flush is superior to a heparin lock. The urokinase significantly reduces both catheter thrombosis and catheter-related bloodstream infections.[52] This may relate to the removal of the platelet fibrin layer that builds up on the internal surface of catheters, creating a site for bacterial adhesion.

SUMMARY

These are just a few of the unanswered questions pertinent to patients on long-term parenteral nutrition. This therapy has opened a window on many fundamental biologic processes, most recently the role of tuftsin in splenic function.[53] Because no single nutritional support program follows enough HPN patients to address many of these research questions, future multicenter cooperation will be important.

REFERENCES

1. Shils ME, Wright WL, Turnbull A, et al: Long term parenteral nutrition through external anteriovenous shunt. N Engl J Med 283:341–344, 1970.
2. Oley Foundation celebrates 20 years on TPN [Editorial]. *In* Lifeline Letter May–June. Albany, NY, Oley Foundation, 1995, p 1.
3. Shils ME: Home TPN Registry annual reports. New York, New York Academy of Medicine, 1978 to 1983.
4. Broviac JN, Scribner BH: Prolonged parenteral nutrition in the home. Surg Gynecol Obstet 139:24–28, 1974.
5. Fleming CR, McGill DB, Berkner S: Home parenteral nutrition as primary therapy in patients with extensive Crohn's disease of the bowel and malnutrition. Gastroenterology 73:1077–1081, 1977.
6. Heizer WD, Orringer EP: Parenteral nutrition at home for 5 years via arteriovenous fistulae. Gastroenterology 72:527–532, 1977.
7. Jeejeebhoy KN, Zohrab WJ, Langer B, et al: Total parenteral nutrition at home for 23 months, without complication and with good rehabilitation. Gastroenterology 65:811–820, 1973.
8. Jeejeeboy KN, Langer B, Tsallas G, et al: Total parenteral nutrition at home: Studies in patients surviving 4 months to 5 years. Gastroenterology 71:943–953, 1976.
9. Steiger E, Srp F: Morbidity and mortality related to home parenteral nutrition in patients with gut failure. Am J Surg 145:102–105, 1983.
10. Howard L: Home parenteral and enteral nutrition in cancer patients. Cancer 72:3531–3541, 1993.
11. Howard L, Ament M, Fleming CR, et al: Current use and clinical outcome of home parenteral and enteral nutrition therapies in the United States. Gastroenterology 109:355–365, 1995.
12. Howard L, Hassan N: Home parenteral nutrition—25 years later. Gastroenterol Clin North Am 27:481–512, 1998.
13. North American Home Parenteral and Enteral Nutrition Patient Registry: Annual reports. Albany, NY, Oley Foundation, 1986–1994.
14. Van Gossum A, Bakker H, Bozzetti F, et al: Home parenteral nutrition in adults: A European multicentre survey in Europe in 1997. ESPEN–Home Artificial Nutrition Working Group. Clin Nutr, in press.
15. Elia M: An international perspective on artificial nutrition support in the community. Lancet 345:1345–1349, 1995.
16. Reddy P, Malone M: Cost and outcome analysis of home parenteral and enteral nutrition. JPEN J Parenter Enteral Nutr 22:302–310, 1998.
17. Curtas S, Hariri R, Steiger E: Case management in home total parenteral nutrition: A cost identifica-
tion analysis. JPEN J Parenter Enteral Nutr 20:113–119, 1998.
18. Kusserow KP: Fraud Alert, Joint Venture Arrangement. OIG-89-04 (US GRP: 0-235-622). Baltimore, Office of Inspector General, 1989.
19. Burrows WP, Fernandez H: Patient Referrals. Health law update. Washington, DC, Bond, Schoeneck and King, 1992.
20. Richards DM, Irving MH: Cost utility analysis of home parenteral nutrition. Br J Surg 83:1226–1229, 1996.
21. Van Gossum A, Bakker H, De Francesco, et al: Home parenteral nutrition in adults: A multicentre survey in Europe in 1993. ESPEN–Home Artificial Nutrition Working Group. Clin Nutr 15:53–59, 1996.
22. Howard L, Malone M: The usage and clinical outcome of elderly patients in the US receiving home parenteral and enteral nutrition. Am J Clin Nutr 66:1364–1370, 1997.
23. Messing B, Lamann M, Landais P, et al: Prognosis of patients with nonmalignant chronic intestinal failure receiving long term home parenteral nutrition. Gastroenterology 108:1005–1010, 1995.
24. Takagi Y, Okada A, Sato T, et al: Report on the first annual survey of home parenteral nutrition in Japan. Surg Today 25:193–201, 1995.
25. Jones L, Ramsey Stewart G, Storey D: Home parenteral nutrition: The Royal Prince Alfred Hospital Experience. Aust J Adv Nurs 12(4):22–25, 1995.
26. Smith CE: Quality of life in long term total parenteral nutrition patients and their family caregivers. JPEN J Parenter Enteral Nutr 17:501–506, 1993.
27. Smith CE: Clinical outcomes of patients helping patients. Abstract presented at Midwest Research Society, 1996.
28. Richards DM, Irving MH: Assessing the quality of life of patients with intestinal failure on home parenteral nutrition. Gut 40:218–222, 1997.
29. Elia M, Micklewright A, Shaffer J, et al: The 1997 Annual Report of the British Artificial Nutrition Survey (BANS). Cambridge, England, 1998.
30. American College of Physicians: Position paper: Parenteral nutrition in patients receiving cancer chemotherapy: A meta-analysis. Ann Intern Med 110:734, 1989.
31. McCann RM, Hall WJ, Groth-Juncker A: Comfort for terminally ill patients. JAMA 272:1263–1266, 1994.
32. Flynn MB, Leighty FF: Preoperative outpatient nutritional support of patients with squamous cancer of the upper aero-digestive tract. Am J Surg 154:359–362, 1987.
33. Abu-Elmagd KM, Reyes J, Fung JJ, et al: Evolution of clinical intestinal transplantation: Improved outcome and cost effectiveness. Transplant Proc 31:1–3, 1999.
34. Buchman AL, Dubin M, Dendren D, et al: Lecithin increases plasma free choline and decreases hepatic steatosis in long-term total parenteral nutrition patients. Gastroenterology 102:1363–1370, 1992.
35. Sokol RJ, Taylor SF, Devereaux MW, et al: Hepatic oxidant injury and glutathione depletion during total parenteral nutrition in weanling rats. Am J Physiol 270:g691–g700, 1996.
36. Buchman AL, Dubin MD, Moukarzel AA, et al: Choline deficiency: A cause of hepatic steatosis during parenteral nutrition that can be reversed with intravenous choline supplementation. Hepatology 22:1399–1403, 1995.

37. Berner YN, Lachian WA, Lowry SF, et al: Low plasma carnitine in patients on prolonged total parenteral nutrition: Association with low plasma lysine. JPEN J Parenter Enteral Nutr 14:255–258, 1990.

38. Guertin F, Roy CC, Lepage G, et al: Effect of taurine on total parenteral nutrition–associated cholestasis. JPEN J Parenter Enteral Nutr 15:247–251, 1991.

39. Spagnuolo MI, Iorio R, Vegnente A, et al: Ursodeoxycholic acid for treatment of cholestasis in children on long-term parenteral nutrition: A pilot study. Gastroenterology 111:716–719, 1996.

40. Lidor C, Schwartz I, Freund U, et al: Successful high-dose calcium treatment of aluminum-induced metabolic bone disease in long-term home parenteral nutrition. JPEN J Parenter Enteral Nutr 15:202–206, 1991.

41. Fell JME, Reynolds AP, Meadows N, et al: Manganese toxicity in children receiving long-term parenteral nutrition. Lancet 347:1218–1221, 1996.

42. Knowles JB, Cussion G, Smith M, Sitrin MD: Pulmonary deposition of calcium phosphate crystals as a complication of home total parenteral nutrition. JPEN J Parenter Enteral Nutr 13:209–213, 1989.

43. Hill SE, Heldman LS, Goo EDH: Fatal microvascular pulmonary emboli from precipitation of a total nutrient admixture solution. JPEN J Parenter Enteral Nutr 20:81–89, 1996.

44. FDA Safety Alert: Hazards of precipitation associated with parenteral nutrition. Washington, DC, Department of Health and Human Services, April 18, 1994.

45. Maki DG, Stolz S, McCormick R, Spiegel C: Possible association of a commercial needleless system with central venous catheter–related bacteremia [Abstract]. 34th International Conference on Antimicrobial Agents and Chemotherapy, 1997.

46. Danzig LE, Short LJ, Collins K, et al: Bloodstream infections associated with a needleless intravenous infusion system in patients receiving home infusion therapy. JAMA 272:1862–1864, 1995.

47. Kellerman S, Shay DK, Howard J, et al: Blood stream infections in home infusion patients: The influence of race and needless intravascular access devices. J Pediatr 129:711–717, 1996.

48. Do A, Ray B, Banerjee SN, Illian AF, et al: Bloodsteam infection associated with needleless device use and the importance of infection-control practices in the home health care setting. J Infect Dis 179:422–448, 1999.

49. Monturo CA, Dickerson RN, Mullen JL: Efficacy of thrombolytic therapy for occlusion of long term catheters. JPEN J Parenter Enteral Nutr 14:312–314, 1990.

50. Mailloux RJ, Delegge MH, Kirby DF: Pulmonary embolism as a complication of long term total parenteral nutrition. JPEN J Parenter Enteral Nutr 17:578–582, 1993.

51. Bern MM, Lokich JJ, Wallach SR, et al: Very low doses of warfarin can prevent thrombosis in central venous catheters. JPEN J Parenter Enteral Nutr 10:49–57, 1986.

52. Fraschini G, Jadeja J, Lawson M, et al: Local infusion of urokinase for the lysis of thrombosis associated with permanent central venous catheters in cancer patients. J Clin Oncol 5:672–678, 1987.

53. Zoki G, Corazza GR, Wood S, et al: Impaired splenic function and tuftsin deficiency in patients with intestinal failure or long term intravenous nutrition. Gut 43:759–762, 1998.

26

◆ Home Parenteral Nutrition: Finances

Carolyn D. Viall, R.N., M.S.N.

The challenges of providing nutritional support services in the home setting are not limited to the physiologic, educational, and environmental criteria that need to be met. The financial reimbursement for providing parenteral nutrition (PN) outside the acute care setting has seen dramatic changes since the mid-1990s. No longer is the identification of a disease process that would benefit from treatment with PN a sufficient justification for the extended use of PN. Payers, in particular the federal government, have developed more criteria for PN in the outpatient setting and have also adjusted their payment rates for the provision of this therapy. These changes have been due to several factors in the home care industry during the 1990s. The charges associated with the provision of home PN have been large, and the industry has been questioned about the reasonableness of these charges. Another reason, partially owing to the high cost of the therapy, is the appropriateness of certain patient populations' receiving PN for an extended period because of their disease. The payers are seeking more evidence on which to base the long-term administration of PN to patients in the outpatient setting, which places the burden of proof on the provider to meet a new set of criteria before discharging the patient from the acute care setting.

The need to carefully evaluate a patient for home parenteral nutrition (HPN) has placed inpatient providers in the position of collaborating with outpatient suppliers to maximize the resources and reimbursement for both the supplier and the patient. There is increasing emphasis on accountability, requiring the provider of health care services to provide information and data that justify the use of PN in the outpatient setting, and the supplier is also accountable for ongoing communication with the provider and the payer regarding the patient's continued need for PN. The business practices of both providers and suppliers are under scrutiny, necessitating their compliance with federal regulations in the administration of the Medicare program.

This chapter provides an overview of the issues related to the financial reimbursement for PN in the outpatient setting. It reviews information, current at the time of this writing on the criteria and payment methods for PN under the Medicare program. The coverage criteria for state and commercial payers are also discussed. Nutritional support practitioners must understand the ramifications of these changes in reimbursement for providers, suppliers, and patients so that the best plans of care can be established for their patients.

◆ MEDICARE

The largest payer of health care services in the United States is the federal government for the Medicare program. Administered by the Health Care Financing Administration (HCFA), the Medicare program has covered HPN since 1981 for specific patient diagnoses and pathologic conditions. Under the Medicare program, the hospitalized patient requiring PN does not fall under the same coverage criteria as HPN patients, and reimbursement for in-hospital services is obtained through the hospital billing of Medicare for the patients demonstrating medical necessity. In 1983, the Medicare program reimbursement for hospitalized patients was revised to a payment system dependent on specified payment rates based on the patient's primary diagnosis, known as the diagnosis-related group (DRG) system. This payment system has predetermined rates for specified primary diagnoses, essentially placing the hospital provider in a modified capitated system.

Payment for services provided to Medicare beneficiaries is made under two parts of the Medicare system, part A and part B. Part A encompasses payments made to hospitals for services provided to patients, based on the DRG system, and covers medication costs and some equipment costs for the therapies. The amount of payment a hospital receives is predetermined by the DRG system, with some additional reimbursement possible on identification of comorbidity diagnoses that may have caused an increased length of stay and complications in the course of treatment.[1] The implementation of the DRG system has placed the hospital provider of services at risk and encourages the provider to use health care resources wisely when providing services to the Medicare beneficiary.

Patients with length of stay that is longer than that usually found in that DRG class or patients with costs that also exceed the average costs associated with a particular DRG class are called *outliers*. If a hospital finds that a patient is an outlier because of the previously stated reasons, the hospital can receive additional payments for the hospital stay, dependent on the decision after a review by a peer review organization. The identification of comorbidities or complications can increase a hospital's reimbursement for a DRG class because of their association with longer hospital lengths of stay. A comorbidity must be identified as being present on admission, whereas a complication is generally considered as occurring during the hospitalization. Protein-calorie malnutrition and kwashiorkor are two examples of nutritional comorbidities that may be relevant to the patient requiring HPN and are usually assessed early in the patient's admission and course of treatment.

Medicare part B covers the nonhospital costs of supplies and services that a patient may receive. This includes physician services, durable medical equipment, and supplies. In 1981, HCFA chose to cover parenteral and enteral nutrition (PEN) services. These services were outlined in the *Coverage Issues Appendix* and can still be found in the since-renamed *Coverage Issues Manual*, which communicates the current conditions of coverage for the Medicare program. The coverage for PEN services was placed under the prosthetic device benefit, which uses the rationale that PEN is needed to replace a malfunctioning or absent body part that would normally allow food to pass through and be absorbed in the digestive tract.

The claims for Medicare beneficiaries are processed by the durable medical equipment regional carriers (DMERCs). There are

Table 26–1. Durable Medical Equipment Regional Carriers

DMERC	States in Region
Region A: MetraHealth (Travelers)	Connecticut, Delaware, Maine, Massachusetts, New Hampshire, New Jersey, New York, Pennsylvania, Rhode Island, and Vermont
Region B: AdminaStar Federal Inc.	District of Columbia, Illinois, Indiana, Maryland, Michigan, Minnesota, Ohio, Virginia, West Virginia, and Wisconsin
Region C: Palmetto Government Benefits Administrators	Alabama, Arkansas, Colorado, Florida, Georgia, Kentucky, Louisiana, Mississippi, New Mexico, North Carolina, Oklahoma, Puerto Rico, South Carolina, Tennessee, Texas, and the Virgin Islands
Region D: CIGNA	Alaska, Arizona, California, Guam, Hawaii, Idaho, Iowa, Kansas, Missouri, Montana, Nebraska, Nevada, North Dakota, Oregon, South Dakota, Utah, Washington, and Wyoming

DMERC, durable medical equipment regional carrier.

four DMERCs designated by HCFA, and part of their responsibility is to issue medical policy and clarify or expand on the detail of the Medicare Coverage Policy. The medical policy regarding PN can be found in the DMERC's most recent issue of Regional Medical Review Policy, which updates previously published policy or provides information related to new policies.[2] The current DMERCs are listed in Table 26–1.

Medicare's *Coverage Issues Manual, 65-10* defines the most current criteria for coverage for PN. The manual addresses what is covered in equipment, nutrients, and supplies. It is specifically directed toward the supplier of the equipment, nutrients, and supplies and does not include any provision for the services of the health care professionals involved in the planning, administration, or monitoring of the PN plan of care through the supplier.

Medicare Parenteral Nutrition Coverage

The formal requirement for coverage of PN in the outpatient setting is that the patient have a permanently nonfunctional internal body organ or a permanent impairment of the alimentary tract that does not allow the absorption of sufficient nutrients to maintain weight and strength commensurate with the patient's general condition. The test of permanence is that the condition be of a long and indefinite duration, which is considered to be at least 90 days. The physician must document in the medical record the evidence that supports the clinical diagnosis and document that the condition meets the test of permanence. If the condition is considered a temporary impairment, coverage will be denied by Medicare.

The *Coverage Issues Manual* describes two criteria for the coverage of outpatient PN. Effective July 1, 1996, the Regional Medical Review Policy was revised, and patients requiring HPN must now meet more stringent criteria than previously established. Under the Medicare program, a patient with either (1) a condition involving the small intestine that significantly impairs the absorption of nutrients or (2) a disease of the stomach and/or intestine that is a motility disorder and impairs the ability of nutrients to be transported through the gastrointestinal tract would be considered eligible. Not only does the health care provider need to document the medical necessity for PN, but there must be objective evidence of the need for PN to treat the pathologic condition and that other means of nutritional support are not viable options for the patient to maintain his or her health. The outcomes that need to be demonstrated for HPN are the failure of the patient to maintain adequate strength and weight when maintained on either an oral or an enteral diet or a combination of both. The documentation in the medical record must include the physical signs, symptoms, and specific test results indicating a severe abnormality of the gastrointestinal tract.

The Regional Medical Review Policy also addresses the medical treatment approaches that are expected to be tried on patients to prove their inability to maintain their nutritional status without PN. The patients' health status must require intravenous nutrition that was not possible using either a modification of the nutrient composition of their enteral diet (e.g., lactose-free; gluten-free; modification of long-chain triglycerides or substitution of medium-chain triglycerides; the provision of protein as either peptides or amino acids) or pharmacologic means (e.g., pancreatic enzymes, prokinetic medications for motility disorders, antibiot-

ics for bacterial overgrowth). The revised policy further defines unresponsiveness to prokinetic medication as the presence of daily symptoms of nausea and vomiting while taking maximal doses.

The policy defines PN as covered in any of the following situations:

A. The patient has undergone recent (within the last 3 months) massive small bowel resection leaving 5 ft or less of small bowel beyond the ligament of Treitz.

B. The patient has a short bowel syndrome that is severe enough that the patient has net gastrointestinal fluid and electrolyte malabsorption such that on an oral intake of 2.5 to 3 L/day the enteral losses exceed 50% of the oral and/or enteral intake and the urine output is less than 1 L/day.

C. The patient requires bowel rest for at least 3 months and is receiving intravenously 20 to 35 kcal/kg/day for the treatment of symptomatic pancreatitis with or without pancreatic pseudocyst, severe exacerbation of regional enteritis, or a proximal enterocutaneous fistula in which tube feeding distal to the fistula is not possible.

D. The patient has complete mechanical small bowel obstruction in which surgery is not an option.

E. The patient is significantly malnourished (10% weight loss over 3 months or less and serum albumin levels of 3.4 g/dl or less) and has very severe fat malabsorption (fecal fat exceeds 50% of the oral and/or enteral intake on a diet of at least 50 g of fat per day as measured by a standard 72-hour fecal fat test).

F. The patient is significantly malnourished (10% weight loss over 3 months or less and a serum albumin level of 3.4 g/dl or less) and has a severe motility disturbance of the small intestine and/or stomach that is unresponsive to prokinetic medication as demonstrated either (1) scintigraphically (a solid meal gastric emptying study demonstrates that the isotope fails to reach the right colon by 6 hours after ingestion), or (2) radiographically (barium or radiopaque pellets fail to reach the right colon by 6 hours after administration). These studies must be performed when the patient is not acutely ill and is not on any medication that would decrease bowel motility.

As seen in these criteria, the policy is clear and specific about the conditions that must be met to allow reimbursement for HPN. Not only has the policy been clarified as to the types of pathologic conditions that are covered, but it has also specified the types of tests and measures that must be performed to either prove or disprove a patient's ability to be maintained on alternative methods of nutritional support other than PN. These conditions, according to the policy, must be severe enough that the patient would not be able to maintain weight or strength on an oral diet or enteral tube feeding. The policy does contain language regarding those patients requiring long-term PN who may not meet the specific criteria listed but do meet the previous criteria regarding modification of diet and pharmacologic intervention as long as they also meet one of the following criteria:

G. The patient is malnourished (10% weight loss over 3 months or less and a serum albumin level of 3.4 gm/dl or less).
H. A disease and clinical condition has been documented as being present, and it has not responded to altering the manner of delivery of appropriate nutrients (e.g., slow infusion of nutrients through a tube with the tip located in the stomach or jejunum).

These examples of what the policy refers to as *moderate abnormalities* require a failed trial of enteral tube feeding before PN is covered. Once again, the policy is very explicit in its definition of a tube trial and criteria that would indicate a failed tube trial. The procedure for a tube trial is listed in Box 26–1.

◆ **Box 26–1**
Enteral Tube Feeding Trial Definition

- Concerted effort must be made to place enteral feeding tube
- For gastroparesis, tube placement must be postpyloric, preferably in jejunum
- Placement of tube must be verified objectively by fluoroscopy or radiographic studies
- Placement by endoscopy or surgery may be used

◆ **Box 26–1**
Enteral Tube Feeding Trial Definition
(Continued)

- Use of double lumen should be considered
- Enteral nutrition must be administered with appropriate dilution of enteral formula, rate of administration, and use of alternative enteral formulas to prevent or address side effects of diarrhea

---

Examples of a failed tube trial according to the Regional Medical Review Policy are listed in Box 26–2.

◆ **Box 26–2**
Examples of Failed Enteral Tube Feeding Trial

- Patient vomits after tube is placed postpylorically, and radiographic recheck shows tube tip to have returned to stomach.
- Tip of tube is in jejunum, enteral feeding is administered for 1–2 days, and patient experiences vomiting and abdominal distention.
- Tube is placed appropriately postpylorically and remains in place. Enteral nutrition is administered with rate and concentration of formula gradually increased. After course of 3–4 wk, attempts to increase rate and/or concentration or to alter formula result in patients being unable to reach target nutritional intake; patient also experiences increased diarrhea and abdominal distention and is unable to meet weight goals (maintenance or weight gain).
- After attempt to place the tube postpylorically (5–6 h), tip remains in stomach or duodenum. Attempt to slowly infuse appropriate enteral formula is made, but vomiting results when rate is increased.

The Regional Medical Review Policy has described examples of situations in which PN will not be covered. Awareness of these examples is essential for the nutritional support practitioner because many of these examples are clearly patient situations that were covered by Medicare in prior years. These examples, as defined by the policy, are listed in Box 26–3.

◆ **Box 26–3**
Conditions for Noncoverage for Home Parenteral Nutrition under Medicare Program

Parenteral nutrition is not covered for patients with a functioning gastrointestinal tract and the following conditions:
- Swallowing disorder
- Psychological disorder impairing food intake (e.g., depression)
- Temporary defect in gastric emptying (e.g., metabolic or electrolyte disorder)
- Metabolic disorder inducing anorexia (e.g., cancer)
- Physical disorder impairing food intake (e.g., dyspnea of severe pulmonary disease or cardiac disease)
- Side effect of medication
- Renal failure or dialysis

The use of PN in patients concurrently receiving intradialytic parenteral nutrition (IDPN) has been controversial since the mid-1990s.[3] The policy, effective July 1, 1996, has also clarified those situations in which IDPN would be covered by Medicare. The criteria for coverage for IDPN do not differ from the criteria for coverage for PN from any other patient situation, as stated in current policy. The patient must have a permanently impaired gastrointestinal tract with insufficient absorption of nutrients to maintain adequate weight and strength. Documentation in the medical record needs to include evidence that the patient cannot be maintained on an oral diet or enteral tube feedings and that the patient must receive PN due to severe abnormality of the gastrointestinal tract. The PN must not be considered supplemental to a deficient diet or deficiencies caused by dialysis. IDPN patients must also meet the criteria listed previously regarding diet modifications and pharmacologic means to attempt to maintain the pa-

tient's nutritional status before the use of HPN.

It is possible to have a patient who is on partial oral and/or enteral nutrition and PN in the home setting and is still considered eligible by Medicare. To be eligible, the patient must meet the following criteria, which refer to criteria A through H listed previously:

(1a) A permanent condition of the gastrointestinal tract is present that has been deemed to require parenteral therapy because of its severity (criteria A through F); or

(1b) A permanent condition of the gastrointestinal tract is present that is unresponsive to standard medical management (criterion H); and

(2) The person is unable to maintain weight and strength (criterion G).

Medicare Certification and Claims

The initial certification for home PN must be specific regarding the patient's abnormality and signs and symptoms, and the results of attempts at other methods of nutritional support. The patient must have a recertification for continued HPN 6 months after the initial certification. Each of the coverage criteria has specific documentation that must accompany the recertification citing the justification for continued PN. The documentation for the criteria is listed in Table 26–2. The ordering physician is expected to see the patient within 30 days before the initial certification and required recertifications. If the physician does not see the patient within this time frame, there must be documentation in the medical record of why the patient was not seen, and the physician must describe the methods that were used to evaluate the patient's status and PN needs. After the recertification at 6 months, further recertifications are not needed but may be requested at the discretion of the DMERC. A revised certification is needed when either nutrients with a different code are ordered or the number of days per week that the PN is administered is decreased. A revised certification does not change the date for the required recertification.

The 6-month recertification must include the physician's documentation of the continued need for PN. For some of the criteria, the statement should also include the pa-

Table 26–2. Coverage Criteria for Recertification of Home Parenteral Nutrition

Medicare Coverage Criteria	Documentation to Be Provided
Criterion A or B (short bowel syndrome)	Documentation that adequate small bowel adaptation has not occurred that would permit enteral or oral feedings
Criterion C (requires bowel rest; pancreatitis; regional enteritis; proximal enterocutaneous fistula)	Documentation of worsening of underlying condition during attempts to resume oral feeding
Criterion D (complete mechanical small bowel obstruction)	Documentation of persistence of condition
Criteria E–H (significant malnutrition; severe fat malabsorption; motility disorders; lack of response to prokinetic medications or modification of oral or enteral diet)	Documentation that improvement of physical condition has not occurred; coverage continues if PN therapy has demonstrated improvement in patient's status by improvement in weight and/or serum albumin level

tient's most recent serum albumin level (within 2 weeks of recertification) and the most recent weight with the date of each. If the patient demonstrates malnutrition based on the results of the weight and serum albumin level, the physician's statement should include the justification for continued PN in addition to any changes in the therapeutic regimen to address the ongoing malnutrition.

Once the coverage criteria are met, Medicare will cover the nutrients, supplies for the administration of PN, and equipment. The policy defines the nutrients, equipment, and supplies that are covered. The total daily caloric intake, including parenteral, enteral, and oral intake, is expected to range from 20 to 35 kcal/kg/day to achieve or maintain an appropriate body weight. Any caloric intake outside this range requires documentation of the medical necessity by the physician, and the documentation must be made available to the DMERC on their request. The protein intake may range from 0.8 to 1.5 g/kg/day, and orders outside this range must be medically necessary and documented in the medical record. The use of dextrose concentrations less than 10% or lipid use greater than 15 units of 20% solution or 30 units of a 10% solution per month must be medically necessary and also documented in the medical record by the ordering physician. Special parenteral formulas, according to policy, are rarely medically necessary. If the need for the special formulas is not substantiated in the medical record, reimbursement will be given only for the medically appropriate formula.

Documentation

The certificate of medical necessity (CMN) must be included in the initial certification for PN. Additional documentation demonstrating the need for PN must also be included with the first claim. The information requested for the initial certification according to the coverage criteria is listed in Table 26–3. The supplier must keep a copy of the CMN on file. The CMN may be completed by someone other than the ordering physician, but it may not be the supplier. The ordering physician is responsible for reviewing the completed CMN and signing and dating it before submission.

Because of the more subjective nature of coverage criteria E through H, a nutritional assessment by a physician, dietitian, or qualified professional is necessary within 1 week before the initiation of PN. The nutritional assessment must include the following information:

1. The current weight with the date, and the weight 1 to 3 months before the initiation of PN
2. The estimated daily calorie intake during the prior month and by what route (i.e., tube or oral)
3. A statement of whether there were caloric losses from vomiting or diarrhea and whether these estimated losses are reflected in the calorie count
4. A description of any dietary modifications made or supplements tried during the prior month (i.e., low fat, increased medium-chain triglycerides)

One stationary intravenous pump is covered for patients in whom PN is also covered. Additional intravenous pumps will be denied as medically unnecessary. There is a differentiation in the payment for pumps used in the home setting and those used in

Table 26–3. Documentation for Initial Certification for Home Parenteral Nutrition

Medicare Criteria for Home PN	Additional Documentation for Initial Certification
Criteria A–D (short bowel syndrome, bowel rest, complete mechanical small bowel obstruction)	Copies of operative report and/or hospital discharge summary and/or x-ray reports and/or physician letter that documents condition and need for therapy
Criteria E and H (if applicable)	Dates and results of fecal fat test
Criteria F and H (if applicable)	Copy of report of small bowel motility study
	List of medications patient received at time of test
Criteria E through H	Dates and results of serum albumin tests (within 1 wk prior to initiation of PN)
	Copy of nutritional assessment within 1 wk before initiation of PN
Criterion H	Statement from physician
	Copies of objective studies
	Excerpts of medical record including following:
	Specific cause of gastroparesis, small bowel dysmotility, or malabsorption
	Detailed description of enteral tube trial
	Copy of x-ray report or procedure report documenting placement of tube in jejunum
	Prokinetic medications used, dosage, and dates of use
	Nondietary treatment given during prior month directed at cause of malabsorption
	Any medications that might impair GI tolerance to enteral feedings or that might interfere with test results and statement explaining need for these medications

GI, gastrointestinal; PN, parenteral nutrition.

an outpatient facility. The pump and pole in an outpatient facility are not to be denied in an individual claim because they can be used for multiple patients in that setting, so they would not be considered rental items. One supply kit and one administration kit are covered for each day that PN is administered if they are considered medically necessary for the patient and if they are, in fact, used by the patient. Only 1 month's supply of PN, equipment, and supplies is allowed for 1 month's prospective billing. If the supplier is submitting claims retroactively, the supplier can include multiple months.

Claims for PN are submitted to one of the designated DMERCs listed in Table 26–1. The DMERCs process Medicare claims submitted by the provider based on the geographic residence of the Medicare beneficiary. In addition to handling claims for PEN, the DMERCs also process claims submitted for durable medical equipment, orthoses, prostheses, and other medical supplies.

The claims process requires the provider to complete form HCFA-1500 for PEN. The form uses a coding system developed by HCFA, referred to as the common procedure coding system (HCPCS) and has standard procedural codes for processing Medicare claims. The three levels of codes in the HCPCS system use procedural codes, item and service codes, and local codes. Level I is a five-digit numeric code that uses the Current Procedural Terminology (CPT) coding system and does not include the supplies and materials and some services normally associated with PN therapy. Level II uses a letter followed by four numbers that are designated nationally for items and services, including those associated with PN therapy. Level III codes are for items used in local situations and have two letters followed by three numbers. Both enteral and parenteral therapies are classified in codes B4000 through B9999.

The actual reimbursement for PN is currently based on reasonable charges. Medicare part B payments currently reimburse at the lesser of the prevailing charge, the customary charge, the actual charge, and the lowest charge level (since 1986). The prevailing charge is generally set at the 75th percentile of the range of the customary charges in an area for a particular service or item, whereas the customary charge is considered that of the particular supplier for the specific service or item. PEN is currently the only item set at the lowest charge level method of reimbursement. This level is set at the 25th percentile of all charges submitted for an item or service during the quarter for which data are analyzed. After the reasonable charge levels are determined by the DMERCs, charges submitted by the suppliers of PEN services may not exceed the lowest charge levels that are widely accepted unless a specific exception is made.

The charge levels are recalculated every year, but the payment increases may not exceed the inflation increase percentage determined by the consumer price index for urban customers. Also, Congress has frozen payments for PEN supplies, equipment, and nutrients and other therapies several times since the mid-1990s. The Balanced Budget Act of 1997 (BBA) resulted in a plan to reduce $116 billion from the Medicare budget over the 5-year period beginning in 1998 through 2002. In effect, reimbursement levels for PEN therapies are frozen at the same reimbursement levels as seen in 1995.

The BBA has had far-reaching ramifications for all sectors of the health care industry, including PEN services. HCFA has the authority, through Congress and the BBA, to develop a fee schedule for any item or service provided to a covered individual in the Medicare program. HCFA is currently working on a fee schedule for PEN services that may be issued in 1999.

Congress also gave HCFA the authority to revise the reimbursement system to one using "inherent reasonableness," which would allow the DMERCs to decrease reimbursement up to 15% annually for any non-physician item or service that is covered under part B of the Medicare program.[4] This method would give HCFA the ability to modify any payment level that was identified as either grossly excessive or deficient. In the past, HCFA would have had this authority only after a full regulatory process and comment period; however, Section 4316 of the BBA gave HCFA the ability to adjust payment rates of 15% or less without the full regulatory process. HCFA now has the authority to develop payment rates for part B services of the Medicare program on an annual basis. It is anticipated that this method will be applied by HCFA and the DMERCs for PEN services in the very near future.[5]

The BBA has also had some other implications for the patient receiving HPN services that must be taken into consideration by the hospital and acute care practitioners and the home care supplier. The BBA has set forth guidelines that limit the Medicare beneficiary's liability for paying for items that are not covered by Medicare, which places the provider of these services at increased risk of reduced payment. Under the Medicare program, the provider of those services must give the covered individual an advance beneficiary notice to notify the covered individual of the likelihood that Medicare will deny payment for a particular claim for a specific reason.[6] Diagnostic laboratories have been particularly affected by this ruling because there have been a number of blood tests and panels of tests that are no longer considered acceptable practice. Specific blood and other diagnostic tests are now designated as appropriate for specific ICD-9 codes according to the patient's diagnosis.

Also, the selection of home health providers must be demonstrated to be a fair choice on the part of the patient and the provider. As of November 3, 1997, all hospitals are required to provide patients with a list of the Medicare-certified home health agencies that serve the patient's geographic area.[7] Patients must be given a choice of the agency that would provide their home health services after discharge from the hospital. Failure to provide this choice to Medicare patients will subject the hospital to severe fines and penalties.

The Medicare program is planning to enroll members in its second generation of a Medicare managed care program.[8] Named Medicare + Choice, the program will offer what are seemingly irresistible options for Medicare beneficiaries. There will be no deductibles, no balance billing, and no claims submission for the enrollee. There will also be no premiums for most plans, and the benefits will equal current parts A, B, and supplemental coverage levels. This program is anticipating widespread appeal with this offering. The financial aspects of managed care programs and its ramifications to home PN are discussed later in this chapter.

Physician Reimbursement for Home Parenteral Nutrition

Under the Medicare program, there are three areas in which the physician may be reimbursed for management of the patient on HPN: case management, coding for services provided in the home, and care plan oversight.[9] The reimbursement for any of these services is not liberal and is fairly burdensome with paperwork, to the extent that many physicians report that it is not worth the effort. Physicians managing HPN patients can be reimbursed for their time in coordinating care and monitoring the patients' response to the PN therapy. The physicians must submit claims to Medicare for services for home patients using specific codes identified in the *Physicians' Current Procedural Terminology CPT '98*, published by the American Medical Association.

Medicare considers physician case management to be a process whereby a physician is responsible for coordinating the care of a patient, which includes the identification and initiation of services by other health care service providers. Case management also includes controlling access to health care services. There are two levels of case management: conferences with health care professionals or family members regarding a specific patient and telephone calls, which may vary in length and complexity, for the medical management of a patient. The definitions of case management services are listed in Table 26–4.

Services provided by a physician in a patient's home may be reimbursed by Medicare. The level of service (minimal, brief, limited, intermediate, and extended) is defined in the *Current Procedural Terminology*

Table 26–4. Physician Case Management Coding

Level of Service	Case Management Activities
Simple or brief	Clarify or alter previous instructions Report on tests and laboratory results Adjust therapy Incorporate new information from other health care disciplines into treatment plan
Intermediate	Initiate therapy by phone Discuss laboratory tests in detail Advise established patient on new problem Coordinate medical management of new problem of established patient Initiate new plan of care
Complex or lengthy	Detailed discussion with family of seriously ill patient Lengthy counseling session with distraught patient Detailed and lengthy communication with several health professionals involved in care plan of patient

Table 26–5. Physician Current Procedural Terminology Coding for Services Provided in the Patient's Home

Patient Status	Level of Service	CPT Code
New patient, initial visit	Problem focus	99341
New patient, initial visit	Expanded focus	99342
New patient, initial visit	Detailed home care	99343
Established patient	Problem focus	99351
Established patient	Expanded focus	99352
Established patient	Detailed focus	99353

Problem focus: service confined to examination of a single organ system. Includes documentation of complaint, present illness, examination, review of medical data, plan of treatment.

Expanded focus: examination and evaluation of an organ system, partial review of medical history, recommendations for care, and generation of a report.

Detailed focus: Evaluation of problems, but does not need a comprehensive evaluation of the patient. Documentation of history of the chief complaint, past medical history, relevant physical examinations, development of a plan for investigating the complaint or therapeutic regimen to treat the complaint and generation of a report.

CPT, current procedural terminology.

From *Physicians Current Procedural Terminology CPT '98.* Chicago, American Medical Association.

manual, and the code that is selected should take the level into consideration. Some extremely debilitated or severely ill HPN patients may require a home visit by the physician. This does not apply to a majority of the HPN population. The six categories that apply to home care are listed in Table 26–5.

Care plan oversight has been defined by HCFA as reimbursement to a physician for oversight services that require 30 or more minutes of physician time per month. Only one physician per patient may be compensated for care plan oversight, even if there are multiple physicians caring for a particular Medicare beneficiary. Care plan oversight is intended for patients with complex medical problems receiving home health or hospice services who require a physician to spend time coordinating complex and/or multidisciplinary care. The codes and guidelines for their use are listed in Table 26–6.

◆ MEDICAID

Medicaid programs are administered and funded jointly by the states and the federal government. There is tremendous variability between states on how their programs are

Table 26-6. Coding for Physician Care Plan Oversight

Care Plan Oversight Codes	Services for Coding
99375	Care plan oversight services 30–60 min
99376	Care plan oversight services greater than 60 min (not reimbursed by Medicare)
Services to be provided	Development of care plan by physician
	Review of laboratory reports, other studies, and subsequent reports of patient's status and response to therapy
	Communications with other health care professionals involved in patient's care
	Adjustment of treatment plan

administered. This is because the federal government establishes certain minimal standards that must be met by the states for covered services that must be provided and groups of individuals that must be covered. Beyond meeting those minimal requirements, the state is free to structure its program as it wishes. A state may even seek waivers from the federal government to give the state more latitude in how it structures its program, including covered services and payment methods. These variances can be readily observed when assessing the PEN services and coverage offered by several states.

PEN services are generally covered under the pharmacy benefit of the Medicaid programs for many states. Some states use a pharmacy formulary system for PEN therapies, requiring the prescribing physician to use the formulary, in particular for enteral nutrition formulas. Prior authorization for HPN may be required, depending on the state's regulations, and many states have adopted coverage eligibility criteria similar to Medicare's for HPN.

Reimbursement for HPN under the Medicaid program also varies widely. A state program may use a method covering nutrients on an average wholesale price basis, plus a small percentage (usually 5 to 10%), and possibly a small dispensing fee (ranging from $3 to $4). Supplies and equipment may be paid according to a fee schedule or on a per-diem basis. It is of paramount importance that the nutritional support clinician understand the coverage criteria of the resi-

dential state of the covered individual to maximize the patient's benefits.

◆ DEPARTMENT OF VETERANS AFFAIRS

The Department of Veterans Affairs (VA) is a system based primarily on hospitals and acute care settings as opposed to an ambulatory practice setting. The VA system provides services to eligible veterans of military service through their medical centers, domiciliaries, outpatient services, community services, outreach clinics, and nursing homes. The services are provided more as a closed panel capitated system in which the VA facilities receive a fixed payment for each patient that they serve. The system provides no reimbursement for outpatient PN unless the veteran has supplemental health care coverage that would cover HPN.

◆ THIRD-PARTY PAYERS

Third-party payers, or what some may refer to as *commercial insurance services*, provide health care benefits for a large number of Americans. The traditional fee-for-service health plans that were prevalent for many years are rapidly being replaced by managed care plans. Many payers now offer several product lines to their customers to meet the customers' needs; the plans range in flexibility and cost in proportion to the freedom of choice of health care providers that the plans provide. The options of health plans differ due to costs (deductibles, out-of-pocket limits, co-pays) or vary as widely as the health care benefits that each plan offers. For a patient requiring HPN, the nutrition support clinician may find it a challenge to ascertain the patient's health care benefit coverage and the suppliers who may provide these services both safely and cost-effectively.

Definitions

To better understand the coverage of most health plans, it is useful to discern the meanings of some of the terms that the payers use to describe the various parties involved in health care services. The beneficiary of a health plan is also referred to as the *enrollee* or *subscriber*. The *payer* is the health plan, which may be traditional insurance company, or some type of managed care organization. The term *provider* covers a broad range of health care personnel and facilities. Providers encompass any party that may bill for services rendered and include physicians, hospitals, home health nursing agencies, durable medical equipment suppliers, pharmacies, diagnostic centers, laboratories, hospices, and skilled nursing facilities. The preferred providers of a managed care organization are those who have negotiated a contract for the pricing of services to members of the managed care organization.[10]

Product Lines

Payers have diversified their health plan offerings to their customers to attempt to reduce costs for both the customer and the health plan. Many managed care organizations offer more than one product line to appeal to the customers' needs. Generally, providing less choice of providers is believed to control costs. In the evolution of health care plans, the public has seen a number of hybrid plans develop that are trying to incorporate the advantages of one type of managed care plan and still give the patient-subscriber some options for choice in the selection of health care providers. Although this chapter does not cover all types of health plans that exist today, it provides an overview of the basic types of plans available and some of the spinoffs that have resulted.

Fee-for-Service Plans

Long considered the basic health plan for many Americans, fee-for-service health plans, also known as *indemnity insurance*, are quickly being replaced with managed care plans across the country. The Blue Cross and Blue Shield Association predicted that by 2000, 80% of their members would be in a managed care plan instead of a fee-for-service plan. A fee-for-service plan establishes a fee schedule that is considered the usual, customary, and reasonable fee for services, referred to as the UCR, based on charges of providers for similar services in a locale. The subscriber to the health plan is then responsible for the payment of any

charges higher than the determined UCR. Before the UCR is paid by the payer, the subscriber is responsible for a deductible amount that is also predetermined by the payer. These deductible amounts are contracted or established when the subscriber first enrolls in the health plan, and in many cases, the enrollee has more than health plan deductible options to choose. A larger deductible amount in the plan results in a lower premium for the subscriber. Most fee-for-service plans also have an "out-of-pocket" limit for the subscriber, which does not include UCR excess, and a limit for payer coverage less than 100%. This is an amount that limits the cash expenditures of subscribers for their health care under the coverage limitations of the health plan. The health plan reimburses partial to full coverage of charges, subject to UCR limits and the patient's out-of-pocket limits.

A fee-for-service plan does not have limitations on the choice of health care providers. The subscriber may choose to receive services from any provider, within the limitations of the descriptions of the types of health providers stated in the health plan, with reimbursement levels for charges as stated within the contract. This allows tremendous freedom of choice for the subscriber and does not limit the ongoing use of services in either frequency or duration. With no limitations on the use of services, it has long been held that this freedom has caused an overuse of services on the part of the subscriber and the health care provider. With the total national costs of health care expenditures steadily increasing, many health plans responded by developing managed care plans to limit the use of health care services and the resultant costs.

Managed Fee-for-Service Plans

An early attempt by the payers to control the costs of health care was to place some mechanisms in place to either prospectively or concurrently address the use of services. In a managed fee-for-service health plan, the subscribers continued to have the ability to choose their provider of health care services as they did in the traditional indemnity plan. The use of precertification for hospitalizations or for expensive procedures (e.g., magnetic resonance imaging studies) was one of the methods used by the payers. The rationale behind this strategy was to have a proactive approach to reviewing the need for these services before they occurred and to possibly deny those services that were deemed unnecessary, or to suggest alternative services.

Second opinions, particularly for certain surgical procedures, was another strategy used in managed fee-for-service plans. When a patient was recommended for certain surgical procedures, for example, cardiac bypass grafting, the health plan might have required a second opinion from another physician before the procedure was performed. Utilization review was another technique used by payers to concurrently review the use of services, in particular, hospitalizations. In utilization review, the hospital and the payers reviewed a patient's current status during the hospitalization and projected the continued need for these services. This may have enhanced communication with the payers, and there were certainly concerns by the health care provider, in particular, the hospital about further reimbursement from the payer beyond certain time periods during a hospitalization. Whether the precertification, second-opinion, or utilization review methods were effective in reducing services is not known, but one would surmise they were insufficient because of the next stage of managing health care that evolved.

Preferred Provider Organizations

In an effort to put more controls on the options of providers used by the subscriber, many health plans developed preferred provider organizations (PPO), which grew steadily in the 1980s and early 1990s. The PPO was developed as a network of health care providers, both inpatient and outpatient services, that agree to accept for their services prenegotiated rates that are usually a percentage of their usual fees or a per-diem rate. The PPO organization contracts with a large number of providers in a locale, also including specialists, and markets its provider networks to purchasers of health care plans, which is generally employers.

The subscriber to a PPO is encouraged to use the health care providers within the network to maximize the discounts that have been negotiated. The use of specialists is permitted, and the subscribers can select their specialty care from those listed in the provider directory. Other providers, for ex-

ample, home health nursing agencies, home infusion suppliers, pharmacies, durable medical equipment providers, and laboratory and diagnostic services, are also negotiated and listed in the provider directory. If the subscriber uses an out-of-network provider, the subscriber is then held responsible for the increased costs associated with using a noncontracted provider. There continues to be some reimbursement for the services of an out-of-network provider, but at a substantially reduced rate. Obviously, this practice is to encourage subscribers to stay within the network developed at contracted rates and control costs, while still offering some choices.

PPOs continue to be a popular product line for payers and subscribers. They continue to offer the consumer a wide array of choices in providers, including specialists, yet offer the payer some control of the expenditures. The premiums for these plans are generally less than those of the fee-for-service plans, therefore offering another cost saving to the employer or purchaser of the plan.

The advantages of the PPOs have resulted in health care providers' themselves getting involved in the financial side of health care reimbursement. Many physician groups have developed their own organizations, some using the term *physician services organization,* to negotiate their rates for services directly with the payers and hospitals. Another version of this type of organization is the *physician hospital organization,* which has developed in areas of the country where competition for the health care dollar is fierce. With mergers and integrated health care systems developing rapidly in some areas of the country, some health care providers and hospitals feel the pressure to remain competitive and cost-effective and have reacted by developing their own plans and networks. In some instances, some of these plans have actually become the payers.

Health Maintenance Organizations

Although believed by many to be a recent addition to the health care plan playing field, the health maintenance organization (HMO) has been in existence since the 1940s in the United States. Kaiser Foundation Health Plan has long been recognized as a leader in the HMO area and was in existence long before many of the organizations that are around today. The growth of HMOs has been steadily increasing since 1980, when the U.S. HMO enrollment was 9.1 million. In 1997, according to *The Interstudy Competitive Edge HMO Industry Report,* the total HMO enrollment in the United States was over 70.6 million.[11] This figure excludes all specialty HMOs, for example, vision and dental plans.

Several models of HMOs exist today. The staff model HMO, of which Kaiser Foundation Health Plan is best known, hires its own physicians and manages its own facilities, that is, hospitals, clinics, and ancillary services. Even these staff model plans have altered their methods of operating over the years and developed more of a network model, contracting some of their services with other providers, including using other hospital facilities rather than their own buildings. The most popular form of HMOs today is the independent practice association, which contracts with primary care physicians in independent practices. These physicians, many times in group practices, agree to accept the HMO's contracted reimbursement rates for services rendered to their patients. A primary care physician can be a member of several PPOs and HMOs at the same time, causing quite a challenge to the physician and staff to track the specific rules of participation for each payer.

To control costs, HMOs use several strategies that focus on reducing the use of health care services by their members. The first strategy is for each enrollee to receive the bulk of the health care through a primary care physician. Any service from a specialist is authorized only after a referral is made by the primary care physician for a particular subscriber. Specialists are those who also are approved or preferred providers through the HMO. The use of any specialists outside of HMO network may cause coverage to be denied unless prior authorization has been given by the HMO.

HMOs negotiate pricing contracts with their providers through a number of strategies. They may negotiate percentage discounts from the usual charges, much as a PPO may do. Many HMOs negotiate per-diem rates for services, particularly for hospitalizations. This has the consequence of placing the provider at increased risk in the reimbursement. Obviously, if a particular patient's use of health care services and length of hospitalization exceed the per-

diem reimbursement that the facility will receive, then the hospital will lose money caring for this patient. This is similar to the effect that DRGs have had on hospitals since their enactment.

The use of capitated payments is another method for reimbursement used by HMOs for many of their services in various parts of the country. A capitated payment is a per-member-per-month rate paid to the HMO's preferred providers for services they render to the HMO's members. This also places the provider at extreme financial risk. If there are a large number of members in the HMO and low utilization of health care services, the provider may fare well financially. However, if the HMO members use a large number of health care services, or very costly services, then the provider may operate at a financial loss. Utilization of services is to be controlled by the primary care physician, and some HMOs have incentive plans to reward physicians in the low use of health care services. This has been a controversial practice because of the concern that patients are being withheld necessary health care services to maintain HMO profit margins.

Variations of HMO plans that are more appealing to the consumer have been developed. Point-of-service plans allow some use of predetermined specialists by the subscriber without the prior authorization of the primary care physician. This returns some of the autonomy to consumers in selecting their health care providers, and several plans have been developed along these lines that have greater appeal to those who would traditionally have objected to enrolling in an HMO.

Probably the most significant feature of HMO plans to control costs and actively monitor services is case management. Although other types of health care plans have adopted case management to facilitate care and control costs, HMOs have long been known to use this method as part of their system. Case managers, usually registered nurses, are responsible for assessing a patient's health care service needs primarily during a hospitalization and planning the most appropriate and cost-effective means to meet those needs with the providers. Other health care disciplines are entering case management roles, for example, social workers and dietitians. Some diagnoses prompt immediate involvement of the case manager, for example, solid organ and bone marrow transplantations or diagnosis of human immunodeficiency virus infection or acquired immunodeficiency syndrome, because of the anticipation of high health care expenditures to treat the disease.

The case manager's role is to identify the short- and long-term health care service needs and collaborate with the physician providers to develop a plan to meet the current needs of the patient, in addition to developing a plan to reduce future hospital admissions, reduce or prevent complications, and identify other providers to be involved in the patient's care. The case manager may mandate the use of contracted preferred providers for health care services, and the health care team must be aware of the capabilities and services of these providers as they plan the patient's ongoing care.

◆ DISCHARGE PLANNING FOR HOME PARENTERAL NUTRITION

Gone are the days when the nutrition support practitioner in the acute care setting could plan for a patient to be discharged on HPN without worrying about reimbursement for HPN by health care insurers. Although reimbursement had been an issue for nutrition support practitioners since the time that the first patient was discharged on HPN, the need to be aware of each patient's financial reimbursement coverage, or lack thereof, is an essential part of the discharge-planning process. The practitioner must also rely on accurate information from others to guide decisions on the treatment plan and must routinely justify the use of an expensive therapy. Nutritional support practitioners have been accustomed to being the decision makers about a specialized and complex therapy being administered in the home setting, and demonstrating its need to others has not been part of their routine. Managed care organizations have illustrated to health care providers that the managed care organizations have the control of the health care dollar and intend to exert that control in as many aspects of the provision of health care services that they find possible.

Once HPN is identified as a viable option for a patient, the nutritional support physician needs to work collaboratively with the hospital team and the home care providers,

in addition to the payer. For Medicare patients, the physician should ensure that the patient meets the coverage criteria for HPN as established in the Regional Medical Policy Review issued by the DMERCs. If the patient needs additional tests done to demonstrate that the criteria are met, this should be done before the patient's discharge. Gastric emptying studies, fecal fat analysis, the use of enteral or oral diet modifications, pharmacologic modalities, and enteral tube feeding trials may be necessary in some cases to demonstrate the abnormality and symptoms that necessitate PN. The supplier of HPN will also benefit from all measures taken to demonstrate the need for HPN because it could be denied reimbursement if the claim is found to be unsubstantiated by the DMERC. Communication between the physician and the home care supplier is indispensable in preventing denied claims and facilitating the patient's discharge. Members of other disciplines, such as dietitians, nurses, pharmacists, and social workers, are essential for a successful discharge. Their input is invaluable in gathering data that will substantiate the need for PN.

For the patient requiring HPN whose health plan coverage is provided through a fee-for-service program, there are generally no issues related to who provides the services in the home setting. In this case, the hospital should work with the patient and the family to determine the most appropriate home care supplier who would best suit their needs on discharge. A factor that must be taken into consideration is the patient's deductible and out-of-pocket expenses for the therapy. Health plan benefits differ widely on covered services between the hospital setting and home care. Some plans may not provide any home care benefit or may place the PN solution under the pharmacy benefit but have limited or no coverage for the home health nursing that may be required. Interpretations of the covered benefits should be ascertained before discharge. Usually the home care supplier takes much of the responsibility for determining the benefit level before admitting a patient to its service, but the physician and hospital team should determine with the home care supplier who would be responsible for communicating any coverage issues with the patient, so the patient can make an informed choice.

With the managed fee-for-service payer,

an HPN patient has the ability, just as with an indemnity plan, to have freedom of choice in the selection of providers. There may be some need for second opinions, depending on the needs of the plan. Some managed fee-for-service plans also use independent case managers to negotiate fees and services for patients requiring extensive services.

Subscribers to a PPO who require HPN are limited to a choice of home care suppliers and nursing agencies that are selected as preferred providers through the PPO. The prescribing physician and the rest of the health care team need to be aware of the capabilities of these providers and generate a plan of care that takes this into consideration. Nonpreferred providers are generally not an option for the patient unless the prescribing physician can delineate issues specific to the patient that would mandate a different provider. Case managers are used extensively by PPOs, and the health care team will find that most of their contacts with the payer are through the case manager.

Like an enrollee in a PPO, the HPN patient who is an HMO subscriber is subject to provisions of the HMO preferred provider network. The use of nonproviders subjects the patient to additional expenses for services provided unless the nonprovider has negotiated with the HMO. The HMO usually has a smaller network of home care providers than that of a PPO. Knowledge of the capabilities of these providers empowers the health care team to make decisions that maximize the patient's health care benefits and facilitate services in the home.

The Medicaid patient who requires HPN presents a different set of care-planning demands on the nutritional support practitioner. Reimbursement to HPN suppliers is not very liberal, so finding a home care supplier willing to accept the Medicaid reimbursement can be difficult in some states. The prescribing physician needs to be familiar with the coverage criteria for the patient's residential state before prescribing HPN. As stated earlier, many states have adopted coverage criteria similar to Medicare's criteria, compelling practitioners to apply the same criteria to the Medicaid population.

Many Medicaid programs have now placed some of their enrollees in managed care plans. The Medicaid managed care subscribers select an HMO from the participating payers, and their care is comparable to that of any patient enrolled in the HMO, managed through a primary care physician. The HMO receives payment from the state Medicaid program for managing the patient's care, with the goal of reducing the patient's overall utilization of health care services and a focus on preventive care that may not have been received before under the traditional Medicaid program. If the patient is enrolled in a managed Medicaid program, then the same concerns that were addressed in the discussion of HMOs apply to this patient.

Also, Medicare has a significant number of patients enrolled in managed care programs. The nutritional support clinician should pursue this with any Medicare patient. At times, patients may not be fully aware of the ramifications of the types of health care insurance coverage they have and may unwittingly lead the health care team to believe that they are covered under a traditional Medicare program.

Once the payer source and coverage benefits for HPN are ascertained and the patient is prepared for discharge, the health care team needs to plan what follow-up will be needed, in addition to what services will be required in the home setting besides the nutrients, equipment, and supplies. Patients may need more than one provider of these services, and this needs to be coordinated with the payer and the home care providers. Any additional patient education, training, or reinforcement of training is generally not a reimbursable service to the home care provider, with some exceptions. Home health nursing agencies can usually bill Medicare for some additional education of the patient in the home setting, but the number of these visits is fairly limited.

MCOs commonly "bundle" services for a patient receiving home care therapies. An HPN patient may require additional training or home health nursing support for the first few days of therapy at home or may need nursing visits for venipunctures for laboratory work. Frequently, the payer negotiates bundling of these services in the per-diem rate of which they reimburse the HPN supplier for the nutrients, equipment, and supplies. Because most HPN suppliers have nurses on staff to train and follow patients, the supplier could provide these services in addition to the supplies, and the payer would not have to reimburse a home health agency separately. Although this is not an issue for the prescribing physician from a reimbursement perspective, it is a concern for the HPN supplier in the amount of financial risk it carries with a patient who may need considerable support from nursing services after discharge.

◆ APPEALS

Even with the best efforts to document the need for HPN, claims may occasionally be denied by any payer. With the federal and state plans, knowing their coverage criteria and meeting their expectations concerning documentation is the best method to prevent denied claims. Medicare, in particular, is fairly specific about the types of documentation it expects and the forms that need to be submitted.

With the managed care plans, the appeals process may be murky. The case manager is usually the first individual encountered within the PPO and HMO when coverage issues arise. PPOs have not regularly hired medical directors in the past, but more PPOs are doing so. If there is a medical director, this is the individual who may be making decisions, on a case-by-case basis, about the interpretation of the subscriber's covered health care. Some PPOs use a panel of health care professionals and administrators to determine benefit levels in cases of appeal. For the HMO enrollee, a medical director is the decision maker for appeals after the case manager has interpreted the covered benefits.

Appeals of denied claims or coverage issues should be filed by the enrollee, although many patients are unaware of this avenue. Once they appeal a decision of the payer, the enrollees require documentation and substantiation of their physical symptoms and the expected outcomes of the therapy. It is beneficial for the prescribing physician to state not only the expected outcomes of the intervention with HPN but also the expected outcomes if the patient does not receive HPN. The nutritional support practitioner plays a key role in providing the documentation necessary for the payer to make an informed decision.

◆ OUTCOMES

Outcomes measurement has become a health care buzzword that has been difficult

for some to define. Payers and consumers want best outcomes of the health care interventions to be delivered, but they also want to know what the value of that outcome is, that is, the cost to achieve the outcome. Nutritional support providers can clarify the expectations of payers regarding the outcomes of nutritional support. These outcomes include the physical outcomes, that is, weight gain or maintenance, improved protein and caloric intake, improved nutritional status through biochemical markers, improved immune system function, wound healing, a decreased hospital length of stay, and improved morbidity and mortality. The functional outcomes are also relevant to payers and consumers and can be described with the patient's physical condition and ability to function at an optimal level. The psychosocial outcomes of nutritional support, although more difficult to measure, are also essential to be determined for both the payers and the consumers. The benefits of an improved functional status and the ability to achieve an improved quality of life are positive psychosocial outcomes that should be investigated.

In a health care environment that constantly commands its providers to prove the worth of their interventions, nutritional support practitioners will need to continually evaluate the effects of their intercessions with patients. The health care dollar will increasingly become more elusive to a number of providers as purchasers of health care continue to compress the number of services that can be squeezed out of that same dollar, putting the providers at increased financial risk. With increasing payer consolidation, economists predict that there will be fewer purchasers determining how the health care dollars are spent, but there will also continue to be a consumer-driven market to maintain our current level of quality in health care in the United States. As the United States enters an era in which the "baby boomers" will need more health care as they age, they will drive the demand for health care. What the country can afford to provide will continue to be the debate.

REFERENCES

1. Parver AK, Lubinsky CA: Reimbursement issues in nutrition support. *In* Crocker KJ (ed): The ASPEN

Nutrition Support Practice Manual. Silver Spring, Md, The American Society for Parenteral and Enteral Nutrition, 1998, pp 1–15.

2. Region C DMERC: Regional Medical Review Policy. Palmetto Government Benefits Administrators, April, 1996.
3. Tallon RW: IDPN: The controversy continues. Infusion 1(12):22–26, 1994.
4. Federal Register, January 7, 1998.
5. On the books. Infusion 4(11):13, 1998.
6. On the books. Infusion 4(10):50, 1998.
7. Federal Register, December 19, 1997.
8. Rollins G: Medicare + Choice. Infusion 4(10):41–44, 1998.
9. Physicians' Current Procedural Terminology—CPT 2000. Chicago, American Medical Association, 2000.
10. Viall CD: Reimbursement for nutrition support under managed care. *In* Merritt RJ (ed): The ASPEN Nutrition Support Practice Manual. Silver Spring, Md, The American Society for Parenteral and Enteral Nutrition, 1998.
11. The Interstudy Competitive Edge HMO Industry Report. Minneapolis, Hospitals and Health Networks, 1998.

27

◆ Transplantation

Jeanette Hasse, Ph.D., R.D., L.D., F.A.D.A., C.N.S.D.
Susan Roberts, M.S., R.D., L.D., C.N.S.D.

Transplantation of solid organs, bone marrow, and peripheral blood stem cells presents unique challenges to nutritional support professionals. Patients undergoing transplantation often are malnourished and experience metabolic changes owing to the transplant and immunosuppressive medications. Conditions such as rejection and graft-versus-host disease (GVHD) are specific complications that affect nutrient needs and delivery. Because there are several differences between the solid organ and bone marrow transplantation populations, this chapter discusses the nutritional care of these groups in two parts.

◆ ORGAN TRANSPLANTATION

Organ transplantation has become an accepted therapy for the treatment of end-stage organ disease. Transplantation involves replacing failed organs with healthy donor organs in recipients who would otherwise die or require long-term artificial replacement (e.g., insulin, dialysis, parenteral nutrition). Organ transplantation, therefore, offers a second chance at life for thousands of individuals each year.

Organ transplantation presents unique nutritional challenges because both the pre-transplantation and the post-transplantation status must be considered when providing nutritional support. First, there are nutrient and metabolic aberrations associated with organ failure in the pretransplantation state. During the post-transplantation phase, surgical complications, organ rejection, infections, and side effects of immunosuppressant medications are major factors influencing nutrient needs and delivery. For optimal success after transplantation, an organized strategy to evaluate and implement nutritional assessment and treatment is vital.

Nutritional Status

A complete initial nutritional assessment should be conducted on each transplant recipient. The goal of the assessment is to (1) determine the current nutritional status, (2) predict the future status based on current conditions, and (3) identify appropriate therapy. Because malnutrition affects transplantation outcomes, nutritional interventions should be implemented to treat or prevent nutritional problems.

Determining Nutritional Status

Assessing the nutritional status of a patient who has undergone transplantation can be complicated by many factors including organ function and complications from transplantation (Table 27–1).[1–8]

A carefully performed physical examination and patient history are imperative to determine the patient's nutritional status. The physical examination may reveal signs of muscle wasting, subcutaneous fat loss, fluid retention (edema and/or ascites), skin breakdown and fragility, hair loss, or other signs of malnutrition.

Historical facts regarding a patient's weight changes, appetite, and activity level provide important information about the nutritional status. A detailed history can reveal the adequacy of the dietary intake and the presence of symptoms influencing the intake, such as nausea, vomiting, diarrhea, early satiety, and dysgeusia.[3] The interviewer should also obtain information about psychosocial issues such as the patient's ability to buy and obtain food and ability to prepare the food. Patients may lack the energy or physical ability to prepare food even if they can purchase it.

Malnutrition

The cause of malnutrition in transplantation candidates is multifactorial (Table 27–2).[1, 4,

Table 27–1. Post-transplantation Factors That Affect Nutritional Assessment

Factor	How Factor Alters Interpretation of Nutritional Assessment Parameters
Altered liver function	Decreases visceral protein concentrations due to decreased synthesis Alters nitrogen balance when ammonia is not converted to urea and excreted Affects immune function tests
Renal failure or insufficiency	Alters nitrogen balance owing to decreased excretion of nitrogen Affects immune function tests Causes overhydration resulting in falsely depressed visceral protein levels If a dialysis graft is in place, anthropometric measurements cannot be accurately measured on that arm
Fluid retention	Increases body weight Dilutes visceral protein levels Affects anthropometric measurements
Immunosuppressive medication	Alters total lymphocyte count Affects skin test antigens
Bleeding	Affects serum protein levels

Data from references 1 through 8.

[5, 7, 9–14] Malnutrition, which is often present before transplantation, results in poor post-transplantation outcomes and has been demonstrated in several studies to reduce post-transplantation survival rates. Among 52 heart transplant recipients, the mortality rate was 50% in severely malnourished patients, 23% in marginally compromised patients, and 21% in adequately nourished patients.[11] Pikul and colleagues reported a trend toward increased post-transplantation mortality in malnourished liver transplant recipients.[15] In addition, among these 68 subjects, malnutrition was associated with prolonged ventilatory support, placement of a tracheostomy, and an increased length of stay in the hospital.

Harrison and colleagues categorized liver transplantation patients into two groups based on midarm circumference and triceps skin fold thickness.[16] Patients with measurements below the 25th percentile had significantly more bacterial infections than patients with measurements greater than the 25th percentile. There was also a trend for increased 6-month mortality in malnour-

ished patients (13% mortality) compared with well-nourished patients (0% mortality). Reduced post-transplantation survival was reported in another study; patients with a body cell mass less than 35% of their body

Table 27–2. Factors Contributing to Malnutrition in Organ Transplantation Candidates

Organ Transplanted	Factors Contributing to Malnutrition
All solid organs	Anorexia Nausea, vomiting Difficulty chewing or swallowing Limited access to food Depression Fatigue Restricted diets Hypermetabolic state due to disease and/or surgery Drug-nutrient interactions
Heart	Poor nutrient delivery to tissue due to impaired waste removal secondary to ↓ circulatory function Cardiac cachexia ↓ nutrient intake ↓ gastrointestinal absorption ↑ stool and urine loss ↑ cardiac and pulmonary energy expenditure Ascites and early satiety (when hepatic congestion occurs)
Intestine	Complications of TPN Metabolic bone disease Trace mineral deficiencies Cholestasis Cholelithiasis Hepatic dysfunction Portal hypertension Splenomegaly Urolithiasis
Kidney	Glucose intolerance Hypertriglyceridemia Abnormal metabolism of calcium, phosphorus, vitamin D, and aluminum Urea causes insulin-stimulated protein synthesis and ↑ protein degradation
Liver	Protein, fluid, electrolyte abnormalities Nutrient malabsorption and steatorrhea Esophageal strictures and dysphagia Mental alteration Early satiety due to ascites ↑ intestinal losses of protein Impaired hepatic protein synthesis Altered intermediary metabolism ↑ energy expenditure Malabsorption due to ↓ bile salt levels Small bowel dysfunction due to portal hypertension or lymphostasis Pancreatic insufficiency
Lung	↑ work of breathing and resting energy expenditure Hyperinflation resulting in early satiety ↑ energy expenditure due to chronic infections (cystic fibrosis)
Pancreas	Nephropathy Gastroparesis Cardiovascular disease

TPN, total parenteral nutrition.
Data from references, 1, 4, 5, 7, 9 through 14.

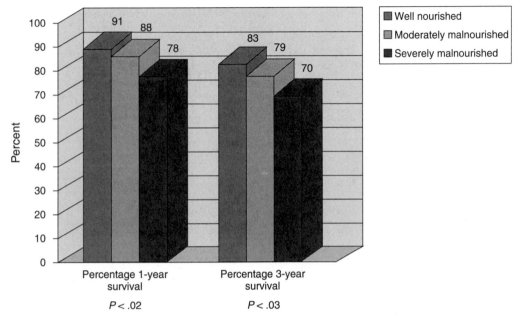

Figure 27–1. Survival in 573 patients who underwent liver transplantation from 1992 to 1996 at a single center. (From Hasse JM, Gonwa TA, Jennings LW, et al: Malnutrition affects liver transplant outcomes [Abstract]. Transplantation 66:553, 1998.)

weight had reduced post-transplantation survival.[17]

In our own experience, malnutrition reduces post–liver transplantation survival.[18] Among 573 liver transplant recipients with at least 1 year of follow-up who received transplants between 1992 and 1996, severely malnourished patients had 1- and 3-year survival rates of 78% and 70% compared with 91% and 83% in well-nourished patients (Fig. 27–1). This contrasted to an analysis of our liver transplantation population from 1985 to 1991 in which malnutrition adversely influenced the hospital length of stay but did not significantly alter the survival. The difference was explained by the fact that the median time waiting for a transplant increased from 13 days for patients evaluated during the first period (1985 to 1991) to 115 days for patients evaluated during the second period (1992 to 1996). Therefore, increased mortality associated with malnutrition appears to be pronounced when waiting times for transplantation are prolonged.

Nutritional Therapy Following Transplantation

Ideally, nutritional therapy should be provided during the pretransplantation phase when patients are waiting for transplantation (see other chapters in this book for guidelines on nutritional therapy for patients with organ failure). Unfortunately, the consequences of organ failure limit the ability to repair the body and restore depleted stores. If the factors causing malnutrition cannot be overcome to allow nutritional repletion, the goal of nutritional therapy is to maintain a patient's current status. However, once a transplantation has been performed and the organ is working well, repletion of depleted nutrient stores should occur.

Few studies have been done to evaluate the benefit of pretransplantation nutritional support. We studied the effect of aggressive pretransplantation oral nutritional support in patients awaiting liver transplantation; preliminary data are reported here.[19] Patients were randomized in a 1:2:2 fashion to receive oral diet alone (n = 9) or in combination with special hepatic (n = 19) or standard casein (n = 18) supplements. The supplements were given in the amount of 0.5 g of protein per kilogram of ideal body weight per day. The patients recorded their dietary intakes three times per week. The patients underwent monthly pretransplantation evaluations by a dietitian and physician and were followed for 4 months after transplantation to assess nutritional and mental

Table 27–3. Effect of Nutritional Supplementation in Patients Awaiting Liver Transplantation

Group	Mean Kilocalories Ingested per Kilogram of Body Weight	Mean Grams of Protein Ingested per Kilogram of Body Weight	Number of Hospitalizations per Patient per Month
Hepatic supplement (n = 9)	33.9 ± 2.6	1.3 ± 0.1*	0.2 ± 0.2‡
Standard supplement (n = 14)	34.6 ± 2.1	1.3 ± 0.1†	0.4 ± 0.2
Control group (no supplement) (n = 6)	26.8 ± 4.3	0.9 ± 0.1	0.7 ± 0.3

*Hepatic versus control, $P = .008$
†Standard versus control, $P = .009$
‡Hepatic versus standard, $P = .007$
From Hasse J, Crippin J, Blue L, et al: Does nutrition supplementation benefit liver transplant candidates with a history of encephalopathy [Abstract]? JPEN J Parenter Enteral Nutr 21:516, 1997.

status and anthropometric measurements. The median days in the study until transplantation or withdrawal from the transplantation list were 143 days (hepatic group), 141 days (casein group), and 64 days (control group). Patients who drank the hepatic formula spent fewer days in the hospital before transplantation compared with other groups. Results from the study are summarized in Table 27–3.

Delivery of Nutritional Support

The preferred method of nutrient delivery in transplantation patients is the oral route. This is, in fact, the reason people with intestinal failure undergo small bowel transplantation—to end dependence on total parenteral nutrition (TPN). Enteral tube feeding is the second choice for pre- and post-transplantation nutritional support; TPN is reserved for situations in which the gastrointestinal (GI) tract is not functional (Fig. 27–2).

Indications for Parenteral Nutrition

The use of TPN is low among organ transplant recipients and is reserved for post-transplantation complications affecting gut function. Severe esophagitis or gastritis (often caused by cytomegalovirus or other infection) may be severe enough to warrant the use of TPN. Pancreatitis can occur after pancreas transplantation, as a side effect of azathioprine therapy, or from biliary tree manipulation. Other complications such as fistulas, small bowel obstruction, and GI

tract bleeding occur occasionally, and TPN may be the only safe method to provide nutrition. Chylous ascites following liver transplantation has been resolved using a combination of TPN and somatostatin[20] or a fat-free oral diet and elemental tube feeding formula.[21] Small bowel transplant recipients require TPN during the immediate post-transplantation phase (1 to 2 weeks) until there is output from the terminal ileostomy signaling gut function.[22, 23] During small bowel graft rejection or infection, TPN is usually indicated.

Benefits of Parenteral Nutrition

The primary and most obvious benefit from TPN is that nutrition can be provided when enteral forms of nutrition are not tolerated. Other theorized benefits include a reduction in nitrogen loss, the provision of adequate nutrients to promote healing and recovery, and the replenishment of depleted nutrient stores.

Nitrogen loss is high in the post-transplantation period owing to surgical stress and the administration of corticosteroids to blunt the immune and rejection response.[24–28] Providing nitrogen via TPN should improve nitrogen balance.

Adequate nutrients are necessary to promote healing and recovery from transplantation surgery. Parenteral nutrition can provide the necessary protein, vitamins, and minerals associated with wound healing. Dextrose and lipid provide energy that is required for basic metabolic processes and physical activity.

Finally, TPN can be a vehicle to help re-

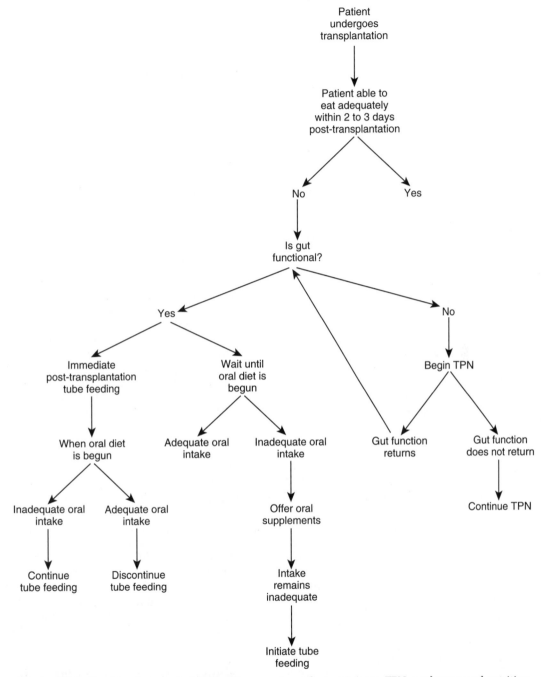

Figure 27–2. Nutritional support algorithm for organ transplant recipients. TPN, total parenteral nutrition.

place nutrients lacking as a result of increased losses, poor intake, and increased utilization due to disease. As mentioned earlier, patients with chronic organ failure often have depleted nutrient stores that can be completely replaced only when organ function returns.

Three studies have evaluated the effects of TPN in the post–liver transplantation period.[29-31] Reilly and colleagues compared two types of TPN to intravenous (IV) fluid during the immediate post-transplantation recovery phase after liver transplantation.[29] Patients were randomized to receive a 1-week infusion of TPN with standard amino acids (n = 8), TPN with branched-chain

Table 27–4. Post–Liver Transplantation Energy Expenditure as Measured by Indirect Calorimetry

Researchers	Design	Results
Delafosse et al.[25]	REE measured in eight patients on first two post-transplantation days	REE was 36–38% above predicted energy expenditure using Harris-Benedict equation
Shanbhogue et al.[26]	REE measured in 11 post-transplantation patients	REE was 7% higher than Harris-Benedict equation using actual weight
Plevak et al.[28]	REE measured in 28 patients before transplantation and on post-transplantation days 1, 3, 5, 14, and 28	REE did not change over time; Harris-Benedict equation (using ideal weight) plus 20% met energy needs in most patients
Hasse et al.[24]	REE measured in 31 patients on post-transplantation days 2, 4, 7, and 12	REE rose gradually in the first 12 post-transplantation days; the peak mean REE was 27% above the Harris-Benedict equation using the patient's lowest recent weight

REE, resting energy expenditure.
From Hasse JM: Solid organ transplant. *In* Matarese LE, Gottschlich MM (eds): Contemporary Nutrition Support Practice: A Clinical Guide. Philadelphia, WB Saunders, 1998, pp 547–560.

amino acids (BCAAs) (n = 10), or IV fluid (n = 10). The TPN in both groups provided 35 kcal/kg body weight and 1.5 g of protein per kilogram of body weight. For both TPN groups, nitrogen balance was improved and the time in the intensive unit decreased. This study should be interpreted with caution because the length of stay is significantly less today that when this study was conducted.

Mehta and colleagues retrospectively compared 63 enterally fed adult liver transplantation patients with 21 adult patients who received TPN.[30] Compared with TPN patients, enterally fed patients began oral diets sooner (1.7 ± 0.9 vs. 3 ± 1.7 days) and met oral diet goals sooner (19.5 ± 11 vs. 38.6 ± 24.6 days). In addition, the frequency of postoperative ileus was significantly higher in TPN patients (33%) compared with enterally fed patients (8.3%).

In a final study, TPN was compared with tube feeding.[31] Liver transplantation patients were randomized to receive TPN (n = 10) through a central IV line or tube feeding (n = 14) through a nasojejunal tube. The TPN solution initiated 24 to 60 hours after surgery consisted of amino acids, dextrose, lipids, vitamins, and minerals. Tube feeding was initiated 12 to 18 hours after surgery with a 1-kcal/mL whole-protein formula. When the oral dietary intake met 70% of the estimated needs, the TPN and tube feeding were discontinued. There were no differences between the groups in the number of days for patients to begin eating (median = 4 days) and to achieve adequate oral intake (median = 5 days). Intestinal permeability

and absorptive capacity were measured at 14 hours, 3 days, and 10 days after transplantation and were found to be similar in both groups. Fourteen episodes of infection (six gut-related) occurred in 10 patients (71%) in the tube-fed group. Seven (70%) of patients in the TPN group had 10 episodes of infection (six gut-related). However, TPN was 10 times more costly than tube feeding.

Parenteral Nutrition Considerations Unique to Transplantation

Some TPN administration concerns are unique to transplantation patients. Because these patients are immunosuppressed, they are at increased risk of infection. Centrally placed IV lines are a likely source of infection, so there should be careful attention to the care of the line, including frequent line and dressing changes. The other transplantation-specific TPN concerns relate to the solution composition because of metabolic and nutrient changes due to transplantation.

Metabolic Changes Associated with Organ Transplantation

Energy

Post-transplantation energy requirements are increased because of surgical stress. In addition, energy demands escalate as patients become ambulatory and participate in physical therapy. Because many patients are malnourished at the time of transplantation, additional calories are required to allow repletion of body weight and fat stores. Imme-

Table 27–5. Nitrogen Loss in the Short-Term Post–Liver Transplantation Phase

Researchers	Design	Results
Hasse et al.[24]	UUN measured in 17 non–tube-fed and 14 tube-fed patients on post-transplantation days 2, 4, 7, and 12	Daily UUN losses for non–tube-fed patients ranged from 9.6 ± 5.1 g to 11.7 ± 6.3 g; UUN losses for tube-fed patients ranged from 2.9 ± 4.3 g to 15.0 ± 7.7 g
Delafosse.[25]	UUN measured in eight patients on the first two post-transplantation days	Post-transplantation day 1: 20.1 g Post-transplantation day 2: 24.6 g
Shanbhogue et al.[46]	UUN measured in 11 post-transplantation patients	Mean UUN excretion was 12.9 ± 4.4 g on post-transplantation day 3
O'Keefe et al.[27]	Evaluated nitrogen losses in 42 transplantation patients	A relatively stable nitrogen state was achieved on the fourth post-transplantation day, with a mean nitrogen loss of 14.4–16 g/day
Plevak et al.[28]	Nitrogen balance measured in 28 patients before transplantation and on post-transplantation days 1, 3, 5, 14, and 28	UUN excretion increased after transplantation, peaking at post-transplantation day 3; nitrogen losses returned to preoperative level by day 28; despite nutritional support, mean nitrogen balance was negative during study period

UUN, urinary urea nitrogen.

From Hasse JM: Solid organ transplant. *In* Matarese LE, Gottschlich MM (eds): Contemporary Nutrition Support Practice: A Clinical Guide. Philadelphia, WB Saunders, 1998, pp 547–560.

diate post-transplantation energy needs are usually estimated to be 130 to 150% of the basal energy expenditure (determined by the Harris-Benedict equation) or 35 kcal/kg of body weight.[1, 11, 13, 25, 26, 32–35] This estimate is partially based on studies that measured resting energy expenditure in post-liver transplantation patients (Table 27–4).

Protein

Protein requirements are estimated to be 1.5 to 2 g/kg of body weight in the immediate post-transplantation phase (Table 27–5). Ad-

equate protein is required during this phase for wound healing and body defenses to fight infection. There must also be adequate protein to cover excess losses from surgical drains, fistulas, dialysis, and wounds. Corticosteroids also increase protein requirements by accelerating the protein catabolic rate.[36–39] Corticosteroid doses are highest in the first few days after transplantation or during treatment for rejection (Table 27–6). As corticosteroid doses increase, so do protein requirements.

Adequate protein intake during the acute post-transplantation phase may help reduce

Table 27–6. Sample Corticosteroid Protocol for Liver Transplantation Immunosuppression

	As Part of Tacrolimus-Based Immunosuppression Regimen	As Part of Cyclosporine-Based Immunosuppression Regimen
Preoperative	50 mg methylprednisolone (Solu-Medrol)	50 mg methylprednisolone
Intraoperative	1 g hydrocortisone (Solu-Cortef)	1 g hydrocortisone
Postoperative day 1	100 mg methylprednisolone	200 mg methylprednisolone
Postoperative day 2	80 mg methylprednisolone	160 mg methylprednisolone
Postoperative day 3	60 mg methylprednisolone	120 mg methylprednisolone
Postoperative day 4	40 mg methylprednisolone	80 mg methylprednisolone
Postoperative day 5	20 mg prednisolone	40 mg methylprednisolone
Postoperative day 6	20 mg prednisolone	20 mg prednisolone
Postoperative day 14	15 mg prednisolone	20 mg prednisolone
Postoperative day 21	12.5 mg prednisolone	20 mg prednisolone
Postoperative day 28–30	10 mg prednisolone	15 mg prednisolone
Postoperative day 60	7.5 mg prednisolone	10 mg prednisolone
Postoperative day 90	5 mg prednisolone	5 mg prednisolone

From Klintmalm, G: Liver Transplantation Immunosuppression Protocol. Dallas, Baylor Institute of Transplantation Sciences, Baylor University Medical Center, 1999.

nitrogen turnover and improve muscle mass. When TPN was given to adult liver transplantation patients with 27 kcal/kg of ideal body weight as glucose and 0.25 g of nitrogen per kilogram, there was a balanced plasma amino acid pattern and body nitrogen turnover.[40] This contrasted with TPN solutions containing only 0.12 and 0.18 g of nitrogen per kilogram, during the infusion of which many serum amino acid levels were low or at a lower range of normal.

Muscle mass increased in 16 kidney transplant recipients when a diet containing 1 to 1.5 g of protein per kilogram of body weight was given.[36] This occurred despite increased protein oxidation due to corticosteroids. In this same study, insulin-like growth factor levels increased 60% compared with healthy matched controls. It is unknown whether this reflects increased growth hormone secretion responding to protein catabolism from corticosteroids or whether it is due to increased dietary protein intake. This study also suggested that protein and carbohydrate were preferential fuels when glucocorticoids were administered.[36]

Conversely, there are instances when protein intake should be limited. Renal insufficiency is a common occurrence due to the nephrotoxic effect of the immunosuppressive drugs cyclosporine and tacrolimus. Protein may need to be limited when severe azotemia occurs. If renal replacement therapy is initiated, protein requirements are adjusted to 1.2 to 1.5 g/kg of body weight.

Special protein or amino acid combinations have been proposed to improve transplantation outcomes in animal models. It has been theorized that nucleotide-free diets will enhance immunity in transplant recipients.[41–43] Rats fed chow, a nucleotide-free casein-based diet, or diet supplemented with 0.25% yeast ribonucleic acid (RNA), underwent heterotopic heart transplantation and were followed for graft survival.[43] Rats given nucleotide-free diet and cyclosporine had increased survival compared with the cyclosporine-treated chow or RNA-supplemented diet groups. In a mouse model, the nucleotide-free diet and cyclosporine created a synergistic effect that was ablated when adenine or uracil was added.[43]

Finally, supplemental arginine may improve post-transplantation survival. Rats undergoing heart transplantation and fed diets supplemented with 2% or 5% arginine had improved survival rates.[44] Arginine may also improve blood pressure after transplantation.[45] Arginine also has been evaluated in combination with fish oil and is discussed in a later section.

Glucose

Glucose metabolism is altered by transplantation. In a study comparing 16 kidney transplant recipients with healthy controls, glucose oxidation increased more than 45% in transplantation patients compared with controls during the second post-transplantation month.[36]

Hyperglycemia is a common metabolic aberration following transplantation and can inhibit wound healing and increase infection rates. When infection rates were compared between diabetic kidney transplantation recipients and nondiabetic recipients, infection rates were 50% higher in diabetic patients.[46]

A sudden increase in serum glucose levels in a pancreas transplant recipient often signals ischemia or rejection.[47] Surgical stress, infection, and the administration of corticosteroids can also alter metabolic responses to neurohormonal and cytokine-mediated stimuli and cause hyperglycemia.[48] In addition, corticosteroids induce insulin resistance, and cyclosporine and tacrolimus inhibit pancreatic islet cell function and insulin release.[47]

Transient post-transplantation hyperglycemia is usually treated with regular insulin dosed on a sliding scale. However, chronic post-transplantation diabetes mellitus develops in 3 to 46% of transplantation patients.[49] The incidence reported varies with the type of transplant, criteria used to diagnose diabetes mellitus, and time that has elapsed since transplantation.[49] Factors other than immunosuppressive drugs that contribute to the development of post-transplantation diabetes mellitus are obesity, a family history of diabetes mellitus, a cadaveric renal transplant, advanced age, and black or Hispanic ethnicity.[50]

Parenteral nutrition solutions for transplant patients typically contain 70% of nonprotein calories as glucose. When hyperglycemia is significant or a patient is diabetic, the glucose content should be limited to 200 g/day and insulin administered (possibly by insulin drip) until euglycemia is achieved. Protocols for the initiation of TPN in diabetic patients suggest starting with 1 mg of glucose per kilogram of body weight per minute (or 200 mg/day) and increasing glucose by 50 g/day when euglycemia is achieved.[51] Suggested initial insulin doses for diabetic patients receiving TPN are 0.1 U of insulin per gram of dextrose.[52]

Close monitoring of serum glucose levels is necessary during the post-transplantation period. When corticosteroids are administered once daily in the morning, serum glucose levels peak in the afternoon. Therefore, while a fasting serum glucose level in the morning may be within normal limits, it could be high in the evening. Glucose levels usually decline when corticosteroid doses decrease. Conversely, when corticosteroid doses are increased to treat rejection (see Table 27–6), it is important to resume blood glucose monitoring because glucose levels often mimic increases in corticosteroid doses.

Lipids

Lipid Abnormalities

Although protein and glucose oxidation increase after transplantation, fat oxidation decreases. The effect appears to be transient because when 16 kidney transplant recipients were studied, lipid oxidation decreased 42 days after transplantation but increased over 15 subsequent months.[36] The mean prednisone dose was correlated with fuel oxidation.

Long-term hyperlipidemia occurs in more than 60% of kidney and heart transplant recipients and 30% of liver transplant recipients.[53] Abnormalities include elevated serum levels of very low density lipoprotein cholesterol, low-density lipoprotein (LDL) cholesterol, total cholesterol, and triglycerides with a concomitant decrease in high-density lipoprotein (HDL) cholesterol concentrations.[53–63] In kidney transplantation patients, increased oxidation of LDL cholesterol has been demonstrated,[64] along with an altered HDL content and its associated altered protective effect,[65] and along with intermediate-density lipoprotein accumulation.[63] In liver transplantation patients, elevated serum cholesterol concentrations have been associated with increased serum levels of triglycerides, total bilirubin, γ-glutamyltransferase, and alkaline phosphatase.[57]

Post-transplantation hyperlipidemia contributes to atherosclerotic vascular disease but also contributes to transplant graft vasculopathy.[53] In heart transplant recipients, this can lead to coronary heart disease; in renal transplantation patients, to chronic rejection; and in liver transplantation patients, to vanishing bile duct syndrome.

Post-transplantation lipid abnormalities can be attributed to several factors.[53, 55, 61] Genetic predisposition plays a role; however, several controllable factors predispose to hyperlipidemia, including body weight, dietary intake, and activity level. Diabetes mellitus, renal dysfunction, and proteinuria also contribute to post-transplantation hyperlipidemia. Finally, antihypertensive drugs and immunosuppressive medications alter lipid levels. Specifically, cyclosporine increases hepatic lipase activity and depresses lipoprotein lipase activity, bile acid synthesis from cholesterol, and transport of cholesterol to the intestines. Cyclosporine also binds to LDL-cholesterol receptors.[53, 56] Corticosteroids increase acetyl-CoA carboxylase, free fatty acid synthetase, and 3-hydroxy-3-methylglutaryl-CoA reductase activity. The synthesis of very low density lipoprotein cholesterol is enhanced by corticosteroids, and LDL-receptor activity and lipoprotein lipase are inhibited.[53, 56]

Dietary Lipid

In TPN solutions, about 30% of nonprotein calories are provided as lipid. When hyperglycemia is problematic in transplant recipients, lipid can temporarily provide up to 50% of nonprotein calories.

Most parenteral lipid emulsions contain n-6 fatty acids. Some studies suggest that providing n-3 fatty acids may be beneficial for transplant recipients. Because n-3 fatty acids produce eicosanoids that have less potency for inducing cellular responses than those derived from n-6 fatty acids, one would expect a decreased inflammatory response.[66] It is theorized that a reduction in leukotriene B$_4$ and thromboxane A$_2$ production would decrease leukosequestration and platelet aggregation and renal dysfunction due to cyclosporine.[48]

Some animal studies support the benefit of n-3 fatty acids in transplantation. One study compared rats pair-fed diets with either 20% fish oil or 20% corn oil.[67] Diets were fed for 4 weeks and cyclosporine administered for 2 weeks. Compared with corn oil–fed animals, the fish oil–fed group exhibited a reduced increase in thromboxane A_2 levels and a decrease in the vasodilators prostaglandin E_2 and I_2 in kidney and peritoneal macrophages. By competitively inhibiting cyclooxygenase metabolites, n-3 fatty acids preserved renal function by preventing cyclosporine from increasing thromboxane A_2 levels.

Fish oil and high–oleic acid oils also have been found to induce long-term functional transplant tolerance in transplanted animals by working synergistically with cyclosporine.[66] A study comparing renal function in groups of rats fed cyclosporine in either olive oil or fish oil found that cyclosporine in fish oil improved renal function and morphology, and renal cortical thromboxane B_2 levels were decreased.[68] Substituting fish oil as a vehicle for cyclosporine has not been shown to compromise cyclosporine's immunosuppressive properties.[69]

In other studies, rats administered n-3 fatty acids before and after heart transplantation survived longer than transplanted rats given n-6 fatty acids.[70, 71] Kelley and associates also demonstrated that n-3 fatty acids enhanced immunosuppression in rats undergoing cardiac transplantation.[69] Alexander and colleagues randomized rats undergoing heart transplantation to one of 10 groups.[44] Control rats were classified as (1) untreated; (2) cyclosporine and 2% glycine; (3) donor-specific transfusion (DST); or (4) DST and cyclosporine. Experimental groups were classified as (5) cyclosporine and 2% arginine; (6) cyclosporine and 10% fish oil; (7) DST, cyclosporine, and 2% arginine; (8) DST, cyclosporine, and 5% arginine; (9) DST, cyclosporine, and 10% fish oil; and (10) DST, cyclosporine, 5% arginine, and 10% fish oil. Survival rates of groups 7 through 10 were significantly greater than rates in groups 1 through 5. Fish oil and arginine improved survival but through different mechanisms.

Fish oil supplementation has also been found to decrease serum triglyceride levels, platelet aggregation, and blood pressure as well as improve renal graft function and decrease cyclosporine's adverse effects on the kidney.[69, 72–76]

Renal hemodynamics were improved in liver transplantation patients maintained on cyclosporine and given fish oil.[77] Thirteen liver transplantation patients maintained on cyclosporine received 12 g of corn oil per day (controls), and 13 patients received an equal amount of fish oil per day for 2 months. Control patients had no change in renal parameters. In study patients, the renal plasma flow increased 22%, the glomerular filtration rate 33%, and the renal blood flow 17%. In addition, the calculated total renal vascular resistance decreased 20%.[77] The beneficial effects of fish oil are believed to be caused by a more vasodilatory state due to different eicosanoids produced by fish oil.

Although fish oil does not appear to have an effect on reducing the incidence of rejection, when rejection occurs, organ function may recover better. When kidney transplantation patients given fish oil were compared with patients receiving equal amounts of coconut oil, renal function after rejection recovered better in the fish oil group.[75]

Fluid

The volume status should be monitored carefully in transplant recipients because fluid changes can occur rapidly, resulting in over- or underhydration. For example, if a newly transplanted kidney does not make urine immediately after transplantation, a patient can become fluid overloaded and require renal replacement therapy. Likewise, many drugs administered to transplant recipients, including cyclosporine and tacrolimus, are nephrotoxic and can cause renal insufficiency and decreased urine output.

Conversely, there are circumstances that cause dehydration because fluid losses exceed intakes. Pancreas transplantation patients with pancreatic-urinary drainage can lose as much as 2 to 3 L of pancreatic secretions daily.[78] Small bowel transplant recipients may have ostomy outputs of up to 4 L/day.[79] Kidney transplant recipients who have oliguria can experience excess fluid losses. Chest tubes, nasogastric tubes, surgical drains, biliary drains, wounds, and fistulas are other sites of potential fluid losses.[80] Finally, fluid losses due to diarrhea or procedures such as para- or thoracentesis can contribute to dehydration.[80]

A general guideline for fluid requirements in a euvolemic patient is to provide 1 mL/kcal. Volume-depleted patients require additional fluid to match losses, and volume-overloaded patients should receive only about 1 to 1.5 L/day.

Table 27–7. Electrolyte Disorders in Transplant Recipients: Causes and Suggested Treatments

Electrolyte Abnormality	Possible Cause(s)	Suggested Treatment
Hypernatremia	Dehydration	Increase fluid intake
	Excess sodium intake	Decrease sodium intake
Hyponatremia	Overhydration	Restrict fluid intake
	Total body sodium deficit	Increase sodium intake if there is total body sodium deficit
Hyperkalemia	Tacrolimus, cyclosporine	Restrict potassium intake
	Potassium-sparing diuretics	Administer potassium binder
	Renal insufficiency	
	Metabolic acidosis	
Hypokalemia	Potassium-wasting diuretics	Increase dietary potassium intake
	Refeeding syndrome	Administer supplements
	Diarrhea	
	Fistula	
	Inadequate potassium intake	
Hyperphosphatemia	Renal insufficiency	Restrict phosphorus intake
		Administer phosphate binders
Hypophosphatemia	Refeeding syndrome	Increase intake of high-phosphorus foods
	Glucocorticoids	Administer phosphorus supplements
Hypocalcemia	Chelation of calcium secondary to citrate in stored blood	Administer calcium supplements
Hypermagnesemia	Renal insufficiency	Limit magnesium intake
Hypomagnesemia	Cyclosporine	Increase intake of high-magnesium foods
	Refeeding syndrome	Administer magnesium supplements
	Diabetic ketoacidosis	
	Diuretics	
	Diarrhea	
Decreased bicarbonate	Increased exocrine drainage (pancreas transplant)	Administer bicarbonate supplements
	Intestinal drainage (intestinal transplant)	If patient is receiving TPN, provide acetate

TPN, total parenteral nutrition.
From Hasse JM: Recovery after organ transplantation in adults: The role of postoperative nutrition therapy. Top Clin Nutr 13(2):15–26, 1998.

Electrolytes

Electrolyte abnormalities are common in the early post-transplantation phase. Renal dysfunction, medication side effects, and refeeding syndrome are some of the causes of electrolyte disorders. In addition, exocrine pancreatic drainage in pancreas transplant recipients and ostomy drainage in small bowel transplantation patients contribute to bicarbonate deficiency. Table 27–7 summarizes common electrolyte abnormalities, causes, and suggested treatment.

Vitamins and Minerals

There have been no comprehensive studies evaluating vitamin and mineral requirements of transplant recipients. However, there are multiple conditions in the perioperative phase that can contribute to a deficiency or an excess of certain vitamins and minerals (Table 27–8).

Other Transplantation Concerns

Immunosuppression

Long-term requirements for immunosuppression result in a unique circumstance for organ transplant recipients. Many of the immunosuppressive drugs have food and nutrient interactions that will be lifelong. Table 27–9 summarizes the major immunosuppressive drugs, their actions, and their side effects.

Obesity

Severe obesity may be a contraindication for transplantation. In heart and kidney transplant recipients, severe obesity is associated with adverse outcomes. If a heart transplant recipient is more than 120% of ideal body weight, it is considered an increased surgical risk.[11]

Several studies reported adverse effects when obese patients received kidney trans-

Table 27–8. Conditions That Contribute to Vitamin and Mineral Abnormalities in Organ Transplantation Patients

Condition (Transplanted Organ)	Nutrient Alterations
Alcoholism	Vitamins A, B_6, and B_{12}; niacin; thiamine; folate; magnesium; and zinc levels are decreased
Antibiotics	Vitamins E and K and folate levels are decreased
Bile drainage (liver)	Copper loss is increased
Biliary obstruction, Wilson's disease (liver)	Copper levels are increased
Bleeding	Iron loss is increased
Cyclosporine	Magnesium loss is increased
Glucocorticoids	Vitamin D and phosphorus levels are decreased
	Urinary loss of calcium is increased
Hemochromatosis (liver)	Iron stores are increased
Liver failure (liver)	Ability to activate vitamin D is decreased
	Vitamin K level is decreased
Ostomy loss (small bowel) or diarrhea	Zinc loss is increased
Refeeding syndrome	Magnesium, phosphorus, and potassium levels are decreased
Renal failure	Vitamin D, calcium, and phosphorus metabolism are abnormal
	Iron levels are decreased owing to depressed erythropoietin levels
	Vitamin A level is increased
	Vitamin C, phosphorus, and potassium levels are decreased owing to dialysis
	Excretion of magnesium and zinc is decreased
	Zinc levels may be decreased in dialysis patients
Steatorrhea	Levels of vitamins A, D, E, and K are decreased
	Calcium level is decreased
Wound	Need for vitamin C and zinc is increased to aid with healing

Data from Hasse JM: Solid organ transplant. *In* Matarese LE, Gottschlich MM (eds): Contemporary Nutrition Support. Philadelphia, WB Saunders, 1998, pp 547–560; and Hasse JM: Recovery after organ transplantation in adults; the role of postoperative nutrition therapy. Top Clin Nutr 13(2):15–26, 1998.

plants. Merion and colleagues classified 263 renal transplant recipients as obese (>120% ideal weight, n = 40) or nonobese (n = 223).[81] Obese patients had higher rates of wound infection and greater 1-year post-transplantation weight gain compared with nonobese patients. In another study comparing 46 obese with 50 nonobese renal transplant recipients, obesity reduced immediate graft function and patient and graft survival and increased the rate of wound complications, intensive care unit admissions, reintubations, and new-onset diabetes mellitus.[82] Finally, 118 of 584 renal transplant recipients classified as obese (body mass index >27.5 kg/m²) developed more urologic and wound complications than nonobese subjects.[83] Those patients who had a body mass index greater than 30 had a greater chance of delayed graft function and immunologic graft loss due to acute rejection than patients with lower body mass.

Severe short-term adverse effects of obesity have not been demonstrated in liver transplant recipients. When 18 severely or morbidly obese liver transplantation patients were evaluated, it was determined that they had higher rates of wound infection, diabetes mellitus, and hypertension than nonobese patients, but those complications were manageable.[84]

Another study evaluated the effect of obesity in liver transplantation patients.[85, 86] Patients were divided into categories based on body mass index: underweight (n = 128), acceptable weight (n = 707), overweight (n = 221), and severely or morbidly obese (n = 189). Weight did not affect liver function tests, serum cholesterol concentrations, or the prevalence of new-onset diabetes mellitus within the first post-transplantation year. Serum triglyceride levels were significantly higher in overweight patients (259 ± 190 mg/dL) at 1 year after transplantation compared with acceptable-weight patients (218 ± 173 mg/dL). The 1-, 3-, and 5-year survival rates and the incidence of rejection were similar between the groups.[85] Increased wound infection rates were the only significant finding; within the first 3 post-transplantation months, 10.7% of the severely or morbidly obese patients had at least one infection compared with 4.3% in acceptable-weight patients.[86]

This study was similar to one by Braunfeld and colleagues.[87] Forty morbidly obese (body mass index >30 kg/m²) liver transplantation patients were compared with 61 time-matched controls. Obese patients had more hypoxemia, an increased rate of diabetes mellitus, increased creatinine levels, and

Table 27–9. Immunosuppressive Medications, Mechanisms of Action and Side Effects

Drug	Mechanism of Action	Side Effects
Cyclosporine (Sandimmune, Neoral)	Inhibits response of cytotoxic T cells to interleukin-2 (IL-2) and prevents T helper lymphocytes from producing IL-2	Nephrotoxicity Neurotoxicity (e.g., headache, tremor, seizure) Hypertension Hyperglycemia Hyperlipidemia Hyperkalemia Hypomagnesemia Gingival hyperplasia
Tacrolimus (Prograf, FK-506)	Inhibits proliferation of cytotoxic T cells and synthesis of IL-2	Nephrotoxicity Neurotoxicity Hypertension Hyperglycemia (diabetogenic effects) Hyperkalemia Nausea and vomiting Gastrointestinal symptoms (e.g., diarrhea)
Corticosteroids (prednisone, prednisolone, methylprednisolone [Solu-Medrol], hydrocortisone [Solu-Cortef])	Anti-inflammatory response at arterial site inhibits IL-1 and decreases IL-2, which suppresses lymphocyte proliferation and decreases circulating lymphocytes	Altered fluid or electrolyte balance Hypertension Adrenal axis suppression Mood swings (depression, euphoria) Peptic ulcer disease Hyperphagia Hyperglycemia Osteoporosis Hyperlipidemia Poor wound healing Cataracts
Azathioprine (Imuran)	Inhibits RNA and DNA synthesis to prevent cytotoxic T and B cell proliferation and antibody production	Bone marrow suppression (leukopenia, thrombocytopenia, pancytopenia, macrocytic anemia) Nausea and vomiting Diarrhea Macrocytic anemia Hepatotoxicity
Mycophenolate mofetil (CellCept, RS-61443)	Decreases lymphocyte activation and replication by suppressing enzymes in the purine salvage pathway, creating a purine deficiency and thus inhibiting T and B cell proliferation Also suppresses antibody formation	Gastrointestinal symptoms (e.g., nausea, vomiting, diarrhea) Leukopenia
Antithymocyte globulin (Atgam)	Decreases circulating lymphocytes	Anaphylactic reaction Fever and chills Nausea and vomiting Leukopenia
Muromonab-CD3 (OKT3)	Binds to mature T cells to decrease their effector function	Anaphylactic reaction Pulmonary edema (usually first dose only) Severe flu-like symptoms Headache Increased incidence of lymphoproliferative disorders
Sirolimus (rapamycin)	Inhibits T and B cell proliferation while not affecting IL-2 production	Possible hyperglycemia and hyperlipidemia Possible gastrointestinal symptoms
Gusperimus (15-deoxyspergualin)	Inhibits T and B lymphocytes	Leukopenia Thrombocytopenia Gastrointestinal symptoms

From Hasse J, DiCecco SR: Solid organ transplantation. *In* Skipper A (ed): Dietitian's Handbook of Enteral and Parenteral Nutrition, 2nd ed. Gaithersburg, Md, Aspen, 1998, pp 295–323.

an increased incidence of surgery for wound problems than controls. Hospital stays and survival rates were similar.

Donor Nutritional Status

One area that is not clear is what role the nutrient intake of the donor has on the outcome of the recipient. Animal studies suggest that supplying nutrition to the donor benefits the recipient. Sadamori and colleagues compared outcomes in pigs undergoing liver transplantation who received donations from other pigs who were (1) fasting, (2) taking an oral diet, or (3) receiving 20% glucose solution intravenously.[88] The glycogen content of the donor liver after cold preservation in groups 2 and 3 was well preserved compared with group 1. The ATP content after reperfusion depleted more rapidly in groups 1 and 2 compared with group 3. Survival was highest in group 3 (37.2 ± 5.5 days) compared with groups 1 (5.8 ± 0.7 days) or 2 (9.8 ± 2.0 days). The authors concluded that oral feeding may adversely affect the function of Kuppfer cells, thereby increasing reperfusion injury, and IV glucose infusion was thus more effective than enteral feeding in donor pigs.

In another study, donor pigs were fed either orally or with IV glucose before liver donation.[89] The pigs receiving livers from glucose-infused pigs had significantly longer survival (34.8 ± 5.5 days) compared with pigs with orally fed donors (9.8 ± 2.0 days). Donor livers from pigs fed with IV glucose also had less reperfusion injury, necrosis, and hepatocyte degeneration; lower aspartate aminotransferase values 24 hours after reperfusion; and decreased serum hyaluronic acid levels. The study also suggested that serum free fatty acids provide an important energy source during early reperfusion.

A final study suggested that an increased donor liver glycogen content influenced graft survival with 24- and 36-hour preservations.[90] Donor rats were either fed with a high-carbohydrate, low-protein diet or fasted. Livers in fed donor rats had an increased glycogen content, and the decline in the glycogen content after cold storage was less in fed donors compared with fasted ones. After 24- and 36-hour preservation, survival rates were higher in rats that received livers from fed donors compared with fasted ones.

The glycogen content of donor livers can also be increased by a glucose-insulin infusion.[91] The glycogen is used the most during reperfusion, least during cold ischemia, and intermediately during warm ischemia. Well-glycogenated livers were protected from injury during periods of prolonged warm ischemia.[91]

Future Research

The field of transplantation continues to broaden as limits are pushed. There are new medical procedures, expanded patient populations, and new drugs. These changes affect nutrient needs and the delivery of nutrition.

Areas for further research include defining the nutritional status and specific nutrient needs of transplant recipients. The effects on nutritional interventions and the effect of specific nutrients such as glutamine, arginine, and fatty acids should be evaluated. In addition, there is little research regarding the nutritional status of the transplant donor. Other areas of potential research are the involvement of nutrients such as vitamin E, glutamine, N-acetylcysteine, and folic acid in their roles as free radical scavengers.[48]

◆ BONE MARROW AND PERIPHERAL BLOOD STEM CELL TRANSPLANTATION

Bone marrow transplantation (BMT) and peripheral blood stem cell transplantation (PBSCT) are performed to treat a variety of disease states including malignant and nonmalignant hematologic disorders, solid tumors such as breast and testicular cancers, lymphomas, and genetic disorders.[92–94] The use of PBSCT in autoimmune diseases is now under investigation[95, 96]; however, most adults receive BMT or PBSCT because of the presence of a malignant disease. BMT and PBSCT are employed to treat cancers for two reasons. First, the intensive therapy before transplantation, high-dose chemotherapy with or without total body irradiation (TBI) to obtain more tumor kill than that achieved with standard doses, can be administered without regard for the lethal myelosuppression produced by these high doses of therapy. The reinfusion of marrow or blood stem cells leads to repopulation of the marrow and sustained hematopoietic function.[94] Second, allogeneic transplants also provide an antitumor effect, referred to as the *graft-versus-tumor effect*, separate from that of the intensive chemotherapy and TBI.[97, 98]

Marrow and stem cells can be obtained from the patient (autologous), an identical twin (syngeneic), or a matched donor (allogeneic—family member [usually a sibling] or an unrelated donor). The source of marrow or stem cells is mostly determined by the disease state. For example, leukemias and other hematologic disorders are typically treated with allogeneic transplants, whereas solid tumors are most often treated using autologous marrow or stem cells.

The normal course of treatment is as follows: administration of high-dose chemotherapy with or without TBI (often referred to as the *conditioning* or *preparative* regimen); IV infusion of marrow or stem cells (referred to as *day zero*); neutropenia; engraftment and early recovery; and long-term recovery. Figure 27–3 illustrates the phases of BMT and PBSCT as well as the key events occurring within each phase. Patients receiving autologous marrow or stem cells have either bone marrow harvest or stem cell collection before the initiation of treat-

ment. The autologous marrow or stem cells are cryopreserved until the day of transplantation. Autologous PBSCT is now more common than autologous BMT because PBSCT, in combination with hematologic growth factors, typically leads to a more rapid recovery of neutrophils.[99] Bone marrow is more commonly used in syngeneic and allogeneic transplantations, although allogeneic PBSCT is becoming more prevalent. Donors' marrow is normally harvested the day of transplantation and does not require any cryopreservation. Throughout this chapter, the term *BMT* is used more often than *PBSCT*, but the terms should be considered interchangeable.

Nutritional Assessment

Nutritional Status

An initial nutritional assessment should be performed on all BMT patients to identify those who are malnourished or underweight and to establish goals for the maintenance of the nutritional status in well-nourished individuals. A study conducted by Deeg and colleagues analyzed survival in relation to patient weight in 1662 adults through 150 days after transplantation.[100] Adults who

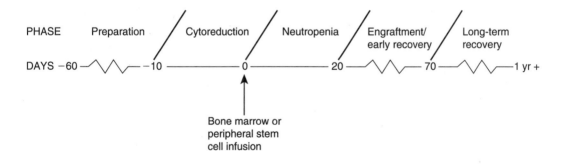

Figure 27–3. Bone marrow transplantation and peripheral blood stem cell transplantation can be characterized by events that occur in five general phases or time periods. The day of transplant is referred to as day zero. GI, gastrointestinal; GVHD, graft-versus-host disease; VOD, veno-occlusive disease. (From Lenssen P: Bone marrow and stem cell transplantation. *In* Matarese LE, Gottschlich MM [eds]: Contemporary Nutrition Support Practice: A Clinical Guide. Philadelphia, WB Saunders, 1998, pp 561–581.)

were 95% to more than 145% of their ideal body weight were found to have similar survival rates, whereas those who were less than 95% of their ideal body weight had significantly lower survival rates. This study illustrates that the initial nutritional status impacts the outcome of BMT patients.

Even well-nourished individuals are at high risk for nutritional depletion owing to the common and often prolonged period of GI toxicities and inadequate oral intake. Weisdorf and colleagues evaluated the effect of prophylactic TPN in a group of BMT patients compared with a control group who received IV hydration with a 5% dextrose solution containing electrolytes, vitamins, minerals, and trace elements.[101] All study patients had a normal nutritional status at the beginning of the study. Parenteral nutrition was initiated 1 week before the BMT. The majority of the control patients (40 of 66) ultimately were also given TPN because of documented nutritional depletion. Overall survival, disease-free survival, and the time to disease relapse were significantly better in the TPN group compared with the control group. The investigators suggested that the prophylactic TPN may have had an effect on graft and immune function, which led to the improved outcomes in the TPN group.[101] The results of this study have led to the very common use of TPN for BMT patients.

Patients are usually not able to take in adequate nutrients during the conditioning regimen before transplantation and for approximately 1 month after the transplantation.[102] Table 27–10 lists common GI complications associated with BMT and their possible causes.[103] In addition to inadequate oral nutrient intake, patients experience nutrient losses due to GI complications and often require nutritional support.

Objective Nutritional Assessment Parameters

In the BMT setting, many factors influence the reliability of objective nutritional assessment tools. Objective parameters at baseline (before the initiation of chemotherapy and TBI) are usually reliable and along with subjective information can be used to judge the nutritional status of the BMT patient. However, once the intensive therapy begins, the objective parameters are often confounded by other circumstances.

Table 27–10. Nutritional Complications of Bone Marrow and Peripheral Blood Stem Cell Transplantation and Their Causes

Gastrointestinal Side Effects	Possible Causes
Nausea and vomiting	Chemotherapy/TBI, medications, dehydration, electrolyte imbalances, mucositis, GI GVHD, GI infections, high serum glucose or amino acid levels
Oral mucositis and esophagitis	Chemotherapy, TBI, infections, GVHD, methotrexate (used for GVHD prophylaxis)
Xerostomia	TBI, antiemetics, chronic GVHD, narcotics
Early satiety	Decreased gastric motility due to prolonged absence of enteral nutrition, narcotics, high-dose chemotherapy
Thick, viscous saliva	TBI, intensive chemotherapy
Dysgeusia	TBI, intensive chemotherapy, antibiotics, narcotics
Diarrhea and steatorrhea	TBI, intensive chemotherapy, antibiotics, GI and liver GVHD, intestinal infections
Anorexia	Disease state, intensive chemotherapy, TBI, drug toxicities, infections, fluid and electrolyte imbalances, psychological and environmental factors
Micronutrient abnormalities	Medications, vomiting, diarrhea, decreased oral intake, altered absorption

GI, gastrointestinal; GVHD, graft-versus-host disease; TBI, total body irradiation.

From Roberts SR: Bone marrow and peripheral blood stem cell transplantation. *In* Lysen LK (ed): Quick Reference to Clinical Dietetics. Gaithersburg, MD, Aspen, 1997, pp 162–168. © Aspen Publishers, Inc.

Visceral Protein Levels

Levels of visceral proteins such as albumin, prealbumin (PA), transferrin, and retinol-binding protein can be influenced by nonnutritional factors, such as the inhibition of protein synthesis seen after intensive chemo- and radiotherapy, the fluid status, fever, infection, blood transfusions, high-dose corticosteroid therapy, hepatic and renal function, albumin infusions, and GVHD.[102–111] Serum albumin levels are commonly affected by the hydration status as well as blood transfusions and are not, in general, a good indicator of nutritional status in the early post-transplantation period.

Muscaritoli and colleagues studied the validity of PA and transferrin levels in the nutritional assessment of 16 adult BMT patients.[106] They found that both parameters decreased significantly from baseline to post-transplantation day 15 and attributed these changes to liver dysfunction, the inflammatory process, tissue injury, and the acute-phase response. This study concluded that serum PA and transferrin concentrations are not reliable indicators of nutritional status in the short-term period after transplantation. Another study in 42 children undergoing BMT found that serum transferrin levels correlated well with decreases in muscle protein reserves, whereas serum albumin and PA concentrations did not reflect the decreases in muscle mass.[105] Cheney and colleagues monitored serum PA levels in 40 adult BMT patients receiving TPN; levels fell to a nadir at 2 weeks after transplantation and returned to baseline level by 4 weeks after transplantation.[110] Patients with fever had lower PA levels, which led the investigators to conclude that PA is affected by the acute stress following transplantation rather than nutrient intake or nitrogen balance.[110]

Other investigators have found PA and retinol-binding protein to be useful indicators of nutritional status.[112] A study of 25 children receiving BMT for leukemia found that PA and retinol-binding protein levels responded to nutritional support with TPN even in the acute catabolic phase following BMT.[112] The investigators cautioned that these parameters were not reliable in study patients with multiorgan failure, sepsis, liver dysfunction, or renal impairment.

In summary, visceral protein concentrations can be affected by non-nutritional factors. The clinician must take into account the presence of these factors when using these laboratory values. Monitoring levels of transferrin, PA, and retinol-binding protein has been shown to be useful, whereas most investigators agree that serum albumin levels do not reflect the short-term nutritional status of the BMT patient.

Anthropometric Measurements

Anthropometric measurements can also be unreliable for nutritional assessment in the early post-transplantation period because of fluid shifts. Body weight is normally obtained daily during the acute post-transplantation period for the monitoring of fluid status. Increases in body weight are common because of the large volumes of IV fluids provided, including TPN, as well as capillary leak syndrome and organ dysfunction. Once the patient has engrafted and is clinically stable, weight is a more dependable gauge of nutritional status.

Several investigators have evaluated the use of midarm circumference and triceps skin fold measurements in BMT patients.[106, 109, 112, 113] Both Uderzo and coworkers[112] and Muscaritoli and associates[106] reported that weight, midarm circumference, and triceps skin fold were stable throughout a short study period of less than 30 days. Cunningham and colleagues[113] studied the effect of physical therapy on muscle protein losses in 30 BMT patients receiving TPN. Patients were randomized to a control group (no physical therapy), physical therapy three times per week, or physical therapy five times per week. Body weight, arm muscle area, and arm fat area did not change significantly over the 35-day post-transplantation study period in any of the groups. Although the amount of the decrease was not statistically significant, the arm muscle area decreased only in the control group. Another finding of the study was that the patients who received calories that more closely met their energy needs experienced less muscle loss. However, changes in arm muscle area were not related to the protein intake.

Cheney and colleagues used anthropometric measurements in combination with isotope dilution to assess body composition and fluid changes in nine BMT patients receiving TPN during the first 4 post-transplantation weeks.[109] This study determined that decreases in arm muscle area, lean body mass, and body cell mass correlated well. Body weight, which did not change significantly over the study period, did not correlate with decreased body cell mass or the observed shift of fluid from the intracellular compartment to the extracellular space. Changes in the arm fat area did not correlate well with the results from the isotope dilution and instead correlated with fluid shifts. Calorie and protein intakes were also not correlated with the changes in body composition.

Although measurements of the arm muscle area may be helpful in assessing the nutritional status of patients in the early post-transplantation period, baseline (before transplantation) and serial (after the first month of transplantation) measures of mid-arm circumference and triceps skin fold are more beneficial in determining changes in body composition.

Other Parameters

Other objective parameters used in the nutritional assessment of BMT patients include nitrogen balance, creatinine excretion, and 3-methylhistidine excretion.[102, 104, 109, 113–116] Negative nitrogen balance occurs in BMT patients despite adequate nutritional support, and it may be unrealistic to attempt to obtain a positive nitrogen balance in the early post-transplantation period.[107] Keller and colleagues assessed protein breakdown using plasma leucine kinetics in six patients five times within a 14-day study period, which included both the chemoradiotherapy phase and the post-transplantation phase.[115] The results indicated that negative nitrogen balance occurred in these patients because of an increased breakdown of protein and not because of a decline in protein synthesis as reported by other investigators.[117] Geibig and coworkers compared the metabolic effects of a high-nitrogen TPN formula with a standard protein TPN formula in 28 BMT patients.[116] The high-nitrogen TPN group received 330 mg of nitrogen per kilogram per day and the standard TPN group received 267 mg of nitrogen per kilogram per day. The high-nitrogen TPN group maintained a more positive nitrogen balance than the standard TPN group without deleterious metabolic changes.

In another study, Cheney and associates investigated the differences in nitrogen balance between 21 men and 19 women undergoing BMT.[114] Nitrogen balance decreased significantly over the 14-day post-transplantation period in both men and women but was more negative in the group of men than in the women, suggesting that men may have higher nutrient needs during a catabolic period.

Alterations in urinary creatinine and 3-methylhistidine excretion have also been shown in the BMT population.[113, 114] It is assumed that the amount of creatinine excretion is associated with muscle mass.[118] Cunningham and associates found a significant decrease in creatinine excretion in a group of patients receiving TPN but no physical therapy when compared with patients receiving TPN and physical therapy.[113]

Cheney and associates evaluated 3-methylhistidine excretion in men versus women and found that both groups experienced an increase in 3-methylhistidine excretion. The men experienced an average rise of 23%, whereas the women's increase was 11%.[114]

These tests demonstrate that protein losses are occurring in the BMT patient, but the clinician must be cognizant of other factors that may affect these tests. Nitrogen balance studies can be affected by renal function, protein intake, diuretic use, the presence of diarrhea and vomiting, and significant GI losses of protein seen in BMT patients after transplantation.[103, 104, 111] Creatinine excretion can be altered by renal and hepatic function, aging, protein intake, diarrhea, and fever.[102, 103] Aging, sex, protein intake, renal status, and infection may modify urinary 3-methylhistidine excretion.[102, 113]

Total lymphocyte count and skin antigen testing are rendered useless in the BMT setting owing to the profound immunosuppression after the conditioning regimen as well as to immunosuppressive medications.

Subjective Nutritional Assessment Parameters

The following is a suggested list of information to obtain from the patient before BMT[102, 103]:

- Current appetite and recent appetite changes
- Usual weight and recent weight loss or gain
- GI complications currently present or present with previous oncologic treatments
- Vitamin and mineral and alternative nutritional therapy supplementation
- Food allergies and intolerances
- Special dietary requirements
- Recent activity level
- Use of oral nutritional supplements
- Diabetes history
- Recent or current medications
- Previous need for nutritional support therapy
- Physical examination to determine the presence of muscle loss and energy reserves

This information in conjunction with objective assessment parameters should allow an accurate determination of the patient's nutritional status before transplantation.

Nutrient Requirements

Energy

The BMT patient population tends to have normal nutritional status before BMT. Therefore, the usual goal of nutritional therapy is the maintenance of the nutritional status and the lean body mass.

Szeluga and colleagues determined the energy requirements in the first 30 days after the transplantation of 91 BMT patients receiving TPN.[119] A simple linear model (nitrogen balance vs. energy intake) was employed to determine the predicted energy needs of each patient. From the linear model, adult and adolescent BMT patients required 30 to 50 kcal/kg/day. Higher energy requirements were seen in patients with GVHD and in those who required a larger percentage of their energy needs to be provided by TPN. Other investigators used 40 kcal/kg/day but found this to be excessive and recommended 30 to 35 kcal/kg/day as an adequate energy intake for BMT patients.[120]

Based on these studies, most BMT centers provide patients with 30 to 35 kcal/kg/day, or 1.3 to 1.5 times the predicted basal energy expenditure as determined by the Harris-Benedict equation.[104, 106, 115, 121, 122] Indirect calorimetry is also useful in determining energy requirements and may be most beneficial in BMT patients who are critically ill, have GVHD, or require long-term TPN because these are the patients at most risk for nutritional depletion and complications associated with over- or underfeeding.

Carbohydrate

The provision of 50 to 60% of total calories in a TPN solution as carbohydrate or dextrose is acceptable. However, both autologous and allogeneic BMT recipients experience impaired glucose tolerance.[104, 123–125] Impaired glucose tolerance in allogeneic patients is typically related to the use of immunosuppressive medications, such as corticosteroids, cyclosporine, and tacrolimus. Autologous patients with normal glucose levels before transplantation may develop impaired glucose tolerance after transplanta-tion because of diminished pancreatic beta cell function after BMT.[124]

Patients who have diabetes mellitus may have an increased rate of complications. A study of nine patients with diabetes mellitus or impaired glucose tolerance receiving autologous BMT for lymphoid malignancies determined that the incidence of complications and organ failure was higher than expected in this group. The investigators theorized that the presence of diabetes and glucose intolerance predisposed these patients, whose performance status and organ function were good before BMT, to more complications.[125] Because of the possibility of a higher complication rate in patients with glucose intolerance, it is important to adjust TPN regimens, possibly by increasing the lipid component of the solutions and adjusting insulin therapy to control blood glucose levels.

Protein

Protein needs are elevated in BMT patients because of the high-dose chemotherapy and TBI, the need for tissue repair and generation, and the very common incidence of infection after transplantation. As discussed in the nutritional assessment section, negative nitrogen balance and decreased visceral protein levels are present after transplantation and do not reverse to a positive state in the first 2 to 4 weeks after transplantation, even with the provision of adequate calories and protein via TPN.[101, 105, 106, 109, 110, 113, 114, 116] Most centers recommend 1.5 to 2 g of protein per kilogram of body weight for the repletion of protein stores as well as tissue repair.[102, 104, 106, 107, 109, 115, 116] Because catabolic surgical patients have been shown to benefit from BCAA-enriched solutions, Lenssen and colleagues evaluated in 40 BMT patients the effect of BCAAs on nitrogen balance, the ratio of urinary 3-methylhistidine to creatinine levels, upper arm anthropometry, PA levels, and the time to engraftment.[126] Patients were randomized to a 45% or a 23% BCAA solution. Protein was provided at 1.5 g/kg of ideal body weight in both groups. No significant differences were seen between the two groups, and the investigators concluded that there is not a routine indication for the use of BCAA solutions in BMT patients.

Other factors that influence protein needs are high-dose steroid therapy for the treatment of GVHD (a major complication after allogeneic BMT) and organ dysfunction. The combination of GVHD and high-dose corticosteroid therapy leads to increased protein losses, and adequate protein intake is important to avoid severe protein wasting.[102, 104, 120, 127, 128] Impairment of the kidneys, liver, or neurologic system may require a lower protein level to avoid worsening of organ and metabolic function.

The use of glutamine-supplemented TPN in BMT patients has been evaluated because of glutamine's possible status as a "conditionally essential" amino acid during catabolic stress.[129–135] A double-blind randomized trial involving 45 BMT patients provided a standard amino acid TPN solution to the control group and a glutamine-supplemented TPN solution to the treatment group. Glutamine was supplemented at 0.57 g/kg of body weight per day. Calories were provided at 1.5 times the basal energy expenditure, and protein was given at 1.5 g/kg to both groups. The investigators found improved nitrogen balance, fewer clinical infections, a decreased length of stay in the hospital, and an improved mood state in the patients receiving glutamine-supplemented TPN.[130, 133]

In a retrospective study of a subset of 20 patients in this same trial, the glutamine-supplemented patients displayed an increase in total lymphocytes, greater amounts of total lymphocytes, and higher CD4$^+$ and CD8$^+$ T lymphocytes in peripheral blood, compared with patients given standard TPN (i.e., glutamine-free).[132] A criticism of the trial is that a difference existed in the amino acid composition between the two groups, with the control group receiving more essential amino acids than the glutamine-supplemented group.

Another, more recent study by Schloerb and colleagues evaluated both enteral and parenteral glutamine supplementation in BMT patients.[136] Sixty-six patients were randomized, double-blinded, to either oral glutamine or a glycine control at a dose of 10 g three times per day. Patients in the treatment group who required TPN were given glutamine-supplemented TPN with a glutamine dose of 0.57 g/kg of body weight per day. The control group received isocaloric, isonitrogenous, standard TPN. These investigators found no benefit from glutamine supplementation in relation to hospital stay, number of days on TPN, engraftment, infec-

tion rate, sepsis mucositis, diarrhea, or incidence of acute graft-versus-host disease. A suggestion of improved survival seen in the glutamine-treated group prompted the investigators to encourage more study of the long-term effects of glutamine on BMT patients.

Possible mechanisms by which glutamine may benefit BMT patients include improved gut integrity and improvements in immune function. Because glutamine-supplemented TPN is not currently available in the United States, the use of glutamine-supplemented TPN has not become widespread. Additionally, more controlled trials are needed to further determine glutamine's efficacy and mechanisms of action in the BMT patient.

Lipid

Clemans and colleagues showed that BMT patients develop essential fatty acid deficiency when fed a fat-free parenteral nutrition solution.[137] These same investigators demonstrated that a 10% fat emulsion providing 10% of total calories as fat and 5% as linoleic acid was adequate to prevent essential fatty acid deficiency in BMT patients.[138] The provision of calories to BMT patients by lipid emulsions is common and appears to be well tolerated. Researchers investigating various aspects of TPN use in BMT patients report a range of 15 to 40% of calories from lipids.[106, 107, 114, 122, 139]

IV lipid emulsions have been associated with a depressed immune function,[140] and concern regarding their use in the BMT population is not surprising in light of the high incidence of infectious complications in this group of patients. Two preliminary studies suggested an increased infection risk in BMT patients receiving IV lipids.[141, 142] In another study, Lenssen and colleagues investigated the relationship between IV lipids and infections in 512 allogeneic and autologous BMT patients.[143] Patients were randomized to a low IV lipid dose (6 to 8% of total calories) or a standard IV lipid dose (25 to 30% of total calories). The incidence of bacteremia and fungemia within the first 30 days after transplantation or until discharge was the primary end-point. The incidence of infection was not different between the groups, leading the researchers to conclude that the standard IV lipid dose does not lead to an increased rate of infections in the BMT patient.[143]

Hypertriglyceridemia is common in the allogeneic BMT patient because of the use of immunosuppressive medications. Cyclosporine and corticosteroids are known to raise lipid levels.[144, 145] One study of allogeneic BMT recipients found a 58% incidence of hypertriglyceridemia.[146] Of all the variables evaluated (age, sex, hyperglycemia, TPN, corticosteroids, estrogen, and cyclosporine), only cyclosporine was significantly related to the development of elevated triglyceride levels. The common presence of hypertriglyceridemia in the allogeneic patient presents a problem for the clinician when deciding doses of IV lipids to provide. In our experience, patients with significantly elevated triglyceride levels often have multiorgan dysfunction or failure, and the elimination of IV lipids does not result in a significant decrease in the triglyceride level. However, because there are possible adverse side effects seen with elevated triglyceride levels, when a triglyceride level is greater than 500 mg/dL, it may be advisable to withhold the IV lipids for 1 to 2 days and then add a smaller dose, 100 to 200 mL of 20% lipid daily. Another option is to provide a minimum of 250 mL of 20% IV lipid two times per week to avoid essential fatty acid deficiency. Slow, continuous infusions of IV lipid (over 16 to 24 hours) tend to be better tolerated and lead to less hypertriglyceridemia.[147]

Two studies, one in mice and the other in humans, have demonstrated that IV lipids have an effect on the immune system in BMT.[148, 149] Tezuka and colleagues showed that the administration of 20% lipids to recipient mice decreased genetic resistance to bone marrow grafts and natural killer cell activity.[148] Muscaritoli and colleagues investigated two different TPN nutrient mixtures, a 100% glucose–based TPN solution compared with an 80% lipid and 20% glucose–based TPN solution, in 60 allogeneic BMT patients.[149] Outcomes evaluated were the time to engraftment, the incidence of sepsis and metabolic complications (hyperglycemia and hypertriglyceridemia), the incidence of acute GVHD and relapse, the survival at 18 months, and the frequency of deaths from acute GVHD and relapse. Hyperglycemia occurrence was significantly higher in the glucose-based TPN group than in the lipid-based TPN group (32% vs. 3.4%). The other significant finding was five deaths from acute GVHD in the glucose-

based TPN group compared with no deaths due to acute GVHD in the lipid-based group. There was also a trend toward improved survival at 18 months after transplantation in the lipid-based TPN group compared with the glucose-based TPN group (62% vs. 42%). The other outcomes were not significantly different between the groups. The researchers hypothesized that the higher dose of IV lipids resulted in changes in the immune response and the production of cytokines, prostaglandins, and leukotrienes, which contribute to the development of GVHD. These findings warrant further research regarding the association of IV lipids and immune response in allogeneic BMT patients.

Vitamins, Minerals, Trace Elements, and Electrolytes

Research regarding vitamin and mineral needs in BMT patients is limited. Deficiencies of vitamins, minerals, and trace elements have been reported in case reports or small clinical trials.[150–156] Side effects of the pretransplantation conditioning regimen as well as medications and post-transplantation organ dysfunction contribute to these deficiencies.

There have been reports of B vitamin deficiencies in some patients after BMT. Leukemia patients undergoing allogeneic BMT have been found to have decreased vitamin B_{12} absorption through the ileum, and normal absorption did not return until 2 months after transplantation.[150] Wernicke's encephalopathy due to thiamine deficiency occurred in eight patients at one center.[151] The patients were receiving TPN with a multivitamin (MVI) additive that was understood to contain 50 mg of thiamine. However, for an unknown length of time, the MVI solution did not contain thiamine. All eight patients developed a "raspberry tongue" and severe metabolic acidosis before death. Another single-case report documents severe lactic acidosis due to thiamine deficiency in a child undergoing BMT for leukemia.[152] The patient was receiving thiamine via an oral MVI supplement only, and the acidosis was corrected by an intramuscular injection of 100 mg of thiamine. These two reports emphasize the need to adequately supplement thiamine in the BMT population. Body stores of thiamine can be depleted in a short time, 10 days or less, in a catabolic patient receiving large glucose loads such as those found in TPN.[151, 152] A malnourished and/or catabolic patient may require more thiamine than is provided in a standard parenteral MVI solution.

Vitamin K deficiency has been reported in one child after allogeneic BMT.[153] BMT patients are susceptible to vitamin K deficiency in the post-transplantation period due to their minimal oral intake and the use of antibiotics for the prevention and treatment of infections. A 10-mg dose of vitamin K should be provided once weekly in TPN solutions. Patients with a prolonged prothrombin time may require more vitamin K supplementation to correct the deficiency.[153]

One investigator reported a significant decrease in plasma vitamin E and β-carotene levels in 19 BMT patients after the conditioning regimen.[154] The patients were receiving TPN at the time the decreased levels were observed, suggesting that the amount of vitamin E present in parenteral MVI preparations is not adequate for BMT patients. β-Carotene is not available in commercial parenteral MVI solutions. The investigator attributed these results to damage caused by the conditioning regimen and proposed further studies to determine the effect of supplementation of high-dose β-carotene and vitamin E on toxicities associated with intensive chemotherapy and radiotherapy.

Another study compared the effect of high-dose vitamin C (25 g) and vitamin E (1000 IU) added to TPN on peroxidation and free radical activity after BMT in 10 supplemented patients compared with 10 controls.[157] Levels of plasma lipoperoxides, vitamin C, and vitamin E were measured before and for 6 weeks after BMT. The amount of lipoperoxides was increased significantly in both groups after the conditioning regimen compared with baseline levels. The blood levels of vitamins C and E were depleted in both groups but returned to a normal level more quickly in the supplemented group.

The conditioning regimens, TBI and alkylating chemotherapy agents, used in the BMT patient are therapies that destroy cells via oxidative damage. An essential question is whether high doses of antioxidant supplements during the conditioning therapy will interfere with tumor destruction by protecting cancer cells as well as healthy cells.[158, 159] Therefore, caution is recommended with high-dose supplementation of antioxidants during the conditioning regimen until further research is available with information not only about short-term toxicities but also regarding the long-term disease status. After the conditioning regimen is completed, antioxidant supplementation could still be harmful because vitamin C acts as a pro-oxidant in a high-iron environment as seen with frequent blood transfusions, and megadoses of vitamin E can be prohemorrhagic.[160] The provision of parenteral MVI to meet the recommended daily allowance and weekly vitamin K supplementation are recommended, with possibly increased needs for thiamine.

Trace element disturbances may be seen in the BMT population due to medication side effects as well as organ dysfunction because trace element homeostasis is regulated by either the kidneys or the liver. One study found that with the exception of zinc, routine trace element supplementation is adequate in BMT patients.[155] Another study in pediatric BMT patients found zinc depletion to be more prevalent in patients with longer febrile episodes, positive blood cultures, and more diarrhea.[156] Additional zinc supplementation may be necessary in individuals with large volumes of diarrhea due to the conditioning regimen or GVHD or in those with infectious complications. Because manganese and copper are excreted through bile via the liver, cholestasis, common in the BMT patient, may necessitate elimination or decreased levels of these two trace elements in TPN solutions. Manganese toxicity, resulting in a Parkinson-like syndrome, has been reported in a BMT patient.[161, 162] Copper levels were not found to be elevated in a small number of cholestatic allogeneic BMT patients,[162] possibly because it is also excreted in the urine. Monitoring of the trace element status is difficult in the clinical setting because serum levels may not accurately reflect tissue stores.[163–165] When providing trace elements to the BMT patient, one should supplement to meet the recommended daily allowance and be aware of conditions that may change the patient's requirements.

Electrolyte needs and replacement are directed by the clinical status and serum electrolyte levels (Table 27–11). Electrolyte levels should be monitored daily in patients receiving TPN. With the exception of potassium and magnesium, usual daily electro-

Table 27–11. Common Electrolyte Alterations and Potential Causes in Bone Marrow Transplantation Recipients

Electrolyte Abnormality	Potential Causes
Hypokalemia[103, 163]	Vomiting, diarrhea Diuretics, corticosteroids, amphotericin B, aminoglycosides
Hyperkalemia[164]	Nephrotoxicity usually associated with cyclosporine or tacrolimus
Hypomagnesemia[105, 165]	Cyclosporine or tacrolimus Poor oral intake Malabsorption Amphotericin B and aminoglycosides
Hypocalcemia	Hypoalbuminemia
Hyponatremia	Alterations in fluid status due to administration of large amounts of intravenous fluids and diuretics

lyte provisions generally meet the requirements of BMT patients.

Complications of Bone Marrow and Peripheral Stem Cell Transplantation Impacting Nutritional Status and Needs

Several common complications after BMT and PBSCT influence patients' nutrient needs and the route of administration of nutrition.

Infection and Sepsis

Post-transplantation infectious complications are common because of profound neutropenia occurring for approximately 2 weeks after transplantation, damage to mucosal linings, and the necessity for continued immunosuppression in the allogeneic patient to prevent and treat GVHD. All types of infectious agents (bacterial, fungal, and viral) are seen in BMT patients.[166, 167] Cytomegalovirus infections occur in 70 to 80% of allogeneic BMT recipients.[167] The presence of the infection in combination with the appropriate antimicrobial therapy often has a negative influence on the patient's oral intake. Depending on the GI function at the time of the infection, TPN may or may not be appropriate. As with other septic patients, the provision of TPN to the septic BMT patient requires attention to the patient's clinical condition, organ function, metabolic derangements, and volume status.

Hepatic Veno-occlusive Disease

Hepatic veno-occlusive disease (VOD) is a clinical syndrome that develops within the first 20 days after transplantation, with the following features: hepatomegaly, jaundice, weight gain, and painful ascites.[168] Elevated bilirubin levels and liver function tests are also seen. The reported incidence ranges from 10 to 60% and depends on a number of factors, such as the patient population and pretransplantation conditioning regimens.[169] Cytoreductive therapy, chemotherapy, and TBI are the causative factors. They damage the endothelial cells, sinusoids, and hepatocytes in zone 3 of the liver acinus, the area encircling the terminal hepatic venules.[170] This damage leads to narrowing of the hepatic venules, congestion of sinusoids, and intrahepatic portal hypertension.[171] Veno-occlusive disease can vary in severity from a mild reversible form to an irreversible form leading to multiorgan failure and death. Risk factors for the development of VOD include pretransplantation elevated transaminase levels, the use of vancomycin or acyclovir during the conditioning regimen, specific cytoreductive therapies, persistent fevers after transplantation, and the use of either a mismatched or an unrelated allogeneic donor.[170] Medical management of the VOD patient focuses on the avoidance of fluid overload to prevent pulmonary edema and ascites and intravascular volume depletion because hepatorenal syndrome is common in this setting.[102, 170]

Nutritional management of VOD can be complex as well. Because fluid and sodium restrictions are often required, TPN solutions must be altered to comply with medical goals. The contribution of sodium from all sources should be considered, including oral intake, IV fluids, TPN, and medications. Overfeeding of calories may contribute to hepatic complications and should be avoided in the setting of VOD. Often, because of the high nutrient requirements of BMT patients and the need for fluid restrictions in VOD, underfeeding of calories and protein is more common than overfeeding. Indirect calorimetry to obtain a more accurate energy requirement may be warranted.

Table 27–12. Nutrient Considerations and Recommendations for Bone Marrow Transplantation Patients with Veno-occlusive Disease

Specific Nutrient	Considerations	Recommendations
Protein	Goal is to provide adequate protein to avoid or lessen contribution of catabolism to encephalopathy BCAA solutions not shown to affect mental status in small study of nine VOD patients[173]	Provide 1–1.5 g protein/kg/day Use of BCAA solutions in TPN may be warranted in patients with hepatic encephalopathy
Carbohydrate	Hepatic dysfunction may contribute to hyperglycemia Composition of TPN solution may help control hyperglycemia	Provide dextrose at rate of 3–5 mg/kg/min to avoid exceeding liver's oxidative capacity Provide insulin therapy Change TPN solution to higher lipid content, if tolerated
Lipid	Lipid clearance may be decreased in BMT patients with hepatic dysfunction Balanced TPN solutions, including lipid, help prevent hepatic complications associated with TPN Numerous causes of hypertriglyceridemia in BMT patient (see lipid metabolism and needs)	Provide lipids, if clearance is acceptable, at 15–40% of total calories
Trace elements	Copper and manganese excretion via bile impaired in presence of cholestasis and decreased bile excretion	Eliminate copper and manganese from TPN solution when bilirubin level reaches 10–15 mg/dL Add other trace elements separately
Antioxidants	Tissue injury, such as VOD, possibly related to decreased antioxidant levels and increased free radical production Case study of one patient with VOD suggested oral vitamin E (400 mg/day) and glutamine (20 g/day) supplementation was beneficial in treatment of VOD[177]	More research needed to confirm this single case study report Consider patient's platelet function before provision of megadoses of vitamin E

BCAA, branched-chain amino acids; TPN, total parenteral nutrition; VOD, veno-occlusive disease.

Table 27–12 gives specific nutrient concerns and recommendations for the BMT patient with VOD.[154, 157, 160, 172–177] The decision regarding the use of cyclic TPN in VOD depends greatly on the clinical status of the patient. If fluid status is tenuous, a slow, continuous TPN infusion may be better tolerated. A long cycle of 16 to 18 hours, to provide the liver a "rest" from TPN, could be tried if the patient's fluid and overall clinical status allow it.

Graft-Versus-Host Disease

GVHD, a major complication after allogeneic BMT, is classified as either acute or chronic; the two types manifest themselves in different ways.

Acute Graft-Versus-Host Disease

Acute GVHD presents in the first 100 days after transplantation and is a syndrome that affects the skin, GI tract, and liver. The development of acute GVHD is attributed to the donor T cells' recognizing the host (patient) as foreign. The incidence and severity of acute GVHD depend on a number of factors, with the degree of human leukocyte antigen (HLA) disparity playing the biggest role. Other factors include gender mismatching, donor parity, age (young patients have a reduced incidence), immunosuppressive therapy, and the incidence of infection after transplantation.[178, 179] Acute GVHD occurs in 25 to 60% of HLA genotypically identical transplantation patients. Approximately 50% of patients who develop moderately severe to severe acute GVHD die, usually because of infectious complications.[180] Acute GVHD is graded (grades I through IV) based on the sites affected and the clinical features present. Grade I is the mildest form, has a good prognosis, and usually does not require treatment. In contrast, Grade IV GVHD is usually fatal.[179] Table 27–13 shows

Table 27–13. Clinical Staging of Acute Graft-Versus-Host Disease

Stage	Skin	Liver Bilirubin (mg/dL)	Gut
+	Maculopapular rash <25% body surface	2–3	Diarrhea, 500–1000 mL/day
+ +	Maculopapular rash 25–50% body surface	3–6	Diarrhea, 1000–1500 mL/day
+ + +	Generalized erythroderma	6–15	Diarrhea, >1500 mL/day
+ + + +	Desquamation and bullae	>15	Pain or ileus

From Sullivan KM: Graft-versus-host disease. *In* Forman SJ, Thomas ED (eds): Bone Marrow Transplantation. Boston, Blackwell Scientific, 1994, pp 339–362.

the clinical staging of acute GVHD. The prevention and treatment of GVHD include the use of immunosuppressive medications such as cyclosporine, tacrolimus, methotrexate, corticosteroids, mycophenolate mofetil, muromonab-CD3, and antithymocyte globulin (ATG).

The nutritional management of acute GVHD varies depending on the affected sites and the severity. GVHD increases energy and protein requirements.[119, 181–183] Patients with significant acute GVHD may require up to 50 kcal/kg for the form of TPN.[119, 181] Treatment of acute GVHD with high-dose corticosteroids and the protein losses that occur through the intestinal tract can result in protein needs that may be as high as 2 g/kg.[102, 182]

Skin GVHD is characterized by a maculopapular rash appearing first on the palms, soles, ears, and trunk. It can progress to generalized erythroderma with desquamation and bullae, resembling a burn injury.[177, 180] Patients with acute GI GVHD may experience secretory diarrhea (often liters per day); guaiac-positive stools; abdominal cramping and pain; anorexia; nausea and vomiting; GI protein-losing enteropathy; hypoalbuminemia; and ileus.[104, 128, 180, 182] Patients with acute GI GVHD and large volumes of diarrhea should be given TPN. Acute GVHD of the liver results in elevated liver function tests and bilirubin levels, cholestasis, and malabsorption and in severe cases can lead to ascites, encephalopathy, and decreased synthesis of clotting factors.[177, 179]

Table 27–14 outlines other nutritional recommendations for patients with acute

GVHD.[103] It is often difficult to provide adequate calories and protein to patients with moderate to severe GVHD because of the metabolic and organ dysfunction that often accompany GVHD. Patients may have significant pulmonary, hepatic, or renal impairment due to infections, which is common in GVHD, or related to medications used to treat GVHD and infections. Additionally, hypertriglyceridemia and hyperglycemia are common and related to the immunosuppressive medications employed to treat GVHD. The care of a patient with acute GVHD is challenging and complex. The clinician should strive to meet the nutrient requirements of the patient without further compromising the clinical status and organ function.

Chronic Graft-Versus-Host Disease

Researchers describe chronic GVHD as either a late phase of acute GVHD or a distinct autoimmune-like process.[178, 179] Chronic

Table 27–14. Nutritional Recommendations for Patients with Acute Graft-Versus-Host Disease

Targeted Organ Site	Recommendations
Skin (severe rash)	Increase energy and protein intake Increase fluid intake Possibly provide additional vitamin C and zinc supplementation for healing
Gastrointestinal system	Increase energy and protein intake Maintain NPO status until diarrhea is <1 L/day and GI symptoms following oral intake are manageable Maintain serum albumin level >2 g/dL Control GI symptoms with antiemetics, antidiarrheals, and H₂ blockers as needed Once an oral diet is begun, restriction of fat, fiber, lactose, acidic foods, and gastric irritants may be needed initially
Liver	Avoid overfeeding with TPN Monitor tolerance of IV lipids Decrease or remove copper and manganese from TPN solution Provide adequate vitamin K Restrict fluid and sodium if needed BCAA solutions may be useful in presence of encephalopathy

GI, gastrointestinal; IV, intravenous; NPO, nothing by mouth; TPN, total parenteral nutrition.

GVHD develops after 100 post-transplantation days, and its incidence is variable, depending on the type of transplant received. Recipients of HLA-identical sibling transplants have a 33% incidence of chronic GVHD, whereas 49% of HLA-nonidentical transplant recipients develop chronic GVHD. Matched unrelated donor transplant recipients and one-antigen–mismatched donor recipients have an incidence of 64% and as high as 80%, respectively.[179] Obviously, chronic GVHD is a prevalent problem in the allogeneic BMT population. Other factors that can influence the incidence of chronic GVHD are prior acute GVHD and increasing patient age.[178, 179]

The clinical features of chronic GVHD can include skin changes, hepatic cholestasis, ocular sicca, xerostomia, oral sensitivity to acidic or spicy foods, oral lesions, bronchiolitis obliterans, physical debilitation, and esophageal strictures.[179] The skin is the main organ involved in chronic GVHD and can present either as lichenoid changes similar to lichen planus or as sclerodermatous alterations resembling scleroderma. Initially, plaques and areas of desquamation are seen. Eventually, either hypo- or hyperpigmentation and skin and joint contractures develop.[178] Extensive chronic skin GVHD can be very debilitating. Infectious complications are also common in patients with chronic GVHD owing to multiple immune defects.

Table 27–15 outlines the clinicopathologic classification of chronic GVHD. Chronic GVHD is classified as either limited or extensive. As expected, patients with limited chronic GVHD have a better prognosis than those with extensive disease. A study of 85 patients with chronic GVHD reported a 42% survival rate at 6 years after transplantation.[184] The treatment of chronic GVHD usually includes prednisone, cyclosporine, or tacrolimus in combination with prednisone, and more recently mycophenolate mofetil. Both ATG and thalidomide have been employed to treat chronic GVHD as well.[179] Most patients also require antimicrobial prophylaxis because of the immunodeficiency seen in chronic GVHD.

Nutrition-related problems are common in patients with chronic GVHD.[185] Lenssen and colleagues conducted a retrospective chart review of 192 allogeneic adult and pediatric patients to determine the incidence of nutrition-related problems.[185] Oral sensi-

Table 27–15. Clinicopathologic Classification of Chronic Graft-Versus-Host Disease

Limited chronic GVHD
  Either or both
    1. Localized skin involvement
    2. Hepatic dysfunction due to chronic GVHD
Extensive chronic GVHD
  Either
    1. Generalized skin involvement or
    2. Localized skin involvement and/or hepatic dysfunction due to chronic GVHD
  Plus
    3a. Liver histologic examination showing chronic aggressive hepatitis, bridging necrosis, or cirrhosis, or
    b. Involvement of eye (Schirmer's test with <5 mm wetting), or
    c. Involvement of minor salivary glands or oral mucosa demonstrated on labial biopsy, or
    d. Involvement of any other target organ

GVHD, graft-versus-host disease.
From Shulman HM, Sullivan KM, Weiden PL, et al: Chronic graft-versus-host syndrome in man. A long-term clinicopathologic study of 20 Seattle patients. Am J Med 69:204–217, 1980.

tivity and xerostomia were the most prevalent problems and occurred in 23 and 18% of the patients, respectively. Weight loss occurred in 28% of the patients. As expected, those with extensive chronic GVHD experienced the highest incidence of nutrition-related problems when compared with those with no chronic GVHD or limited chronic GVHD. In addition, because nutrition-related problems were more common in patients with extensive disease, inadequate intake of calories (<85% of estimated needs) and poor nutritional status were seen more frequently in this group when compared with patients without GVHD or with limited GVHD. Recommendations from the investigators include screening allogeneic BMT patients for the presence of chronic GVHD at 3 months after transplantation, frequent weight evaluations, and referral for a complete nutritional evaluation in patients with weight loss or eating problems. This study underlines the need for continual monitoring of BMT patients with chronic GVHD. The provision of nutritional support, either enteral or parenteral, may be needed in patients unable to gain or maintain body weight through oral intake.

Parenteral Nutritional Support
Indications

The use of TPN support in the allogeneic BMT patient is accepted as beneficial in terms of limiting nutritional deficits and improving survival and is appropriate in light of the complications such as GVHD, infections, and prolonged inadequate oral intake often seen in this group of patients.[101, 112] Once an allogeneic BMT patient has had an inadequate oral intake for 3 to 5 days, the use of TPN should be considered. A more controversial question is whether the autologous BMT recipient benefits from the provision of TPN. There are no published studies available to answer this question, and the use of TPN in the autologous patient varies from center to center. In either patient group, the goal of nutritional support is to avoid the depletion of nutrient stores, specifically lean body mass, and to support tissue healing and regeneration.

At our center, a group of 55 breast cancer patients undergoing autologous BMT were prospectively randomized either to TPN beginning at day 1 or to an oral diet.[186] The patients were followed until post-transplantation day 30. The patients in the oral diet group were given TPN after 10 consecutive days of oral intake meeting less than 40% of their estimated needs. Half of this group required TPN after 10 consecutive days of inadequate oral intake related to moderate to severe mucositis. The patients who received early nutritional support had significantly less weight loss and decrease in midarm muscle circumference, so it appears that early TPN preserved the nutritional status better than delayed TPN or an oral diet. Other nutritional outcomes, such as changes in triceps skin fold measurements, serum albumin levels, and the number of post-transplantation days to achieve an oral intake meeting more than 66% of estimated needs were not different. Clinical outcomes such as the days to engraftment, length of stay, and number of positive blood cultures were not different between the groups. The 2-year survival and disease-free survival rates were not different between the groups.

If the preparative regimen does not cause significant toxicities to the GI tract, both allogeneic and autologous patients who are well nourished and able to take in adequate nutrients orally can avoid TPN. It is appropriate to provide TPN to a stressed individual whose oral intake will be inadequate because of GI dysfunction for more than 7 to 10 days. Typically, patients with an early onset of severe mucositis or intractable nausea and vomiting and/or diarrhea require TPN. In addition, patients who are malnourished on admission for BMT, those with complicated post-transplantation courses, as seen with sepsis and organ failure, and patients with GI GVHD are also candidates for nutritional support.

Monitoring

Because metabolic abnormalities are not uncommon in the BMT patient, careful monitoring is necessary so that TPN solutions can be altered to avoid or correct any problems. The following parameters should be obtained on a daily basis: body weight (for monitoring of the fluid status); calorie and protein intake (oral and TPN); and serum concentrations of electrolytes, glucose, urea nitrogen, and creatinine. Two or three times per week, liver function tests and serum levels of calcium, phosphorus, magnesium, albumin, and bilirubin should be evaluated. Serum turbidity and triglyceride level should be checked weekly for the evaluation of IV lipid tolerance. Other tests that may be beneficial include serum concentrations of prealbumin, transferrin, copper, zinc, and manganese; nitrogen balance studies; creatinine excretion; and anthropometric measurements.[103, 108] As discussed earlier, many factors are present that may affect these parameters.

Discontinuing Total Parenteral Nutrition

Most BMT patients begin to tolerate oral intake once recovery of the marrow occurs and mucositis resolves. These two events, which usually occur 10 to 14 days after transplantation, allow the discontinuation of many medicines, such as antibiotics and narcotics, which can negatively affect the oral intake. Additionally, the recovery of the immune system allows healing of the entire GI tract, resulting in a decreased incidence of nausea, vomiting, and diarrhea. However, many patients continue to complain of other eating problems, including xerostomia, anorexia, early satiety, and dysgeusia. It can take 4 to 8 weeks after transplantation, even in the autologous BMT patient, for the oral intake to be adequate. At the same time, if the patient is not experiencing any adverse medical problems, such as infection or GVHD, the patient's nutritional demands have decreased compared with the neutropenic period immediately after transplantation.[102] A dietitian familiar with the eating problems of BMT patients is helpful in counseling patients and families on ways to improve their oral intake during this time.

A double-blind randomized study examined the effect of home TPN versus IV hydration on the resumption of oral intake, body weight, hospital readmissions, relapse of disease, and survival during the first 28 days after transplantation.[187] Eligible patients were defined as those 2 years of age or older, less than 65 days after transplantation, meeting less than 70% of their caloric needs orally at the time of discharge, and requiring 10 units or less of insulin per liter of TPN. The provision of outpatient TPN delayed adequate oral intake (defined as ≥85% of estimated caloric needs by 6 days) compared with the IV hydration group. The weight loss during the 4-week study period was mild in both groups but significantly higher in the IV hydration group (4.63%) compared with the TPN group (1.27%). However, the other outcomes were not different between treatment groups. The researchers concluded that the use of IV hydration in place of outpatient TPN does not lead to adverse outcomes and is recommended unless a patient has GI GVHD.[187]

Future Research Areas

Areas that warrant further research in the BMT area have been discussed in more detail earlier in this chapter. These include the effect of antioxidants on short-term toxicities and long-term survival, the role of IV lipids in relation to GVHD and survival, and glutamine's effects on the BMT patient. Another area of interest not discussed in this chapter is the use of early enteral nutritional support in conjunction with or in place of TPN.

CONCLUSION

Organ and BMT patients experience a range of nutritional problems that make them susceptible to malnutrition. TPN may to be beneficial in limiting or preventing nutritional deficits. TPN may also improve survival in the BMT population. Close monitoring of the nutritional status and nutritional support are crucial in the early post-transplantation period. In addition, transplant recipi-

ents are prone to chronic nutritional problems and often require long-term follow-up and nutritional intervention.

REFERENCES

1. Poindexter SM: Nutrition support in cardiac transplantation. Top Clin Nutr 7(3):12–16, 1992.
2. DiCecco SR, Wieners EJ, Wiesner RH, et al: Assessment of nutritional status of patients with end-stage liver disease undergoing liver transplantation. Mayo Clin Proc 64:95–102, 1989.
3. Hasse J, Strong S, Gorman MA, Liepa GU: Subjective global assessment: Alternative nutritional assessment technique for liver transplant candidates. Nutrition 9:339–343, 1993.
4. Hasse JM: Solid organ transplant. In Matarese LE, Gottschlich MM (eds): Contemporary Nutrition Support. Philadelphia, WB Saunders, 1998, pp 547–560.
5. Porayko MK, DiCecco S, O'Keefe SJ: Impact of malnutrition and its therapy on liver transplantation. Semin Liv Dis 11:305–314, 1991.
6. Baron P, Waymack JP: A review of nutrition support for transplant patients. Nutr Clin Pract 8:12–18, 1993.
7. Lowell JA, Beindorff ME: Nutritional assessment and therapy in abdominal organ transplantation. In Shikora S, Blackburn G (eds): Nutrition Support: Theory and Therapeutics. Glasgow, Scotland, Chapman & Hall, 1997, pp 422–448.
8. Akerman PA, Jenkins RL, Bistrian BR: Preoperative nutrition assessment in liver transplantation. Nutrition 9:350–356, 1993.
9. Rosenberg ME, Hostetter TH: Nutrition. In Toledo-Pereya LH (ed): Kidney Transplantation. Philadelphia, FA Davis, 1988, pp 169–186.
10. Mitch WE, May RC, Maroni BJ: Mechanisms for abnormal protein metabolism in uremia. J Am Coll Nutr 8: 305–309, 1989.
11. Frazier OH, Van Buren CT, Poindexter SM, Waldenberger F: Nutritional management of the heart transplant recipient. J Heart Transplant 4:450–452, 1985.
12. Grady KL, Herold LS: Comparison of nutritional status in patients before and after heart transplantation. J Heart Transplant 7:123–127, 1988.
13. Evans MA, Shronts EP, Fish JA: A case report: Nutrition support of a heart-lung transplant recipient. Support Line 14(1):1–8, 1992.
14. Poindexter SM: Nutrition in heart transplantation. Support Line 14(1):8–9, 1992.
15. Pikul J, Sharpe MD, Lowndes R, Chent CN: Degree of preoperative malnutrition is predictive of postoperative morbidity and mortality in liver transplant recipients. Transplantation 57:469–472, 1994.
16. Harrison J, McKiernan J, Neuberger JM: A prospective study on the effect of recipient nutritional status on outcome in liver transplantation. Transpl Int 10:369–374, 1997.
17. Selberg O, Böttcher J, Tusch G, et al: Identification of high- and low-risk patients before liver transplantation: A prospective cohort study of nutritional and metabolic parameters in 150 patients. Hepatology 25:652–657, 1997.
18. Hasse JM, Gonwa TA, Jennings LW, et al: Malnu-

trition affects liver transplant outcomes [Abstract]. Transplantation 66:553, 1998.

19. Hasse JM, Crippin JS, Blue LS, et al: Does nutrition supplementation benefit liver transplant candidates with a history of encephalopathy [Abstract]? JPEN J Parenter Enteral Nutr 21:516, 1997.

20. Shapiro AMJ, Bain VG, Sigalet DL, Kneteman NM: Rapid resolution of chylous ascites after liver transplantation using somatostatin analog and total parenteral nutrition. Transplantation 61:1410–1411, 1996.

21. Wall WJ: Chylous ascites after liver transplantation. Transplantation 58:368–369, 1994.

22. Reyes JD, Tzakis AG, Todo S, et al: Post-operative care of small bowel transplant recipients. Care Crit Ill 9:193–194, 196–198, 1993.

23. Todo S, Tzakis A, Abu-Elmagd K, et al: Clinical intestinal transplantation. Transplant Proc 25:2195–2197, 1993.

24. Hasse JM, Blue LS, Liepa GU, et al: Early enteral nutrition support in patients undergoing liver transplantation. JPEN J Parenter Enteral Nutr 19:437–443, 1995.

25. Delafosse B, Faure JL, Bouffard Y, et al: Liver transplantation—Energy expenditure, nitrogen loss, and substrate oxidation rate in the first two postoperative days. Transplant Proc 21:2453–2454, 1989.

26. Shanbhogue RLK, Bistrian BR, Jenkins RL, et al: Increased protein catabolism without hypermetabolism after human orthotopic liver transplantation. Surgery 101:146–149, 1987.

27. O'Keefe SJ, Williams R, Calne RY: "Catabolic" loss of body protein after human liver transplantation. BMJ 280:1107–1108, 1980.

28. Plevak DJ, DiCecco SR, Wiesner RH, et al: Nutritional support for liver transplantation: Identifying caloric and protein requirements. Mayo Clin Proc 69:225–230, 1994.

29. Reilly J, Mehta R, Teperman L, et al: Nutritional support after liver transplantation: A randomized prospective study. JPEN J Parenter Enteral Nutr 14:386–391, 1990.

30. Mehta PL, Alaka KJ, Filo RS, et al: Nutrition support following liver transplantation: A comparison of jejunal versus parenteral routes. Clin Transplant 837–840, 1995.

31. Wicks C, Somasundaram S, Buarnason I, et al: Comparison of enteral feeding and total parenteral nutrition after liver transplantation. Lancet 344:837–840, 1994.

32. Ragsdale D: Nutritional program for heart transplantation. J Heart Transplant 6:228–233, 1987.

33. Edwards MS, Doster S: Renal transplant diet recommendations: Results of a survey of renal dietitians in the United States. J Am Diet Assoc 90:843–846, 1990.

34. Zabielski P: What are the calorie and protein requirements during the acute postrenal transplant period? Support Line 14(1)11–13, 1992.

35. Kowalchuk D: Nutritional management of the pancreas transplant patient. Support Line 14(1):10–11, 1992.

36. Steiger U, Lippuner K, Jensen EX, et al: Body composition and fuel metabolism after kidney grafting. Eur J Clin Invest 25:809–816, 1995.

37. Seagraves A, Moore EE, Moore, FA, Weil R: Net protein catabolic rate after kidney transplantation: Impact of corticosteroid immunosuppression. JPEN J Parenter Enteral Nutr 10:453–455, 1986.

38. Hoy WE, Sargent JA, Freeman RB, et al: The influence of glucocorticoid dose on protein catabolism after renal transplantation. Am J Med Sci 291:241–247, 1986.

39. Hoy WE, Sargent JA, Hall D, et al: Protein catabolism during the postoperative course after renal transplantation. Am J Kidney Dis 5(3):186–190, 1985.

40. Iapichino G, Radrizzani D, Bonetti G, et al: Early metabolic treatment after liver transplant: Amino acid tolerance. Intensive Care Med 21:802–807, 1995.

41. Van Buren CT, Kulkami A, Rudolph F: Synergistic effect of a nucleotide-free diet and cyclosporine on allograft survival. Transplant Proc 15(Suppl 1):2967–2968, 1983.

42. Van Buren CT, Kulkami AD, Schandle VB, Rudolph FB: The influence of dietary nucleotides on cell-mediated immunity. Transplantation 36:350–352, 1983.

43. Van Buren CT, Kim E, Kulkami AD, et al: Nucleotide-free diet and suppression of immune response. Transplant Proc 19(4, Suppl 5):57–59, 1987.

44. Alexander JW, Levy A, Custer D, et al: Arginine, fish oil, and donor-specific transfusions independently improve cardiac allograft survival in rats given subtherapeutic doses of cyclosporine. JPEN J Parenter Enteral Nutr 22:152–155, 1998.

45. Alexander JW, Dreyer D, Greenberg N, et al: Oral L-arginine with and without canola oil modulates blood pressure and renal function in patients following kidney transplantation [Abstract]. JPEN J Parenter Enteral Nutr 23:519, 1999.

46. Eckstrand AV, Eriksson JG, Gronhagen-Riska C, et al: Insulin resistance and insulin deficiency in the pathogenesis of posttransplantation diabetes in man. Transplantation 53:563–569, 1992.

47. Jindal RM: Posttransplant diabetes mellitus—A review. Transplantation 58:1289–1298, 1994.

48. Driscoll DF, Palombo JD, Bistrian BR: Nutritional and metabolic considerations of the adult liver transplant candidate and organ donor. Nutrition 11:255–263, 1995.

49. Hasse J, DiCecco SR: Solid organ transplantation. In Skipper A (ed): Dietitian's Handbook of Enteral and Parenteral Nutrition. Gaithersburg, MD, Aspen, 1998, pp 295–323.

50. Friedman EA, Shyh T, Beyer MM, et al: Posttransplant diabetes in kidney transplant recipients. Am J Nephrol 5:196–202, 1985.

51. Babineau TJ, Borlase BC, Blackburn GL: Applied total parenteral nutrition in the critically ill. In Rippe JM, Irwin RS, Alpert JS, Fink MP, (eds): Intensive Care Medicine, 2nd ed. Boston, Little, Brown, 1991. pp 1675–1691.

52. McMahon M, Manji N, Driscol DF, et al: Parenteral nutrition in patients with diabetes mellitus: Theoretical and practical considerations. JPEN J Parenter Enteral Nutr 13:545–553, 1989.

53. Kobashigawa JA, Kasiske BL: Hyperlipidemia in solid organ transplantation. Transplantation 63:331–338, 1997.

54. Imagawa DK, Dawson S, Holt CD, et al: Hyperlipidemia after liver transplantation. Natural history and treatment with the hydroxy-methylglutaryl-coenzyme A reductase inhibitor pravastatin. Transplantation 62:934–942, 1996.

55. Moore R, Thomas D, Morgan E, et al: Abnormal

lipid and lipoprotein profiles following renal transplantation. Transplant Proc 25:1060–1061, 1993.

56. Perez R: Managing nutrition problems in transplant patients. Nutr Clin Pract 8:28–32, 1993.

57. Mathe D, Adam R, Malmendier C, et al: Prevalence of dyslipidemia in liver transplant recipients. Transplantation 54:167–170, 1992.

58. Mor E, Facklam D, Hasse J, et al: Weight gain and lipid profile changes in liver transplant recipients: Long-term results of the American FK506 multicenter study. Transplant Proc 27:1126, 1995.

59. Munoz SJ: Hyperlipidemia and other coronary risk factors after orthotopic liver transplantation: Pathogenesis, diagnosis and management. Liver Transpl Surg 1(5, Suppl 1):29–38, 1995.

60. Munoz SJ, Deems RO, Moritz MJ, et al: Hyperlipidemia and obesity after orthotopic liver transplantation. Transplant Proc 23:1480–1483, 1991.

61. Palmer M, Schaffner F, Thung SN: Excessive weight gain after liver transplantation. Transplantation 51:797–800, 1991.

62. Stegall MD, Everson G, Schroter G, et al: Metabolic complications after liver transplantation. Transplantation 60:1057–1060, 1995.

63. Arnadottir M, Berg AL: Treatment of hyperlipidemia in renal transplant recipients. Transplantation 63:330–345, 1997.

64. Ghanem H, van den Dorpel MA, Weimar W, et al: Increased low density lipoprotein oxidation in stable kidney transplant recipients. Kidney Int 49:488–493, 1996.

65. Ettinger WH, Bender WL, Goldberg AP, et al: Lipoprotein lipid abnormalities in healthy renal transplant recipients: Persistence of low HDL_2 cholesterol. Nephron 47(1):17–21, 1987.

66. Alexander JW: Immunonutrition: The role of ω-3 fatty acids. Nutrition 14:7–8, 627–633, 1998.

67. Rogers TS, Elzinga L, Bennett WM, Kelley VE: Selective enhancement of thromboxane in macrophages and kidneys in cyclosporine-induced nephrotoxicity. Transplantation 45:153–156, 1988.

68. Elzinga L, Kelley VE, Houghton DC, Bennett WM: Model of experimental nephrotoxicity with fish oil as the vehicle for cyclosporine. Transplantation 43:271–274, 1987.

69. Kelley VE, Kirkman RL, Bastos M, et al: Enhancement of immunosuppression by substitution of fish oil for olive oil as a vehicle for cyclosporine. Transplantation 48:98–102, 1989.

70. Perez RV, Waymack JP, Munda R, Alexander JW: The effect of donor specific transfusions and dietary fatty acids on rat cardiac allograft survival. J Surg Res 42:335–340, 1987.

71. Otto DA, Kahn DR, Hamm HW, et al: Improved survival of heterotopic cardiac allografts in rats with dietary omega-3 polyunsaturated fatty acids. Transplantation 50:193–198, 1990.

72. Homan van der Heide JJ, Bilo HJ, Tegzess AM, Donker AJ: The effects of dietary supplementation with fish oil on renal function in cyclosporine-treated renal transplant recipients. Transplantation 43:523–527, 1990.

73. Sweny P, Wheeler DC, Lui SF, et al: Dietary fish oil supplements preserve renal function in renal transplant recipients with chronic vascular rejection. Nephrol Dial Transplant 4:1070–1075, 1989.

74. Homan van der Heide JJ, Bilo HJG, Donker AJM, et al: Dietary supplementation with fish oil modifies renal reserve filtration capacity in postoperative, cyclosporin A–treated renal transplant recipients. Transplant Int 3:171–175, 1990.

75. Homan van der Heide JJ, Bilo HJG, Donker AJM, et al: The effects of dietary supplementation with fish oil on renal function and the course of early postoperative rejection episodes in cyclosporine-treated renal transplant recipients. Transplantation 54:257–263, 1992.

76. Homan van der Heide JJ, Bilo HJG, Donker JM, et al: Effect of dietary fish oil on renal function and rejection in cyclosporine-treated recipients of renal transplants. N Engl J Med 329:769–773, 1993.

77. Badalamenti S, Salerno F, Lorenzano E, et al: Renal effects of dietary supplementation with fish oil in cyclosporine-treated liver transplant recipients. Hepatology 22:1695–1701, 1995.

78. Bartucci MR, Loughman KA, Moir EJ: Kidney-pancreas transplantation: A treatment option for ESRD and type I diabetes. Am Nephrol Nurs Assoc J 19:467–474, 1992.

79. Reyes J, Tzakis AG, Todo S, et al: Nutritional management of intestinal transplant recipients. Transplant Proc 25:1200–1201, 1993.

80. Hasse JM: Recovery after organ transplantation in adults: The role of postoperative nutrition therapy. Top Clin Nutr 13(2):15–26, 1998.

81. Merion RM, Twork AM, Rosenberg L, et al: Obesity and renal transplantation. Surg Gynecol Obstet 172:367–376, 1991.

82. Holley JL, Shapiro R, Lopatin WB, et al: Obesity as a risk factor following cadaveric renal transplantation. Transplantation 49:387–389, 1990.

83. Pirsch JD, Armbrust MJ, Knechtle SJ, et al: Obesity as a risk factor following renal transplantation. Transplantation 59:631–633, 1995.

84. Keeffe EB, Gettys C, Esquivel CO: Liver transplantation in patients with severe obesity. Transplantation 57:309–311, 1994.

85. Hasse JM, Testa G, Gonwa TA, et al: Is pre-liver transplant obesity a risk factor for posttransplant metabolic complications [Abstract]? Transplantation 66:553, 1998.

86. Testa G, Hasse JM, Jennings LW, et al: Morbid obesity is not an independent risk factor for liver transplantation [Abstract]. Transplantation 66:535, 1998.

87. Braunfeld MY, Chan S, Pregler J, et al: Liver transplantation in the morbidly obese. J Clin Anesth 8:585–590, 1996.

88. Sadamori H, Tanaka N, Yagi T, et al: The effects of nutritional repletion on donors for liver transplantation in pigs. Transplantation 60:317–321, 1995.

89. Ishikawa T, Yagi T, Ishine N, et al: Energy metabolism of the grafted liver and influence of preretrieval feeding process on swine orthotopic liver transplantation. Transplant Proc 29:397–399, 1997.

90. Adam R, Astarcioglu I, Gigou M, et al: The influence of the glycogen content of the donor liver on subsequent graft function and survival in rat liver transplantation. Transplantation 54:753–756, 1992.

91. Cywes R, Greig PD, Sanabrid JR, et al: Effect of intraportal glucose infusion on hepatic glycogen content and degradation, and outcome of liver transplantation. Ann Surg 216:235–247, 1992.

92. Appelbaum FR: The use of bone marrow and peripheral blood stem cell transplantation in the treatment of cancer. CA Cancer J Clin 46:142–164, 1996.

93. Ringden O: Allogeneic bone marrow transplantation for hematological malignancies—Controversies and recent advances. Acta Oncol 36:549–564, 1997.

94. Territo M: The use of autologous transplantation in the treatment of malignant disorders. J Rheumatol 48S:36–40, 1997.

95. Thomas ED: Pros and cons of stem cell transplantation for autoimmune disease. J Rheumatol 48S:100–102, 1997.

96. Brooks PM: Hematopoietic stem cell transplantation for autoimmune diseases. J Rheumatol 48S:19–22, 1997.

97. Barrett AJ: Mechanisms of the graft-versus-leukemia reaction. Stem Cells 15:248–258, 1997.

98. Fefer A: Graft-versus-tumor responses: Adoptive cellular therapy in bone marrow transplantation. *In* Forman SJ, Blume KG, Thomas ED (eds): Bone Marrow Transplantation. Boston, Blackwell Scientific, 1994, pp 231–241.

99. Bensinger W, Singer J, Appelbaum, et al: Autologous transplantation with peripheral blood mononuclear cells collected after administration of recombinant granulocyte stimulating factor. Blood 81:3158–3163, 1993.

100. Deeg HJ, Seidel K, Bruemmer B, et al: Impact of patient weight on non-relapse mortality after marrow transplantation. Bone Marrow Transplant 15:461–468, 1995.

101. Weisdorf SA, Lysne J, Wind D, et al: Positive effect of prophylactic total parenteral nutrition on long-term outcome of bone marrow transplantation. Transplantation 43:833–838, 1987.

102. Aker SN: Bone marrow transplantation: Nutrition support and monitoring. *In* Bloch AS (ed): Nutrition Management of the Cancer Patient. Rockville, MD, Aspen, 1990, pp 199–225.

103. Roberts SR: Bone marrow and peripheral blood stem cell transplantation. *In* Lysen LK (ed): Quick Reference to Clinical Dietetics. Gaithersburg, MD, Aspen, 1997, pp 162–168.

104. Herrmann VM, Petruska PJ: Nutrition support in bone marrow transplant recipients. Nutr Clin Pract 8:19–27, 1993.

105. Taskinen M, Saarinen UM: Skeletal muscle protein reserve after bone marrow transplantation in children. Bone Marrow Transplant 18:937–941, 1996.

106. Muscaritoli M, Conversano L, Cangiano C, et al: Biochemical indices may not accurately reflect changes in nutritional status after allogeneic bone marrow transplantation. Nutrition 11:433–436, 1995.

107. Weisdorf SA, Schwarzenberg SJ: Nutritional support of bone marrow transplant recipients. *In* Forman SJ, Blume KG, Thomas ED (eds): Bone Marrow Transplantation. Boston, Blackwell Scientific, 1994, pp 327–336.

108. Tomalis L, Sigley P, Kennedy MJ, et al: Nutritional outcome of women undergoing autologous bone marrow transplantation [Abstract]. A.S.P.E.N. 18th Clinical Congress, San Antonio, Texas, February 1994.

109. Cheney CL, Abson KG, Aker SA, et al: Body composition changes in marrow transplant recipients receiving total parenteral nutrition. Cancer 59:1515–1519, 1987.

110. Cheney CL, Lenssen P, Aker SN: Prealbumin as a nutritional marker in marrow transplantation [Abstract]. J Am Coll Nutr 7:415, 1988.

111. Papadopoulou A, Lloyd DR, Williams MD, et al: Gastrointestinal and nutritional sequelae of bone marrow transplantation. Arch Dis Child 75:208–213, 1996.

112. Uderzo C, Rovelli A, Bonomi M, et al: Total parenteral nutrition and nutritional assessment in leukaemic children undergoing bone marrow transplantation. Eur J Cancer 27:758–762, 1991.

113. Cunningham BA, Morris GM, Cheney CL, et al: Effects of resistive exercise on skeletal muscle in marrow transplant recipients receiving total parenteral nutrition. JPEN J Parenter Enteral Nutr 10:558–563, 1986.

114. Cheney CL, Lenssen P, Aker SA, et al: Sex differences in nitrogen balance following marrow grafting for leukemia. J Am Coll Nutr 6:223–230, 1987.

115. Keller U, Kraenzlin ME, Gratwohl A, et al: Protein metabolism assessed by 1-^{13}C leucine infusions in patients undergoing bone marrow transplantation. JPEN J Parenter Enteral Nutr 14:480–484, 1990.

116. Geibig CB, Owens JP, Mirtallo JM, et al: Parenteral nutrition for marrow transplant recipients: Evaluation of an increased nitrogen dose. JPEN J Parenter Enteral Nutr 15:184–188, 1991.

117. Herrmann VM, Sarnick MB, Moore FD, et al: Effect of cytotoxic agents on protein kinetics in patients with metastatic cancer. Surgery 90:381–387, 1981.

118. Heymsfield SB, Arteaga C, McManus C, et al: Measurement of muscle mass in humans: Validity of the 24 hour creatinine method. Am J Clin Nutr 37:478–479, 1983.

119. Szeluga DJ, Stuart RK, Brookmeyer R, et al: Energy requirements of parenterally fed bone marrow transplant recipients. JPEN J Parenter Enteral Nutr 9:139–143, 1985.

120. Guiot HFL, Biemond J, Klasen E, et al: Protein loss during acute graft-versus-host disease: Diagnostic and clinical significance. Eur J Haematol 38:187–196, 1987.

121. Szeluga DJ, Stuart RK, Brookmeyer R, et al: Nutritional support of bone marrow transplant recipients: Randomized clinical trial comparing total parenteral nutrition to an enteral feeding program. Cancer Res 47:3309–3316, 1987.

122. Lenssen P, Bruemmer BA, Bowden RA, et al: Intravenous lipid dose and incidence of bacteremia and fungemia in patients undergoing bone marrow transplantation. Am J Clin Nutr 67:927–933, 1998.

123. Ost L, Tyden G, Fehman I: Impaired glucose tolerance in cyclosporine-prednisone treated renal graft recipients. Transplantation 46:370–372, 1988.

124. Smedmyr B, Wibbell L, Simonsson B, et al: Impaired glucose tolerance after autologous bone marrow transplantation. Bone Marrow Transplant 6:89–92, 1990.

125. Schouten HC, Maragos D, Vose J, et al: Diabetes mellitus or an impaired glucose tolerance as a potential complicating factor in patients treated with high-dose therapy and autologous bone marrow transplantation. Bone Marrow Transplant 6:333–335, 1990.

126. Lenssen P, Cheney CL, Aker SA, et al: Intravenous branched chain amino acid trial in marrow transplant recipients. JPEN J Parenter Enteral Nutr 11:112–118, 1987.

127. Gauvreau J, Lenssen P, Cheney CL, et al: Nutritional management of patients with intestinal graft-versus-host disease. J Am Diet Assoc 79:673–677, 1981.

128. Cohen D: Nutrition management of gastrointestinal graft-versus-host disease following bone marrow transplantation. Support Line 28:13–15, 1996.

129. Lacey JM, Wilmore DW: Is glutamine a conditionally essential amino acid? Nutr Rev 48:297–309, 1990.

130. Ziegler TR, Young LS, Benfell K, et al: Clinical and metabolic efficacy of glutamine-supplemented parenteral nutrition after bone marrow transplantation. Ann Intern Med 116:821–828, 1992.

131. Scheltinga MR, Young LS, Benfell K, et al: Glutamine-enriched intravenous feedings attenuate extracellular fluid expansion after a standard stress. Ann Surg 214:385–395, 1991.

132. Ziegler TR, Bye RL, Persinger RL, et al: Effects of glutamine supplementation on circulating lymphocytes after bone marrow transplantation: A pilot study. Am J Med Sci 315:4–10, 1998.

133. Young LS, Bye R, Scheltinga M, et al: Patients receiving glutamine-supplemented intravenous feedings report an improvement in mood. JPEN J Parenter Enteral Nutr 17:422–427, 1993.

134. MacBurney M, Young LS, Ziegler TR, et al: A cost-evaluation of glutamine-supplemented parenteral nutrition in adult bone marrow transplant patients. J Am Diet Assoc 94:1263–1266, 1994.

135. Schloerb PR, Amare M: Total parenteral nutrition with glutamine in bone marrow transplantation and other clinical applications (a randomized, double-blind study). JPEN J Parenter Enteral Nutr 17:407–413, 1993.

136. Schloerb PR, Skikne BS: Oral and parenteral glutamine in bone marrow transplantation: A randomized double-blind study. JPEN J Parenter Enteral Nutr 23:117–122, 1999.

137. Clemans GW, Yamanaka W, Flournoy N, et al: Plasma fatty acid patterns of bone marrow transplant patients primarily supported by fat-free parenteral nutrition. JPEN J Parenter Enteral Nutr 5:221–225, 1981.

138. Yamanaka WK, Tilmont G, Aker SA: Plasma fatty acids of marrow transplant recipients on fat-supplemented parenteral nutrition. Am J Clin Nutr 39:607–611, 1984.

139. Ignoffo RJ: Parenteral nutrition support in patients with cancer. Pharmocotherapy 12:353–357, 1992.

140. Wan JMF, Teo TC, Babayan VK, et al: Invited comment: Lipids and the development of immune dysfunction and infection. JPEN J Parenter Enteral Nutr 12:43S–48S, 1988.

141. Cheney CL, Lenssen P, Aker SN: Association of iv lipid emulsion with risk of infection [Abstract]. J Am Coll Nutr 9:532, 1990.

142. Desai TK, Luk GD, Ehrinpreis MN: Intralipid infusions and septicemia in bone marrow transplant recipients [Abstract]. Gastroenterology 98a:409, 1990.

143. Lenssen P, Bruemmer BA, Bowden RA, et al: Intravenous lipid dose and incidence of bacteremia

144. Ballantyne CM, Podet EJ, Patsch WP, et al: Effects of cyclosporine therapy on plasma lipoprotein levels. JAMA 262:53–56, 1989.

145. Hasse J: Nutritional implications of perioperative medications used in liver transplantation. Dietitians Nutr Support 11:2,7,11, 1989.

146. Carreras E, Villamor JC, Reverter J, et al: Hypertriglyceridemia in bone marrow transplant recipients: Another side effect of cyclosporin A. Bone Marrow Transplant 4:385–388, 1989.

147. Sacks GS: Is IV lipid emulsion safe in patients with hypertriglyceridemia? Nutr Clin Pract 12:120–123, 1997.

148. Tezuka H, Sawada H, Sakoda H, et al: Suppression of genetic resistance to bone marrow grafts and natural killer cell activity by administration of fat emulsion. Exp Hematol 16:609–612, 1988.

149. Muscaritoli M, Conversano L, Torelli GF, et al: Clinical and metabolic effects of different parenteral nutrition regimens in patients undergoing allogeneic bone marrow transplantation. Transplantation 66:610–616, 1998.

150. Milligan DW, Quick A, Barnard DL: Vitamin B_{12} absorption after allogeneic bone marrow transplantation. J Clin Path 40:1472–1474, 1987.

151. Bleggi-Torres LF, de Medeiros BC, Ogasawara VSA, et al: Iatrogenic Wernicke's encephalopathy in allogeneic bone marrow transplantation: A study of eight cases. Bone Marrow Transplant 20:391–395, 1997.

152. Rovelli A, Bonomi M, Murano A, et al: Severe lactic acidosis due to thiamine deficiency after bone marrow transplantation in a child with acute monocytic leukemia. Hematologica 75:579–581, 1990.

153. Carlin A, Walker WA: Rapid development of vitamin K deficiency in an adolescent boy receiving total parenteral nutrition following bone marrow transplantation. Nutr Rev 49:179–183, 1991.

154. Clemans MR, Ladner C, Ehninger G, et al: Plasma vitamin E and β-carotene concentrations during radiochemotherapy preceding bone marrow transplantation. Am J Clin Nutr 51:216–219, 1990.

155. Antila HM, Salo MS, Kirvelä O, et al: Serum trace element concentrations and iron metabolism in allogeneic bone marrow transplant recipients. Ann Med 24:55–59, 1992.

156. Papadopoulou A, Nathavitharana K, Williams MD, et al: Diagnosis and clinical associations of zinc depletion following bone marrow transplantation. Arch Dis Child 74:328–331, 1996.

157. Hunnisett A, Davies S, McLaren-Howard J, et al: Lipoperoxides as an index of free radical activity in bone marrow transplant recipients. Biol Trace Elem Res 47:125–132, 1995.

158. Sweetman SF, Strain JJ, Mc-Kelvey-Martin VJ: Effect of antioxidant vitamin supplementation on DNA damage and repair in human lymphoblastoid cells. Nutr Cancer 27:122–130, 1997.

159. Meister A: Glutathione, ascorbate, and cellular protection. Can Res 54(Suppl):1969s–1975s, 1994.

160. Herbert V: The antioxidant supplement myth. Am J Clin Nutr 60:157–158, 1994.

161. Fredstrom S, Rogosheke J, Gupta P, et al: Extrapyramidal symptoms in a BMT recipient with hyperintense basal ganglia and elevated manganese. Bone Marrow Transplant 15:989–992, 1995.

and fungemia in patients undergoing bone marrow transplantation. Am J Clin Nutr 67:927–933, 1998.

162. Fredstrom SF: Trace element toxicities in parenteral nutrition during BMT. Marrow Transpl Nutr Network Newslett 3:1, 4, 1996.
163. Weinstein D: Electrolyte, trace element, and vitamin requirements of marrow transplant patients. Marrow Transpl Nutr Network Newslett 3:2, 1996.
164. McCauly J, Fung J, Jain A, et al: The effects of FK 506 on renal function after liver transplantation. Transplant Proc 22s:17–20, 1990.
165. June CH, Thompson CB, Kennedy MS, et al: Profound hypomagnesemia and renal magnesium wasting associated with the use of cyclosporine for marrow transplantation. Transplantation 41:47–51, 1985.
166. Wingard JR: Prevention and treatment of bacterial and fungal infections. *In* Forman SJ, Blume KG, Thomas ED (eds): Bone Marrow Transplantation. Boston, Blackwell Scientific, 1994, pp 363–375.
167. Zaia JA: Cytomegalovirus infection. *In* Forman SJ, Blume KG, Thomas ED (eds): Bone Marrow Transplantation. Boston, Blackwell Scientific, 1994, pp 376–403.
168. McDonald GB, Hinds MS, Fisher LD, et al: Venoocclusive disease of the liver and multiorgan failure after bone marrow transplantation: A cohort study of 355 patients. Ann Intern Med 118:255–267, 1993.
169. McDonald GB: Veno-occlusive disease of the liver following marrow transplantation. Marrow Transpl Rev: Issues Hematol Oncol Immunol 3:49–54, 1994.
170. Shuhart MC, McDonald GB: Gastrointestinal and hepatic complications. *In* Forman SJ, Blume KG, Thomas ED (eds): Bone Marrow Transplantation. Boston, Blackwell Scientific, 1994, pp 454–481.
171. Shulma HM, Hinterberger W: Hepatic veno-occlusive disease—Liver toxicity syndrome after bone marrow transplantation. Bone Marrow Transplant 10:197–214, 1992.
172. Andris DA, Krzywda EA: Nutrition support in specific diseases: Back to the basics. Nutr Clin Pract 9:28–32, 1994.
173. Lenssen P, Spencer GD, McDonald GB: A randomized trial of FreAmine vs HepatAmine vs placebo in acute hepatic coma [Abstract]. Gastroenterology 92:5, 1987.
174. Miller JE: Hepatic veno-occlusive disease: A challenging complication of bone marrow transplantation. Support Line 19(7):10–13, 1997.
175. Hager LA: Hepatic complications associated with total parenteral nutrition. Support Line 16(3):1–6, 1994.
176. Habeck A: Nutrition management of VOD. Marrow Transpl Nutr Network Newslett 4:3, 1997.
177. Nattakom TV, Charlton A, Wilmore DW: Use of vitamin E and glutamine in the successful treatment of severe veno-occlusive disease following bone marrow transplantation. Nutr Clin Pract 10:16–18, 1995.
178. Klingebiel T, Schlegel PG: GVHD: Overview on pathophysiology, incidence, clinical and biological features. Bone Marrow Transplant 21:S45–S49, 1998.
179. Sullivan KM: Graft-versus-host disease. *In* Forman SJ, Blume KG, Thomas ED (eds): Bone Marrow Transplantation. Boston, Blackwell Scientific, 1994, pp 339–362.
180. Deeg HJ, Storb R: Acute and chronic graft-versus-host disease: Clinical manifestations, prophylaxis, and treatment. J Natl Cancer Inst 76:1325–1328, 1986.
181. Ringwald-Smith K, Williams R, Horwitz E, et al: Determination of energy expenditure in the bone marrow transplant patient. Nutr Clin Pract 13:215–218, 1998.
182. Gauvreau JM, Lenssen P, Cheney CL, et al: Nutritional management of patients with intestinal graft-versus-host disease. J Am Diet Assoc 79:673–677, 1981.
183. Guiot HFL, Biemond J, Klasen E, et al: Protein loss during acute graft-versus-host disease: Diagnostic and clinical significance. Eur J Haematol 38:187–196, 1987.
184. Wingard JR, Piantadosi S, Vogelsang GB, et al: Predictors of death from chronic graft versus host disease after bone marrow transplantation. Blood 74:1428–1435, 1989.
185. Lenssen P, Sherry ME, Cheney CL, et al: Prevalence of nutrition-related problems among long-term survivors of allogeneic marrow transplantation. J Am Diet Assoc 90:835–842, 1990.
186. Roberts SR, Miller JM, Pineiro LA: Is total parenteral nutrition beneficial in breast cancer patients after autologous marrow or blood transplantation [Abstract]? Presented at Discovery Days BMT Conference, Dallas, Texas, March 1997.
187. Charuhas PM, Fosberg LF, Bruemmer B, et al: A double-blind randomized trial comparing outpatient parenteral nutrition with intravenous hydration: Effect on resumption of oral intake after marrow transplantation. JPEN J Parenter Enteral Nutr 21:157–161, 1997.

28

◆ Nutrient Pharmacotherapy

Carolyn R. Jonas, Ph.D., R.D.
Daniel P. Griffith, R.Ph., B.C.N.S.P.
Glen F. Bergman, M.M.Sc., R.D., C.N.S.D.
Lorraine M. Leader, M.D., C.N.S.P.
Thomas R. Ziegler, M.D., C.N.S.P.

It has become apparent that conventional parenteral nutrition (PN) may be less efficacious than has been previously assumed.[1] The provision of conventional amounts of macro- and micronutrients in current PN solutions clearly is beneficial in individuals with severe protein-energy malnutrition and for the correction or prevention of specific nutrient deficiencies.[2] Classic signs of micronutrient deficiency in patients receiving specialized nutrition in the hospital or home environments are now uncommon. Body weight may be maintained and loss of body protein attenuated in patients on nutritional support compared with patients receiving limited or no dietary intake.[3] However, the clinical efficacy of PN in well-nourished or mildly malnourished patients unable to be fed enterally, and in patients with critical illness, is less well documented. Blinded randomized trials are relatively few and often include small study populations and/or incorporate inadequate study design. Further, the true metabolic requirements and the adequacy of doses of specific nutrients provided are largely unknown in many patient groups routinely administered PN. Data suggest that PN formulations may provide certain nutrients in excess (e.g., manganese)[4] or in insufficient amounts (e.g., glutamine).[5] Further, PN is associated with significant complications including sepsis, venous thrombosis, liver and renal dysfunction, metabolic bone disease, and frequent alterations in serum electrolyte levels.

Therapeutic strategies designed to enhance the efficacy of specialized enteral and parenteral nutrition are increasingly being investigated around the world.[6] These include (1) the increased use of enteral feeding in hospitalized patients; (2) modulation of enteral tube feeding formulas to provide in-creased amounts of specific macro- and micronutrients (e.g., n-3 fatty acids derived from fish oil; arginine; glutamine; antioxidants); (3) the use of recombinant growth factors and anabolic steroids to enhance the efficiency of nutrient utilization (e.g., growth hormone, oxandrolone); (4) the increased provision of apparently conditionally essential nutrients (e.g., glutamine), nutrient antioxidants (e.g., vitamins C and E), and new lipid products (n-3 fatty acids, medium-chain triglycerides, structured lipids); and (5) combinations of these approaches.[6, 7]

The term *nutriceutical* has been coined to describe the specific nutrients that are provided in larger-than-usual or "pharmacologic" amounts.[8] In many cases, these substances, or the doses being administered, are in the early stages of clinical investigation. In addition to nutrient pharmacotherapy's clinical and metabolic effects, information on nutrient pharmacotherapy is generally lacking with regard to the effects of age, gender, illness, underlying nutritional status, medications, and concomitant nutritional support. Some of the relevant specific nutrients and metabolites being evaluated in clinical research are listed in Table 28–1. This chapter focuses on findings from the exciting new area of nutrient pharmacology, concentrating primarily on clinical studies in patients receiving intravenous feeding.

◆ NUTRIENT PHARMACOTHERAPY

Amino Acids and Peptides

Glutamine

The amino acid glutamine, classically considered a nonessential amino acid, has been the most intensively studied nutriceutical in

Table 28–1. Selected Agents Under Clinical Investigation as Nutrient Pharmacotherapy

Amino acids and peptides
  L-Amino acids (e.g., glutamine, arginine, branched-chain amino acids, cyst[e]ine)
  Glutathione (L-glutamyl-L-cysteinylglycine)
  Dipeptides (L-alanyl-L-glutamine, glycyl-L-tyrosine)
Lipids
  Fish oils (n-3 fatty acids)
  Short-chain fatty acids
  Short- and medium-chain triglycerides
  Structured lipids
Micronutrients
  Vitamin C
  Vitamin E
  Selenium
  Copper
  Zinc
  Thiamine
Miscellaneous compounds
  Ornithine–α-ketoglutarate
  α-Ketoglutarate
  Nucleotides
  Carnitine
  Choline

clinical trials. A substantial body of work in animal models and increasing clinical trials on glutamine supplementation of PN and enteral feeding suggest that it probably becomes conditionally essential during catabolic stress.[9, 10] Glutamine accounts for more than 60% of the skeletal muscle free amino acid pool and 20% of the plasma free amino acid pool. In addition to its importance in many key metabolic processes (e.g., gluconeogenesis, acid-base homeostasis, and nucleic acid biosynthesis), glutamine is used as a major substrate by intestinal mucosal cells and by cells of the immune system.[9, 10] Data in animal stress models indicate that glutamine is a key substrate for tissue production of the critical antioxidant glutathione[11, 12] and may also enhance insulin-mediated glucose uptake.[13]

Glutamine is adequately synthesized to meet metabolic needs during health. However, during illness, skeletal muscle exports large amounts of glutamine into the blood (>35% of all amino acid nitrogen). This provides glutamine for tissues such as the gut, at the expense of decreased glutamine levels in muscle, negative nitrogen balance, and ultimately decreased muscle mass and, presumably, function. Eventually, plasma glutamine concentrations decline if the catabolic stress persists. Concomitant with muscle glutamine efflux, glutamine-utilizing tissues (kidney, gut, immune cells) markedly increase glutamine uptake and metabolism during illness. The provision of conventional nutritional support without supplemental glutamine does not appear to support glutamine requirements adequately during severe illness. Thus, during stress, atrophy and decreased function of tissues such as the intestinal mucosa may be due in part to relative glutamine deficiency.[9]

This model of conditional glutamine deficiency is supported by numerous animal studies of glutamine supplementation published during the 1990s. Although some studies show no beneficial effects, either L-glutamine or glutamine dipeptides given at doses constituting 15 to 40% of administered amino acids in PN solutions and enteral diets enhanced gut mucosal growth and repair, upregulated immune cell numbers, decreased infectious morbidity, and reduced mortality in models of catabolic stress.[9, 10] In animal models, PN is associated with marked intestinal mucosal atrophy compared with the effects of enteral feeding. Unfortunately, relatively few human data exist on gut mucosal changes during PN.[14] In rodent and pig models, glutamine added to otherwise complete PN formulations attenuates mucosal small bowel and colonic atrophy, improves gut barrier function, decreases mucosal inflammatory responses, improves gut glutathione levels, and decreases gut-origin sepsis (reviewed in Ziegler and associates[9]).

Physicochemical properties of poor solubility and heat instability have limited L-glutamine provision in clinical care, and the commercial availability of PN solutions enriched in L-glutamine is limited. As an alternative, synthetic glutamine peptides such as alanylglutamine (Ala-Gln) and glycylglutamine (Gly-Gln) confer both heat stability and solubility in solution and are rapidly hydrolyzed in plasma.[9] Several clinical studies indicate that both enteral and parenteral glutamine supplementation exert beneficial metabolic and clinical effects in certain patient groups (Table 28–2). In these carefully controlled trials, glutamine has been well tolerated clinically and biochemically, even with large intravenous loads approaching 40% of administered protein. Diet-controlled and blinded trials in postoperative or bone marrow transplantation patients receiving PN demonstrated that nitrogen balance is significantly improved with

Table 28-2. Beneficial Effects of Glutamine Supplementation in Clinical Trials

Improved nitrogen retention (IV Gln in postoperative, BMT, trauma patients)

Increased rates of protein synthesis (IV Gln in postoperative patients)

Maintained skeletal muscle glutamine concentrations (IV Gln in postoperative patients)

Increased systemic lymphocyte cell number (IV and enteral Gln in postoperative, BMT, trauma patients)

Attenuated extracellular fluid expansion (IV Gln in BMT patients)

Maintained jejunal villus height and gut barrier function during PN (IV Gln in stable PN-dependent patients)

Decreased oral mucositis (enteral Gln in BMT patients)

Improved D-xylose absorption (IV Gln in critically ill ICU patients)

Improved intestinal nutrient absorption (combined with a modified diet and growth hormone (IV + enteral Gln in SBS patients)

Decreased rates of bacteremia (enteral Gln in premature infants, trauma patients)

Decreased incidence of hospital infection (enteral Gln in trauma patients, IV Gln in BMT patients)

Shortened length of hospital stay (IV Gln in BMT and postoperative patients)

Improved 6-mo survival after ICU discharge (IV Gln in critically ill ICU patients)

BMT, bone marrow transplantation; Gln, glutamine; ICU, intensive care unit; IV, intravenous; PN, parenteral nutrition; SBS, short bowel syndrome.

---

supplementation of Ala-Gln, Gly-Gln, or L-glutamine (12–40 g of glutamine per day).[15, 16] These protein-anabolic effects are associated with significantly increased glutamine concentrations in plasma and skeletal muscle, improved rates of protein synthesis, and decreased rates of protein degradation. In contrast, nitrogen balance or protein kinetics did not improve and plasma glutamine levels did not increase with the administration of L-glutamine–enriched tube feedings in short-term trials in critically ill patients.[17] In a clinical trial comparing routes of glutamine administration, isonitrogenous L-glutamine–enriched tube feeding or PN was given for 5 days postoperatively in patients undergoing gastric or pancreatic operation for cancer.[18] Plasma glutamine levels did not increase over time in the tube-fed patients but rose significantly in the parenteral group after 5 days.[18]

Several investigations support the concept that glutamine or glutamine dipeptides are trophic to human gut mucosal cells. The addition of both L-glutamine and the dipep-tide Ala-Gln increased cellular proliferation in cells isolated ex vivo from ileal and proximal and distal colonic mucosal biopsies from healthy adults.[19] PN-dependent patients given Gly-Gln supplementation demonstrated significantly reduced intestinal sugar permeability and increased duodenal villus height compared with those given standard PN.[20] Critically ill intensive care unit (ICU) patients given Ala-Gln–enriched PN showed markedly improved D-xylose absorption (194% increase) compared with clinically similar patients receiving glutamine-free PN.[21] Thus, the available limited data suggest that PN-enriched glutamine is a trophic nutrient for human intestinal mucosa. Additional trials on this issue are under way in other types of catabolic patients.

Macrophages and lymphocytes use glutamine at a high rate, especially when activated by mitogens. In a double-blind clinical trial, intravenous L-glutamine given in balanced PN solutions significantly increased the total lymphocyte, T lymphocyte, CD4 helper, and CD8 suppressor cell recovery after bone marrow transplantation.[22] Gly-Gln–supplemented PN increased T lymphocyte proliferative responses in postoperative patients[23] and decreased the mononuclear cell release of the cytokine interleukin 8 in patients with acute pancreatitis.[24] Thus, available clinical data indicate that dietary glutamine supplementation may regulate human immune cell number and possibly function.

Studies demonstrate that glutamine-supplemented nutrition improves other relevant clinical outcomes (see Table 28-2). In the first double-blind outcome study, we demonstrated that patients undergoing allogeneic bone marrow transplantation and receiving L-glutamine–enriched PN (0.57 g/kg/day) had lower rates of microbial colonization and clinical infection and a shortened length of stay in the hospital compared with patients receiving nonenriched PN.[18] In postoperative adults, another double-blind trial demonstrated a 6-day reduction in the hospital length of stay, concomitant with improved nitrogen balance and lymphocyte recovery, in patients receiving Ala-Gln–enriched PN (0.3 g/kg/day) compared with controls who received isonitrogenous glutamine-free solutions.[25] In a large controlled and blinded trial in adult ICU patients requiring PN, patients receiving L-glutamine–enriched feeding demonstrated significantly improved 6-month survival compared with the controls (24/42 vs. 14/42).[26]

L-Glutamine–supplemented tube feedings (0.2 to 0.3 g/kg/day) given to very low birth weight premature infants was well tolerated, resulted in better enteral feeding tolerance, and was associated with a marked reduction in bacteremia compared with controls (11% vs. 30%).[27] A double-blind trial demonstrated that multitrauma patients receiving tube feedings with L-glutamine supplementation (approximately 30% of dietary protein) had significantly less pneumonia, bacteremia, and gut-origin sepsis than controls receiving standard low-glutamine feedings.[28] In another randomized double-blind placebo-controlled study, L-glutamine or placebo (L-glycine) at a swish-and-swallow dose of 1 g/m^2 four times daily (6 to 9 g/day) was administered from admission until day 28 in 193 autologous or allogeneic bone marrow transplantation patients.[29] No significant differences in PN use, rate of cancer relapse or progression, antibiotic use, graft-versus-host-disease, or days of hospitalization were observed in either autologous or allogeneic transplant recipients. However, in autologous marrow transplantation patients (n = 87), glutamine use was associated with significantly less severe mucositis, whereas in allogeneic patients the day-28 survival was improved in the glutamine-treated group.[29]

Several studies suggest that the anabolic and tissue-specific trophic effects of dietary glutamine are enhanced by exogenous growth factors (insulin-like growth factor I, epidermal growth factor, or growth hormone) in a synergistic or additive fashion (reviewed in Ziegler and coworkers[6]). In a series of studies, Byrne and colleagues studied combined effects of intravenous or enteral L-glutamine, parenteral growth hormone, and a modified enteral diet in PN-dependent adult patients with gastrointestinal failure due to short gut syndrome.[30, 31] Significantly improved intestinal absorption of protein, carbohydrate, calories, sodium, and water occurred with the combined therapy.[30] A larger group of patients was given the combined nutrient–growth factor therapy for 3 weeks and then maintained on a glutamine-supplemented modified diet indefinitely. Therapy was associated with an 80% elimination or reduction in PN needs after an average of 1 year of follow-up.[31] A crossover study in eight patients confirmed

improved electrolyte but not macronutrient absorption with this therapeutic approach, although different dietary and medical treatment methods were used.[32] Further, the gastric emptying time was decreased, and over half the individuals studied demonstrated markedly improved nitrogen and fat absorption with active therapy.[32] Additional blinded trials of diet, growth factors, and glutamine are in progress in this patient population to define clinical effects and underlying mechanisms of action of these approaches as methods to improve human intestinal growth and function.

Branched-Chain Amino Acids

The use of PN solutions enriched in the branched-chain amino acids (BCAAs) leucine, isoleucine, and valine was an early example of nutrient pharmacotherapy.[33] A fairly extensive literature on the effects of BCAA-enriched PN in human liver failure, trauma, and sepsis is available, whereas additional trials have examined BCAA supplementation in respiratory failure and as a modulator of food intake and gastric emptying.

Interest in the BCAAs initially derived from studies performed in vitro or in animal models suggesting that BCAAs (especially leucine) or their ketoacids have a regulatory and anabolic role in protein metabolism by increasing rates of skeletal muscle protein synthesis and/or decreasing rates of protein degradation.[34] In addition, patients with hepatic failure demonstrate decreased circulating BCAA levels and accumulation of aromatic amino acids (phenylalanine, tyrosine, and tryptophan) and methionine in the blood.[35] It was theorized that an increased ratio of aromatic amino acids to BCAAs may increase tryptophan uptake across the blood-brain barrier, increase cerebral serotonin levels, and precipitate encephalopathy. Thus, the provision of amino acid solutions designed to correct this imbalance was suggested as a method to improve hepatic encephalopathy and also to enhance nitrogen balance.[34]

BCAA-enriched PN has been extensively investigated as a method to improve nitrogen retention in critical illness and as therapy in patients with hepatic encephalopathy. Standard amino acid solutions provide approximately 15 to 25% of amino acids as BCAAs, and the BCAA-enriched formulations studied provided approximately 35 to 50% of total protein as BCAAs. The initial studies showed improvement in the low levels of plasma BCAAs with enriched solutions, concomitant with decreased hepatic encephalopathy in cirrhosis.[34, 35] In contrast, several other appropriately controlled studies showed minimal or no effect of BCAA-enriched PN on hepatic encephalopathy.[36–39] The results of a meta-analysis of randomized clinical trials of BCAA-enriched PN in hepatic encephalopathy were published by Naylor and associates in 1989.[40] The authors concluded that slight, but significant, improvements in hepatic encephalopathy may occur in cirrhotic patients given parenteral BCAA-enriched solutions, which thus may allow larger amounts of protein to be administered. However, effects on clinical outcomes are discrepant among the trials, and these were primarily short-term studies.[40] The clinical guidelines of the American Society for Parenteral and Enteral Nutrition suggest that BCAA-enriched PN should be used in hepatic encephalopathy only when, in spite of standard medical care (lactulose and/or neomycin), the encephalopathy makes it impossible to provide adequate protein to the patient.[2]

Randomized trials in critically ill patients without hepatic disease comparing BCAA-enriched PN versus standard parenteral formulas have demonstrated variable effects on clinical and metabolic outcomes. There have now been more than 17 studies of the efficacy of BCAA supplementation on protein metabolism in stress and septic patients, and the results remain controversial. Some uncontrolled studies in postoperative patients receiving hypocaloric support supplemented with BCAAs have reported nitrogen-sparing effects.[41, 42] In a randomized prospective double-blind multicenter study in 87 patients, the six-center study reported increased nitrogen retention with BCAA-enriched versus standard amino acid solutions.[43] However, other studies did not find a difference in nitrogen retention between standard amino acid or BCAA-enriched formulas.[44–46] Chiarla and colleagues reported that BCAA enrichment (47% of PN amino acids) improved nitrogen economy and increased plasma levels of anti-inflammatory acute-phase proteins and formed coagulation elements in post-traumatic sepsis.[47] Cerra and colleagues[48] and Nuwer and co-workers[49] demonstrated an elevation in the absolute lymphocyte count and a reversal of anergy to recall skin test antigens with BCAA supplementation.

The study by Garcia-de-Lorenzo and associates is the only one demonstrating a difference in mortality with BCAA in ICU patients.[50] This was a prospective randomized multicenter study in ICUs in seven university hospitals in Spain. A total of 69 septic patients requiring PN were randomized to three clinically matched groups; two study groups received PN enriched in BCAAs (45% of amino acids as BCAAs, and either 1.5 or 1.1 g of protein per kilogram per day), and the control group received 1.5 g of protein per kilogram per day (23% BCAAs). Plasma prealbumin and retinol-binding protein levels increased in the BCAA-enriched groups. The length of stay in the ICU did not change between the groups. However, the mortality rate in the control group (41%) was significantly higher than that of the two groups of patients receiving BCAA supplementation (8% and 23% mortality, respectively).[50] In 1993, the American Society for Parenteral and Enteral Nutrition clinical guidelines stated that because proven effects on clinical outcomes are lacking, BCAA-supplemented diets cannot be routinely advocated during critical illness.[2] Of note, no adverse effects specifically attributable to the BCAA component of parenteral diets have been published.

Both the composition and the quantity of protein intake have significant effects on respiration.[51] Infusion of L-amino acids has been shown to increase minute ventilation, the ventilatory response to hypoxia, oxygen consumption, and the ventilatory response to hypoxia and hypercarbia.[51–55] Compared with standard amino acid solutions, the administration of BCAA-enriched PN formulas was shown to magnify the respiratory stimulation induced by intravenous amino acids in ICU patients.[54] In an open crossover study, the effects of increased amounts of PN BCAAs (53% vs. 30%) on respiratory function and episodes of apnea in premature infants was examined.[55] Ten premature infants at 34 weeks of gestation or less were observed. The high-BCAA solution significantly increased dynamic pulmonary compliance and specific dynamic compliance and decreased total pulmonary resistance and peak-to-peak pressure. In 4 of 10 infants with significant apnea, the incidence of apneic episodes decreased from 58 during standard PN to 11 with the enriched solution infusion during matched 12-hour periods.[55] Thus, BCAA supplementation may improve aspects of pulmonary function in this specific patient population. Further studies need to be done to define the exact mechanisms of action and the pulmonary disease subgroups that may benefit from BCAA administration.

Conventional PN has been demonstrated by Gil and coworkers to suppress ad libitum oral food intake in humans, but intake was improved during the infusion of BCAAs.[56] The mechanism of this effect is not completely defined. Bursztein-De Myttenaere and associates demonstrated that PN attenuated gastric emptying compared with hydration fluid alone; gastric emptying of a standardized meal was significantly increased when subjects were given a PN formula enriched with BCAAs (as 50% of administered amino acids) compared with a solution providing standard amounts of amino acids.[57] These findings have clinical potential as a method to facilitate oral intake and accelerate the conversion from a parenteral to an oral diet.

Arginine

Arginine has been extensively studied as an enterally administered nutriceutical (reviewed in Ziegler and Young[58]), but few data are published on its effects when given intravenously in humans. Arginine is an intermediary metabolite in the urea cycle, is indirectly linked to the citric acid cycle, is involved in polyamine synthesis, and is a critical substrate for in vivo and in vitro nitric oxide (NO) production by conversion to citrulline by the arginine deaminase pathway.[58] Arginine is a known secretagogue for several peptide hormones, including growth hormone, insulin, prolactin, and glucagon, although the magnitude and importance of this effect in healthy persons are unclear.[59] A large number of animal studies suggest that arginine-supplemented enteral feeding has stimulating effects on immune cell number and/or function. In addition, arginine-enriched diets attenuate thymic atrophy,[60] improve animal survival to septic challenge,[61] and enhance wound healing.[62, 63] Several animal studies indicate that arginine-supplemented intravenous solutions also improve nitrogen balance, immune cell responses, and wound healing.[64–66]

Human data on arginine's potential benefits are limited; however, several published studies suggest that enteral supplementation with arginine may be an important dietary component in catabolic patients, primarily as an immune-stimulating agent and also in wound healing.[67–69] In the first study reported with intravenous arginine in humans, Elsair and coworkers gave PN-treated patients 3 days of supplemental arginine hydrochloride infusion (15 g/day) after cholecystectomy.[70] Improved nitrogen retention was noted in the supplemented patients in comparison with controls receiving isonitrogenous PN. In the only other intervention study, Sigal and associates gave 30 patients either 20 g of parenteral arginine per day or an isonitrogenous amino acid solution (3.7 g of arginine per day) alone for 7 days after major gastrointestinal operations.[71] No differences in nitrogen balance were observed, but the mean total number of circulating T cells increased in the arginine group on day 7. In general, this study did not document improved indices of immunity in these patients with intravenous arginine compared with a more balanced amino acid mixture.[71] Thus, arginine may need to be administered with an adequate substrate background in order to exert effects on immune function. In burn patients, Yu and coworkers demonstrated increased arginine catabolism proportional to whole-body protein turnover in patients fed high-nitrogen total PN (0.39 g/kg/day).[72] Conversion of citrulline to arginine was not elevated above baseline conditions found in healthy adults, leading to negative arginine balance. The authors suggest that exogenous arginine (above the level in present amino acid infusions) may be required to maintain arginine homeostasis in burn injury. Of note, enteral administration of L-glutamine has been demonstrated to increase plasma arginine levels in healthy subjects and in catabolic patients, probably via the conversion of gut-derived citrulline to arginine by the kidney.[28, 58] Although L-arginine is required for NO synthesis and thus may potentially affect vascular tone, to date no adverse effects on blood pressure or hemodynamic stability have been reported in humans with enteral or parenteral arginine administration in nutrient infusions.

A few additional studies suggest theoretical benefits of arginine supplementation. Vosatka and colleagues reported depressed plasma arginine levels in infants with persistent pulmonary hypertension of the newborn compared with control infants.[73] Administration of exogenous NO has been used in the management of this condition but may consume arginine. Providing amino acids at an infusion of 2.5 g/kg/24 h to 10 infants with persistent pulmonary hypertension of the newborn resulted in significantly increased plasma arginine levels 3 to 4 days after the initiation of infusion.[73] Because most of the patients began to improve clinically before intravenous feeding, no conclusion could be reached regarding the positive or negative effects of arginine-containing PN. The authors propose that intravenous arginine may support the elevated NO synthesis required in this condition to minimize pulmonary hypertension.[73]

The ability of arginine to generate NO has been suggested as a potential benefit in the treatment of two diseases caused by *Escherichia coli* O157:H7.[74] This strain of *E. coli* has been implicated as the cause of hemolytic uremic syndrome and thrombotic thrombocytopenic purpura. Conventional antibiotic treatment often worsens the course of the disease by increasing the release of toxin from the bacteria. The stimulation of NO production by intravenous arginine supplementation may impede the excessive platelet aggregation that occurs in hemolytic uremic syndrome and thrombotic thrombocytopenic purpura, minimizing the renal damage that results from severe blood clotting.[74] Clinical trials based on these theoretical concepts may be warranted. With regard to currently administered arginine doses, pediatric amino acid products provide 730 to 860 mg of arginine per 100 mL, and commercial amino acids for adult PN typically supply arginine at concentrations of 810 to 1470 mg/100 mL; thus, conventional PN prescriptions for adults provide about 5 to 10 g of L-arginine per day.[75]

Effects of Other Amino Acids and Peptides

In enteral nutrient solutions, amino acids are provided in the form of intact proteins (e.g., milk, egg white solids); partially hydrolyzed proteins (e.g., whey, casein, lactalbumin) containing peptides of various lengths; dipeptides; or, less commonly, crystalline L-amino acids. These formulations provide known adequate amounts of essential amino acids for stressed patients but as

noted previously may be limited in some conditionally essential amino acids. The overall amino acid composition of enteral formulas are probably more complete and of higher biologic value than current parenteral amino acid solutions.[76] The possible clinical implications of these differences between parenteral and enteral amino acid composition are unclear and require further study.

All the intravenous solutions available in the United States also contain L-histidine, which is essential for infants and may be semiessential for older children and adults.[2] Neonates, especially those with low birth weight or prematurity, appear to require cyst(e)ine and taurine,[77] whereas healthy infants appear to require additional histidine and tyrosine.[2, 78] The immaturity of enzyme systems in low-birth-weight infants inhibits the normal conversion of methionine to cysteine and taurine and inhibits the conversion of phenylalanine to tyrosine.[2, 78–80] L-Cysteine HCl, as a single amino acid supplement for neonates and preterm infants, can be admixed with intravenous solutions containing mixed amino acids.

Taurine is beginning to receive more interest as a potentially important amino acid in nutritional and metabolic support in adults. Taurine is the most abundant intracellular free amino acid in the human body but is not incorporated into body protein.[80] Taurine is important in bile acid conjugation, cell volume regulation, neural and retinal function, and platelet aggregation and as an antioxidant, among other functions.[81, 82] Low plasma and urinary taurine levels occur in adults with cancer[82] and in adults after operative injury,[82] burns,[83] and chemotherapy and/or irradiation,[84] suggesting total body taurine depletion in these disorders. The rate-limiting enzyme for taurine synthesis from methionine or cysteine, cysteine sulfinic acid decarboxylase, may be inhibited during catabolic illness.[84] In one study by Mequid and colleagues, intravenous taurine supplementation (8.6 mg/kg/day) in PN corrected low plasma taurine levels in 12 malnourished patients after 10 days of infusion.[81]

Current intravenous amino acid formulas may provide limiting and/or excessive amounts of certain amino acids depending on the patient subgroup.[77, 78] Amino acid levels are in a dynamic state, and are influenced by the nutritional status, nutrient intake, disease type, severity of illness, age, and sex. It is therefore difficult to determine amino acid requirements or amino acid "deficiency" by the use of plasma levels or free amino acid levels in tissues.[77, 78] Low plasma and/or intracellular free histidine, serine, taurine, threonine, tyrosine, and valine levels occur in uremic patients, and low cyst(e)ine, taurine, and tyrosine levels occur in cirrhotic patients receiving PN, suggesting possible conditional deficiency of these amino acids.[76–78] Some amino acids are totally lacking in standard parenteral amino acid formulations (taurine, cyst[e]ine, and glutamine) or are present in very small amounts (tyrosine).[77, 78] Poor solubility (in the case of cystine, tyrosine, and glutamine) or instability in solution (with cyst[e]ine) may limit their use in the free form in parenteral diets.[76, 77] However, dipeptide forms, for example in combination with glutamine or alanine, represent new heat-stable and soluble substrates for PN therapy.[85]

Gazzaniga and associates studied the effects of a complete PN solution containing a pediatric amino acid formula in stable adults.[86] The formula contained 33% BCAAs; increased amounts of histidine, tyrosine, and arginine; and taurine. Patients received this PN formulation with or without added cysteine HCl (0.5 mmol/kg/day), and a total protein dose of 1.5 g/kg/day for at least 6 days. A significant positive correlation between the increase in taurine levels in plasma and improved nitrogen balance in the group receiving intravenous cysteine was found.[86] A positive correlation between improved nitrogen balance and plasma levels of cystine, total cysteine plus cystine, tyrosine, and ornithine was seen.[65] These findings suggest possible benefits in adults with amino acid solutions tailored initially for infants and children. Further clinical study is needed on the efficacy of new combinations of parenteral amino acid formulations in organ failure and other clinical conditions. In this regard, it may be of interest to study novel formulations that mimic the amino acid efflux from muscle during stress.

Use of α-Ketoglutarate Salts

The use of ornithine α-ketoglutarate (OKG) and α-ketoglutarate (AKG) in enteral and parenteral nutrition has received considerable research attention.[87] OKG is a salt formed of one AKG molecule and two ornithine molecules. AKG is a key intermediary in the Krebs cycle, and ornithine is a central amino acid in the urea cycle. After intravenous or enteral administration, OKG dissociates readily into ornithine and AKG.[87–89] OKG has been shown to stimulate growth hormone and insulin release, and ornithine is important in polyamine synthesis.[87] Both substances serve as glutamine biosynthetic precursors by conversion to glutamate in the body and then metabolism to glutamine by the enzyme glutamine synthetase.[87] Both OKG and AKG appear to be well tolerated when provided in enteral and parenteral feedings.

A number of trials evaluated the enteral administration of OKG.[87–92] OKG given at a dose of 20 g/day significantly improved wound healing, nitrogen balance, and serum protein levels in patients with moderate-sized burns, compared with isonitrogenous placebo.[90] Trauma patients given enteral tube feedings supplemented with OKG (approximately 16 g/day) demonstrated enhanced nitrogen balance and increased plasma glutamine, growth hormone, and insulin-like growth factor I levels compared with controls receiving OKG-free isonitrogenous tube feedings.[91] Intravenous OKG and AKG administration in postoperative and critically ill patients induces metabolic and protein-sparing effects very similar to those produced by glutamine administration.[87, 91] Both OKG- and AKG-enriched intravenous nutrient solutions attenuate the loss of skeletal muscle intracellular glutamine and preserve muscle protein synthesis (measured by skeletal muscle polyribosome concentration).[91] In a study in children with growth retardation secondary to short bowel syndrome, PN enriched with OKG (15 g/day) was associated with increased height growth rate and increased plasma glutamine and insulin-like growth factor I levels.[92]

Lipid Substrates

Intravenous lipid emulsions have routinely been used clinically in nutritional support since the mid-1970s to prevent essential fatty acid deficiency and to provide energy.[58] More recently, the regulatory role of parenteral lipids in physiologic functions, including immune function and inflammatory responses, is increasingly being elucidated and has potentially important clinical applications.[93] The fatty acid composition of exogenous lipid sources is known to influence fatty acid metabolism and the incorporation of phospholipids into the cell membrane, thus modulating eicosanoid synthesis and the function of biomembranes. Modifications of lipid emulsion formulations that alter inflammatory and immune functions may offer an opportunity to improve the metabolic support and clinical outcomes in PN-dependent patients.[85, 93] An extensive review of lipid therapy is covered in Chapter 3.

Long-chain triglycerides (LCTs) derived from soybean and/or safflower oils are the predominant lipid source in emulsions used in the United States as standard-of-care PN support. LCT emulsions, primarily composed of polyunsaturated fatty acids, contain large amounts of linoleic acid and relatively small amounts of α-linolenic acid. These essential fatty acids, linoleic and α-linolenic, are metabolized through carbon elongation and desaturation to form the derivatives eicosapentaenoic acid (EPA), docosahexaenoic acid (DHA), and arachidonic acid (AA).[58] The n-3 polyunsaturated fatty acids (α-linolenic acid, EPA, and DHA) and n-6 polyunsaturated fatty acids (linoleic acid and AA) serve as precursors for eicosanoid synthesis, prostaglandins (PGs), thromboxanes, and leukotrienes (LTs), which have important physiologic functions, including vascular and homeostatic actions and critical inflammatory, allergic, and immune responses in humans.[85, 93] The eicosanoids derived from AA (PGE$_2$, thromboxane A$_2$, LTB$_4$) are important inflammatory mediators and regulators of cytokine production, whereas n-3 fatty acid (EPA and DHA)–derived metabolites competitively inhibit AA conversion to eicosanoids and form less biologically active mediators (PGE$_3$, thromboxane A, LTB$_5$).[85–93]

The administration of LCT emulsions in critically ill patients prevents essential fatty acid deficiency, improves nitrogen balance and can diminish triglyceride accumulation.[94] However, the administration of LCT emulsions with a high n-6 fatty acid content has been associated with impairment of reticuloendothelial system functions, impairment of neutrophil and macrophage functions, and reduced clearance rates during sepsis.[95] In critically injured patients, the immunosuppressive effects of intravenous LCT infusions have been considered to be a possible contributor to increased patient morbidity, including infection, pulmonary dysfunction, and delayed recovery.[94, 96] Thus, the use of alternative lipid substrates that do not facilitate proinflammatory eicosanoid synthesis and amplify inflammatory responses is actively being investigated in the parenteral support of critically ill patients. There is mounting evidence that n-3 fatty acid administration, which alters cell membrane composition and substrate availability for eicosanoid production, and the use of alternative triglycerides, such as medium-chain triglycerides (MCTs) or structured lipids, may be particularly beneficial to patients with inflammatory or immunologic diseases.[97–100]

n-3 Fatty Acids

The administration of fish oils that are rich in n-3 fatty acids or n-3 fatty acid supplementation of enteral formulas has shown therapeutic benefit in a number of patient subgroups with inflammatory disease processes and immunologic dysfunction, including rheumatoid arthritis, psoriasis, asthma, lupus, and ulcerative colitis.[101, 102] Studies in critically ill patients demonstrate conflicting results regarding the clinical benefits of enteral formulas enriched in n-3 fatty acids in combination with arginine and nucleotides.[85, 93, 103–105] Several studies showed improved clinical outcomes, including reduced septic complications, incidences of systemic inflammatory responses, and multiple organ failures, that were associated with improved immune function.[103–105] Oral supplementation of fish oil or EPA alone has improved the clinical course in a variety of patient groups, including those undergoing renal transplantation and upper gastrointestinal surgery[106, 107] and those with ulcerative colitis.[108]

Less is known about the potential therapeutic use of intravenous n-3 fatty emulsions in patients requiring PN. The administration of parenteral n-3 fatty acid emulsions has been shown to be safe and well tolerated, even for prolonged periods up to 4 weeks, by healthy volunteers and critically ill and stable cystic fibrosis patients.[97, 98] The effect of modifying the n-6/n-3 ratio to improve inflammatory and immunologic responses in patients appears to be a result of altering the types of PGs, LTs, and thromboxanes synthesized, by EPA's competing with AA as a substrate, thus reducing AA conversion to proinflammatory mediators (PGE$_2$, thromboxane A$_2$, LTB$_4$).[99] In addition, n-3 fatty acids also exert physiologic effects by decreasing the production of proinflammatory cytokines interleukin 1α, interleukin 1β, interleukin 6, and tumor necrosis factor; this appears to be related to changes in eicosanoid metabolism.[99, 109]

Studies of n-3 fatty acid infusion in trauma and surgical patients demonstrate that eicosanoid and cytokine production by leukocytes is altered within 5 days of fish oil administration.[85, 97, 100] Administration of 0.15 g of fish oil per kilogram per day via PN for 5 days resulted in significantly higher n-3 fatty acid (EPA and DHA) incorporation into circulating leukocytes in postoperative trauma patients.[97] Synthesis of LTB$_5$ and LTC$_5$ by leukocytes isolated from these patients was markedly increased, suggesting that n-3 fatty acid infusion can increase EPA conversion to less potent eicosanoids in vivo.[97] A study by Wachtler and associates showed similar increases in LTB$_5$ production by circulating leukocytes after 5 days of fish oil–enriched PN in patients undergoing major intestinal surgery.[100] In surgical patients receiving PN, oral supplementation of EPA ethyl ester (1.8 g/day) decreased the production of the proinflammatory cytokine interleukin 6 and improved cell-mediated immunity, as measured by lymphocyte proliferation, natural killer activity, and the CD4/CD8 ratio.[110] The immunomodulatory effects of administered n-3 fatty acids observed in critically ill patients is consistent with a study in patients with active Crohn's disease.[101] In this trial, PN-dependent Crohn's patients given fish oil (EPA 0.6 g/day) for 2 weeks showed increased LTB$_5$ generation by activated leukocytes. An increased LTB$_5$/LTB$_4$ ratio in these patients may be important to disease activity and recovery from acute inflammations, as the potent proinflammatory form (LTB$_4$) is an important mediator of colonic mucosal inflammation in Crohn's patients.[101] Current studies demonstrate the safety of n-3 fatty acid infusion and provide sound preliminary evidence for immunomodulatory action of n-3 fatty acids in certain patient populations. Additional randomized trials are needed to evaluate whether intravenous n-3 fatty acid administration improves clinical outcomes and represents a valuable adjunct to PN support.

Medium-Chain Triglycerides

MCTs are triacylglycerols that contain saturated fatty acids of 6 to 12 carbon atoms; they are derived from the fractionated coconut and palm kernel oils.[95] The administration of intravenous MCT emulsions offers several advantages to the metabolic support of critically ill patients. MCTs are more water soluble than LCTs and are more efficiently cleared from the blood and metabolized when administered parenterally.[95, 111] MCTs are more efficiently oxidized and do not require carnitine for transport into mitochondria and subsequent oxidation. MCTs do not accumulate as storage in adipose tissue or in the liver.[95]

MCT use in enteral nutritional support has proved clinically valuable to patients with impaired fat digestion or diminished absorptive capacity or lymphatic transport, because MCTs are rapidly hydrolyzed in the intestinal lumen and do not require bile for pancreatic lipase secretion or micelle formation for absorption.[94] Thus, enteral formulas containing MCTs are routinely used in patients with pancreatitis, liver dysfunction, and short bowel syndrome. Preparations of MCTs for intravenous administration are not commercially available in the United States but are in routine use in Europe and other countries. MCTs are delivered for parenteral support in emulsions containing a physical mixture of MCTs and LCTs, or, more recently, as a component of synthetic structured lipids.[112] The published clinical experience with parenteral MCT preparations has included patients with critical illness, pulmonary disease, liver disease, and immunosuppression.[94, 95] MCT-based lipid emulsions may have an advantage over LCT emulsions in these clinical settings because they are more efficiently oxidized, do not influence eicosanoid synthesis or availability, are rapidly cleared from the blood, and are metabolized independently of carnitine.[94, 95]

The safety and efficacy of MCT-LCT infusion has been demonstrated in critically ill patients administered a 50:50 MCT-LCT emulsion.[113] Increased plasma ketone and glycerol concentrations and improved nitrogen balance were demonstrated in patients provided the MCT-LCT emulsion compared with those given the LCT infusion.[113] These findings suggest that MCTs represent an excellent substrate that is rapidly oxidizable for patients who are often insulin resistant and possibly carnitine deficient. The rapid clearance and the efficient oxidation of MCTs also suggest potential therapeutic value in patients with impaired hepatic lipid metabolism, such as those with cirrhotic liver disease. A preliminary study by Balderman and coworkers in 14 patients demonstrated no change in liver fat infiltration by ultrasonography after MCT-LCT administration for 7 days, but increased fatty infiltration and liver size were associated with LCT infusion.[114] In patients with respiratory insufficiency, the administration of lipids provides important nonprotein calories owing to its lower carbon dioxide production during oxidation. Interest in MCT infusion in patients with pulmonary disease is based on the potential modulation of eicosanoid synthesis by LCTs, which may increase prostaglandin levels and worsen pulmonary hemodynamics and respiratory gas exchange.[115, 116] However, studies have not demonstrated consistent improvements in pulmonary hemodynamics and in gas exchange parameters by MCT-LCT administration when compared with LCTs.[115–118] There is evidence that the alterations in respiratory function are also related to the quantity and rate of lipid administration and not the lipid emulsion composition alone.[118]

Evaluation of the potential immunomodulatory effects of MCT-LCT emulsions in immunocompromised patients remains limited. A randomized crossover study in malnourished patients undergoing surgery for gastric cancer showed no change in monocyte function and modestly decreased neutrophil bacterial killing after 48 hours of MCT-LCT infusion.[119] A study by Gelas and associates evaluated the administration of MCT-LCT emulsions for 6 days in malnourished acquired immunodeficiency syndrome patients; the study demonstrated adequate tolerance of MCT-LCT emulsion and maintenance of normal lymphocyte function when compared with LCT infusion.[120] These initial evaluations of parenteral MCT-LCT administration in various disease states demonstrate their safety and suggest that MCTs may be an important component in PN support of patients with inflammatory or immune dysfunction. Further trials of MCTs are necessary to identify the duration, timing, and dose required for optimal nutritional and metabolic support of patients requiring PN.

Structured Lipids

Structured lipids are triacylglycerols synthesized by the random esterification of fatty acids to a glycerol backbone to produce triglycerides containing different medium- and long-chain fatty acid compositions.[85, 121] The use of pure MCT solutions is limited because of their potential to induce metabolic acidosis; further, MCTs lack essential linoleic and linolenic fatty acids.[121] Structured lipids with MCT-LCT physical mixtures may reduce the risk of potential MCT adverse effects.[94] Novel structured lipid substrates have become commercially available for clinical studies. A study conducted in healthy subjects and patients undergoing elective surgery demonstrated that the infusion of a structured lipid emulsion for 6 days was well tolerated and was more rapidly oxidized and cleared from the plasma compared with LCT infusion but did not alter nitrogen balance as did LCTs.[121]

Administration of Nutrient Antioxidants

Antioxidants provide the body with critical protection against oxidizing free radicals produced during normal metabolic processes and during active disease. Increased free radical generation occurs in a variety of clinical conditions, including inflammatory disorders, trauma, sepsis, surgical insult, and the catabolic state in general.[6, 122] Reactive oxygen species (ROS) play an important role in AA metabolism, immune cell activation, and cytokine production during catabolic illness. However, ROS are believed to mediate cellular injury and organ dysfunction during critical illness through damage of DNA, protein, and cell membrane polyunsaturated fatty acids. There is substantial evidence that plasma and tissue antioxidants that quench and deactivate ROS are depleted in critically ill patients.[6, 9] Compromised antioxidant status may exacerbate oxidative injury and tissue dysfunction. Approaches to adjunctive nutritional therapies have included antioxidant supplementation in patients with impaired antioxidant defenses or increased exposure to ROS.

The body's endogenous antioxidant system consists of enzymatic and nutrient antioxidants. The enzymatic antioxidants—superoxide dismutase, glutathione peroxidase, and catalase—detoxify ROS and are dependent on the nutrient trace elements selenium, copper, zinc, and manganese. Nonenzymatic nutrient antioxidants, including α-tocopherol, ascorbic acid, β-carotene, cysteine, and taurine, also provide protection against ROS in aqueous and lipophilic environments. The tripeptide glutathione (GSH) is composed of cysteine, glutamate, and glycine and is considered to be an important antioxidant that maintains other cellular proteins in the reduced state.[6] In addition, GSH is intimately related to vitamin E and vitamin C metabolism. GSH is capable of regenerating reduced vitamin E by reduction of vitamin C to its functional form. Vitamin C (ascorbic acid) reduces the vitamin phenoxyl radical to the phenolic form, thus regenerating reduced vitamin E for further ROS detoxification.[123]

Substantial clinical evidence indicates that critically ill patients requiring nutritional support have impaired antioxidant defenses.[122–125] However, only a limited number of clinical trials have evaluated the efficacy of antioxidant supplementation.[124, 125] Strategies to augment antioxidant defenses have included the administration of antioxidant nutrients (α-tocopherol, ascorbic acid, β-carotene, and acetylcysteine), trace elements required for antioxidant enzyme function (i.e., selenium, copper, zinc, and manganese), or oxygen radical scavengers (e.g., allopurinol).

Significant depletion of nutrient antioxidants has been demonstrated in several ICU patient populations.[124–130] A study in ICU patients with septic shock and secondary organ failure showed markedly reduced levels of α-tocopherol, β-carotene, and lycopene in plasma and elevated lipid peroxidation.[129] Similarly, patients with sepsis-induced adult respiratory distress syndrome have depleted serum concentrations of α-tocopherol and GSH and concomitantly increased levels of lipid peroxides.[128, 129] A study in critically ill patients demonstrated very low plasma ascorbic acid concentrations that were directly related to the severity of illness.[127] Decreased ascorbic acid and α-tocopherol levels in association with increased levels of oxidants have been observed in the plasma of blunt trauma patients.[125] In these patients, intravenous administration of ascorbic acid and α-tocopherol (500 mg of ascorbic acid, 50 mg of dl-α-tocopherol) for 7 days improved neu-

trophil function.[125] In burn injury patients, trace mineral nutrients with antioxidant properties, that is, copper, selenium, and zinc, are depleted as evidenced by low plasma and urine concentrations.[124, 130] When provided large intravenous doses of copper (4.5 mg), selenium (190 μg), and zinc (40 mg) daily, these burn patients had increased plasma copper, selenium, and zinc concentrations and an improved clinical outcome with regard to grafting requirements.[124, 130] There are only limited data demonstrating the efficacy of antioxidant nutrient administration in ICU patients. Further clinical studies are needed to determine the potential benefits of antioxidant supplementation and the most appropriate antioxidant mixtures for specific ICU patient populations demonstrating antioxidant deficiencies.

Compromised antioxidant status has been reported in surgical patients. Patients undergoing coronary artery bypass surgery, vascular surgery, organ transplantation, and bowel obstruction surgery are subjected to ischemia-reperfusion injury. Ischemia followed by reperfusion results in excessive generation of ROS through xanthine oxidase activity, which is thought to cause tissue injury, oxidative stress, and loss of organ function.[122] Patients undergoing coronary artery bypass grafting and revascularization operations show increased oxidative stress during reperfusion,[131, 132] and this was shown to be proportional to the severity of the ischemic period.[131] The administration of oral vitamin E (600 mg/day), vitamin C (2 g/day), and allopurinol (600 mg/day) for 2 days before and 1 day after coronary artery bypass grafting decreased complications and improved cardiac function after surgery in stable patients.[133] Intravenous supplementation of antioxidants by a "cocktail" containing 5 mg of α-tocopherol, 500 mg of vitamin C, 5.5 mg of vitamin A (retinol palmitate) and B complex (thiamine, riboflavin, nicotinamide, pyridoxine) prevented the increase in plasma lipid peroxides and reduced the limb swelling associated with ischemia-reperfusion injury during limb salvage operations.[132] Antioxidant therapy that ameliorates reperfusion injury may represent an important adjunct to the nutritional support of surgical patients.

Patients recovering from liver and kidney transplantation, also subject to ischemia-reperfusion injury, show significantly lower plasma concentrations of antioxidants and higher levels of lipid peroxidation products.[134, 135] One controlled trial of nutrient antioxidant administration has been conducted in solid organ transplantation patients. Intravenous administration of a multivitamin mixture (containing 5 mg of vitamin E, 500 mg of vitamin C, 5.5 mg of vitamin A and B complex) to kidney transplantation patients before reperfusion reduced lipid peroxide appearance in the plasma and improved post-transplantation renal function.[136] Trials in pancreatic or liver transplantation patients have not been published. Antioxidant therapy delivered in the absence of other nutrients must be evaluated to clarify the specific role of antioxidant support alone in improving clinical outcomes, and further clinical trials in transplantation patients are indicated.

Inflammatory diseases, as seen in pancreatitis and inflammatory bowel disease patients, are known to be mediated in part by increased oxidant production. The loss of plasma and tissue antioxidant capacity has been well documented in pancreatitis and inflammatory bowel disease patients.[137] Acute and chronic pancreatitis is associated with severe depletion of plasma vitamin E, ascorbic acid, β-carotene, and GSH, and elevated levels of lipid peroxidation products have been consistently reported as an early feature of the disease.[137, 138] In a case report of a patient with acute necrotizing pancreatitis and multiple organ failure treated with intravenous N-acetylcysteine (an amino acid precursor for GSH), respiratory and renal function significantly improved after 3 days.[139] The use of nutrient antioxidant therapy has been evaluated in patients with recurrent (both acute and chronic) pancreatitis.[140] Oral supplementation with 600 μg of selenium, 9000 IU of β-carotene, 270 IU of vitamin E, and 2 g of L-methionine for 20 weeks improved pain and prevented relapse of pancreatitis regardless of the disease's cause or severity.[140] Well-controlled studies of nutrient antioxidant administration in pancreatitis patients are indicated as the available evidence indicates a benefit from the repletion of plasma antioxidant stores during active pancreatitis.

Patients receiving chemotherapy for solid or hematologic malignancies show evidence of increased ROS formation and oxidative stress induced by chemotherapeutic agents.[141] Increased requirements for antioxidant nutrients during this therapy are suggested by increased plasma levels of lipid peroxides and decreased plasma levels of vitamin C, α-tocopherol, and β-carotene.[141, 142] There is evidence that standard PN formulas do not maintain plasma antioxidant concentrations of GSH and α-tocopherol in patients receiving high-dose chemotherapy during bone marrow transplantation.[143, 144] Despite the provision of precursor amino acids (glycine, glutamate, and methionine) needed for GSH synthesis and 20 mg of α-tocopherol per day, we demonstrated marked declines in plasma GSH and α-tocopherol concentrations in bone marrow transplantation patients.[143] However, intravenous administration of vitamin C in large dosage (700 mg/day) was associated with normal levels of plasma vitamin C concentrations after high-dose chemotherapy. These data suggest the possible need for increased or even pharmacologic doses of certain antioxidants in such patients.[143, 144] One randomized trial in bone marrow transplantation patients demonstrated that oral supplementation with α-tocopherol, ascorbic acid, and β-carotene for 3 weeks before high-dose chemotherapy and bone marrow transplantation can increase plasma α-tocopherol and β-carotene concentrations and decrease lipid peroxide levels.[145] Antioxidants may play an important role in protecting normal host tissue from cytotoxic injury. The administration of topical vitamin E (oral 400 mg/day) significantly improved the healing of oral lesions in patients with chemotherapy-induced mucositis.[146] A pilot study in patients with advanced gastric cancer showed that vitamin E, vitamin C, and N-acetylcysteine supplementation reduced the cardiotoxic effects of chemotherapy and irradiation.[147] Based on these limited findings, further randomized trials of antioxidant nutrient therapy are needed to determine the appropriate timing, dosage, and combination of antioxidant nutrient supplementation for cancer chemotherapy patients.

Low plasma levels of circulating antioxidants, including vitamin C, selenium, and β-carotene, have been reported in patients with chronic Crohn's disease.[148] It is possible that compromised antioxidant defenses related to both mucosal oxidative stress and poor nutritional status may increase susceptibility to further gut mucosal injury and impair patients' recovery from acute inflammatory episodes.[5, 6] In this regard, the administration of the gut-trophic amino acid glutamine may be of particular benefit as a method to improve antioxidant and GSH redox capacity. Glutamine may serve as a GSH precursor (through interconversion to glutamate) and/or may alter GSH levels by decreasing tissue requirements for GSH or other antioxidants.[9] In animal models, glutamine-enriched PN given after intestinal ischemia-reperfusion injury, chemotherapy, or hepatic injury induced by acetaminophen markedly increased gut mucosal and circulating GSH concentrations and decreased tissue damage, bacterial translocation, and levels of lipid peroxidative products.[10–12] No human data on glutamine supplementation and antioxidant capacity in patients requiring PN have been published. Based on the animal data, however, clinical trials to determine whether glutamine improves the redox status systemically and in tissues appear warranted.

Thiamine

Evidence suggests that thiamine deficiency may not be uncommon in patients with chronic heart failure receiving diuretics such as furosemide that increase urinary thiamine losses.[149–151] In addition to precipitation of encephalopathy and lactic acidosis in association with refeeding syndrome (especially with high-carbohydrate diets),[2] thiamine depletion is known to adversely affect cardiac function. Peripheral vasodilation, with secondary arteriovenous shunting and salt and water retention, contributes to biventricular heart failure in some patients with thiamine deficiency (wet beriberi).[149] Of note, two studies have demonstrated that the administration of intravenous thiamine followed by oral thiamine (200 mg/day via each route) for several weeks to adult patients with moderate to severe congestive heart failure was beneficial. Thiamine administration normalized the diuretic-associated depressed plasma thiamine status, and significantly improved left ventricular ejection fraction (22% improvement). Thus, pending additional efficacy trials in patients requiring specialized feeding, consideration should be given to monitoring of the plasma thiamine status and the pharmacologic administration of thiamine in malnourished patients requiring chronic diuretic therapy.

REFERENCES

1. Klein S, Kinney J, Jeejeebhoy K, et al: Nutrition support in clinical practice: Review of published data and recommendations for future research directions. JPEN J Parenter Enteral Nutr 21:133–156, 1997.
2. ASPEN Board of Directors: Guidelines for the use of parenteral and enteral nutrition in adult and pediatric patients. JPEN J Parenter Enteral Nutr 17:1sa–52sa, 1993.
3. Fleming CR, Jeejeebhoy KN: Advances in clinical nutrition. Gastroenterology 106:1365–1373, 1994.
4. Van Gossum A, Neve J: Trace element deficiency and toxicity. Curr Opin Clin Nutr Metab Care 1:499–507, 1998.
5. Ziegler TR: Glutamine supplementation in catabolic illness. Am J Clin Nutr 64:645–647, 1996.
6. Ziegler TR, Leader LM, Jonas CR, Griffiths DP: Adjunctive therapies in specialized nutrition support. Nutrition 9(Suppl):64s–72s, 1997.
7. Souba WW: Nutritional support. N Engl J Med 336:41–48, 1997.
8. Grimble RF, Grimble GK. Immunonutrition: Role of sulfur amino acids, related amino acids, and polyamines. Nutrition 14:605–610, 1998.
9. Ziegler TR, Szeszycki EE, Estívariz CF, et al: Glutamine: From basic science to clinical applications. Nutrition 12(Suppl):s2–s4, 1996.
10. Griffiths RD: Glutamine: Establishing clinical indications. Curr Opin Clin Nutr Metab Care 2:177–182, 1999.
11. Hong RW, Rounds JD, Helton WS, Wilmore DW: Glutamine preserves liver glutathione after lethal hepatic injury. Ann Surg 215:114–119, 1992.
12. Harward TRS, Coe D, Souba WW, et al: Glutamine preserves gut glutathione levels during intestinal ischemia/reperfusion. J Surg Res 56:351–355, 1994.
13. Borel MJ, Williams PE, Jabbour K, et al: Parenteral glutamine infusion alters insulin-mediated glucose metabolism. JPEN J Parenter Enteral Nutr 22:280–285, 1998.
14. Buchman AL, Moukarzel AA, Bhuta S, et al: Parenteral nutrition is associated with intestinal morphologic and functional changes in humans. JPEN J Parenter Enteral Nutr 19:453–460, 1995.
15. Ziegler TR, Young LS, Benfell K, et al: Clinical and metabolic efficacy of glutamine-supplemented parenteral nutrition following bone marrow transplantation: A randomized, double-blind, controlled study. Ann Intern Med 116:821–828, 1992.
16. Stehle P, Zander J, Mertes N, et al: Effect of parenteral glutamine peptide supplements on muscle glutamine loss and nitrogen balance after major surgery. Lancet 1:231–233, 1989.
17. Long CL, Borghesi L, Stahl R, et al: Impact of enteral feeding of a glutamine-supplemented formula on the hypoaminoacidemic response in trauma patients. J Trauma 40:97–102, 1996.
18. Fish J, Sporay G, Beyer K, et al: A prospective randomized study of glutamine-enriched parenteral compared with enteral feeding in postoperative patients. Am J Clin Nutr 65:977–983, 1997.
19. Scheppach W, Loges C, Bartram P, et al: Effect of free glutamine and alanyl-glutamine dipeptide on mucosal proliferation of the human ileum and colon. Gastroenterology 107:429–434, 1994.

20. Van der Hulst RRW, van Kreel BK, von Meyenfeldt MF, et al: Glutamine and the preservation of gut integrity. Lancet 341:1363–1365, 1993.

21. Tremel H, Kienle B, Weilemann LS, et al: Glutamine dipeptide supplemented TPN maintains intestinal function in the critically ill. Gastroenterology 107:1595–1601, 1994.

22. Ziegler TR, Bye RL, Persinger RL, et al: Effects of glutamine-enriched intravenous nutrition on circulating lymphocytes after bone marrow transplantation: A pilot study. Am J Med Sci 315:4–10, 1998.

23. O'Riordain MG, Fearon KCH, Ross JA, et al: Glutamine-supplemented total parenteral nutrition enhances T-lymphocyte response in surgical patients undergoing colorectal resection. Ann Surg 220:212–221, 1994.

24. De Beaux AC, O'Riordan MG, Ross JA, et al: Glutamine-supplemented total parenteral nutrition reduces blood mononuclear cell interleukin-8 release in severe acute pancreatitis. Nutrition 14:261–265, 1998.

25. Morlion B, Stehle P, Siedhoff H, et al: Glutamine dipeptide (L-alanyl-L-glutamine)–supplemented total parenteral nutrition improves nitrogen balance and shortens hospitalization in surgical patients. Ann Surg 227:302–308, 1998.

26. Griffiths RD, Jones C, Palmer TE: Six-month outcome of critically ill patients given glutamine-supplemented parenteral nutrition. Nutrition 13:295–302, 1997.

27. Neu J, Roig JC, Meetze WH, et al: Enteral glutamine supplementation for very low birth weight infants decreases morbidity. J Pediatr 131:691–699, 1997.

28. Houdijk AP, Rijnsburger ER, Jansen J, et al: Randomised trial of glutamine-enriched enteral nutrition on infectious morbidity in patients with multiple trauma. Lancet 352:772–776, 1998.

29. Anderson PM, Ramsay NK, Shu XO, et al: Effect of low-dose oral glutamine on painful stomatitis during bone marrow transplantation. Bone Marrow Transplant 22:339–344, 1998.

30. Byrne TA, Morrissey TB, Nattakom TV, et al: Growth hormone, glutamine and a modified diet enhance nutrient absorption in patients with the severe short bowel syndrome. JPEN J Parenter Enteral Nutr 19:296–302, 1995.

31. Byrne TA, Persinger RL, Young LS, et al: A new treatment for patients with the short-bowel syndrome: Growth hormone, glutamine and a modified diet. Ann Surg 222:243–255, 1995.

32. Scolapio JS, Camilleri M, Fleming CR, et al: Effect of growth hormone, glutamine, and diet on adaptation in short-bowel syndrome: A randomized, controlled study. Gastroenterology 113:1074–1081, 1997.

33. Furst P, Kuhn K, Ziegler TR: Amino acids and proteins—New definitions and requirements, hormonal interactions, methodological advances and pitfalls. Curr Opin Clin Nutr Metab Care 2:5–8, 1999.

34. Freund HR, Dienstag J, Lehrich et al: Infusion of branched-chain amino acid solution in patients with hepatic encephalopathy. Ann Surg 196:209–220, 1982.

35. Cerra FB, Chung NK, Fischer JE, et al: Disease-specific amino acid infusion (F080) in hepatic encephalopathy: A prospective, randomized, double-blind controlled trial. JPEN J Parenter Enteral Nutr 9:288–295, 1985.

36. Fiaccadori F, Ghinelli F, Pedretti G, et al: Branched-chain enriched amino acid solution in the treatment of hepatic encephalopathy: A controlled trial. Ital J Gastroenterol Hepatol 17:5–10, 1985.

37. Wahren J, Denis J, Desurmont P, et al: Is intravenous administration of branched chain amino acids effective in the treatment of hepatic encephalopathy? A multicenter study. Hepatology 3:475–480, 1983.

38. Michel H, Bories P, Aubin JP, et al: Treatment of acute hepatic encephalopathy in cirrhotics with a branched-chain amino acids enriched versus a conventional amino acids mixture. Liver 5:282–289, 1985.

39. Vilstrup H, Gluud C, Hardt F, et al: Branched chain enriched amino acids versus glucose treatment of hepatic encephalopathy. A double-blind study of 65 patients with cirrhosis. J Hepatol 10:291–296, 1990.

40. Naylor CD, O'Rourke K, Detcky AS, Baker JP: Parenteral nutrition with branched-chain amino acids in hepatic encephalopathy. A meta-analysis. Gastroenterology 97:1033–1042, 1989.

41. Echenique MM, Bristrian BR, Moldawer LL, et al: Improvement in amino acid use in the critically ill patient with parenteral formulas enriched with branched chain amino acids. Surg Gynecol Obstet 159:233–241, 1984.

42. Desai SP, Bristain BR, Palombo JD, et al: Branched-chain amino acid administration in surgical patients. Arch Surg 122:760–764, 1987.

43. Cerra F, Hirsch J, Mullen K, et al: The effect of stress level, amino acid formula, and nitrogen dose on nitrogen retention in traumatic and septic stress. Ann Surg 205:282–287, 1987.

44. Vander Woude P, Morgan R, Kosta JM, et al: Addition of branched-chain amino acids to parenteral nutrition of stressed critically ill patients. Crit Care Med 14:685–688, 1986.

45. Lenssen P, Cheney CL, Aker SN, et al: Intravenous branched chain amino acid trial in marrow transplant patients. JPEN J Parenter Enteral Nutr 11:112–118, 1987.

46. Scholten DJ, Morgan RE, Davis AT, Albrecht RM: Failure of BCAA supplementation to promote nitrogen retention in injured patients. J Am Coll Nutr 9:101–106, 1990.

47. Chiarla C, Siegel JH, Kidd S, et al: Inhibition of post-traumatic septic proteolysis and ureagenesis and stimulation of hepatic acute-phase protein production by branched-chain amino acid TPN. J Trauma 28:1145–1171, 1988.

48. Cerra FB, Mazuski JE, Chute E, et al: Branched chain metabolic support. A prospective, randomized, double-blind trial in surgical stress. Ann Surg 199:286–291, 1984.

49. Nuwer N, Cerra FB, Shronts EP, et al: Does modified amino acid total parenteral nutrition alter immune-response in high level surgical stress. JPEN J Parenter Enteral Nutr 7:521–524, 1983.

50. Garcia-de-Lorenzo A, Ortiz-Leyba C, Planas M, et al: Parenteral administration of different amounts of branch-chain amino acids in septic patients: Clinical and metabolic aspects. Crit Care Med 25:418–423, 1997.

51. Wilson DO, Rogers RM, Hoffman RM: Nutrition

and chronic lung disease. Am Rev Respir Dis 132:1347–1352, 1985.

52. Van den Berg B, Stram H, Hop WCF: Effects of dietary protein content on weaning from the ventilator. Clin Nutr 8:207–212, 1989.

53. Askanazi J, Weissman C, LaSala PA, et al: Effect of protein intake on ventilatory drive. Anesthesiology 60:106–110, 1984.

54. Takala J, Askanazi J, Weissman C, et al: Changes in respiratory control induced by amino acid infusions. Crit Care Med 16:465–469, 1988.

55. Blazer S, Reinersman GT, Askanazi J, et al: Branched-chain amino acids and respiratory pattern and function in the neonate. J Perinatol 14:290–295, 1994.

56. Gil KM, Skeie B, Kvetan V, et al: Parenteral nutrition and oral intake: Effect of branched chain amino acids. Nutrition 6:291–295, 1990.

57. Bursztein-De Myttenaere S, Gil KM, Heymsfield SB, et al: Gastric emptying in humans: Influence of different regimens of parenteral nutrition. Am J Clin Nutr 60:244–248, 1994.

58. Ziegler TR, Young LS: Therapeutic effects of specific nutrients. In Rombeau JL, Rolandelli RH (eds): Clinical Nutrition: Enteral and Tube Feeding, 3rd ed. Philadelphia, WB Saunders, 1996, pp 112–137.

59. Barbul A: Arginine: Biochemistry, physiology and therapeutic implications. JPEN J Parenter Enteral Nutr 10:227–238, 1986.

60. Gianotti L, Alexander JW, Payles T, et al: Arginine-supplemented diets improve survival in gut-derived sepsis and peritonitis by modulating bacterial clearance—The role of nitric oxide. Ann Surg 217:644–654, 1993.

61. Barbul A, Rettura G, Levenson S, et al: Wound healing and thymotrophic effects of arginine: A pituitary mechanism of action. Am J Clin Nutr 37:786–794, 1983.

62. Kirk SJ, Barbul A: Role of arginine in trauma, sepsis and immunity. JPEN J Parenter Enteral Nutr 14:226s–229s, 1990.

63. Gonce SJ, Peck MD, Alexander JW, et al: Arginine supplementation and its effect on established peritonitis in guinea pigs. JPEN J Parenter Enteral Nutr 14:237–244, 1990.

64. Barbul A, Wasserkrug HL, Yoshimura N, et al: High arginine levels in intravenous hyperalimentation abrogate post-traumatic immune suppression. J Surg Res 36:620–624, 1984.

65. Barbul A, Fishel RS, Shimazu S, et al: Intravenous hyperalimentation with high arginine levels improves wound healing and immune function. J Surg Res 38:328–334, 1985.

66. Barbul A, Wasserkrug HL, Penberthy LT, et al: Optimal levels of arginine in maintenance intravenous hyperalimentation. JPEN J Parenter Enteral Nutr 8:281–284, 1984.

67. Barbul A, Rettura G, Wasserkrug HL, et al: Arginine stimulates lymphocyte immune responses in healthy humans. Surgery 90:244–251, 1981.

68. Daly JM, Reynolds J, Thom A, et al: Immune and metabolic effects of arginine in the surgical patient. Ann Surg 208:512–523, 1988.

69. Kirk SJ, Hurson M, Regan MC, et al: Arginine stimulates wound healing and immune function in elderly human subjects. Surgery 114:155–160, 1993.

70. Elsair J, Poey J, Isaad H, et al: Effect of arginine chlorhydrate on nitrogen balance during the three days following routine surgery in man. Biomed Press 29:312–317, 1978.

71. Sigal RK, Shou J, Daly JM: Parenteral arginine infusion in humans: Nutrient substrate or pharmacologic agent? JPEN J Parenter Enteral Nutr 16:423–428, 1992.

72. Yu Y-M, Ryan CM, Burke JF, et al: Relations among arginine, citrulline, ornithine, and leucine kinetics in adult burn patients. Am J Clin Nutr 62:960–968, 1995.

73. Vosatka RJ, Kashyap S, Trifletti RR: Arginine deficiency accompanies persistent pulmonary hypertension of the newborn. Biol Neonate 66:65–70, 1994.

74. Jaradat ZW, Marquardt RR: L-Arginine as a therapeutic approach for the verotoxigenic Escherichia coli–induced hemolytic uremic syndrome and thrombotic thrombocytopenic purpura. Med Hypothesis 49:277–280, 1997.

75. Dickerson RN, Brown RO, White KG: Parenteral nutrition solutions. In Rombeau JL, Caldwell MD (eds): Parenteral Nutrition: Clinical Nutrition, 2nd ed. Philadelphia, WB Saunders, 1993, pp 310–333.

76. Furst P, Kuhn K, Ziegler TR: Amino acids and proteins—New definitions and requirements, hormonal interactions, methodological advances and pitfalls. Curr Opin Clin Nutr Metab Care 2:5–8, 1999.

77. Fürst P, Stehle P: Are we giving unbalanced amino acid solutions? In DW Wilmore, Carpentier YA (eds): Metabolic Support of the Critically Ill Patient. Berlin, Springer-Verlag, 1993, pp 119–136.

78. Zelikovic I, Chesney RW, Friedman AL, et al: Taurine depletion in very low birthweight infants receiving prolonged total parenteral nutrition: Role of renal immaturity. J Pediatr 116:301–306, 1990.

79. Laidlaw SA, Kopple JD: Newer concepts of the indispensable amino acids. Am J Clin Nutr 46:593–605, 1987.

80. Wright CE, Tallan HH, Lin YY: Taurine: Biological update. Annu Rev Biochem 55:427–436, 1986.

81. Gray GE, Landel AM, Mequid MM: Taurine-supplemented total parenteral nutrition and taurine status of malnourished cancer patients. Nutrition 10:11–15, 1994.

82. Paauw JD, Davis AT: Taurine concentrations in serum of critically injured patients and age- and sex-matched healthy control subjects. Am J Clin Nutr 52:657–660, 1990.

83. Martensson J, Larson J, Schildt BO: Metabolic effects of amino acid solutions in burned patients: With emphasis on sulfur amino acid metabolism and protein breakdown. J Trauma 25:427–432, 1985.

84. Desai TK, Maliakkal J, Kinzie JL, et al: Taurine deficiency after intensive chemotherapy and/or radiation. Am J Clin Nutr 55:708–711, 1992.

85. Fürst P: Old and new substrates in clinical nutrition. J Nutr 128:789–796, 1998.

86. Gazzaniga AB, Waxman K, Day AT, et al: Nitrogen balance in adult hospitalized patients with the use of a pediatric amino acid model. Arch Surg 123:1275–1281, 1988.

87. Cynober L: The use of alpha-ketoglutarate salts in clinical nutrition and metabolic care. Curr Opin Clin Nutr Metab Care 2:33–37, 1999.

88. Cynober L, Saizy R, Nguyen DF, et al: Effect of

enterally administered ornithine alpha-ketogluta-rate on plasma and urinary levels after burn injury. J Trauma 24:590–596, 1984.

89. Leander U, Fürst P, Vesterberg K, et al: Nitrogen sparing effect of Ornicetil® in the immediate post-operative state: Clinical biochemistry and nitrogen balance. Clin Nutr 4:43–51, 1985.

90. Cynober L, Lioret N, Coudray-Lucas C, et al: Action of ornithine alpha ketoglutarate on protein metabolism in burn patients. Nutrition 3:187–191, 1987.

91. Wernerman J, Hammarqvist F, Von der Decken A, et al: Ornithine–alpha ketoglutarate improves skeletal muscle protein synthesis as assessed by ribosome analysis and nitrogen use after surgery. Ann Surg 206:674–678, 1987.

92. Moukarzel A, Goulet O, Sala JS, et al: Growth retardation in children receiving long term total parenteral nutrition: Effects of ornithine alpha-ketoglutarate. Am J Clin Nutr 60:408–413, 1994.

93. Calder PC, Deckelbaum RJ: New metabolic pathways and role for lipids and lipid emulsions. Curr Opin Clin Nutr Metab Care 1:139–141, 1998.

94. Chan S, McCowen KC, Bistrian B: Medium chain triglyceride and n-3 polyunsaturated fatty acid–containing emulsions in intravenous nutrition. Curr Opin Clin Nutr Metab Care 1:163-169, 1998.

95. Ulrich H, Pastores SM, Katz DP, Kvetan V: Parenteral use of medium-chain triglycerides: A reappraisal. Nutrition 12: 231-238, 1996.

96. Battistella FD, Widergren JT, Anderson JT, et al: A prospective, randomized trial of intravenous fat emulsion administration in trauma victims requiring total parenteral nutrition. J Trauma 43:52–57, 1997.

97. Morlion BJ, Torwesten E, Lessire H, et al: The effect of parenteral fish oil on leukocyte membrane fatty acid composition and leukotriene-synthesizing capacity in patients with postoperative trauma. Metabolism 45:1208–1213, 1996.

98. Katz DP, Manner T, Fürst P, Askanazi J: The use of an intravenous fish oil emulsion enriched with omega-3 fatty acids in patients with cystic fibrosis. Nutrition 12:334–339, 1996.

99. Hwang D: Essential fatty acids and immune responses. FASEB J 3:2052–2061, 1989.

100. Wachtler P, Konig W, Senkal M, et al: Influence of a total parenteral nutrition enriched with ω-3 fatty acids on leukotriene synthesis of peripheral leukocytes and systemic cytokine levels in patients with major surgery. J Trauma 42:191–198, 1997.

101. Ikehata A, Hiwatashi N, Kinouchi Y, et al: Effect of intravenously infused eicosapentaenoic acid on the leukotriene generation in patients with active Crohn's disease. Am J Clin Nutr 56:938–942, 1992.

102. Calder PC: Immunomodulatory and anti-inflammatory effects of n-3 polyunsaturated fatty acids. Proc Nutr Soc 55:737–745, 1996.

103. Kudsk KA, Minard G, Corce MA, et al: A randomized trial of isonitrogenous enteral diets after severe trauma. An immune-enhancing diet reduces septic complications. Ann Surg 224:531–543, 1996.

104. Weimann A, Bastian L, Bischoff WE, et al: Influence of arginine, omega-3 fatty acids and nucleotide-supplemented enteral support on systemic inflammatory response syndrome and multiple organ failure in patients after severe trauma. Nutrition 14:165–172, 1998.

105. Braga M, Gianotti L, Cestari A, et al: Gut function and immune and inflammatory responses in patients perioperatively fed with supplemented enteral formulas. Arch Surg 131:125–165, 1996.

106. Homan van der Heide JJ, Bilo HJ, Donker JM, et al: Effect of dietary fish oil on renal function and rejection in cyclosporine-treated recipients or renal transplants. N Engl J Med 329:769–773, 1993.

107. Swails WS, Kenler AS, Discoll DF, et al: Effect of fish oil structured lipid–based diet on prostaglandin release from mononuclear cells in cancer patients after surgery. JPEN J Parenter Enteral Nutr 21:266–274, 1997.

108. Stenson WF, Cort D, Rodgers J, et al: Dietary supplementation with fish oil in ulcerative colitis. Ann Intern Med 116:609–614, 1992.

109. Meydani SM, Endres S, Woods MM, et al: Oral (n-3) fatty acid supplementation suppresses cytokine production and lymphocyte proliferation: Comparison between young and older women. J Nutr 121:547–555, 1991.

110. Tashiro T, Yamamori H, Takagi K, et al: n-3 versus n-6 polyunsaturated fatty acids in critical illness. Nutrition 14:551–553, 1998.

111. Sato N, Decklbaum RJ, Neeser G, et al: Hydrolysis of mixed lipid emulsions containing medium-chain and long-chain triacylglycerol with lipoprotein lipase in plasma-like medium. JPEN J Parenter Enteral Nutr 18:122–118, 1994.

112. Hyltander A, Sandstrom R, Lundholm K: Metabolic effects of structured triglycerides in humans. Nutr Clin Pract 10:91–97, 1995.

113. Ball MJ: Parenteral nutrition in critically ill: Use of a medium chain triglyceride emulsion. Intens Care Med 19:89–95, 1993.

114. Balderman H, Wicklmayer M, Rett K, et al: Changes in hepatic morphology during parenteral nutrition with lipid emulsions containing LCT or MCT/LCT quantified by ultrasound. J Parenter Enteral Nutr 15:601–603, 1991.

115. Smirniotis V, Kostopanogiotou D, Vassiliou J, et al: Long chain versus medium chain lipids in patients with ARDS: Effects on pulmonary haemodynamics and gas exchange. Intens Care Med 24:1029–1033, 1998.

116. Planas N, Masclans JR, Iglesia R, et al: Eicosanoids and fat emulsions in acute respiratory distress syndrome patients. Nutrition 13:202–205, 1997.

117. Radermacher P, Santak B, Strobach H, et al: Fat emulsions containing medium chain triglycerides in patients with sepsis syndrome: Effects on pulmonary hemodynamics and gas exchange. Intens Care Med 18:231–234, 1992.

118. Masclans JR, Iglesia R, Bermejo B, et al: Gas exchange and pulmonary haemodynamic responses to fat emulsions in acute respiratory distress syndrome. Intens Care Med 24:218–223, 1998.

119. Waitzberg DL, Bellinati-Pires R, Salgado MM, et al: Effect of total parenteral nutrition with different lipid emulsions on human monocyte and neutrophil functions. Nutrition 13:128–132, 1997.

120. Gelas P, Cotte L, Poitevin-Later F, et al: Effect of parenteral medium- and long-chain triglycerides on lymphocyte subpopulations and functions in patients with acquired immunodeficiency syndrome: A prospective study. JPEN J Parenter Ent Nutr 22:67–71, 1998.

121. Sandstrom R, Hyltander A, Korner U, Lundholm K: Stuctured triglycerides were well tolerated and

induced whole body fat oxidation compared with long-chain triglycerides in post-operative patients. JPEN J Parenter Enteral Nutr 19:381–386, 1995.

122. Ziegler TR: Glutamine supplementation in catabolic illness. Am J Clin Nutr 64:645–647, 1996.

123. Bray TM, Taylor CG: Enhancement of tissue glutathione for antioxidant and immune function in malnutrition. Biochem Pharmacol 47:2113–2119, 1994.

124. Berger MM, Cavadini C, Chiolero R, et al: Influence of large intakes of trace elements on recovery after major burns. Nutrition 10:327–334, 1994.

125. Maderazo EG, Woronick CL, Hickingbotham N, et al: A randomized trial of replacement antioxidant vitamin therapy for neutrophil locomotory dysfunction in blunt trauma. J Trauma 31:1142–1150, 1991.

126. Goode HF, Cowley HC, Walker BE, et al: Decreased antioxidant status and increased lipid peroxidation in patients with septic shock and secondary organ dysfunction. Crit Care Med 23:646–651, 1995.

127. Schorah CJ, Downing C, Piripitsi A, et al: Total vitamin C, ascorbic acid, and dehydroascorbic acid concentrations in plasma of critically ill patients. Am J Clin Nutr 63:760–765, 1996.

128. Bernard GR. *N*-Acetylcysteine in experimental and clinical acute lung injury. Am J Med 91:54s–59s, 1991.

129. Richard C, Lemonnier F, Thibault M: Vitamin E deficiency and lipoperoxidation during adult respiratory distress syndrome. Crit Care Med 18:4–9, 1990.

130. Berger MM, Shenkin A: Trace elements in trauma and burns. Curr Opin Clin Nutr Metab Care 1:513–518, 1998.

131. Ferrari R, Alfieri O, Curello S, et al: Occurrence of oxidative stress during reperfusion of the human heart. Circulation 81:201–211, 1990.

132. Rabl H, Khoschsorur G, Petek W: Antioxidative vitamin treatment: Effect on lipid peroxidation and limb swelling after revascularization. World J Surg 19:738–744, 1995.

133. Sisto T, Paajanen H, Metsa-Ketela T, et al: Pretreatment with antioxidants and allopurinol diminishes cardiac onset events in coronary artery bypass grafting. Ann Thorac Surg 59:1519–1523, 1995.

134. Galley HF, Richardson N, Howdle PD, et al: Total antioxidant capacity and lipid peroxidation during liver transplantation. Clin Sci 89:329–332, 1995.

135. Goode HF, Webster NR, Howdle PD, et al: Reperfusion injury, antioxidants and hemodynamics during orthotopic liver transplantation. Hepatology 19:3544–3559, 1994.

136. Rabl H, Khoschsorur G, Colombo T, Esterboum H:

137. Schoenberg MH, Birk D, Beger HG: Oxidative stress and chronic pancreatitis. Am J Clin Nutr 62:1306s–1314s, 1995.

138. Braganza JM, Scott P, Bilton D, et al: Evidence for early oxidative stress in acute pancreatitis. Int J Pancreatol 17:69–81, 1995.

139. Braganza JM, Holmes AM, Morton AR, et al: Acetylcysteine to treat complications of pancreatitis. Lancet 20:914–915, 1986.

140. Uden S, Schofield S, Miller PF, et al: Antioxidant therapy for recurrent pancreatitis: Biochemical profiles in a placebo-controlled trial. Aliment Pharmacol Ther 6:229–240, 1992.

141. Weijl NI, Leton FJ, Osanto S: Free radicals and antioxidants in chemotherapy-induced toxicity. Cancer Treat Rev 197; 23:209–240, 1992.

142. Clemens MR, Ladner C, Ehninger G: Plasma vitamin E and B-carotene concentrations during radiochemotherapy preceding bone marrow transplantation. Am J Clin Nutr 51:216–219, 1990.

143. Jonas CR, Puckett AB, Kurtz JC, et al: High dose chemotherapy decreases plasma glutathione in patients undergoing bone marrow transplantation. FASEB J 11:A649, 1997.

144. Jonas CR, Ziegler TR: Nutrition support and antioxidant defenses: A cause for concern? Am J Clin Nutr 68:765–767, 1998.

145. Clemens MR, Waladkhani AR, Bublitz K, et al: Supplementation with antioxidants prior to bone marrow transplantation. Wien Klin Wochenschr 109:771–776, 1997.

146. Wadleigh RG, Redman RS, Graham ML, et al: Vitamin E in the treatment of chemotherapy-induced mucositis. Am J Med 92:481–484, 1992.

147. Wagdi P, Fluri M, Aeschbacher B, et al: Cardioprotection in patients undergoing chemo- and/or radiotherapy for neoplastic disease. A pilot study. Jpn Heart J 37:353–359, 1996.

148. Geerling BJ, Badart-Smook A, Stockbrugger RW, Brummer RJM: Comprehensive nutritional status in patients with long-standing Crohn disease currently in remission. Am J Clin Nutr 67:919–926, 1998.

149. Leslie D, Gheorghiade M: Is there a role for thiamine supplementation in the management of heart failure? Am Heart J 131:1248–1250, 1996.

150. Seligmann H, Halkin H, Rauchfleisch S, et al: Thiamine deficiency in patients with congestive heart failure receiving long term furosemide therapy: A pilot study. Am J Med 91:151–155, 1991.

151. Shimon I, Almog S, Vered Z, et al: Improved left ventricular function after thiamine supplementation in patients with congestive heart failure receiving long-term furosemide therapy. Am J Med 98:485–490, 1995.

29

◆ Peripheral Parenteral Nutrition

Jesus M. Culebras, M.D., Ph.D.
A. Garcia-de-Lorenzo, M.D., Ph.D.
A. Zarazaga, M.D., Ph.D.
F. Jorquera, M.D., Ph.D.

Total parenteral nutrition (TPN) has completely changed the medical and surgical management of patients with intestinal insufficiency or intestinal failure. Long-term maintenance of patients with irreversible intestinal failure is now possible with an acceptable quality of life. In addition, the successful treatment of severe malnutrition during the preoperative period offers new possibilities to complex operations and the control of severe complications. These are some examples of a technology that can be applied in a variety of clinical situations and in all patient populations. The use of TPN can also involve some difficulties and lead to complications. To circumvent difficulties and avoid complications, the practitioner must have a deep fund of knowledge and constantly analyze the situation critically. Because TPN is costly, the financial implications of its use should also be taken into consideration.

Typically, TPN is delivered through a vein with sufficient flow to allow the infusion of hypertonic solutions without risking phlebitis or thrombosis. Access to these large-caliber veins (central veins) and the subsequent management may lead to serious, and even lethal, complications (Table 29–1). Administration of TPN solutions can produce important metabolic changes as well as complications unrelated to the insertion of a central line.[1] Thus, highly specialized medical and nursing personnel are required to administer TPN.

Peripheral parenteral nutrition (PPN) is an alternative to TPN that has been employed for several decades. When used in properly selected patients, PPN diminishes many of the complications of TPN and is less expensive. However, the patients for whom PPN should be the form of parenteral nutrition of choice still remain to be defined objectively. Some of its indications have not been well established, and other known indications are now being questioned.

PPN can supply through a peripheral vein a nitrogen and calorie mix that is very similar to that administered in TPN. For the purpose of this chapter, when we mention TPN we refer to the administration of hypertonic nutrient mixtures, with a high osmolarity, deliverable only through a central vein, even though PPN can also supply a complete nutrient mix.

Before embarking on the discussion of the clinical applications of PPN, we define various terms used in the context of administering nutrients via peripheral veins.

Peripheral parenteral nutrition is the generic term for this type of therapy. It is applied to the intravenous administration of nutrients without specifying the formulation (usually amino acids, carbohydrates, and lipids) as long as the osmolarity remains within the limits of tolerance of peripheral veins (maximum 800 to 850 mOsm/L).

Hypocaloric peripheral parenteral nutrition (HPPN) is more restrictive than the previous term. It usually refers to commercial formulations containing amino acids and carbohydrates in a single bottle, with an osmolarity tolerable for peripheral veins and with a caloric content of less than 1000 kcal over a 24-hour period of administration.

Perioperative peripheral parenteral nutri-

Table 29–1. Complications of Central Catheters for Parenteral Nutrition

---

Mechanical complications related to
   central catheter placement
Arterial puncture
Pneumothorax
Air embolism
Catheter sepsis
Central vein thrombophlebitis
Pulmonary thromboembolism

---

tion (PPPN) refers to the use of nutritive mixtures through a peripheral route immediately before and/or after surgical procedures.

◆ USE OF PERIPHERAL PARENTERAL NUTRITION

The concept of PPN is not new. Blackburn and colleagues in 1973 administered only amino acids through a peripheral vein to patients in different clinical situations of stress and fasting, demonstrating improved nitrogen balance.[2] However, compared with current formulations, there were differences in the amount of amino acids infused.[3]

A review of 1261 patients conducted by the Spanish Society of Intensive Care and Coronary Units showed that 18.2% received PPN, 38.5% received TPN, and 53.3% received enteral nutrition.[4] Medical patients received nutrition through the enteral route in a significantly higher proportion than surgical patients. In a review on the use of parenteral nutrition in the United Kingdom, Payne-James and Khawaja showed that in 1988 only 7% of patients were on PPN, whereas in 1991 this figure rose to 15% and in some centers up to 60%.[5] In children, these figures were even higher, with the reported use of PPN ranging between 60 and 70% of all parenteral nutrition being used.[6]

◆ INDICATIONS FOR PERIPHERAL PARENTERAL NUTRITION

There are some indications for PPN in which there is no doubt about its effectiveness.[6] However, there are other indications in which routine PPN, despite a large body of data suggesting its efficacy, has not been unequivocally validated by prospective studies. This is partly because there are multiple factors that confound the interpretation of outcome data when PPN is used in clinical practice.[7]

Some of these factors deserve special mention. First, the nutritional status is an important factor because of the inherent difficulties in objectively assessing it to enable a meaningful statistical comparison. Second, the nature of the disease is also a common problem when analyzing outcome studies. We can clearly establish two large patient populations: cancer patients and noncancer patients. In the cancer patient population, the anatomic location of the tumor, host and tumor metabolic interactions, and immune response to the tumor are all highly variable among patients receiving PPN.

The American Society for Parenteral and Enteral Nutrition has provided some guidelines on the use of PPN.[8] According to these guidelines, PPN is *not* the optimal choice for patients with significant malnutrition, severe metabolic stress, large nutrient or electrolyte needs, fluid restriction, and/or a need for prolonged intravenous nutrition.

◆ COMPARISON OF PERIPHERAL PARENTERAL NUTRITION AND TOTAL PARENTERAL NUTRITION

In order to compare PPN and TPN, one should know the purported advantages and potential risks of each. The main advantages of TPN over PPN are the possibility of use during long periods of time and the assurance of administering every nutrient necessary for complete nutrition, in both quality and quantity. However, this is achieved at the expense of potentially severe complications, and these risks should not be overlooked. The placement of a central venous line has a rate of adverse effects of 5.7%.[9, 10] In up to 9% of patients, there is inadvertent migration of the catheter or venous thrombosis. In 6.5% of patients, catheter sepsis may occur.[11, 12]

Conversely, although the nutrient requirements are usually met by PPN, the types of complications associated with PPN are less morbid, and their incidence is lower. Thrombophlebitis is the main complication associated with PPN, and its incidence seems to correlate with the length of the time a catheter remains within a peripheral vein. If nutritional requirements are covered while the incidence of thrombophlebitis is kept at a low rate, then PPN would be considered the nutritional therapy of choice in a great number of patients. In order to define who these patients would be, that is, the best candidates for PPN, we have developed a matrix that includes the degree of metabolic stress, energy requirements, nitrogen requirements, calorie-to-nitrogen ratio, need for intestinal rest, and nutritional status (Ta-

Table 29–2. Indications for Peripheral Parenteral Nutrition in Relation to Metabolic Stress

Indication	Degree of Metabolic Stress	Energy Requirements	g N₂	Ratio kcal np/g N₂	Bowel Rest	Nutritional State
No indication	3 / 2		+ / 16 g	80–100:1 / 100:1 / 120:1	>7 days	Well nourished / Malnourished
Indication	1 / 0	1500 kcal			>2 days / <7 days	
Doubtful indication	0		−	150:1	<2 days	

g N₂ = grams of nitrogen; np/g N₂ = nonprotein calories/gram of nitrogen.

ble 29–2). As depicted in this table, a select group of patients have a "probable indication" for PPN, whereas in others the indication is doubtful, or there is no indication.

The rationale for the inclusion of these parameters in the matrix is as follows. Energy requirements are related to the degree of metabolic stress. Patients with an indication for PPN would be in groups 0 or 1 of metabolic stress, and their energy requirements range between 1500 and 2000 kcal/day as long as they do not develop sepsis.[13] PPN has usually been recommended in patients considered to require nutritional support for periods under 7 days. Present trends have increased this figure to 14 days, as long as nutritional requirements are well covered. This can be achieved by adding lipids and administering a total amount of 2200 to 2300 kcal/day. This is important because in most patients TPN is used for less than 14 days, and in one fourth of them is used for less than 7 days.[14] PPN is not recommended for periods longer than 14 days. PPN can supply 75 to 105 g of amino acids (13.5 to 16.2 g of nitrogen) in a volume of 2500 to 3000 ml. This amount is within the range of grams of amino acids per kilogram per day recommended in stress situations (1.1 to 1.7 g of amino acids per kilogram per day). The nonprotein calorie–nitrogen ratio is a limiting factor for the use of PPN. Ratios of 150:1 are impossible to achieve with PPN unless a large quantity of lipids is used.

Integrating all these parameters, we find a broad spectrum of indications for PPN (Table 29–3). The advantages of PPN are lower cost, easier handling, and fewer and less severe complications. However, this saving is not worthwhile unless protein catabolism is diminished and protein synthesis is increased in both muscle and viscera.[15]

◆ PARTIAL PARENTERAL NUTRITION FORMULATIONS

Protein administration with PPN, although slightly decreased when compared with central TPN, is placed within the required limits in minimal degrees of metabolic stress, but the calorie-to-nitrogen ratio is clearly reduced (40:1). If ready-to-use preparations are used (e.g., glucose and/or polyols with amino acids), it is not possible to increase this ratio without increasing the osmolarity to levels that are not tolerated by a peripheral vein. The question is then whether it is possible to reduce protein catabolism with this low calorie-to-nitrogen ratio.

A multicenter study conducted in Europe in 1994 by Jiménez and coworkers studied the effect of three types of HPPN with 9.2, 9.4, and 8.4 g of nitrogen and 654, 500, and 650 kcal, respectively.[16] The study was conducted in 75 malnourished patients during the first 5 postoperative days compared with a control group maintained on 5% dex-

Table 29–3. Indications for Peripheral Parenteral Nutrition in Relation to the Clinical Situation

Indication	Degree of Metabolic Stress	Bowel Rest	Nutritional State		Typical Clinical Examples
No indication	3 2	>7 days			Fulminant pancreatitis Critically ill surgical patients Surgical complications Multiple organ failure

Indication	1
	 0
		>2 days
		 <7 days
			Well nourished	Malnourished	Postoperative period
					   Gastric resections
					   Peritonitis
					   Intestinal obstruction
					   Inflammatory bowel disease
					   Acute pancreatitis (uncomplicated)

Doubtful indication	0	<2 days			Cholelithiasis Bowel resection (uncomplicated) Acute appendicitis

trose and saline solutions. The serum levels of proteins with a short half-life improved, the nitrogen balance was less negative, and the urinary 3-methylhistidine excretion significantly diminished in all three groups receiving HPPN. No statistical differences were shown among HPPN groups. This study shows the advantage of HPPN during the postoperative period but at an additional cost.

Lipids are other substrates with a high concentration of calories that can be administered through a peripheral vein. Are lipids a good nutritional alternative to carbohydrates? Their use in PPN is still debated.

The long-chain fatty acids linoleic acid and linolenic acid are considered essential fatty acids. Both are included in long-chain triglyceride (LCT), medium-chain triglyceride (MCT)-LCT, LCT–n-3, and LCT–n-9 emulsions. Lipid particles administered intravenously with fat emulsions are cleared in 1 to 2 hours in normal humans, depending on the amount infused. Maximal triglyceride-clearing capacities are 3.8 g of lipid per kilogram per day after 15 hours of fasting and 5.6 g/kg/day after 36 hours of fasting. The rate of elimination rises to 11 g/kg/day after a surgical operation.[17] We can conclude that in stress situations, lipid clearance is enhanced, and this would support its use in the critically ill patient.[18] In addition, the lowering of the respiratory quotient in pulmonary patients being weaned off mechanical ventilation suggests that fat emulsions are a good substrate in this patient population.[19]

There is both clinical and experimental evidence of the efficacy and safety of lipid emulsions in parenteral nutrition. It is also recognized that the combined use of fat and carbohydrate (dual system) is the most physiologic method of supplying energy (Table 29–4). Even in patients with liver disease, in whom their use was previously questioned, fat emulsions have been shown to be safe, convenient, and effective.[20]

The use of lipids through a peripheral vein provides another advantage: its lower osmolarity and physiologic pH reduce the incidence of phlebitis.[21]

In patients receiving TPN, it is recommended to use a minimum of 15 g of fats per day in order to optimize the utilization of glucose and proteins and to meet the pa-

Table 29–4. Beneficial Effects of Energy Supply with Simultaneous Administration of Fat and Carbohydrates

Is more physiologic
Does not affect liver function
Prevents and reverses liver steatosis
Is less hyperglycemic
Prevents saturation of oxidative pathways of carbohydrates
Prevents and corrects essential fatty acid deficiency
Improves immune system
Promotes lean body mass
Reduces metabolic stress
Prevents water overload
Reduces respiratory stress
Reduces risk of hypophosphatemia
Allows peripheral nutrition with adequate caloric supply

tient's needs for essential fatty acids. However, the rapid administration of lipids over a rate of 1 kcal/kg/h can impair the function of the reticuloendothelial system, producing an overload of fats in macrophages and diminishing their phagocytic capacity, obviously an undesirable effect in the critically ill patient.[22] Other authors have questioned this impairment of the reticuloendothelial system by lipids.[23–25] Hamaway and associates reported a study on septic rats in which the clearance of inoculated bacteria was higher when an MCT-LCT emulsion was given compared with LCT alone.[22] Lipid combinations such as LCT-MCT, n-3–LCT or n-9–LCT offer the advantage of supplying essential fatty acids and energy substrates that are easier to oxidate.

In summary, lipid emulsions are an excellent source of energy in PPN formulations, especially when used in patients under stress and in those with respiratory failure. Lipid administration is acceptable in pancreatic disease except in hyperlipidemic situations (types I and V). Lipids also reduce gastric and pancreatic secretions.[26–28]

Waxman and coworkers studied 34 surgical patients, some with multiple trauma, who received a PPN formula based on glycerol and amino acids with the addition of either a 10% (group 1) or a 20% (group 2) lipid emulsion. Daily doses were 1.35 g of amino acids per kilogram plus 1.35 g of glycerol and 500 mL of lipid emulsion per day. The most interesting finding was an improvement in nitrogen balance in group 1 (−0.3 g/day) compared with group 2 (−4.1 g/day). A better nitrogen balance when using less fat seems paradoxical and can only be explained by a limitation in the clearance of fats in these situations. Stokes and Hill found that a PPN solution with lipids administered in the form of soybean emulsion, egg yolk lecithin, and glycerol, supplying 1000 kcal, offered the same functional improvement as a standard TPN solution.[30]

In Europe, there are ready-to-use all-in-one preparations containing amino acids, glucose, fats, and electrolytes (Kavimix) to which vitamins and oligoelements can be added. These solutions provide 57 g of amino acids, 100 g of lipids, and 150 g of glucose, all in a volume of 2500 mL, with an osmolarity of 695 mOsm/L, 1830 kcal, and at a reasonable cost. Because they are ready to use, their administration does not require highly skilled personnel. A disad-

vantage is the low protein supply and the high proportion of calories supplied in the form of fats, resulting in a high calorie-to-nitrogen ratio of 178, a figure higher than recommended. The lipid content of these formulations does not include MCTs. MCTs are of particular interest because of their easier hydrolysis with rapid oxidation and less incorporation into tissue lipids. Furthermore, MCTs given in conjunction with LCTs seem to lessen the deleterious effect of LCTs on the reticuloendothelial system.[31]

◆ THROMBOPHLEBITIS AND PERIPHERAL PARENTERAL NUTRITION

The incidence of phlebitis in patients receiving PPN varies between 2.3% and 70%.[32, 33] This broad range is partially due to the various criteria used to define phlebitis. The causes of PPN-induced thrombophlebitis are multifactorial (Table 29–5).[4] One of the most important factors is the nature of the solution being infused. Both osmolarity and pH have a clear influence. Therefore, the solutions to be infused must not have an osmolarity higher than 600 mOsm/L and must remain within a pH range of 7.2 to 7.4.[4] The catheter material is also important. With polyurethane catheters the incidence of phlebitis is reduced significantly. Silicone elastomer catheters are also quite safe, but the polyurethane cathe-

Table 29–5. Factors Associated with the Risk of Thrombophlebitis and Possible Prophylactic Measures

Possible etiologic factors
Catheter size
Catheter material
Bacterial colonization of catheters
Infused drugs
Length of infusion
Nature of solution infused
Particles present in infusion
Site of catheter placement
Trauma related to venopuncture
Vein size
Prophylactic measures against thrombophlebitis
Buffer solutions
Glycerol
Local nitrites
Heparin-hydrocortisone
Lipids
Local anti-inflammatory drugs
Nutritional support teams

ters have the advantage of a higher internal gauge with the same external diameter. Other factors are the catheter placement site, with a higher incidence of phlebitis in flexures, and the size of cannulated veins, with a higher incidence of phlebitis in smaller veins.[4] A factor shown to increase the incidence of phlebitis is the presence of particles in the solution. For this reason, some authors recommend the use of filters in the infusion tubing.[34, 35] Bacterial colonization seems to be another factor; however, the presence of skin saprophytic bacteria in the catheter tip on removal does not seem to correlate with thrombophlebitis.

In order to reduce the incidence of thrombophlebitis, it is important to establish a strict protocol for the management of catheters inserted through peripheral veins. There are several measures that have proved to be important (see Table 29–5). The addition of buffer solutions such as 1% bicarbonate seems to reduce the incidence of phlebitis. The high osmolarity of solutions containing glucose can be reduced, in part, by adding glycerol or lipids as an alternative source of calories. Energy requirements can then be met while osmolarity and, consequently, phlebitis, are reduced. The addition of corticosteroids to PPN formulas is based on their effects on inhibiting the action of phospholipase and eicosanoid synthesis, producing fewer inflammatory stimuli. Heparin has also been used to reduce phlebitis. Heparin has the disadvantage that it renders the all-in-one solutions unstable by forming calcium-heparin-lipid complexes. Topical medications are of interest because of their easy application and lack of adverse effects. Transdermal trinitrate applied topically promotes an in situ vasodilation and stimulates the synthesis of prostacyclin, which is a potent inhibitor of platelet aggregation. Other substances for topical use are nonsteroidal anti-inflammatory drugs.

◆ PRESENT USE OF PERIPHERAL PARENTERAL NUTRITION

The addition of lipids to parenteral nutrition solutions ensures an adequate content of calories with an outstanding reduction in osmolarity. This allows the use of peripheral veins for complete solutions, notably reducing the complications of classic TPN. Another advantage is a reduction in and simplification of work for nurses and physicians and the lowering of the cost. Easy preparation procedures for PPN solutions and the availability of all-in-one solutions make them sterile and stable, allowing an immediate source of nutritional support. Most of the patients requiring nutritional support require it for periods shorter than 10 to 14 days. In these patients, PPN offers adequate nutritional support with the previously mentioned advantages.

If the ultimate goal of any form of nutritional support is its efficacy, and this can be achieved with PPN, we must concentrate our efforts on counteracting the frequency and severity of its most important complication, thrombophlebitis. Usually, PPN is administered satisfactorily following certain protocols. Catheter placement must be performed under strict aseptic technique. Catheters must be thin, preferably made of polyurethane or silicone elastomers, and placed in a vein of adequate size. Nitrites or topical anti-inflammatory drugs may be of use in the prevention of thrombophlebitis, but at the moment signs of thrombophlebitis appear, a new catheter must be placed in a different location. The most effective measures in preventing complications are to reduce the osmolarity by adding lipids and to avoid manipulation of the infusion system by using all-in-one solutions whenever possible. When the total number of patients who receive PPN is considered and the cost of treating complications is divided by the entire group at risk, the estimated cost of treating the complications associated with PPN was $12.50 per patient in 1985 in the United States. The decreased cost of PPN administration that has occurred since then in combination with acceptably low complication rates associated with this form of therapy have tipped the cost-effectiveness scales in favor of PPN use.[36]

The role of HPPN remains to be defined. This type of nutritional support improves several biochemical parameters but without correlations in morbidity and mortality. However, HPPN continues to be used during the perioperative period until oral nutrition is resumed. It has also been indicated as a bridge toward TPN when TPN is soon to be prescribed or when its administration is delayed due to technical reasons. It seems that on many occasions, HPPN is used just as an attempt to "do something for the patient" from a nutritional point of view without risking the potential complications of TPN.

When nutritional support for a patient is planned, the enteral route is always the first choice. If enteral nutrition is not feasible, the patient has a moderate stress situation, and the expected length of nutritional support is less than 10 to 14 days, PPN can be the next choice. A proof of the efficacy and safety of PPN is that it is the first choice in newborns and children and is capable of maintaining their nutritional status and promoting growth even though the nutritional requirements of children are proportionally higher than those of adults. For the moment, hypercaloric nutrition, recommended in situations of stress, must always be administered through a central vein, that is, TPN. A solution containing 30% lipids has been introduced into the market and will improve caloric support without increasing osmolarity. The ultimate evaluation of these solutions remains to be determined.

REFERENCES

1. Jorquera F, Culebras JM, González-Gallego J: Influence of nutrition on liver oxidative metabolism. Nutrition 12:442–447, 1996.
2. Blackburn GL, Flatt JP, Clowes GH: Protein sparing therapy during periods of starvation with sepsis or trauma. Ann Surg 177:588–592, 1973.
3. Shizgal HM, Knowles JB: Peripheral amino acids. In Fischer JE (ed): Total Parenteral Nutrition. Boston, Little, Brown, 1991, pp 389–402.
4. Planas M, Nutritional and metabolic working group of the Spanish Society of Intensive Care and Coronary Units (SEMIUC): Artificial nutrition support in intensive care units in Spain. Intensive Care Med 21:842–846, 1995.
5. Payne-James JJ, Khawaja HT: First choice for total parenteral nutrition: The peripheral route. JPEN J Parenter Enteral Nutr 17:468–478, 1993.
6. Pencharz PB, Zlotkin SH: Peripheral and parenteral nutrition: Preliminary report on its efficacy and safety. JPEN J Parenter Enteral Nutr 17:588–589, 1993.
7. Garcia de Lorenzo A, Zarazaga A, Culebras JM: Nutrición parenteral periférica: ¿Mito o realidad? Nutr Hosp 8:1–21, 1993.
8. ASPEN Board of Directors: Guidelines for the use of parenteral and enteral nutrition in adult and pediatric patients. JPEN J Parenter Enteral Nutr 17:9SA, 1993.
9. Wolfe BM, Ryder MA, Nishikawa RA, et al: Complications of parenteral nutrition. Am J Surg 152:93–99, 1986.
10. Culebras JM: Complicaciones derivadas de la utilización de catéteres venosos centrales. Nutr Hosp 6:143–144, 1991.
11. Sitzmann JV, Townsend TR, Siler MC, et al: Septic and technical complications of central venous catheterization. Ann Surg 202:766–770, 1985.
12. Mughal MM: Complications of intravenous feeding catheters. Br J Surg 76:15–21, 1989.
13. MacFie J: Active metabolic expenditure of gastroenterological surgical patients receiving intravenous nutrition. JPEN J Parenter Enteral Nutr 8:371–376, 1984.
14. Payne-James J, de Gara C, Grimble G, et al: Nutritional support in hospitals in the United Kingdom; National Survey 1988. Health Trends 22:9–13, 1990.
15. Schwartz S: Aminoácidos. In Net A, Sánchez JM, Benito S (eds): Nutrición artificial en el paciente grave. Barcelona, Doyma, 1989, pp 198–204.
16. Jiménez FJ, Ortiz C, Jiménez L, García MS: Estudio de la nutrición parenteral periférica hipocalórica en pacientes postquirúrgicos (proyecto Europan) (II). Nutr Hosp 9:139–154, 1994.
17. Hallberg D: Studies on the elimination of exogenous lipids from the blood stream. The kinetics of the elimination of a fat emulsion studied by single injection technique in man. Acta Physiol Scand 64:306–313, 1965.
18. Carpentier YA: Are present fat emulsions appropriate? In Wilmore DW, Carpentier YA (eds): Metabolic support of the critically ill patient. Berlin, Springer-Verlag, 1993, pp 157–171.
19. Elwyn DH, Kinney JM, Gump FE, et al: Some metabolic effects of fat infusions in depleted patients. Metabolism 29:125–132, 1980.
20. Jorquera F, Villares C, Culebras JM: Nutrición artificial en las hepatopatías. In Culebras JM, González-Gallego J, Garcia-de-Lorenzo A (eds): Nutrición por la vía enteral. Madrid, Grupo Aula Médica, 1994, pp 187–198.
21. Matsusue S, Nishimura S, Koizumi S, et al: Preventive effect of simultaneously infused lipid emulsion against thrombophlebitis during postoperative peripheral parenteral nutrition. Surg Today 25:667–671, 1995.
22. Hamaway KJ, Moldawer LL, Georgieff M, et al: The effect of lipid emulsions on reticuloendothelial system function in the injured animal. JPEN J Parenter Enteral Nutr 9:559–565, 1985.
23. Ota DM, Jessup JM, Babcock GB, et al: Immune function during intravenous administration of a soybean oil emulsion. JPEN J Parenter Enteral Nutr 9:23–27, 1985.
24. Rasmusses A, Hessou I, Segel E: The effect of intralipid on polymorphonuclear leucocytes. Clin Nutr 7:37–41, 1988.
25. Nishiwari H, Iriyama K, Asami H, et al: Influence of an infusion of lipid emulsion on phagocytic activity on cultured Kupffer's cells in septic rats. JPEN J Parenter Enteral Nutr 10:614–616, 1986.
26. Varner AA, Isenberg JL, Elashoff JD, et al: Effect of intravenous lipid on gastric acid secretion stimulated by intravenous amino acids. Gastroenterology 79:873–876, 1980.
27. Bivins BA, Bell RM, Rapp RP, et al: Pancreatic exocrine response to parenteral nutrition. JPEN J Parenter Enteral Nutr 8:34–36, 1984.
28. Sánchez JM: Nutrición en la pancreatitis aguda severa. In Net A, Sánchez JM, Benito S (eds): Nutrición artificial en el paciente grave. Barcelona, Doyma, 1989, pp 58–68.
29. Waxman K, Day AT, Stellin GT, et al: Safety and efficacy of glycerol and amino acids in combination with lipid emulsion for peripheral parenteral nutrition support. JPEN J Parenter Enteral Nutr 16:374–378, 1992.

30. Stokes MA, Hill GL: Peripheral parenteral nutrition: A preliminary report on its efficacy and safety. JPEN J Parenter Enteral Nutr 17:145–147, 1993.

31. Kuse ER, Kemnitz J, Kotzerke J, et al: Fat emulsions in parenteral nutrition after liver transplantation: The recovery of the allografts and histological observations. Clin Nutr 9:331–336, 1990.

32. Tager IB, Ginsber MB, Simchem E, et al: Rationale and methods for a statewide prospective surveillance system for the identification and prevention of nosocomial infection. Rev Infect Dis 3:683–693, 1981.

33. Sakajaa T, Dahl J, Jensen JK, et al: Frekvensen af overfladiske trombophlebitterefter intravenos infusion. Nord Med 66:1447–1451, 1961.

34. Romero JA, Ibañez GC, Correa M, et al: Incidencia de flebitis en pacientes con enfermedad inflamatoria intestinal sometidos a nutrición parenteral periférica. Nutr Hosp 11:63–65, 1996.

35. Falchuk KH, Peterson L, McNeil BJ: Microparticulate-induced phlebitis. N Engl J Med 312:78–82, 1985.

36. Berry SM, Lacy JA: Critical evaluation of results: Cost and benefit of nutrition support. *In* Fischer JE (ed): Nutrition and metabolism in the surgical patient. Boston, Little, Brown, 1996, pp 779–795.

30

◆ Ethical Issues and Parenteral Nutrition

Timothy O. Lipman, M.D.*

> It appears to me that in Ethics . . . the difficulties and disagreements, of which history is full, are mainly due to a very simple cause: namely to the attempt to answer questions, without first discovering precisely *what* question it is you desire to answer.
>
> *George Edward Moore*
> *1873–1958*
> Principia Ethica (1903), Preface

Genetic engineering, brain death, cloning, persistent vegetative states, abortion, living wills, right to life, in vitro fertilization, physician-assisted suicide, euthanasia: individuals and society struggle daily with a host of ethical issues brought on by advances in medical care and technology and the fact that we can keep people alive longer. Medical ethics allows the analysis of these difficult issues by putting them in the framework of competing value systems. Parenteral nutrition is associated with a variety of difficult issues: end-of-life care and terminal care, refusal of care, informed consent, and allocation of limited resources. I attempt to discuss these issues in this chapter.

◆ ETHICS OVERVIEW [1–3]

Ethics is a branch of philosophy with many schools of thought, a long tradition and history, and a scope far beyond a simple textbook chapter. A simplistic definition for purposes here states that ethics is "a branch of philosophy that deals with morality. . . . [*and*] is concerned with distinguishing between good and evil in the world, between right and wrong human actions, and be-

tween virtuous and non-virtuous characteristics of people."[4] Ethical thinking embodies "good" behavior and "idealistic" goals. In the past 50 to 100 years, ethical analysis has emphasized the application of ethical thinking to practical problems.

Medical ethics is the study of human values as they relate to the practice of medicine. What are the values and beliefs about what is right and what is wrong in the practice of medicine? The idea sounds easy, but deciding what is right and what is wrong can be quite complicated. Medical practice involves a number of stated and unstated relationships and/or commitments—to individual patients, to other patients, to families, to society, and to ourselves. As clinicians, patients, family, and society, we have different religious, cultural, and philosophic beliefs, which often lead to disagreement and dissent regarding clinical practice and our various commitments. Ethical dilemmas occur when these various commitments conflict; we have values in collision.[5] Competing values and value systems mandate the need for ethical analysis. Medical ethics and medical ethical decision making are a form of practical, situational, or case-based ethics—principles are applied to specific situations, and competing values are analyzed in a rational fashion.

Some basic ethical principles and concepts are key to understanding ethical analysis. The first of these is *autonomy*—a second half of the 20th century principle that has replaced *beneficence* as the paramount ethical principle in medicine. Autonomy—that a competent patient capable of making decisions has the right to determine his or her own destiny by accepting or refusing any and all medical care—is probably the most

---

*I am not an ethicist but rather a clinician asked to ponder and present the ethical issues associated with the delivery of parenteral nutrition. I became interested in medical ethics several years ago when asked to discuss the ethical issues involved with terminating enteral nutrition at the end of life. Since then, I have read some and become an active member of our Medical Center Ethics Committee. For this chapter I have tried to present concepts and approaches that are understandable and appropriate to the practicing clinician. I hope the clinician can appreciate the competing and strongly felt dilemmas arising from ethical conflicts.

fundamental current principle in medical ethics. Autonomy, or self-determination, simply holds that medical care or intervention cannot be delivered without consent. An autonomous patient can deliberate about choices and act on the basis of these deliberations; the patient is capable of self-governance. Patient autonomy means that clinician-patient relationships are less paternalistic and authoritarian. Patient autonomy is often uncomfortable for the clinician because it challenges the clinician's authority, means that the clinician cannot decide what is good for the patient without input from the patient, and mandates a dialogue between the patient and the clinician.

Beneficence and *nonmaleficence* are principles that address the ethical issue of doing good and right for the patient and preventing harm. Beneficence holds that one ought to promote good and prevent evil or harm. Nonmaleficence is the parallel principle, which holds that one ought not to inflict evil or harm. Until about 25 years ago, beneficence was the paramount principle in medical ethics, holding that the need to do good is more important than the patient's right to decide, that beneficence takes precedence over patient autonomy. Hence, a paternalistic approach to patient care is grounded in the ethical principle of beneficence.

Associated with beneficence and nonmaleficence are the related concepts of *benefits* and *burdens*. Does an intervention provide a net good for the patient and/or will it cause harm? The potential benefits of any proposed intervention must be balanced with the potential for harm; the benefit should outweigh the harm. Obviously, collisions may occur if a clinician's attempt to apply the principle of beneficence conflicts with a patient's autonomy, or if the assessment of possible benefits conflicts with potential burdens.

Justice is the ethical principle that deals with fairness and relationships with the community rather than with the individual per se. Justice considers how benefits and burdens for an individual should be equitably and fairly distributed within the community. The ethical principle of justice attempts to determine what is due an individual—what that individual deserves and what he or she can legitimately claim. For the physician, justice recognizes that ethical problems may be posed by multiple responsibilities—to a single patient, to other patients, to other members in the community, to oneself, or to one's family. How should multiple responsibilities be prioritized, or what should be done when duties to an individual patient appear to conflict with duties to others?

Futility is a key concept that is important to any medical ethics discussion.[6–9] It is a simple, yet incredibly complex concept, with lectures and monographs devoted to the subject. From the dictionary, futility is "useless, ineffectual, vain . . . lacking in purpose . . . serving no useful purpose." Despite dictionary definitions, there is no consensus in medicine about a definition of futility. In medicine, we wish to know whether a planned intervention would be futile. Usually, this is taken to mean that the intervention would have no effect, or even if there were an effect, there would be no benefit.

In practice, defining medical futility is difficult. Definitions of futility have been attempted by quantification, qualification, or hierarchical examples. A definition by quantification has suggested that if an intervention has not worked in the past 100 times, it is unlikely, although not impossible, that it will work the next time. This definition encompasses probability—the probability is either low or high that an effect can be achieved.[10] A qualitative definition usually implies value judgments—the condition being treated is not a state that anyone would desire, or historical and contemporary goals of medicine would not support such a condition.[2] Hierarchical definition by example consists of the following: A truly futile intervention is one in which it would be impossible to achieve a desired effect, for example, mechanical ventilation to restore life in the dead or antibiotic use to eradicate a viral infection. At the next level, medical futility may involve accomplishing a physiologic effect without reversing an underlying disorder; for example, oxygenating a brain-dead individual would not restore cerebral function. Finally, at still another level, there may be some functional benefit from an intervention, but it is unlikely to alter the progression of the disease, for example, blood replacement in a patient whose gastrointestinal bleeding cannot be stopped—the hematocrit may be maintained, but the transfusion will not stop the bleeding.[11] In all of these examples, one needs to establish the goal by which success will be measured in order to assess futility.

It is generally agreed in the ethics literature that a clinician is not required to provide futile care. Problems and ethical dilemmas obviously arise if in an individual case, consensus cannot be achieved concerning the appropriate definition of futility—my assessment of the probability of an outcome or my assessment of the quality of a clinical condition may differ from yours. When issues of futility are confronted, disagreement and discomfort arise from (1) trying to decide if an intervention is truly futile, (2) addressing levels of futility, and (3) deciding whose opinion counts when there is disagreement. Additionally, problems may occur because of competing ethical principles—patient autonomy versus clinician assessment of futility, that is, the patient's desire for care versus the clinician's assessment that such care would be futile.

For the rest of the chapter, I assess the interactions among these ethical principles and concepts of autonomy, beneficence and nonmaleficence, justice, and futility and the delivery of parenteral nutrition. I examine potential ethical issues and conflicts, their analysis, and their potential resolution using these concepts.

◆ PARENTERAL NUTRITION AT THE END OF LIFE

End-of-life care using parenteral nutrition is far less common than the use of enteral nutrition. Enteral nutrition is often used in coma, persistent vegetative states, and neurologic disorders with dementia and neuropharyngeal dysphagia. Parenteral nutrition is rarely considered for these conditions, other than short-term use in acute settings. However, our own nutritional support team occasionally receives a request for parenteral nutrition in a terminal cancer or acquired immundeficiency syndrome patient with, or sometimes without, a functioning gastrointestinal tract. The request is made because it is "unethical" to let someone starve to death. Buried in this statement are two assumptions: (1) that parenteral nutrition is the same as food and (2) that allowing starvation is, a priori, a malevolent act resulting in patient maleficence.

The use of the term *nutrition* in parenteral nutrition does not mean that parenteral nutrition is equivalent to food. A host of psychosociocultural characteristics associated with food and eating cannot be attached to parenteral nutrition. The relation of parenteral nutrition to the digestive tract is akin to that of dialysis to the kidneys, mechanical ventilation to the lungs, or heart-lung bypass to the heart. Parenteral nutrition is a technological, pharmacologic, and invasive therapy that provides defined nutrients in an artificial manner with accompanying significant risks. Parenteral nutrition provides known essential nutrients but lacks the wide variety of known and unknown "nonessential" nutrients contained in food. Parenteral nutrition bypasses cephalic, gastric, and intestinal phases of digestion and bypasses intestinal and hepatic *first-pass* metabolism of nutrients. Parenteral nutrition can support life for years in patients with a short gut, but it is associated with a host of well-documented acute and chronic complications that are not associated with normal food ingestion. Intervention with parenteral nutrition should be viewed in the same way as intervention with mechanical ventilation or dialysis—potential benefits and burdens need to be assessed in the context of the individual patient. In and of itself, parenteral nutrition cannot be considered to provide a net benefit or a net burden, but its use must be considered with reference to the clinical situation and management goals.

The term *starvation* conjures up powerful images. However, the use of the term *starvation* when dealing with patients dying from their underlying disease has been termed *sloganism*[12] and considered a distortion that impairs analysis.[13] Starvation must be taken in context. Starvation may have several meanings, including to be malnourished, to experience hunger, or to die or be killed by withholding food. Certainly, it is this latter meaning—the gruesome death scenario with associations of concentration camps and famines—that is visually disturbing. However, hunger strikes may be a form of political protest; for example, the great Indian leader Mahatma Gandhi protested by fasting—a form of self-induced starvation. Fasting, as a form of ideologic protest, may be considered heroic, moral, and spiritual; it is a form of starvation that should be considered in a totally different context.

Further examination of terminology illustrates how language influences our thought processes and potential approaches to a clinical situation. For example, consider the terms *food* and *feeding*, usually regarded as a priori "goods." The symbolic aspects of feeding, food, and eating are multiple.[14] Food represents nurturing; it represents happiness and joyous occasions; it may define us religiously or culturally. From this perspective, consider the term *forced feeding*; certainly, forced feeding is not necessarily an inherent "good." Forced feeding has negative connotations, from animal husbandry (force feeding a goose to produce *pâté de foie gras* or force feeding a calf to produce tender veal) to human situations (force feeding a prisoner or a political protestor undergoing a hunger strike). Forced feeding suggests coercion, perhaps brutal force. I am not sure that there is any context in which forced feeding engenders tender, nurturing, or positive thoughts.

Perhaps the best terminology that I have found that frames issues of feeding in neutral terms speaks of *volitional* and *nonvolitional* feeding.[15] If we eat, we undergo volitional feeding. Eating is putting food into our mouth, chewing, swallowing, and deriving the pleasures and benefits from food. We find forcibly preventing volitional feeding— concentration camps, famines—horrific. If we do not eat but are provided parenteral nutrition—artificial nutrition and hydration—we undergo a form of forced feeding or, in less pejorative terms, we undergo nonvolitional nutrition. Although nonvolitional feeding provides nutrition and may be therapeutic and life sustaining, it does not provide the other physiologic phenomena and social pleasures associated with eating. Parenteral nutrition is not eating, and withholding or withdrawing nonvolitional feeding is not the same as withholding volitional feeding.[16] The proper choice of words helps us understand what we are doing and places potential ethical dilemmas in more neutral contexts.

Death without food and water—starvation at the end of a terminal disease—is not necessarily a painful and terrible death. The phenomenon has been termed *terminal dehydration*. There is now a moderate literature from the hospice movement documenting what occurs when food and water are not forced. Anecdotal reports and case series document pain-free, peaceful, and comfortable deaths when food and water are provided only for comfort. Many patients are

not hungry. Conversion to a ketone economy from the metabolism of endogenous body fat is an important factor in blocking hunger in these patients. In addition, insisting that the patient eat when food is not wanted, or forcing food, may cause abdominal discomfort, nausea, and occasionally vomiting. Hospice workers have often observed that terminal dehydration leads to decreased secretions and excretions, thereby reducing respiratory problems, vomiting, and urinary and fecal incontinence. The azotemia, hypernatremia, and hypercalcemia that occur with terminal dehydration contribute to the analgesia, sedation, and occasionally euphoria experienced by patients. Thirst is a frequent problem at the end of life when patients do not eat or drink; a dry and cracked mouth as well as sore gums may also occur. Thirst, however, is not synonymous with dehydration and may occur in the absence of dehydration. Thirst and other mouth problems may be treated with sips of water and other fluids, ice chips, petroleum jelly to the lips and gums, and good mouth care.[17-23]

With an understanding of language and terminal dehydration, one can approach our original clinical problem—a request for parenteral nutrition for a terminal patient— with an appropriate ethical framework. For ethical analysis, a range of questions must be answered. The clinical situation must be known: What is the prognosis? What is the performance status? What is the quality of life? What are treatment options? We then consider the ethical principles of autonomy, beneficence, and futility. What does the patient want? Does he or she want to be kept alive at all costs? Does the patient value the quality of life? What is the patient's definition of quality of life? Where and how does the patient want to spend the final days? What benefit is the treatment going to provide? Will it prolong life? Will it improve the quality of life? Will it enable a patient to come to terms with his or her own mortality—to spend final time with the family? Are there risks—of infection, discomfort, immobility, costs? Is the intervention with nonvolitional feeding futile? What is the evidence that the intervention will prolong life, decrease morbidity, or ease pain and discomfort? The answers to these questions need to be assessed in the ethical framework of autonomy, beneficence, nonmaleficence, and futility. Our nutritional support team's approach in this clinical

Table 30–1. Guidelines for TPN in Dying Patients

Prognosis (est. Survival)	Consider TPN	Provide TPN
<3 mo	No	No
>3 but <6 mo	Yes	No
>6 mo	Yes	Yes

TPN, total parenteral nutrition.
From Hammes BJ: Total parenteral nutrition: An ethical assessment. Nutrition 6:402–404, 1990.

scenario—the terminal patient without a chance of recovery—has been to regard nonvolitional parenteral nutrition as a futile intervention without benefit and with a potential for causing harm.

One institution has established time guidelines for the consideration of nonvolitional feeding—parenteral nutrition for dying patients.[13] Parenteral nutrition is not initiated if the estimated survival is less than 3 months because the parenteral nutrition is not considered to increase survival, improve the quality of life, or decrease suffering. These guidelines are illustrated in Table 30–1. Thus, by understanding the clinical condition and applying ethical fundamentals, one can address the ethical issues in difficult situations.

◆ PARENTERAL NUTRITION AS A SUBSTITUTE FOR ENTERAL NUTRITION

Occasionally case reports in the literature or at conferences as well as consultations with our nutritional support team have presented several clinical scenarios: A competent patient refuses enteral nutrition or, more often, an incompetent patient recurrently removes the feeding tube. Parenteral nutrition is requested as a substitute, usually with the thought that the patient will not object to, or pull out, a central line. This line of reasoning has always bothered me; it raises issues of autonomy, beneficence, and justice. By virtue of the ethical principle of autonomy, the competent patient has the right to refuse a medical intervention. It is the obligation of the clinician to attempt to explain the purpose and benefits of the intervention—in this case, enteral nutrition—but it remains the prerogative of the patient to refuse. Reference to patient autonomy is

more problematic with an incompetent patient. The incompetent or incapacitated patient may have lost autonomy; the patient can no longer self-govern and is incapable of making clinical decisions. Under such circumstances, either the patient's surrogate must act in the patient's behalf, permitting what the patient would have permitted, or the clinician needs to act with beneficence, doing what is best for the patient. However, I have taken the view that the patient is expressing a form of functional autonomy—the patient is telling the clinician that the feeding tube is burdensome and bothersome. The incompetent patient might otherwise be tied down and restrained to keep a feeding tube in place—a burden that many would consider excessive.

Under either of these clinical situations—a competent autonomous patient or an incapacitated questionably autonomous patient—is parenteral nutrition an acceptable or appropriate alternative? Although I have argued that the evidence generally does not exist to support the thesis that enteral nutrition is preferable to parenteral nutrition,[24] most clinicians probably disagree. Certainly, parenteral nutrition is more expensive, has more long-term complications, and may have greater short-term complication risks. Parenteral nutrition would be contraindicated if the patient accepted enteral nutrition. Virtually all clinicians would think that parenteral nutrition is a less preferable therapy to enteral nutrition and is never the treatment of choice with a functioning gastrointestinal tract. Giving parenteral nutrition when enteral nutrition is refused runs the risk of maleficence—doing harm. A less efficacious, more expensive, perhaps riskier therapy is being used because the appropriate therapy is refused. It is questionable, at best, to provide inappropriate therapy when the appropriate therapy is refused. Issues of justice—fair allocation of societal resources—should also be raised. Given increasingly limited resources, similar concerns hold; should a more expensive, perhaps riskier, and probably less effective therapy use up scarce resources? Our nutritional support team's approach in this clinical scenario is to consider the principles of autonomy, nonmaleficence, and justice; we do not think that nonindicated therapy should be substituted for the refusal of appropriate therapy.

◆ INFORMED CONSENT AND PARENTERAL NUTRITION

Informed consent in nutritional support, if obtained at all, usually consists of a stranger asking the patient to sign a sheet of paper. Discussion, questions, and treatment goals are not a part of the process. Many years ago, the old Veterans Administration (now the Department of Veterans Affairs) required that written informed consent be obtained from patients before the initiation of parenteral nutrition. At that time, I thought that this was an absurd requirement because informed consent was not necessary for other intravenous lines, including central lines, and was not necessary for chemotherapy, which was far more toxic and dangerous than parenteral nutrition. I thought that parenteral nutrition would be delayed or not given because patients, in their ignorance, would refuse. I was wrong in my belief, as I discuss in the next two paragraphs.

Informed consent speaks to the changing paradigm of the relationship between the clinician and the patient—from the former beneficence-based, paternalistic approach of the clinician to the current autonomy-based approach in which the patient is involved as a partner in health care decisions.[25] Because an autonomous patient can accept or refuse any intervention, there must be a dialogue between the patient and the clinician that is informative and educational about the procedure, its risks and benefits, alternatives, and possible outcomes. Patients should be told in their own terms and language about the intervention, and opportunity should be available to ensure that the patient understands and comprehends. The autonomous patient should have freedom of choice. Autonomy, self-determination, and communication are the underlying vocabulary of informed consent. Elements of disclosure and dialogue in the informed consent should include the patient's current medical status and likely course if left untreated; the interventions that might improve the prognosis, including the potential benefits and risks as well as an estimate of associated probabilities and uncertainties; a professional opinion as to other potential treatment options; and finally, a recommendation based on best judgment.[3]

The ideal informed consent is a standard that is probably impossible to meet given the current stresses on clinicians' time and resources. The prevailing lack of true informed consent with the provision of parenteral nutrition is certainly no worse than that with any other intervention in medicine. In practice, lip service is given to the concept. Nonetheless, with the wide potential for short-term and long-term parenteral nutrition–associated mechanical, vascular, infectious, and metabolic complications, plus a lack of evidence documenting efficacy in many clinical situations,[26] we are, I think, not fulfilling our ethical duties to our patients every time we arrange for a piece of paper to be signed anonymously without incorporating the contemporary elements of informed consent.

◆ PARENTERAL NUTRITION AND ISSUES OF JUSTICE

Many nutritional support clinicians have confronted the situation in which a patient has the medical indications for parenteral nutrition, usually long-term home parenteral nutrition, but lacks insurance. The patient and the clinician are then faced with the problem of who is going to pay for the expensive therapy. A second scenario may involve a similar patient, again usually without financial resources, but also without the psychosocial resources to handle this treatment. In this latter case, the patient may not have motor skills, cognitive understanding, family, or other support. The patient may miss appointments, demonstrate an inability for self-care in other ways, or exhibit destructive behavior. Should such an individual be started on a resource-intensive therapy when there is a high likelihood of failure?

Such questions deal with the relationship of the patient or the clinician and the community at large rather than the relationship between the individual and the clinician.[27] My discussions of prior ethical issues have centered around the responsibility of the clinician to the patient. Now we are concerned not only with this relationship, but with relationships to others. If there is only a finite "pot of gold" available for treatment, to whom does it go? What are the responsibilities to other patients? If all my energies are devoted to issues of a single patient, do others that I am responsible for suffer? These issues of justice, or macroallocation of resources, often have responses that differ from issues of personal relationships. The ability to act in the best interest of an individual patient may be limited by policies set by others on a more global scale. Unfortunately, in my reading I have found that the descriptions of these issues are clear, but the resolutions may be unsatisfactory.

The ethical dilemma arises from multiple responsibilities of the clinician—to the individual patient, to other patients, to a more global community of payers. The conflict arises when it is unclear how to prioritize responsibilities or when duties to the patient conflict with duties to others. Justice is the relevant ethical principle because it deals with the fair and equitable distribution of burdens and benefits within a community. The clash and sometimes unsatisfactory resolution derive from the conflict between the individual and the community—between autonomy-beneficence and justice.

When these conflicts arise, the following ethical guidelines should prevail, although, admittedly, they may be difficult or impossible to follow. In the first clinical scenario—when there is a lack of financial resources—medical indications and patient preferences retain priority. Every effort should be made by the clinician and the support staff to obtain appropriate funding for necessary therapy. The primary elements of patient-clinician relationships should be preserved, and within the clinician's ability and power, the clinician should remain the patient's advocate within the "system." The clinician should strive to preserve or introduce a just allocation of resources within the system, but the obligation to the individual patient—to try to make things work—goes beyond the obligation to the system to maintain a fair allocation of resources. With reference to the second scenario, in which there are both concerns regarding the patient's ability to comply with therapy and concerns that the intervention represents a misuse of resources, clinical decisions should be made about what is in the best interest of the patient. Then efforts should be made to implement the appropriate clinical care to the best of one's ability. A medical decision may be made that intervention in such circumstances represents futile care with the potential for maleficence. No matter what the clinical decision, from an ethical perspective, the potential for misuse of resources should not be part of the clinical decision.

Table 30–2. A Procedure for Clinical Ethical Decision Making

1. Gather relevant available information and identify facts of case
   Medical information
      Diagnosis
      Prognosis
      Care management and treatment goals
      Decision-making capacity
   Patient preferences
      Values
      Care management goals
      Advanced care planning
      Health care agent or surrogate
   Quality of life
      Suffering
      Pain
      Psychosocial
      Cultural
      Spiritual
   Contextual issues
      Economic
      Legal
      Administrative
2. Identify ethical issues
3. Specify implications for relevant ethical concepts or moral values
      Appeal to nonmaleficence and/or beneficence
      Appeal to rights (autonomy)
      Appeal to virtues
      Appeal to justice
      Appeal to consequences
4. Identify convergence and conflict(s) between and among relevant ethical concepts and values
5. Decide among practical alternatives
6. Provide argument to show how conflict should be resolved
7. Advise those involved as to preferred course of action
8. Review outcome
9. Consider: how could the ethical conflict(s) have been prevented?

Prepared by Joanne Joyner, R.N., Ph.D., Chair of the Washington, DC, Veterans Affairs Medical Center Clinical Ethics Committee. Adapted from work prepared by the faculty of the Center of Medical Ethics and Health Policy, Baylor College of Medicine, Houston, Texas, and references 3, 30–32.

◆ THE HOSPITAL ETHICS COMMITTEE

I have tried in this chapter to provide an insight and overview of ethical issues involved with the delivery of parenteral nutrition. Many of these issues are complex, and in dealing with individual patients, the conflict of values, ideology, and goals may be overwhelming. For these and other reasons, every hospital in the United States is now mandated to have an ethics committee available to act in consultation for assistance with these difficult issues.[3, 28–32] Members of the committee should be familiar with the literature and methodology of bioethics and be able to provide neutral consultation when clinical issues arise. The hospital ethics committee can be a valuable resource when these ethical dilemmas arise in the care of parenteral nutrition patients. Table 30–2 outlines a procedure for clinical ethical decision making that has been developed at our medical center.

♦ ETHICAL ISSUES AND THE INTERNET

The Internet has become a useful and often utilized resource for both patients and clinicians.[33] One can go to any search engine (e.g., Yahoo, AltaVista, HotBot, Excite) and search under the term *bioethics*. Thousands of sites are available. By the nature of the Internet, some sites are nonfunctional and new sites appear daily. Listed in Table 30–3 are a very few selected sites that I have found useful in performing ethics consultations and preparing for this chapter.

SUMMARY

Ethical conflicts arise in medicine because of competing value systems and differing goals. I have tried to present some of the more common issues as they relate to parenteral nutrition and some that are less recognized. Some ethical conflicts may be easily solvable, and others may lack any satisfactory resolution. At the least, the clinician should remember the ethical concepts of autonomy, beneficence, nonmaleficence, and futility. The hospital ethics committee should be a valuable resource in understanding and resolving ethical conflicts.

ACKNOWLEDGMENT

I thank JoAnne Joyner, Henry Lipman, and Doris Strader for their thoughtful and useful critiques of this manuscript.

REFERENCES

1. Dunn PM, Gallagher TH, Hodges MO, et al: Medical ethics: An annotated bibliography. Ann Intern Med 121:627–632, 1994.
2. Loewy EH: Textbook of Healthcare Ethics. New York, Plenum Press, 1996.
3. Jonsen AR, Siegler M, Winslade WJ: Clinical Ethics, 3rd ed. New York, McGraw-Hill, 1992.
4. Hirsch ED Jr, Kett JF, Trefil J: The Dictionary of Cultural Literacy. Boston, Houghton Mifflin, 1988, p 90.
5. Burck R: Feeding, withdrawing, and withholding: Ethical perspectives. Nutr Clin Pract 11:243–253, 1996.
6. Paris JJ, Schreiber MD, Statter M, et al: Beyond autonomy—physicians refusal to use life-prolonging extracorporeal membrane oxygenation. N Engl J Med 329:354–358, 1993.
7. Tomlinson T, Brody H: Futility and the ethics of resuscitation. JAMA 264:1276–1280, 1990.
8. Truog RD, Brett AS, Frader J: The problem with futility. N Engl J Med 326:1560–1564, 1992.
9. McCamish MA, Crocker NJ: Enteral and parenteral nutrition support of terminally ill patients: Practical and ethical perspectives. Hospice J 9:107–129, 1993.
10. Schneiderman LJ, Jecker NS, Jonsen AR: Medical futility: Its meaning and ethical implications. Ann Intern Med 112:949–954, 1990.
11. Gillon R: Persistent vegetative state and withdrawal of nutrition and hydration. J Med Ethics 19:67–68, 1993.
12. Ahronheim JC, Gasner MR: The sloganism of starvation. Lancet 335:278–279, 1990.
13. Hammes BJ: Total parenteral nutrition: An ethical assessment. Nutrition 6:402–404, 1990.
14. Slomka J: What do apple pie and motherhood have to do with feeding tubes and caring for the patient? Arch Intern Med 155:1258–1263, 1995.
15. Chapman G: An oncology patient's choice to forgo nonvolitional nutrition support: Ethical considerations. Nutr Clin Pract 11:265–268, 1996.
16. Lipman TO: Ethics and nutrition support. Nutr Clin Pract 11:241–242, 1996.
17. Sullivan RJ Jr: Accepting death without artificial nutrition or hydration. J Gen Intern Med 8:220–224, 1993.
18. McCann RM, Hall WJ, Groth-Juncker A: Comfort care for terminally ill patients: The appropriate use of nutrition and hydration. JAMA 272:1263–1266, 1994.

Table 30–3. Selected Bioethics Sites on the Internet

- Bioethics Internet project
  The Center for Bioethics, University of Pennsylvania
  www.med.upenn.edu/bioethic/
  or
  http://bioethics.net
- Choice in dying (for living wills, etc)
  www.choices.org
- "Five Wishes" project
  A new type of living will
  www.agingwithdignity.org
- Ethics in medicine
  University of Washington School of Medicine
  http://eduserv.hscer.washington.edu/bioethics
- Bioethics line (bibliographic retrieval)
  via Internet Grateful Med
  http://igm.nlm.nih.gov/

19. Printz LA: Terminal dehydration: A compassionate treatment. Arch Intern Med 152:697–700, 1992.
20. Zerwekh JV: The dehydration question. Nursing 13:47–51, 1983.
21. Oliver D: Terminal dehydration. Lancet 2:631, 1984.
22. Andrews MR, Levine AM: Dehydration in the terminal patient: Perception of hospice nurses. Am J Hospice Care Jan-Feb:31–34, 1989.
23. Miller FG, Meier DE: Voluntary death: A comparison of terminal dehydration and physician-assisted suicide. Ann Intern Med 128:559–562, 1998.
24. Lipman TO: Grains or veins: Is enteral nutrition really better than parenteral nutrition? A look at the evidence. JPEN J Parenter Enteral Nutr 22:167–182, 1998.
25. Corsino B: Informed Consent: Policy and Practice. Washington, DC, Department of Veterans Affairs National Center for Clinical Ethics, 1966.
26. Klein S, Kinney J, Jeejeebhoy K, et al: Nutrition support in clinical practice: Review of published data and recommendations for future research directions. JPEN J Parenter Enteral Nutr 21:133–156, 1997.
27. Knowles JB, Gilmore N: Discontinuation of total parenteral nutrition in a patient with acquired immunodeficiency syndrome: A Canadian perspective. Nutr Rev 52:271–274, 1994.
28. Fletcher JC, Quist N, Jonsen AR (eds): Ethics Consultation in Health Care. Ann Arbor, MI, Health Administration Press, 1989.
29. La Puma J, Toulmin SE: Ethics, consultants and ethics committees. Arch Intern Med 149:1109–1112, 1989.
30. Durnan RJ, Nelson WA: Ethical Issues at the End of Life: An Ethical Educational Package. Videotape and Facilitator's Guide. White River Junction, VT, and Northport, NY, Regional Medical Education Center and the VA National Center for Clinical Ethics, 1995.
31. Purtillo RB: Ethical Dimensions in the Health Professions, 2nd ed. Philadelphia, WB Saunders, 1993.
32. Nelson WA: Using ethics advisory committees to cope with ethical issues. Mo Med 89:827–830, 1992.
33. Peters R, Sikorski R: Navigating to knowledge: Tools for finding information on the Internet. JAMA 277:505–506, 1997.

◆ Index

Page numbers is *italics* refer to illustrations; numbers followed by t indicate tables.

ISBN 0-7216-8120-4

90038

9 780721 681207